Priorities in Critical Care Nursing

seventh edition

Linda D. Urden
DNSc, RN, CNS, NE-BC, FAAN
Professor and Director
Master's and International Programs
Hahn School of Nursing and Health Science
University of San Diego
San Diego, California

Kathleen M. Stacy
PhD, RN, CNS, CCRN, PCCN, CCNS
Clinical Associate Professor
Hahn School of Nursing and Health Science
University of San Diego
San Diego, California

Mary E. Lough
PhD, RN, CNS, CCRN, CNRN, CCNS
Critical Care Clinical Nurse Specialist
Stanford Health Care
Clinical Assistant Professor
Stanford University
Stanford, California

With approximately 180 Illustrations

ELSEVIER

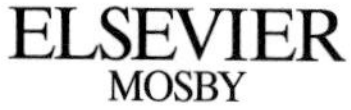

3251 Riverport Lane
St. Louis, Missouri 63043

PRIORITIES IN CRITICAL CARE NURSING ISBN: 978-0-323-32085-6

Notice

Knowledge and best practice in this field are constantly changing. As new research and experience broaden our knowledge, changes in practice, treatment, and drug therapy may become necessary or appropriate. Readers are advised to check the most current information provided (i) on procedures featured or (ii) by the manufacturer of each product to be administered, to verify the recommended dose or formula, the method and duration of administration, and contraindications. It is the responsibility of the practitioner, relying on their own experience and knowledge of the patient, to make diagnoses, to determine dosages and the best treatment for each individual patient, and to take all appropriate safety precautions. To the fullest extent of the law, neither the Publisher nor the Authors assume any liability for any injury and/or damage to persons or property arising out or related to any use of the material contained in this book.

The Publisher

Library of Congress Control Number: 2015932034

Executive Content Strategist: Lee Henderson
Content Development Manager: Jean Fornango
Associate Content Development Specialist: Melissa Rawe
Project Manager: Sukanthi Sukumar
Marketing Manager: Anne Mundloch
Publishing Services Manager: Hemamalini Rajendrababu
Designer: Julia Dummitt

Printed in Canada

Last digit is the print number: 9 8 7 6 5 4 3 2

CONTRIBUTORS

Caroline Arbour, PhD, RN
Post-Doctoral Fellow in Neuroscience
Université de Montréal
Center for Advanced Research in Sleep Medicine (CARSM)
Hôpital du Sacré-Cœur de Montréal
Montréal, Quebec, Canada
Chapter 8, Pain and Pain Management

Barbara Buesch, MSN, RN, CNS
District Stroke Coordinator
Palomar Health
Escondido, California
Chapter 18, Neurologic Disorders and Therapeutic Management

Darlene M. Burke, MS, MA, RN
Adjunct Nursing Faculty
MiraCosta College
Oceanside, California &
San Diego State University
San Diego, CA
Consultant and Educator
Professional Source Nursing Consulting
Carlsbad, California
Chapter 17, Neurologic Clinical Assessment and Diagnostic Procedures

Beverly Carlson, PhD, RN, CNS, CCRN
Lecturer, School of Nursing
San Diego State University
San Diego, California
Chapter 26, Shock, Sepsis, and Multiple Organ Dysfunction Syndrome

Kelly K. Dineen, BSN, JD
Assistant Dean for Academic Affairs and Instructor of Health Law
Saint Louis University School of Law
St. Louis, Missouri
Chapter 2, Ethical and Legal Issues

Joni L. Dirks, MS, RN-BC, CCRN
Manager, Clinical Educators
Nurse Educator
Adult Intensive Care Units
Providence Healthcare
Spokane, Washington
Chapter 13, Cardiovascular Therapeutic Management

Caroline Etland, PhD, RN, CNS, AOCN, ACHPN
Director of Education, Research and Professional Practice
Department of Nursing
Bioethics Consultant
Sharp Chula Vista Medical Center
Chula Vista, California
Chapter 10, End-of-Life Care

Céline Gélinas, PhD, RN
Associate Professor
Ingram School of Nursing
McGill University
Researcher
Center for Nursing Research and Lady Davis Institute for Medical Research
Jewish General Hospital
Montreal, Quebec, Canada
Chapter 8, Pain and Pain Management

Annette Haynes, MS, RN, CNS, CCRN, CCNS
Cardiology Clinical Nurse Specialist
Stanford Health Care
Stanford, California
Chapter 12, Cardiovascular Disorders

Lourdes Januszewicz, MSN, RN, CNS, CCRN
Clinical Nurse Specialist
Intensive Care/Intermediate Care
Palomar Health
Poway, California
Chapter 18, Neurologic Disorders and Therapeutic Management

Sheryl E. Leary, MS, RN, CCNS, CCRN, PCCN
Progressive Care Clinical Nurse Specialist
VA San Diego Healthcare System
San Diego, California
Chapter 22, Gastrointestinal Disorders and Therapeutic Management

Mary E. Lough, PhD, RN, CNS, CCRN, CNRN, CCNS
Critical Care Clinical Nurse Specialist
Stanford Health Care
Clinical Assistant Professor
Stanford University
Stanford, California
Chapter 9, Sedation, Agitation and Delirium Management
Chapter 11, Cardiovascular Clinical Assessment and Diagnostic Procedures
Chapter 19, Kidney Clinical Assessment and Diagnostic Procedures
Chapter 20, Kidney Disorders and Therapeutic Management
Chapter 23, Endocrine Clinical Assessment and Diagnostic Procedures
Chapter 24, Endocrine Disorders and Therapeutic Management
Chapter 25, Trauma

Jeanne M. Maiden, PhD, RN, CNS
Professor
School of Nursing
Point Loma Nazarene University
San Diego, California
Chapter 14, Pulmonary Clinical Assessment and Diagnostic Procedures

Kasuen Mauldin, PhD, RD
Assistant Professor
Department of Nutrition & Food Science
San José State University
San José, California
Chapter 6, Nutritional Alterations

Barbara Mayer, MS, PhD, RN-BC
Director of Nursing Quality
Stanford Health Care
Stanford, California
Chapter 3, Patient and Family Education

Mary Russell, MSN, RN, CNS, CCRN, FNP (c)
Clinical Nurse Specialist
Acute Surgical Unit
Surgical Progressive Unit
Trauma Intensive Care Unit
Palomar Pomerado Health
Escondido, California
Chapter 27, Hematologic Disorders and Oncologic Emergencies

Kathleen M. Stacy, PhD, RN, CNS, CCRN, PCCN, CCNS
Clinical Associate Professor
Hahn School of Nursing and Health Science
University of San Diego
San Diego, California
Chapter 5, Sleep Alterations
Chapter 14, Pulmonary Clinical Assessment and Diagnostic Procedures
Chapter 15, Pulmonary Disorders
Chapter 16, Pulmonary Therapeutic Management
Chapter 21, Gastrointestinal Clinical Assessment and Diagnostic Procedures

Carol A. Suarez, MSN, RN, CNS, PHN, FNP
Clinical Nurse Specialist
Orthopaedic Medical/Surgical Acute Care, NeuroSciences Progressive Care, Intermediate Care Units
Palomar Health
Escondido, California
Chapter 27, Hematologic Disorders and Oncologic Emergencies

Linda D. Urden, DNSc, RN, CNS, NE-BC, FAAN
Professor and Director
Master's and International Programs
Hahn School of Nursing and Health Science
University of San Diego
San Diego, California
Chapter 1, Caring for the Critically Ill Patient
Chapter 2, Ethical and Legal Issues

Julie M. Waters, MS, RN, CCRN
Clinical Educator
Cardiac Intensive Care Unit
Providence Healthcare
Spokane, Washington
Chapter 13, Cardiovascular Therapeutic Management

Fiona Winterbottom, MSN, RN, APRN, ACNS-BC, CCRN
Clinical Nurse Specialist for Critical Care
Ochsner Medical Center-New Orleans
New Orleans, Louisiana
Chapter 7, Gerontological Alterations

Valerie J. Yancey, PhD, RN, CHPN, HNC
Associate Professor
Department of Nursing
Southern Illinois University Edwardsville
Edwardsville, Illinois
Chapter 4, Psychosocial and Spiritual Alterations and Management

REVIEWER

James Graves, PharmD
Staff Pharmacist, Certified Immunizer
St. Mary Health Center
Jefferson City, Missouri

To Nurses who care for the critically ill.

LDU

To Linda and Mary—thank you for the successful partnership making a difference!

KMS

To Madeleine Lough-Stevens
For staying strong during adversity, for not giving up and for being a bright light for everyone else

MEL

ACKNOWLEDGMENTS

The talent, hard work, and inspiration of many people have produced the Seventh Edition of *Priorities in Critical Care Nursing.* We appreciate the assistance of the editorial teams that worked with us on this edition: Tamara Myers at the beginning and Lee Henderson and Melissa Rawe who saw us through to publication. We are also grateful to our project manager, Sukanthi Sukumar, for her scrupulous attention to detail.

PREFACE

We are grateful to the many students, nurses, and educators who made the first six editions of *Priorities in Critical Care Nursing* successful. The emphasis continues to be on priorities for the critical care nurse. We believe that prioritizing conditions and issues will assist critical care nurses in quickly assessing and intervening in the most efficient and effective manner.

ORGANIZATION

The book is comprised of nine major units, with two appendices. The chapter content of Unit One, *Foundations of Critical Care Nursing,* forms the basis of practice regardless of the physiologic alterations of the critically ill patient. Unit Two, *Common Problems in Critical Care,* examines potential critical care practice problems. Unit Three, *Cardiovascular Alterations,* and Unit Four, *Pulmonary Alterations,* are each organized according to the three-chapter format of Clinical Assessment and Diagnostic Procedures, Disorders, and Therapeutic Management. Unit Five, *Neurological Alterations;* Unit Six, *Renal Alterations;* Unit Seven, *Gastrointestinal Alterations;* and Unit Eight, *Endocrine Alterations,* are each organized according to the two-chapter format of Clinical Assessment and Diagnostic Procedures and Disorders and Therapeutic Management. Unit Nine, *Multisystem Alterations,* addresses disorders that affect multiple body systems and necessitate discussion as a separate category: Trauma; Shock, Sepsis, and Multiple Organ Dysfunction Syndrome; and Hematological Disorders and Oncological Emergencies.

Appendix A, *Nursing Management Plans of Care,* contains the core of critical care nursing practice in a nursing process format: signs and symptoms, nursing diagnosis, outcome criteria, and nursing interventions. The Nursing Management Plans of Care are referenced throughout the book within the *Nursing Diagnosis Priorities* boxes. Appendix B, *Physiologic Formulas for Critical Care,* features common hemodynamic and oxygenation formulas and other calculations presented in easily understood terms.

EVIDENCE-BASED PRACTICE AND RESEARCH

The power of research-based critical care practice has been incorporated into nursing interventions. To foster critical thinking and decision making, a boxed menu of nursing diagnoses complete with specific etiologic or related factors accompanies each medical disorder and major medical treatment discussion and directs the learner to the section of the book where appropriate nursing management is detailed.

SEVENTH EDITION CONTINUING FEATURES

In keeping with the emphasis on priorities in critical care, *Nursing Diagnosis Priorities* boxes list the most urgent potential nursing diagnoses to be addressed. To facilitate student learning, the *Nursing Management Plans of Care* (Appendix A) incorporate nursing diagnoses, etiologic or related factors, clinical manifestations, and interventions with rationales. These *Plans of Care* are cross-referenced throughout the book. *Concept Maps* appearing throughout the book link pathophysiological processes, clinical manifestations, and medical and nursing interventions. *Case Studies* with critical thinking questions consist of a brief patient history, clinical assessment, diagnostic procedures, and medical diagnosis(es). Questions follow that correspond with key points of the case.

NEW TO THIS EDITION

New to this edition are *QSEN* boxes that alert the nurse to special evidence-based considerations to specific practices and interventions that ensure safe patient care and best outcomes. Also new to this edition are the Internet Boxes which guide the reader to additional resources on chapter content. *Patient Education Priorities* boxes appear where key content is a priority for educating patients and families.

EVOLVE RESOURCES FOR *CRITICAL CARE NURSING*

We are pleased to offer additional new and updated resources for students and instructors on our companion site, Evolve Resources for *Priorities in Critical Care Nursing.*

Student Resources

Student Resources are available at http://evolve.elsevier.com/Urden/priorities/ and include the following:

- Self-assessment opportunities, including
- NCLEX® Review Questions
- CCRN Review Questions
- PCCN Review Questions
- Evolve Glossary
- Concept Map Creator
- Audio Clips
- Critical Care Procedures from Mosby's Nursing Skills Online

Instructor Resources

Instructor Resources, available at http://evolve.elsevier.com/Urden/priorities/, provide a variety of aids to enhance classroom instruction. Instructors have access to all of the Student Resources listed above, as well as the following:

- TEACH for Nurses—a brand new feature that replaces the Instructor Manual. TEACH for Nurses consists of detailed lesson plans that offer:
- Objectives and Teaching Focus
- Nursing Curriculum Standards (QSEN, BSN Essentials, Concepts from Concept-Based Curriculum, CCRN, and PCCN)
- List of all student and instructor chapter resources found on Evolve
- Teaching Strategies that present a chapter outline, content highlights, and learning activities
- New Case Study for select chapters
- Answers to the textbook Case Study provided for select chapters
- Test Bank of approximately 700 questions

- PowerPoint presentation by chapter. New to the presentations for this edition are lecture notes on most slides, more images from the book, and audience response questions.
- Image Collection containing all of the images from the text

Priorities in Critical Care Nursing, Seventh Edition, represents our continued commitment to bringing you the best in all things a textbook can offer: the best and brightest in contributing and consulting authors, the latest in scientific research, a logical organizational format that exercises diagnostic reasoning skills, and artwork that enhances student learning. We pledge our continued commitment to excellence in critical care education.

Linda D. Urden
Kathleen M. Stacy
Mary E. Lough

CONTENTS

UNIT ONE Foundations in Critical Care Nursing

CHAPTER 1

Caring for the Critically Ill Patient

Linda D. Urden

Be sure to check out the bonus material, including review questions, on the Evolve website at http://evolve.elsevier.com/Urden/priorities/.

CONTEMPORARY CRITICAL CARE

Modern critical care is provided to patients by an interprofessional team of health care providers who have in-depth education in the specialty field of critical care. The team consists of physician intensivists, specialty physicians, registered nurses, advanced practice nurses, specialty nurse clinicians, pharmacists, respiratory therapy practitioners, other specialized therapists and clinicians, social workers, and clergy. Critical care is provided in specialized units or departments, and importance is placed on the continuum of care, with an efficient transition of care from one setting to another.

Critical care patients are at high risk for actual or potential life-threatening health problems. Critical care nurses practice in a variety of settings: adult, pediatric, and neonatal critical care units; step-down, telemetry, progressive, or transitional care units; cardiac catheterization laboratories, and postoperative recovery units.[1] Nurses are now considered to be knowledge workers because they are highly vigilant and use their intelligence and cognition to go past tasks in order to quickly pull together multiple data to make decisions regarding subtle and/or deteriorating conditions. Nurses work technically with theoretical knowledge.[2]

A growing trend in acute care settings is the designation of progressive care units, considered to be part of the continuum of critical care. In past years, patients who are placed on these units would have been exclusively in critical care units. However, with the use of additional technology and monitoring capabilities, newer care delivery models, and additional nurse education, these units are considered the best environment. The patients are less complex, more stable, have a decreased need for physiologic monitoring, and more self-care capabilities. They can serve as a bridge between critical care units and medical-surgical units, while providing high quality and cost-effective care at the same time.[3] Additionally, these progressive units can be found throughout the acute care setting, thus leaving critical care unit beds for those who need the highest level of care and monitoring.[4]

CRITICAL CARE NURSING ROLES

Nurses provide and contribute to the care of critically ill patients in a variety of roles. The most prevalent role for the professional registered nurse is that of direct care provider. The American Association of Critical-Care Nurses (AACN) created Standards for Acute and Critical Care Nurses.[5] (See Box 1-4.)

Expanded-Role Nursing Positions

Expanded-role nursing positions interact with critical care patients, families, and the health care team. Nurse case managers work closely with the care providers to ensure appropriate, timely care and services and to promote continuity of care from one setting to another. Other nurse clinicians, such as patient educators, cardiac rehabilitation specialists, physician office nurses, and infection control specialists, also contribute to the care. The specific types of expanded-role nursing positions are determined by patient needs and individual organizational resources.

Advanced Practice Nurses

Advanced practice nurses (APNs) have met educational and clinical requirements beyond the basic nursing educational requirements for all nurses. The most commonly seen APNs in critical care are the clinical nurse specialist (CNS) and the nurse practitioner (NP) or acute care nurse practitioner (ACNP). APNs have a broad depth of knowledge and expertise in their specialty area and manage complex clinical and systems issues. The organizational system and existing resources of an institution determine what roles may be needed and how the roles function.

CNSs serve in specialty roles that use their clinical, teaching, research, leadership, and consultative abilities. They work in direct clinical roles and systems or administrative roles and in various other settings in the health care system. CNSs work closely with all members of the health care team, mentor staff, lead quality teams, and consult on complex patients. They are instrumental in ensuring that care is evidence-based and that safety programs are in place. They may be organized by specialty, such as cardiovascular care, or by function, such as cardiac rehabilitation. CNSs also may be designated as case managers for specific patient populations.

NPs and ACNPs manage direct clinical care of a group of patients and have various levels of prescriptive authority, depending on the state and practice area in which they work. They also provide care consistency, interact with families, plan for patient discharge, and provide teaching to patients, families, and other members of the health care team.[6]

CRITICAL CARE PROFESSIONAL ACCOUNTABILITY

The nursing organization most closely associated with critical care nurses is the American Association of Critical-Care Nurses (AACN). It is the world's largest specialty nursing organization and was created in 1969. The top priority of the organization is education of critical care nurses. AACN publishes numerous materials, evidence-based practice summaries, and practice alerts related to the specialty. AACN is at the forefront of setting professional standards of care for critical care nursing.

AACN serves its members through a national organization and many local chapters. The AACN Certification Corporation, a separate company, develops and administers many critical care specialty certification examinations for registered nurses. The examinations are provided in specialties such as neonatal, pediatric, and for those who practice in diverse settings, such as critical care, progressive care, "virtual" ICU, or remote monitoring (e-ICU).[7] Certification is considered one method to maintain high quality of care and to protect consumers of care and services. Research has demonstrated more positive outcomes when care is delivered by health care providers who are certified in their specialty.[8] AACN also recognizes critical care and acute care units who achieve a high level of excellence through its *Beacon Award for Excellence.* The unit that receives this award has demonstrated exceptional care through improved outcomes and greater overall satisfaction. It reflects on a supportive overall environment, teamwork and collaboration, and distinguishes itself with lower turnover and higher morale.[9]

Professional organizations support critical care practitioners by providing numerous resources and networks. The Society of Critical Care Medicine (SCCM) is a multidisciplinary, multispecialty, international organization. Its mission is to secure the highest quality, cost-efficient care for all critically ill patients.[10] Numerous publications and educational opportunities provide cutting-edge critical care information to critical care practitioners.

EVIDENCE-BASED NURSING PRACTICE

The dramatic and multiple changes in health care and the ever-increasing presence of managed care in all geographic regions have placed greater emphasis on demonstrating the effectiveness of treatments and practices on outcomes. Emphasis is on greater efficiency, cost-effectiveness, quality of life, and patient satisfaction ratings. It has become essential for nurses to use the best evidence available to make patient care decisions and carry out the appropriate nursing interventions.[11-12] By using an approach employing a scientific basis, nurses are able to provide research-based interventions with consistent, positive outcomes. The content of this book is research-based, with the most current, cutting-edge research abstracted and placed throughout the chapters as appropriate to topical discussions.

Evidence-based nursing practice considers the best research evidence on the care topic, along with clinical expertise of the nurse, and patient preferences. For instance, when determining the frequency of vital sign measurement, the nurse would use available research, nursing judgment (stability, complexity, predictability, vulnerability, and resilience of the patient),[13] along with the patient's preference for decreased interruptions and the ability to sleep for longer periods of time. At other times the nurse will implement an evidence-based protocol or procedure that is based on evidence, including research. An example of an evidence-based protocol (EBP) is one in which the prevalence of indwelling catheterization and incidence of hospital-acquired catheter-associated urinary tract infections in the critical care unit can be decreased.[14]

The AACN has promulgated several EBP summaries in the form of a "Practice Alert." These alerts are short directives that can be used as a quick reference for practice areas (e.g., oral care, noninvasive blood pressure monitoring, ST segment monitoring). They are succinct, supported by evidence, and address both nursing and multidisciplinary activities. Each alert includes the clinical information, followed by references that support the practice.[15]

HOLISTIC CRITICAL CARE NURSING

Caring

The high technology–driven critical care environment is fast-paced and directed toward monitoring and treating life-threatening changes in patients' conditions. For this reason, attention is often focused on the technology and treatments necessary for maintaining stability in the physiologic functioning of the patient. Concern has been voiced about the diminished emphasis on the caring component of nursing in this fast-paced, highly technologic health care environment.[16-17] The critical care nurse must be able to deliver high-quality care skillfully, using all appropriate technologies, while incorporating psychosocial and other holistic approaches as appropriate to the time and condition of the patient.

Individualized Care

The differences between nurses' and patients' perceptions of caring point to the importance of establishing individualized care that recognizes the uniqueness of each patient's preferences, condition, and physiologic and psychosocial status. It is clearly understood by care providers that a patient's physical condition progresses at fairly predictable stages, depending on the presence or absence of comorbid conditions. What is not understood as distinctly is the effect of psychosocial issues on the healing process. For this reason, special consideration must be given to determining the unique interventions that can positively affect each person and help the patient progress toward the desired outcomes.

An important aspect in the care delivery to and recovery of critically ill patients is the personal support of family members and significant others. The value of patient- and family-centered care should not be underestimated.[18,19] It is important for families to be included in care decisions and to be encouraged to participate in the care of the patient as appropriate to the patient's personal level of ability and needs.

Cultural Care

Cultural diversity in health care is not a new topic, but it is gaining emphasis and importance as the world becomes more accessible to all as the result of increasing technologies and interfaces with places and peoples. Diversity includes not only ethnic sensitivity but also sensitivity and openness to differences in lifestyles, opinions, values, and beliefs. More than 28% of the U.S. population is made up of racial and ethnic minority groups.[20] The predominant minorities in the United States are Americans of African, Hispanic, Asian, Pacific Island, Native American, and Eskimo descent. Significant differences exist among their cultural beliefs and practices and the level of their acculturation into the mainstream American culture.[21]

Cultural competence is one way to ensure that individual differences related to culture are incorporated into the plan of care.[22-24] Nurses must possess knowledge about biocultural, psychosocial, and linguistic differences in diverse populations to make accurate assessments. Interventions must then be tailored to the uniqueness of each patient and family. See Box 1-3 for select multicultural Web resources.

COMPLEMENTARY AND ALTERNATIVE THERAPIES

Consumer activism has increased, and consumers are advocating for quality health care that is cost-effective and humane. They are asking whether options other than traditional Western medical care exist for treating various diseases and disorders. The possibilities of using centuries-old practices that are considered alternative or complementary to current Western medicine have been in demand.[25,26] These types of therapies can be seen in all health care settings, including the critical care unit. Complementary therapies offer patients, families, and health care providers additional options to assist with healing and recovery.[27] The term *complementary* was proposed to describe therapies that can be used to complement or support conventional treatments.[27] The remainder of this section includes a brief discussion about nontraditional complementary therapies that have been used in critical care areas.

Guided Imagery

One of the most well-studied complementary therapies is guided imagery, a mind-body strategy that is frequently used to decrease stress, pain, and anxiety.[28] Additional benefits of guided imagery are 1) decreased side effects, 2) decreased length of stay, 3) reduced hospital costs, 4) enhanced sleep, and 5) increased patient satisfaction.[28] Guided imagery is a low-cost intervention that is relatively simple to implement. The patient's involvement in the process offers a sense of empowerment and accomplishment and motivates self-care.

Massage

Back massage as a once-practiced part of routine care of patients has been eliminated for various reasons, including time constraints, greater use of technology, and increasing complexity of care requirements. However, there is a scientific basis for concluding that massage offers positive effects on physiologic and psychologic outcomes. A comprehensive review of the literature revealed that the most common effect of massage was reduction in anxiety, with additional reports of a significant decrease in tension. There was also a positive physiologic response to massage in the areas of decreased respiratory and heart rates and decreased pain.

Animal-Assisted Therapy

The use of animals has increased as an adjunct to healing in the care of patients of all ages in various settings. Pet visitation programs have been created in various health care delivery settings,[29] including acute care, long-term care, and hospice. In the acute care setting, animals are brought in to provide additional solace and comfort for patients who are critically or terminally ill. Fish aquariums are used in patient areas and family areas because they humanize the surroundings. Scientific evidence indicates that animal-assisted therapy results in positive patient outcomes in the areas of attention, mobility, and orientation. Other reports have shown improved communication and mood in patients.[30]

TECHNOLOGY IN CRITICAL CARE

The growth in technologies has been seen throughout health care, especially in critical care settings. All providers are challenged to learn new equipment, monitoring devices, and related therapies that contribute to care and services. Take, for example, the evolving electronic health record (EHR) that was originally designed to capture data for clinical decision making and to increase the efficiency of health care providers. There are complexities inherent in providing a "user-friendly" EHR. Thus, one that meets the needs and reflects the thought processes and actual work flow of diverse clinicians has been greatly lacking. Add to that the fact that staff-created "workarounds" to some of the software/procedures have not significantly reduced errors or increased productivity.

A more recent opportunity for critical care nurses is working in a role that encompasses the Tele-ICU. Telemedicine was initially employed in outpatient areas, remote, rural geographic locations, and areas where there was a dearth of medical providers. Currently, there are Tele-ICUs in areas where there are limited resources on site. However, there are experts (critical care nurses, intensivists) located in a central distant site. Technologies relay continuous surveillance with monitoring information and communication among care providers. Each Tele-ICU varies in size and location; the key component is the availability of back-up experts. Goran describes competencies for critical care nurses who practice in a Tele-ICU.[31]

INTERPROFESSIONAL COLLABORATIVE PRACTICE

The growing managed care environment has placed emphasis on examining methods of care delivery and processes of care by all health care professionals. Collaboration and partnerships have been shown to increase quality of care and services while containing or decreasing costs.[32-39] It is more important than ever to create and enhance partnerships, because the resulting interdependence and collaboration among disciplines is essential to achieving positive patient outcomes.

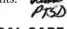

BOX 1-1 Core Competencies for Interprofessional Collaborative Practice

Values/Ethics for Interprofessional Practice
- Work with individuals of other professions to maintain a climate of mutual respect and shared values.

Roles/Responsibilities for Collaborative Practice
- Use the knowledge of one's own role and the role of other professions to assess and address the health care needs of the patients and populations served appropriately.

Interprofessional Communication
- Communicate with patients, families, communities, and other health professionals in a responsive and responsible manner that supports a team approach to maintaining health and treatment of disease.

Interprofessional Teamwork and Team-Based Care
- Apply relationship-building values and principles of team dynamics to perform effectively in different team roles to plan and deliver patient/population-centered care that is safe, timely, efficient, effective, and equitable.

Researchers reported findings from a study in which physician-nurse relationships improved collaboration after meeting together to create a method to change the unit culture. They met together to examine collaboratively what the issues were and create strategies to resolve them. There were higher scores on openness of communication within groups, between groups, accuracy between groups, and overall collaboration.[40]

The Interprofessional Education Collaborative (IEC) published their *Core Competencies for Interprofessional Collaborative Practice*. The IEC sponsors include the American associations of nursing, dentistry, medicine, osteopathy, public health, and pharmacy. Their goal was to establish a set of competencies to serve as a framework for professional socialization of health care professionals. They also intended to assess the relevance of the competencies and develop an action plan for implementation.[41] These competencies are especially important at this time as we move forward with health care reform and explore innovative care delivery models using the skill sets of all health care providers in the most effective and efficient manner. Box 1-1 delineates the four core competencies.

INTERPROFESSIONAL CARE MANAGEMENT TOOLS

Many quality improvement tools are available to providers for care management. The four evidence-based tools addressed in this chapter are clinical algorithm, practice guideline, protocol, and order sets.[42] These tools may also be embedded in the EHR.

Algorithm

An *algorithm* is a stepwise decision-making flowchart for a specific care process or processes. Algorithms guide the clinician through the "if, then" decision-making process, addressing patient responses to particular treatments. Well-known examples of algorithms are the advanced cardiac life support (ACLS) algorithms published by the American Heart Association. Weaning, medication selection, medication titration, individual practitioner variance, and appropriate patient placement algorithms have been developed to give practitioners additional standardized decision-making abilities.

Practice Guideline

A *practice guideline* is usually created by an expert panel and developed by a professional organization (e.g., AACN, Society of Critical Care Medicine, American College of Cardiology, government agencies such as the Agency for Health Care Research and Quality [AHRQ]). Practice guidelines are generally written in text prose style rather than in the flowchart format of algorithms.

Protocol

A *protocol* is a common tool in research studies. Protocols are more directive and rigid than guidelines, and providers are not supposed to vary from a protocol. Patients are screened carefully for specific entry criteria before being started on a protocol. There are many national research protocols, such as those for cancer and chemotherapy studies. Protocols are helpful when built-in *alerts* signal the provider to potentially serious problems. Computerization of protocols assists providers in being more proactive regarding dangerous medication interactions, abnormal laboratory values, and other untoward effects that are preprogrammed into the computer.

Order Set

An *order set* consists of preprinted provider orders that are used to expedite the order process after a standard has been validated through analytic review of practice and research. Order sets complement and increase compliance with existing practice standards. They can also be used to represent the algorithm or protocol in order format.

QUALITY, SAFETY, AND REGULATORY ISSUES IN CRITICAL CARE

Quality and Safety Issues

In critical care units, errors may occur because of the hectic, complex environment, where there is little room for error and safety is essential.[43,44] In this environment, patients are particularly vulnerable because of their compromised physiologic status, multiple technologic and pharmacologic interventions, and multiple care providers who frequently work at a fast pace. It is essential that care delivery processes that minimize the opportunity for errors are designed and that a "safety culture" rather than a "blame culture" is created.[45] One author discussed results of a research study in which nurses were hesitant to report medication errors or unsafe practices so that they would not be ridiculed or "talked about" by their peer nurses. This uncivil behavior was thought to continue to contribute to an unsafe environment and one in which true error or unsafe practices and systems were greatly unreported.[46]

Medication administration continues to be one of the most error-prone nursing interventions for the critical care nurse.[47] Frith conducted a comprehensive literature review and concluded that "…stress, high workloads, knowledge deficits, and performance deficits are associated with medication errors…factors such as frequent interruptions, communication problems and poor fit of health information technology to the workflow of providers…"[48, p 389] also contributed to the errors. Various interventions have been created in an attempt to decrease medication errors. One article reported establishing a "no interruption zone" for medication safety in a critical care unit. In this pilot study, there was a 40% decrease in interruptions from the baseline measurement. Although researchers questioned the feasibility of sustaining this decrease in interruptions in the future,[49] this is an example of an approach that could be used to increase medication safety in the critical care unit.

When an injury or inappropriate care occurs, it is crucial that health care professionals promptly give an explanation of how the injury or mistake occurred and the short- or long-term effects on the patient and family. They should be informed that the factors involved in the injury will be investigated so that steps can be taken to reduce or prevent the likelihood of similar injury to other patients.

It has been shown that intimidating and disruptive clinician behaviors can lead to errors and preventable adverse patient outcomes. Verbal outbursts, physical threats, and more passive behaviors such as refusing to carry out a task or procedure are all under this category. Unfortunately, these types of behavior are not rare in health care organizations. If these behaviors go unaddressed, it can lead to extreme dissatisfaction, depression, and turnover. There also may be systems issues that lead to or perpetuate these situations, such as push for increased productivity, financial constraints, fear of litigation, and embedded hierarchies in the organization.[45]

Technologies are both a solution to error-prone procedures and functions, and another potential cause for error. Consider bar-code medication administration procedures, multiple bedside testing devices, computerized medical records, bedside monitoring, computerized physician order entry (CPOE), and many other technologies now in development. Each in itself can be a great assistance to the clinician but must be monitored for effectiveness and accuracy to ensure the best in outcomes as intended for specific use.[47]

Quality and Safety Regulations

There are numerous regulations governing health care, including local, state, national, Medicare/Medicaid, and payer requirements. However, for purposes of this chapter, key regulations and accreditation standards impacting the majority of critical care areas will be discussed.

The Joint Commission (TJC) is an independent organization that certifies more than 19,000 health care organizations in the United States. Its goal is to evaluate these health care entities using their pre-established standards of performance to ensure high levels of care are provided in these entities. Annually, it establishes National Patient Safety Goals (NPSGs)[50] that are to be implemented in health care organizations. The 2014 NPSGs are the following:

- Identify patients correctly.
- Improve staff communication.
- Use medicines safely.
- Use alarms safely.
- Prevent infection.
- Identify patient safety risks.
- Prevent mistakes in surgery.

TJC has also mandated a "Do Not Use" List. This consists of abbreviations that may be confused with other similar ones. For instance, do not use "U", "u" (unit); instead, write out "unit". Another example is do not use "IU (International Unit); instead write out "International Unit". Refer to TJC for a complete "Do Not Use" List.[51]

The Safe Medical Device Act (SMDA) requires that hospitals report serious or potentially serious device-related injuries or illness of patients and/or employees to the manufacturer of the device, and if death is involved, to the U.S. Food and Drug Administration (FDA). In addition, implantable devices must be documented and tracked.[52] This reporting serves as an early warning system so that the FDA can obtain information on device problems. Failure to comply with the act will result in civil action.

The U.S. Food and Drug Administration (FDA) requires that a drug company place a boxed warning on the labelling of a prescription drug or in literature describing it. This boxed warning (also known as a "black box warning") signifies that medical studies indicate that the drug carries a significant risk of serious or even life-threatening adverse effects.[53] Some examples include Warfarin, Celebrex, Avandia, Cipro. Alerts are published as soon as a drug is found to meet the criteria. Providers are to use caution when using the medications and to consider alternative medications that carry less adverse effects.

Quality and Safety Resources

The Institute for Safe Medication Practices (ISMP) is a not-for-profit organization dedicated to medication error prevention and safe medication use. It has numerous tools to assist care providers, including newsletters, education programs, safety alerts, consulting, patient education materials, error reporting system, and more. One newsletter is devoted specifically to nurses. It offers a very comprehensive array of tools.[54]

The Quality and Safety Education for Nurses (QSEN) project established standards for educating registered nurses at the baccalaureate and master levels of academic education. In this model, the knowledge, skills, and attitudes (KSAs) were created so that nurses would be able to continuously improve the quality and safety of the health care systems for which they work. There are six major categories that delineate the KSAs for each section (Box 1-2).[55] Boxes that address the QSEN competencies will be presented throughout the book, with the QSEN icon QSEN appearing in them. Box 1-3 lists the website addresses of quality, safety, and regulatory resources.

The transfer of appropriate and accurate information from one care provider to another is an essential component of communication in health care. This point of information exchange is most commonly termed "handoff". It occurs between shifts, handover to a new clinician on the case, transfer to another unit/level of care/procedure department, and discharge. During an effective handoff, critical information, continuity of care and treatment is maintained. Ineffective handoffs lead to adverse events and patient safety risks. Clinical environments are dynamic and complex, presenting multiple challenges for communication among care providers. Specialized care units, shortened hospital stays, complex

BOX 1-2 Quality and Safety (QSEN) Education for Nurses Competencies

- Patient-Centered Care
  - Recognize the patient or designee as the source of control and full partner in providing compassionate and coordinated care based on respect for patient's preferences, values, and needs.
- Teamwork and Collaboration
  - Function effectively within nursing and interprofessional teams, fostering open communication, mutual respect, and shared decision making to achieve quality patient care.
- Evidence-Based Practice
  - Integrate best current evidence with clinical expertise and patient/family preferences and values for delivery of optimal health care.
- Quality Improvement
  - Use data to monitor the outcomes of care processes and use improvement methods to design and test changes to improve the quality and safety of health care systems continuously.
- Safety
  - Minimizes risk of harm to patients and providers through both system effectiveness and individual performance.
- Informatics
  - Use information and technology to communicate, manage knowledge, mitigate error, and support decision making.

From Cronenwett L, et al: Quality and safety education for nurses, *Nursing Outlook* 55(3):122, 2007.

conditions and treatment plans requiring multiple specialist clinicians also add to the potential for unclear and missing communication. For nursing, the greatest number of hand-offs occur daily during the exchange of patient information at change of shift. Many procedures, guidelines, and communication tools have been developed that facilitate an effective handoff.[56]

HEALTHY WORK ENVIRONMENT

There is an increasing amount of evidence that unhealthy work environments lead to medical errors, suboptimal safety monitoring, ineffective communication among health care providers, and increased conflict and stress among care providers. Synthesis of research in the area of work environment has demonstrated that a combination of leadership styles and characteristics contributes to the development and sustainability of healthy work environments.[57]

The AACN has formulated standards for establishing and sustaining healthy work environments (HWE).[58] The intent of the standards is to promote creation of environments that will have a positive impact on nursing and patient outcomes. Evidence-based and relationship-centered principles were used to create the standards of professional performance. A summary of the six standards is provided in Box 1-4. Figure 1-1 illustrates the interdependence of each standard and the ultimate impact on optimal patient outcomes and clinical excellence.

BOX 1-3 INTERNET RESOURCES

- American Association of Critical Care Nurses (AACN): http://www.aacn.org
- Healthcare Information and Management Systems Society (HIMSS): http://www.himss.org
- Institute for Healthcare Improvement (IHI): http://www.ihi.org
- Institute of Medicine (IOM): http://www.iom.gov
- Institute for Safe Medicine Practices (ISMP): http://www.ismp.org
- The Joint Commission (TJC): http://www.jointcommission.org
- National Database of Nursing Quality Indicators (NDNQI): http://www.nursingquality.org
- National Quality Forum (NQF): http://www.nqf.org
- Quality and Safety Education for Nurses (QSEN): http://www.qsen.org
- Society of Critical Care Medicine (SCCM): http://www.sccm.org
- Multicultural Resources
  - Ethnomed: www.ethnomed.org
  - Refugee Health Information Network: http://www.rhin.org
  - Culture Clues: http://depts.washington.edu/pfes/CultureClues.htm
  - Medline Plus: Health Information in Multiple Languages: http://www.nlm.nih.gov/medlineplus/languages/languages.htlm
  - Selected Patient Information Resources in Asian Languages: htpp://spiral.tufts.edu; Spanish Languages: http://www.nlm.nih.gov/medlineplus/spanish

BOX 1-4 Healthy Work Environment Standards

Standard I: Skilled Communication
Nurses must be as proficient in communication skills as they are in clinical skills.

Standard II: True Collaboration
Nurses must be relentless in pursuing and fostering true collaboration.

Standard III: Effective Decision Making
Nurses must be valued and committed partners in making policy, directing and evaluating clinical care, and leading organizational operations.

Standard IV: Appropriate Staffing
Staffing must ensure the effective match between patient needs and nurse competencies.

Standard V: Meaningful Recognition
Nurses must be recognized and must recognize others for the value each brings to the work of the organization.

Standard VI: Authentic Leadership
Nurse leaders must fully embrace the imperative of a healthy work environment, authentically live it, and engage others in its achievement.

From American Association of Critical-Care Nurses (AACN). Standards for establishing and sustaining healthy work environments. Aliso Viejo, CA, 2005, AACN.

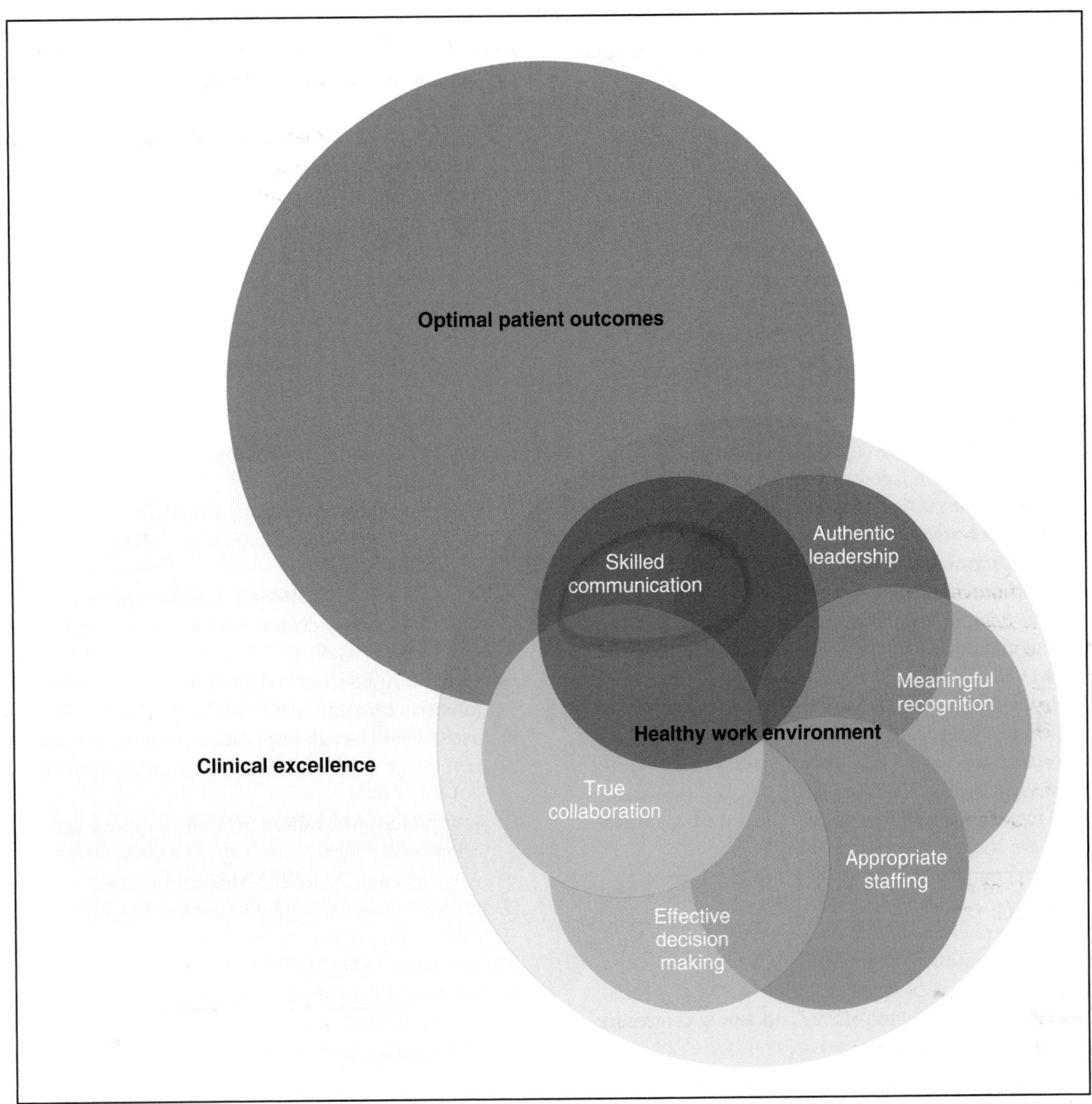

FIG 1-1 Interdependence of Healthy Work Environment, Clinical Excellence, and Optimal Patient Outcomes. (From American Association of Critical-Care Nurses [AACN]. Standards for establishing and sustaining healthy work environments. Aliso Viejo, CA, 2005, AACN.)

Everyone has a role in creating and sustaining a healthy work environment. Although the manager has a major role in establishing the culture, it is the staff who greatly impact the culture by mentoring new staff, role-modeling behaviors, and leading interdisciplinary teams. It is this peer pressure that has the most impact on all other staff.[59,60] Bylone discussed her experience of talking with many staff members about how they think that they can influence the work unit culture. She recommends asking them how they influence each of the HWE standards, thus making it a personal experience and journey in achieving the HWE.[61] Kupperschmidt and colleagues posed a five-factor model for becoming a skilled communicator: 1) becoming aware of self-deception, 2) becoming authentic, 3) becoming candid, 4) becoming mindful, and 5) becoming reflective, all of which lead to being a skilled communicator, thus creating a healthy work environment.[62] An additional approach for implementing the HWE model was offered by Blake, who suggested five steps: 1) rallying the team, 2) surveying the team, 3) establishing work groups, 4) setting goals and developing action steps, and 5) celebrating successes along the way.[63] Whatever approach taken will depend on the passion and commitment of the team.

REFERENCES

1. American Association of Critical Care Nurses: About critical care nursing. http://www.aacn.org. Accessed June 2012.
2. Jost SG, Bonnell M, Chako SJ, Parkinson DL: Integrated primary nursing: a care delivery model for the 21st-century knowledge worker, *Nurs Admin Q* 34(3):208, 2010.
3. Stacy KM: Progressive care units: different but the same, *Crit Care Nurse* 31(3):77, 2011.
4. American Association of Critical Care Nurses: Progressive care unit fact sheet. http://www.aacn.org. Accessed June 2012.

5. American Association of Critical-Care Nurses (AACN): *Standards for acute and critical care nursing practice*, Aliso Viejo, California, 2008, AACN.
6. American Association of Critical Care Nurses: About critical care nursing. http://www.aacn.org. Accessed June 30, 2014.
7. Williams LM, Hubbard KE, Daye O, Barden C: Telenursing in the intensive care unit: transforming nursing practice, *Crit Care Nurse* 32(6):62, 2012.
8. American Association of Critical Care Nurses: Value of certification resource center. http://www.aacn.org. Accessed June 2012.
9. American Association of Critical Care Nurses: Welcome to the beacon award for excellence. http://www.aacn.org. Accessed June 2012.
10. Society of Critical Care Medicine: About SCCM: *History of critical care*. http://www.sccm.org. Accessed June 2012.
11. Makic MB, VonRueden KT, Rauen CA, Chadwick J: Evidence-based practice habits: putting more sacred cows out to pasture, *Crit Care Nurse* 31(2):38, 2011.
12. Cullen L, Adams SL: Planning for implementation of evidence-based practice, *JONA* 42(4):222, 2012.
13. Schulman CS, Staul L: Standards for frequency of measurement and documentation of vital signs and physical assessments, *Crit Care Nurse* 30(3):74, 2010.
14. Gray M: Reducing catheter-associated urinary tract infection in the critical care unit, *AACN Adv Crit Care* 21(3):247, 2010.
15. American Association of Critical Care Nurses: Practice alert. http://www.aacn.org. Accessed Sept 2012.
16. Panting K: Intensive care/intensive cure: the future of critical care? *Crit Care Nurse* 15(12):100, 1995.
17. Miller KL: Keeping the care in nursing care: our biggest challenge, *J Nurse Adm* 25(11):29–32, 1995.
18. Warren NA: The phenomenon of nurses' caring behaviors as perceived by the critical care family, *Crit Care Nurs Q* 17(3):67, 1994.
19. Powers PH, et al: The value of patient- and family-centered care, *Am J Nurs* 100(5):84, 2000.
20. Collins KS, Hall A: *U.S. minority health: a chart book*, 1999, Commonwealth Fund.
21. Bushy A: Social and cultural factors affecting health care and nursing practice. In Lancaster J, editor: *Nursing: issues in leading and managing change*, St. Louis, 1999, Mosby.
22. Gonzales R, et al: Eliminating racial and ethnic disparities in health care, *Am J Nurs* 100(3):56, 2000.
23. Leonard B, Plotnikoff GA: Awareness: the heart of cultural competence, *AACN Clin Issues* 11(1):51, 2000.
24. Schnall JG, Fowler M: Multicultural web resources, *AJN* 114(6):63, 2014.
25. Lindquist R, Kirksey K: Preface, *AACN Clin Issues* 11(1):1, 2000.
26. Lindquist R, et al: Challenges of implementing a feasibility study of acupuncture in acute and critical care settings, *AACN Adv Crit Care* 19(2):202, 2008.
27. Kreitzer MJ, Jensen D: Healing practices: trends, challenges, and opportunities for nurses in critical care, *AACN Clin Issues* 11(1):7, 2000.
28. Tusek DL, Cwynar RE: Strategies for implementing guided imagery program to enhance patient experience, *AACN Clin Issues* 11(1):68, 2000.
29. McKenney C, Johnson R: Unleash the healing power of pet therapy, *Am Nurse Today* 3(5):29, 2008.
30. Cole K, Fawlinski A: Animal-assisted therapy: the human-animal bond, *AACN Clin Issues* 11(1):139, 2000.
31. Goran SF: A new view: Tele-intensive care unit competencies, *Crit Care Nurse* 31(5):17, 2011.
32. Wheelan SA, et al: The link between teamwork and patients' outcomes in intensive care units, *Am J Crit Care* 12(6):527, 2003.
33. Boyle DK, Kochinda C: Enhancing collaborative communication of nurse and physician leadership in two intensive care units, *J Nurs Adm* 34(2):60, 2004.
34. Falise JP: True collaboration: interdisciplinary rounds in nonteaching hospitals—it can be done! *AACN Adv Crit Care* 18(4):346, 2007.
35. Golanowski M, et al: Interdisciplinary shared decision making—taking shared governance to the next level, *Nurs Admin Q* 31(4):341, 2007.
36. Reina ML, et al: Trust: the foundation for team collaboration and healthy work environments, *AACN Adv Crit Care* 18(2):103, 2007.
37. Manojlovich M, Antonakos C: Satisfaction of intensive care unit nurses with nurse-physician communication, *JONA* 38(5):237, 2008.
38. Blot S, Afonso E, Labeau S: Insights and advances in multidisciplinary critical care: a review of recent research, *AJCC* 23(1):70, 2014.
39. Garland A: Effect of collaborative care on cost variation in an intensive care unit, *AJCC* 22(3):232, 2013.
40. Tschannen D, et al: Implications of nurse-physician relations: report of a successful intervention, *Nurs Econ* 29(3):127, 2011.
41. Interprofessional Education Collaborative Expert Panel: *Core competencies for interprofessional collaborative practice*, 2011, Association of American Medical Colleges.
42. D'Arcy Y: Practice guidelines, standards, consensus statements, position papers: what they are, how they differ, *Am Nurse Today* 2(10):23, 2007.
43. White GB: Patient safety: an ethical imperative, *Nurs Econ* 20(4):195, 2002.
44. Henneman EA, et al: Strategies used by critical care nurses to identify, interrupt, and correct medical errors, *AJCC* 19(6):500, 2010.
45. The Joint Commission: Behaviors that undermine a culture of safety, *Sentinel Event Alert* (40), 2008. http://www.jointcommission.org/sentinel_event.aspx. Accessed June 30, 2014.
46. Covell CL: Can civility in nursing work environments improve medication safety? *JONA* 40(7/8):300, 2010.
47. Henneman EA: Patient safety and technology, *AACN Adv Crit Care* 20(2):128, 2009.
48. Frith KH: Medication errors in the intensive care unit, *AACN Adv Crit Care* 24(4):389, 2013.
49. Anthony K, et al: No interruptions please: impact of a no interruption zone on medication safety in intensive care units, *Crit Care Nurse* 30(3):21, 2010.
50. The Joint Commission: 2014 Hospital National Patient Safety Goals. http://www.jointcommission.org. Accessed June 30, 2014.
51. The Joint Commission: Facts about the official "Do Not Use" List. http://www.jointcommission.org.
52. *Medical Device Reporting (MDR)*. http://www.fda.gov/MedicalDevices/Safety/ReportaProblem/default.htm. Accessed June 30, 2014.
53. U.S. Department of Health and Human Services, Food and Drug Administration: Warnings for Industry: Warnings and

precautions, contraindications, and boxed warning sections of labeling for human prescriptive drug and biological products-content and format, October 2011. http://www.fda.gov/Drugs/GuidanceComplianceRegulatoryinformation/Guidances/default.htm. Accessed June 30, 2014.

54. Institute for Safe Medication Practices: About ISMP. http://www.ISMP.org. Accessed June 30, 2014.
55. Quality Safety Education for Nurses. http://www.QSEN.org. Accessed June 30, 2014.
56. Friesen MA, White SV, Byers JF: Chapter 34: Handoffs: implications for nurses. *Patient Safety and Quality: An Evidence-Based Handbook for Nurses Vol 2.* http://www.NCbi.NLM.NIH.gov/books. Accessed June 30, 2014.
57. Pearson A, et al: Comprehensive systematic review of evidence on developing and sustaining nursing leadership that fosters a healthy work environment in healthcare, *Int J Evid Based Health* 5:208–253, 2007.
58. American Association of Critical-Care Nurses (AACN): AACN standards for establishing and sustaining healthy work environments. http://www.aacn.org. Accessed June 2012.
59. Bylone M: Healthy work environments: whose job is it anyway? *AACN Adv Crit Care* 20(4):325, 2009.
60. Bylone M: I think they are talking about me!! *AACN Adv Crit Care* 20(2):137, 2009.
61. Bylone M: Health work environment 101, *AACN Adv Crit Care* 22(1):19, 2011.
62. Kupperschmidt B, et al: A healthy work environment: it begins with you, *Online J Issues Nurs* 15(1):manuscript 3, 2010. http://nursingworld.org/mainmenucategories/ANAMarketplace/ANAPeriodicals/OJIN. Accessed February 17, 2010.
63. Blake N: Practical steps for implementing healthy work environments, *AACN Adv Crit Care* 23(1):14, 2012.

2 CHAPTER

Ethical and Legal Issues

Linda D. Urden, Kelly K. Dineen

Be sure to check out the bonus material, including review questions, on the Evolve website at http://evolve.elsevier.com/Urden/priorities/.

ETHICAL ISSUES

Differences between Morals, Ethics, and Ethical Problems

Morals are traditions of belief about what is right or wrong in human behavior. Informed by individual and group values, morality is comprised of standards of conduct that include moral principles, rules, virtues, rights, and responsibilities. Moral norms form the basis for right action and provide a framework for the evaluation of behavior through a system of ethics.[1-3]

Ethics is a generic term for the reasoned inquiry and understanding of a moral life. Different theories or systems of ethics identify which moral norms should be used and how they should be prioritized to evaluate whether conduct is ethical.[1,2] Applied ethics, of which health care ethics is a branch, is the attempt to use moral norms to evaluate conduct and to resolve particular ethical problems in context.[1] Although only the extreme situations at the end or beginning of life garner attention, health care providers, and especially nurses, act repeatedly in small ethical or unethical ways each day that impact patient care. Day-to-day decisions fall within the realm of ethics if they 1) pertain to things within our control and 2) will show respect or fail to respect human beings.[4] Most of the time, there is a right thing to do, and it can be done without conflict or resulting harm.

Nurses and Moral Distress

Nurses face multiple challenges on a daily basis: emergency situations, tension from conflict with others, complex clinical cases, new technologies, increasing regulatory requirements, acquisition of new skills/knowledge, staffing issues, financial constraints, challenging emotional and behavioral responses from patients and coworkers, and workplace violence, to name a few. This has led to an increasingly complex moral environment and frequent ethical dilemmas.[6] These factors as well as feelings of powerlessness and lack of control can contribute to detachment from the ethical impact of day-to-day decisions and contribute to professional "burn out."[6,7]

Moral distress has recently been widely discussed in the literature as a serious problem for nurses.[6-9] Moral distress occurs when a person knows the ethically appropriate action but feels unable to act on it because of one or more barriers. These barriers can include the medical plan of care, workplace dynamics, organizational rules, imbalanced power dynamics, interpersonal conflict, or even individual psychosocial processes. Moral courage is the strength to act ethically despite the barriers that cause moral distress.

It is crucial that nurses recognize moral distress and actively seek strategies to address the issue through institutional, personal, and professional organizational resources. The AACN has created a framework—*The 4A's to Rise Above Moral Distress*—to support nurses who are experiencing moral distress (Figure 2-1).[10-13] ASK, the first stage, is a self-awareness and reflection period in which one becomes more aware of the distress and its effects on oneself. Specific areas to address are physical, spiritual, emotional, and behavioral responses. During stage two, AFFIRM, one affirms the distress and makes a commitment to take care of oneself. In stage three, ASSESS, one needs to identify the timing and context of when the stressors occur, determine the severity of the distress, and examine one's readiness to act. The final stage, ACT, consists of preparation, the action itself, and maintaining the desired change. Although the model was created by AACN, it is a framework that can be used in diverse settings and by various health care professionals.[11-12]

HEALTH CARE ETHICS AND PRINCIPLES

As mentioned before, moral norms form the basis of ethics. In health care, certain principles and corresponding rights form the basis of the most prevalent ethical frameworks. Principles are general guidelines that govern conduct, provide a basis for reasoning, and direct actions.[15] Decisions at the bedside often reflect adherence to a principle or principles while overriding another. This must be resolved by justifying the decision for overriding one or more principles and specifying the conditions under which it may occur.[1] The six ethical principles that are discussed in this chapter are respect for persons/autonomy, beneficence, non-maleficence, veracity, fidelity, and justice.

Respect for Persons/Autonomy

In health care, respect for persons requires individuals to honor the patient's right to autonomy or to self-determine a course of action[15] without coercion or undue interference from others. Autonomy is a basic human right and is subject to compromise in the context of health care decision making. Autonomy is also the foundation of the legal and ethical

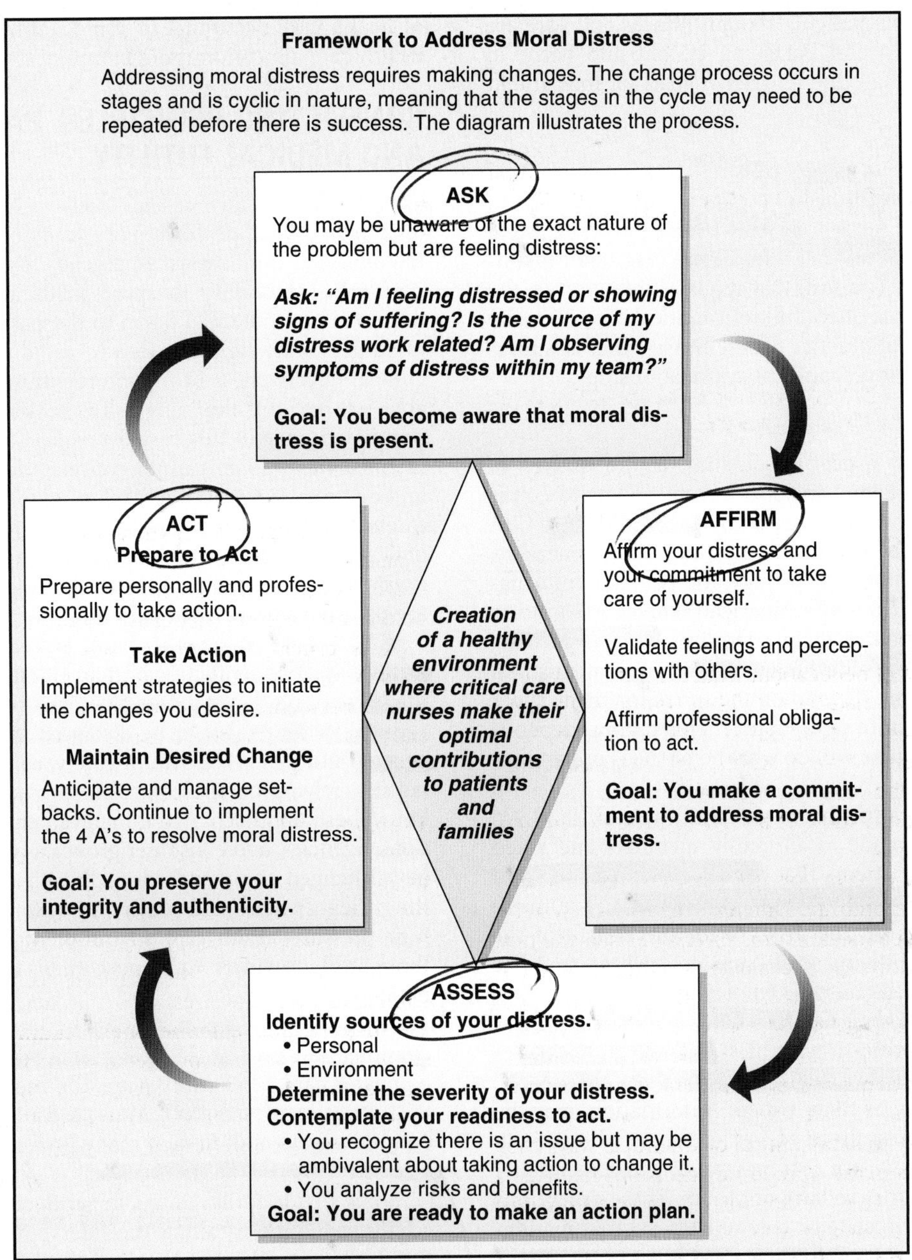

Framework to Address Moral Distress
Addressing moral distress requires making changes. The change process occurs in stages and is cyclic in nature, meaning that the stages in the cycle may need to be repeated before there is success. The diagram illustrates the process.
ASK
You may be unaware of the exact nature of the problem but are feeling distress:
Ask: "Am I feeling distressed or showing signs of suffering? Is the source of my distress work related? Am I observing symptoms of distress within my team?"
Goal: You become aware that moral distress is present.
AFFIRM
Affirm your distress and your commitment to take care of yourself.
Validate feelings and perceptions with others.
Affirm professional obligation to act.
Goal: You make a commitment to address moral distress.
ASSESS
Identify sources of your distress.
• Personal
• Environment
Determine the severity of your distress.
Contemplate your readiness to act.
• You recognize there is an issue but may be ambivalent about taking action to change it.
• You analyze risks and benefits.
Goal: You are ready to make an action plan.
ACT
Prepare to Act
Prepare personally and professionally to take action.
Take Action
Implement strategies to initiate the changes you desire.
Maintain Desired Change
Anticipate and manage setbacks. Continue to implement the 4 A's to resolve moral distress.
Goal: You preserve your integrity and authenticity.
Creation of a healthy environment where critical care nurses make their optimal contributions to patients and families

FIG 2-1 The ACCN 4 A's to Rise above Moral Distress. (From American Association of Critical-Care Nurses. *Position Statement: Moral Distress.* Aliso Viejo, CA: AACN; July 8, 2004.)

requirement of informed consent and includes the right to refuse some or all treatments.[1]

Promoting autonomous decision making is a crucial and sometimes difficult responsibility of nurses in critical care. Emergency situations may require action without consent. Even in non-emergent situations, critically ill patients may not have capacity, and family, friends, or others must act as surrogate decision-makers (through formal powers of attorney or pursuant to state laws). Patients and families must have all of the relevant information and the ability to understand and weigh options before they can make a decision that is consistent with the patient's values. This is where the nurse is a most important member of the health care team—as patient advocate, the nurse provides and clarifies information, encourages reflection, and provides support during the decision-making process.

Beneficence and Nonmaleficence

The ethical principles of beneficence and nonmaleficence require actions that maximize good and minimize harm to the patient, often in a delicate balance. The principle of beneficence presupposes compassion and requires the promotion of others' well-being through positive action and the desire to do good.[15] In contrast, nonmaleficence dictates that nurses prevent and minimize harm and correct harmful situations. Benefits must be maximized and harms minimized. In critical care practice, every inaction as well as procedure and intervention holds the serious potential for harm even though the intent is to benefit the patient. Thoughtfulness and care are necessary in defining and balancing benefit and harm in terms of both immediate and long-term goals for the patient.

Veracity

Veracity, the quality of being truthful, is a principle that underlies a trusting relationship between nurse and patient. Veracity requires the nurse to disclose the appropriate information fully in a manner that minimizes biases and misunderstandings.[7,15] This is a task that requires intention in the midst of the chaos that often infiltrates critical care. Veracity must guide all areas of practice for the nurse—that is, supervisor, colleague, employee, and patient relationships.

Fidelity

Fidelity, an essential aspect of nursing, is the quality of keeping commitments and includes commitments to confidentiality and privacy; it is based on the virtue of caring.[15] In critical care especially, patients and families are vulnerable; they surrender much of their privacy and personal information while receiving care. The American Nurses Association (ANA) states that this principle requires loyalty, fairness, truthfulness, advocacy, and dedication to our patients. All patients in critical care depend on the nurse for many types of physical care and emotional support. This support depends upon trust that the nurse will do what he or she is professionally required to do.

Fidelity also supports the nurse-family relationship. An implicit promise is made to all family members and loved ones of critically ill patients that they will be kept informed in a timely fashion of any changes or concerns. The nurse must follow through on the promise for the benefit of the patient, family, the nursing profession as a whole, and the institution in which the nurse is employed.

Confidentiality and *privacy* are elements of fidelity in traditional health care professional ethics. Confidentiality relates to information or data while privacy relates to the person. Confidentiality requires that patient information may be shared only with those involved in the care of the patient. Exceptions to this only occur if maintaining confidentiality *seriously* jeopardizes the welfare of others. These exceptions are usually reflected in state or federal laws, such as mandatory reporting laws. *Privacy* is closely aligned with confidentiality of patient information but relates to the person. Nurses must minimize violations of patient privacy by, for example, ensuring that doors and curtains are closed during interactions and taking extra steps to keep the patient covered during procedures.

Justice

The principle of justice means that there is an equitable distribution of limited resources. The most common example of the principle of justice is the allocation of organs for transplant. Another is access to health care, which is an issue of social justice although it is not a constitutional right in the United States. Countless studies have demonstrated the negative impact of the U.S. system of care delivery on the health status of U.S. residents. In fact, the Affordable Care Act attempts to improve the just distribution of health care access by increasing the availability health insurance for many Americans. At the same time, escalating health care costs, expanded technologies, an aging population, and a scarcity of health care personnel in some settings make the issue of health care allocation more complex.

CONFLICTING PRINCIPLES, PATERNALISM, AND MEDICAL FUTILITY

Conflict between principles is common and usually does not lead to an ethical problem. For example, suppose a patient is unconscious and needs emergency surgery for suspected peritonitis secondary to appendicitis and rupture. Surgery does real and potential harm to the patient, but the benefits of surgery outweigh the need to avoid harm because of the clinical effectiveness of the intervention and lack of reasonable, less harmful alternatives. The balance of beneficence and nonmaleficence in this case overrides autonomy because the unconscious patient cannot consent, time is of the essence, and delay will increase the likelihood of harm. It is justifiable to override autonomy here because of the competing reality of death in a patient with a treatable condition. Two common examples of the unethical resolution of conflicting principles are paternalism and medical futility.

Paternalism, on the other hand, is an example of an unethical resolution of conflicting principles. Paternalism exists when the nurse or physician makes a decision for the patient without consulting the patient or by disregarding the patient's preferences. Until the 1970s, health care was almost entirely paternalistic, relying on the control of providers under a "doctor knows best" approach. Active involvement by various organizations, agencies, and consumer groups as well as legal decisions have changed the standards in health care to deference to the patients' values and preferences. However, fast-paced and high-pressure health care environments may lead less-than-thoughtful providers to impose their recommendations on patients.

The concept of *medical futility* has resulted in various discussions and proposed criteria or formulas to predict outcomes of care.[16-19] Futility generally means there will be no useful result to an action. Medical futility has been defined countless ways and, in fact, many prefer the terms medically ineffective or non-beneficial care.[16]

Some divide futility into categories such as physiologic or scientific futility, meaning the intervention cannot treat the problem.[2,16] The classic example of physiologic futility is administering antibiotics for a viral infection. A closely related concept is quantitative or probabilistic futility, which means, based on statistical evidence, "any effort to achieve a result that is possible but that reasoning or experience suggests is highly improbable and that cannot be systematically reproduced."[17] However, there is a lack of generalizable research as well as conflicting thresholds for treatments to be considered futile.[16,19]

Futility is also described as qualitative, which is more appropriate in the context of critical care, although it also lacks consistency in agreement.[18] *Ethical futility* is treatment that will not serve the underlying interests, values, and preferences of the patient.[2] Perhaps a useful way to think about futility in the context of critical care is as an unethical balance of the principles of beneficence and nonmaleficence (doing harm with no balancing or overriding benefit) or as paternalism (imposing the provider's idea of benefit contrary to the values and preferences of the patient).

In critical care, futility is most often discussed in the context of end-of-life interventions. This is a pervasive ethical problem in the United States. According to Hofmann and Schneiderman, "death is not necessarily a medical failure; a bad death is not only a medical failure, but also an ethical breakdown."[20] Too many people in the United States experience a bad death. In general, providers fail to discuss death with patients, fail to refer to programs such as hospice or even palliative care appropriately, and persist in aggressively treating patients in high tech settings far past the appropriate time. Critical care nurses are on the forefront of this reality and can educate patients and families about options, clarify the realities associated with coding patients, and work with health care colleagues to foster thoughtfulness about the goals of care. Moral distress is extremely common among nurses who feel compelled to provide continued, painful, invasive care that will not benefit the patient or is contrary to the patient's wishes.

PROFESSIONAL NURSING ETHICS

A professional ethic forms the framework for any profession[21] and is based on three elements: 1) the professional code of ethics, 2) the purpose of the profession, and 3) the standards of practice of the professional. The code of ethics developed by the profession is the delineation of its values and relationships with and among members of the profession and society. The need for the profession and its inherent promise to provide certain duties form a contract between nursing and society. The professional standards describe specifics of practice in a variety of settings and subspecialties. Nursing professionals must stay consistent with their values and ethics and ensure that the ethical environment is maintained wherever nursing care and services are performed.[22-23] Each element is dynamic, and ongoing evaluations are necessary as societal expectations change, technologies increase, and the profession evolves.

Nursing Code of Ethics

The nursing code of ethics contains statements and directives for ethical nursing behavior.[24] The ANA Code of Ethics for Nurses provides the major source of ethical guidance for the nursing profession.[24] The nine statements of the code are found in Box 2-1. Further delineation of each of the provisions along with in-depth discussion and examples of application can be found on the ANA website, www.nursingworld.org. The Code of Ethics is a dynamic document and changes when "nursing and its social context changes."[25]

BOX 2-1 ANA Code of Ethics for Nurses

1. The nurse, in all professional relationships, practices with compassion and respect for the inherent dignity, worth, and uniqueness of every individual, unrestricted by considerations of social or economic status, personal attributes, or the nature of health problems.
2. The nurse's primary commitment is to the patient, whether an individual, family, group, or community.
3. The nurse promotes, advocates for, and strives to protect the health, safety, and rights of the patient.
4. The nurse is responsible and accountable for individual nursing practice and determines the appropriate delegation of tasks consistent with the nurse's obligation to provide optimum patient care.
5. The nurse owes the same duties to self as to others, including the responsibility to preserve integrity and safety, to maintain competence, and to continue personal and professional growth.
6. The nurse participates in establishing, maintaining, and improving health care environments and conditions of employment conducive to the provision of quality health care and consistent with the values of the profession through individual and collective action.
7. The nurse participates in the advancement of the profession through contributions to practice, education, administration, and knowledge development.
8. The nurse collaborates with other health professionals and the public in promoting community, national, and international efforts to meet health needs.
9. The profession of nursing, as represented by associations and other members, is responsible for articulating nursing values, for maintaining the integrity of the profession and its practice, and for shaping social policy.

From American Nurses Association. *Guide to the Code of Ethics for Nurses.* Washington, DC: ANA; 2008.

Situational and Organizational Ethical Decision Making in Critical Care

As discussed earlier, the critical care nurse encounters ethical issues on a daily basis. Pavlish and colleagues studied nurses involved in ethical problems, their early indicators and risk factors, nurse actions, and outcomes. From this study, they derived risk factors for patients, families, health care providers, and health care organizations. Additionally, they delineated early indicators for ethical dilemmas in six areas (Box 2-2).[28]

BOX 2-2 Early Indicators of Ethical Dilemmas

- Conflict among or between health care (HC) team members and patient/family members
- Patient suffering
- Nurse distress
- Ethics violation
- Unrealistic expectations
- Poor communication

Neglect of ethical problems or inadequate process or resolution at the individual or systems level results in harm to more than patients; this often results in poor staff morale, moral distress, increased operational and legal costs, negative public relations, and loss of trust in the profession. Because the nurse is on the front line of health care ethics and especially in the critical care setting, he or she has a unique and essential role in the resolution of ethical problems. Box 2-3 presents a sample of ethics-related Internet resources.

Resolving Ethical Problems

Ethical problems are ubiquitous in critical care and often related to conflicts surrounding the use of technology, including the withdrawal of technology. As mentioned earlier, ethical problems in critical care occur when there is 1) conflict between the right action and the ability to take it, 2) uncertainty about the right action, or 3) conflict about which of several right actions is most ethical.[4] Dealing with an ethical problem effectively requires those involved to pause,

BOX 2-3 ETHICS INTERNET RESOURCES

American Association of Critical-Care Nurses (AACN): www.aacn.org
- Joint Position Statement on ICU Overflow Patients
- Acute and Critical Care Choices—Guide to Advanced Directives
- Clinical Practice Guidelines for Quality Palliative Care
- Clinical Practice Guideline on Shared Decision Making in the Appropriate Initiation of Withdrawal from Dialysis
- Last Acts: Precepts of Palliative Care
- Pain Assessment in Nonverbal Patients

American Journal of Bioethics: www.bioethics.net
- Bioethics news and blog

American Nurses Association (ANA): www.nursingworld.org
- Multiple position statements on ethical issues in nursing (examples below)
- Nursing Care and Do Not Resuscitate (DNR) and Allow Natural Death Decisions
- Reduction of Patient Restraint and Seclusion in Health Care Settings
- Forgoing Nutrition and Hydration
- Registered Nurses' Roles and Responsibilities in Providing Expert Care and Counseling at End of Life
- The Nurses' Role in Ethics and Human Rights: Protecting and Promoting Individual Worth, Dignity, and Human Rights in Practice Settings
- Active Euthanasia

American Society for Bioethics and the Humanities (ASBH): www.asbh.org
- Not-for-profit organization committed to education and research in clinical ethics
- Core Competencies for Clinical Ethics Consultants
- Code of Ethics for Clinical Ethicists
- Nursing ethics interest group (affinity group)

Catholic Health Care Association of the United States: http://www.chausa.org/ethics/overview
- Catholic health care facilities are the largest group of non-profit health care in the United States and require consideration of additional ethical norms, the Ethical and Religious Directives for Catholic Health Care, in delivering care and resolving problems.

The Hastings Center: www.thehastingscenter.org
- Independent, nonpartisan, nonprofit bioethics research institute
- Provides educational resources and conferences, publications, and ethics consultation

International Council of Nurses (ICN): www.icn.org
- International Code of Ethics for Nurses

Presidential Commission for the Study of Bioethical Issues: http://www.bioethics.gov/
- Advisory panel of U.S. leaders in health care, science, law, and ethics that seeks to develop policies to foster the socially and ethically responsible delivery of health care and technology development.

United States Department of Veterans Affairs: www.ethics.va.gov
- Created ISSUES Preventative Ethics Model
- Preventative Ethics tools, educational resources, and toolkit for implementing the model
  - Integrated Ethics Program materials available

expand group consciousness about the issue, validate assumptions, look for patterns of thoughts or behaviors, and facilitate reflection and inquiry prior to making any decision.[33]

Steps in Ethical Decision Making

To facilitate the ethical decision-making process, a model or framework must be used so that all involved will consistently and clearly examine the multiple ethical issues that arise in critical care. There are numerous ethical decision-making models in the literature.[1,4,16,34-35] Box 2-4 lists steps in an ethical decision-making model used in this chapter.

BOX 2-4 Steps in Ethical Decision Making

1. Identify the *health problem.*
2. Define the *ethical issue(s).*
3. Gather *additional information.*
4. Identify the *stakeholders* and delineate the *decision maker.*
5. Examine ethical *norms* and other relevant norms.
6. Explore alternative *options.*
7. Implement decisions/*Act.*
8. *Evaluate and modify* actions.

Step One–Identify Health Problems

The major aspects of the medical and health problems must be identified. This includes the patient's history, diagnoses, potential sequelae, prognosis, and all data relevant to the health status. This should include the degree and invasiveness of care involved and the probability of success, including the patient's level of expected long-term function.

Step Two–Define the Ethical Issue(s)

The ethical problem must be clearly delineated from other types of problems. Is there uncertainty about the right action or conflicting ideas of right action? What ethical principles are in conflict? Is the problem something that can be addressed by correcting an underlying issue? Distinguish ethical problems from systems or social problems.

Step Three–Gather Any Relevant Additional or Previously Missing Information

Any relevant information missing in the initial problem presentation, as well as contextual data, should be obtained. Long-term prognosis is critical, and demographic data—age, ethnicity, religious preference, and educational and economic status—may be useful in the decision-making process. The role of the family or extended family and other support systems must be examined. It is essential to ascertain any patient values that are relevant as well as desires the patient might have expressed about treatment decisions.

Step Four–Identify the Stakeholders and Decision Maker

The patient is the primary decision maker and autonomously makes decisions after receiving information about the alternatives and sequelae of treatments or lack of treatments. However, in many ethical dilemmas, the patient lacks decision-making capacity because of a decreased level of consciousness or serious cognitive changes. It is in these situations that surrogate decision makers are relied upon. It is essential to have accurate information about any existing advanced directives, living wills, appointed durable powers of attorney for health care as well as state law regarding surrogate decision making. All stakeholders, including family and other support systems, nurses, physicians, social workers, clergy members, and others need to be identified.

Step Five–Examine Ethical and Legal Norms and Other Relevant Norms

Personal values, beliefs, and moral convictions of all involved in the decision process should be examined as they may inappropriately influence decisions away from the values and preferences of the patient. What ethical principles are in conflict? In the context of this patient, does beneficence balance out the necessary harm, or is the harm greater than benefit? Are the wishes of the patient in conflict with beneficence? What action most appropriately balances the various conflicting norms and most importantly, why? Are there legal requirements that conflict with an ethical option? Is the professional code of ethics in conflict with current or proposed actions?

Step Six–Options

After the identification of alternative options, the outcome of each action must be predicted in the specific context of the patient's situation. The short-range and long-range consequences of each action must be examined, and new or creative actions must be encouraged. Is there an option of taking a small action and reevaluating in a few days? Maintaining the status quo or doing nothing is always an option. This analysis helps eliminate inappropriate and identify ethically viable options. The nurse's problem-solving abilities will be important in arriving at appropriate and creative solutions.

Step Seven–Act or Implement the Decision

A decision is reached, usually after much thought and consideration, and the decision is implemented. Close attention to detail of the agreed-upon plan is essential. All members of the health care team must be updated, along with the family. Ongoing accurate communication is essential, as is support for the family and caregivers.

Step Eight–Evaluate

Evaluation of the decision provides a basis for future ethical decisions. If outcomes are not as predicted, it may be possible to modify the plan or implement an alternative. The case can then be reviewed for implications in future ethical interventions and education of the health care team.

CASE STUDY Patient with Ethical Dilemma

Brief Patient History

Mr. X is a 67-year-old obese male. He has a 2-year history of emphysema (100 packs/year history of tobacco abuse in the past) with two recent hospitalizations for pneumonia that required ventilatory support. Mr. X states that he does not want to be placed on a ventilator again but does not want to suffer either. He was involved in a motor vehicular accident (MVA) and sustained blunt trauma to his trunk and lower extremities, with bilateral femur fractures. Although his condition is critical, he is expected to recover. Mr. X received morphine 5 mg by intravenous push in the emergency department, with minimal pain relief; however, he has experienced new-onset confusion. Mr. X's spouse and children express concern about the risk of respiratory depression due to pain medication. They state that they would rather Mr. X experience pain than have him placed on the ventilator again.

Clinical Assessment

Mr. X is admitted to the critical care unit from the emergency department with blood transfusions in progress. Buck's traction (5 pounds) has been applied to both lower extremities. He is awake, alert, and oriented to person, time, place, and situation. Mr. X is breathing through his mouth, taking shallow breaths. He complains of right upper quadrant abdominal pain when taking a deep breath. His skin is warm and dry. Mr. X is able to move his toes on command, and lower extremity sensation to touch is intact; however, he is complaining of severe bilateral lower extremity pain with restlessness.

Diagnostic Procedures

Arterial blood gases: PaO_2, 55 mm Hg; $PaCO_2$, 28 mm Hg; pH, 7.35; HCO_3^-, 24 mEq/L; O_2 saturation, 88%.

Hematocrit, 24%; hemoglobin, 8 g/dL. Patient reports pain as a 10 on the Baker-Wong Faces Scale. Riker Sedation-Agitation Scale score = 5.

Medical Diagnosis

Mr. X is diagnosed with a hepatic hematoma and bilateral femur fractures from an MVA.

Questions

1. What major outcomes do you expect to achieve for this patient?
2. What problems or risks must be managed to achieve these outcomes?
3. What interventions could be initiated to monitor, prevent, manage, or eliminate the problems and risks identified?
4. Assuming the patient consents, what interventions could be initiated to promote optimal functioning, safety, and well-being of the patient?
5. What possible learning needs would you anticipate for this patient?
6. What cultural and age-related factors might have a bearing on the patient's plan of care?

LEGAL ISSUES

Overview

This section will highlight some of the laws and legal systems that figure prominently in nursing practice, including 1) administrative law (illustrated by the regulation of the profession by state boards of nursing), 2) tort law (lawsuits brought by patients for the actions or inactions of nurses), 3) constitutional law (illustrated through a discussion of the legal rights of patients to make decisions to accept or refuse treatment), and 4) federal and state health care statutory laws (illustrated through self-determination laws and select federal laws).

ADMINISTRATIVE LAW: PROFESSIONAL REGULATION

Functions of Boards of Nursing

The regulation of nursing practice is intended to protect the health and safety of citizens by 1) regulating the conditions of licensure, 2) regulating the scope of practice, 3) establishing a framework of standards of nursing practice, 4) removing incompetent or unsafe practitioners through disciplinary actions, and 5) prohibiting unlicensed persons from providing services reserved for licensed individuals. In addition, the regulation of nursing can enhance the professional status and public's trust of nurses.

Scope of Practice

BONs maintain expectations for and limits of nursing practice in each state through licensure and also through challenges to non-nurses engaged in professional activities that intrude upon the nursing scope of practice.[36-38] The scope of practice generally refers to the broad range of activities that nurses perform and manage in the delivery of care. Scope of practice is framed broadly to account for the many professional nursing settings and roles but also to account for activities that are reserved for professional nurses or, as appropriate, their delegatees with nursing supervision.

Standards of Practice

NPAs establish the scope of nursing practice, while BONs usually develop standards of practice at the state level through administrative rulemaking. These standards of practice communicate the expectations of safe and effective nursing practice within the scope of practice. State standards of practice also assist BONs in evaluating the ongoing practice of nursing. Thus, to understand the expectations for and limits of nursing fully in any particular state, it is necessary to review both the NPA and the rules or regulations of the BON.

In addition to standards developed by BONs, many specialty nursing organizations have developed standards of practice. While the BON standards establish broad expectations of safety and efficacy, specialty standards are more targeted and aimed at fostering excellence in the specialized field. An example of specialty standards are those developed by the American Association of Critical-Care Nurses (AACN).[39]

Nursing standards developed by professional and specialty nursing organizations complement BON standards, provide detail and specificity, and are typically drafted to promote excellence in clinical practice. Foundational organizations such as the American Nurses Association (ANA) and the AACN publish standards of practice and standards of care.[39-40] These specialty standards are helpful in establishing and measuring quality care and often reflect a consensus opinion of experts in the particular specialty of appropriate nursing care.

The extent to which specialty standards are introduced in a legal context varies widely from state to state. It is critical to understand that the legal term of art, "standard of care," is not the same as the standards of practice. In some cases, specialty standards of practice or care have been introduced in court to help establish a legal "standard of care," but not all courts will consider these. The legal standard of care and the use of specialty standards will be discussed further in the Tort Law section.

TORT LAW: NEGLIGENCE AND PROFESSIONAL MALPRACTICE, INTENTIONAL TORTS

Many civil lawsuits for injuries fall under the legal heading of torts. Anyone can find themselves as a party in such a lawsuit. Torts are civil lawsuits based on unintentional acts (failure to act or negligence that results in harm) or intentional acts, such as assault, battery, or defamation. For the lay public, the standard of behavior for negligence is based on reasonableness, or what a reasonably prudent person would do in the same situation. This is also known as ordinary negligence.

In a professional capacity, individuals are judged based on their professional standard of care. Nurses caring for acutely and critically ill patients may be alleged to have acted in a manner that is inconsistent with standards of care or standards of professional practice, and they may find themselves involved in civil litigation that focuses in whole or in part on the alleged failure. This is professional malpractice or negligence law applied to professional behavior. This chapter will focus on negligence and professional malpractice, intentional torts of assault and battery, and some cases based on specific clinical circumstances.

Ordinary Negligence

Generally, the standard for negligence is failing to act as a reasonably prudent person would under similar circumstances. There are four criteria or elements for all negligence cases: 1) duty to another person, 2) breach of that duty, 3) harm that would not have occurred in the absence of the breach (causation), and 4) damages that have a monetary value. All four elements must be satisfied for a case to go forward. Negligence in the professional health care context differs in that expert testimony is needed to establish the standard of care. These cases are referred to as professional negligence or professional malpractice.

Professional Malpractice

Whereas negligence claims may apply to anyone, malpractice requires the alleged wrongdoer to have special standing as a professional. If a nurse caring for acutely and critically ill patients is accused of failing to act in a manner consistent with the standard of care, that nurse is subject to liability for professional malpractice (negligence applied to a professional). Just as in ordinary negligence, the person bringing the lawsuit must prove the elements of negligence. In the health care context, patient/plaintiffs (person[s] bringing the lawsuit) must prove 1) that the nurse had a duty to care for the patient, 2) that the nurse breached that duty by deviating from the standard of care, 3) that the breach caused harm that would not have occurred in the absence of negligence, and 4) that the plaintiff should be compensated for the resulting damages.

In civil cases alleging wrongdoing by health care professionals, the terms "malpractice" and "negligence" are used interchangeably, although there are courts that distinguish between the two causes of action. The legal standard of care for nurses is established by expert testimony and is generally "the care that an ordinarily prudent *nurse* would perform under the same circumstances."[41] The standard of care determination focuses more on accepted practice of competent nurses rather than best practice of excellent nurses (which may be reflected in some specialty standards of practice). This is sometimes interpreted as the knowledge and skills of an average nurse, applied with reasonable care.[42] In addition to expert testimony, courts may rely on multiple types of evidence to establish the standard of care.

Duty

Duty to the injured party is the first element of a malpractice case and is premised on the existence of a nurse-patient relationship. Nurses assume a duty to the patient to provide care that is consistent with the standard of care when the nurse-patient relationship is established. Cases from a number of states recognize the nurse-patient relationship as a separate and distinct relationship[43] and as a prerequisite for determining whether a nurse owes the patient a duty to provide care in accordance with the requisite standard of care. If a nurse shows that he or she was either 1) not assigned to that particular patient or 2) not working on the date that the negligence allegedly occurred, no duty will be imposed on the nurse. Because no duty is imposed on the nurse, negligence allegations will fail.[44]

Breach

Breach is the failure to act within applicable standards of care. For a nurse to be found negligent, the patient-plaintiff must establish that the nurse failed to provide care consistent with those standards. A breach does not exist if the standard of care is met. The other elements of duty to the patient, causation of harm, and resulting damages must also be proven.

Documents or policies specific to the nurse's employer or practice setting may also be used to inform the appropriate standard of care. For example, a nurse's job description or employment contract may contain provisions that require a nurse to act or to refrain from acting in a specific manner and within a specific period of time. Failure to adhere to those provisions could give rise to negligence causes of action wherein the patient-plaintiff asserts that the nurse failed to act in accordance with his or her job description or employment contract. Accordingly, job descriptions and employment contracts must be reflective of the standard of care, clear and accurate.

Nurses caring for acutely and critically ill patients are required to act in a manner that is consistent with organizational policies, procedures, protocols, and clinical pathways. Failure to do so may result in liability if a patient is harmed because of the failure. For example, in *Teffeteller v University of Minnesota*,[45] a nurse's failure to follow an established protocol resulted in a critically ill pediatric patient's death from narcotic toxicity.

Harm Caused by the Breach

Patients must also prove that the breach actually caused the harm suffered. If patient-plaintiffs fail to establish that some act or omission directly resulted in the harm, or if something else can be shown to have caused the harm, recovery will be denied. In *McMullen v Ohio State University Hospitals*,[46] 3 days after a patient was intubated and placed on a ventilator, her oxygen saturation and blood pressure suddenly dropped, and she became cyanotic and dyspneic. The nurse heard a squeak and thought it was a cuff leak on the endotracheal tube. The nurse believed that the patient was dying and paged the on-call physician "stat." Before the physicians arrived, the nurse removed the patient's endotracheal tube. Successful reintubation took twenty minutes. The patient never resumed consciousness and died 7 days later. The case went to trial, through several appeals and eventually to the Ohio Supreme Court. The court held the nurse's act of removing the endotracheal tube was negligent and directly caused a chain of events that resulted in the patient's death.

Damages

The fourth element of negligence is damages. Damages must be in the form of money and are derived from the harm or injury suffered by the patient. Patient-plaintiffs in a malpractice case can usually point to additional medical bills associated with their injuries and continuing care needs to satisfy this element.

The number of nurses being named defendants in these cases is increasing, and this is especially true for advanced practice nurses. Accordingly, nurses caring for acutely and critically ill patients need to consider carefully whether to purchase professional liability insurance and, if so, the amount and type of coverage that is needed. Most institutions will provide some level of malpractice insurance coverage for nurses, but the amount and circumstances under which each nurse is covered are important considerations.

Professional Malpractice and the Nursing Process

Malpractice claims may be premised on care delivered at any point from the moment a nurse-patient relationship is established to patient discharge. What constitutes reasonable care has been the focus of many cases filed against health care professionals and the hospitals in which they practice. For nurses, there seems to be an emerging trend. If the nurse reasonably executes every component of the nursing process by assessing, planning, implementing, and evaluating the care in accordance with the requisite standard of care, reasonable care will have been provided. However, if the nurse fails with regard to a single component of the nursing process, care provided to an acutely or critically ill patient will be deemed insufficient, unreasonable, and negligent. Expert testimony is required to establish the standard of care. The following cases are just a few examples of malpractice resulting from failures in particular stages of the nursing process.

Assessment failure: failure to assess and analyze the level of care needed by the patient. Nurses caring for acutely and critically ill patients have a duty to assess and analyze the level of care needed by their patients. Where a nurse allegedly fails to fulfill this responsibility, liability for negligence may be threatened. Brandon HMA, Inc. v Bradshaw[47] demonstrates how courts handle nurses' failure to assess and analyze the level of care needed. In Brandon, the patient, Bradshaw, sustained permanent injuries from an anoxic episode caused by negligence of the nursing staff during a hospitalization for bacterial pneumonia. Shortly after a chest tube was inserted, her nurse failed to take vital signs between 11:00 PM and 3:30 AM. At 3:30 AM, Ms. Bradshaw was disoriented, sweating profusely, and unable to follow verbal commands. Ten minutes later she arrested, a code was called and CPR initiated. The code team arrived and successfully resuscitated her, but she suffered anoxic brain injury. The night nurse's failure to assess Bradshaw for over 4 hours and to act immediately on her symptoms at 3:30 AM was the cause of the preventable deterioration. Bradshaw was awarded $9,000,000 by a jury.

Assessment failure: failure to ascertain a patient's wishes with regard to self-determination. Nurses caring for acutely and critically ill patients have a legal and ethical obligation to act in accordance with a patient's wishes with regard to self-determination. The patient's rights are discussed further in the Constitutional Law section below, but nurses must determine and abide by those wishes or risk facing disciplinary action and civil liability.

Anderson v St. Francis-St. George Hospital[48] demonstrated a failure to assess and implement the patient's wishes. Mr. Winter was admitted to the hospital for chest pain and fainting. After discussing treatment options with Mr. Winter, his physician, Dr. Russo, entered a "no code" order in Mr. Winter's chart. Three days later, a nurse defibrillated Mr. Winter for ventricular tachycardia, contrary to the "no code" order that reflected the patient's wishes. Two days later, Mr. Winter suffered a stroke that paralyzed his right side for the remainder of his life. Mr. Winter sued the hospital, alleging that it was negligent in failing to obey the "no code" order that had been issued. The Ohio Supreme Court eventually heard the case and concluded that the nurse's failure to honor Mr. Winter's wishes constituted a breach of care.

Implementation failure: failure to take appropriate action and failure to document. Cases from across the country continue to affirm that it is the nurse's responsibility to take affirmative action when action is indicated. *Garcia v United States*[49] is one such case. Failure to take appropriate action in cases involving acutely and critically ill patients has included not only physician-notification issues but also failure to follow physician orders,[50-51] failure to treat properly,[52] and failure to administer medication appropriately.[52-54] To avoid allegations of failure to take appropriate action, nurses caring for acutely and critically ill patients need to recognize signs and symptoms of complications and patient compromise and act on them appropriately. Patient findings, interventions and actions taken, and patient responses to those interventions must be documented.

Implementation failure: failure to preserve patient privacy and confidentiality. Nurses have a duty to preserve patient's privacy and confidentiality. State and federal statutes and case law affirm this duty. In *Doe v Ohio State University Hospital and Clinics,*[55] a nurse taking care of a human immunodeficiency virus (HIV) positive patient wrote "HIV +" on the "other test" section of a lab requisition form ordering a complete blood count and a serum potassium level. This was reportedly done to alert laboratory personnel of the patient's HIV status; however, the laboratory staff interpreted the notation as an instruction to perform an HIV screen, despite a hospital policy requiring physician-obtained informed consent. The patient was outraged that the HIV testing had been done without his consent and filed a malpractice action.

The case was ultimately dismissed, but it serves as a reminder to guard the privacy of every patient. Nurses must ensure that the privacy of acutely and critically ill patients is protected through professional behavior, such as restricting patient-specific discussions to the immediate care team and only in a non-public setting. Privacy and confidentiality provisions at the institutional, state, and federal level set minimum levels of conduct for nurses. Laws such as the Health Insurance Portability and Accountability Act (HIPAA)[56] as well as institutional policies and procedures are in place to protect patients.

Evaluation failure: failure to act as a patient advocate. From admission to discharge, nurses have a duty to act as a patient advocate. For nurses caring for acutely and critically ill patients, this duty imposes the responsibility to evaluate the care that is being given to patients. The landmark failure to advocate case was *Darling v Charleston Community Memorial Hospital,*[57] in which an 18-year-old athlete with a complicated leg fracture was hospitalized, placed in traction and casted. Shortly after the cast was applied, Dorrence began to complain of severe pain in his leg, and his exposed toes were swollen, discolored, cold, and insensitive to touch. Nonetheless, the cast remained in place for days despite these physical findings as well as a noxious odor and significant drainage from the cast. Dorrence lost his leg as a result of the prolonged ischemia.

According to the court, if the nursing staff had promptly recognized and acted on the circulatory compromise, the damage may have been reversible. The nurses should have exercised their duty to advocate for the patient and prevent the loss of his leg. The hospital was liable for their failure. Courts consistently hold that all nurses have a nondelegatable duty to act as patient advocate. Failure to act as patient advocate exposes the nurse to substantial liability and, more importantly, exposes patients to avoidable life-altering and life-ending complications.

Wrongful Death

Wrongful death cases are a variation of negligence action in which the harm is the actual death of the individual. Like ordinary negligence, wrongful death claims can also be brought against non-professionals. However, in the professional health care context, these claims are a form of professional negligence and are filed by the survivors of patients who allege that the patient died because of the negligence of health care organizations or health care professionals. The elements are the same as professional negligence: 1) duty, 2) breach, 3) causation of harm, and 4) damages, but the harm is always death.

Assault and Battery

Assault and battery are examples of intentional torts that are frequently brought against health care providers. Although they are often used together, they are actually two separate torts. Assault is any intentional act that creates *reasonable fear* of immediate harmful or offensive contact. With assault, no actual contact is necessary. Battery, on the other hand, is any intentional act that brings about actual harmful or offensive contact.

In health care cases, patient consent is a defense to these claims. Assault occurs if a patient fears harmful or offensive touching. For example, the act of telling a patient that they will be restrained may be assault. Battery occurs if the health care professional actually touches the patient in an unauthorized manner. The act of restraining a patient without consent is battery. Another defense to assault and battery is an emergency situation. Thus, cutting a patient's throat to create an emergency tracheostomy may be justified, while cutting a patient's neck on the wrong side for surgery in opposition to the informed consent may be battery.

CONSTITUTIONAL LAW: PATIENT DECISION MAKING

The right of competent adult patients to refuse treatment is well-established in state and federal constitutional law. This right has evolved from the common law doctrine of informed consent, the laws of assault and battery (the right to be free from fear of harm and unwanted touching), and the common law right to self-determination.[58]

A competent adult patient has the right to refuse even life-sustaining treatment for any reason at all, without regard for that individual's motivations. *Bouvia v Superior Court*[59] is representative of this principle. In *Bouvia*, a young woman with significant mobility disabilities refused to eat and accept treatment except comfort care. The facility in which she resided subjected her to countless psychiatric evaluations, all of which indicated she was fully competent (or had decision-making capacity). The court held that because she was a competent adult who understood the consequences of her decisions, she could not be compelled to accept even food against her wishes.

Patients without Decision-Making Capacity and Advanced Directives

Patients without decision-making capacity include individuals who were previously competent (those who reached adulthood but lost competence), those who were never competent (those born with severe-to-profound cognitive disabilities), those who are not yet competent (primarily children under 18), and those with fluctuating competence, such as individuals with cyclical disorders such as bipolar disorder that can seriously impair decision making. When a patient lacks capacity, a surrogate decision maker must make treatment decisions. The law imposes standards of judgment for surrogate decision makers to guide and evaluate decisions. The legal requirements and analyses are more stringent for decisions that may directly impact life, including decisions to forgo or withdraw treatment at the end of life.

Advanced Directives allow patients to provide clear direction themselves before losing capacity. These documents commonly include the living will, a statement of health care directives, and the durable power of attorney for health care. Many states also have Physician's or Medical Orders for Life-saving Treatment (POLST or MOLST forms) that implement wishes directly in the form of a valid physician's order. Some states also have out-of-hospital DNR forms.

These are legally binding documents that allow individuals to specify a variety of preferences, particular treatments they want to avoid, and circumstances in which they wish to avoid them. The *living will* specifies that if certain circumstances occur, such as terminal illness, the patient will decline specific treatments. They are of marginal use because of common limitations based on life expectancy, pregnancy status, and in some states, nutritional support may not be declined through a living will. Advanced statements of directives based on treatments quickly become outdated as technology and practice changes. The most effective advanced directive is the appointment of a *durable power of attorney for health care (DPOA)*. The DPOA is a surrogate, or agent, designated by the patient, who must make decisions for the patient based on the patient's values. The DPOA is obligated to use the patient's values and preferences to make the decision the patient would make if he or she were able to do so. This is not an easy task, and individuals are urged to consider carefully their choice of agent. Each state has requirements for advance directives and how they must be created and validly executed. Once a patient creates a valid advance directive in their own state, other states must honor it. Advanced directives emerged in response to highly publicized legal cases over decision making.

Previously Competent Patients

Several highly publicized cases beginning in the 1970s concerned the withdrawal of treatment in young women who were previously competent. In each of these cases, the patient had sustained devastating neurologic injury, and a legal challenge was presented to their families' ability to withdraw treatment, including nutrition and hydration.[58-61] In each case, those same family members were entrusted for years with medical decisions for complex and life-threatening procedures, but the request to withdraw care or artificial nutrition or hydration was met with years of struggle in the legal system. This was, in part, because of state interests in protecting citizens and life in the absence of direct statements from the patient. These cases also established that in the absence of specific directions from the patient but with knowledge of the patient's previously expressed values and preferences, surrogate decision makers should use the substituted judgment standard. This means they must use the patient's values to decide what the patient would have wanted. The surrogate decision maker's own judgment about what should be done may differ; he or she must assume the preferences and values of the patient in making the decision. This is an enormous responsibility as well as a difficult task. To the extent patients can make their wishes known in advance, the agony already associated with these difficult decisions can be lessened.

Never and Not Yet Competent Patients

Competent adults can refuse treatment for any reason at all, even if others believe it is in opposition to their best interests. On the other hand, in the absence of a competent adult decision maker, directives, or a known set of values and preferences, the law requires decisions made in the best interest of the patient. This is true for adults born with neurologically devastating disabilities or incapacitated adults without family or friends. For never competent adults who are still able to evidence preferences, those should at least be considered in decision making.

Children under 18 do not have capacity for decision making. The law also imposes a best interest standard on children. This is most straightforward for very young children. As a child matures, there are increased legal obligations to involve the patient in developmentally and situationally appropriate ways.

The Patient Self-Determination Act

The Patient Self-Determination Act of 1990 is an example of a federal statute that impacts practice. It was designed to encourage competent patients to consider what they would want in the event of serious illness and to facilitate completion of advance directives.[62] All providers who accept federal funds (Medicare, Medicaid) must have policies and procedures 1) to inform all adult patients at initiation of treatment of their right to execute an advance directive, 2) to document in the medical record whether an individual has executed an advance directive, 3) *not* to condition care and treatment or otherwise discriminate on the basis of whether a patient has an advance directive, 4) to comply with state laws on advance directives, and 5) to provide information and education to staff and the community on advance directives.

Futile Treatment and Orders Not to Resuscitate

Sometimes the most appropriate clinical action is to stop aggressive treatment in favor of supportive care and comfort. Critical care nurses observe and deliver care at some point that seems useless, unnecessary, and even unkind. Futile care means care that will not serve the underlying interests, values, and preferences of the patient. Nurses play a crucial role in the health care team by advocating for the best interest of the patient in a holistic way. This is incredibly valuable in an area where providers focus heavily on particular disease processes. Nurses may be responsible for reminding the team of the "big picture" and the need to provide quality of life and compassionate care to the patient.

Many providers have reported moral distress in situations in which they feel obligated to continue treating patients in the absence of any reasonable chance of improvement. There is no legal obligation to provide care that is not, in the provider's judgment, reasonably calculated to improve the patient's condition or symptoms. Although patients have a legal right to refuse treatment, there is no corresponding right to receive treatment. Nonetheless, some states have recently created state statutes that provide protection from liability for providers refusing to provide futile care. The Texas Futile Care Act[63] creates a specific process for providers withdrawing or refusing to provide futile care, even over the objections of the patient.

Policies that address orders to withhold or withdraw treatment should exist in all critical care units. Institutional policies on *do not resuscitate (DNR) orders* should be well-established and tested after decades of implementation. These policies should include, but are not limited to, the following: 1) DNR orders should be entered in the patient's record with full documentation by the responsible physician about the patient's prognosis and the patient's agreement (if he or she is capable) or, alternatively, the family's consensus; 2) patients with capacity must give their informed consent; 3) for patients without capacity, that incapacity must be thoroughly documented, along with any prior evidence of patient wishes, the diagnosis, prognosis, and family consensus; 4) if applicable, DNR orders should be consistent with advance directives, or if not, the reasons for those differences should be documented and explained; 5) if required by state law, DNR orders should require concurrence of another physician as standard policy, and 6) policies should specify that orders are reviewed periodically (some policies require daily review).

Other orders to withhold or withdraw treatment may involve any intervention. These may include mechanical ventilation, oxygen, IV vasoactive agents or other medications, serial labs, imaging tests, pulmonary artery catheters, and other invasive monitoring. One of the most contested areas is the withdrawal of artificial nutrition and hydration. The legal and ethical implications of these orders for each patient must be carefully considered in light of state law, hospital mission, and patient preferences and values. Hospital policies should exist to guide the withdrawal of care in light of state and federal legal constraints. In addition, hospital ethicists and ethics committees can play a valuable role to providers negotiating the complexities of these decisions.

CASE STUDY **Patient with Legal Issues**

Brief Patient History

Mr. A is an 87-year-old man. He has a history of aortic stenosis; however, he has been relatively healthy until recent episodes of syncope. Mr. A lives in an assisted living facility because of forgetfulness but was independent in activities of daily living before this hospitalization.

Clinical Assessment

Mr. A was admitted to the critical care unit yesterday, after undergoing aortic valvuloplasty. Mr. A has not received any opioids or benzodiazepines since yesterday's interventional procedure. The night nurse reported that Mr. A was confused to place when awakened during the night but commented that this is normal for an 87-year-old. This morning, Mr. A was oriented to person, time, place, and situation. He is easily aroused but dozes off and on when unstimulated. Although Mr. A is able to follow simple commands, he requires repeated instructions. The nurse failed to document or report the patient's mental status change or the abnormal serum electrolyte findings to the physician.

Diagnostic Procedures

Mr. A's baseline vital signs are blood pressure, 110/62 mm Hg; heart rate, 82 beats/min (sinus rhythm); respiratory rate, 18 breaths/min; and temperature, 98.4° F. The chest radiograph is normal; O_2 saturation (pulse oximetry) is 96% on room air. Results from serum electrolyte analysis include the following: sodium, 120 mmol/L; potassium, 4.1 mmol/L; chloride, 95 mmol/L; CO_2, 25 mEq/L; blood urea nitrogen, 60 mg/dL; and creatinine, 2 mg/dL.

Medical Diagnosis

Mr. A is diagnosed with delirium secondary to hyponatremia.

Questions

1. What major outcomes do you expect to achieve for this patient?
2. What problems or risks must be managed to achieve these outcomes?
3. What interventions must be initiated to monitor, prevent, manage, or eliminate the problems and risks identified?
4. What interventions should be initiated to promote optimal functioning, safety, and well-being of the patient?
5. What possible learning needs would you anticipate for this patient?
6. What cultural and age-related factors might have a bearing on the patient's plan of care?

REFERENCES

1. Beachump TL, Childress JF: *Principles of biomedical ethics*, ed 5, 2001, Oxford University Press.
2. Furrow B, et al: *Bioethics: health care law and ethics*, ed 7, 2013, West Publishing.
3. Thompson IE, Melia KM, Boyd KM, Horsburgh D: *Nursing ethics*, ed 4, London, 2006, Churchill Livingston.

4. DuBois J: *A framework for analyzing ethics cases, ethics in mental health research*, New York, NY, 2008, Oxford Press, also available at Ethics in Mental Health Research website at: https://sites.google.com/a/narrativebioethics.com/emhr/home. Accessed June 12, 2014.
5. Purtilo RB, Doherty RF: *Ethical Decisions in the Health Professions*, ed 5, St. Louis, 2011, Saunders.
6. LaSala CA, Biarnason D: Creating workplace environments that support moral courage, *OJIN* 15(3), 2010.
7. Cummings CL: Moral distress and the nursing experience, *Nurse Leader* 2010.
8. Epstein EG, Delgado S: Understanding and addressing moral distress, *OJIN* 15(3):Manuscript 1, 2010.
9. Gallagher A: Moral distress and moral courage in everyday nursing practice, *OJIN* 16(2), 2010.
10. AACN: Position statement: moral distress. http://www.aacn.org. Accessed July 9, 2012.
11. AACN: The 4A's to rise above moral distress. http://www.aacn.org. Accessed July 7, 2012.
12. McCue C: Using the AACN framework to alleviate moral distress, *OJIN* 16(1), 2010.
13. Lachman VD, Murray JS, Iseminger K, Ganske KM: Doing the right thing: pathways to moral courage, *Am Nurse Today* 7(5):24, 2012.
14. Murray JS: Moral courage in healthcare: acting ethically even in the presence of risk, *OJIN* 15(3):2010.
15. ANA: Short definitions of ethical principles and theories. http://www.nursingworld.org. Accessed July 7, 2012.
16. Jonsen A, et al: *Clinical ethics: a practical approach to ethical decisions in clinical medicine*, ed 6, 2006, McGraw-Hill.
17. Schneiderman LJ, et al: Medical futility: its meaning and ethical implications, *Ann Intern Med* 112(12):949, 1990.
18. McIntosh B: Medical futility: *DCMS Online, Northeast Florida Supplement*. 2008. Accessed July 9, 2010.
19. Bernat JL: Medical futility: definition, determination, and disputed in critical care, *Neurocrit Care* 2(2):198, 2005.
20. Hofmann PB, Schneiderman LJ: Physicians should not always pursue a good clinical outcome, *Hastings Cent Rep* 37(3), 2007.
21. Lachman VD: Practical use of the nursing code of ethics: part I, *Medsurg Nurs* 18(1):55, 2009.
22. Curtin L: Ethics for nurses in everyday practice, *Am Nurse Today* 5(2), 2010.
23. Murray JS: Creating ethical environments in nursing, *Am Nurse Today* 2(10):48, 2007.
24. Fowler DM, editor: *Guide to the code of ethics for nurses*, Silver Springs, MD, 2008, American Nurses Association.
25. American Nurses Association: Code of Ethics for Nurses. http://www.nursingworld.org. Accessed June 12, 2014.
26. Benner P: Relational ethics of comfort, touch, and solace—endangered arts? *Am J Crit Care* 13(4):346, 2004.
27. Lachman VD: Applying the ethics of care to your nursing practice, *Medsurg Nurs* 21(2):112, 2012.
28. Pavlish C, et al: Early indicators and risk factors for ethical issues in clinical practice, *J Nursing Scholarship* 43(1):13, 2011.
29. *United States Department of Veterans Affairs*: Preventative ethics. http://www.ethics.va.gov. Accessed July 12, 2010.
30. Epstein EG: Preventative ethics in the intensive care unit, *AACN Advanced Critical Care* 23(2):217, 2012.
31. Rushton CH: Ethics of nursing shift report, *AACN Advanced Critical Care* 21(4):380, 2010.
32. White DB, Jonsen A, Lo B: Ethical challenge: When clinicians act as surrogates for underepresented patients, *AJCC* 21(3):202, 2012.
33. Rushton CH: Ethical discernment and action: the art of pause, *AACN Adv Crit Care* 20(1):108, 2009.
34. Rushton CH, Penticuff JH: A framework for analysis of ethical dilemmas in critical care nursing, *AACN Adv Crit Care* 18(3):323, 2007.
35. Clark AP: A model for ethical decision making in cases of patient futility, *Clin Nurse Spec* 24(4):189, 2010.
36. *Sermchief v Gonzales*, 660 SW2d 683 (Mo 1983).
37. *Marion Ob/Gyn v State Med. Bd.*, 137 Ohio App. 3d 522 (Ohio Ct. App., Franklin County 2000).
38. *State Bd. of Nursing v Ruebke*, 259 Kan. 599 (Kan. 1996).
39. American Association of Critical-Care Nurses (AACN): Standards for Acute and Critical Care Nursing Practice, Aliso Viejo, California, 2008, AACN.
40. American Nurses Association (ANA): Nursing: Scope and Standards of Practice, Washington, DC, 2004, ANA.
41. Painter L, et al: The nurse's role in the causation of compensable injury, *J Nurs Care Qual* 26(4):311–319, 2011.
42. *Gould v New York City Health and Hospital Corp.*, 490 NYS.2d 87 (1985).
43. For example, California: *Ybarra v Spangard*, 154 P.2d 687 (Cal. 1944); Colorado: Wood v Rowland, 592 P.2d 1332 (Colo. 1978); Delaware: *Larrimore v Homeopathic Hospital Association*, 176 A.2d 362 (Del. 1962); Minnesota: *Plutshack v University of Minnesota Hospital*, 316 NW2d 1 (Minn. 1982); Montana: *Hunsaker v Bozeman Deaconess Foundation*, 588 P.2d 493 (Mont. 1978); Pennsylvania: *Baur v Mesta Machine Co.*, 176 A.2d 684 (Pa. 1962); Texas: *Childs v Greenville Hospital Authority*, 479 S.W.2d 399 (Tx. 1972); and Washington: *Stone v Sisters of Charity of the House of Providence*, 469 P.2d 229 (Wash. 1970).
44. *Clough v Lively*, 387 SE2d 573 (Ga. 1989).
45. *Teffeteller v University of Minnesota*, 645 NW2d 420 (Minn. 2002).
46. *McMullen v Ohio State University Hospitals*, 725 NE2d 1117 (Ohio 2002).
47. *Brandon HMA, Inc. v Bradshaw*, 809 So.2d 611 (Miss. 2001).
48. *Anderson v St. Francis-St. George Hospital*, 671 NE2d 225 (Ohio 1996).
49. *Garcia v United States*, 697 F.Supp. 1570 (Colo. 1988).
50. *Keyser v Garner*, 922 P.2d 409 (Idaho 1996).
51. *Long v Methodist Hospital of Indiana*, 699 NE2d 1164 (Ind. 1998).
52. *Richardson v Miller*, 44 SW3d 1 (Tenn. 2000).
53. *Ginsberg v St. Michaels Hospital*, 678 A.2d 271 (N.J. 1996).
54. *G.S. v Dep't of Human Servs.*, Div. of Youth & Family Servs., 723 A.2d 612 (N.J. 1999).
55. *Doe v Ohio State Univ. Hosp. & Clinics*, 663 NE2d 1369 (Ohio 1995).
56. The Health Insurance Portability and Accountability Act of 1996 (HIPAA), Public Law 104-191, enacted on August 21, 1996.
57. *Darling v Charleston Comm. Mem. Hosp.*, 211 NE2d 614 (Ill. 1965).
58. *Cruzan v Director*, Missouri Department of Mental Health, 497 U.S. 261 (1990).
59. *Bouvia v Superior Court*, 179 Cal. App. 3d 1127, 225 Cal. Rptr. 297, 1986 Cal. App. LEXIS 1467 (Cal. App. 2d Dist. 1986).
60. *In re Quinlan*, 70 N.J. 10 (N.J. 1976).
61. *In re Schiavo*, 851 So.2d 182 (Fla. Ct. App. 2003).
62. *Patient Self Determination Act*, Omnibus Budget Reconciliation Act of 1990, Pub.L. 101-508 (1990).
63. *For example, the Texas Futile Care Law*, Texas Health and Safety Code, Section 166 (1999).

3 CHAPTER

Patient and Family Education

Barbara Mayer

Be sure to check out the bonus material, including review questions, on the Evolve website at http://evolve.elsevier.com/Urden/priorities/.

The Education Process

The education process follows the same framework as the nursing process: assessment, diagnosis, goals or outcomes, interventions, and evaluation.[1] Although this chapter discusses these steps individually, in practice, they may occur simultaneously and repetitively. The teaching-learning process is a dynamic, continuous activity that occurs throughout the entire hospitalization and may continue after the patient has been discharged. This process is often envisioned by the nurse as a time-consuming task that requires knowledge and skills to accomplish. Whereas knowledge and skills can be obtained, time in the critical care unit is a scarce commodity. The nurse must recognize that teaching occurs during every moment of a nurse-patient encounter.[2] Instructions for how to use the call bell or explanations of events and sensations to expect during a bed bath can be considered an education session. It is the nurse's role to recognize that education, no matter how brief or extensive, affects the daily lives of each person with whom he or she comes in contact.

STEP 1: ASSESSMENT

Learning needs can be defined as gaps between what the learner knows and what the learner needs to know, such as survival skills, coping skills, and the ability to make a care decision. Identification of actual and perceived learning needs directs the health care team to provide need-targeted education. Need-targeted or need-to-know education is directed at helping the learner to become familiar with the current situation.

Strategic questioning provides an avenue for the nurse to determine whether the patient or family has any misconceptions about the environment, their illness, self-management, or medication schedule. Health care providers use the term *noncompliant* to describe a patient or family members who do not modify behaviors to meet the demands of the prescribed treatment regimen, such as following the rules of a low-fat diet or medication dosing. However, the problem behind noncompliance may not be a conscious desire to defy the treatment plan but instead be a misunderstanding of the importance of the medication or how to take the medication. Generally, with practice and effort, educational needs can quickly be determined without much disruption in the routine care of the patient.

Age-Specific Considerations

The critical care patient population differs culturally, by age and by stages of human development. Older adult patients may have more difficulty reading patient educational materials or the label on the bottle of prescription medication than younger adults. Printed materials with larger fonts may be needed for these patients. Older adults were not exposed to technology during their youth and may find it difficult to navigate the fragmented maze of modern health care. Because of multiple medical conditions associated with advanced age, this population of adults may have prescriptions for multiple drug therapies necessitating education to prevent adverse drug reactions.[3] Older adults may also be coping with end-of-life issues and are in need of information to make informed decisions. Young adults may struggle with the issue of how to incorporate intimacy into their lives without feeling isolated from the mainstream social scene. The need for privacy and peer support may be required to assist the young adult in coping with the current situation. The practitioner must recognize these age-specific issues and incorporate them into the education plan.[4]

Adult Learners

Adults learn in large part through lived experiences, and the motivation to learn is internal and problem-oriented, focusing on life events. Malcolm Knowles described these principles of adult learning in a model known as *andragogy.* Adult learning theory stresses concepts of individualism, self-assessment, self-direction, motivation, experience, and autonomy. Adults tend to have a strong sense of self-concept, are goal-oriented learners, and like to make their own decisions.[5] They take responsibility and accountability for their own learning and want to be respected as individuals, as well as recognized for accomplished life experiences. Adults have individualized learning styles and often lack confidence in their ability to learn. Education is resisted when the information given is perceived to be in conflict with the individual's self-image.

Physiologic Factors

Physiologic alterations in heart rate and blood pressure can be measured and taken into consideration during the teaching-learning encounter.[6] Sources of physiologic stress in the critically ill include medications, pain, hypoxia, decreased cerebral and peripheral perfusion, hypotension, fluid and electrolyte imbalances, infection, sensory alterations, fever, and neurologic deficits.[7] Experiencing one or more of these stressors may completely consume all the patient's available energy and thoughts, affecting his or her ability to interact, comprehend, and respond to teaching.

Health Literacy

Patients and families may be ready and willing to learn but lack the ability to comprehend and act upon the information presented to them.[8]

Shame has been cited as one of the most common emotions associated with low health literacy.[9] Behaviors such as handing a form to a family member to complete, claiming to be too tired, or "forgetting" their glasses are a few behaviors that may be used by individuals to hide their limitations. In some cases, asking a direct question can elicit an individual's level of health literacy. For example, how the individual answers questions such as "How comfortable are you in reading medicine labels?" or "How well do you understand your disease process?" may help the practitioner gain insight into the level of health literacy and plan appropriate educational interventions. Additional behaviors that may provide clues to a patient's health literacy are listed in Box 3-1.

BOX 3-1 Behavioral Cues Indicating Low Health Literacy

- Requests family always to be present.
- Opens a medication bottle to identify a medicine.
- Makes excuses:
  I forgot my glasses.
  I want my son to read it first.
  I'll take it home with me.
- Refers to medications by shape or color rather than name.
- Cannot teach-back.
- Frequently misses appointments.
- Postpones decision making.
- Watches or mimics behavior or responses of others.
- Pretends to read material—eyes wander over page, slow to read.
- Does not complete forms or asks staff or family to complete.

Psychologic Factors

When confronted with life-altering situations such as admission to a critical care unit, patients and families may experience anxiety and emotional stress. Anxiety and fear disrupt the normalcy of daily life. Sources of emotional stress include fear of death, uncertain prognosis, role change, self-image change, social isolation, disruption in daily routine, financial concerns, and unfamiliar critical care environment.[6,10] These intense emotions can lead to a crisis situation and alter the ability of the patient and family to cope.[11,12] During the critical illness, an individual's ability to process or retain information and ability to participate in the treatment plan could be altered.[13]

STEP 2: EDUCATION PLAN DEVELOPMENT

Education must be ongoing, interactive, and consistent with the patient's plan of care, ability to comprehend, and education level.[4] The nurse must consider the patient's physical and emotional status when setting education priorities. Ability, willingness, and readiness to learn are factors that influence acceptance of new information and add to the complexity of the teaching-learning encounter. These factors should be recognized by the nurse before implementation of teaching. The plan of care should include the nursing diagnosis for deficient knowledge and a written teaching plan should identify the learning needs, goals, or expected outcomes of the teaching-learning encounter, interventions to meet that outcome, and appropriate teaching strategies.

Research and accepted national guidelines or standards can be used to assist the practitioner in developing an evidence-based plan for education. Examples of organizations that offer education standards are the American Association of Critical-Care Nurses, American Heart Association Guidelines for Practice, and the Society of Critical Care Medicine. These evidence-based interventions and outcomes assist the nurse in providing consistent outcomes and interventions from nurse to nurse, shift to shift, and discipline to discipline.

Determining What to Teach

The multiple learning needs of patients in the critical care unit, the progressive care, or the telemetry setting can be separated into four different categories to help set teaching priorities during each phase of the hospitalization (Table 3-1).

TABLE 3-1 Categories of Educational Needs in Critical Care

PHASE	EDUCATIONAL NEEDS
Initial contact or first visit, with a focus on immediate needs	Preparation for the visit: patient representatives or nurses can prepare the family and patient for the first visit. What to expect in the environment How long the visit will last What the patient may look like (e.g., tubes, IV lines) Orientation to the unit or environment: call light, bed controls, waiting rooms, unit contact numbers Orientation to unit policies and hospital policies HIPAA, advanced directives, visitation policies Equipment orientation: monitors, IV pumps, pulse oximetry, pacemakers, ventilators

Continued

TABLE 3-1 **Categories of Educational Needs in Critical Care—cont'd**

PHASE	EDUCATIONAL NEEDS
	Medications: rationale, effects, side effects What to do during the visit: talk to the patient, hold the patient's hand, monitor length of visits (if applicable) Patient status: stable or unstable and what that terminology means What treatments and interventions are being done for the patient Upcoming procedures When the doctor visited or is expected to visit Disciplines involved in care and the services they provide Immediate plan of care (next 24 hours) Mobilization of resources for crisis intervention
Continuous care	Day-to-day routine: meals, laboratory visits, doctor visits, frequency of monitoring (VS), nursing assessments, daily weights, and shift routines Explanation of any procedures: expected sensations or discomforts (e.g., chest tube removal, arterial sheath removal) Plan of care: treatments, progress, patient accomplishments (e.g., extubation) Medications: name, why the patient is receiving them, side effects to report to the nurse or health care team Disease process: what it is and how it will affect life, symptoms to report to health care team How to mobilize resources to assist the patient and family in coping with stress and crisis: pastoral care, social workers, case managers, victim assistance, domestic violence counseling Gifts: When a loved one is ill, it is traditional to send flowers, balloons, or cards. If your unit has restrictions on gifts, make the family aware. Begin teaching self-management skills and discuss aftercare information.
Transfer to a different level of care	**Sending Unit** Acknowledge positive move out of critical care When the transfer will occur Why the transfer is occurring What to expect in the different unit Name of the new caregiver Availability of care provider Visiting hours Directions for how to get there; the new room number and phone number **Receiving Unit** Orientation to environment, visitation policies, visitors Unit routine, meals, shift changes, doctor visits Expectations about patient self-care; ADLs Medication and diagnostic testing routine times
Planning for aftercare, discharge planning	Self-care management: symptom management, medication administration, diet, activity, durable medical equipment, tasks or procedures What to do for an emergency What constitutes an emergency or when to call the physician How to care for incisions or procedure sites
Completed throughout the hospital stay	Return appointment: name of physician practice, practice phone numbers and contacts Obtaining medications: prescriptions, pharmacy, special medication ordering information Required lifestyle changes: mobility and safety issues for the paraplegic or stroke victim, activities of daily living issues relative to medications or symptoms Potential risk modifications: smoking cessation, diet modifications, exercise Resources: cardiac rehabilitation, support groups, home care agencies
End-of-life care	End-of-life care: participation in care, services available, mobilizing resources Palliative care Hospice

ADLs, Activities of daily living; *HIPAA*, Health Insurance Portability and Accountability Act; *IV*, intravenous; *VS*, vital signs.

Learning needs during the initial contact or first hours of hospitalization can be predicted. Education during this time frame should be directed toward the reduction of immediate stress, anxiety, and fear rather than future lifestyle alterations or rehabilitation needs. Interventions are targeted to promote comfort and familiarity with the environment and surroundings.[14] The plan should focus on survival skills, orientation to the environment and equipment, communication of prognosis, procedure explanations, and the immediate plan of care.

As the hospital length of stay increases, patients and families begin to adapt to the situation, and learning needs change.

Patient Education Priorities boxes are displayed in order to assist the nurse in meeting the most immediate education interventions.

Developing Interventions

Interventions describe how a nurse will become involved in providing education to the patient or the family, and determining education interventions is part of clinical decision making.[15] Nurse-initiated interventions are based on clinical knowledge and judgment and have a direct impact on the outcome of the teaching encounter.[16] Although physiologic problems occupy most of the nursing plan of care, it is essential to incorporate teaching interventions into the daily plan to create positive patient outcomes.

Standardized Education Plans

Standardized education plans provide the health care team with consistent outcomes and interventions. Even though standardized plans are easy to implement, they must be individualized to meet the specific needs of each patient or family. Examples of standardized plans of care include clinical pathways, traditional nursing care plans for Deficient Knowledge. Examples of nursing management plans for Deficient Knowledge are included in Appendix A.

STEP 3: IMPLEMENTATION

After the assessment is completed and the education plan is developed, need-targeted education can commence. Beginning practitioners differ from experienced practitioners in their skills of implementing the education plan of care. Experienced practitioners use their intuition and knowledge base to anticipate learning needs and form a mental list of interventions and possible outcomes.[17] Those just starting in the profession need the concrete education plan that has been developed to guide the teaching-learning encounter.[17]

Setting Up the Environment

The optimal environment for learning is one that is nonthreatening, comfortable, open, and honest. Many factors concerning the critical care environment can be threatening or anxiety- producing, and the practitioner must assess for these distractions and control them as much as possible. Providing the family with open visitation and access to the patient and health care providers can help decrease their anxiety level and improve satisfaction with care.[2] The following is a list of strategies the practitioner can implement to facilitate learning[18]:

- Show empathy and concern. Actively listen to the learner and acknowledge lived experiences and ideas.
- Use language and nonverbal communication to enhance choice and promote problem solving.
- Reduce language that is controlling, criticizing, guilt provoking, judgmental, or punishing.
- Provide rationale for self-management behaviors: the importance of changing lifestyle to manage symptoms.

Teaching Strategies

Bedside nurses are in a unique position to facilitate, mentor, and coach patients through the endless maze of information presented in the critical care arena. Information overload can often occur, and the information taught can easily be forgotten, resulting in patients and families asking the same questions many times. Although health care providers would like patients and families to retain 100% of information given, in reality, learning does not take place in one session or may not occur at all. An individual may be able to remember only two to three pieces of information in one education session.

Nurses are continuously interacting with patients and discussing their progress, updating them on treatment plans, and describing procedures. With that in mind, every patient contact can be thought of as a brief teaching-learning encounter. The nurse must use every teachable moment and take advantage of the patient's readiness and willingness to learn. When educating adults, a combination of teaching strategies should be used to facilitate giving and receiving information.[19,20] Each individual has a different learning style: visual, auditory, or tactile. Common strategies include discussion, demonstration, and use of media. The nurse must use different teaching strategies and techniques and modify them frequently according to the situation and the patient's or family's response to the education.

Discussion

Informal discussion can take place anywhere and at any time. Focus on what the patient or family wants or *needs* to know at that moment, rather than on what might be *nice* to know. Obtaining and maintaining the learner's attention during the discussion may be challenging. The following strategies are used to maintain a positive teaching-learning encounter:

- Addressing the patient and family members by name
- Clearly stating the purpose of the education encounter
- Getting and keeping them involved in the learning process
- Maintaining eye contact during the encounter
- Keeping the encounter brief and to the point
- Giving positive reinforcement
- Communicating with professionals in other disciplines about the progress and additional learning needs of the patient and family[1,19]

Demonstration and Practice

Demonstration and practice are the best strategies for teaching technical skills. Adults learn best when they are able to participate in the learning process. Involving the learner, providing consistent step-by-step instructions, and presenting a visual demonstration of the skill to be performed are important strategies to achieve successful task acquisition. By allowing the patient or family to practice the skill in a simulated or real situation, the outcome of the teaching encounter can be evaluated. This strategy allows the nurse to offer positive reinforcement and constructive feedback during the learning encounter, thereby building learner confidence in performing the newly acquired skill.

Audiovisual Media

The use of media in mainstream patient education is becoming more prevalent as a first-line teaching strategy. Media are excellent tools to relay information to persons with any one of the three learning styles. Pamphlets, videos, and anatomic pictures or models are the most common types of audiovisual aids. This teaching strategy supplies the learner with a large amount of information in a relatively short period. Videos and written materials enable different nurses to distribute information that remains consistent from patient to patient and family to family. The use of media can assist practitioners to obtain informed consent and to communicate current and future prescribed treatment plans.[21,22]

Written Materials

Written media, such as brochures, pamphlets, patient pathways, and booklets, are common in outpatient and inpatient areas of health care. They usually are inexpensive and offer opportunities for a wide range of education: disease process education, risk factor modification information, procedure education, medication education, and use of medical equipment in the home setting. Written materials address multiple learning styles and offer learner-centered teaching with concrete, basic information that can be placed at the learner's fingertips for immediate review, as well as future review any time the learner desires. Several factors should be considered when choosing printed materials for patient education: readability, cultural considerations, age-specific considerations, primary language, and literacy.[23]

Readability is an important factor in the consideration of printed educational materials. *Readability* refers to how easy or hard the literature is to read. Nearly 20% of the U.S. adult population have low literacy skills and read at or below the fifth-grade reading level.[24] Typical patient educational materials are written at or above the eighth- or ninth-grade reading level and may be out of reach for many readers.[23,25] If the patient or family is unable to read the material or understand its meaning, he or she cannot perform self-management tasks to maintain health.

Providing written educational materials at the appropriate reading level is important, if the information is to be easily read and understood by most patients and families. To assist the nurse in overcoming literacy-related barriers to health education, it is recommended that patient educational materials be printed at or below the fifth-grade reading level.[23,25] Samples of health-related instructions at different reading levels are provided in Box 3-2.

Computer-Assisted Instruction

Computer-assisted instruction is a relatively new strategy for providing patient and family education.[26] Even though personal computers have become common, they may not be suitable because comfort levels with the technical aspects of the computer vary from person to person. Software programs can be accessed through a single hard drive or through a server for multiple computer sites. Computer screens may be placed in every patient's room at the bedside for easy access to education videos or the Internet. Bedside computers provide the patient and family with an avenue to receive education on demand whenever they are ready, willing, and able.

BOX 3-2 Samples of Reading Levels

College Reading Level
Consult your physician immediately at the onset of chest discomfort, shortness of breath, or increased perspiration.

Twelfth-Grade Reading Level
Call your physician immediately if you experience chest discomfort, shortness of breath, or increased sweatiness.

Eighth-Grade Reading Level
Call your doctor immediately if you start having chest pain or shortness of breath or you feel sweaty.

Fourth-Grade Reading Level
Call your doctor right away if you start having chest pain, cannot breathe, or feel sweaty.

BOX 3-3 INTERNET RESOURCES

- HealthFinder
  http://www.healthfinder.gov/Familydoctor.org
- FamilyDoctor
  http://familydoctor.org/familydoctor/en.html
- HealthyWomen
  http://www.healthywomen.org/
- AHRQ Men Stay Healthy at Any Age
  http://www.ahrq.gov/ppip/healthymen.htm
- NIH Senior Health
  http://nihseniorhealth.gov/

Internet Sites

Patients and families often use websites to research information about the illness or condition about which they are concerned.[27] Information on the Internet is generally presented on an eighth-grade reading level.[2] Websites contain a wealth of information. However, the information is not regulated or controlled for reliability or validity,[27] and not all information provided on every website is accurate. The nurse must advise the patient and family about this concern and ask them to print out and bring in such material so it can be discussed. Government websites and those of professional organizations, reputable health care organizations, and consumer health groups offer trustworthy information for the practitioner and the public.[27] See Box 3-3 for Internet resources.

Communication

Speaking slowly, clearly, and avoiding the use of slang or medical jargon are essential. Even when the patient and family speak English, the stress of hospitalization, fear of health outcomes, and difficulty speaking of personal issues with a stranger can present a challenge to providing patient education. When the patient or family has limited English proficiency (LEP), the challenge becomes even greater. In many instances a family member is called upon to serve in the role of interpreter. Although this may seem like an ideal solution, the family member may not have any better

BOX 3-4 Tips for Using an Interpreter

- Speak directly to the patient not the interpreter.
- Position yourself so that you can maintain eye contact with the patient.
- Introduce the interpreter and clarify roles of others in the room.
- Nothing should be said that the patient shouldn't hear.
- Pause after each complete thought to give interpreter time to translate.
- Plan ahead; let the interpreter know exactly the content and purpose of the session.
- Use the teach-back method to evaluate learning.
- Listen to the interpreter, who may identify cultural practice or norms that impede understanding.

From Techniques for educating with the aid of an interpreter, *Patient Educ Manag* 7:77, 2007.

comprehension of the material being taught and thus is unable to relay the information adequately. The use of professional interpreter services is preferable when the message is vital to a patient's health and well-being. Interpreter services are available through a variety of modes.[28] Telephonic interpretive services are offered by many vendors, and special phones with dual handsets are available for use. Emerging technology has given rise to video-on-demand interpretive services such as those offered through the Language Access Network. Whichever method is used, interpretation can be a frustrating process. Box 3-4 describes helpful techniques to enhance the experience.[29]

Special Considerations

The Older Adult

As individuals age, cognitive, physiologic, and psychological changes occur that must be considered when planning and implementing a teaching plan. It is the nurse's responsibility to understand the effects of aging and adjust teaching strategies to accommodate them.[30]

Cognitive effects of aging. Cognitive effects include processing information more slowly, a decrease in the ability to take in multiple messages, and difficulty understanding the abstract. When teaching the older adult, nurses should provide information slowly and deliberately to allow the patient time to process each concept. Information should be presented in two to three essential points and reviewed frequently. Nurses should avoid using vague terms such as "several times a day" or "until better." Instead, they must be very specific with amounts, times, and frequencies.

Physical effects of aging. Presbyopia, cataracts, glaucoma, and macular degeneration affect the vision of many older adults. Although additional lighting is necessary, it is also necessary to avoid direct sunlight, harsh lights, and using glossy paper. Colors in the blue end of the spectrum are difficult for the older adult to distinguish because of yellowing of the lens of the eye. When using written instructions or color-coded dosing, blues, greens, and purples should not be used.

High-pitched tones become more difficult to hear as an individual ages. Female nurses will need to make an effort to modulate their voices into the lower register so the older adult can hear better. In addition, careful enunciation of words containing higher-pitched sounds like "f", "s", "k", and "sh" may be necessary. Providing audio and video recordings will help reinforce learning.[31]

Aging and associated co-morbidities may result in fatigue, joint pain, or decreased dexterity. Learning can be facilitated by scheduling teaching sessions early in the day, keeping sessions short, and managing pain prior to learning.

Psychologic effects of aging. Older adults often suffer from depression. Learning can be enhanced by selecting content that holds value and relevance to the individual. Nurses should choose content that is perceived by the learner as important in maintaining quality of life and should try to relate what they are teaching to the individual's previous life experiences.

Sedated and Unconscious Patients

Patient education should not be reserved for the conscious and coherent patient only; it should be provided to the unconscious or sedated patient as well. Addressing the learning needs of this critically ill population of patients is challenging. Although it is truly not known what the unconscious or sedated patient hears or remembers, it is known that some sedated patients undergoing surgery remember discussions that took place among physicians and staff during the procedure. Therefore, one should not ignore unconscious or sedated patients during the education process. These patients may not be able to respond or participate, and the effectiveness of the teaching process cannot be evaluated, but providing information regarding environment, procedures, sensations, and time of day is benevolent and may help to decrease immediate physiologic stress.

The Noncompliant Patient

Noncompliance, or an unwillingness to learn, does not necessarily mean that the patient is consciously choosing not to participate in their care or follow medical instructions. There are many other issues that can lead to noncompliance. The nurse must be alert for barriers that may prevent a willing patient from being compliant. Factors that may contribute to noncompliance or unwillingness to learn[32] include the following:

- Limited English Proficiency (LEP)
- Lack of education
- Cultural or ethnic beliefs
- Financial constraints
- Lack of adequate tools or supplies
- Lack of family support

STEP 4: EVALUATION

Techniques such as verbalization of information, return demonstration, and physiologic measurement are common evaluation methods to determine the effectiveness of a teaching-learning encounter. Evaluation of knowledge retention can be completed by verbally questioning the learner. This method is known as teach-back. Teach-back is an interactive process that assists the nurse in determining whether the learner has retained the information taught.[33] The nurse may ask the patient if he or she is able to list signs and symptoms of heart failure. Verbal questioning should occur immediately after the teaching event and throughout the hospitalization to assess knowledge retention. For example, the physician orders a new medication for the patient today, and the nurse educates that patient on the effects and side effects; the next day, the nurse may assess retention by asking the patient if he or she remembers the reason for taking the new medication. Common items that patients and families are asked to verbalize are reportable signs and symptoms, how to manage symptoms at home, when to take medication, how often the medication should be taken, and who to call for questions or concerns.

Observation and return demonstration is the evaluation of choice for the skills-learning domain. For the patient and family members to be "checked off" on a particular skill, they should be able to perform it independently, using the nurse only as a resource for questions. Endotracheal suctioning, placing condom catheters, and performing dressing changes are examples of common tasks that patients and families may be asked to learn. Because of the increasingly complex care that patients require at home after discharge, these skills may be the entire focus of teaching before discharge. Not every teaching moment is a success, and the nurse need not feel guilty or like a failure when the learner has not achieved the desired objective. Revisiting and revising the goals and objectives during the teaching-learning session may be necessary to meet the ever-changing needs of the patient or family.

STEP 5: DOCUMENTATION

Documentation of education is necessary to communicate educational efforts to members of the health care team, patients and families, and regulatory agencies. The nurse should recognize that informal teaching at the bedside is education. It is important to record any information given to the patient on formal documents approved for use by each health care institution. In most institutions, formal education records are used to document education rendered by practitioners of any discipline involved in the care of a particular patient and family. These forms are communication tools used to indicate progress in the teaching-learning process from shift to shift, day to day, and discipline to discipline. Documentation should include education from admission to discharge on topics ranging from orientation to the environment to acquisition of self-management skills for home care.

Documentation of the education assessment should include learning preferences; factors that impair ability, readiness, and willingness to learn, and actual or perceived learning needs. Information should be recorded on the interaction, material taught, supplemental materials distributed, response to the education, achievement of outcome, and any follow-up education or resources needed.

INFORMATIONAL NEEDS OF FAMILIES IN CRITICAL CARE

Family members and significant others of critically ill patients are integral to the recovery of their loved ones. When planning for the overall care of patients, nurses and other caregivers need to consider the informational and emotional support needs of this group.[34] Families of critically ill patients report their greatest need is for information.[34] Flexible visiting hours and informational booklets regarding the critical care experience are recommended to meet this need.[35]

PREPARATION OF THE PATIENT AND FAMILY FOR TRANSFER FROM CRITICAL CARE

When patients are more stable, requiring less hemodynamic monitoring and close observation, they are frequently transferred to another level of care in a different geographic hospital setting. They may be transferred to an intermediate care unit (i.e., step-down unit, intermediate care area, or telemetry). While on these units, patients receive optimal care to their level of requirement, a lower nurse-to-patient ratio, and less expensive technologic monitoring in a quieter environment.[24,36]

Preparation for transfer should start after the patient has been stabilized and the life-threatening event that resulted in hospitalization has subsided. Explanations about where the patient will be transferred, the reason for transfer, and the name of the nurse who will be providing care should be offered as soon as known. Before transfer, information about changes in care, expectations for self-care, and visiting hours should be provided to the patient and family. Family members should be contacted concerning exactly when the patient will be transferred so they can be present during the transfer or made aware of the patient's new location (Box 3-5).

BOX 3-5 Education Components for Patient Transfer to Another Unit

Sending Unit

- Acknowledge positive move out of critical care.
- When the transfer will occur
- Why the transfer is occurring
- What to expect in the different unit
- Name of the new caregiver
- Availability of care provider
- Visiting hours
- Directions for how to get there; the new room number and phone number

Receiving Unit

- Orientation to environment, visitation policies, visitors
- Unit routine, meals, shift changes, doctor visits
- Expectations about patient self-care, activities of daily living
- Medication and diagnostic testing routine times

CASE STUDY Patient and Family Education

Brief Patient History

Mr. S is a 30-year-old Vietnamese-American man who is employed as a fisherman. Mr. S is married and has three children younger than 5 years. He was diagnosed a few months earlier with type 1 diabetes mellitus after a 30-pound weight loss and a change in visual acuity. He has had two admissions for diabetic ketoacidosis in the past month.

Clinical Assessment

Mr. S was admitted to the critical care unit with diabetic ketoacidosis 2 days ago. His condition has been stabilized, and he is ready to be transferred to a nursing unit today. Mr. S states that he does not understand why "this keeps

CASE STUDY Patient and Family Education—cont'd

happening" because he takes his insulin if he plans on eating but does not always eat. Mr. S's wife states that his blood sugar seems to be okay when he is at home but that he gets into trouble when offshore.

Diagnostic Procedures

These laboratory results were obtained on admission: blood glucose level of 620 mg/dL, carbon dioxide concentration of 11 mEq/L, and pH of 7.25. Ketones were identified in the urine and blood.

Assessment of learning needs identified a deficit in understanding regarding glucose monitoring and insulin requirements while away from home.

Medical Diagnosis

Mr. S is diagnosed with diabetic ketoacidosis resulting from noncompliance.

Questions

1. What major outcomes do you expect to achieve for this patient?
2. What problems or risks must be managed to achieve these outcomes?
3. What interventions must be initiated to monitor, prevent, manage, or eliminate the problems and risks identified?
4. What interventions should be initiated to promote optimal functioning, safety, and well-being of the patient?
5. What possible learning needs do you anticipate for this patient?
6. What cultural and age-related factors may have a bearing on the patient's plan of care?

REFERENCES

1. Bastable S: *Nurse as educator: principles of teaching and learning for nursing practice*, ed 3, Boston, 2008, Jones and Bartlett Publishers.
2. Burkhead V, et al: Enter: a care guide for successfully educating patients, *J Nurses Staff Dev* 19(3):143, 2003.
3. Blount KA, Moore LA: Medications and the elderly, *Crit Care Nurs Clin North Am* 14(1):111, 2002.
4. The Joint Commission: *2012 Comprehensive accreditation manual for hospitals*, Oakbrook Terrace, IL, 2014, The Joint Commission.
5. Knowles MS: *The modern practice of adult education: from pedagogy to andragogy*, New York, 1980, Cambridge Books.
6. Leske J: Comparison of family stresses, strengths, and outcomes after trauma surgery, *AACN Clin Issues Crit Care* 14(1):33, 2003.
7. Phillips LD: Patient education: understanding the process to maximize time and outcomes, *J Intraven Nurs* 22(1):19, 1999.
8. Jordan J, et al: The Health Literacy Management Scale (HeLMS): A measure of an individual's capacity to seek, understand and use health information within the healthcare setting, *Patient Educ Couns* 91(2):228–235, 2014.
9. Moore V: Assessing health literacy, *J Nurse Pract* 8(3):243, 2012.
10. Institute of Medicine: *Health literacy: a prescription to end confusion*, Washington, DC, 2004, National Academies Press.
11. Naveen S, Anice G: The Perceived Communication Barriers and Attitude on Communication among Staff Nurses in Caring for Patients from Culturally and Linguistically Diverse Background, *Int J Nurs Educ* 5(1):141–146, 2013.
12. VanHorn E, et al: Family interventions during the trajectory of recovery from cardiac event: an integrative literature review, *Heart Lung* 31(3):186, 2002.
13. Davis N, et al: Improving the process of informed consent in the critically ill, *JAMA* 289(15):1963, 2003.
14. Happ MB, et al: Nurse-Patient Communication Interactions in the Intensive Care Unit, *AJCC* 20(2):e28–e40, 2011.
15. White M, et al: Is "Teach-Back" Associated With Knowledge Retention and Hospital Readmission in Hospitalized Heart Failure Patients? *J Cardiovasc Nurs* 28(2):137–146, 2013.
16. Bulechek GM, editor: *Nursing Interventions Classification (NIC)*, ed 6, St. Louis, 2013, Mosby.
17. Benner C, et al: *From beginner to expert: excellence and power in clinical nurse practice*, Menlo Park, 1984, Addison-Wesley.
18. Clark P, Dunbar S: Family partnership intervention: a guide for family approach to care of patients with heart failure, *AACN Clin Issues* 14(4):467, 2003.
19. Marcus C: Strategies for improving the quality of verbal patient and family education: a review of the literature and creation of the EDUCATE model, *Health Psychol Behav Med* 2(1):482–495, 2014.
20. Rankin S, Stallings K, London F: *Patient education in health and illness: issues, principles and practice*, ed 5, Philadelphia, 2005, JB Lippincott.
21. Houts P, et al: The role of pictures in improving health communication: a review of research on attention, *Patient Educ Couns* 61:173, 2006.
22. Peregrin T: Picture this: visual cues enhance health education messages for people with low literacy skills, *J ADA* 110(5):S28, 2010.
23. Wei H, Camargo C: Patient education in the emergency department, *Acad Emerg Med* 7(6):710, 2000.
24. Obringer K, et al: Needs of adult family members of intensive care unit patients, *J Clin Nurs* 21:11–12, 2012.
25. Kingbeil C, et al: Readability of pediatric patient education materials, *Clin Pediatr* 34(2):96, 1995.
26. Doak C, et al: Improving comprehension for cancer patients with low literacy skills: strategies for clinicians, *CA Cancer J Clin* 38(3):151, 1998.
27. Street R, et al: *Health promotion and interactive technology: theoretical applications and future directions*, New York, 2009, Routledge.
28. Dragan I: The Role of the Internet on Patient Knowledge Management, Education, and Decision Making, *Telemed e-Health* 16(6):664–669, 2010.
29. Mikkelson H: The art of working with interpreters: a manual for health care professionals. http://www.acebo.com/papers/artintrp.htm. Accessed April 28, 2012.
30. Techniques for educating with the aid of an interpreter, *Patient Educ Manag* 77, 2007.
31. Speros C: More than words: promoting health literacy in older adults, *Online J Issues Nurs* 14(3), 2009.
32. Kane R, et al: *Essentials of clinical geriatrics*, ed 7, Columbus, OH, 2013, McGraw Hill Education.
33. Thomas M: Lack of compliance may mean patients don't understand, *Case Manag Advisor* 20(8):85, 2009.
34. Russell C, Freiburghaus M: Heart transplant patient teaching documentation, *Clin Nurs Spec* 17(5):249, 2004.
35. Doering LV, et al: Recovering from cardiac surgery: what patients want to know, *Am J Crit Care* 11(4):333, 2002.
36. White SK, Edwards RJ: Visitation guidelines promote safe satisfying environments, *Nurs Manage* 37(8):21, 2006.

4 CHAPTER

Psychosocial and Spiritual Alterations and Management

Valerie J. Yancey

Be sure to check out the bonus material, including review questions, on the Evolve website at http://evolve.elsevier.com/Urden/priorities/.

Patients are admitted to critical care units because they need physiologic rescue. Life or death depends on restoring physiologic homeostasis through the use of highly technical interventions carried out by a competent critical care team. When a person is seriously ill or injured, however, it is not just the body that suffers. An experience of critical illness impacts the whole person—body, mind, and spirit. While not as readily measured as physical parameters, psychological and spiritual variables significantly impact outcomes in physically compromised and vulnerable patients. Psychological and spiritual interventions have the power to engage a patient's hope, energy, will to survive, and his or her ability to meet life's challenges.[1] This chapter provides a discussion of the psychosocial-spiritual challenges encountered by critically ill patients and offers holistic nursing interventions for helping patients and family members cope effectively and thrive during a stressful experience.

STRESS AND PSYCHONEUROIMMUNOLOGY

The term "stress" is often used to indicate a negative experience or internal tension. While living with chronic stress can contribute to numerous health problems over time,[2,3,4] an acute stress response is an essential, protective, inherent reaction to a stressor, designed to mobilize the body's response to threats, actual or perceived, for purposes of survival. Stress is a non-specific response to any demand placed on a person to adapt or change and can come from physical, emotional, social, spiritual, cultural, chemical, or environmental sources.[5,6]

To respond appropriately to patients at risk for stress overload, nurses must first become aware of the many stressors patients in critical care units face (Box 4-1). Normal life patterns are disrupted, and patients experience alterations in their bodily functions, social roles, job status, and finances. They are in strange, frightening, and restrictive environments. Patients report distressing bodily reactions, deprivation of control, fear of medical equipment, loss of meaning, and relationship disturbances during and after treatment in a critical care unit.[7] They are subjected to painful procedures, abrupt or continual noises, loss of privacy, sleep interruptions, pain, medications, isolation, and minimal contact with loved ones.[8,9] Lack of sleep and interrupted sleep-wake cycles depress mood and immune functions.[10] Sources of stress overload described in the literature include worry about life events, illness, social factors, low educational level or lack of education, poverty, severe emotional responses, lack of resources, and environmental threats.[11]

Stress Response

Stress of any type—whether positive or negative, biologic, psychological, spiritual, or social—elicits the same physical responses.[6] Classic stress theorists describe stress as a stimulus, a response, and a transaction.[12-15] Selye, in his pioneering work,[12] described the body's responses to a stressor as the "general adaptation syndrome" (GAS), characterized by three stages: alarm reaction, resistance, and exhaustion. An alarm reaction is initiated by the hypothalamus, which upon receiving sensory and chemical information regarding the presence of a stressor, signals the release of corticotrophin-releasing factor (CRF). The pituitary gland, signaled by CRF, releases two stress hormones, cortisol and aldosterone. The sympathetic nervous division of the autonomic nervous system (ANS) releases neurotransmitters and endocrine hormones associated with an acute stress response. Known as the "fight or flight" response, an alarm reaction triggers highly integrated cardiovascular and endocrine changes, evidenced by elevations in blood pressure, respiratory rate, heart rate, systemic vascular resistance, glucose production, and sweating, tremors, and nausea. During the resistance stage, the person's systems fight back, leading to adaptation and a return of normal functioning. If the stressors continue, exhaustion occurs, a stage in which the person's reserves have been depleted. Reversal of stress exhaustion can be accomplished by restoration of one's reserves through the use of medications, nutrition, and other stress-reduction measures.

BOX 4-1 Common Stressors for Patients in Critical Care Units

- Threat of death
- Uncertainty about future and fear of permanent residual health deficits
- Pain, discomfort, and physical restrictions
- Lack of sleep
- Loss of autonomy and control over one's body, environment, privacy, and daily activities
- Unfamiliar environments with excessive light, noises, alarms, and distressing events
- Worry about finances, potential job loss, and stress on loved ones
- Separation from family, friends, and meaningful social roles and work
- Loss of dignity, embarrassing exposures, and a sense of vulnerability
- Boredom broken only by brief visits, threatening stimuli, and procedural touch
- Loss of ability to express oneself verbally when intubated
- Unfamiliar bodily sensations due to bed rest, medications, surgery, or symptoms
- Unanswered spiritual questions and concerns about meaning of the events and life

Individual response to stressors depend on

- Individual's perception of the stressors
- Acute or chronic nature of the stressors
- Cumulative effect of multiple stressors
- Effectiveness of the person's usual coping strategies and style
- Degree of social support

POST-TRAUMATIC STRESS REACTIONS

Increasingly, clinicians and researchers have begun to describe the frequency and nature of acute stress reactions, panic attacks, or post-traumatic stress disorder (PTSD) experienced by patients after discharge from critical care units.[16,17,18] Labeling post-traumatic stress reactions a "disorder" misrepresents the true nature of the phenomenon. As with stress overload, PTSD is not a disordered response to stress resulting from a failure of a person's will, strength, endurance, or courage. The stress response is automatic and essential for survival. If threats to survival are multiple and relentless, without adequate recovery time, it is difficult for brain and body chemistry to adjust quickly. PTSD should be thought of as a "normal" response to abnormal and impossible demands. Post-traumatic stress responses, however, manifest as multiple distressing symptoms.

Even though post-traumatic reactions occur from several weeks to years after an event, critical care nurses should be aware of the possibility of post-traumatic stress reactions after a critical care experience for purposes of reducing all unnecessary stressors during a patient's stay, being alert to those patients who might be at higher risk for developing PTSD, and by using psychosocial-spiritual interventions to reduce the occurrence of post-traumatic stress reactions in the critical care patient population. A patient may survive a critical illness, only to face an even greater challenge on the road to recovery after leaving the critical care unit.

The actual incidence and nature of PTSD symptoms in the critical care population has not yet been fully determined. The problem is serious enough, however, to demand the attention of critical care professionals. Published studies report a wide range, from 5%-63%, of critical care patients experiencing PTSD symptoms of varying degrees.[19] Numerous studies indicate that patients with PTSD are at risk for developing other mental health problems and physical illnesses.[19,20]

Family members are also at risk for developing post-traumatic stress reactions[21,22] related to prolonged periods of uncertainty, anxious waiting, disrupted sleep patterns, financial concerns, witnessing emergency interventions, and confronting fears of loss and death. Kross et al.[23] report both depression and higher rates of PTSD in family members of patients who die during a critical care admission. Also at higher risk are family members of younger patients and those for whom mechanical ventilation is not withdrawn.

Critical care nurses can engage in health-promotion activities related to preventing post-traumatic stress reactions in patients and family members. Being aware of the possibility for stress overload in critical care settings is the first step. Care providers should take steps to manage or eliminate as many of those stressors as possible. Often patients are unaware or uncertain of what has happened to them and their bodily function. Nurses should engage in encouraging but realistic discussions of the patient's experiences, explain events carefully, and talk openly about recovery timelines and the gradual process of regaining strength.

Patient and family members usually recall and interpret the events, decisions, and time sequences involved in a critical care stay differently. Keeping a diary with photographs taken during a patient's stay in the critical care unit can help patients and family members reach a degree of shared common ownership of the experience. Having a family member keep a journal for later review often helps patients understand what happened so they can better come to terms with their illness and their recovery process.[24,25] In learning to live with the memories of critical care, patients benefit when they can construct a meaningful story.[26] The interventions described in this chapter not only support patients while they are in the unit but can also support patients' well-being over time, preparing them for the challenges of rehabilitation and recovery.

ANXIETY

Anxiety is a normal and common subjective human response to a perceived or actual threat, which can range from a vague, generalized feeling of discomfort to a state of panic and loss of control. Feelings of anxiety are common in critically ill patients but are often undetected by care providers.[27]

The physiologic effects of anxiety can produce negative effects in critically ill patients by activating the sympathetic nervous system and hypothalamic-pituitary-adrenal axis. Anxiety elicits changes in the neurohumoral release patterns involving the neurotransmitters in the brain that regulate mood—including acetylcholine, norepinephrine, dopamine, and serotonin and gamma-aminobutyric acid (GABA)—and their corresponding receptors. As anxiety levels increase, a patient experiences the physiologic effects of sympathetic nervous system stimulation with feelings of excitement and heightened awareness, followed by a diminishment of his or her perceptual field, problem-solving abilities, and coping skills. Panic attacks, a manifestation of severe anxiety not uncommon in critical care patients, can produce an acute stress response with tachycardia, hyperventilation, and dyspnea. Pharmacologic interventions for acute anxiety include the use of benzodiazepines, antihistamines, noradrenergic agents, antidepressants, and anxiolytics.[17]

The stressful experiences of having an acute or chronic illness, facing a real or anticipated loss, being admitted or discharged from a critical care unit, or requiring mechanical ventilation can trigger high degrees of patient anxiety.[29,30,31] Research also suggests that women, patients with minimal social support, and those with longer critical care lengths of stay are at higher risk for developing anxiety upon transfer out of the unit to a less intense level of care.[31,32] Whether the causes of anxiety are biochemical, genetic, emotional, or driven by the threats inherent in the situation, the critical care nurse should consider all contributing factors if interventions are to be effective.

Although rates of moderate to high anxiety exist in critical care patients, leading to higher complication rates,[33] valid and reliable methods to assess anxiety have not been put into practice. Critical care nurses most often rely on behavioral indicators such as agitation and restlessness and physiologic parameters such as increased heart rate and blood pressure.[34] Behavioral or vital sign changes do not provide consistently reliable indicators of anxiety and may lead to underestimation of the extent of anxiety in critical care patients.[32] The literature on anxiety in critical care patients cites over 50 clinical indicators, many of which are nonspecific or can be associated with multiple causes.[34] Using valid scales for evaluating patients' self-perceived anxiety levels can be helpful in determining the level and extent of anxiety.[27,33,34] See also Appendix A, Nursing Management Plan: Anxiety.

Anxiety and Pain

Of particular importance in the critical care setting is the cyclic relationship between levels of anxiety and perceptions and tolerance of pain. Pain triggers anxiety, and increased anxiety intensifies pain experiences. This reciprocal relationship varies, depending on whether pain is produced by disease processes or invasive procedures, is acute or chronic in nature, or if the pain is anticipated. In critical care, pain experiences arise from many sources, including injured tissues, immobility, pre-existing and chronic pain conditions, intubation, diagnostic or treatment procedures, bright lights, excessive noise, and interrupted sleep. When pain or a discomfort such as nausea is severe enough, patients try to conserve energy and focus inwardly to gain control of their pain and anxiety. They may startle easily, become irritable, display anger, be vigilant and wary of caregivers, or may be perceived as demanding. An overwhelmed patient often withdraws from interpersonal contact.[28,35] In situations of pain-induced anxiety, the nurse must identify the source of the pain, validate observations with the patient, and initiate pain-management strategies. Medications such as theophylline, anticholinergics, dopamine, levodopa, salicylates, and steroids can also contribute to feelings of anxiety.[35,36]

SPIRITUAL CHALLENGES IN CRITICAL CARE

Many of the psychosocial issues already discussed are rooted in the spiritual dimension of life, the seat of a person's deepest meanings and ground of being. One's spiritual dimension encompasses those elements of life that provide meaning, purpose, hope, and connectedness to others and a higher power.[37,38,39] Providing spiritual care is essential for patient recovery in critical care units.

Spiritual Distress

Spiritual distress has been defined as a disruption in the life principle that pervades a person's entire being and that integrates and transcends one's biologic and psychosocial nature.[37] Threats of physiologic or psychological illness, prolonged pain, and suffering can challenge a person's spirituality. Separation from one's meaningful religious or spiritual practices and rituals, coupled with intense suffering, can induce spiritual distress for patients and their families. Patients experiencing spiritual distress may question the meaning of suffering and death in relation to their personal belief system. They may wonder why the illness or injury has happened to them or may fear that what they have believed in has failed them in the time of greatest need. Some individuals in spiritual despair may question their existence, verbalize a wish to die, or display anger toward religious traditions. Unresolved spiritual distress is interpreted in the body as a stressor. Prolonged spiritual distress may lead to a sense of hopelessness, unwillingness to seek further treatment, or refusal to consent to helpful therapeutic interventions or regimens.[37]

Hope and Hopelessness

Hope is a subjective, dynamic internal process essential to life. Considered to be a spiritual process, hope is an energy that arises out of a sense of being meaningfully connected to one's self, others, and powers greater than the self. With hope, a person is able to transition from a state of vulnerability to a point of being able to live as fully as possible.[40] The need for hope is stimulated by a demand to adapt or change in unexpected situations, as is the case for people who are critically ill. The desire to maintain hope underlies many coping mechanisms. When people have hope and belief in their goals, they are empowered to engage in their own recovery with a sense of internal peace and freedom. While hope has a future orientation, it also has a present orientation that impacts people in the here and now.[41] We have come to understand, through observations of people in extreme circumstances, that an element of hope must be maintained for survival[42] and is an essential component in the successful treatment of illness.[43]

By contrast, hopelessness is a subjective state in which an individual sees extremely limited or no alternatives and is unable to mobilize energy on his or her own behalf.[35,37] Feelings of hopelessness can greatly hinder recovery. Conditions that increase a person's risk for feeling hopeless include a loss of dignity, long-term stress, loss of self-esteem, spiritual distress, and isolation, all of which can be present in a critical care experience. Patients who feel hopeless may be less involved in their recovery, may withdraw from the support of others, and lack the energy and initiative to engage in increasing degrees of self-care.[37]

Loss of Control and Powerlessness

Many patients admitted to a critical care unit have experienced a rapid onset of illness or an injury and have not had time to adjust to the limits of their changed circumstances. They have to adapt quickly to a loss of control. The loss of control in critical care hospitalization can be as minor as not getting a preferred food or as serious as experiencing a radical loss of a sense of self. Control, a person's ability to determine the use of time, space, and resources, becomes compromised in the critical care unit. On admission to a hospital, people forfeit much of their independence as they become patients. Choice of clothing and use of other personal belongings are usually restricted in a critical care unit. Patients cannot decide who enters the room, who provides personal care, or who intrudes with painful treatments. Hospital rules are usually not open to modification.

Rotter's early research[44] on human behavior and perception of control has been helpful in explaining the wide range of responses people have in situations in which they must give up control. Rotter suggests that a person's locus of control is internally or externally focused. Individuals who have an internal locus of control perceive themselves to be responsible for the outcome of events. Individuals with an external locus of control believe that their actions will have no effect on the outcome of a situation. Furthermore, as with any highly individualized concept, people vary in the amount of control they prefer.

Patients who have a pervasive sense that they can do nothing to change or control their circumstances are at risk for feeling powerless.[37] Critically ill people experience powerlessness due to the constraints of their health and the care environment, a loss of meaningful interpersonal interactions with their usual support system, inability to maintain cultural or religious beliefs and practices, or by adopting a helpless coping style. The degree of powerlessness a person experiences depends on his or her perceived sense of control, the type of loss that was experienced, and the availability of social support. Powerlessness can be manifested by a refusal to participate in decision making, disengagement from the plan of care, expressions of self-doubt, or a seeming lack of interest in recovery. Frustration, anger, and resentment over being dependent on others often occur and are exhibited in verbal expressions regarding dissatisfaction with care.[37] Poor interactions with health care providers who are perceived as imposing restrictions can make the situation worse. Patients may react aggressively, may try bargaining, or may refuse to comply with diagnostic and treatment regimens. Patients may lose sight of those areas of life over which they still maintain some influence because so much control has been taken from them. See Appendix A, Nursing Management Plan: Powerlessness.

COPING WITH STRESS AND ILLNESS

Coping mechanisms are intentional processes used to adjust, adapt, and successfully meet life stressors. Each patient's response to stress is unique and depends on a variety of environmental factors and individual differences, including cognitive variables, one's place in the life cycle, degree of social support, and the person's perception of the nature of the stressor or loss.[28]

If a patient is coping effectively, he or she appears relatively comfortable with self and others, is able to form a valid appraisal of stressors, makes decisions consistent with his or her own preferences and values, and has access to needed resources. Effective coping mechanisms help a person maintain a perception of an acceptable degree of control, empower him or her to take necessary actions, share concerns, use healthy denial, and manage troublesome life challenges and uncertainties. Most people have a repertoire of coping mechanisms to manage stressful situations and life challenges. Coping mechanisms are learned and practiced over a lifetime and are based on the person's sense of the effectiveness of any given strategy for adapting to the stressor.[45]

Ineffective coping is defined as the impairment of a person's adaptive behaviors and problem-solving abilities when meeting life's demands and necessary roles. Manifestations of ineffective coping in critical illness include verbalization of an inability to cope, anxiety, and being unable to meet basic needs. The patient exhibits inappropriate use of defense mechanisms and has diminished problem-solving abilities. The patient may display apathy or destructive behavior toward self and others.

Use of Psychological Defense Mechanisms

The overuse of psychological defense mechanisms may give evidence of ineffective patient or family coping. Defense mechanisms are automatic self-protective measures developed in response to an internal or external stressor and may be evident when patients or family members feel out of control and unable to cope.[41] Unrelenting anger, excessive protectiveness, distrust of others, extreme dependence or regression, psychological withdrawal, denial, or apathy concerning treatment goals may suggest that the stressors of the critical care experience have outstripped a person's coping abilities. Use of maladaptive measures may temporarily minimize anxiety but does not effectively or permanently resolve the conflict. Two common defense mechanisms especially evident in critical care settings include regression and denial.

Regression

Regression is an unconscious defense mechanism characterized by a retreat, in the face of stress, to behaviors characteristic of an earlier developmental level.[28] Regression allows a patient to give up his or her usual role, autonomy, and privacy to become the passive recipient of medical and nursing care. Admittedly, patients in critical care settings are expected to relinquish control and rely on others for even the most basic needs. To resist the care that others provide can jeopardize a patient's outcome. On the other hand, favorable patient outcomes and a speedy recovery can be threatened when patients regress to the point of relinquishing all control and responsibility for themselves to others and become excessively dependent. Behaviors such as whining, clinging to staff, needing the nurse constantly at the bedside, and giving evidence of an inability to self-modulate feelings of anxiety or fear can interfere with patient recovery and negatively affect nurse-patient relationships.

When expectations related to patient or family participation in self-care must be challenged or changed, patients are best served when limits and responsibilities are mutually determined and set in a supportive manner. Responses to patients will be more therapeutic when nurses recall that regression has been encouraged and expected at certain phases of a critical care stay, fear and anxiety have been reinforced in critical care experiences, and usual coping mechanisms have been abandoned. Although regressive behaviors can be frustrating to caregivers, avoid confrontations or reprimands. Threatening responses from staff may worsen a situation in which the patient is already struggling with issues of dependence, autonomy, and self-worth.

Denial

Denial is defined as the "conscious and unconscious attempts to disavow knowledge or the meaning of an event to reduce anxiety and fear."[46] Critically ill patients or their family members may use denial as a defense mechanism to protect against and manage an overwhelming sense of threat brought on by illness, injury, or impending death. As Weisman[47] describes in his classic work, denial has both protective and potentially detrimental functions.

The degree to which denial is used varies from person to person or may vary in the same person at different times. An inability to face the realities of a potential health problem leads some people to deny various aspects of their illness or the significance of potentially serious symptoms. Denial can lead to delayed treatment or lack of awareness of the danger of a symptom. Family members, unable to cope with a loved one's serious, irreversible illness, may focus only on the possibility of a full recovery. They resist having realistic discussions concerning goals of care, insist on repeated resuscitation attempts, or invest in home remodeling in anticipation of a homecoming. They may regard caregivers who try to discuss anything other than a full recovery as being negative or untrustworthy people.

While it is common to be alert to the potentially negative aspects of ineffective denial, denial often serves as a valuable defense mechanism for people unable to absorb the full force of a loss or significant life change at a given time. Denial is protective, in that sense, and gives a person the psychological space and time needed to process and accept the realities of a highly distressing loss.

Nurses may find it particularly difficult to communicate with people who seem to be using denial to their own detriment. It may seem to the caregiver that the person would cope better by facing the realities of a situation and by taking the steps needed to go on with life. Depending on the need people have to protect against their changing realities, they may or may not be readily influenced by information that contradicts their beliefs. Patients or family members who give evidence of firm or fixed denial are best supported by caregivers who understand that their denial is protective at this time and who watch for cues that indicate a readiness to accept the reality of their situation. See Appendix A, Nursing Management Plan: Compromised Family Coping.

HOLISTIC PSYCHOSOCIAL-SPIRITUAL CARE

In addition to having sophisticated knowledge of anatomy and physiology, the pathophysiology of disease processes, and appropriate nursing interventions, the holistic critical care nurse also needs the knowledge, wisdom, and skills to interpret the internal human responses to experiences of serious illness or injury. Attention to the whole patient is the ultimate goal of nursing care and is vitally important for critical care patients, families, and nurses. Nightingale believed that it was "unthinkable to consider sick humans as mere bodies who could be treated in isolation from their minds and spirits."[48] Essential skills that underlie nursing interventions for psychosocial-spiritual care include communicating with compassion and care, practicing dignity-enhancing care, supporting patient coping, using a family-centered focus, and engaging spiritual resources.

COMMUNICATE WITH COMPASSION AND CARE

Caring, compassionate verbal and nonverbal communication patterns give substance to nursing activities that promote expert psychosocial-spiritual care interventions. Nelson et al.[49] describe the top challenges to caregivers working in critical care areas, especially with the very seriously ill. None of the top challenges concerned the technical issues of medical management. Instead, the top challenges include inadequate patterns of communication between the critical care team and family members, insufficient staff knowledge of effective communication, unrealistic family and provider expectations, family disagreements, lack of advance directives, voiceless patients, and suboptimal space for having meaningful conversations. Patients and family members rank their needs for communication with health care providers as one of the most important aspects of feeling cared for in the critical care setting,[50] especially in nonspeaking patients.[51,52] Interviews with patients after a critical care stay revealed that they believed that a nurse's caring attitude led to more positive memories of their experience. Patients also reported less stress when they perceived nurses to be caring, warm, and competent, and when they communicated respect.[53] Many patients interpret a nurse's expressions of empathy and physical contact as evidence of caring and support.[54]

Many times sharing concerns with a caring and understanding listener can relieve emotional or spiritual distress. Patients are consoled knowing that they are not alone and when they sense that someone knows and cares about their feelings and experiences. Although the patient may share concerns with family members, she or he may be reluctant to upset loved ones and find that talking to a nurse seems more appropriate and emotionally safer. A patient who copes by talking to others will benefit from a nurse who recognizes when the patient needs to talk and who knows how to listen.[55,56]

Nurses should not avoid difficult conversations. Many patients need to talk about their fears and prefer conversations that balance their needs for honesty with their need to maintain hope.[54,58] It is also important to remember cultural differences in communicating with patients and family members. Many people in Western and American culture expect and value honesty and truth-telling in difficult situations. Patients and family members from other cultures may have taboos surrounding what should be discussed regarding the diagnosis and prognosis in serious illness.[58,59] Careful medical and nursing assessments, use of family and team conferences to foster communication, and enlisting the assistance of a spiritual counselor can facilitate fruitful, understanding conversations in crisis and decision-making situations. Patients and family members in critical care areas need careful nurse-patient communication strategies (Box 4-2).

BOX 4-2 Strategies for Communicating with Patients and Family Members

- Be patient. What is routine for caregivers can be stressful and new to patients and family members.
- Repeat information as many times as necessary. Stress reduces concentration, memory, and comprehension, especially in unfamiliar situations.
- Assess patient and family knowledge level and prior experience with critical care.
- Use understandable language and interpret medical terms, without talking down.
- Ask clarifying questions to help validate understanding.
- Use a welcoming, open communication style. Critical care units can feel intimidating to people unfamiliar with the environment.
- Offer frequent updates regarding patient's condition, even if not asked.
- Engage in conversations of meaning with patients and family members, even if brief. Often critical care conversations are reduced to conveying only technical aspects of care.
- Honor privacy and provide space for family conferences.
- Speak to patients, even if they are unconscious. This conveys caring to family, and words may comfort the patient, even if there is no response.
- Use communication boards or other devices with patients unable to speak.
- Give patients time to respond and ask questions patient can likely answer easily.
- Speak slowly and look at patients when communicating. Gestures, lip movements, and facial expressions convey important messages.

Trust

Effective verbal and nonverbal communication is essential for the development of trust in a nurse-patient relationship.[55] Trust manifests itself in critical care patients' belief that the people they depend on will get them through the illness and will be able to manage any untoward event that might occur. A patient needs to trust the nurse's competence in the physical and technical aspects of care and rely on what the nurse says. Patients are keen observers of their caregivers and read them well. Trust and hope are easily lessened when inappropriate information is given or nurses do not follow through on what they say. See also Appendix A, Nursing Management Plan: Impaired Verbal Communication.

PRACTICE DIGNITY-ENHANCING CARE

"The capacity to give one's attention to a sufferer is a very rare and difficult thing; it is almost a miracle; it is a miracle."[60] The practice of dignity-enhancing care is anchored in authentic human presence, the giving of one's whole attention and being to another person in a given moment. When authentically present, the nurse is able to go beyond relying only on scientific information and attunes him- or herself to patient needs, experiences, and emotions in a way that facilitates the patient's healing.[61]

Dignity-enhancing perspectives include the need a person has to maintain a continuity of the self, one's roles and legacy, and a sense of pride, hopefulness, control, acceptance, and resiliency. Dignity-enhancing care has four components: attitude, behaviors, compassion, and dialogue.[62] Caregivers' first step in providing dignity-conserving care involves reflecting on the attitudes and assumptions they hold about other people and their situations. The nurse's attitudes, worldviews, and beliefs about a patient or family member influence his or her openness and ability to develop a trusting relationship.

Dignity-enhancing care is manifest in behaviors. Attending to the patient's physical appearance affirms the person's self-esteem and a healthy body image. Cleanliness and absence of body odors give patients a sense of worth. When providing physical care, provide privacy, respect social boundaries, and ask permission before touching when possible. Validate the patient by giving importance to the things that he or she cares about. Spending time with patients as they share their life stories helps the nurse know them better and facilitates the development of individualized interventions. Show respect for patients by calling them by their preferred names or titles to help reinforce the patient's self-concept and identity. Obtain the patient's permission to include others in private conversations.

Compassion refers to the awareness of another person's suffering, coupled with a sincere intention to alleviate the suffering. In compassion, caregivers are able to identify with another person and recognize a shared humanity. Showing compassion can be quite simple, in acts of consideration, kindness, or a simple touch. Critical care nurses frequently touch people in the completion of procedures and caregiving activities. Keeping in mind individual and cultural differences, nurses should include nonprocedural touch in their care. The use of touch intended to communicate care and comfort can be an important part of patient healing and interpersonal connection. Compassion is also evidenced in dialogue, the fourth element of dignity-conserving care. At the most basic level, patients and family members need timely updates, explanations, repetition of unfamiliar information, and thorough information sharing. At a deeper level, patients need to feel that they are heard by their caregivers and know that their personhood is valued and respected.[62]

SUPPORT PATIENT COPING

A goal of expert psychosocial-spiritual care is to promote patient and family flourishing, empowering them to experience as much control and predictability as possible. As noted above, coping is a dynamic process involving cognitive and behavioral efforts to manage specific internal or external demands that are perceived to exceed the person's resources. The key to effective coping is to encourage the use of the best mix of strategies appropriate for a given situation.

Most adults cope by relying on their previously developed conscious and unconscious coping strategies and defense mechanisms, which are automatically triggered in a stressful situation. Teaching new coping skills to people who are experiencing acute psychological stress may be unrealistic. However, by using active listening skills and initiating conversations with patients and family members, the nurse can identify those coping resources, skills, and preferences that may be most helpful.

Helping Patients Maintain Control

Research suggests that one of the most effective ways to decrease the stress of being in a critical care environment is to give patients as much control over their care and the environment as possible.[53] Allow patients to make decisions as they are able, such as how and when to administer personal hygiene, diet preferences, and the timing of nursing interventions. Inform patients and family members about daily activities, tests, or therapies, their purpose, and anticipated effects. Critical care patients are often unable to see or turn around to witness what is going on in their environments. During treatments and procedures, provide the patient with explanations, brief discussions on what to expect, the anticipated time of a procedure, and descriptions of what is happening during an intervention. The patient for whom control is important should be helped to maintain control in as many areas of his or her life as possible. On the other hand, a patient must be given the opportunity not to exercise control if having too many choices provokes even greater stress.

Support Patient-Preferred Complementary Therapies

Patients and families enter health care settings with well-established practices and beliefs about managing stress, maintaining wellness, balance, and harmony in their lives and know what methods best facilitate their bodies' own healing responses. Integrative health care practices involve a blending of allopathic medical health care methods with patient-identified complementary therapies.[63]

The type of complementary or integrative therapies used depends on a patient's preferences, coping style, physical capabilities, and personality type. Music therapy, relaxation, guided imagery, therapeutic massage, visualization, prayer, biofeedback, and mindfulness meditation are potentially useful for critical ill patients.[64,65] Significant decreases in anxiety and symptom distress have been attributed to tactile touch. Although more research is needed to support the value of complementary therapies on selected outcomes in critically ill hospitalized patients, early studies support their potential as therapeutic nursing interventions (see Chapter 1).

Creating Healing Environments

People are continuous with their environments. Alterations in the physical environment of critical care units can provide a sense of calm, enhance patient coping, and facilitate healing.[66] Nurses can make environmental changes to give patients a greater sense of comfort and familiarity while they are in the unit. Critical care areas are bright, loud, and busy. Close patient doors to adjacent areas, use sound dampening panels, turn off unnecessary noisy equipment, and decrease noise at workstations. Nurse call interruptions can be minimized with the use of smart phones. Music can be used to produce therapeutic sound in critical care areas. Control lighting for individual patient preference, allow for natural sunlight if possible, and position patients so that they can see out of windows.[66] Within the limits of unit policy, familiarize patient rooms by displaying photographs, cards, drawings, and favored items. Sleep deprivation is a serious concern in critical care environments. To prevent light exposures that awaken patients, nurses should group care activities to limit nighttime interruptions and collaborate with lab personnel to decrease sleep interruptions.[53,67]

Visiting Policies

While practices vary among critical care units, a more relaxed visitation policy humanizes the environment and facilitates healing. The American Association of Critical-Care Nurses' AACN Practice Alert[68] recommends giving unrestricted access of hospitalized patients to a chosen support person. Giving family members access to their loved ones enhances patient and family satisfaction and improves safety of care. Family members have insight into the patient's behaviors and preferences, especially with patients who are unable to communicate. Interactions with family members reduce patient anxiety and enhance a sense of control.[69] Including patients and family members in critical care interdisciplinary rounds has been shown to improve perceptions of accessibility and communication.[70]

PROVIDE FAMILY-CENTERED CARE

Family-centered care, endorsed by the AACN as a practice standard for critical care, formalizes the patient and family as the unit of care. Family-centered care is based on the belief that patients and families should participate in decisions together and that patients need their families for love, understanding, and support while coping with critical illness.[71] The nurse's observable support of family members gives the patient comfort.

The elements essential to family-centered care include respect, collaboration, and support. Research had demonstrated that family members of critical care patients want information, reassurance, and proximity to their loved ones. They also want accurate information, communicated in an understandable manner, and they need room for hope.[57] The majority of family members who were able to help with caregiving had a more positive outlook.

Family members, themselves in a time of crisis, are particularly sensitive to a nurse's words and actions, making it essential that the nurse convey understanding and acceptance. Although the critical care nurse rarely has the time or opportunity to perform a full family assessment or give ongoing support to all family members, he or she can observe the quality of the patient-family interaction and formulate interventions that will aid the family in supporting the patient.[62] The patient determines who counts as "family." Regard non-biologic or non-legal partners as full members of the patient's family or support system if that is the nature of the patient's relationships. The critical care nurse provides interventions aimed at supporting family members throughout the patient's stay in the unit.

ENGAGE SPIRITUAL RESOURCES

A time of crisis can also lead to a time of positive spiritual renewal and readiness for an enhanced spiritual life. Spiritual and religious beliefs and practices often give patients and family members some measure of acceptance of an illness, a sense of mastery and control, strength to endure the stressors of illness, and a source of hope and trust beyond what medical interventions can provide.

Transformative spiritual care strategies are particularly helpful in times of crisis and uncertainty. When faced with significant life challenges, people need resources to transcend their circumstances and know that no matter what happens, they will endure. Spiritual resources include faith in a higher power, support communities, a sense of hope and meaning in life, and religious practices. Patient and family spirituality affects their ability to cope with loss.[72]

While distinctions between spiritual and religious concerns are important to highlight,[39] many people find spiritual strength in their adherence to a particular religious tradition. They get inspiration to endure, hope, comfort, assurance, and confidence from the texts, rituals, and beliefs of their faith communities. Facilitate patient access to religious rituals, prayer, and scripture reading as hope-sustaining activities and help patients make connections to their spiritual or cultural communities. Collaborate with the hospital's spiritual care department when you sense that a person has unmet or unaddressed spiritual questions or needs. Often a professional spiritual care provider is the best person to assess spiritual needs and plan helpful interventions. Spiritual and religious leaders can also provide valuable insights when discussing ethical decisions that may have implications for the person's values and beliefs. Religious, spiritual, or philosophical practices can also directly inform diet, hygiene practices, and rituals surrounding birth, death, and medical interventions.

PATIENTS WITH MENTAL HEALTH CO-MORBIDITIES

Not infrequently, patients admitted to critical care settings have a pre-existing mental health condition. Chronic depression, bipolar disorders, substance addiction, and self-destructive behaviors, including suicide attempts, can also be the primary cause of a critical care hospitalization. The critical care team should make every effort to continue medications for mental health conditions during the critical care stay unless medically contraindicated. If the patient is unable to take oral medications, attempt to find an alternative route, if possible. If psychotropic medications have been discontinued for medical reasons, discuss the need to resume those medications with the health care providers receiving the patient after discharge from the critical care unit.

Alcohol Withdrawal in Critical Care Settings

Nurses in any acute care setting must be alert to the symptoms of withdrawal from chemical substances, including alcohol, which can complicate recovery from the admitting diagnosis. Not infrequently, in emergency admissions to a critical care unit, a full patient history of substance use has not been elicited. Investigators estimate that 1 in 4 patients admitted to general hospitals meet criteria for alcohol dependence.[73] Without treatment, withdrawal from an alcohol addiction progresses to delirium tremens and can occur from 3 hours up to 7 days after the last alcohol consumption. Peak withdrawal time is 48-72 hours after last alcohol consumption in a person with alcohol addiction.[74]

The signs and symptoms of alcohol withdrawal syndrome (AWS) are easily confused with other conditions. Patient with AWS exhibit altered concentration, tremulousness, autonomic hyperarousal, hallucinations, disorientation, psychosis, tachycardia, hypertension, low-grade fever, agitation, diaphoresis, and delirium tremens.

Caring for Patients after Attempted Suicide

Nurses in critical care settings not infrequently care for patients who have attempted suicide. It is especially important to practice dignity-enhancing care in these situations. Nurses should carefully consider their own attitudes concerning people who engage in self-destructive behaviors. Patients who have attempted suicide are often stigmatized, and caregivers can resent caring for a person whose critical condition is self-inflicted. A suicide attempt indicates, however, that the patient was experiencing personal and spiritual distress to the point of wanting to end his or her life. A suicidal behavior resides at the extreme, maladaptive end of a continuum of self-protective responses to life's challenges.[28] Usually a person who has attempted suicide is quickly transferred out of the unit for further evaluation and mental health care when they are medically stable. While the patient is in the unit, however, primary nursing interventions include validating the patient's worth and self-esteem, helping him or her regulate emotional states and behaviors, and mobilizing the patient's social support, necessary for long-term recovery.[28,45]

Nurses also care for family members of persons who have attempted suicide. They are often undergoing a significant family crisis and can have feelings of shame, guilt, or anger concerning the suicide attempt. Talk to family members in a private setting and establish an atmosphere of interested concern for their loved one. Before the patient is discharged from the unit or hospital, gather assessment data from family members, including information about the patient's medical and psychiatric history, history of previous suicide attempts, presence of a trigger for self-destructive behavior (recent disagreement with someone or anniversary of a loss), presence of acute stressors, and availability of support systems. Family members should be encouraged to inform health care providers if the patient has stopped taking prescribed psychotropic medications or seeing a mental health provider and begin to make a plan for immediate follow-up care after discharge from the unit.[75]

NURSE SELF-CARE

Critical care nurses do amazing, life-giving work. In the words of poet John O'Donohue, nurses "stand like a secret angel between the bleak despair of illness and the unquenchable light of spirit that can turn the darkest destiny towards dawn."[76] Critical care nurses possess the knowledge, wisdom, and power to help others in situations of uncertainty and suffering.

Remembering always critical care nurses' life-giving work, it is also important to recognize the need for consistent, intentional self-care. A nurse cannot give fully engaged, compassionate care to others when he or she feels depleted or does not feel cared for him- or herself. In critical care settings, nurses rarely have time to recover from one emotionally draining situation before they are called upon to respond to another. They often witness prolonged, concentrated suffering on a daily basis, leading to feelings of frustration, anger, guilt, sadness, or anxiety. Frequent, intense, or prolonged exposure to grief and loss places nurses at risk for developing compassion fatigue, a physical, emotional, and spiritual exhaustion accompanied by emotional pain. The stressors of caregiving can lead to a decreased capacity to show compassion or empathize with suffering people.[77] Nurses, too, are at risk for developing STRESS reactions due to the relentless stress and psychologically difficult work of caring for others in extreme situations.

To avoid the extremes of either becoming overly involved in patients' suffering or detaching from them, nurses can use self-care activities to maintain balance. Nurses should first use self-reflection when they feel overwhelmed, considering the possible reasons for their feelings. There are often multiple causes for feeling overwhelmed: sadness about a particular patient, overwork, lateral hostility at work,[78] and disruptions in one's personal life. Reflection is an important first step because without awareness, it is difficult to identify possible solutions. Talking with friends, a spiritual care provider, or a close colleague can help the nurse recognize his or her own grief and reflect on the meaning of work.

Stress-management techniques help to restore energy and enjoyment in caring for patients. In some instances, nurses choose to work temporarily in less emotionally stressful settings. Nurses who practice self-care are more likely to experience professional and personal growth and find much meaning in their work. Maintain physical health by eating well, exercising, engaging in relaxing activities, laughing, and by getting enough sleep. Promote emotional health by participating in calming activities such as meditation, daily gratitude reflections, deep breathing, walking, or listening to music.[79,80] Use self-transcendence (spiritual awareness) activities, such as journal writing, sharing stories, recognizing one's own positive contributions and unique gifts, and connecting with one's self.[81] Given the ongoing demands of critical care nursing, balance time at work with time for recreation and relaxation. Invest time in those people and activities that nurture the spirit. Learn from the courage exhibited by patients and family members, and with good self-care, find joy and fulfillment in being a critical care nurse.

CASE STUDY Patient with Psychosocial Needs

Brief Patient History

Ms. T is a 17-year-old woman who took an acetaminophen overdose after her boyfriend broke up with her. She states that she did not want to kill herself but just wanted to scare her boyfriend. Ms. T is having difficulty facing the need for a psychiatric evaluation and the potential for severe liver damage.

Clinical Assessment

Ms. T was admitted to the critical care unit from the emergency department in stable condition. She is awake, alert, and oriented to person, time, place, and situation. She is irritable, withdrawn, and wants to be left alone. Her parents stay at her bedside and share with the nurse their intense feelings of fear, confusion, and uncertainty concerning their daughter's serious psychological and physical condition.

Diagnostic Procedures

A psychiatric evaluation was completed, with the recommendation that Ms. T receive inpatient psychiatric care when medically stable.

Medical Diagnosis

Ms. T is diagnosed with acetaminophen toxicity and risk for hepatic failure.

Questions

1. What major outcomes do you expect to achieve for this patient?
2. What problems or risks must be managed to achieve these outcomes?
3. What interventions must be initiated to monitor, prevent, manage, or eliminate the problems and risks identified?
4. What interventions should be initiated to promote optimal functioning, safety, and well-being of the patient?
5. What possible learning needs do you anticipate for this patient?
6. What cultural and age-related factors may have a bearing on the patient's plan of care?

REFERENCES

1. Chochinov H: Dignity-conserving care–a new model for palliative care: helping the patient feel valued, *JAMA* 287(17):2253, 2002.
2. Cropley M, Steptoe A: Social support, life events and physical symptoms: a prospective study of chronic and recent life stress in men and women. Psychology, *Health Med* 10:317, 2005.
3. Lloyd C, et al: Stress and diabetes: a review of the links, *Diabetes Spectrum* 18:121, 2005.
4. Neilsen N, et al: Self-reported stress and risk of breast cancer, *Br Med J* 331:548, 2005.
5. Lovallo W: *Stress and health: biological and psychological interactions*, Thousand Oaks, CA, 2005, Sage.
6. Seaward BL: *Managing stress: principles and strategies for health and wellbeing*, ed 5, Sudbury, MA, 2009, Jones and Bartlett.
7. Fredriksen ST, Ringsberg K: Living the situation stress-experiences among intensive care patients, *Internat Crit Care Nurs* 23:124, 2007.
8. Pang P, Suen L: Stressors in the ICU: a comparison of patients' and nurses' perception, *J Clin Nurs* 17:2681, 2008.
9. Rattray J, et al: Patients' perceptions of and emotional outcome after intensive care: results from a multicenter study, *Nurs Crit Care* 15(2):86, 2010.
10. Ganz F: Sleep and immune function, *Crit Care Nurs* 32(2):19, 2012.
11. Lunney M: Stress overload: a new diagnosis, *Internat J Nurs Term Classif* 17(4):165, 2006.
12. Selye H: *Stress in health and disease*, Boston, 1976, Butterworth.
13. Lazarus R, Lazarus B: *Passion and reason: making sense of emotions*, New York, 1994, Oxford University.
14. Lazarus R, Folkman S: *Stress, appraisal, and coping*, New York, 1984, Springer.
15. Neurberger P: *Freedom from stress: a holistic approach*, Honesdale, PA, 1981, The Himalayan International Institute of Yoga Science and Philosophy.
16. Davydow D, et al: Posttraumatic stress disorder in general intensive care unit survivors: a systematic review, *Gen Hosp Psychiatry* 30:421, 2008.
17. Tedstone J, Tarrier N: Posttraumatic stress disorder following medical illness and treatment, *Clin Psych Rev* 23:409, 2003.

18. Wallen K, et al: Symptoms of acute posttraumatic stress disorder after intensive care, *Am J Crit Care* 17(6):534, 2008.
19. Jackson JC, et al: Posttraumatic stress disorder and posttraumatic stress symptoms following critical illness in medical ICU patients: assessing the magnitude of the problem, *Criti Care* 11:R27, 2007.
20. Jones C, et al: Precipitants of post-traumatic stress disorder following intensive care: a hypothesis generating study of diversity in care, *Intensive Care Med* 33:978, 2007.
21. Azoulay E, et al: Risk of post-traumatic stress symptoms in family members of intensive care patients, *Am J Resp Crit Care Med* 171:987, 2005.
22. Pillai L, et al: Can we predict intensive care relatives at risk for posttraumatic stress disorder? *Indiana J Crit Care Med* 14(2):83, 2010.
23. Kross E, et al: ICU care associated with symptoms of depression and posttraumatic stress disorder among family members of patients who died in the ICU, *Chest* 139(4):795, 2011.
24. Combe D: The use of patient diaries in the intensive care unit, *Nurs Crit Care* 10:31, 2005.
25. Phillips C: Use of patient diaries in critical care, *Nurs Stand* 26(11):35, 2011.
26. Williams S: Recovering from the psychological impact of intensive care: how constructing a story helps, *Nurs Crit Care* 14(6):281, 2009.
27. Perpina-Galvan J, Richart-Martinez M: Scales for evaluating self perceived anxiety levels in patients admitted to intensive care units: a review, *Am J Crit Care* 18(6):571, 2009.
28. Stuart G: *Principles and practices of psychiatric nursing*, ed 9, St. Louis, 2009, Mosby.
29. Khalaila R, et al: Communication difficulties and psychoemotional distress in patients receiving mechanical ventilation, *Am J Crit Care* 20(6):470, 2011.
30. Chlan L, Savik K: Patterns of anxiety in critically ill patients receiving mechanical ventilator support, *Nurs Res* 60(3S):S50, 2011.
31. Brodsky-Israeli M, Ganz F: Risk factors associated with transfer anxiety among patients transferring from the intensive care unit to the ward, *J Adv Nurs* 67(3):510, 2011.
32. Moser D: The rust of life: impact of anxiety on cardiac patients, *Am J Crit Care* 16(4):361, 2007.
33. Ruz M, et al: Evidence that the brief symptom inventory can be used to measure anxiety quickly and reliably in patients hospitalized for acute myocardial infarction, *J Cardiovascular Nurs* 25(2):117, 2010.
34. Frazier S, et al: Critical care nurses' assessment of patients' anxiety: reliance on physiological and behavioral parameters, *Am J Crit Care* 11(1):57, 2002.
35. Doenges ME, Murr A, Moorhouse MF: *Nurse's pocket guide: diagnoses, interventions, and rationales*, ed 12, Philadelphia, 2010, FA Davis.
36. Pasacreta JV, Minarik P, Nield-Anderson L: Anxiety and depression. In Ferrell B, Coyle N, editors: *Textbook of palliative nursing*, ed 3, New York, 2010, Oxford University Press.
37. Ackley B, Ladwig G, editors: *Nursing diagnosis handbook: an evidence-based guide to planning care*, St. Louis, 2011, Mosby.
38. Griffin A, Yancey V: Spiritual dimensions of the perioperative experience: theoretical and practical concerns, *J AORN* 89(5):875, 2009.
39. Puchalski C: Spirituality and the care of patients at the end of life: an essential component of care, *Omega (Westport)* 56(1):33, 2007-2008.
40. Arnaert A, et al: Stroke patients in the acute care phase: role of hope in self-healing, *Holist Nurs Prac* 20(3):137, 2006.
41. Cutcliffe J, Hearth K: The concept of hope in nursing 5: hope and critical care nursing, *Br J Nurs* 11(18):1190, 2002.
42. Frankl V: *Man's search for meaning*, New York, 1959, Washington Square Press.
43. Miller JF: Hope: a construct central to nursing, *Nurs Forum* 42(1):12–19, 2007.
44. Rotter JB: Generalized expectancies for internal versus external control of reinforcement, *Psychol Monogr* 80(1):1, 1966.
45. Varacarolis E, Halter M, editors: *Foundations of psychiatric mental health nursing: a clinical approach*, ed 6, St. Louis, 2010, Elsevier.
46. NANDA International: *Nursing diagnosis: definitions and classification 2012-2014*, Philadelphia, 2011, Wiley-Blackwell.
47. Weisman A: *On dying and denying: a psychiatric study of terminality*, Mourning Heights, NY, 1972, Behavioral Publications.
48. Dossey B: Body-mind-spirit: attention to holistic care, *Am J Nurs* 98(8):35, 1998.
49. Nelson JE, et al: End of life care for the critically ill: a national intensive care unity survey, *Crit Care Med* 34:2547, 2006.
50. Batty S: Communication, swallowing and feeding in the intensive care unit patient, *Nurs Crit Care* 14(4):175, 2009.
51. Happ M, et al: Nurse-patient communication interactions in the intensive care unit, *Am J Crit Care Nurs* 20(2):e28, 2011.
52. Grossbach I: Promoting effective communication for patients receiving mechanical ventilation, *Crit Care Nurs* 31(3):46, 2011.
53. Lusk B, Lash A: The stress responses, psychoneuroimmunology, and stress among ICU patients, *Dim Crit Care Nurs* 24(1):25, 2005.
54. Stajduha K, et al: Patient perceptions of helpful communication in the context of advanced cancer, *J Clin Nurs* 19:2039, 2010.
55. Watson J: *Caring science as sacred science*, Philadelphia, 2005, F A Davis.
56. Lowey S: Communication between the nurse and family caregiver in end of life care: a review of the literature, *J Hosp Pall Nursing* 10(1):35, 2008.
57. Verhaeghe S, et al: How does information influence hope in family members of traumatic coma patients in intensive care unit? *J Clin Nurs* 16:1488, 2007.
58. Johnstone L, Kanitsaki O: Ethics and advance care planning in a culturally diverse society, *J Transcult Nurs* 20(4):405, 2009.
59. Erichsen E, et al: A phenomenological study of nurses' understanding of honesty in palliative care, *Nurs Ethics* 17(1):39, 2010.
60. Lipson M, Lipson A: Psychotherapy and the ethics of attention, *Hast Cent Rep* 26(1):17, 1996.
61. Newman M: *Transforming presence: the difference that nursing makes*, Philadelphia, 2008, F.A. Davis.
62. Tulsky J: Interventions to enhance communication among patients, providers, and families, *J Palliat Med* 8(S 1):S95, 2005.

63. Henricson M, et al: The outcome of tactile touch on stress parameters in intensive care: a randomized controlled trial, *Compl Ther Clin Prac* 14:244, 2008.
64. Caine R: Psychological influences in critical care: perspectives from psychoneuroimmunology, *Crit Care Nurs* 23(2):60, 2003.
65. Austin D: The psycholophysiological effects of music therapy in intensive care units, *Paediatric Nurs* 22(3):14, 2010.
66. Bazuin D, Cardon K: Creating healing intensive care unit environments: physical and psychological considerations in designing critical care areas, *Crit Care Nurs* 24(4):259, 2011.
67. Dunn H, et al: Nighttime lighting in intensive care units, *Crit Care Nurs* 30(3):31, 2010.
68. AACN Practice alert: *Family visitation in the adult ICU*, 2011, AACN.
69. Black P, et al: The effect of nurse-facilitated family participation in the psychological care of the critically ill patient, *J Adv Nurs* 67(5):1091, 2011.
70. Jacobowski N, et al: Communication in critical care: family rounds in the intensive care unit, *Am J Crit Care* 19(5):421, 2010.
71. Mitchell M, et al: Positive effects of a nursing intervention on family-centered care in adult critical care, *Am J Crit Care* 18(6):543, 2009.
72. Hermann C: The degree to which spiritual needs of patients near the end of life are met, *Onc Nurs Forum* 34(1):70, 2007.
73. Repper-DeLisi J, et al: Successful implementation of an alcohol withdrawal pathway in a general hospital, *Psychomatics* 39(4):292, 2008.
74. York L, Rayback S: Behavioral and psychological factors in critical care. In Ahrens T, Prentice D, Kleinpell R, editors: *Critical care nursing certification*, New York, 2010, McGraw Hill.
75. National Suicide Prevention Lifeline: After attempt: a guide for taking care of your family member after treatment in the emergency department. http://www.suicidepreventionlifeline.org. Accessed September 20, 2012.
76. O'Donahue J: *To bless the space between us: a book of blessings*, New York, 2008, Doubleday.
77. Bush N: Compassion fatigue: are you at risk? *Onc Nurs Forum* 26(1):24, 2009.
78. Alspach G: Lateral hostility between critical care nurses: a survey report, *Crit Care Nurs* 28(2):13, 2008.
79. Showalter S: Compassion fatigue: what is it? why does it matter? recognizing the symptoms, acknowledging the impact, developing the tools to prevent compassion fatigue, and strengthen the professional already suffering from the effects, *Am J Hosp Palliat Med* 27(4):239, 2010.
80. Wilson L: Getting a self-care tune-up, *Beginnings* 28(1):8, 2008.
81. Hunnibell L, et al: Self-transcendence and burnout in hospice and oncology nurses, *J Hosp Palliat Nurs* 10(3):172, 2008.

CHAPTER 5

Sleep Alterations

Kathleen M. Stacy

ⓔ Be sure to check out the bonus material, including review questions, on the Evolve website at http://evolve.elsevier.com/Urden/priorities/.

NORMAL HUMAN SLEEP

Nurses who have an appreciation of the importance of sleep place a higher priority on protection of patients' sleep.[1] Health care providers interrupt patients' sleep for assessment, treatments, or interventions, and environmental noise, pain, or anxiety can also disturb it.[2] Although prioritizing care is essential, the consequence of sleep interruptions is not merely sleep-deprived patients; alterations in sleep patterns can result in chronic sleep problems, poor recovery, and decreased quality of life.[1]

Sleep Physiology

Humans spend about one-third of their lives engaged in a process known as *sleep.* Although little is now known about the physiologic process or the depths to which it affects us, researchers are learning more about sleep every day. The behavioral definition of sleep is a reversible behavioral state of perceptual disengagement from and unresponsiveness to the environment.[3] Sleep is a basic human need, just as food and water are. For patients to regain and maintain their optimal physical and emotional health, they must be able to get adequate amounts of quality sleep. To help patients obtain their optimal amount of sleep, a nurse must first understand what constitutes normal sleep and how the nursing plan of care can contribute to accomplishing this goal.

Polysomnography (PSG) is the collection of multiple channels of physiologic data to assess sleep and its disorders using various electrodes.[4] Electroencephalographic (EEG) electrodes are attached to the patient's scalp to measure brain waves. Changes in the EEG frequency (number of waveforms) and amplitude (height of waveform) over the course of the study allow the sleep to be scored into stages. Sleep stages are distinguished primarily by the EEG waveforms they produce. Sleep is scored by each 30-second epoch or segment of the tracing. The criteria for scoring sleep in infants differ from those used for adults.[4]

Electrooculography (EOG) measures eye movement activity. The study can help to determine when the patient is in rapid eye movement (REM) sleep; it also can establish when sleep onset occurs as reflected by slow, rolling eye movements.[4] Electromyography (EMG) involves leads placed over various muscle groups. When placed over the chin, the leads can help detect muscle atonia associated with REM sleep. Intercostal leads detect respiratory effort, whereas leads over the anterior tibialis detect leg movements that may be causing the patient to arouse. The electrocardiogram (ECG) shows any cardiac abnormalities, oximetry monitors the oxygen saturation levels, and piezoelastic bands around the chest and abdomen detect respiratory disorders such as apnea. Thermocouples are used to monitor airflow through the nose and mouth.[4]

Sleep Stages

Humans experience three states of being. They are awake, in REM sleep, or in non-rapid eye movement (NREM) sleep. NREM sleep usually occupies 70% to 75% of the sleep cycle, with REM sleep comprising 20% to 25%.[5] Some theorize that NREM sleep is a restorative period that relieves the stresses of waking activities, whereas REM sleep serves to refuel creative brain stores.

Non-Rapid Eye Movement Sleep

NREM sleep can be further divided into stages 1 through 3 (N1-N3), with each stage being a progressively deeper sleep state. Adults usually enter sleep through NREM stage N1 sleep, which is a transitional, lighter sleep state from which the patient can be easily aroused by light touch or by softly calling his or her name.

Stage N1 comprises 2% to 5% of a night's sleep and is demonstrated by an EEG pattern of low-voltage, mixed-frequency waveforms with vertex sharp waves.[5] The EOG during stage N1 may demonstrate slow, side-to-side eye movements. A patient with severely disrupted sleep may experience an increase in the amount of stage N1 sleep throughout the sleep cycle. As a patient makes the transition from awake to asleep, a brief memory impairment may occur.[4] As a result, the patient may not remember educational or care instructions given by the nurse during the transition between sleep and wake states. Stage N2 sleep occupies about 45% to 55% of the night, with sleep deepening and a higher arousal threshold being required to awaken the patient. Changes seen in the EEG pattern include sleep spindles and K complexes.[5] As stage N2 continues, high-voltage, slow-wave activity begins to appear.[4] When these slow waves represent 20% of the EEG activity per page, the criteria are met for stage N3 sleep, which constitutes 15% to 20% of the cycle.[5] In stage N3 sleep, slow waves continue to develop until 50% of the EEG waveforms are slow wave. This stage of sleep is often referred to as *slow-wave sleep.*[5]

NREM sleep is dominated by the parasympathetic nervous system. The body tries to maintain a homeostatic regulation, and this causes a decreased level of energy expenditure. Blood pressure, heart and respiratory rates, and the metabolic rate return to basal levels. EMG levels are lower in NREM as opposed to wake states but not as low as in REM sleep. Sweating or shivering that a patient may experience with temperature extremes occurs during NREM sleep but ceases during REM sleep.[3] During slow-wave sleep, 80% of the total daily growth-stimulating hormone is released, which works to stimulate protein synthesis while sparing catabolic breakdown. The release of other hormones, such as prolactin and testosterone, suggests that anabolism is occurring during slow-wave sleep. Cortisol release peaks during early morning hours, whereas melatonin is released only during darkness, and thyroid-stimulating hormone is inhibited during sleep. The activities associated with stage N3 sleep include protein synthesis and tissue repair, such as the repair of epithelial cells and specialized cells of the brain, skin, bone marrow, and gastric mucosa.[6]

Rapid Eye Movement Sleep

REM sleep occupies about 20% to 25% of the night in healthy young adults and is sometimes known as the *dream stage.* However, dreaming is not the exclusive property of any one stage. REM can be viewed as a highly active brain in a paralyzed body and is frequently referred to as a *paradoxic sleep.* The paradox is that some areas of the brain remain very active, whereas others are suppressed. EEG waveforms are relatively slow voltage, and sawtooth waves are present. Increased cortical activity occurs, with the EEG pattern resembling those of the wake state. Synchronized bursts of rapid, side-to-side eye movements with suppressed EMG activity (muscle atonia) are seen, indicating functional paralysis of the skeletal muscles.[7]

The sympathetic nervous system predominates during REM sleep. Oxygen consumption increases, and blood pressure, cardiac output, and respiratory and heart rates become variable. The body's response to decreased oxygen levels and increased carbon dioxide levels is lowest during REM sleep. An increase in premature ventricular contractions and tachydysrhythmias may be associated with respiratory pauses during REM sleep and can lead to oxygen reduction, particularly in patients with pulmonary or cardiac disease. Arterial pressure surges and increases in heart rate, coronary arterial tone, and blood viscosity may cause the combination of plaque rupture and hypercoagulability in persons with cardiac disease.[7]

Sleep Cycles

NREM and REM sleep cycles alternate throughout the night. Sleep onset usually occurs in stage N1 sleep, progressing through stages N2 and N3, then going back to stage N2, at which time the person usually enters REM. This first cycle typically takes about 70 to 100 minutes, with later cycles lasting 90 to 120 minutes. Four to five cycles are completed during normal adult sleep. NREM sleep predominates during the first third of the night, whereas REM is more prominent during the last third. Brief episodes of wakefulness (usually less than 5%) tend to intrude later into the night and are usually not remembered the next morning.[5]

The amount of sleep required is uncertain. No set number of hours has been established, and sleep length may be determined by many factors, including genetic predisposition. A sufficient amount of sleep has been achieved when one awakens without external stimuli and gets through the day without feeling sleepy.

Sleep Regulation

Sleep is not merely a response to fatigue. A complex group of interacting systems determines the timing and depth of sleep. The following section reviews circadian and homeostatic processes and theories of sleep regulation.

Circadian System

Many body systems cycle within approximately a 24-hour period.[8] Among these systems is the sleep-wake rhythm. A bundle of cells in the anterior hypothalamus, known as the *suprachiasmatic nucleus,* functions as the pacemaker for these rhythms. The circadian system facilitates cycling of the prescribed functions within a predictable period, but the functions are also influenced by other conditions, such as social activity, posture, and physical environment.[8]

Under normal conditions, a person's rhythms interact and influence one another. For example, when body temperature is becoming lower, a person is more likely to sleep, and as the body temperature rises in early morning hours, people awaken. Another example is the melatonin cycle, which tends to run in synchrony with the sleep-wake cycle.[8]

External influences such as posture, exercise, and light also influence the sleep circadian rhythm. These external influences, known as *zeitgebers,* can shift the rhythm, causing it to peak at different times, or fragment it. Light is the most influential zeitgeber for sleep;[8] critical care nurses therefore need to limit the light in the environment during nocturnal hours to facilitate sleep and circadian continuity in their patients.[9]

Homeostatic Mechanism

The recent history of the sleep obtained by an individual also influences timing and depth of sleep. Known as the *homeostatic process of sleep regulation,* this determinant of sleep is linked to how much sleep the individual has had previously. Essentially, someone who is sleep-deprived will sleep more readily, regardless of circadian phase, whereas someone who is well- rested will not fall asleep readily.[10,11] The amount of slow-wave sleep (stage N3) reflects sleep intensity, and individuals recovering from sleep deprivation have increased amounts of slow-wave sleep.[11]

PHARMACOLOGY

Hypnotic benzodiazepines remain the medications of choice to treat insomnia. Insomnia is a patient complaint of inability to initiate or maintain sleep, and prescriptions for treatment of insomnia cost more than $1 billion annually.[12] Acute stress, such as admission to a critical care unit, may cause some patients to experience acute sleep-onset insomnia. Hypnotics tend to promote lighter sleep stages and have a higher lipophilicity, which can cause the elderly to experience an increased drug half-life.[12] Care should be used in the administration and dosage of hypnotics in the elderly. This age group may experience night terrors, nightmares, and increased agitation. The metabolism of hypnotics in elderly patients can be inhibited by the use of steroids, or it can be accelerated in those who smoke. Hypnotics may also produce anterograde amnesia, which is a memory failure of information processed after the medication is consumed. Patients with normal ventilation should not be affected by the mild respiratory depression caused by hypnotics, although patients with chronic obstructive pulmonary disease (COPD) or sleep-disordered breathing may be affected.[13]

Patients with illness may respond differently to medications than do healthy patients. Patients may come to the critical care unit with impaired sleep or poor cognitive function. Beta-blockers, a commonly used class of medications in critical care, are known to produce nightmares and have disruptive effects on sleep quality in some individuals.[14] The effect of various drug combinations are not well known. The critical care nurse should assess the patient's need for sedative and analgesic medications. The nurse has a responsibility to administer these medications in the most efficient manner to promote sleep and to monitor effectiveness. This can be achieved through assessment, including a medication history, diagnostic test results, and review of the patient's medical history. Information from that assessment assists the nurse in formulating a nursing diagnosis with outcome criteria and interventions. Evaluation of the patient ensures attainment of the desired outcomes.[15]

SLEEP PATTERN DISTURBANCE

Description

Sleep disturbance in critically ill patients is defined as insufficient duration or stages of sleep that results in discomfort and interferes with quality of life. When ill, most people need more sleep than usual, and sleep seems to promote recovery. Studies have demonstrated that the nocturnal sleep of patients in critical care units is severely disturbed, even though many receive medications to promote sleep.[1,16,17]

Sleep disturbance in critically ill patients may stem from psychologic stress associated with critical illness and the critical care environment, surgical stress, noise, interruptions for care, painful procedures or physiologic processes, excessive bright light, and muscular and joint discomfort resulting from bed rest.[18] Of 84 patients' recollections about sleep-disturbing factors in the critical care unit, the most frequently mentioned factors included an inability to get comfortable or lie comfortably (recalled by 70% of patients), inability to perform one's usual routine before going to sleep (57%), anxiety (55%), and pain (54%).[19] The stressful nature of the critical care environment and uncertainty and worry regarding the outcomes of a critical illness may explain why some patients have such difficulty sleeping while hospitalized.

Bright nocturnal light, excessive noise, and frequent interruptions for care procedures also may disturb sleep in critically ill patients. In a study of light and sound levels and interruptions to sleep in medical and respiratory critical care units, light levels maintained a day-night rhythm, with peak levels dependent on window orientation. Peak sound levels were extremely high in all areas and exceeded recommendations of the Environmental Protection Agency as acceptable for a hospital. Patient interruptions for care procedures tended to be variable but ubiquitous, leaving little time for condensed sleep.[1,2,18]

Pathophysiology

Normal sleep is a period of decreased physiologic workload for the cardiovascular system. Insufficient sleep in acutely and critically ill patients has been associated with physiologic and psychologic exhaustion and may delay recovery from illness. These effects include mental status changes resulting in delirium.[20] A general consensus among sleep experts and researchers is that sleep deprivation results in psychologic alterations such as changes in mood and performance, fatigue, increased irritability, and feelings of persecution.[1,18]

The intensification of pain related to sleep disturbance is a significant problem in acutely and critically ill patients. Sunshine and colleagues related a potential theory for pain alleviation from massage therapy that is linked to quiet or restorative sleep. During deep sleep, somatostatin is normally released. Without this substance, pain is experienced. Substance P is released when an individual is deprived of deep sleep, and substance P is noted for causing pain. When people are deprived of deep sleep, they may have less somatostatin and increased substance P, which results in greater pain and more sleep disruption.[21]

Assessment and Diagnosis

Assessment of the patient on admission to the critical care unit includes a description of multiple sleep-related factors: the normal sleep pattern, including awakenings, naps, normal bedtime, and waking time; customary habits that enhance sleep (e.g., number of pillows, extra blankets, bedtime rituals, medications); any recent changes in the patient's normal sleep pattern resulting from the acute illness; recent history of difficulty falling asleep or staying asleep, snoring, gasping for breath at night, stopping breathing at night, or excessive daytime sleepiness; frequency and duration of daytime naps; and the severity, duration, and history of chronic illnesses and disturbances that may disrupt sleep, such as COPD, arthritis, nocturnal angina, reflux esophagitis, or nocturia.

The patient's psychologic response to admission to the critical care unit needs to be assessed, along with the noise level in the patient's immediate environment. The critical care nurse needs to elicit any history of snoring because of its relationship to sleep apnea and sleep disturbances. One effective way to assess the quality of the patient's sleep is for the nurse to ask the patient how his or her sleep in the hospital compares with sleep at home. Because individuals differ in their sleep behaviors and requirements, a flexible, individualized plan of care must be formulated to promote rest and sleep.

Compiling a record of a patient's sleep for 48 to 72 hours may assist in assessing actual quantity of sleep as well as necessary and unnecessary awakenings. The sleep record includes the date and time, whether the patient was awake or asleep, and any procedures that necessitated waking the patient. A 24-hour flow sheet, commonly used in critical care units, could include an area for documentation of sleep. Just as nurses document other data relevant to the patient's recovery, sleep periods of more than 90 minutes in duration, number and length of awakenings, and total possible sleep time should be recorded and evaluated.

Medical Management

Medical management of sleep pattern disturbance in critically ill patients consists of the administration of sedative-hypnotics. The nonbenzodiazepine short-acting hypnotics zolpidem and zaleplon have few side effects and little effect on sleep architecture. Because of their short half-life, they may be repeated once during the night. Although hypnotics may assist the patient in falling asleep, it is a nursing responsibility to provide an environment and care procedures that promote sleep and allow patients to stay asleep.

Nursing Management

If one of the primary causes of the sleep pattern disturbance for a patient hospitalized in the critical care unit is a state of heightened anxiety and discomfort, nursing interventions, such as massage, that promote relaxation and comfort may be effective. In a review of 22 articles investigating the effects of massage on relaxation, comfort, and sleep, massage consistently reduced anxiety and pain.[22] Another research-based intervention is playing audio of ocean sounds or other relaxing auditory sounds. Williamson found that an audiotape of the ocean or the rain significantly increased sleep quality in patients in a progressive care unit.[23] Providing a relaxed, caring environment that encourages confidence in care providers may also assist the patient to relax. Allowing close family members to sit quietly at the bedside while the patient rests may comfort the family and the patient and allow the patient to rest better. Stanchina and colleagues found that white noise machines in patient rooms decreased the variance in peak noises and increased arousal thresholds for patients.[24]

Nurses should limit interruptions for care procedures and should coordinate the care among other disciplines to allow patients time for consolidated nocturnal sleep and a daytime nap. Draperies or blinds should be opened during the day to allow patients to receive bright natural light and to help orient them to time of day, with lights dimmed at night. Noise from staff, squeaky carts, alarms, televisions, slamming doors, and ringing phones should be minimized. Offering the patient earplugs may help decrease noise and promote sleep. Outcomes of these nursing interventions can be assessed and documented on the 24-hour flow sheet. One group reported that an enforced afternoon quiet time resulted in benefits for patients as well as the multidisciplinary team.[25]

SLEEP APNEA SYNDROME

Sleep apnea syndrome, sometimes called *sleep-disordered breathing*, occurs when airflow is absent or reduced. Apnea during sleep can be divided into three types: 1) obstructive, 2) central, and 3) mixed. In obstructive apnea, the absence of airflow is caused by an obstruction in the upper airway. Complete obstruction lasting 10 seconds or longer is referred to as an *obstructive apnea*, whereas a partial obstruction is known as a *hypopnea*. In central apnea, airflow is absent because of lack of ventilatory muscle effort. The third type of sleep apnea syndrome, mixed apnea, occurs when a combination of obstructive and central patterns occurs in a single apneic event.

Obstructive Sleep Apnea

Description and Etiology

OSA syndrome occurs when at least five apnea or hypopnea events per hour of sleep occur as the result of an obstruction in the upper airway. In the general population, between 3% and 7% of people have severe OSA.[26] The incidence of OSA is believed to increase with age. Consequences include chronic hypoventilation syndrome; arousals that fragment sleep; cardiovascular changes such as hypertension, stroke, ischemic heart disease, insulin resistance, ventricular hypertrophy, and nocturnal angina.[27] Because of the cardiovascular complications and accidents caused by sleepiness, OSA is a significant condition that should be effectively evaluated.

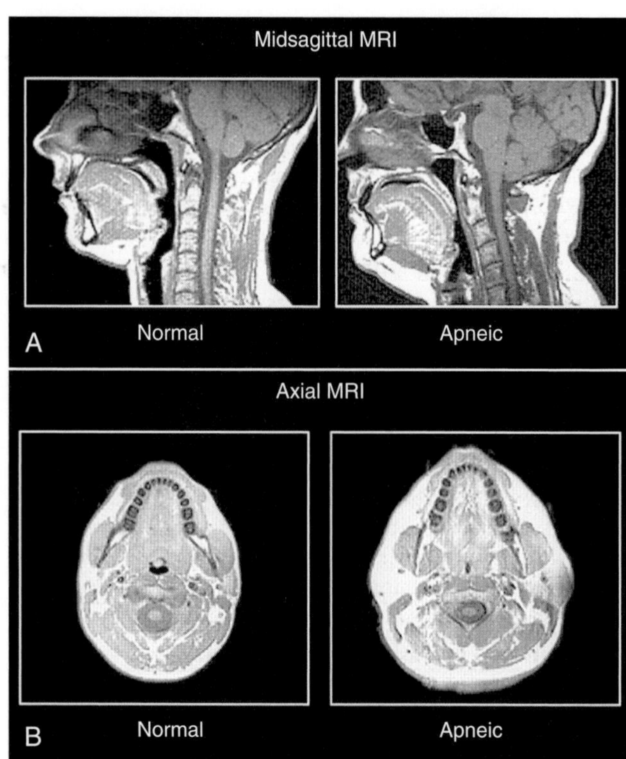

FIG 5-1 Midsagittal magnetic resonance imaging of a normal subject *(left)* and a subject with sleep apnea *(right)*. Notice the narrowing of the trachea and the elongated soft palate. (From Kryger MH, et al, eds. *Principles and Practice of Sleep Medicine*. 5th ed. St. Louis: Saunders; 2011.)

The cause of OSA is not entirely understood; however, upper airway structure, hormonal balance, and neural control are implicated. Factors that contribute to OSA are 1) anatomic narrowing of the upper airway, 2) increased compliance of the upper airway tissue, 3) reflexes affecting upper airway caliber, and 4) pharyngeal inspiratory muscle function.[28] Computed tomographic studies of awake subjects have shown that patients with OSA have narrower airways than normal subjects do. The narrower the airway, the more easily it may become obstructed (Figure 5-1).

Upper airway patency is also affected by upper airway function, which is under the control of the respiratory motor neurons. During sleep, this control varies and causes decreased neural activity, thereby narrowing the airway. This effect is especially prevalent during REM sleep, when the motor neurons are hypotonic. Unstable control of the respiratory nerves of the diaphragmatic, intercostal, and upper airway muscles can cause sleep apneas.[28] Hypothyroidism can alter respiratory controls and thereby contribute to OSA. Other contributing disorders are exogenous obesity, kyphoscoliosis, and autonomic dysfunction.[29]

Pathophysiology

The patient with OSA develops cycles of hypoxemia, hypercapnia, and acidosis with each episode of apnea until he or she is aroused and airflow resumes. Alveolar hypoventilation accompanies each episode of apnea and results in hypercapnia. Between episodes, alveolar ventilation improves so that overall there is no retention of carbon dioxide (CO_2).

With obstruction, inspiratory subatmospheric intrathoracic pressures are abnormally elevated. This leads to a tendency for airways to collapse, resulting in hemodynamic and electrocardiographic changes. The extremely elevated pressures that occur in individuals with OSA who have apneic episodes in REM and NREM stages cause systemic and pulmonary hypertension. Systemic pressures of 200/120 mm Hg (awake control: 130/80 mm Hg) and pulmonary artery pressures of 80/54 mm Hg (awake control: 30/20 mm Hg) have been reported.[30] Cardiac dysrhythmias associated with obstructive apnea include bradycardias, sinus arrest, and occasionally, second-degree heart blocks. After resumption of airflow, tachycardias commonly occur. Bradycardia-tachycardia syndrome is associated with OSA.[31]

Assessment and Diagnosis

Careful monitoring of oxygen saturation and breathing patterns can help the critical care nurse identify patients with this syndrome and assist in its diagnosis and treatment. Patients at risk for OSA may have the following symptoms: snoring; obesity; short, thick neck circumference; cardiovascular disease; systemic hypertension; pulmonary hypertension; sleep fragmentation; gastroesophageal reflux; and an impaired quality of life. Apneas may occur in people whose throats are abnormally small or collapsible. Muscles that would normally hold the throat open relax while the patient is asleep. Snoring is caused when those soft tissues in the throat vibrate. Snoring often precedes the complaint of daytime sleepiness, and the intensity increases with weight gain and alcohol ingestion.[29]

OSA episodes frequently end in brief EEG arousals. Patients may experience hundreds of arousals and not even realize they awaken hundreds of times during the night. These arousals cause sleep fragmentation and daytime sleepiness, which can lead to irritability, poor job performance, troubled relationships, depression, and impaired quality of life. The definitive diagnosis of OSA syndrome is made with PSG during an overnight sleep study. PSG is used to determine the number and length of apnea episodes and sleep stages, number of arousals, airflow, respiratory effort, and oxygen desaturation.

Medical Management

For patients with mild OSA, weight loss, sleeping on the side if apneas are associated with sleeping on the back, avoidance of sedative medications and alcohol before bedtime, and avoidance of sleep deprivation may be all that is necessary. Oral appliances may be prescribed to stabilize the jaw or retain the tongue. These devices must be fitted by a dentist and are not always as effective as continuous positive airway pressure (CPAP). Moderate to severe levels of apnea may be treated with mechanical, surgical, or pharmacologic therapy. Treatment can vary depending on the type and severity of illness.

CPAP via nasal mask is the treatment of choice. CPAP machines are simply pressure generators with the effective pressure being determined during the titration part of the PSG. This holds the airway open and prevents collapse. The patient wears a small, triangle-shaped mask over the nose or uses nasal pillows if the mask is not tolerated. CPAP treats the obstruction and the snoring, choking, and gasping that accompany it, and it provides cardiovascular benefits. Although CPAP is the treatment of choice, it is only effective if the patient is compliant with therapy. If a patient cannot tolerate the continuous pressure of CPAP, bimodal positive airway pressure (BiPAP), which provides separate pressures for inspiration and expiration, may be tried.[32]

Various surgical interventions are available for the treatment of apnea and snoring. Patients with mild OSA or snoring alone may undergo an outpatient procedure called *laser uvulopalatopharyngoplasty (LAUP)*, which uses lasers to remove excess tissue at the soft palate level. For patients who snore but do not have apnea, somnoplasty may provide relief. Somnoplasty involves inserting a small electrode into the soft palate and heating the tissue, causing the area to shrink and tighten.[33] Uvulopalatopharyngoplasty (UPPP) was one of the earlier surgeries used to treat OSA. Essentially, a large tonsillectomy is performed, and all redundant tissue is removed. Reports of success from UPPP vary widely, with 40% to 80% of patients experiencing sleep apnea improvement.[34] Complications include speech impairment, inability to eat, postoperative bleeding, and infection. Severe pain after UPPP is documented and may continue well into the postoperative period.[34] UPPP patients are not usually admitted to critical care areas, because the postoperative recovery does not require critical care.

Although tracheostomy was the original surgery procedure used to treat OSA, it is now used only in the most severe cases of apnea that do not respond to other treatments. Bariatric surgery is an effective means to facilitate weight loss and subsequent improvement in OSA.[35]

Treatment of OSA with medication is usually a last resort and has proved to be very disappointing. Protriptyline has been shown to decrease apnea and reduce excessive daytime sleepiness by decreasing sleep apnea frequency that increases during REM sleep. Oxygen may be used to lower hypoxemia and nocturnal desaturations.

Central Sleep Apnea

Description and Etiology

Central sleep apnea (CSA) can be seen on PSG as an absence of airflow and respiratory effort for at least 10 seconds. A complete loss of electromyographic activity by the respiratory muscles would be expected, because CSA is defined as a pause in respiration without ventilatory effort.[36] CSA may result from many physiologic or pathophysiologic events.[37] Possible causes of nonhypercapnic CSA include periodic breathing at high altitude, renal or metabolic disturbances, and idiopathic central apnea seen at sea level. Hypercapnic CSA can occur in many neuromuscular conditions such as spinal cord or brain injury, encephalitis, brainstem neoplasm or infarcts, muscular dystrophy, myasthenia gravis, bulbar poliomyelitis, and postpolio syndrome.[38]

Pathophysiology

A chemoreceptor sensitive to the levels of CO_2 resides within the brain. When CO_2 levels become excessive, ventilatory efforts are increased to blow off the excess CO_2. This negative-feedback loop exists to provide a homeostatic balance in the carbon dioxide and oxygen levels of the body. Whereas OSA results from an obstructed or collapsed airway, patients with CSA suffer from a lack of ventilatory effort. This can be observed in patients with cardiopulmonary disease (e.g., COPD) or heart failure, because their chemoreceptors have become adjusted to an increased CO_2 level.[38] However, the uniting factor is cessation of breathing momentarily during sleep due to the transient withdrawal of central nervous system drive to the muscles of respiration.[37] It is not uncommon for a patient who experiences CSA also to have some obstructive events.

Assessment and Diagnosis

Clinical characteristics of hypercapnic CSA include respiratory failure, cor pulmonale, peripheral edema, polycythemia, daytime sleepiness, and snoring. Patients with nonhypercapnic CSA have clinical features very similar to those of OSA. Nonhypercapnic CSA characteristics include daytime sleepiness, insomnia or poor sleep, mild or intermittent snoring, and awakenings accompanied by choking or feeling short of breath; frequently, the patients are of normal body weight. Diagnosis is made by overnight PSG or sleep study, which will determine the respiratory and sleep patterns of the patient.[37]

Medical Management

Because there are two types of CSA, there are two therapeutic approaches depending on the cause of the apnea. The hypercapnic patient who has worsening hypoventilation during sleep is best served by nocturnal ventilation. Most such patients experience some respiratory muscle failure. One treatment for the nonhypercapnic or heart failure patients is nasal CPAP, which also may provide a beneficial cardiovascular effect. Nocturnal oxygen supplementation may be effective as well. If CPAP is not tolerated, pharmacologic management may be tried. Medroxyprogesterone, a respiratory stimulant, may improve ventilation in selected patients. Acetazolamide, a carbonic anhydrase inhibitor that can result in metabolic acidosis, also may decrease the frequency of apneic episodes. Several studies have reported the development of obstructive apnea in patients successfully treated for central apnea.[39]

Nursing Management

Nursing management of the patient with sleep apnea incorporates a variety of diagnoses (Box 5-1). **Nursing priorities are directed toward 1) optimizing oxygenation and ventilation, 2) providing comfort and emotional support, 3) maintaining surveillance for complications, and 4) educating the patient and family.**

 **BOX 5-1 NURSING DIAGNOSIS PRIORITIES**

Sleep Apnea

- Ineffective Breathing Pattern related to musculoskeletal fatigue or neuromuscular impairment, p. 598
- Decreased Cardiac Output related to alterations in preload, p. 579
- Disturbed Sleep Pattern related to fragmented sleep, p. 587
- Disturbed Body Image related to functional dependence on life-sustaining technology, p. 586
- Deficient Knowledge related to lack of previous exposure to information, p. 584 (see Patient Education, Box 5-2)

Optimizing Oxygenation and Ventilation

Nasal CPAP is most effective when patients are properly fitted with the nasal mask and have clear instructions regarding its use. Several types and sizes of masks are available, including one type called a *nasal pillow*, which does not cover the nose but instead fits into the nostrils. If patients are admitted to the critical care unit with a history of sleep apnea, they need to use their home CPAP mask and equipment as part of their regular sleep routine. The nurse can enhance compliance with the CPAP system. Nursing care includes ensuring proper fit of the CPAP mask, with no air blowing into the patient's eyes, correct airway pressure, no pressure sores from the mask, and no gastric insufflation.

Maintaining Surveillance for Complications

The nurse needs to monitor and assess the respiratory status of the patient carefully. Monitoring of patients should include assessment of the breathing patterns, hours of sleep, and pulse oximetry. Cautious administration of narcotics to patients with sleep apnea is suggested because of the potential for respiratory depression. The nurse needs to address any fear or anxiety about going to sleep.

Educating the Patient and Family

The nurse's role in the management of sleep apnea includes educating the patient and family about the syndrome and the consequences of noncompliance with treatment regimens (Box 5-2). Nurses also need to caution patients to avoid alcohol and sedative medications. This education may also include preoperative teaching for any surgical procedures.

BOX 5-2 PATIENT EDUCATION PRIORITIES

Sleep Apnea

- Pathophysiology of the disease specific to the patient and type of apnea
- Modification of risk factors, such as weight loss, abstaining from alcohol, establishing a program of sleep hygiene, lateral body positioning during sleep
- Importance of compliance with continuous positive airway pressure (CPAP)
- Consequences of untreated apnea, such as vascular hypertension, coronary artery disease, cerebrovascular disease, arrhythmias, pulmonary hypertension, diabetes, daytime sleepiness, death

CASE STUDY Patient with Sleep Alterations

Brief Patient History

Mr. D is a 43-year-old, severely obese, self-employed man. His medical history includes excessive daytime sleepiness, hypertension, and sinus dysrhythmia. He received a diagnosis of obstructive sleep apnea (OSA) 2 years ago, and his health care provider prescribed nasal continuous positive airway pressure (CPAP) for use at night. However, Mr. D has been, for the most part, noncompliant because of reported discomfort and interference with his sex life.

CASE STUDY Patient with Sleep Alterations—cont'd

Mr. D's hypertension has required increasing medication, and he has begun to develop cardiomegaly. His business suffers from his inability to stay awake and focus. He and his wife have started sleeping in separate rooms because of his snoring. These circumstances have prompted Mr. D's physician to recommend surgical correction of Mr. D's airway. He refused to consider a tracheostomy but agreed to uvulopalatopharyngoplasty (UPPP) despite the 50% chance of success. Mr. D and his spouse understand that endotracheal intubation may be necessary for 24 to 48 hours because of the severity of his condition.

Clinical Assessment

Mr. D is admitted to the surgical critical care unit after a very complicated surgical procedure with an oral endotracheal tube connected to supplemental oxygen with spontaneous respiration. He is awake and follows commands; however, he is having periods of restlessness and pulling at tubes.

Diagnostic Procedures

Mr. D's vital signs include blood pressure of 160/72 mm Hg, heart rate of 120 beats/min (sinus tachycardia), respiratory rate of 20 breaths/min, and temperature of 97.8° F. The chest radiograph is clear. Arterial blood gases were obtained: pH of 7.38, PaO_2 of 90 mm Hg, $PaCO_2$ of 35 mm Hg, HCO_3^- level of 24%, and O_2 saturation of 98%. Mr. D indicates that his pain is a 5 on the Baker-Wong faces scale by pointing. The Riker Sedation-Agitation Scale score is 5.

Medical Diagnosis

Mr. D is diagnosed with OSA.

Questions

1. What major outcomes do you expect to achieve for this patient?
2. What problems or risks must be managed to achieve these outcomes?
3. What interventions must be initiated to monitor, prevent, manage, or eliminate the problems and risks identified?
4. What interventions should be initiated to promote optimal functioning, safety, and well-being of the patient?
5. What possible learning needs do you anticipate for this patient?
6. What cultural and age-related factors may have a bearing on the patient's plan of care?

REFERENCES

1. Matthews EE: Sleep disturbances and fatigue in critically ill patients, *AACN Adv Crit Care* 22:204, 2011.
2. Boyko Y, et al: Sleep disturbances in critically ill patients in ICU: how much do we know? *Acta Anaesthesiol Scand* 56:950, 2012.
3. Carskadon MA, Dement WC: Normal human sleep: an overview. In Kryger MH, et al, editors: *Principles and practice of sleep medicine*, ed 5, St Louis, 2011, Saunders.
4. Jafari B, Mohsenin V: Polysomnography, *Clin Chest Med* 31:287, 2010.
5. Collop NA, et al: Normal sleep and circadian processes, *Crit Care Clin* 24:449, 2008.
6. Ganz FD: Sleep and immune function, *Crit Care Nurse* 32(2):e19, 2012.
7. Siegel JM: REM sleep. In Kryger MH, et al, editors: *Principles and practice of sleep medicine*, ed 5, St Louis, 2011, Saunders.
8. Czeisler CA, Buxon OM: The human circadian timing system and sleep-wake regulation. In Kryger MH, et al, editors: *Principles and practice of sleep medicine*, ed 5, St Louis, 2011, Saunders.
9. Hardin KA: Sleep in the ICU: potential mechanisms and clinical implications, *Chest* 136:284, 2009.
10. Brandon SL, Zee PC: Neurobiology of sleep, *Clin Chest Med* 31:309, 2010.
11. Achermann P, Borbely AA: Sleep homeostasis and models of sleep regulation. In Kryger MH, et al, editors: *Principles and practice of sleep medicine*, ed 5, St Louis, 2011, Saunders.
12. Mendelson W: Hypnotic medications: mechanisms of action and pharmacologic effects. In Kryger MH, et al, editors: *Principles and practice of sleep medicine*, ed 5, St Louis, 2011, Saunders.
13. Roux FJ, Kryger MH: Medication effects on sleep, *Clin Chest Med* 31:397, 2010.
14. Schweitzer PK: Drugs that disturb sleep and wakefulness. In Kryger MH, et al, editors: *Principles and practice of sleep medicine*, ed 5, St Louis, 2011, Saunders.
15. Ahmed AQ: Effects of common medications used for sleep disorders, *Crit Care Clin* 24:493, 2008.
16. Nicolas A, et al: Perception of nighttime sleep by surgical patients in an intensive care unit, *Nurs Crit Care* 13:25, 2008.
17. Ugras GA, Oztekin SD: Patient perception of environmental and nursing factors contributing to sleep disturbances in a neurosurgical intensive care unit, *Tohoku J Exp Med* 212:299, 2007.
18. Salas RE, Gamaldo CE: Adverse effects of sleep deprivation in the ICU, *Crit Care Clin* 24:461, 2008.
19. Simpson T, et al: Patients' perceptions of environmental factors that disturb sleep after cardiac surgery, *Am J Crit Care* 5:173, 1996.
20. Stuck A, et al: Preventing intensive care unit delirium, *Dimen Crit Care Nurs* 30:315, 2011.
21. Sunshine W, et al: Massage therapy and transcutaneous electrical stimulation effects on fibromyalgia, *J Clin Rheumatol* 2:18, 1997.
22. Richards KC, et al: Effects of massage in acute and critical care, *AACN Clin Issues* 11:77, 2000.
23. Williamson JW: The effects of ocean sounds on sleep after coronary artery bypass graft surgery, *Am J Crit Care* 1:91, 1992.
24. Stanchina JL, et al: The influence of white noise on sleep in subjects exposed to ICU noise, *Sleep Med* 6:423, 2005.
25. Lower J, et al: High-tech high-touch: mission possible? *Dimens Crit Care Nurs* 21:201, 2002.
26. Punjabi NM: The epidemiology of adult obstructive sleep apnea, *Proc Am Thorac Soc* 5:136, 2008.
27. Krieger S, Caples SM: Obstructive sleep apnea and cardiovascular disease: implications for clinical practice, *Cleve Clin J Med* 74:853, 2007.
28. Yaggi HK, Strohl KP: Adult obstructive sleep apnea/hypopnea syndrome: definitions, risk factors, and pathogenesis, *Clin Chest Med* 31:179, 2010.

29. Ulualp SO: Snoring and obstructive sleep apnea, *Med Clin N Am* 94:1047, 2010.
30. Young T, et al: Systemic and pulmonary hypertension in obstructive sleep apnea. In Kryger MH, et al, editors: *Principles and practice of sleep medicine*, ed 5, St Louis, 2011, Saunders.
31. Somers VK, Javaheri S: Cardiovascular effects of sleep-related breathing disorders. In Kryger MH, et al, editors: *Principles and practice of sleep medicine*, ed 5, St Louis, 2011, Saunders.
32. Freedman N: Treatment of obstructive sleep apnea syndrome, *Clin Chest Med* 31:187, 2010.
33. Friedman M, Wilson MN: Surgical therapy for sleep breathing disorders, *Sleep Med Clin* 5:153, 2010.
34. Carpenter JM, LaMear WR: Uvulopalatopharyngoplasty: results of a patient questionnaire, *Ann Otol Rhinol Laryngol* 117:24, 2008.
35. Buchwald H, et al: Bariatric surgery: a systematic review and meta-analysis, *JAMA* 292:1724, 2004.
36. Wellman A, White DP: Central sleep apnea and periodic breathing. In Kryger MH, et al, editors: *Principles and practice of sleep medicine*, ed 5, St Louis, 2011, Saunders.
37. Ekhert DJ, et al: Central sleep apnea: pathophysiology and treatment, *Chest* 131:595, 2007.
38. Javaheri S: Central sleep apnea, *Clin Chest Med* 31:235, 2010.
39. Buysse DJ, et al: Clinical pharmacology of other drugs used as hypnotics. In Kryger MH, et al, editors: *Principles and practice of sleep medicine*, ed 5, St Louis, 2011, Saunders.

CHAPTER 6

Nutritional Alterations

Kasuen Mauldin

Be sure to check out the bonus material, including review questions, on the Evolve website at http://evolve.elsevier.com/Urden/priorities/.

Nutrition support is an essential component of providing comprehensive care to the critically ill patient. Nutrition screening must be conducted on every patient, and a more thorough nutrition assessment completed on any patient screened to be nutritionally at risk. Malnutrition can be related to any essential nutrient or nutrients. Malnutrition is associated with a variety of adverse outcomes, such as wound dehiscence, infections, pressure ulcers, respiratory failure requiring ventilation, longer hospital days, and death. The purpose of this chapter is to provide an overview of nutrient metabolism, nutritional status assessment, and implications of malnutrition for the sick or stressed patient. Specifically, nutrition for each of the system alterations will be discussed along with nursing management.

NUTRIENT METABOLISM

Nutrients are chemical substances found in foods that are needed for human life, growth, maintenance, and repair of body tissues. The main nutrients in foods are carbohydrates, proteins, fats, vitamins, minerals, and water. The process by which nutrients are used at the cellular level is known as *metabolism.* The energy-yielding nutrients or macronutrients are carbohydrates, proteins, and fats. For proper metabolic functioning, adequate amounts of micronutrients, such as vitamins, minerals (including electrolytes), and trace elements also must be supplied to the human body.

ASSESSING NUTRITIONAL STATUS

In the United States, The Joint Commission mandates nutrition screening be conducted on every patient within 24 hours of admission to an acute care center.[1] A brief questionnaire to be completed by the patient or significant other, the nursing admission form, or the physician's admission note usually provides enough information to determine whether the patient is at nutritional risk (Box 6-1). Any patient judged to be nutritionally at risk needs a more thorough nutrition assessment.

Nutrition assessment involves collection of four types of information: 1) anthropometric measurements, 2) biochemical (laboratory) data, 3) clinical signs (physical examination), and 4) diet and pertinent health history. This information provides a basis for 1) identifying patients who are malnourished or at risk of malnutrition, 2) determining the nutritional needs of individual patients, and 3) selecting the most appropriate methods of nutrition support for patients with or at risk of developing nutritional deficits. Nutrition support is the provision of specially formulated or delivered oral, enteral, or parenteral nutrients to maintain or restore optimal nutrition status.[3] The nutrition assessment can be performed by or under the supervision of a registered dietitian or by a nutrition care specialist (e.g., nurse with specialized expertise in nutrition). Figure 6-1 shows the route of administration of specialized nutrition support.

Anthropometric Measurements

Height and current weight are essential anthropometric measurements, and they should be measured rather than obtained through a patient or family report. The most important reason for obtaining anthropometric measurements is to be able to detect changes in the measurements over time (e.g., track response to nutritional therapy). The patient's measurements may be compared with standard tables of weight-for-height or standard growth charts for infants and children. Another simple tool for gauging appropriateness of weight-for-height for adults and older adolescents is the body mass index (BMI):

$$\text{BMI} = \text{weight} \div \text{height}^2$$

Weight is measured in kilograms and height in meters. BMI values are independent of age and gender and are used for assessing health risk. It may be impossible to measure the height of some patients accurately. Total height can be estimated from arm span length or recumbent length.[3,4] In addition to height and weight data, other measurements such as arm muscle circumference, skin fold thickness, and body composition (proportion of fat and lean tissue, determined by bioelectric impedance or other methods) are sometimes performed, but these measurements are of limited use in assessing critically ill patients.[5]

Biochemical Data

A wide range of laboratory tests can provide information about nutritional status. Those most often used in the clinical setting are described in Table 6-1. No diagnostic tests for evaluation of nutrition are perfect, and care must be taken in interpreting the results of the tests.[6]

Clinical or Physical Manifestations

A thorough physical examination is an essential part of nutrition assessment. Box 6-2 lists some of the more common findings that may indicate an altered nutritional state. It is especially important for the nurse to check for signs of muscle wasting, loss of subcutaneous fat, skin or hair changes, and impairment of wound healing.

> **BOX 6-1 Patients Who are at Risk for Malnutrition**
>
> **Adults Who Exhibit Any of the Following**
> - Involuntary weight loss or gain of significant amount of weight (>10% of usual body weight in 6 months, >5% in 1 month), even if the weight achieved by loss or gain is appropriate for height.
> - Chronic disease
> - Chronic use of modified diet
> - Increased metabolic requirements
> - Illness or injury that may interfere with nutritional intake
> - Inadequate nutrient intake for > 7 days
> - Regular use of three or more medications
> - Poverty and/or lack of access to healthy food

Diet and Health History

Information about dietary intake and significant variations in weight is a vital part of the history. Dietary intake can be evaluated in several ways, including a diet record, a 24-hour recall, and a diet history. The diet record, a listing of the type and amount of all foods and beverages consumed for some period (usually 3 days), is useful for evaluating the patient's intake in the critical care setting if the adequacy of intake is questionable. However, such a record reveals little about the patient's habitual intake before the illness or injury. The 24-hour recall of all food and beverage intake is easily and quickly performed, but it also may not reflect the patient's usual intake and has limited usefulness. The diet history consists of a detailed interview about the patient's usual intake, along with social, familial, cultural, economic, educational, and health-related factors that may affect intake. Although the diet history is time-consuming to perform and may be too stressful for the acutely ill patient, it does provide a wealth of information about food habits over a prolonged period and a basis for planning individualized nutrition education if

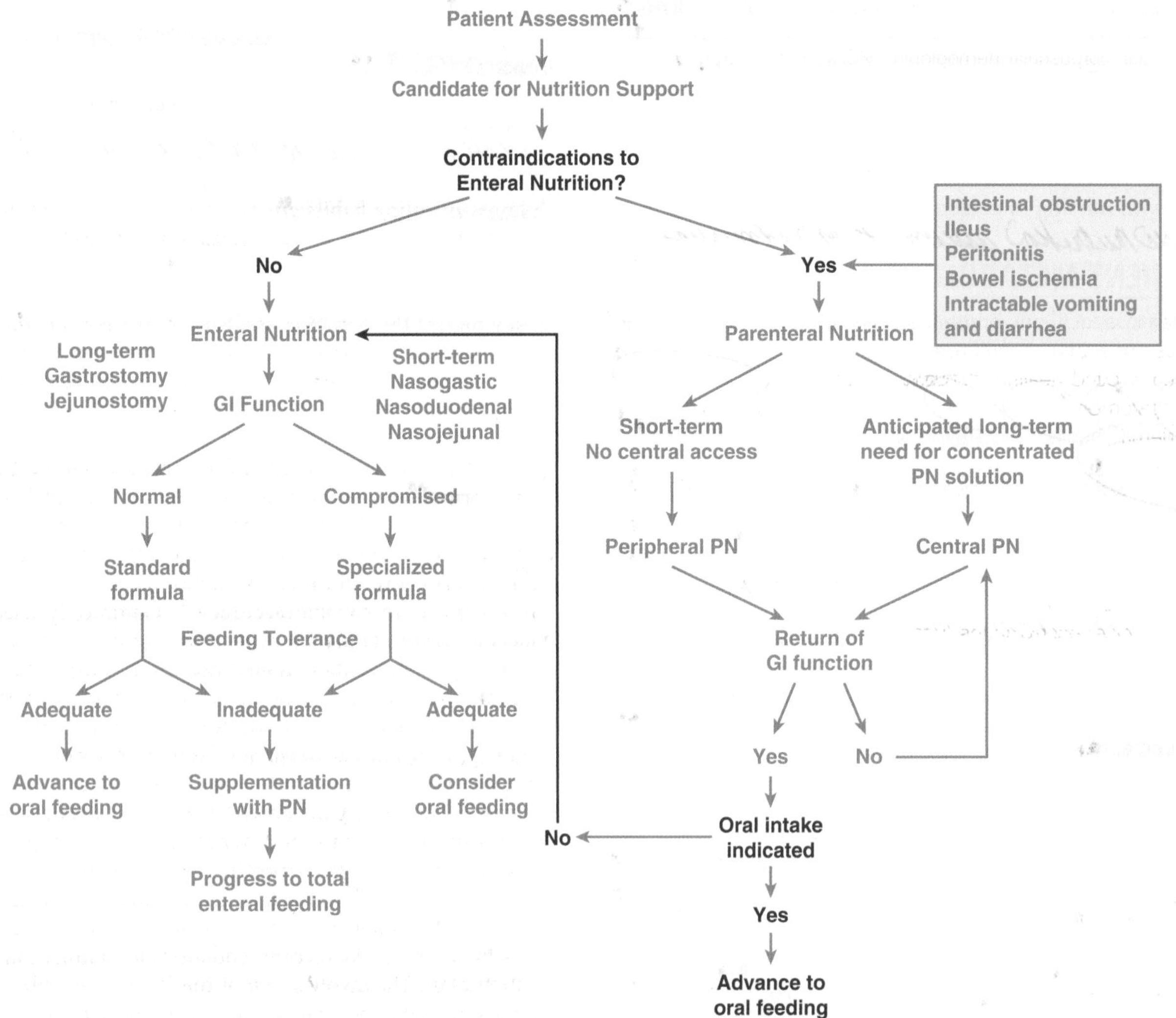

FIG 6-1 Route of Administration of Specialized Nutrition Support. (Redrawn from Ukleja A, et al. Standards for nutrition support. *Nutr Clin Pract* 25(4):403, 2010.)

TABLE 6-1 Common Blood and Urine Tests Used in Nutrition Assessment

TEST	COMMENTS AND LIMITATIONS
Serum Proteins	
Albumin or prealbumin	Levels decrease with protein deficiency and in liver failure. Albumin levels are slow to change in response to malnutrition and repletion. Prealbumin levels fall in response to trauma and infection.
Hematologic Values	
Normocytic Anemia (normal MCV, MCHC)	Common with protein deficiency
Microcytic Anemia (decreased MCV, MCH, MCHC)	Indicative of iron deficiency (can be from blood loss)
Macrocytic Anemia (increased MCV)	Common in folate and vitamin B_{12} deficiency
Lymphocytopenia	Common in protein deficiency

MCH, Mean corpuscular hemoglobin; *MCHC*, mean corpuscular hemoglobin concentration; *MCV*, mean corpuscular volume.

BOX 6-2 Clinical Manifestations of Nutritional Alterations

Manifestations That May Indicate Protein-Calorie Malnutrition
- Hair loss; dull, dry, brittle hair; loss of hair pigment
- Loss of subcutaneous tissue; muscle wasting
- Poor wound healing; decubitus ulcer
- Hepatomegaly
- Edema

Manifestations Often Present in Vitamin Deficiencies
- Conjunctival and corneal dryness (vitamin A)
- Dry, scaly skin; follicular hyperkeratosis, in which the skin appears to have gooseflesh continually (vitamin A)
- Gingivitis; poor wound healing (vitamin C)
- Petechiae; ecchymoses (vitamin C or K)
- Inflamed tongue, cracking at the corners of the mouth (riboflavin [vitamin B_2], niacin, folic acid, vitamin B_{12}, or other B vitamins)
- Edema; heart failure (thiamine [vitamin B_1])
- Confusion; confabulation (thiamine [vitamin B_1])

Manifestations Often Present in Mineral Deficiencies
- Blue sclerae; pale mucous membranes; spoon-shaped nails (iron)
- Hypogeusia, or poor sense of taste; dysgeusia, or bad taste; eczema; poor wound healing (zinc)

Manifestations Often Observed with Excessive Vitamin Intake
- Hair loss; dry skin; hepatomegaly (vitamin A)

BOX 6-3 Nutrition History Information

Inadequate Intake of Nutrients
- Alcohol abuse
- Anorexia, severe or prolonged nausea or vomiting
- Confusion, coma
- Poor dentition
- Poverty

Inadequate Digestion or Absorption of Nutrients
- Previous gastrointestinal operations, especially gastrectomy, jejunoileal bypass, and ileal resection
- Certain medications, especially antacids and histamine H_2-receptor antagonists (reduce upper small bowel acidity), cholestyramine (binds fat-soluble nutrients), and anticonvulsants

Increased Nutrient Losses
- Blood loss
- Severe diarrhea
- Fistulas, draining abscesses, wounds, decubitus ulcers
- Peritoneal dialysis or hemodialysis
- Corticosteroid therapy (increased tissue catabolism)

Increased Nutrient Requirements
- Fever
- Surgery, trauma, burns, infection
- Cancer (some types)
- Physiologic demands (pregnancy, lactation, growth)

changes in eating habits are desirable. Other information to include in a nutrition history is listed in Box 6-3.

Evaluating Nutrition Assessment Findings

A key part of the nutrition assessment process is using gathered patient information to estimate nutrient, specifically calorie or energy, needs. In the in-patient setting, estimated energy needs can be measured or calculated as described below.

Calorie and protein needs of patients are often estimated using formulas that provide allowances for increased nutrient use associated with injury and healing. Although indirect calorimetry is considered the most accurate method to determine energy expenditure, estimates using formulas have demonstrated reasonable accuracy.[7-9] Commonly used formulas for critically ill patients can be found in Appendix B.

The goal of nutrition assessment is to obtain the most accurate estimate of nutritional requirements. Underfeeding and overfeeding must be avoided during critical illness. Overfeeding results in excessive production of carbon dioxide, which can be a burden in the person with pulmonary compromise. Overfeeding increases fat stores, which can contribute to insulin resistance and hyperglycemia. Hyperglycemia increases the risk of postoperative infections in diabetic and nondiabetic individuals.[10] In critical care, it is usually the Registered Dietitian (RD) who will conduct the full nutrition assessment and make recommendations for a nutrition intervention plan. The involvement of the RD is often after nutritional screening and referral from a member of the medical team, frequently the critical care nurse. A systematic, multidisciplinary team approach to nutrition assessment can help avoid delays and failures to diagnose and manage nutrition-related problems.

MALNUTRITION IN THE CRITICAL CARE SETTING: IMPLICATIONS FOR THE SICK OR STRESSED PATIENT

As many as 40% of hospitalized patients are at risk for malnutrition.[11-14] Although illness or injury is the major factor contributing to development of malnutrition, other possible contributing factors are lack of communication among the nurses, physicians, and dietitians responsible for the care of these patients; frequent diagnostic testing and procedures, which lead to interruption in feeding; medications and other therapies that cause anorexia, nausea, or vomiting and thereby interfere with food intake; insufficient monitoring of nutrient intake, and inadequate use of supplements, tube feedings, or parenteral nutrition to maintain the nutritional status of these patients.

Nutritional status tends to deteriorate during hospitalization unless appropriate nutrition support is started early and continually reassessed. Malnutrition in hospitalized patients is associated with a wide variety of adverse outcomes. Wound dehiscence, pressure ulcers, sepsis, infections, respiratory failure requiring ventilation, longer hospital stays, and death are more common among malnourished patients.[15-17] Decline in nutritional status during hospitalization is associated with higher incidences of complications, increased mortality rates, increased length of stay, and higher hospital costs.

It is rare for a patient to exhibit a lack of only one nutrient. Nutritional deficiencies usually are combined, with the patient lacking adequate amounts of protein, calories, and possibly vitamins and minerals.

Energy Deficiency

Protein-Calorie Malnutrition

Malnutrition results from the lack of intake of necessary nutrients or improper absorption and distribution of them, as well as from excessive intake of some nutrients. Malnutrition can be related to any essential nutrient or nutrients, but a serious type of malnutrition found frequently among hospitalized patients is protein-calorie malnutrition (PCM). Poor intake or impaired absorption of protein and energy from carbohydrate and fat worsens the debilitation that may occur in response to critical illness. In PCM, the body proteins are broken down for gluconeogenesis, reducing the supply of amino acids needed for maintenance of body proteins and healing. Malnutrition can be caused by simple starvation—the inadequate intake of nutrients (e.g., in the patient with anorexia related to cancer). It also can result from an injury that increases the metabolic rate beyond the supply of nutrients (hypermetabolism). In the seriously ill patient, if malnutrition occurs, usually it is the result of the combined effects of starvation and hypermetabolism. Two types of PCM are kwashiorkor and marasmus.

Metabolic Response to Starvation and Stress

To understand the development of malnutrition in the hospitalized patient, the nurse must understand the metabolic response to starvation and physiologic stress. Changes in endocrine status and metabolism together determine the onset and extent of malnutrition. Nutritional imbalance occurs when the demand for nutrients is greater than the exogenous nutrient supply. The major difference between a person who is starved and one who is starved and injured is that the latter has an increased reliance on tissue protein breakdown to provide precursors for glucose production to meet increased energy demands. Although carbohydrate and fat metabolism are also affected, the main concern is about protein metabolism and homeostasis.

Critically ill patients are at risk for a combination of starvation and the physiologic stress resulting from injury, trauma, major surgery, or sepsis. Starvation occurs because the person must have nothing by mouth (NPO) for surgical procedures, is unable to eat because of disease-related factors, or is hemodynamically too unstable to be fed. The physiologic stress causes an increased metabolic rate (hypermetabolism) that results in increased oxygen consumption and energy expenditure.

NUTRITION SUPPORT

Nursing Management of Nutrition Support

Nutrition support is an important aspect of the care of critically ill patients. Maintenance of optimal nutritional status may prevent or reduce the complications associated with critical illness and promote positive clinical outcomes.[2] Critical care nurses play a key role in the delivery of nutrition support and must work closely with dietitians and physicians in promoting the best possible outcomes for their patients.

Oral Supplementation

Oral supplementation may be necessary for patients who can eat and have normal digestion and absorption but cannot consume enough regular foods to meet caloric and protein needs. Patients with mild-to-moderate anorexia, burns, or trauma sometimes fall into this category.

Enteral Nutrition

Enteral nutrition or tube feedings are used for patients who have at least some digestive and absorptive capability but are unable or unwilling to consume enough by mouth. When possible, the enteral route is the preferred method of feeding over total parenteral nutrition (TPN). The proposed advantages of enteral nutrition over TPN include lower cost, better maintenance of gut integrity, and decreased infection and hospital length of stay.[2] A review of the literature comparing enteral nutrition and TPN indicates that enteral nutrition is less expensive than TPN and is associated with a lower risk of infection.[2,18]

The gastrointestinal (GI) tract plays an important role in maintaining immunologic defenses, which is why nutrition by the enteral route is thought to be more physiologically beneficial than TPN. Some of the barriers to infection in the GI tract include neutrophils; the normal acidic gastric pH; motility, which limits GI tract colonization by pathogenic bacteria; the normal gut microflora, which inhibit growth of or destroy some pathogenic organisms; rapid desquamation and regeneration of intestinal epithelial cells; the layer of mucus secreted by GI tract cells, and bile, which detoxifies endotoxin in the intestine and delivers immunoglobulin A (IgA) to the intestine.

Patients who are experiencing severe stress that greatly increases their nutritional needs (caused by major surgery, burns, or trauma) often benefit from tube feedings. Table 6-2 lists different enteral formula types and the nutritional indications for using each one. Individuals who require elemental formulas because of impaired digestion or absorption or the specialized formulas for altered metabolic conditions usually require tube feeding because the unpleasant flavors of the free amino acids, peptides, or protein hydrolysates used in these formulas are very difficult to mask if taken in orally.

There are a variety of commercial enteral feeding products, some of which are designed to meet the specialized needs of the critically ill. Products designed for the stressed patient with trauma or sepsis are usually rich in glutamine, arginine, branched amino acids (a major fuel source, especially for muscle), and antioxidant nutrients, such as selenium and vitamins C, E, and A.[19] The antioxidants help to reduce oxidative injury to the tissues (e.g., from reperfusion injury).

Early enteral nutrition, administered within the first 24 to 48 hours of critical illness, has been advocated as a way to reduce septic complications and improve feeding tolerance in critically ill patients. Although studies[20] have shown a lower risk of infection and decreased length of stay with early enteral nutrition, the benefit of early enteral nutrition compared with enteral nutrition delayed a few days remains controversial.[2,21] Current guidelines support the initiation of nutrition support in critically ill patients who will be unable to meet their nutrient needs orally for a period of 5 to 10 days.[2] To avoid complications associated with intestinal ischemia and infarction, enteral nutrition must be initiated only after fluid resuscitation and adequate perfusion have been achieved.[22,23]

Critically ill patients may not tolerate early enteral feeding because of impaired gastric motility, ileus, or medications administered in the early phase of illness. This is particularly true for patients receiving gastric enteral feeding.[24] The assessment of enteral feeding tolerance is an important aspect of nursing care. Monitoring of gastric residual volume is a method used to assess enteral feeding tolerance. However, evidence suggests that gastric residuals are insensitive and unreliable markers of tolerance to tube feeding.[25] There is little evidence to support a correlation between gastric residual volumes and tolerance to feedings, gastric emptying, and potential aspiration. Except in selected high-risk patients, there is little evidence to support holding tube feedings in patients with gastric residual volumes less than 400 mL.[25] The gastric residual volume should be evaluated within the context of other gastrointestinal symptoms. Prokinetic agents, including metoclopramide and erythromycin, have been used to improve gastric motility and promote early enteral nutrition in critically ill patients.[26-28]

Enteral feeding access. Achievement of enteral access is the cornerstone of enteral nutrition therapy. Several techniques can be used to facilitate enteral access. These include surgical methods, bedside methods, fluoroscopy, endoscopy, air insufflation, and prokinetic agents.[5] Placement of feeding tubes beyond the stomach (postpyloric) eliminates some of the problems associated with gastric feeding intolerance. However, placement of postpyloric feeding tubes is time-consuming and may be costly. Tubes with weights on the proximal end are available; they were originally designed for postpyloric feeding in the belief that they would be more likely than unweighted tubes to pass spontaneously through the pyloric sphincter. However, randomized trials with the two types of tubes have shown that unweighted tubes are more likely to migrate through the pylorus than weighted tubes.[29] The weights sometimes cause discomfort while being inserted through the nares. Unweighted tubes therefore may be preferable.

After the tube is placed, correct location must be confirmed before feedings are started and regularly throughout the course of enteral feedings. Radiographs are the most accurate way of assessing tube placement, but repeated radiographs are costly and can expose the patient to excessive radiation. After correct placement has been confirmed, marking the exit site of the tube to check for movement is helpful. Alternative methods for confirming tube placement have been researched and attempt to verify placement in the stomach or small intestine. An inexpensive and relatively accurate alternative method involves assessing the pH of fluid removed from the feeding tube; some tubes are equipped with pH monitoring systems. Assessing the pH and the bilirubin concentration in fluid aspirated from the feeding tube is a newer method for confirming tube placement.[30]

Location and type of feeding tube. Decisions regarding enteral access should be determined based on gastrointestinal anatomy, gastric emptying, and aspiration risk.[2] Nasal intubation is the simplest and most commonly used route for enteral access. This method allows access to the stomach, duodenum, or jejunum. Tube enterostomy—a gastrostomy or jejunostomy—is used primarily for long-term feedings (6 to 12 weeks or more) and when obstruction makes the nasoenteral route inaccessible. Tube enterostomies may also be used for the patient who is at risk for tube dislodgment because of severe agitation or confusion. A conventional gastrostomy or jejunostomy is often performed at the time of other abdominal surgery. The percutaneous endoscopic gastrostomy (PEG) tube has become extremely popular because it can be inserted at the bedside without the use of general anesthetics. Percutaneous endoscopic jejunostomy (PEJ) tubes are also used.

Postpyloric feedings through nasoduodenal, nasojejunal, or jejunostomy tubes are commonly used when there is a high risk of pulmonary aspiration because the pyloric sphincter theoretically provides a barrier that lessens the risk of regurgitation and aspiration.[31] However, some studies have demonstrated that gastric feeding is safe and not associated with an increased risk of aspiration.[32-34] Postpyloric feedings have an advantage over intragastric feedings for patients with delayed gastric emptying, such as those with head injury, gastroparesis associated with uremia or diabetes, or postoperative ileus. Delivery of enteral nutrition into the small bowel is associated with improved tolerance,[35] higher calorie and protein intake,[36] and fewer gastrointestinal complications.[24] Small bowel motility returns more quickly than gastric motility after surgery, and it is often possible to deliver transpyloric feedings within a few hours of injury or surgery.[31] Figure 6-2 shows the locations of tube feeding sites.

Assessment and prevention of feeding tube complications. Nursing care of patients receiving enteral nutrition involves prevention and management of complications associated with the use of feeding tubes. Nursing management of these problems is summarized in Table 6-3. The skin around the feeding tube should be cleaned at least daily and the tape around the tube replaced whenever loosened or soiled. Secure

TABLE 6-2 Enteral Formulas

FORMULA TYPE	NUTRITIONAL USES	CLINICAL EXAMPLES	EXAMPLES OF COMMERCIAL PRODUCTS (MANUFACTURER)
Formulas Used When GI Tract Is Fully Functional			
Polymeric (standard): Contains whole proteins (10%-15% of calories), long-chain triglycerides (25%-40% of calories), and glucose polymers or oligosaccharides (50%-60% of calories); most provide 1 calorie/mL	Inability to ingest food Inability to consume enough to meet needs	Oral or esophageal cancer Coma, stroke Anorexia resulting from chronic illness Burns or trauma	Ensure (Ross) NuBasics (Nestlé) IsoSource (Novartis) PediaSure (Ross), for children 1-10 years old Boost (Mead Johnson)
High-nitrogen: Same as polymeric except protein provides >15% of calories	Same as polymeric plus mild catabolism and protein deficits	Trauma or burns Sepsis	IsoSource HN (Novartis) Osmolite HN (Ross) Ultracal (Mead Johnson)
Concentrated: Same as polymeric except concentrated to 2 calorie/mL	Same as polymeric but fluid restriction needed	Heart failure Neurosurgery COPD Liver disease	Deliver 2.0 (Mead Johnson) TwoCal HN (Ross) Nutren 2.0 (Nestlé)
Formulas Used When GI Function Is Impaired			
Elemental or predigested: Contains hydrolyzed (partially digested) protein, peptides (short chains of amino acids), and/or amino acids, little fat (<10% of calories) or high MCT, and glucose polymers or oligosaccharides; most provide 1 calorie/mL	Impaired digestion and/or absorption	Short bowel syndrome Radiation enteritis Inflammatory bowel disease	Criticare HN (Mead Johnson) Vital High Nitrogen (Ross) Reabilan HN (Nestlé)
Diets for Specific Disease States*			
Renal failure: Concentrated in calories; low sodium, potassium, magnesium, phosphorus, and vitamins A and D; low protein for renal insufficiency; higher protein formulas for dialyzed patients	Renal insufficiency Dialysis	Predialysis Hemodialysis or peritoneal dialysis	Suplena (Ross) Renalcal (Nestlé) Nepro (Ross) Magnacal Renal (Mead Johnson)
Hepatic failure: Enriched in BCAA; low sodium	Protein intolerance	Hepatic encephalopathy	NutriHep (Nestlé) Hepatic-Aid II (B Braun/McGaw)
Pulmonary dysfunction: Low carbohydrate, high fat, concentrated in calories	Respiratory insufficiency	Ventilator dependence	NutriVent (Nestlé) Pulmocare (Ross)
Glucose intolerance: High fat, low carbohydrate (most contain fiber and fructose)	Glucose intolerance	Individuals with diabetes mellitus whose blood sugar is poorly controlled with standard formulas	Glucerna (Ross) Choice DM (Mead Johnson) Diabetisource (Novartis) Glytrol (Nestlé)
Critical care, wound healing: High protein; most contain MCT to improve fat absorption; some have increased zinc and vitamin C for wound healing; some are high in antioxidants (vitamin E, beta-carotene); some are enriched with arginine, glutamine, and/or omega-3 fatty acids	Critical illness	Severe trauma or burns Sepsis	Immun-Aid (B Braun/McGaw) Impact (Novartis) Perative (Ross) Crucial (Nestlé) TraumaCal (Mead Johnson)

BCAA, Branched chain–enriched amino acid; *COPD*, chronic obstructive pulmonary disease; *GI*, gastrointestinal; *MCT*, medium-chain triglyceride.
*These diets may be beneficial for selected patients; costs and benefits must be considered.

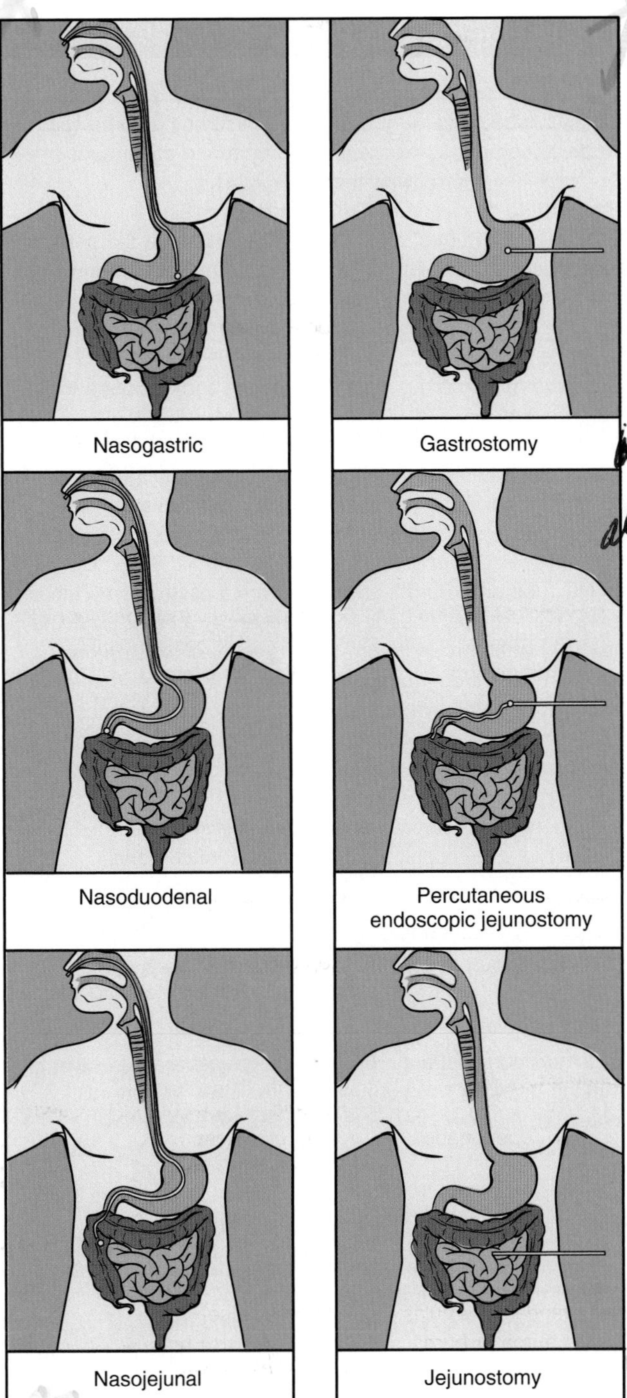

FIG 6-2 Tube Feeding Sites.

taping helps to prevent movement of the tube, which may irritate the nares or oral mucosa or result in accidental dislodgment. The tube must be taped in the dependent position to prevent unnecessary pressure and prevent necrosis. Commercially available attachment devices may be used to avoid inadvertent dislodgment.

Feeding tube occlusion. Regular irrigation helps to prevent feeding tube occlusion. Usually, 20 to 30 mL of warm water every 3 to 4 hours during continuous feedings and before and after intermittent feedings and medication administration can maintain patency.[2] The volume of irrigant may have to be reduced for fluid restriction. Automatic enteral flush pumps are also available. Although cranberry juice or cola beverages are sometimes used in an effort to reduce the incidence of tube occlusion, water is the preferred irrigant because it has been shown to be superior in maintaining tube patency.[37] Tube occlusion may occur as a result of stagnant formula, inadequately crushed pills, or medication interactions with formula. Enteral infusion pumps should be used, and tubes should be flushed before feeding infusions are paused. Liquid medications or elixirs should be used when possible to avoid tube occlusion with pill fragments. The use of pancreatic enzymes in the feeding tube appears to reduce the risk of tube clogging and may be successful in removing a clog after it has formed.[37,38]

Aspiration. Pulmonary aspiration of enteral formulas and subsequent pneumonia are serious complications of enteral feeding in critically ill patients. Risk factors for aspiration of enteral feeding include decreased level of consciousness, supine position, and swallowing disorders.[39] To reduce the risk of pulmonary aspiration of formula during enteral feeding, the nurse must keep the head of the bed elevated unless contraindicated, temporarily stop feedings when the patient must be supine for prolonged periods, position the patient in the right lateral decubitus position when possible to encourage gastric emptying, use postpyloric feeding methods, keep the cuff of the endotracheal tube inflated as much as possible during enteral feeding, if applicable, and be alert to any increase in abdominal distention.

Two bedside methods have been used in the past to detect pulmonary aspiration of enteral feeding. One is the addition of blue dye to the enteral formula and observation of the patient for any dye-tinged tracheal secretions, and the other is glucose testing of tracheal secretions to detect the presence of the glucose-containing enteral formula. The glucose oxidase method may cause false-positive reactions if blood is present. It has a low sensitivity when low-glucose formulas are used, and it has questionable specificity.[40] There is no established protocol for blue dye testing. Although it has been used routinely in clinical practice for several years, there is no evidence to support its efficacy or safety. It lacks sensitivity and specificity in ruling out aspiration. Numerous clinical reports of systemic absorption of blue dye and adverse outcomes have been described.[41-42] Glucose oxidase testing and blue food coloring are not recommended as appropriate methods for detecting aspiration of enteral feedings.[41,43]

Gastrointestinal complications. Diarrhea is common in patients receiving enteral nutrition, with an incidence of 2% to 70%. No single definition has been established for diarrhea. Current definitions include various stool frequencies, volumes, and weights.[44] Diarrhea in enterally fed critically ill patients has many factors. Common causes include medications, malabsorption, formula contamination, or low-fiber formulas. While the cause of diarrhea is being determined, nurses must provide adequate fluid and electrolyte replacement, maintain skin integrity, and administer antidiarrheal agents. To prevent complications, stool must be checked for infection, especially Clostridium difficile, before antidiarrheal medications can be administered.[45] Constipation is a complication of enteral feeding that may result from dehydration, bed rest, opioid administration, or lack of adequate fiber in enteral formulas. Pasty stools are normal in enterally fed patients. Bowel movements should be assessed daily. The

TABLE 6-3 Nursing Management of Enteral Tube Feeding Complications

COMPLICATION	CONTRIBUTING FACTORS	PREVENTION OR CORRECTION
Pulmonary aspiration (signs and symptoms include tachypnea, shortness of breath, hypoxia, and infiltrate on chest radiographs)	Feeding tube positioned in esophagus or respiratory tract	Confirm proper tube placement before administering any feeding; check tube placement at least every 4-8 hr during continuous feedings; consider intermittent feedings.
	Regurgitation of formula	Elevate head to 30-45 degrees during feedings unless contraindicated; if the head cannot be raised, position the patient in lateral (especially right lateral, which facilitates gastric emptying) or prone position to improve drainage of vomitus from the mouth. Consider giving feeding into small bowel rather than stomach in high-risk patients. Metoclopramide may improve gastric emptying and decrease the risk of regurgitation. Evaluate feeding tolerance every 2 hr initially, then less frequently as condition becomes stable. Intolerance may be manifested by bloating, abdominal distention and pain, lack of stool and flatus, diminished or absent bowel sounds, tense abdomen, increased tympany, nausea and vomiting, residual volume >200 mL aspirated from an NG tube or >100 mL aspirated from a gastrostomy tube, although a high residual volume in the absence of other abnormal findings may not be grounds for stopping feedings (measuring residual volumes is a controversial practice; see the section on tube occlusion that follows below in Table 8-5). If intolerance is suspected, abdominal radiographs may be done to check for distended gastric bubble, distended loops of bowel, or air-fluid levels.
Diarrhea	Medications with GI side effects (e.g., antibiotics, digitalis, laxatives, magnesium-containing antacids, quinidine, caffeine, many others)	Evaluate the patient's medications to determine their potential for causing diarrhea and consult the pharmacist if necessary.
	Predisposing illness (e.g., short bowel syndrome, inflammatory bowel disease)	Use continuous feedings; consider a formula with MCT and/or soluble fiber.
	Hypertonic formula or medications (e.g., oral suspensions of antibiotics, potassium, other electrolytes), which can cause dumping syndrome	Evaluate formula administration procedures to ensure that feedings are not being given by bolus infusion; administer the formula continuously or by slow intermittent infusion. Dilute enteral medications well.
	Bacterial contamination of the formula	Use scrupulously clean technique in administering tube feedings; prepare formula with sterile water if there are any concerns about the safety of the water supply or if the patient is seriously immunocompromised; keep opened containers of formula refrigerated and discard them within 24 hr; discard enteral feeding containers and administration sets every 24 hr; hang formula no more than 4-8 hr unless it comes prepackaged in sterile administration sets.
	Fecal impaction with seepage of liquid stool around the impaction	Perform a digital rectal examination to rule out impaction; see guidelines for prevention of constipation that follow below in this table (Table 8-5).
	Lactose intolerance	Use lactose-free formula.
Constipation	Low-residue formula, creating little fecal bulk, lack of fiber	Consider using a fiber-containing formula; ensure fluid intake is adequate; stool softeners may be beneficial.

TABLE 6-3 Nursing Management of Enteral Tube Feeding Complications—cont'd

COMPLICATION	CONTRIBUTING FACTORS	PREVENTION OR CORRECTION
Tube occlusion	Medications administered by tube that physically plug the tube or coagulate the formula, causing it to clog the tube	If medications must be given by tube, avoid use of crushed tablets; consult with the pharmacist to determine whether medications can be dispensed as elixirs or suspensions. Irrigate tube with water before and after administering any medication; never add any medication to the formula unless the two are known to be compatible.
	Sedimentation of formula	Irrigate tube every 4-8 hr during continuous feedings and after every intermittent feeding. If residuals are measured, flush the tube thoroughly after returning the formula to the stomach, since gastric juices left in tube may cause precipitation of formula. Instilling pancreatic enzymes into the tube can remove or prevent some occlusions.
Gastric retention	Delayed gastric emptying related to head trauma, sepsis, diabetic or uremic gastroparesis, electrolyte balance, or other illness	The cause must be corrected if possible. Consult with the physician about use of postpyloric feedings or prokinetic agents to stimulate gastric emptying. Encourage the patient to lie in the right lateral position frequently, unless contraindicated.

GI, gastrointestinal; *NG*, nasogastric.
Modified from Moore MC. *Pocket Guide to Nutritional Assessment and Care.* 6th ed. St. Louis: Mosby; 2009.

nurse must ensure adequate fluid and fiber intake, promote optimal mobility, and administer laxatives and stool softeners as necessary.[46]

Formula delivery. Careful attention to administration of tube feedings can prevent many complications. Very clean or aseptic technique in the handling and administration of the formula can help prevent bacterial contamination and a resultant infection. When using cans of formula transferred to a feeding container, wash hands and tops of cans before opening, hang enough formula for just 8 hours of infusion, and do not add new formula to formula already hanging. Closed systems that use a prefilled sterile container that can be spiked with the enteral tube are also available.

Tube feedings may be administered intermittently or continuously. Bolus feedings, which are intermittent feedings delivered rapidly into the stomach or small bowel, are likely to cause distention, vomiting, and dumping syndrome with diarrhea. Instead of using bolus feedings, nurses can gradually drip intermittent feedings, with each feeding lasting 20 to 30 minutes or longer, to promote optimal assimilation. The question of which feeding schedule—continuous or intermittent—is superior for critically ill patients remains unanswered.

Tubing and catheter misconnections. Examples of misconnection errors include misconnecting an enteric feeding tube into an intravenous catheter or injection of an intravenous fluid into a tracheostomy cuff inflation tube. These misconnection errors are potentially life- threatening, and increased awareness as well as precautions can improve patient safety. The following strategies should be followed to minimize risk for tubing and catheter misconnections:[47]

- Label all tubes and catheters, especially arterial, epidural, and intrathecal catheters.
- Trace lines back to their origins when initiating any new device or infusion.
- Standardize a line reconciliation process with patient handoffs.
- Consider routing tubes and catheters with different purposes in different, standardized directions.
- Never use a standard Luer syringe for oral medications or enteric feedings.

Total Parenteral Nutrition

TPN refers to the delivery of all nutrients by the intravenous route. It is used when the GI tract is not functional or when nutritional needs cannot be met solely through the GI tract. Likely candidates for TPN include patients who have a severely impaired absorption (e.g., short bowel syndrome, collagen vascular diseases, radiation enteritis), intestinal obstruction, peritonitis, or prolonged ileus. Some postoperative, trauma, or burn patients may need TPN to supplement the nutrient intake that they are able to tolerate by the enteral route.

Types of parenteral nutrition. TPN involves administration of highly concentrated dextrose (25% to 70%), providing a rich source of calories. These highly concentrated dextrose solutions are hyperosmolar, as much as 1800 mOsm/L, and therefore must be delivered through a central vein.[48] Peripheral parenteral nutrition (PPN) has a glucose concentration of 5% to 10% and may be delivered safely through a peripheral vein. PPN solution delivers nutrition support in a large volume that cannot be tolerated by patients who require fluid restriction. It provides short-term nutrition support for a few days to less than 2 weeks.

Regardless of the route of administration, PPN and TPN provide glucose, fat, protein, electrolytes, vitamins, and trace elements. Although dextrose–amino acid solutions are commonly thought of as good growth media for microorganisms, they actually suppress the growth of most organisms usually associated with catheter-related sepsis, except yeasts. However, because the many manipulations required to prepare solutions increase the possibility of contamination, TPN solutions are best used with caution. They should be prepared under laminar flow conditions in the pharmacy, with avoidance of additions on the nursing unit. Solution containers need to be inspected for cracks or leaks before hanging, and solutions must be discarded within 24 hours of hanging. An in-line 0.22-micron filter, which eliminates all microorganisms but not endotoxins, may be used in the administration of solutions. Use of the filter, however, cannot be substituted for good aseptic technique.

Nursing management of potential complications. Nursing management of the patient receiving TPN includes catheter care, administration of solutions, prevention or correction of complications, and evaluation of patient responses to intravenous feedings. Table 6-4 describes nursing management of TPN complications. Evaluation of the patient's response is discussed later in this chapter.

Metabolic complications associated with parenteral nutrition include glucose intolerance and electrolyte imbalance. Slow advancement of the rate of TPN (25 mL/hr) to goal rate allows pancreatic adjustment to the dextrose load. Capillary blood glucose should be monitored every 4 to 6 hours. Insulin can be added to the TPN solution or can be infused as a separate drip to control glucose levels. Rapid cessation of TPN may not lead to hypoglycemia; however, tapering the infusion over 2 to 4 hours is recommended.[49]

Serum electrolytes are obtained on starting TPN. During critical illness, levels should be monitored and corrected daily and then weekly or twice weekly after the patient is more stable. The refeeding syndrome is a potentially lethal condition characterized by generalized fluid and electrolyte imbalance. It occurs as a potential complication after initiation of oral, enteral, or parenteral nutrition in malnourished patients.

It is important to anticipate refeeding syndrome in patients who may be at risk. Patients with chronic malnutrition or underfeeding, chronic alcoholism, or anorexia nervosa or those maintained NPO for several days with evidence of stress are at risk for refeeding syndrome.[50] In high-risk patients, nutrition support should be started cautiously at 25% to 50% of required calories and slowly advanced over 3 to 4 days as tolerated. Close monitoring of serum electrolytes before and during feeding is essential. Normal values do not always reflect total body stores. Correction of pre-existing electrolyte imbalances are necessary before initiation of feeding. Continued monitoring and supplementation with electrolytes and vitamins are necessary throughout the first week of nutrition support.[50]

Lipid emulsion. Lipids or fat emulsions provide calories for energy and prevent essential fatty acid depletion. In contrast to dextrose–amino acid solutions, intravenous lipid emulsions provide a rich environment for the growth of bacteria and fungi, including Candida albicans. Lipid emulsions cannot be filtered through an in-line 0.22-micron filter because some particles in the emulsions have larger diameters than this. Lipids may be infused into the TPN line downstream from the filter. No other medications should be infused into a line containing lipids or TPN. Lipid emulsions are handled with strict asepsis, and they must be discarded within 12 to 24 hours of hanging.

Monitoring and Evaluation of Nutrition Support

A multidisciplinary approach is required in evaluating the effects of nutrition support on clinical outcomes. Assessment of response to nutrition support is an ongoing process that involves anthropometric measurements, physical examination, and biochemical evaluation. Daily monitoring of nutritional intake is an important aspect of critical care and is a key element in preventing problems associated with underfeeding and overfeeding. Daily weights and the maintenance of accurate intake-and-output records are crucial for evaluating nutritional progress and the state of hydration in the patient receiving nutrition support. Serum levels of electrolytes, calcium, phosphorus, and magnesium serve as a guide to the amount of these nutrients that must be supplied.

The Society of Critical Care Medicine (SCCM) and the American Society for Parenteral and Enteral Nutrition (A.S.P.E.N.) published *The Guidelines for the Provision and Assessment of Nutrition Support Therapy in the Adult Critically Ill Patient.* The publication is based on evidence from an extensive review of 307 articles and is intended for the care of critically ill adults who require a stay of greater than 3 days in the critical care area. All practitioners who care for this target population are encouraged to become familiar with these evidence-based guidelines.[2]

NUTRITION AND CARDIOVASCULAR ALTERATIONS

Diet and cardiovascular disease may interact in a variety of ways. Excessive nutrient intake—manifested by overweight or obesity and a diet rich in cholesterol, saturated fat, and added sugars—is a risk factor for development of arteriosclerotic heart disease. However, the consequences of chronic myocardial insufficiency can include malnutrition.

Nutrition Assessment in Cardiovascular Alterations

A nutrition assessment provides the nurse and other members of the health care team the information necessary to plan the patient's nutrition care and education. Common findings in the nutrition assessment of the cardiovascular patient are summarized in Box 6-4. The major nutritional concerns relate to appropriateness of body weight and the levels of serum lipids and blood pressure.

Nutrition Intervention in Cardiovascular Alterations

Myocardial Infarction

In the early period after a myocardial infarction (MI), nutrition interventions and education are designed to reduce angina, cardiac workload, and risk of dysrhythmia. Meal size, caffeine intake, and food temperatures are some of the dietary factors that are of concern. Small, frequent snacks are preferable to larger meals for patients with severe myocardial compromise or postprandial angina.

If caffeine is included in the diet, its effects should be monitored. Because caffeine is a stimulant, it may increase heart rate and myocardial oxygen demand. In the United States and in most industrial nations, coffee is the richest source of caffeine in the diet, with about 150 mg of caffeine per 180 mL (6 fluid oz) of coffee. In comparison, the caffeine content of the same volume of tea or cola is approximately 50 mg or 20 mg, respectively. Very hot or very cold foods should be avoided because they can potentially trigger vagal or other neural input and cause cardiac dysrhythmias.

TABLE 6-4 Nursing Management of Total Parenteral Nutrition Complications

COMPLICATION	CLINICAL MANIFESTATIONS	PREVENTION OR CORRECTION
Catheter-related sepsis	Fever, chills, glucose intolerance, positive blood culture	Use aseptic technique when handling catheter, IV tubing, and TPN solutions. Hang a bottle of TPN no longer than 24 hr, lipid emulsion no longer than 12-24 hr. Use an in-line 0.22-micron filter with TPN to remove microorganisms. Avoid drawing blood, infusing blood or blood products, piggybacking other IV solutions into TPN IV tubing, or attaching manometers or transducers through the TPN infusion line, if possible. If catheter-related sepsis is suspected, remove the catheter or assist in changing the catheter over a guidewire and administer antibiotics as ordered.
Air embolism	Dyspnea, cyanosis, apnea, tachycardia, hypotension, "millwheel" heart murmur; mortality estimated at 50% (depends on quantity of air entering)	Use Luer-Lok connections; use an in-line air-eliminating filter. Have the patient perform a Valsalva maneuver during tubing changes; if the patient is on a ventilator, change tubing quickly at end expiration. Maintain occlusive dressing over catheter site for at least 24 hr after removing catheter to prevent air entry through catheter tract. If an air embolism is suspected, place the patient in left lateral decubitus and Trendelenburg positions (to trap air in the apex of the right ventricle, away from the outflow tract) and administer oxygen and CPR as needed; immediately notify physician, who may attempt to aspirate air from the heart.
Pneumothorax	Chest pain, dyspnea, hypoxemia, hypotension, radiographic evidence, needle aspiration of air from pleural space	Thoroughly explain the catheter insertion procedure to the patient, because when a patient moves or breathes erratically, he or she is more likely to sustain pleural damage. Perform x-ray examination after insertion or insertion attempt. If pneumothorax is suspected, assist with needle aspiration or chest tube insertion, if necessary.
Central venous thrombosis	Edema of neck, shoulder, and arm on same side as catheter; development of collateral circulation on chest; pain in insertion site; drainage of TPN from the insertion site; positive findings on venography	Follow measures to prevent sepsis; repeated or traumatic catheterizations are most likely to result in thrombosis. If thrombosis is confirmed, remove the catheter and administer anticoagulants and antibiotics, as ordered.
Catheter occlusion or semi-occlusion	No flow or a sluggish flow through the catheter	If the infusion is stopped temporarily, flush the catheter with saline or heparinized saline. If the catheter appears to be occluded, attempt to aspirate the clot; if this is ineffective, the physician may order a thrombolytic agent such as streptokinase or alteplase (tPA) instilled in the catheter.
Hypoglycemia	Diaphoresis, shakiness, confusion, loss of consciousness	Infuse TPN within 10% of the ordered rate; monitor blood glucose until stable. If hypoglycemia is present, administer oral carbohydrate; if the patient is unconscious or oral intake is contraindicated, the physician may order an IV bolus of dextrose.
Hyperglycemia	Thirst, headache, lethargy, increased urinary output	Administer TPN within 10% of the ordered rate; monitor blood glucose level at least daily until stable. The patient may require insulin added to the TPN if hyperglycemia is persistent; sudden appearance of hyperglycemia in a patient who was previously tolerating the same glucose load may indicate the onset of sepsis.
Hypertriglyceridemia	Serum triglyceride concentrations elevated (especially serious if >400 mg/dL); serum may appear turbid	Monitor serum triglycerides at baseline, 6 hr after lipid infusion, and at least 3 times weekly until stable in patients receiving lipid emulsions; reduce lipid infusion rate or administer low-dose heparin with lipid emulsions as ordered if elevated levels are observed.

CPR, cardiopulmonary resuscitation; *IV*, intravenous; *TPN*, total parenteral nutrition.
Modified from Moore MC. *Pocket Guide to Nutritional Assessment and Care.* 6th ed. St. Louis: Mosby; 2009.

BOX 6-4 Common Findings in the Nutrition Assessment of the Patient with Cardiovascular Disease

Anthropometric Measurements
- Overweight or obesity; underweight (cardiac cachexia)
- Abdominal fat: increased risk of cardiovascular disease with waist measurement >102 cm (>40 inches) for men and >88 cm (>35 inches) for women

Biochemical (Laboratory) Data
- Elevated total serum cholesterol, low-density lipoprotein (LDL) cholesterol, and triglycerides

Clinical Findings
- Wasting of muscle and subcutaneous fat

Diet or Health History
- Sedentary lifestyle
- Excessive intake of saturated fat, cholesterol, salt, added sugar, and/or alcohol
- Angina, respiratory difficulty, or fatigue during eating
- Medications that impair appetite (e.g., digitalis preparations, quinidine)

Heart Failure

Nutrition intervention in heart failure is designed to reduce fluid retained within the body and therefore reduce the preload. Because fluid accompanies sodium, limitation of sodium is necessary to reduce fluid retention. Specific interventions include limiting salt intake, usually to 2 g a day or less, and limiting fluid intake as appropriate.[51] If fluid is restricted, the daily fluid allowance is usually 1.5 to 2 L/day, which includes fluids in the diet and those given with medications and for other purposes (see "Heart Failure" in Chapter 12).

NUTRITION AND PULMONARY ALTERATIONS

Malnutrition has extremely adverse effects on respiratory function, decreasing surfactant production, diaphragmatic mass, vital capacity, and immunocompetence. Patients with acute respiratory disorders find it difficult to consume adequate oral nutrients and can rapidly become malnourished. Individuals who have an acute illness superimposed on chronic respiratory problems are also at high risk. Nearly three-fourths of patients with chronic obstructive pulmonary disease (COPD) have had weight loss.[52] Patients with undernutrition and end-stage COPD, however, often cannot tolerate the increase in metabolic demand that occurs during refeeding. They also are at significant risk for development of cor pulmonale and may fail to tolerate the fluid required for delivery of enteral or parenteral nutrition support. Prevention of severe nutritional deficits, rather than correction of deficits after they have occurred, is important in nutritional management of these patients (see "Acute Respiratory Failure" and "Long-Term Mechanical Ventilator Dependence" in Chapter 15).

Nutrition Assessment in Pulmonary Alterations

Common findings in nutrition assessment related to pulmonary alterations are summarized in Box 6-5. The patient with

BOX 6-5 Common Findings in the Nutrition Assessment of the Patient with Pulmonary Disease

Anthropometric Measurements
Underweight

Biochemical (Laboratory) Data
Elevated PCO_2 related to overfeeding

Clinical Findings
Edema, dyspnea, signs of pulmonary edema related to fluid volume excess

Diet or Health History
Poor food intake related to dyspnea, unpleasant taste in the mouth from sputum production or bronchodilator therapy; endotracheal intubation preventing oral intake

respiratory compromise is especially vulnerable to the effects of fluid volume excess and must be assessed continually for this complication, particularly during enteral and parenteral feeding.

Nutrition Intervention in Pulmonary Alterations

Prevent or Correct Undernutrition and Underweight

The nurse and dietitian work together to encourage oral intake in the undernourished or potentially undernourished patient who is capable of eating. Small, frequent feedings are especially important, because a very full stomach can interfere with diaphragmatic movement. Mouth care should be provided before meals and snacks to clear the palate of the taste of sputum and medications. Administering bronchodilators with food can help to reduce the gastric irritation caused by these medications. Because of anorexia, dyspnea, debilitation, or need for ventilatory support, however, many patients will require enteral tube feeding or TPN.

Avoid Overfeeding

Overfeeding of total calories or of carbohydrate or lipid alone can impair pulmonary function. The production of carbon dioxide (VCO_2) increases when carbohydrate is relied on as the primary energy source. This is unlikely to be significant in the patient who is eating foods. Instead, it is an iatrogenic complication of TPN, in which glucose is often the predominant calorie source, or occasionally of tube feeding in a patient with a very high carbohydrate formula. Excessive calorie intake can raise $PaCO_2$ sufficiently to make it difficult to wean a patient from the ventilator. A balanced regimen with lipids and carbohydrates providing the nonprotein calories is optimal for the patient with respiratory compromise, and the patient needs to be reassessed.

Prevent Fluid Volume Excess

Pulmonary edema and failure of the right side of the heart, which may be precipitated by fluid volume excess, further worsen the status of the patient with respiratory compromise. Maintaining careful intake-and-output records allows for accurate assessment of fluid balance. Usually the patient requires no more than 35 to 40 mL/kg/day of fluid. For the patient receiving nutrition support, fluid intake can be reduced by using 20% lipid emulsions as a source of calories, by using tube feeding formulas that provide at least 2 calories/mL (the dietitian can recommend appropriate formulas), and by choosing oral supplements that are low in fluid.

NUTRITION AND NEUROLOGIC ALTERATIONS

Because neurologic disorders such as stroke and closed head injury tend to be long-term problems, they necessitate good nutritional care to prevent nutritional deficits and promote well-being.

Nutrition Assessment in Neurologic Alterations

Nutrition-related assessment findings vary widely in the patient with neurologic alterations, depending on the type of disorder present. Some common assessment findings are listed in Box 6-6.

Nutrition Intervention in Neurologic Alterations

Prevention or Correction of Nutritional Deficits

Oral feedings. Patients with dysphagia or weakness of the swallowing musculature often experience the greatest difficulty in swallowing foods that are dry or thin liquids, such as water, that are difficult to control. For these patients, the nurse, the dietitian, and the speech therapist can work together to plan suitable meals and evaluate patient acceptance and tolerance (see "Stroke" in Chapter 18).

Soft, moist foods are usually easier to swallow than dry ones. An upright sitting position is preferable during meals, if possible, to allow gravity to facilitate effective swallowing. Water and other thin liquids may be especially difficult for the person with swallowing dysfunction to manage. Beverages may be thickened with commercial thickening products, with infant cereal, or with yogurt if the patient has difficulty swallowing thin fluids. Fruit nectars may be better tolerated than thinner juices.

Tube feedings or total parenteral nutrition. Patients who are unconscious or unable to eat because of severe dysphagia, weakness, ileus, or other reasons require tube feedings or TPN. Prompt initiation of nutrition support must be a priority in the patient with neurologic impairments. Needs for protein and calories are increased by infection and fever, as may occur in the patient with encephalitis or meningitis. Needs for protein, calories, zinc, and vitamin C are increased during wound healing, as occurs in the trauma patient and the patient with pressure ulcers.

Patients with neurologic deficits are at increased risk for certain complications (particularly pulmonary aspiration) during tube feeding and therefore require especially careful nursing management. Patients of most concern are 1) those with an impaired gag reflex, such as some patients with cerebral vascular accident; 2) those with delayed gastric emptying, such as patients in the early period after spinal cord injury and patients with head injury treated with barbiturate coma, and 3) patients likely to experience seizures.

Administering phenytoin with enteral formulas decreases the absorption of the medication and the peak serum level achieved. A problem arises when a patient is receiving continuous enteral feedings and requires anticonvulsant therapy. One way to deal with the problem is to stop the feeding for 1 to 2 hours before and after phenytoin administration.[53] Even when this practice is followed, the patient may require a higher phenytoin dosage than normal to maintain therapeutic serum concentrations. When continuous feedings are discontinued and the patient resumes eating meals or receives intermittent enteral feedings, the phenytoin dosage must be adjusted appropriately. Phenytoin levels should be monitored carefully in patients receiving enteral feedings. The infusion rate may need to be increased to account for the time that the enteral feeding is held for phenytoin administration.

Hyperglycemia is a common complication in patients receiving corticosteroids. Regular monitoring of blood glucose levels is an important part of care of such patients. They may require insulin to control the hyperglycemia.

Prompt use of nutrition support is especially important for patients with head injuries because head injury causes marked catabolism, even in patients who receive barbiturates, which should decrease metabolic demands. Head-injured patients rapidly exhaust glycogen stores and begin to use body proteins to meet energy needs, a process that can quickly lead to PCM. The catabolic response is partly a result of corticosteroid therapy in head-injured patients. However, the hypermetabolism and hypercatabolism are also caused by dramatic hormonal responses to this type of injury.[54] Levels of cortisol, epinephrine, and norepinephrine increase as much as seven times normal. These hormones increase the metabolic rate and caloric demands, causing mobilization of body fat and proteins to meet the increased energy needs. Head-injured patients undergo an inflammatory response and may be febrile, creating increased needs for protein and calories. Improvement in outcome and reduction in complications have been observed in head-injured patients who receive adequate nutrition support early in the hospital course.[54-55]

BOX 6-6 Common Findings in the Nutrition Assessment of the Patient with Neurologic Alterations

Biochemical (Laboratory) Data
- Hyperglycemia (with corticosteroid use)

Clinical Findings
- Wasting of muscle and subcutaneous fat related to disuse or to poor food intake

Diet or Health History
- Poor food intake related to altered state of consciousness, dysphagia or other chewing or swallowing difficulties, or ileus resulting from spinal cord injury or use of pentobarbital
- Hypermetabolism resulting from head injury
- Pressure ulcers

NUTRITION AND RENAL ALTERATIONS

Providing adequate nutrition care for the patient with renal disease can be extremely challenging. Although renal disturbances and their treatments can markedly increase needs for nutrients, necessary restrictions in intake of fluid, protein, phosphorus, and potassium make delivery of adequate calories, vitamins, and minerals difficult. Thorough nutrition

BOX 6-7 Common Findings in the Nutrition Assessment of the Patient with Renal Failure

Anthropometric Measurements
- Underweight (may be masked by edema)

Biochemical (Laboratory) Data
- Electrolyte imbalances
- Hypoalbuminemia related to protein restriction and amino acid losses in dialysis
- Anemia related to inadequate erythropoietin production and blood loss with hemodialysis
- Hypertriglyceridemia related to use of glucose as osmotic agent in dialysis and use of carbohydrates to supply needed calories

Clinical Findings
- Wasting of muscle and subcutaneous tissue (may be masked by edema)

Diet or Health History
- Poor dietary intake related to protein and electrolyte restrictions and alterations in taste

assessment provides the basis for successful nutrition management in patients with renal disease.

Nutrition Assessment in Renal Alterations

Some common assessment findings in individuals with renal disease are listed in Box 6-7.

Nutrition Intervention in Renal Alterations

Nutritional needs of patients with renal disease are complex. The goal of nutrition intervention is to balance adequate calories, protein, vitamins, and minerals, while avoiding excesses of protein, fluid, electrolytes, and other nutrients with potential toxicity.

Protein

When urinary excretion of urea is impaired in acute kidney injury (AKI), BUN rises. Excessive protein intake may worsen uremia. However, the patient with AKI often has other physiologic stresses that increase protein or amino acid needs: losses because of dialysis, wounds, and fistulas; use of corticosteroid medications that exert a catabolic effect; increased endogenous secretion of catecholamines, corticosteroids, and glucagon, all of which can cause or aggravate catabolism; metabolic acidosis, which stimulates protein breakdown, and catabolic conditions, such as trauma, surgery, and sepsis.[56] Patients with AKI need adequate amounts of protein to avoid catabolism of body tissues.

Patients with stable AKI without evidence of fluid overload or electrolyte or acid-base disturbances can often be managed conservatively without dialysis. However, when renal function worsens, some form of renal replacement therapy (RRT) is required to maintain homeostasis and prevent metabolic complications (see Chapter 20). To limit catabolism, patients with AKI on dialysis therapy should receive approximately 1.5 to 2.0 g of protein/kg/day (with a maximum of 2.5 g of protein/kg/day), depending on catabolic rate, renal function, and dialysis losses.[2,57]

Fluid

The patient with renal insufficiency usually does not require a fluid restriction until urine output begins to diminish. Patients receiving hemodialysis are limited to a fluid intake resulting in a gain of no more than 0.45 kg (1 lb) per day on the days between dialysis. This generally means a daily intake of 500 to 750 mL plus the volume lost in urine. With the use of continuous peritoneal dialysis, hemofiltration, or hemodialysis, the fluid intake can be liberalized.[58] This more liberal fluid allowance permits more adequate nutrient delivery by oral, tube, or parenteral feedings. Enteral formulas containing 1.5 to 2 calories/mL or more provide a concentrated source of calories for tube-fed patients who require fluid restriction. Intravenous lipids, particularly 20% emulsions, can be used to supply concentrated calories for the TPN patient.

Energy (Calories)

Energy needs are not increased by renal failure, but adequate calories must be provided to avoid catabolism.[56,58] It is essential that the renal patient receive an adequate number of calories to prevent catabolism of body tissues to meet energy needs. Catabolism reduces the mass of muscle and other functional body tissues, and it releases nitrogen that must be excreted by the kidney. Adults with renal insufficiency need about 30 to 35 calories/kg/day to prevent catabolism and ensure that all protein consumed is used for anabolism rather than to meet energy needs.[53] After renal transplantation, when the patient usually receives large doses of corticosteroids, it is especially important to ensure that caloric intake is adequate (usually 25 to 35 calories/kg/day) to prevent undue catabolism.

Other Nutrients

Certain nutrients such as potassium and phosphorus are restricted because they are excreted by the kidney. The patient has no specific requirement for the fat-soluble vitamins A, E, and K because they are not removed in appreciable amounts by dialysis and restriction generally prevents development of toxicity. Patients with end-stage renal disease may have decreased clearance of vitamin A, and levels should be monitored.[57] The needs for several water-soluble vitamins and trace minerals are increased in the dialysis patient because they are small enough to pass freely through the dialysis filter. Vitamin and minerals should be supplemented as necessary.[58]

NUTRITION AND GASTROINTESTINAL ALTERATIONS

Because the GI tract is inherently related to nutrition, it is not surprising that impairment of the GI tract and its accessory organs has a major impact on nutrition. Two of the most serious GI-related illnesses seen among critical care patients are hepatic failure and pancreatitis, and the following discussion focuses on these disorders.

Nutrition Assessment in Gastrointestinal Alterations

Some common assessment findings in individuals with GI disease are listed in Box 6-8.

BOX 6-8 Common Findings in the Nutrition Assessment of the Patient with Gastrointestinal Disease

Anthropometric Measurements
- Underweight related to malabsorption (from inadequate production of bile salts or pancreatic enzymes), anorexia, or poor intake (because of pain caused by eating)

Biochemical (Laboratory) Data
- Hypoalbuminemia (may result primarily from liver damage and not malnutrition)
- Hypocalcemia related to steatorrhea
- Hypomagnesemia related to alcohol abuse
- Anemia related to blood loss from bleeding varices

Clinical Findings
- Wasting of muscle and subcutaneous fat
- Confusion, confabulation, nystagmus, or peripheral neuropathy related to thiamine deficiency caused by alcohol abuse (Wernicke-Korsakoff syndrome)

Diet or Health History
- Steatorrhea

Nutrition Intervention in Gastrointestinal Alterations

Hepatic Failure

The liver is the most important metabolic organ, and it is responsible for carbohydrate, fat, and protein metabolism, vitamin storage and activation, and detoxification of waste products. Liver failure is associated with a wide spectrum of metabolic alterations. Because the diseased liver has impaired ability to deactivate hormones, levels of circulating glucagon, epinephrine, and cortisol are elevated. These hormones promote catabolism of body tissues and cause glycogen stores to be exhausted. Release of lipids from their storage depots is accelerated, but the liver has decreased ability to metabolize them for energy. The damaged liver cannot clear ammonia from the circulation adequately, and ammonia accumulates in the brain. The ammonia may contribute to the encephalopathic symptoms and to brain edema.[2,59]

Provision of a nutritious diet and evaluation of response to dietary protein. Protein-calorie malnutrition (PCM) and nutritional deficiencies are common in patients with liver failure. The causes of malnutrition are complex and usually are related to decreased intake, malabsorption, maldigestion, and abnormal nutrient metabolism. Nutrition intervention is individualized and based on these metabolic changes. A diet with adequate protein helps to suppress catabolism and promote liver regeneration. Stable patients with cirrhosis usually tolerate 0.8 to 1 g of protein/kg/day. Patients with severe stress or nutritional deficits have increased needs—as much as 1.2 to 2 g of protein/kg/day.[59] Aggressive treatment with medications, including lactulose, neomycin, or metronidazole, is considered first-line therapy in the management of acute hepatic encephalopathy. Chronic protein restriction, which could lead to PCM, is not recommended as a long-term management strategy for patients with liver disease.[2,59]

A diet adequate in calories (at least 30 calories/kg daily) is provided to help prevent catabolism and to prevent the use of dietary protein for energy needs.[60] In cases of malabsorption, medium-chain triglycerides (MCTs) may be used to meet caloric needs. Pancreatic enzymes may also be considered for malabsorption problems.

Pancreatitis

The pancreas is an exocrine and endocrine gland required for normal digestion and metabolism of proteins, carbohydrates, and fats. Food intake stimulates pancreatic secretion, increasing the damage to the pancreas and the pain associated with the disorder. Patients usually present with abdominal pain and tenderness and with elevations of pancreatic enzymes. A mild form of acute pancreatitis occurs in 80% of patients requiring hospitalization, and a severe form of acute pancreatitis occurs in the other 20%.[61] Patients with the mild form of acute pancreatitis do not require nutrition support and generally resume oral feeding within 7 days. Chronic pancreatitis may develop, and it is characterized by fibrosis of pancreatic cells. This results in loss of exocrine and endocrine function because of the destruction of acinar and islet cells. The loss of exocrine function leads to malabsorption and steatorrhea. In chronic pancreatitis, the loss of endocrine function results in impaired glucose intolerance.[61]

Prevention of further damage to the pancreas and preventing nutritional deficits. Effective nutritional management is a key treatment for patients with acute pancreatitis or exacerbations of chronic pancreatitis. The concern that feeding may stimulate the production of digestive enzymes and perpetuate tissue damage has led to the widespread use of TPN and bowel rest. Recent data suggest that for patients with severe pancreatitis, providing enteral nutrition support is more beneficial than prolonged bowel rest and provision of TPN.[2,62] Enteral nutrition infused into the distal jejunum bypasses the stimulatory effect of feeding on pancreatic secretion.

When oral intake is possible, small, frequent feedings of low-fat foods are least likely to cause discomfort,[63] though the level of fat restriction should depend on the level of steatorrhea and abdominal pain the patient experiences.[62] For patients with chronic pancreatitis, pancreatic enzyme replacement therapy may be indicated.[62] Guidelines for the treatment of diabetes (discussed later) are appropriate for the care of the person with glucose intolerance or diabetes related to pancreatitis.

NUTRITION AND ENDOCRINE ALTERATIONS

Endocrine alterations have far-reaching effects on all body systems and affect nutritional status in a variety of ways. One of the most common endocrine problems in the general population and among critically ill patients is diabetes mellitus.

Nutrition Assessment in Endocrine Alterations

Because of the prevalence of patients with non–insulin-dependent diabetes mellitus (type 2 diabetes) among the hospitalized population and the association of type 2 diabetes with overweight, the nutritional problems most commonly identified in patients with endocrine alterations are

BOX 6-9 NUTRITIONAL INTERNET RESOURCES

Academy of Nutrition and Dietetics (AND)	http://www.eatright.org/
American Society of Parenteral and Enteral Nutrition (ASPEN)	http://www.nutritioncare.org/
ASPEN: Malnutrition Awareness tools and resources	http://www.nutritioncare.org/index_malnutrition.aspx?id=7917
American Society for Nutrition (ASN)	http://www.nutrition.org/
USDA Nutrition Evidence Library	http://www.nel.gov/
USDA National Agricultural Library: nutrient database for foods	http://www.nal.usda.gov/
National Institutes of Health Office of Dietary Supplements	http://ods.od.nih.gov/

overweight and obesity. Hyperglycemia and hyperlipidemia are other common findings in the individual with diabetes.

Nutrition Intervention in Endocrine Alterations

Nutrition Support and Blood Glucose Control

Patients with insulin-dependent diabetes mellitus (type 1 diabetes) or endocrine dysfunction caused by pancreatitis often have weight loss and malnutrition as a result of tissue catabolism because they cannot use dietary carbohydrates to meet energy needs. Although patients with type 2 diabetes are more likely to be overweight than underweight, they also may become malnourished as a result of chronic or acute infections, trauma, major surgery, or other illnesses.[64] Nutrition support should not be neglected simply because a patient is obese because malnutrition can develop in these patients. When a patient is not expected to be able to eat for at least 5 to 7 days or inadequate intake persists for that period, initiation of tube feedings or TPN is indicated. No disease process benefits from starvation, and development or progression of nutritional deficits may contribute to complications, such as pressure ulcers, pulmonary or urinary tract infections, and sepsis, which prolong hospitalization, increase the costs of care, and may even result in death. See Chapter 24 for management of glycemic control.

Severe Vomiting or Diarrhea in the Patient with Type 1 Diabetes Mellitus

When insulin-dependent patients experience vomiting and diarrhea severe enough to interfere significantly with oral intake or result in excessive fluid and electrolyte losses, adequate carbohydrates and fluids must be supplied. Nausea and vomiting should be treated with antiemetic medication.[65] Delayed gastric emptying is common in diabetes and may improve with administration of prokinetic agents.[65] See Box 6-9 for nutritional Internet resources.

CASE STUDY Patient with Nutritional Issues

Brief Patient History

Mrs. S is a 49-year-old woman with end-stage cardiomyopathy. She and her husband have been restaurant owners for many years. She is anorexic and finds it difficult to eat solid foods, which is emotionally distressing for her and her family. She has lost 10 pounds in the past month. Mrs. S was placed on the heart transplant list 6 months ago. She has agreed to hospitalization to optimize her medical management and nutritional status.

Clinical Assessment

Mrs. S is admitted to the critical care unit. A central line has been inserted for dobutamine therapy. A nutritional assessment has been completed by the dietitian that includes recommendations for frequent, small, calorie-dense, low-sodium feedings.

Diagnostic Procedures

Mrs. S is 5 feet 2 inches tall and weighs 90 pounds. Her vital signs are as follows: blood pressure of 100/60 mm Hg, heart rate of 80 beats/min (sinus rhythm), respiratory rate of 20 breaths/min, and temperature of 98.2°F. Serum laboratory findings are as follows: hemoglobin level of 8.3 g/dL, prealbumin level of 14 mg/dL, sodium level of 125 mmol/L, potassium level of 3.3 mmol/L, chloride level of 94 mmol/L, carbon dioxide concentration of 26 mEq/L, calcium level of 8 mg/dL, magnesium level of 1.5 mg/dL, and B-type natriuretic peptide concentration of 500 pg/mL.

Medical Diagnosis

Mrs. S is diagnosed with cachexia resulting from end-stage cardiomyopathy.

Questions

1. What major outcomes do you expect to achieve for this patient?
2. What problems or risks must be managed to achieve these outcomes?
3. What interventions must be initiated to monitor, prevent, manage, or eliminate the problems and risks identified?
4. What interventions should be initiated to promote optimal functioning, safety, and well-being of the patient?
5. What possible learning needs do you anticipate for this patient?
6. What cultural and age-related factors may have a bearing on the patient's plan of care?

REFERENCES

1. Joint Commission on Accreditation of Healthcare Organizations: *Comprehensive accreditation manual for hospitals*, Chicago, IL, 2007, Joint Commission on Accreditation of Healthcare Organizations.
2. McClave SA, et al: Society of Critical Care Medicine (SCCM) and American Society for Parenteral and Enteral Nutrition (ASPEN): Guidelines for the provision and assessment of nutrition support therapy in the adult critically ill patient, *J Parenter Enteral Nutr* 33(3):277, 2009.

3. Prins A: Nutritional assessment of the critically ill patient, *South Afr J Clin Nutr* 23(1), 2010.
4. Berger MM, et al: Stature estimation using the knee height determination in critically ill patients, *E Spen Eur E J Clin Nutr Metab* 3(2):e84, 2008.
5. Ravasco P, et al: A critical approach to nutritional assessment in critically ill patients, *Clin Nutr* 21(1):73, 2002.
6. Raguso C, et al: The role of visceral proteins in the nutritional assessment of intensive care unit patients, *Curr Opin Nutr Metab Care* 6:211, 2003.
7. Academy of Nutrition and Dietetics. Evidence Analysis Library: Estimating RMR with predictive equations: what does the evidence tell us? http://www.adaevidencelibrary.com. Accessed April 24, 2012.
8. Academy of Nutrition and Dietetics. Evidence Analysis Library: If indirect calorimetry is unavailable or impractical, what is the best way to estimate resting metabolic rate (RMR) in obese adult critically ill patients? http://www.adaevidencelibrary.com. Accessed April 24, 2012.
9. Academy of Nutrition and Dietetics. Evidence Analysis Library: If indirect calorimetry is unavailable or impractical, what is the best way to estimate resting metabolic rate (RMR) in non-obese adult critically ill patients? http://www.adaevidencelibrary.com. Accessed April 24, 2012.
10. Ramos M, et al: Relationship of perioperative hyperglycemia and postoperative infections in patients who undergo general and vascular surgery, *Ann Surg* 248(4):585, 2008.
11. Pirlich M, et al: Prevalence of malnutrition in hospitalized medical patients: impact of underlying disease, *Dig Dis* 21(3):245, 2003.
12. Kyle UG, et al: Prevalence of malnutrition in 1760 patients at hospital admission: a controlled population study of body composition, *Clin Nutr* 22(5):473, 2003.
13. Barker LA, Gout BS, Crowe TC: Hospital malnutrition: prevalence, identification and impact on patients and the healthcare system, *Int J Environ Res Public Health* 8(2):514, 2011.
14. Joosten KFM, Hulst JM: Malnutrition in pediatric hospital patients: current issues, *Nutrition* 27(2):133, 2011.
15. Braunschweig C, et al: Impact of declines in nutritional status on outcomes in adult patients hospitalized for more than 7 days, *J Am Diet Assoc* 100:1316, 2000.
16. Mathus-Vliegen EMH: Nutritional status, nutrition and pressure ulcers, *Nutr Clin Pract* 16:286, 2001.
17. Rubinson L, et al: Low caloric intake is associated with nosocomial bloodstream infections in patients in the medical intensive care unit, *Crit Care Med* 32:350, 2004.
18. Braunschweig CL, et al: Enteral compared with parenteral nutrition: a meta-analysis, *Am J Clin Nutr* 74(4):534, 2001.
19. Preiser J-C, et al: Enteral feeding with a solution enriched with antioxidant vitamins A, C, and E enhances the resistance to oxidative stress, *Crit Care Med* 28(12):3828, 2000.
20. Marik PE, Zaloga GP: Early enteral nutrition in acutely ill patients: a systematic review, *Crit Care Med* 29(12):2264, 2001.
21. Jeejeebhoy KN: Enteral feeding, *Curr Opin Clin Nutr Metab Care* 5:695, 2002.
22. Zaloga GP, Roberts PR, Marik PE: Feeding the hemodynamically unstable patient: a critical evaluation of the evidence, *Nutr Clin Pract* 18:285, 2003.
23. Moore FA, Weisbrodt NW: Gut dysfunction and intolerance to enteral nutrition in critically ill patients, *Nestle Nutr Workshop Ser Clin Perform Programme* 8:149, 2003.
24. Montejo JC, et al: Multicenter, prospective, randomized, single-blind study comparing the efficacy and gastrointestinal complications of early jejunal feeding with early gastric feeding in critically ill patients, *Crit Care Med* 30(4):796, 2002.
25. McClave SA, Snider HL: Clinical use of gastric residual volumes as a monitor for patients on enteral tube feeding, *JPEN J Parenter Enteral Nutr* 26(Suppl 6):S43, 2002.
26. Berne JD, et al: Erythromycin reduces delayed gastric emptying in critically ill trauma patients: a randomized, controlled trial, *J Trauma* 53(3):422, 2002.
27. Booth CM, et al: Gastrointestinal promotility drugs in the critical care setting: a systematic review of the evidence, *Crit Care Med* 30(7):1429, 2002.
28. Doherty WL, Winter B: Prokinetic agents in critical care, *Crit Care* 7(3):206, 2003.
29. Lord LM, et al: Comparison of weighted vs. unweighted enteral feeding tubes for efficacy of transpyloric intubation, *JPEN J Parenter Enteral Nutr* 17(3):271, 1993.
30. Metheny NA, et al: pH and concentration of bilirubin in feeding tube aspirates as predictors of tube placement, *Nurs Res* 48:189, 1999.
31. Heyland DK, et al: Effect of postpyloric feeding on gastroesophageal regurgitation and pulmonary microaspiration: results of a randomized controlled trial, *Crit Care Med* 29(8):1495, 2001.
32. Esparza J, et al: Equal aspiration rates in gastrically and transpylorically fed critically ill patients, *Intensive Care Med* 27:660, 2001.
33. Neumann DA, DeLegge MH: Gastric versus small-bowel tube feeding in the intensive care unit: a prospective comparison of efficacy, *Crit Care Med* 30(7):1436, 2002.
34. Marik PE, Zaloga GR: Gastric versus postpyloric feeding: a systematic review, *Crit Care* 7(3):R46, 2003.
35. Davies AR, et al: Randomized comparison of nasojejunal and nasogastric feeding in critically ill patients, *Crit Care Med* 30(3):586, 2002.
36. Kearns PJ, et al: The incidence of ventilator-associated pneumonia and success in nutrient delivery with gastric versus small intestine feeding: a randomized clinical trial, *Crit Care Med* 28(6):1742, 2000.
37. Lord LM: Restoring and maintaining patency of enteral feeding tubes, *Nutr Clin Pract* 18:422, 2003.
38. Bourgault AM, et al: Prophylactic pancreatic enzymes to reduce feeding tube occlusions, *Nutr Clin Pract* 18:398, 2003.
39. Metheny NA: Risk factors for aspiration, *JPEN J Parenter Enteral Nutr* 26(6 Suppl):S26, 2002.
40. Metheny NA, et al: A survey of bedside methods used to detect pulmonary aspiration of enteral formula in intubated tube-fed patients, *Am J Crit Care* 8:160, 1999.
41. Maloney JP, Ryan TA: Detection of aspiration in enterally fed patients: a requiem for bedside monitors of aspiration, *JPEN J Parenter Enteral Nutr* 26(6):S34, 2002.
42. Lucarelli MR, et al: Toxicity of food drug and cosmetic blue no. 1 dye in critically ill patients, *Chest* 125(2):793, 2004.
43. McClave SA, et al: North American summit on aspiration in the critically ill patient: consensus statement, *JPEN J Parenter Enteral Nutr* 26(6):S80, 2002.
44. Wiesen P, et al: Diarrhoea in the critically ill, *Curr Opin Crit Care* 12(2):149, 2006.

45. Bernard AC, et al: Defining and assessing tolerance in enteral nutrition, *Nutr Clin Pract* 19(5):481, 2004.
46. Mostafa SM, et al: Constipation and its implications in the critically ill patient, *Br J Anaesth* 91(6):815, 2003.
47. Aust MP: Tubing misconnections, *Am J Crit Care* 20(4):346, 2011.
48. Worthington P, et al: Parenteral nutrition for the acutely ill, *AACN Clin Issues* 11(4):559, 2000.
49. Speerhas R, et al: Maintaining normal blood glucose concentrations with total parenteral nutrition: is it necessary to taper total parenteral nutrition? *Nutr Clin Pract* 18:414, 2003.
50. Hearing SD: Refeeding syndrome, *BMJ* 328(7445):908, 2004.
51. Academy of Nutrition and Dietetics: Nutrition Care Manual website. Nutrition Care > Cardiovascular Disease > Heart Failure > Nutrition Prescription. http://nutritioncaremanual.org. Accessed April 24, 2012.
52. Cochrane WU, Afolabi OA: Investigation into the nutritional status, dietary intake and smoking habits of patients with chronic obstructive pulmonary disease, *J Hum Nutr Diet* 17(1):3, 2004.
53. Dickerson RN, et al: Adverse effects from inappropriate medication administration via a jejunostomy feeding tube, *Nutr Clin Pract* 18:402, 2003.
54. Donaldson J, et al: Nutrition strategies in neurotrauma, *Crit Care Nurs Clin North Am* 12(4):465, 2000.
55. Taylor SJ, et al: Prospective, randomized, controlled trial to determine the effect of early enhanced enteral nutrition on clinical outcome in mechanically ventilated patients suffering head injury, *Crit Care Med* 27(11):2525, 1999.
56. Kapadi FN, et al: Special issues in the patient with renal failure, *Crit Care Clin* 19:233, 2003.
57. Brown RO, Compher C, the American Society for Parenteral and Enteral Nutrition (ASPEN) Board of Directors: A.S.P.E.N. Clinical guideline: nutrition support in adult acute and chronic renal failure, *J Parenter Enteral Nutr* 34(4):366, 2010.
58. Wiggins KL, Harvey KS: A review of guidelines for nutrition care of renal patients, *J Ren Nutr* 12(3):190, 2002.
59. Patton KM, Aranda-Michel J: Nutritional aspects in liver disease and liver transplantation, *Nutr Clin Pract* 17:332, 2002.
60. Florez DA, Aranda-Michel J: Nutritional management of acute and chronic liver disease, *Semin Gastrointest Dis* 13(3):169, 2002.
61. Khokhar AS, Seidner DL: The pathophysiology of pancreatitis, *Nutr Clin Pract* 19:5, 2004.
62. Academy of Nutrition and Dietetics. Nutrition Care Manual website: Nutrition Care > Gastrointestinal Disease > Liver, Gallbladder, and Pancreas Disease > Pancreatitis > Nutrition Intervention. http://nutritioncaremanual.org. Accessed April 27, 2012.
63. Russell MK: Acute pancreatitis: a review of pathophysiology and nutrition management, *Nutr Clin Pract* 19:16, 2004.
64. Woolf SH, et al: Controlling blood glucose levels in patients with type 2 diabetes mellitus: an evidence-based policy statement by the American Academy of Family Physicians and American Diabetes Association, *J Fam Pract* 49(5):453, 2000.
65. Jones MP: Management of diabetic gastroparesis, *Nutr Clin Pract* 19:145, 2004.

CHAPTER 7

Gerontological Alterations

Fiona Winterbottom

Be sure to check out the bonus material, including review questions, on the Evolve website at http://evolve.elsevier.com/Urden/priorities/.

OVERVIEW

Incidence of disease and chronic conditions increases in older adults, and it is important for critical care nurses to differentiate between changes in health caused by physiologic and pathologic processes.[1] The purpose of this chapter is to discuss nursing assessment of normal and abnormal physiologic age-related changes.

CARDIOVASCULAR SYSTEM

Age-Related Changes of the Cardiovascular System

Cardiac and arterial system changes include atherosclerosis, hypertension, myocardial infarction, and stroke. Pathologic alterations of aging include hypertrophy, altered left ventricular (LV) function, increased arterial stiffness, and impaired endothelial function.[2] See Table 7-1.

Age-Related Changes in Electrocardiogram

Electrocardiogram (ECG) changes include decreased R-wave and S-wave amplitude, increased P-R interval, and increased Q-T duration reflective of prolonged rate of relaxation.[3] See Table 7-2. Dysrhythmias increase with age and can be predictive of future cardiac morbidity and mortality.[3] Common dysrhythmias include atrial fibrillation, paroxysmal supraventricular tachycardia, and premature ventricular contractions (PVC). Atrial fibrillation may be related to increased arterial stiffness and reduced LV compliance. Rate control and anticoagulation are recommended for most patients.[4]

Age-Related Changes in Myocardial Structure and Function

Myocardial collagen content increases with age, decreasing compliance and increasing loading of blood vessels. Myocyte function may influence diastolic filling and changes in cardiac structure, increasing systolic blood pressure (SBP).[5]

Myocardial Infarction and Heart Failure

Cardiovascular disease and heart failure (HF) are key contributors to mortality and morbidity worldwide. Expenditure for cardiovascular health care in the United States is expected to triple over the next two decades, increasing costs from $272.5 billion to $818.1 billion.[6] Prevention strategies and advanced therapies have greatly improved life expectancy and morbidity; however, economic costs associated with these advanced therapies have contributed to increased financial and societal burden. Accessibility to advanced therapies, such as transplant and mechanical circulatory support, are limited due to availability of organs for transplant and device-associated costs and resource allocation.[7]

Myocardial infarction (MI) is one of the most common causes of heart failure.[8] Atypical chest pain often occurs in older adults, which is less intense and of short duration. Symptoms may be characterized by dyspnea, confusion, and failure to thrive, resulting in unrecognized signs and symptoms and delays in diagnosis and treatment.[9] Arterial large vessels tend to become less distensible with age, resulting in lengthened systolic contraction, prolonged diastolic relaxation, increased myocardial oxygen demand, and diminished organ perfusion.[3] The LV hypertrophies and thickens with age without significant changes in LV cavity size but may lead to prolonged early diastolic filling and increased cardiac pressures.[3]

Peripheral Vascular System

Aging effects on the peripheral vascular system include a rise in SBP until age 80 years.[9] Diastolic blood pressure (DBP) is less affected by age and generally remains the same or decreases.[9] Determinants of SBP include vascular compliance and blood volume within the system. Endothelial function and compliance of the vasculature are determined by cell type and tissue composition. Arteriosclerosis describes thickening and decreases in compliance in the intimal layer of the large and distal arteries due to increases in smooth muscle cells and connective tissue.[2] Atherosclerosis is the accumulation of lipoproteins and fibrinous products such as platelets, macrophages, and leukocytes within a vessel.[2] Arteriosclerotic and atherosclerotic processes cause arteries to become less distensible and alter the vascular pressure-volume relationship.

Hypertension

Changes in arterial structure and function decrease distensibility of large vessels, reduce forward circulation flow, increase pulse wave velocity, cause late SBP augmentation, increase myocardial oxygen demand, and limit organ perfusion.[4] Older adults with poor BP control have an increased risk of cerebrovascular disease (CVD), coronary artery disease

TABLE 7-1 Age-Related Cardiovascular Changes

PHYSIOLOGIC ALTERATION	MECHANISM	PATHOLOGIC CHANGE
Cardiovascular Structural Remodeling		
↑ Vascular intimal thickness	↑ Migration of and ↑ matrix production by VSMC Possible derivation of intimal cells from other sources	Early stages of atherosclerosis
↑ Vascular stiffness	Elastin fragmentation ↑ Elastase activity ↑ Collagen production by VSMC and ↑ cross-linking of collagen Altered growth factor regulation/tissue repair mechanisms	Systolic hypertension LV wall thickening Stroke Atherosclerosis
↑ LV wall thickness	↑ LV myocyte size with altered Ca^{2+} handling ↑ Myocyte number (necrotic and apoptotic death) Altered growth factor regulation Focal matrix collagen deposition	Retarded early diastolic cardiac filling ↑ Cardiac filling pressure Lower threshold for dyspnea ↑ Likelihood of heart failure with relatively normal systolic function
↑ Left atrial size	↑ Left atrial pressure/volume	↑ Prevalence of lone atrial fibrillation and other atrial arrhythmias
Cardiovascular Functional Changes		
Altered regulation of vascular tone	↓ NO production/effects	Vascular stiffening; hypertension Early atherosclerosis
Reduced threshold for cell Ca^{2+} overload	Changes in gene expression of proteins that regulate Ca^{2+} handling; ↑ PUFA ration in cardiac membranes	Lower threshold for atrial and ventricular arrhythmia Increases myocyte death Increased fibrosis
↑ Cardiovascular reserve		Lower threshold for increased severity of heart failure
Reduced physical activity	Learned lifestyle	Exaggerated age changes in some aspects of cardiovascular structure and function Negative impact on atherosclerotic vascular disease, hypertension, and heart failure

LV, left ventricular; *PUFA*, polyunsaturated fatty acids; *VSMC*, vascular smooth muscle cells.
Adapted from Strait JB, Lakatta EG: Aging-associated cardiovascular changes and their relationship to heart failure, *Heart Failure Clin* 8(1):143, 2012.

TABLE 7-2 Age-Related Changes in Resting Electrocardiographic Variables

ECG VARIABLE	CHANGE WITH AGE
R–R internal	No change
P-wave duration	Minor increase
PR interval	Increase
QRS duration	No change
QRS axis	Leftward shift
QRS voltage	Decrease
QT interval	Minor increase
T-wave voltage	Decrease

Modified from Strait JB, Lakatta EG: Aging-associated cardiovascular changes, *Heart Failure Clin* 8:143, 2012.

(CAD), disorders of LV structure and function, aortic and peripheral arterial disease, chronic kidney disease (CKD), ophthalmologic disorders, and quality-of-life (QOL) issues.[4] Secondary issues related to hypertension include renal artery stenosis, obstructive sleep apnea, primary aldosteronism, and thyroid disorders. Older adults generally have contracted intravascular volumes and impaired baroreflexes, which may be exacerbated by diuretics, sodium, and water depletion, causing orthostatic hypotension. Volume overload is commonly due to excessive salt intake, inadequate kidney function, or insufficient diuretic therapy. An age-related decline in plasma renin activity, tubular function, and glomerular filtration rate affects overall sodium and water homeostasis.[9]

Monitor how they feel

Pharmacologic management of hypertension. Older adults with CAD, hypertension, stable angina, or previous MI should be prescribed a beta-blocker for initial therapy.[4] Long-acting calcium antagonists (CA) may be added to initial therapy for BP control. Angiotensin-converting enzyme inhibitors (ACEI) are indicated if LV ejection fraction is reduced and/or if HF is present. Older adult patients with hypertension and systolic HF should receive a diuretic, beta-blocker, ACEI, and aldosterone antagonist.[4]

Age-Related Changes in Baroreceptor Function

Baroreflex-mediated tachycardia response to depressor agents is also attenuated in older adults.[10] Orthostatic hypotension results from alteration in distribution of blood volume with position change, resulting in a reduction in CO and BP.[10] The

Anticoagulant therapy

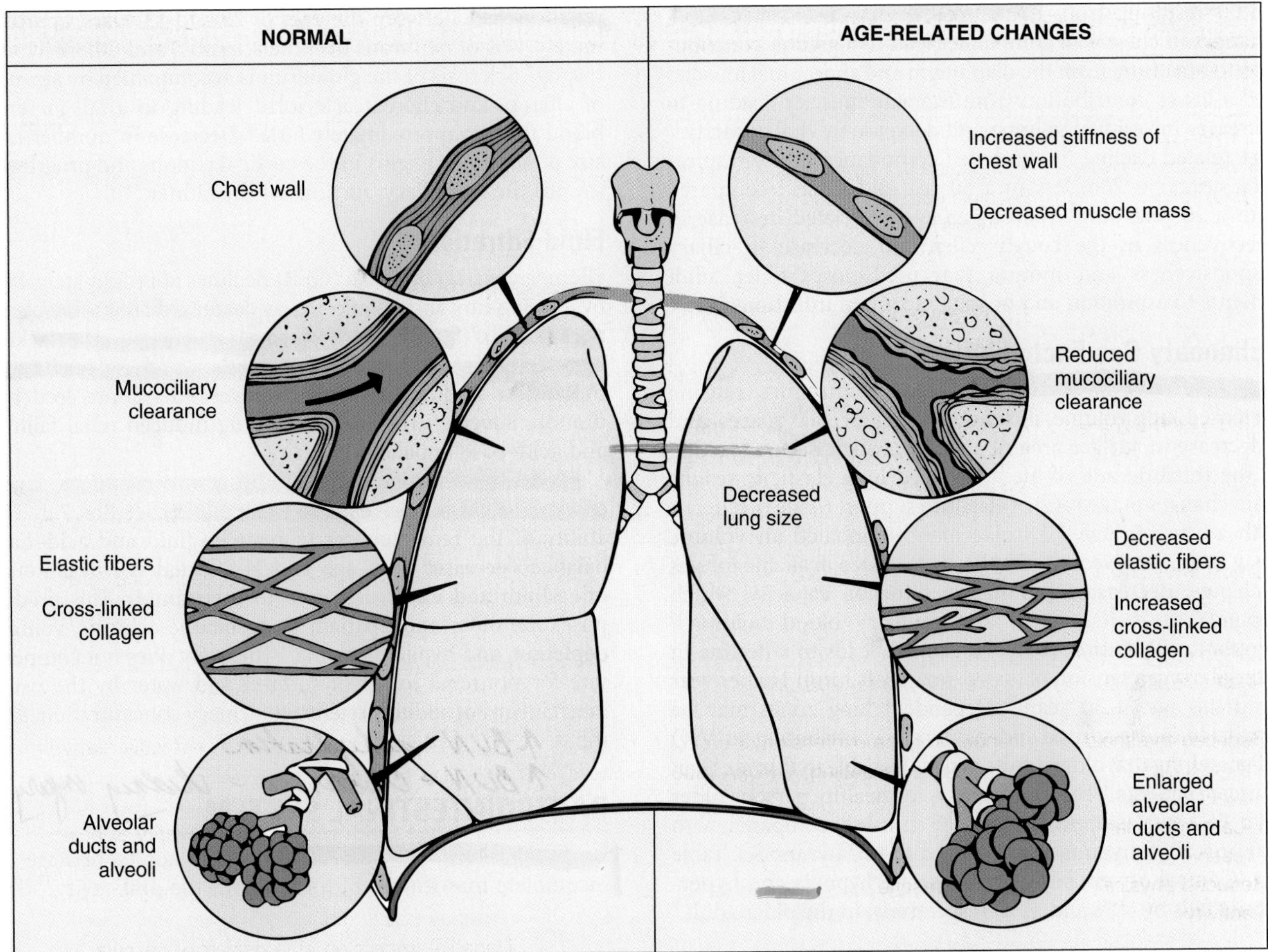

FIG 7-1 Age-related changes occur in the respiratory system. With advancing age, the compliance of the chest wall and lung tissue changes. There is also a reduced clearance of mucus by the cilia that line the pulmonary tree and an enlargement of the alveolar ducts and alveoli.

baroreceptor-reflex response mediates changes in heart rate, peripheral resistance and force of myocardial contraction, offsetting the drop in BP. Prevalence of orthostatic hypotension is greater in geriatric patients; therefore, judicious use of antihypertensive medications is recommended.[10]

Cardiac Medication Considerations in Older Adults

Treatment with medication should be considered when nonpharmacologic interventions are unsuccessful. Hypertension therapy should target a SBP of 140 mm Hg to 145 mm Hg and diastolic of greater than 95 mm Hg in patients older than 80 years of age.[4] Heart rate control can be managed with beta-blockers and calcium channel blockers. Amiodarone can be used for conversion and maintenance of sinus rhythm with atrial fibrillation.[4] Aging increases the risk of major hemorrhage in patients with atrial fibrillation, with or without anticoagulation therapy.[4] Anticoagulation therapy can be complicated by polypharmacy, simultaneous use of antiplatelet medications, uncontrolled hypertension, and poorly controlled anticoagulation therapy.[11] Ventricular dysrhythmias are best managed with cardiac-resynchronization therapy and pharmacologic therapy in patients with advanced HF.[12]

PULMONARY SYSTEM

Many changes in the pulmonary system occur with aging, including changes in compliance of the chest wall, static elastic recoil of the lung, and strength of respiratory muscles.[13] Progressive changes due to age should not alter the older adult's ability to breathe effortlessly; however, factors such as repeated exposure to environmental pollutants and frequent pulmonary infections may accelerate age-related changes. See Figure 7-1.

Thoracic Wall and Respiratory Muscles

The aging thorax has a greater anterior–posterior diameter than in younger adults, and there is some degree of dorsal kyphosis due to osteoporosis.[13] Rib mobility declines due to contractures of intercostal muscles and calcification of costal cartilage, decreases in chest wall compliance, shape of the thorax, and changes in chest wall mechanics leading to deterioration in respiratory function.[13] During aging, skeletal muscle progressively atrophies, and its energy metabolism decreases.[13] Respiratory muscle performance is impaired by geometric modifications of the rib cage, decreased chest wall compliance, and increases in functional residual capacity

(FRC) resulting from decreased elastic recoil of the lung. Changes in chest wall compliance lead to a greater contribution to breathing from the diaphragm and abdominal muscles and a lesser contribution from thoracic muscles, leading to increases in residual volume and decrease in vital capacity.[13] Age-related decline in chest wall compliance of the respiratory system is 20% less in a 60-year-old subject compared with a 20-year-old.[13] There is an age-associated decrease in effectiveness of the cough reflex and decrease in ciliary responsiveness and motion that predisposes older adult patients to aspiration and hospital-acquired infections.[9]

Pulmonary Gas Exchange

Diminished recoil of the lung occurs with aging, causing increased lung volume, distention of the alveolar spaces, and a decrease in surface area of airspace, which occurs starting in the third decade of life.[13] Reduced lung elasticity results from changes in the ratio of elastic to support tissue that occur with advancing age.[14] Displacement of inhaled air volume away from the alveoli limits the surface area available for gas exchange, decreasing pulmonary diffusion capacity, which depends on surface area and capillary blood volume.[14] Ventilation/Perfusion (V/Q) mismatch leads to a decline in arterial oxygen tension of approximately 0.3 mm Hg per year from the age of 30 years.[2] Dependent lung zones may be ventilated and perfused inconsistently, contributing to V/Q mismatching that older adults may be less able to tolerate than younger patients.[9] The typical PaO_2 for healthy persons older than 65 years is approximately 89 mm Hg, compared with 100 mm Hg for younger adults aged 18 to 24 years. See Table 7-3. Control of ventilatory responses to hypoxia and hypercapnia falls by 50% and 40%, respectively, in the older adult.[9]

Lung Volumes and Capacities

Decreased 1-second forced expiratory volume (FEV_1)., maximal expiratory flow rate, and maximal mid-expiratory flow rate are decreased in older adults.[15] Older adults may experience decreased T-cell function, decline in mucociliary clearance, and a reduced swallowing ability with loss of cough reflex, increasing frequency and severity of pneumonia in older adults.

RENAL SYSTEM

Acute kidney injury (AKI) is common in critically ill patients, with a prevalence ranging from 2% to 25%.[16] Age places patients at a higher risk of developing AKI and end-stage renal disease. Between the ages of 25 and 85 years, approximately 40% of nephrons become sclerotic, and others hypertrophy.[9] Sclerosis of the glomeruli is accompanied by atrophy of afferent and efferent arterioles, leading to a fall in renal blood flow of approximately 50%.[9] Decrease in number and size of nephrons begins in the cortical regions and progresses toward the medullary portions of the kidney.[9]

TABLE 7-3 Progressive Changes in Arterial Oxygen Tension and Carbon Dioxide Tension

AGE GROUP (YR)	PaO_2 (mm Hg)	$PaCO_2$ (mm Hg)
≤30	94	39
31-40	87	38
41-50	84	40
51-60	81	39
>60	74	40

$PaCO_2$, Carbon dioxide tension; *PaO_2*, arterial oxygen tension.
Data from Sorbini CA, et al: Arterial oxygen tension in relation to age in healthy subjects, *Respiration* 25:3, 1968.

Fluid Filtration

Glomerular filtration rate (GFR) declines approximately 45% by age 80 years and is reflected as decreased creatinine clearance (CrCl).[9] Decreased GFR in older adults is most likely caused by decreased nephron number and reduced renal blood flow. Reduced GFR predisposes older adults to dehydration, adverse drug reactions, drug-induced renal failure, and acid–base imbalance.[9]

Blood urea nitrogen (BUN) and serum creatinine levels can be normal or decreased in older adults. See Box 7-1. The ability of the renal tubules to regulate fluid and acid–base balance decreases with age and is affected by the amount of sodium and water delivered to the tubules. This predisposes the older adult patient to metabolic acidosis, volume depletion, and hyperchloremia.[9] The body does not compensate for nonrenal losses of sodium and water by the usual mechanisms of sodium retention, urinary concentration, and thirst.

GASTROINTESTINAL SYSTEM

Swallowing may be difficult for older adults because of incomplete mastication of food within the oral cavity.[17] The

BOX 7-1 Effects of Aging on Various Laboratory Values

Values That Do Not Change with Age

- Hemoglobin, hematocrit
- Platelet count
- White blood cell count with differential
- Serum electrolytes
- Coagulation profile
- Liver function tests
- Thyroid function tests
- NC or ↓ Blood urea nitrogen
- NC or ↓ Creatinine

Values That Change with Age but Have Little Clinical Significance

- ↓ Calcium
- ↑ Uric acid

Values That Change with Age and Have Clinical Significance

- ↓ Erythrocyte sedimentation rate
- ↓ Arterial oxygen pressure
- ↑ Blood glucose
- ↓ or ↑ Serum lipid profile
- ↓ Albumin

NC, No change; ↓ decreased; ↑ increased.
From Duthie EH, Abbasi AA: Laboratory testing: current recommendations for older adults, *Geriatrics* 46:41, 1991.

result of deteriorating dentition, diminished lubrication (from salivary dysfunction), ill-fitting dentures, and incomplete mastication can put the older adult patient at risk for aspiration.[2] The number and velocity of peristaltic contractions in the older adult's esophagus decreases, and the number of nonperistaltic contractions increases.[17] These changes in esophageal motility are referred to as *presbyesophagus.* The epithelial layer of mucosa results in esophagitis and gastritis-prevalence in older adults.[17] Aging alters taste, smell, and gastric motility. Dysphagia and alterations in motor and sensory function can lead to silent aspiration and delay in gastric emptying that may contribute to postprandial hypotension and maldigestion. Gag reflex has been reported to be absent in 40% of healthy older adults, and reports have revealed a reduction in esophageal peristalsis, increase in non-propulsive contractions, and reduction in lower esophageal sphincter pressure.[18]

Few age-related changes have been noted in sensory and motor function of the small bowel; however, aging is linked to weakening of colonic muscles and altered rectal sensation. Structure and function of the pelvic floor and anorectum may contribute to constipation, fecal incontinence, and diverticulosis encountered in older adults.[18] Although most vitamins and minerals are normally absorbed, calcium absorption is reduced, fat-soluble vitamin A is increased, and there is the potential for impaired absorption of vitamin D, B_{12}, and folic acid.[19] Thinning of intestinal lining, decreased mucus production, weaker intestinal muscles, and medications mobility may increase risks of constipation and fecal impaction in older adult patients.[19]

Age-Related Changes in the Liver

Mortality ascribed to liver disease may increase four-fold in adults aged 45 to 85 years.[20] Age-related changes in hepatic function include a reduction in synthesis of cholesterol, total bile acid pool, and bile acid from cholesterol. There is also a reduced capacity of the liver for regeneration in response to injury compared with a younger population, which may enhance the progress of hepatic diseases and compromise liver transplantation.[20] Tests of liver function are unaltered with advancing age. The most important age-related change in liver function decreases the liver's capacity to metabolize medications.[20] Polypharmacy is cited as a common cause of adverse medication reactions in the older adult population.[20]

Individuals with alcoholic hepatitis and underlying alcoholic cirrhosis have the highest mortality. Reports suggest that 5% to 15% of older adults over 65 years of age have alcohol-related problems.[21] Hepatocellular carcinoma is the most common complication of liver cirrhosis affecting older adults.[21]

CENTRAL NERVOUS SYSTEM

Cognitive Functioning and Aging

Cognitive functioning has become one of the greatest threats of old age with more than 50% of older adults over the age of 85 years affected by Alzheimer's disease.[22]

Structure and Morphology

The brain decreases approximately 20% in size between 25 and 95 years of age.[23] See Figures 7-2 and 7-3. Neurons are lost from the hippocampus, amygdala, cerebellum, and from areas of the brainstem such as the locus ceruleus, dorsal motor nucleus of the vagus, and substantia nigra. Conversely, very few neurons disappear from the hypothalamus with advancing age.[22] Portions of the cerebral cortex atrophy, predominantly the frontal and temporal cortical association areas (the superior frontal gyrus and superior temporal gyrus, respectively).[22] Cerebral blood flow is influenced by age-related changes in BP, barometric response to positional change, and severity of CVD. Accompanying the loss of neurons are changes in ultrastructure and intracellular structures of the neuron, including decrease of dendrites and axons.

IMMUNE SYSTEM

Infections in older adults are usually more severe and frequent than those in younger adults. Common infections in the older adult are associated with bacterial pneumonia, urinary tract infection, intra-abdominal infections, gram-negative bacteremia, and decubitus ulcers.[24] Increased susceptibility to infection may be due to cell-mediated and humoral-mediated immunity and breakdown in physical barriers, such as the skin and oral mucosa. Adults older than age 65 are hospitalized at more than three times the rate of persons of all ages.[24]

Cell-Mediated and Humoral-Mediated Immunity

Immune system function depends on many cell types with distinct functions. T cells are the primary effector of cell-mediated immunity, whereas bone marrow-derived B cells produce antibodies that are effector cells of humoral-mediated immunity. Cell-mediated immunity declines and T-cell function decreases with aging despite the total number of T cells remaining unchanged.[25] Older adults show deficiencies in the ability to produce appropriate defensive immune responses to pathogens and vaccines, contributing to increased vulnerability to infections and bacterial pathogens. Defects in T-cell function are often found in protective immunity at the cellular and humoral levels. Evidence suggests that T cells from older adult donors are generally slower and of lower amplitude than responses of T cells from younger individuals.

Older patients may have an impaired ability of bone marrow to increase neutrophil production in response to infection, and those with major infections often have normal white blood cell counts, but the differential count usually shows a large proportion of immature forms. Sepsis and septic shock in the older adult may present as acute mental status changes, anorexia, urinary incontinence, falls, or generalized weakness.[24]

INTEGUMENTARY AND MUSCULOSKELETAL SYSTEMS

Older adult conditions of the skin include seborrheic keratosis, xerosis, and Campbell de Morgan spots.[26] Older adults are vulnerable to intrinsic and extrinsic dermatologic conditions resulting from degenerative and metabolic changes occurring throughout the skin layers.[26] Intrinsic aging refers to the skin's natural, metabolic aging process where the skin's upper layers become thin and blood flow is decreased, which leads to a reduced ability to nourish and repair cells. Extrinsic influences describe metabolic reactions to environmental factors

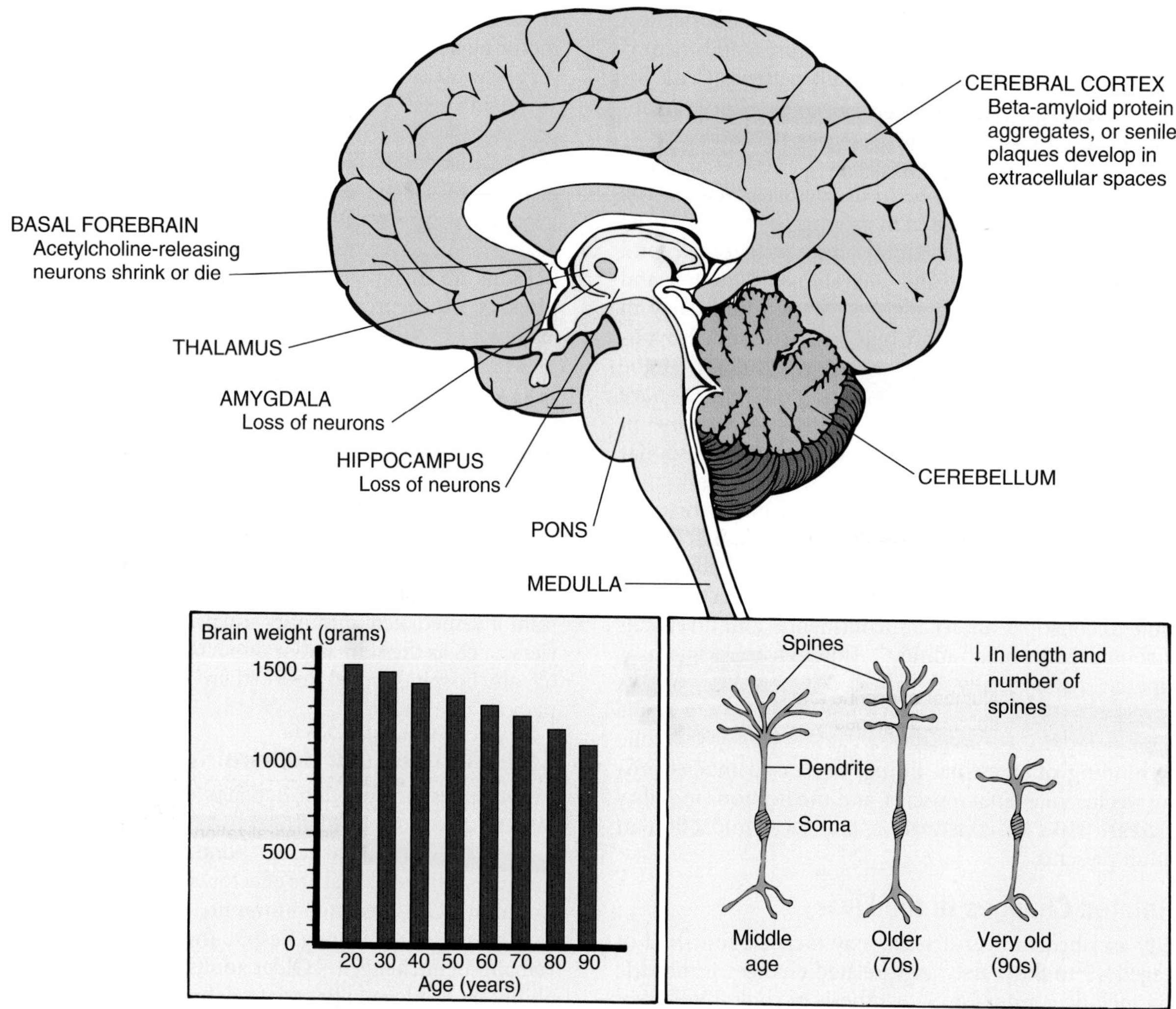

FIG 7-2 Summary of age-related changes in the brain. (From Selkoe DJ: Aging brain, aging mind, *Sci Am* 267:134, 1992.)

such as solar radiation/sun exposure that leads to a decline in dermatologic integrity and skin that easily sags, breaks, bruises, and itches.[26] Alterations in collagen structure reduce overall skin elasticity, and reductions in immune function degrade the skin's ability to protect against bacterial assault and cause the skin to wrinkle.[26] The underlying structures such as veins and muscles are more visible because of skin transparency. Nearly 1 million Americans develop chronic wounds, with annual prevalence of 10% to 35% in frail older adults.[27] Impaired wound healing is affected by disease conditions, comorbidities, environment, genetic factors, and the aging process.[27] There is an increase in body fat, a decrease in lean muscle mass, and a decline in muscle strength due to selective loss of muscle fibers by up to 40% at age 80 years.[9] Energy expenditure decreases with age, with resting energy expenditure decreasing by as much as 15%.[9] Oxygen consumption and energy expenditure after acute illness or injury are approximately 20% to 25% less in patients over 65 years than in younger patients.

Bone demineralization affects both men and women as they age but occurs more often in women than in men, predisposing older adults to fractures.[28] Decreased intake of dietary calcium, immobility, excess glucocorticoid secretion, and smoking all contribute to development of osteoporosis. Physical signs of deformities associated with osteoporosis, such as kyphosis or scoliosis, may place limitations on physical mobility or lead to gait instability. Fractures, particularly hip fractures, are especially devastating in older adults, leading to diminished QOL and increased morbidity and mortality.[28]

PHARMACOLOGIC THERAPY IN OLDER ADULTS

Adverse drug effects and medication interactions may be related to pharmacokinetics or the manner in which the body absorbs, distributes, metabolizes, and excretes a medication.[29] See Table 7-4. The aging process is associated with changes in gastric acid secretion, fat content increases, lean body mass decreases, and total body water decreases, which can alter medication disposition. The senescent liver and kidneys are less able to metabolize and excrete medications, leading to changes in absorption rates, time to peak plasma concentration, and clearance. Table 7-5 lists potentially inappropriate symptom management medications for older adults.

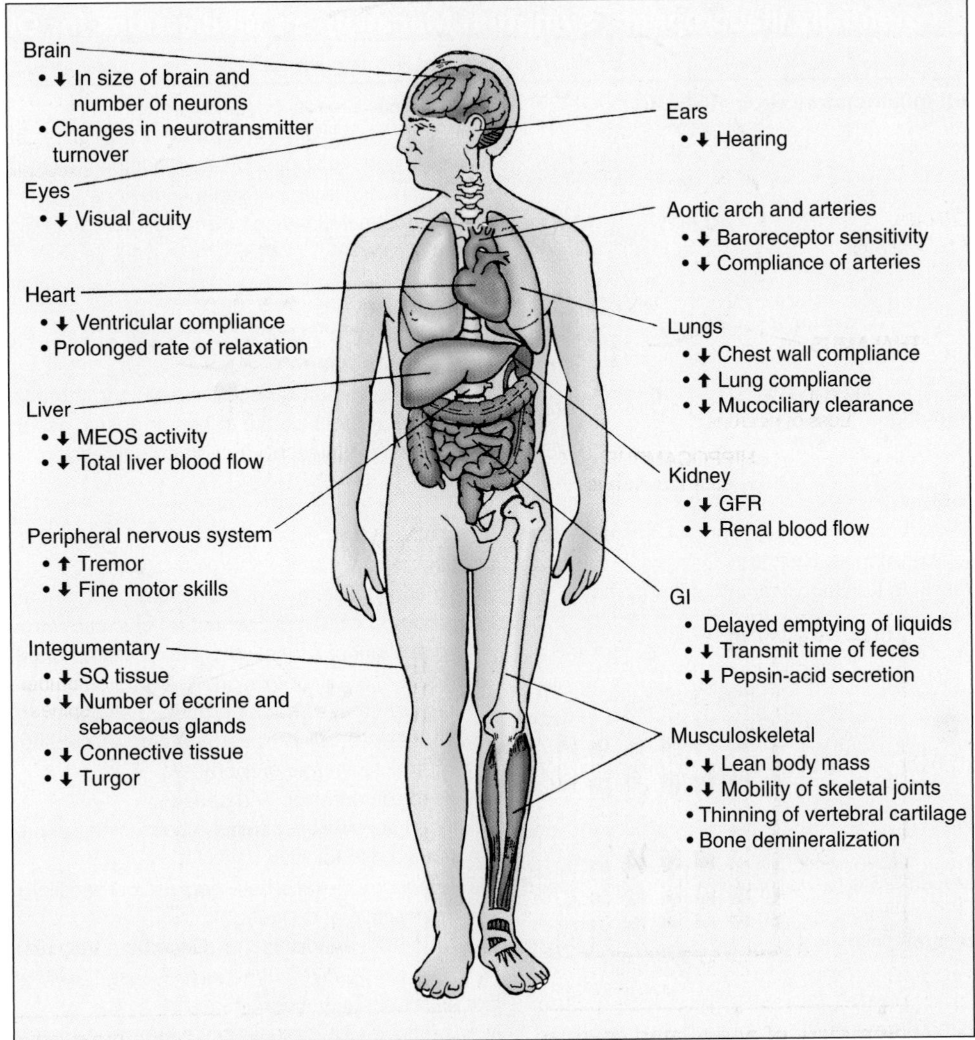

FIG 7-3 Summary of the physiologic changes that occur in all systems and that the critical care nurse must consider in caring for the older adult patient in the critical care unit. *GFR*, Glomerular filtration rate; *GI*, gastrointestinal; *MEOS*, microsomal enzyme oxidative system; *SQ*, subcutaneous.

TABLE 7-4 Age-Related Changes in Pharmacokinetics

PHARMACOKINETIC PARAMETER	DEFINITION	AGE-RELATED CHANGES
Absorption	Receptor-coupled or diffusional uptake of medication into tissue	Decreased absorptive surface area of small intestine Decreased splanchnic blood flow Increased gastric acid pH Decreased gastrointestinal motility
Distribution	Theoretic space (tissue) or body compartment into which free form of medication distributes	Decreased lean body mass and total body water Increased total body fat Decreased serum albumin level Increased alpha$_1$-acid glycoprotein
Metabolism	Chemical change in medication that renders it active or inactive	Decreased liver mass Decreased activity of microsomal medication-metabolizing enzyme system Decreased total liver blood flow
Excretion	Removal of medication through an eliminating organ, often the kidney; some medications are excreted in bile or feces, in saliva, or through the lungs.	Decreased renal blood flow and glomerular filtration rate Decreased distal renal tubular secretory function

TABLE 7-5 Potentially Inappropriate Symptom Management Medications for Older Adults

MEDICATION	POSSIBLE SIDE EFFECT
Nonsteroidal Anti-Inflammatory Drugs (NSAIDs)‡	
Indomethacin	Central nervous system (CNS) effects (highest of all NSAIDs)*
Ketorolac	Asymptomatic gastrointestinal conditions (ulcers*)
Aspirin (>325 mg)	Asymptomatic gastrointestinal conditions (ulcers*)
Naproxen	Gastrointestinal bleeding*; renal failure*; high blood pressure*; heart failure*
Opioids	
Meperidine	Intense side-effect profile for adverse effects, especially CNS effects (seizures) Most critical in individuals with renal compromise*
Morphine, hydromorphone, fentanyl	Intense side-effect profile at higher doses, especially CNS effects (such as somnolence, respiratory depression, and delirium)*
Adjuvant Medications	
Muscle relaxants (methocarbamol, carisoprodol, chlorzoxazone, metaxalone, cyclobenzaprine, baclofen)	Anticholinergic effects*†; sedation*; weakness*; cognitive impairment*
Tricyclic antidepressants (amitriptyline and amitriptyline compounds)	Strong anticholinergic effects*†; may lead to ataxia, impaired psychomotor function, syncope, falls; cardiac arrhythmias (QT interval changes)*; may produce polyuria or lead to urinary incontinence*; may exacerbate chronic constipation
Doxepin	Cardiac arrhythmias*; may produce polyuria or lead to urinary incontinence*; may exacerbate chronic constipation
Antihistamines (diphenhydramine, hydroxyzine, promethazine)	Potent anticholinergic properties*† May lead to confusion and sedation
Benzodiazepines	Increased sensitivity at higher doses with prolonged sedation and increased risk for falls
Short-acting (lorazepam ≥3 mg, oxazepam ≥60 mg, alprazolam ≥2 mg)	May produce or exacerbate depression; smaller doses may be both effective and safer.
Long-acting (diazepam)	CNS effects*; may cause or exacerbate respiratory depression in chronic obstructive pulmonary disease*; may produce polyuria or lead to urinary incontinence*
Selective serotonin reuptake inhibitor antidepressants (fluoxetine, citalopram, paroxetine, sertraline)	May produce CNS stimulation, sleep disturbances, and increasing agitation*; may exacerbate or cause syndrome of inappropriate secretion of antidiuretic hormone or hyponatremia
Decongestants	High level of CNS stimulation, which may lead to insomnia*
CNS stimulants (methylphenidate)	Altered CNS function, leading to cognitive impairment*; appetite-suppressing effect*

Based on data from Fick DM, et al: Updating the Beers criteria for potentially inappropriate medication use in older adults: results of a US consensus panel of experts, *Arch of Intern Med* 163(22):2716-2724, 2003. doi:10.1001/archinte.163.22.2716; Laroche ML, Charmes JP, Merle L: Potentially inappropriate medications in the elderly: a French consensus panel list, *Eur J Clinical Pharmacol* 63(8):725-731, 2007. doi 10.1007/s00228-007-0324-2; Campanelli CM: American Geriatrics Society Updated Beers Criteria for Potentially Inappropriate Medication Use in Older Adults: The American Geriatrics Society 2012 Beers Criteria Update Expert Panel, *J Am Geriatr Soc* 60(4):616, 2012. doi: 10.1111/j.1532-5415.2012.03923.x

*High-severity rating.

†Anticholinergic effects include some of the following symptoms: blurred vision, constipation, drowsiness, sedation, dry mouth, tachycardia, urinary retention, confusion, disorientation, memory impairment, dizziness, nausea, nervousness, agitation, anxiety, facial flushing, weakness, and delirium.

‡May cause or exacerbate gastric or duodenal ulcers, prolonged clotting time and international normalized ratio, and decreased platelet function.

HOSPITAL-ASSOCIATED RISK FACTORS FOR OLDER ADULTS

Pre-existing conditions can be exacerbated with critical illness or hospital encounters. Invasive devices such as central lines or chest tubes and indwelling catheters may threaten suppressed immune systems. Nutritional deficiencies may compound muscle weakness and mood. Older adults require more intense observation and consideration in critical care units because they are less adaptable to stress and illness (Table 7-1).

Care Transitions

Transitions of care are difficult for older adults, increasing fragmentation of care and transfer of information between health care providers.[30] Families and informal caregivers of vulnerable older adults often become the messengers between providers. Older adults without family frequently remain in

CASE STUDY Older Patient with Myocardial Infarction and Anemia

Brief Patient History

Ms. Smith is a 90-year-old woman with a long history of heart disease. Over the past month, Ms. Smith has experienced fatigue, indigestion, and loss of appetite, leading to weight loss and depression.

Clinical Assessment

Ms. Smith is admitted to the critical care unit from the emergency department for hypotension, change in level of consciousness, and electrolyte abnormalities. Nursing assessment findings show dysphagia, weight loss, poor eye sight, and hearing loss. She also has minimal urine output.

Diagnostic Procedures

Ms. Smith's admission laboratory work reveals increased BUN, creatinine, and sodium with baseline vital signs including blood pressure of 85/60 mm Hg, heart rate of 120 beats/min, respiratory rate of 22 breaths/min, and temperature of 99.6° F, with Q waves on ECG.

Medical Diagnosis

Ms. Smith is diagnosed with an old myocardial infarction and dehydration.

Questions

1. What major outcomes do you expect to achieve for this patient?
2. What problems or risks must be managed to achieve these outcomes?
3. What interventions must be initiated to monitor, prevent, manage, or eliminate the problems and risks identified?
4. What interventions should be initiated to promote optimal functioning, safety, and well-being of the patient?
5. What possible learning needs do you anticipate for this patient?
6. What cultural and age-related factors may have a bearing on the patient's plan of care?

higher levels of care for extended time periods, reducing bed availability for others.

REFERENCES

1. Resnick NM, et al: Geriatric medicine. In Kasper D, et al, editors: *Harrison's principles of internal medicine*, ed 16, New York, 2005, McGraw-Hill.
2. North BJ: The intersection between aging and cardiovascular disease, *Circ Res* 110(8):1097, 2012. doi: 10.1161/CIRCRESAHA.111.246876.
3. Strait J, et al: Aging-associated cardiovascular changes and their relationship to heart failure, *Heart Fail Clin* 8(1):143, 2012.
4. Aronow WS, et al: ACCF/AHA 2011 Expert Consensus Document on Hypertension in the Elderly: A Report of the American College of Cardiology Foundation Task Force on Clinical Expert Consensus Documents, *J Am Coll Cardiol* 57(20):2037, 2011.
5. Gazoti Debassa CR, Messiano Maifrino LB, Rodrigues de Souza R: Age-related changes of the collagen network of the human heart, *Mech Ageing Dev* 122(2001):1049, 2001.
6. Heidenreich PA, et al: Forecasting the future of cardiovascular disease in the United States a policy statement from the American Heart Association, *Circulation* 123(8):933–944, 2011.
7. Desai AS, Stevenson LW: Rehospitalization for heart failure predict or prevent? *Circulation* 126(4):501–506, 2012. doi: 10.1161/CIRCULATIONAHA.112.125435.
8. Shih H, et al: The aging heart and post-infarction left ventricular remodeling, *JACC* 57(1):9, 2010.
9. Marik P: Management of the critically ill geriatric patient. In O'Donnell JM, Nacul FE, editors: *Surgical intensive care medicine*, ed 2, New York, 2010, Springer Science.
10. Hajjar I: Postural blood pressure changes and orthostatic hypotension in elderly patients: impact of antihypertensive medications, *Drugs Aging* 22(1):55, 2005.
11. Cooney D, Pascuzzi K: Polypharmacy in the elderly Focus on drug interactions and adherence in hypertension, *Clin Geriatr Med* 25:221, 2009. doi: 10.1016/j.cger.2009.01.005.
12. Moss AJ, et al: Cardiacresynchronization therapy for the prevention of heart failure events, *N Engl J Med* 361:1, 2009.
13. Janssens JP: Aging of the respiratory system: impact on pulmonary function tests and adaptation to exertion, *Clin Chest Med* 26(30), 2005.
14. Bonomo L, et al: Aging and the respiratory system, *Radiol Clin North Am* 46(4), 2008.
15. Fragoso CAV, Gill TM: Respiratory impairment and the aging lung: a novel paradigm for assessing pulmonary function, *J Gerentol A Biol Sci Med Sci* 67A(3):264, 2011. doi: 10.1093/gerona/glr198.
16. Chao CT, et al: Advanced age affects the outcome-predictive power of RIFLE classification in geriatric patients with acute kidney injury, *Kidney Int* 80:1222, 2012. doi: 10.1038/.
17. Clark JA, Coopersmith CM: Intestinal crosstalk: a new paradigm for understanding the gut as the "motor" of critical illness, *Shock* 28:384, 2007.
18. Bitar K, et al: Aging and gastrointestinal neuromuscular function: insights from within and outside the gut, *Neurogastroenterol Motil* 23:490, 2011.
19. Lacasse C: Polypharmacy and symptom management in older adults, *Clin J Oncol Nurs* 15(1):27, 2010. doi: 10.1188/11.CJON.27-30.
20. Schmucker DL: Age-related changes in liver structure and function: Implications for disease? *Exper Gerontol* 40:650, 2005. doi: 10.1016/j.exger.2005.06.009.
21. Floreani A: Liver disorders in the elderly, *Best Pract Res Clin Gastroenterol* 23:909, 2009.
22. Bishop NA, Lu T, Yankner BA: Neural mechanisms of ageing and cognitive decline, *Nature* 464:529, 2010.
23. Quinn J, Kaye J: The neurology of aging, *Neurologist* 7:98, 2001.
24. Htwe TH, et al: Infection in the elderly, *Infect Dis Clin North Am* 21(3):711, 2007.
25. Akha AAS, Miller RA: Signal transduction in the aging immune system, *Curr Opin Immunol* 17(5):486, 2005.
26. Smith DR, Leggat PA: Prevalence of skin disease among the elderly in different clinical environments, *Aust J Ageing* 24(2):71, 2005.
27. Pittman J: Effect of aging on wound healing current concepts, *J WOCN* 34:412, 2007.

28. Black DM, Rosen CJ: Following the bone density trail: a clinical perspective, *J Clin Endocrinol Metab* 97(4):1176, 2012. doi: 10.1210/jc.2012-1528.
29. American Geriatrics Society 2012 Beers Criteria Update Expert Panel: American Geriatrics Society updated Beers Criteria for potentially inappropriate medication use in older adults, *J Am Geriatr Soc* 60(4):616, 2012.
30. Manderson B, et al: Navigation roles support chronically ill older adults through healthcare transitions: a systematic review of the literature, *Health Soc Care Community* 20(2):113, 2012. doi: 10.1111/j.1365-2524.2011.01032.x.

CHAPTER 8

Pain and Pain Management

Céline Gélinas, Caroline Arbour

Be sure to check out the bonus material, including review questions, on the Evolve website at http://evolve.elsevier.com/Urden/priorities/.

Despite national and international efforts, guidelines, standards of practice, position statements, and many important discoveries in the field of pain management in the past 3 decades, critically ill patients suffer from moderate to severe pain which can be experienced at rest or during routine care.[1,2] For instance, chest tube removal, turning, drain removal, and wound care were identified as the most painful procedures by critically ill adults in previous studies.[2-4] Despite this situation, pain remains undertreated in most critically ill patients. Poor treatment of acute pain may lead to the development of serious complications and chronic pain syndromes, which may seriously impact the patient's functioning, quality of life, and well-being. Such evidence reinforces the importance of providing attention to pain in this specific context of care.

IMPORTANCE OF PAIN ASSESSMENT

Appropriate pain assessment is the foundation of effective pain treatment. Because pain is recognized as a subjective experience, the patient's self-report is considered the most valid measure for pain and should be obtained as often as possible.[5] Unfortunately in critical care, many factors such as the administration of sedative agents, the use of mechanical ventilation, and altered levels of consciousness may impact communication with patients. These obstacles make pain assessment more complex. Nevertheless, except for being unable to speak, many mechanically ventilated patients can communicate that they are in pain by using head nodding, hand motions, or by seeking attention with other movements.[4,6]

Self-report pain intensity scales have been used with postoperative mechanically ventilated patients who were asked to point on the scale.[2,7] However, in a study of mechanically ventilated adults with various diagnoses (trauma, surgical, or medical), only one- third of mechanically ventilated patients were able to use a pain intensity scale.[7] With a greater degree of critical illness, providing a pain intensity self-report becomes more difficult because it requires concentration and energy. When the patient is unable to communicate in any way, observable behavioral and physiologic indicators become unique indices for pain assessment as recommended by clinical guidelines.[8,9] Pain is frequently encountered in critical care, and there is increased emphasis on the professional responsibility to manage the patient's pain effectively. The critical care nurse must understand the mechanisms, assessment process, and appropriate therapeutic measures for managing pain.

This chapter provides an understanding of the physiology of pain and discusses indicators of pain assessment and pain management in critically ill patients.

DEFINITION AND DESCRIPTION OF PAIN

Pain is described as an unpleasant sensory and emotional experience associated with actual or potential tissue damage or described in terms of such damage.[10] Specifically, the subjective characteristic implies that pain is whatever the person experiencing it says it is and that it exists whenever the patient says it does.[11] This definition also suggests that the patient is able to self-report. However, in the critical care context, many patients are unable to self-report their pain.

Components of Pain

The experience of pain includes sensory, affective, cognitive, behavioral, and physiologic components:[12]

- *Sensory component:* Perception of many characteristics of pain, such as intensity, location, and quality
- *Affective component:* Negative emotions such as unpleasantness, anxiety, fear, and anticipation that may be associated with the experience of pain
- *Cognitive component:* Interpretation or the meaning of pain by the person who is experiencing it
- *Behavioral component:* Strategies used by the person to express, avoid, or control pain
- *Physiologic component:* Nociception and the stress response

Types of Pain

Pain can be acute or chronic, with different sensations related to the origin of the pain.

Acute Pain

Acute pain has a short duration, and it usually corresponds to the healing process (30 days) but should not exceed 6 months. It implies tissue damage that is usually from an identifiable cause. If undertreated, acute pain may bring a prolonged stress response and lead to permanent damage to the patient's nervous system. In such instance, acute pain can become chronic pain.

use same pain scale
find out an acceptable level of pain

Chronic Pain

Chronic pain persists for more than 6 months after the healing process from the original injury, and it may or may not be associated with an illness.[13] It develops when the healing process is incomplete or when acute pain is poorly managed.[14]

Both acute and chronic pain can have a nociceptive or neuropathic origin.[5]

Nociceptive Pain

Nociceptive pain arises from activation of nociceptors,[5] and it can be somatic or visceral. Somatic pain involves superficial tissues, such as the skin, muscles, joints, and bones. Its location is well-defined. Visceral pain involves organs such as the heart, stomach, and liver. Its location is diffuse, and it can be referred to a different location in the body.[15-17]

Neuropathic Pain

Neuropathic pain arises from a lesion or disease affecting the somatosensory system.[5] The origin of neuropathic pain may be peripheral or central. Neuralgia and neuropathy are examples related to peripheral neuropathic pain, which implies a damage of the peripheral somatosensory system. Central neuropathic pain involves the central somatosensory cortex and can be experienced by patients after a cerebral stroke. Neuropathic pain can be difficult to manage and frequently requires a multimodal approach that combines several pharmacological and/or nonpharmacological treatments.[15]

Physiology of Pain

Nociception

Nociception represents the neural processes of encoding and processing noxious stimuli[5] but are not sufficient for pain. Pain results from the integration of the pain-related signal into specific cortical areas of the brain associated with higher mental processes and consciousness. In other words, pain is the conscious experience that may emerge from nociception. Four processes are involved in nociception[15]:

1. Transduction
2. Transmission
3. Perception
4. Modulation

The four processes are shown in Figure 8-1, which integrates pain assessment with nociception, and in Figure 8-2.

Transduction

Transduction refers to mechanical (e.g., surgical incision), thermal (e.g., burn), or chemical (e.g., toxic substance) stimuli that damage tissues. In critical care, many nociceptive stimuli exist that exacerbate the patients' acute illness including invasive technologies and interventions. These stimuli, also called stressors, stimulate the liberation of chemical substances, such as prostaglandins, bradykinin, serotonin, histamine, glutamate, and substance P. These neurotransmitters stimulate peripheral nociceptive receptors and initiate nociceptive transmission.

Transmission

As a result of transduction, an action potential is produced and is transmitted by nociceptive nerve fibers in the spinal cord that reach higher centers of the brain. This is called transmission, and it represents the second process of nociception. The principal nociceptive fibers are the A-delta and C fibers. Large-diameter, myelinated Aδ fibers transmit well-localized, sharp pain, are involved in "first pain," and lead to reflex withdrawal. Small-diameter, unmyelinated C fibers transmit diffuse, dull, aching pain, often referred to as "second pain."[17] These fibers transmit the noxious sensation from the periphery through the dorsal root of the spinal cord. With the liberation of substance P, these fibers then synapse with ascending spinothalamic fibers to the central nervous system (CNS). These spinothalamic fibers are clustered into two specific pathways: neospinothalamic (NS) and paleospinothalamic (PS) pathways. Generally, the Ad fibers transmit the pain sensation to the brain within the NS pathway, and the C fibers use the PS pathway.[18]

Through synapsing of nociceptive fibers with motor fibers in the spinal cord, muscle rigidity can appear because of a reflex activity.[19] Muscle rigidity can be a behavioral indicator associated with pain. It can contribute to immobility and decrease diaphragmatic excursion. This can lead to hypoventilation and hypoxemia. Hypoxemia can be detected by a pulse oximeter (SpO_2) and by oxygen arterial pressure (PaO_2) monitoring. An intubated patient's activation of alarms or fighting the ventilator may indicate the presence of pain.[20]

Perception

The pain message is transmitted by the spinothalamic pathways to centers in the brain, where it is perceived. Pain sensation transmitted by the NS pathway reaches the thalamus, and the pain sensation transmitted by the PS pathway reaches brainstem, hypothalamus, and thalamus.[18] These parts of the CNS contribute to the initial perception of pain. Projections to the limbic system and the frontal cortex allow expression of the affective component of pain.[21] Projections to the sensory cortex located in the parietal lobe allow the patient to describe the sensory characteristics of pain, such as location, intensity, and quality.[21,22]

Modulation

Modulation is a process by which painful messages that travel from the nociceptive receptors to the CNS may be enhanced or inhibited. A typical example of ascending pain modulation is rubbing an injury site, thus activating large A-beta fibers in the periphery.[18] In the descending pain modulation mechanism, the efferent spinothalamic nerve fibers that descend from the brain can inhibit the propagation of the pain signal by triggering the release of endogenous opioids in the brainstem and in the spinal cord. Serotonin and norepinephrine are important inhibitory neurotransmitters that act in the CNS. These substances are also released by the descending fibers of the descending spinothalamic pathway.[23] The use of distraction, relaxation, and imagery techniques facilitate the release of endogenous opioids and have been shown to reduce the overall pain experience.[24]

PAIN ASSESSMENT

Pain assessment is an integral part of nursing care. It is a prerequisite for adequate pain control and relief. Pain assessment has two major components: 1) nonobservable or subjective and 2) observable or objective. The complexity of pain

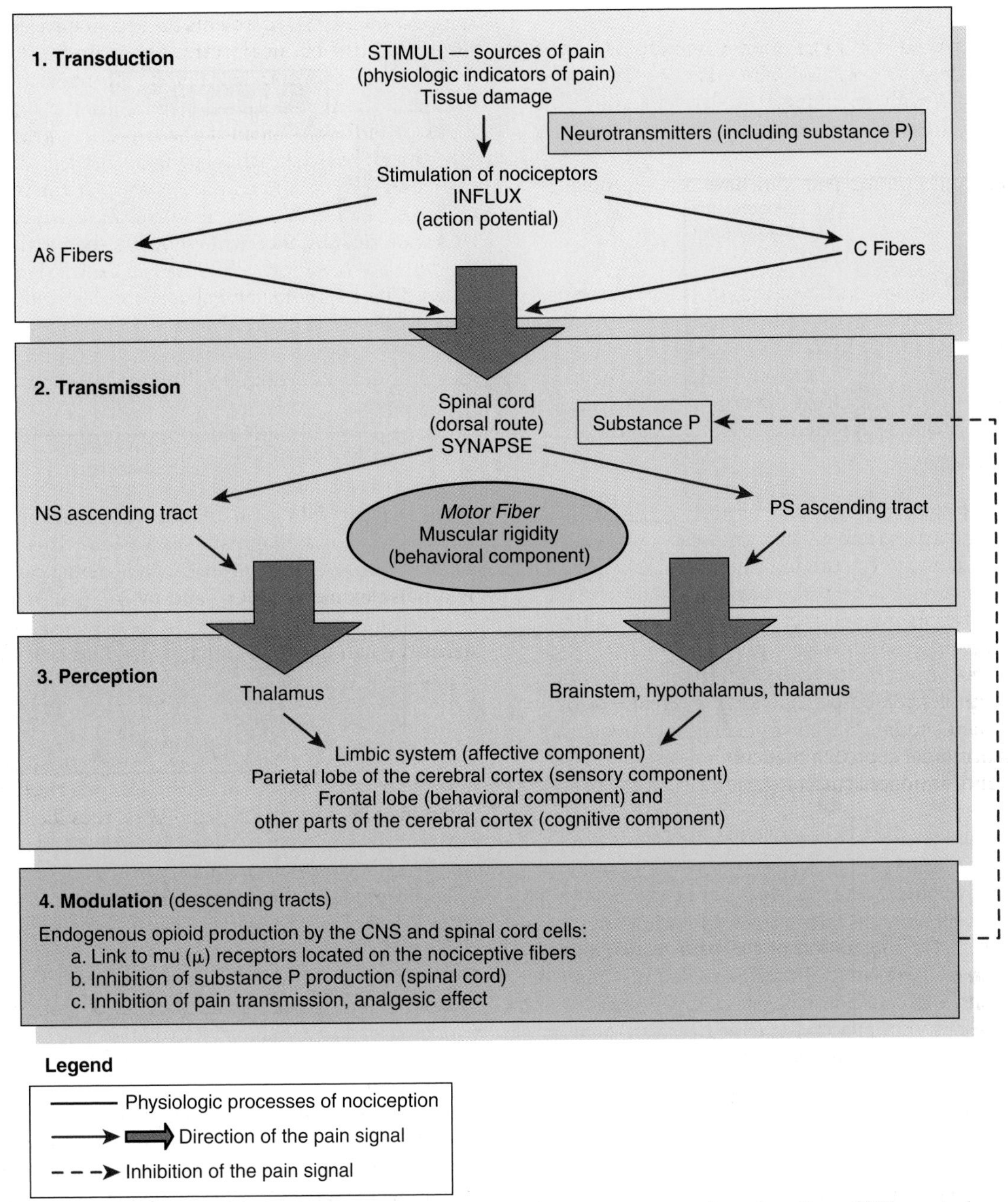

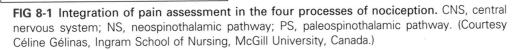

FIG 8-1 Integration of pain assessment in the four processes of nociception. CNS, central nervous system; NS, neospinothalamic pathway; PS, paleospinothalamic pathway. (Courtesy Céline Gélinas, Ingram School of Nursing, McGill University, Canada.)

assessment requires the use of multiple strategies. In the following sections, patient, health professional, and organizational barriers to pain assessment and management are addressed, and recommendations are proposed.

Pain Assessment: The Subjective Component

Pain is a subjective experience. The subjective component of pain assessment refers to the patient's self-report of pain, and this must be obtained whenever possible.[8] A simple yes or no (presence versus absence of pain) is considered a valid self-report. Mechanical ventilation should not be a barrier for nurses to document patients' self-reports of pain. Many mechanically ventilated patients can communicate that they have pain or can use pain scales by pointing to numbers or symbols on the scale.[2,4,7] Sufficient time should be allowed for the patient to respond to the questions.[8]

If sedation and cognition levels allow the patient to give more information about pain, a multidimensional assessment can be documented. Multidimensional pain assessment tools, including the sensorial, emotional, and cognitive components, are available such as the Brief Pain Inventory,[25] the Initial Pain Assessment Tool,[15] and the McGill Pain Questionnaire–Short Form.[26] However, because of the administration of sedative and analgesic agents in mechanically ventilated patients, the tool must be short enough to be completed. For instance, the McGill Pain Questionnaire–Short

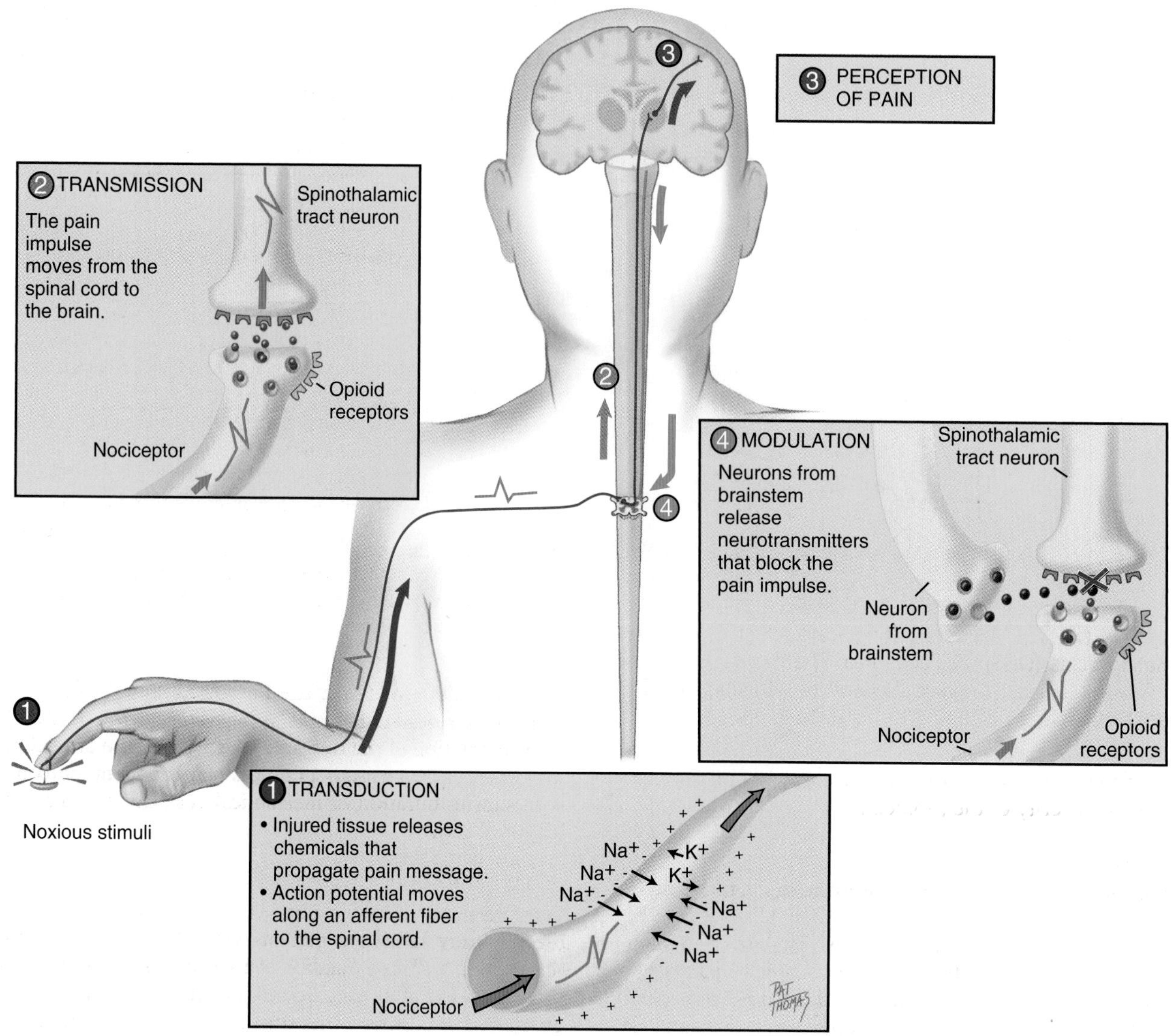

FIG 8-2 The four processes of nociception. (From Jarvis C: *Physical examination & health assessment*, ed 6, Philadelphia, 2011, Saunders.)

Form takes 2 to 3 minutes to complete and has been used to assess mechanically ventilated patients who were in a stable condition.[2]

The patient's self-report of pain can also be obtained by questioning the patient using the mnemonic PQRSTU:[27]

P: provocative and palliative or aggravating factors
Q: quality
R: region or location, radiation
S: severity
T: timing
U: understanding

P: Provocative and Palliative or Aggravating Factors

The P in the mnemonic indicates what provokes or causes the patient's pain, what he or she was doing when the pain appeared, and what makes the pain worse or better.

Q: Quality

Q refers to the quality of the pain or the pain sensation that the patient is experiencing. For instance, the patient may describe the pain as dull, aching, sharp, burning, or stabbing. This information provides the nurse with data regarding the type of pain the patient is experiencing.

R: Region or Location, Radiation

R usually is easy for the patient to identify, although visceral pain is more difficult for the patient to localize.[15] If the patient has difficulty naming the location or is mechanically ventilated, ask that the patient point to the location on himself or herself or on a simple anatomic drawing.

S: Severity

S denotes pain severity or intensity. Many visual analog scales are available, as are the descriptive and numeric pain rating scales often used in the critical care environment (Figure 8-3). Asking the patient to grade pain intensity on a scale of 0 to 10 is a consistent method and helps objectify the subjective nature of the patient's pain.

T: Timing

T refers to documenting the onset, duration, and frequency of pain. This information can help to determine whether the

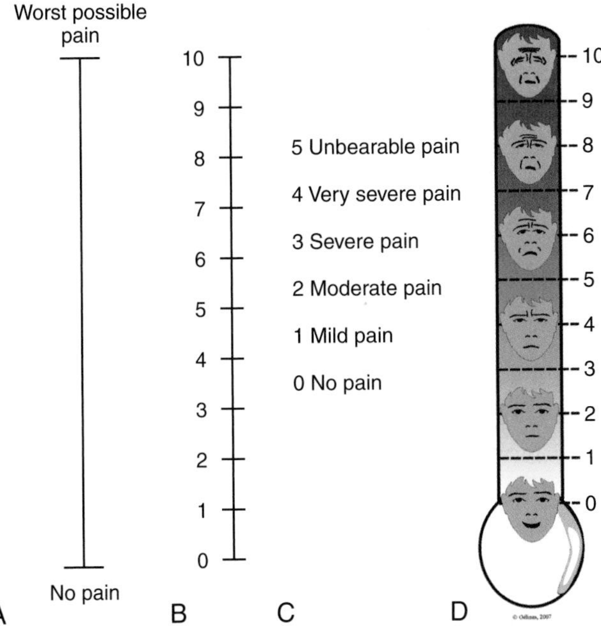

FIG 8-3 **Pain intensity scales (vertical format).** *A*, Visual analog scale (VAS). *B*, Numeric Rating Scale (NRS). *C*, Descriptive Rating Scale (DRS). *D*, Faces Pain Thermometer. (Courtesy Céline Gélinas, Ingram School of Nursing, McGill University, Canada.)

origin of the pain is acute or chronic. Duration of pain can indicate the severity of the problem.

U: Understanding

U is the patient's perception of the problem or cognitive experience of pain.

Begin by asking, "Do you have pain?" The use of a simple yes or no question allows the patient to answer verbally or to indicate by nodding the head or by other signs. It is often easier for mechanically ventilated patients to communicate with clinicians in this way because they cannot express themselves verbally. Pain intensity and location also are necessary for the initial assessment of pain.

Pain Assessment: The Observable or Objective Component

When the patient's self-report is impossible to obtain, nurses can rely on the observation of behavioral indicators, which are strongly emphasized in clinical recommendations and guidelines for pain management in nonverbal patients.[8,9] Similarly, fluctuations in physiologic indicators (i.e., vital signs) can be used as a cue to begin further assessment for pain.

Pain-related behaviors have been described in critically ill patients and were studied in the AACN Thunder Project II.[28] Patients who experienced pain during nociceptive procedures were three times more likely to have tense facial expressions, muscle rigidity, and vocalization than patients without pain. Patients who experienced pain during turning showed significantly more intense facial expressions (e.g., grimacing), muscle rigidity, and less compliance with the ventilator (e.g., fighting the ventilator) compared with patients without pain.[20] Behavioral indicators are strongly recommended for pain assessment in nonverbal patients,[8] and several tools are recommended in guidelines for critically ill adults,[9] including the Behavioral Pain Scale (BPS)[29] and the Critical-Care Pain Observation Tool (CPOT).[30] Implementation of the BPS and the CPOT in the critical care unit has improved pain practices[31] and patient outcomes, with shorter duration of mechanical ventilation and shorter length of stay.[32]

TABLE 8-1 Behavioral Pain Scale (BPS)

ITEM	DESCRIPTION	SCORE
Facial expression	Relaxed	1
	Partially tightened (e.g., brow lowering)	2
	Fully tightened (e.g., eyelid closing)	3
	Grimacing	4
Upper limbs	No movement	1
	Partially bent	2
	Fully bent with finger flexion	3
	Permanently retracted	4
Compliance with ventilation	Tolerating movement	1
	Coughing but tolerating ventilation for most of the time	2
	Fighting ventilator	3
	Unable to control ventilation	4
Total		3 to 12

From Payen JF, et al. Assessing pain in the critically ill sedated patients by using a behavioral pain scale. *Crit Care Med* 29 (12): 2258-2263, 2001.

Behavioral Pain Scale

The BPS shown in Table 8-1 was tested mostly in nonverbal mechanically ventilated patients with altered levels of consciousness.[29,33-36] The validity of its use was supported with significantly higher BPS scores during nociceptive procedures (e.g., turning, endotracheal suctioning, peripheral veinous cannulation) compared with rest or nonnociceptive procedures (e.g., arterial catheter dressing change, compression stocking applications, eye care). The authors of the BPS determined a cut-off score >5 for the presence of pain.

Critical-Care Pain Observation Tool

The CPOT shown in Table 8-2 was tested in verbal and nonverbal, critically ill adult patients.[7,20,30,37] Content validation was supported by expert critical care clinicians, including nurses and physicians.[38] Validity of the CPOT use was supported with significantly higher CPOT scores during a nociceptive procedure (e.g., turning with or without other care) compared with rest or a nonnociceptive procedure (e.g., taking blood pressure). Positive associations were found between the CPOT scores and the patient's self-report of pain.[7,20,30] A cut-off score >2 was established with the CPOT in postoperative adults in critical care unit.[39] Similarly to the BPS, good interrater reliability of CPOT scores was achieved with critical care nurses.[7,30] Feasibility and satisfaction of the CPOT were positively evaluated by nurses at 12-month post-implementation of its use in the critical care unit.[40]

Use of Cutoff Scores

A cutoff score refers to the score on a specific scale associated with the best probability of correctly ruling in or ruling out

TABLE 8-2 Critical Care Pain Observation Tool (CPOT)

INDICATOR	SCORE		DESCRIPTION
Facial expression	Relaxed, neutral	0	No muscle tension observed
	Tense	1	Presence of frowning/brow lowering, orbit tightening and levator contraction or any other change (e.g., opening eyes or tearing during nociceptive procedures)
Relaxed, neutral 0; Tense 1; Grimace 2	Grimacing	2	All previous facial movements plus eyelid tightly closed (the patient may present with mouth open or biting the endotracheal tube)
Body movements	Absence of movements or normal position	0	Does not move at all (doesn't necessarily mean absence of pain) or normal position (movements not aimed toward the pain site or not made for the purpose of protection)
	Protection	1	Slow, cautious movements, touching or rubbing the pain site, seeking attention through movements
	Restlessness/ Agitation	2	Pulling tube, attempting to sit up, moving limbs/thrashing, not following commands, striking at staff, trying to climb out of bed
Compliance with the ventilator (intubated patients) *or*	Tolerating ventilator or movement	0	Alarms not activated, easy ventilation
	Coughing but tolerating	1	Coughing, alarms may be activated but stop spontaneously
	Fighting ventilator	2	Asynchrony: blocking ventilation, alarms frequently activated
Vocalization (nonintubated patients)	Talking in normal tone or no sound	0	Talking in normal tone or no sound
	Sighing, moaning	1	Sighing, moaning
	Crying out, sobbing	2	Crying out, sobbing
Muscle tension	Relaxed	0	No resistance to passive movements
	Tense, rigid	1	Resistance to passive movements
	Very tense or rigid	2	Strong resistance to passive movements, incapacity to complete them
TOTAL		___ / 8	

TABLE 8-2 Critical Care Pain Observation Tool (CPOT)—cont'd

INDICATOR	SCORE	DESCRIPTION

1. The patient must be observed at rest for 1 minute to obtain a baseline value of the CPOT.
   1.1 **Observation of patient at rest (baseline).**
   The nurse looks at the patient's face and body to note any visible reactions for an observation period of 1 minute. She gives a score for all items except for muscle tension. At the end of the one-minute period, the nurse holds the patient's arm in both hands—one at the elbow, and uses the other one to hold the patient's hand. Then, she performs a passive flexion and extension of the upper limb and feels any resistance the patient may exhibit. If the movements are performed easily, the patient is found to be relaxed with no resistance (score 0). If the movements can still be performed but with more strength, then it is concluded that the patient is showing resistance to movements (score 1). If the nurse cannot complete the movements, strong resistance is felt (score 2). This can be observed in patients who are spastic.
2. Then, the patient should be observed during painful procedures (e.g., turning, wound care) to detect any changes in the patient's behaviors.
   2.2 **Observation of patient during a painful procedure.**
   While she's performing a procedure known to be painful, the nurse looks at the patient's face to note any reactions such as brow lowering or grimacing. These reactions may be brief or can last longer. The nurse also looks out for body movements. For instance, she looks for protective movements like the patient trying to reach or touching the pain site (e.g., surgical incision, injury site). In the mechanically ventilated patient, she pays attention to alarms and if they stop spontaneously or require that she intervenes (e.g., reassurance, administering medication). According to muscle tension, the nurse can feel if the patient is resisting the movement or not. A score 2 is given when the patient is resisting against the movement and attempts to get on his/her back.
3. The patient should be evaluated before and at the peak effect of an analgesic agent to assess whether the treatment was effective or not in relieving pain.
4. The patient should be attributed the highest score observed during the observation period.
5. The patient should be attributed a score for each behavior included in the CPOT, and muscle tension should be evaluated last as it may lead to behavioral reactions not necessarily related to pain, but more to the actual stimulation.

Modified from Gélinas C, et al. Validation of the Critical-Care Pain Observation Tool (CPOT) in adult patients, *Am J Crit Care* 15: 420, 2006. Figure of facial expressions a courtesy of Caroline Arbour, RN, BSc, PhD, McGill University, Canada, and redrawn by Elsevier. An online teaching video funded and created by Kaiser Permanente Northern California Nursing Research (KPNCNR) to learn how to use the CPOT at the bedside is available at http://pointers.audiovideoweb.com/stcasx/il83win10115/CPOT2011-WMV.wmv/play.asx.

a patient with a specific condition—in this case, pain. The use of a cutoff score with behavioral pain scales can help to identify when pain is highly likely to be present and guide nurses in determining whether an intervention to alleviate pain is required or not. Also, a cutoff score can help to evaluate the effectiveness of pain management interventions. It is important to highlight that cutoff scores are established using a criterion (i.e., a gold standard in the field). For a case example showing how a cutoff score can be used in practice, refer to Box 8-1.

Physiologic Indicators

When patients cannot react behaviorally to pain, the only possible clues left for the detection of pain are physiologic indicators (i.e., vital signs).[41] Although vital sign values generally increase during painful procedures,[7,20,41,29,36] they are not consistently related to the patient's self-report of pain, nor are they predictive of pain.[7,20] For example, none of the monitored vital signs (heart rate, mean arterial pressure [MAP], respiratory rate, transcutaneous oxygen saturation [SpO_2], and end-tidal CO_2 capnography) predicted the presence of pain in critical care patients.[20]

The American Society for Pain Management Nursing (ASPMN) recommendations emphasize that vital signs should *not* be considered as primary indicators of pain because they can be attributed to other distress conditions, homeostatic changes, and medications. See Box 8-2 for Internet Resources. Changes in vital signs offer a cue to begin further assessment of pain or other stressors.[8]

BOX 8-1 Case Example of Using a Cutoff Score with the CPOT

A patient is admitted to the critical care unit following cardiac surgery. He is mechanically ventilated and too drowsy to communicate effectively with the nurse using signs (i.e., head nodding or pointing on a communication board). However, he seems to be uncomfortable as he becomes agitated each time he's being touched. The nurse in charge is puzzled about the need to administer an analgesic or a sedative—both prescribed on the postoperative care protocol. She first assesses for the presence of pain and gets a score of 4 out of 8 on the CPOT as the patient grimaces and attempts to sit in the bed. Considering that a CPOT score higher than 2 strongly suggests the presence of pain, the nurse gives a dose of subcutaneous analgesic. Thirty minutes after the administration of analgesic, the patient has a relaxed face and is cautiously moving his hand from time to time toward the surgical wound on his chest. The CPOT score is now 1 out of 8, indicating pain relief as it dropped from 4 to 1 (i.e., more than 2 points).

CPOT, Critical Care Pain Observation Tool.

Fifth Vital Sign

Because pain is considered the fifth vital sign, including pain assessment with other routinely documented vital signs may help ensure that pain is assessed and controlled for in all patients on a regular basis. This approach can ensure that pain

hourly + PRN

BOX 8-2 INTERNET RESOURCES

ASPMN	American Society for Pain Management Nursing	http://www.aspmn.org/
APS	American Pain Society	http://www.americanpainsociety.org
SCCM	Society of Critical Care Medicine	http://www.sccm.org/
Pain Agitation Delirium guidelines		http://www.learnicu.org/SiteCollectionDocuments/Pain,%20Agitation,%20Delirium.pdf

is detected and treatment implemented before the patient develops complications associated with unrelieved pain. The use of a pain flow sheet in critical care settings allows for a visible and on-going pain assessment before and after an intervention for pain. This communication tool may be in the electronic health record, or on paper, and should be accessible to all clinicians involved in the assessment and management of pain.[31,42]

Patient Barriers to Pain and Assessment Management

Communication

The most obvious patient barrier to the assessment of pain in the critical care population is an alteration in the ability to communicate. The patient who is mechanically ventilated cannot verbalize a description of the pain. If the patient can communicate in any way, such as by head nodding or pointing, pain can be reported in that manner. If writing is possible, the patient may be able to describe the pain thoroughly. With patients unable to self-report, the nurse relies on behavioral indicators to assess the presence of pain.

The patient's family can contribute significantly in pain assessment. The family is intimately familiar with the patient's normal responses to pain and can assist in identifying clues. A family member's impression of a patient's pain should be considered in the pain assessment process of the critically ill patient.[8]

Altered Level of Consciousness

The patient who is unconscious or has an altered level of consciousness presents a dilemma for all clinicians. Because pain relies on cortical response to provide recognition, the belief that the patient with a brain injury altering higher cortical function has no perception of pain may persist. Conversely, the inability to interpret the nociceptive transmission does not negate the transmission. Interviews with 100 patients, who recalled their experiences from a time when they were unconscious in critical care, revealed that they could hear, understand, and respond emotionally to what was being said.[43] Experts recommend assuming that patients who are unconscious or with an altered level of consciousness have pain and that they be treated the same way as conscious patients are treated when they are exposed to sources of pain.[8] It has been demonstrated that behavioral indicators of pain can be observed in reaction to a painful procedure in critically ill patients, no matter what their level of consciousness.[20] Moreover, it has been shown that some cortical activation related to pain perception is still present in unconscious patients in a neurovegetative state.[44] Knowing this, the critical care nurse can initiate a discussion with the other members of the health care team to formulate a plan of care for the patient's comfort.

Older Patients

Many elderly patients do not complain much about pain. Some misconceptions, such as believing that pain is a normal consequence of aging or being afraid to disturb the health care team, are barriers to pain expression for the elderly.[15] Cognitive deficits or delirium present additional pain assessment barriers. Many elderly patients with mild-to-moderate cognitive impairments and even some with severe impairment are able to use pain intensity scales.[45,46] Vertical pain intensity scales are more easily understood by this group of patients and are recommended[8] (see Figure 8-3). Elderly patients with cognitive deficits should receive repeated instructions and be given sufficient time to respond.[16] More than 24 behavioral tools have been developed for elderly patients with cognitive deficits.[43,46,47] The Pain Assessment Checklist for Seniors with Limited Ability to Communicate (PACSLAC),[48] Doloplus-2,[49] and the Pain Assessment in Advanced Dementia (PAINAD)[50] are promising tools that are recommended by experts.[47,51]

Cultural Influences

Another barrier to accurate pain assessment is cultural influences on pain and pain reporting. Cultural influences are compounded when the patient speaks a language other than that of the health team members. To facilitate communication, the use of a pain intensity scale in the patient's language is vital. The 0 to 10 numeric pain scales have been translated into many different languages.[15]

Lack of Knowledge

A relatively overlooked patient barrier to accurate pain assessment is the public knowledge deficit regarding pain and pain management. Many patients and their families are frightened by the risk of addiction to pain medication. They fear that addiction will occur if the patient is medicated frequently or with sufficient amounts of opioids necessary to relieve the pain. This concern is so powerful for some that they will deny or deliberately underreport the frequency or intensity of pain. It is important to teach the family and the patient about the importance of pain control and the use of opioids in treating pain in critical illness.

Health Professional Barriers to Pain Assessment and Management

The health professional's beliefs and attitudes about pain and pain management are frequently a barrier to accurate and adequate pain assessment. This can lead to poor management practices. Addiction rates for patients in acute pain who receive opioid analgesics are less than 1%. Some of the false beliefs that surround addiction result from a lack of knowledge about addiction and tolerance, and other concerns are related to the possible side effects of opioids.

Addiction and Tolerance

Addiction is defined by a pattern of compulsive drug use that is characterized by an incessant longing for an opioid and the need to use it for effects other than pain relief.

Tolerance is defined as a diminution of opioid effects over time. Physical dependence and tolerance to opioids may develop if the opioid is given over a long period. Physical dependence is manifested by withdrawal symptoms when the opioid is abruptly stopped. If this is an anticipated problem, withdrawal may be avoided by weaning the patient from the opioid slowly to allow the brain to reestablish neurochemical balance in the absence of the opioid.[15]

Respiratory Depression

Another concern of the health care professional is the fear that aggressive management of pain with opioids will cause critical respiratory depression. Opioids can cause respiratory depression, but when used safely, this is a rare phenomenon. The incidence of respiratory depression is less than 2%.[52,53]

PAIN MANAGEMENT

The management of pain in the critically ill patient is as multidimensional as the assessment. It is a multidisciplinary task. The control of pain can be pharmacologic, nonpharmacologic, or a combination of the two therapies. Pharmacologic pain management is predominantly used in critical care.

Pharmacologic Control of Pain

Pharmacologic management of pain has infinite variety in the critical care unit. Although this chapter is not an in-depth discussion of pharmacology, some commonly administered agents are discussed. Pain pharmacology is divided into three categories of action: opioid agonists, non-opioids, and adjuvants. Elements of the Pain Agitation Delirium guidelines of the Society of Critical Care Medicine (SCCM) for pharmacologic interventions in the critically ill adult are presented for each medication. How pain is approached and managed is a progression or combination of the available agents, the type of pain, and the patient response to the therapy.

Opioid Analgesics

The opioids most commonly used and recommended as first-line analgesics are the agonists. These opioids bind to mu (μ) receptors (transmission process) responsible for pain relief. Additional pharmacologic information is presented in Table 8-4. SCCM guidelines for pain management are summarized in Box 8-3, and in the Pain Care Bundle in Figure 8-4.[9]

Morphine. Morphine is the most commonly prescribed opioid in the critical care unit. Because of its water solubility, morphine has a slower onset of action and a longer duration compared with the lipid-soluble opioids (e.g., fentanyl). This makes it and hydromorphone preferred opioids for intermittent therapy.[9] Morphine has two main metabolites: morphine-3-glucuronide (M3G, inactive) and morphine-6-glucuronide (M6G, active). M6G is responsible for the analgesic effect but may accumulate and cause excessive sedation in patients with kidney failure or liver failure.[54] Morphine is available in a variety of delivery methods. It is the standard by which all other opioids are measured. It is also the agent that most closely mimics the endogenous opioids in the human pain modification system.

PAIN

ASSESS

Assess pain ≥ 4x/shift & prn
Preferred pain assessment tools:
- Patient able to self-report → NRS (0-10)
- Unable to self-report → BPS (3-12) or CPOT (0-8)

Patient is in significant pain if NRS > 3, BPS > 5, or CPOT > 2

TREAT

Treat pain within 30 minutes then reassess:
- Non-pharmacologic treatment—e.g., relaxation therapy
- Pharmacologic treatment:
  - — Non-neuropathic pain → IV opioids +/− non-opioid analgesics
  - — Neuropathic pain → gabapentin or carbamazipine, + IV opioids
  - — S/P AAA repair, rib fractures → thoracic epidural

PREVENT

- Administer pre-procedural analgesia and/or non-pharmacologic interventions (e.g., relaxation therapy)
- Treat pain first, then sedate

FIG 8-4 Pain Care Bundle. *AAA,* abdominal aortic aneurysm; *BPS,* Behavioral Pain Scale; *CPOT,* Critical Care Pain Observation Tool; *IV,* Intravenous; *S/P,* Status post; *NRS,* Numeric Rating Scale. (From Barr J, et al: Clinical practice guidelines for the management of pain, agitation, and delirium in adult patients in the intensive care unit, *Crit Care Med* 41:263, 2013.)

Morphine is indicated for severe pain. It has additional actions that are helpful for managing other symptoms. Morphine dilates peripheral veins and arteries, making it useful in reducing myocardial workload. Morphine is also viewed as an antianxiety agent because of the calming effect it produces.

Many side effects have been reported with the use of morphine (see Table 8-3). The hypotensive effect can be particularly problematic in the hypovolemic patient. The vasodilation effect is potentiated in the volume-depleted patient, and the hemodynamic status must be carefully monitored. Volume resuscitation restores blood pressure in the event of a prolonged hypotensive response.

A more serious side effect requiring diligent monitoring is the respiratory depressant effect. Opioids may cause this complication because they reduce the responsiveness of carbon dioxide chemoreceptors in the respiratory center located in the medulla.[55] Risk factors for opioid-induced respiratory depression include advanced age, obesity, sleep apnea, impaired kidney/lung/liver/heart function, patients in whom pain is controlled after a period of poor control, patients who are opioid naïve (i.e., receiving opioids for less

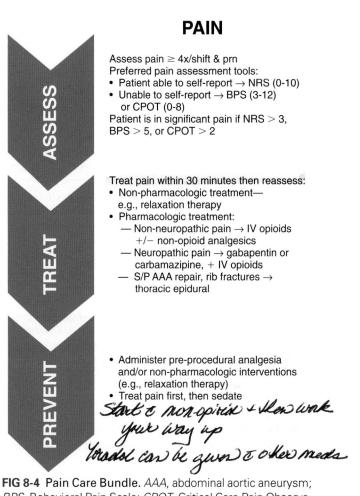

BOX 8-3 Summary of Pain and Analgesia Guidelines

1. Critically ill patients routinely experience pain at rest and with nursing and medical procedures. Pain in cardiac surgery patients, especially women, is poorly treated. Procedural pain is common in critically ill patients.
2. Perform routine pain assessment in all patients. In motoring intact patients unable to self-report, we suggest using behavioral pain scales rather than vital signs to assess pain. The BPS and CPOT are the most valid and reliable behavioral pain scales. Vital signs should only be used as a cue for further pain assessment.
3. For non-neuropathic pain, use intravenous opioids as first-line analgesic therapy; use non-opioid analgesics to reduce opioid side effects, and use either gabapentin or carbamazepine in conjunction with intravenous opioids for neuropathic pain.
4. Suggest preemptively treating procedural pain, especially chest tube removal.
5. Use thoracic epidural analgesia for abdominal aortic surgery and suggest also using for traumatic rib fractures. No evidence guides the use of lumbar epidural analgesia for abdominal aneurysm surgery or thoracic epidural analgesia for either intrathoracic or nonvascular abdominal surgical procedures. No evidence guides the use of regional vs. systemic analgesia in medical critical care patients.

From: Barr J, et al. Clinical practice guidelines for the management of pain, agitation, and delirium in adult patients in the intensive care unit, *Crit Care Med* 41:263, 2013.

TABLE 8-3 Pharmacologic Management: Pain

MEDICATION	DOSAGE	ONSET (min)	DURATION (hr)	AVAILABLE ROUTES	PROPERTIES	SIDE EFFECTS AND COMMENTS
Morphine	1-4 mg IV bolus 1-10 mg IV infusion	5-10	3-4	PO, SL, R, IV, IM, SC, EA, IA	Analgesia, antianxiety	Srandard for comparison Side effects: sedation, respiratory depression, euphoria or dysphoria, hypotension, nausea, vomiting, pruritus, constipation, urinary retention M6G can accumulate in patients with kidney failure or liver failure.
Fentanyl	25-100 μg IV bolus 25-200 μg IV infusion	1-5	0.5-4	OTFC, IV, IM, TD, EA, IA	Analgesia, antianxiety	Same side effects as morphine Rigidity with high doses
Hydromorphone (Dilaudid)	0.2-1 mg IV bolus 0.2-2 mg IV infusion	5	3-4	PO, R, IV, IM, SC, EA, IA	Analgesia, antianxiety	Same side effects as morphine
Codeine	15-30 mg IM, SC	10-20	3-4	PO, IM, SC	Analgesia (mild to moderate pain)	Lacks potency (unpredictable absorption; not all patients convert it to an active form to achieve analgesia) Most common side effects: light-headedness, dizziness, shortness of breath, sedation, nausea, and vomiting
Methadone (Dolophine)	5-10 mg IV	10	4-8	PO, SL, R, IV, SC, IM, EA, IA	Analgesia	Usually less sedating than morphine, but repeated doses can result in accumulation and can cause serious sedation (2-5 days).

TABLE 8-3 Pharmacologic Management: Pain—cont'd

MEDICATION	DOSAGE	ONSET (min)	DURATION (hr)	AVAILABLE ROUTES	PROPERTIES	SIDE EFFECTS AND COMMENTS
Acetaminophen	650 mg Maximum of 4 g/day	20-30	4-6	PO, R	Analgesia, antipyretic	Rare side effects Hepatotoxicity
Ketorolac (Toradol)	15-30 mg IV	<10	6-8	PO, IM, IV	Analgesia, minimum antiinflammatory effect	Short-term use (<5 days) Side effects: gastric ulceration, bleeding Use with care in elderly patients and with kidney failure.

EA, epidural analgesia; IA, intrathecal analgesia; IM, intramuscular; IV, intravenous; M6G, morphine-6-glucuronide; OTFC, oral transmucosal fentanyl citrate; PO, oral; R, rectal; SC, subcutaneous; SL, sublingual; TD, transdermal.

BOX 8-4 PRIORITY MEDICATIONS

Morphine Sulfate

Medication Class: Opioid
Medication Action: Analgesia

Medication Delivery and Medication Dosage

Morphine is administered in many ways. In critical care usual routes are IV bolus, IV continuous infusion, and PCA; also administered PO in tablet or liquid form (see Table 8-3).[9] Morphine may also be administered via continuous IV infusion. Dosage requirements vary widely between individuals depending on whether morphine is used to treat acute pain or chronic pain. Dosage requirements are generally higher in chronic pain related to pain severity and development of opioid tolerance over time. Consultation with a medical pain service to manage chronic pain effectively and enable the transition from IV to oral morphine is often helpful. Morphine is the standard opioid used for opioid comparison and conversion in equianalgesic dosing (see Table 8-4).

Priority Nursing Considerations

The goal is to alleviate pain while minimizing side effects. Morphine has many secondary effects that are unpleasant. The experience of unwanted secondary effects is not the same for everyone. In order of occurrence secondary symptoms include dry mouth, sedation, constipation, anxiety, confusion, nausea, sadness, myoclonus, difficulty urinating, hallucination, and vomiting. Nursing interventions to alleviate unpleasant symptoms include oral care to relieve dry mouth, use of an antiemetic to relieve nausea and vomiting, use of a stool softener and mobility as tolerated to decrease constipation, dosage adjustments or switching opioids to alleviate symptoms of sedation, confusion, hallucination, and myoclonus. If the patient does not have a urinary drainage catheter inserted, assess ability to void urine voluntarily. The risk of respiratory depression is a concern in the non-intubated patient. Monitoring of the respiratory rate, depth, and SpO_2 level to detect hypoventilation and respiratory depression is an essential nursing responsibility.

Clinical Examples

Morphine is used in a variety of clinical situations in critical care. It is successfully used to treat acute pain postoperatively. It is used to manage chronic pain such as severe cancer pain. Morphine is also used to alleviate symptoms of dyspnea and provide comfort at end of life (see Chapter 10). In each case the dose and delivery mechanism can differ. In each situation, the nurse must know the reason the medication is being given, continuously assess for side effects, and re-assess the efficacy of pain control.

than a week), concurrent use of central nervous system depressants, and postoperative day 1 were described.[53] In addition to side effects common to all opioids, morphine may stimulate histamine release from mast cells, resulting in cardiac instability and allergic reactions. See Box 8-4: Priority Medications—Morphine Sulphate.

Fentanyl. Fentanyl is a synthetic opioid preferred for critically ill patients with hemodynamic instability or morphine allergy. It is a lipid-soluble agent that has a more rapid onset than morphine and a shorter duration.[56] The metabolites of fentanyl are largely inactive and nontoxic, which makes it an effective and safe opioid. The use of fentanyl in the critical care unit is growing in popularity, and it is the preferred agent for acutely distressed patients. Fentanyl or hydromorphone are also recommended in hemodynamically unstable patients or patients with kidney impairment.[9] It is available in intravenous, intraspinal, and transdermal forms. The transdermal form is commonly referred to as the *Duragesic patch* or the *72-hour patch.*

Because the side effects of fentanyl are similar to those of morphine, the nurse must monitor hemodynamic and respiratory responses. When fentanyl is given by rapid administration and at higher doses, it has been associated with the additional hazard of bradycardia and rigidity in the chest wall muscles.[54,57] See Box 8-5: Priority Medications—Fentanyl.

BOX 8-5 PRIORITY MEDICATIONS

Fentanyl

Medication Class: Opioid
Medication Action: Analgesia

Medication Delivery and Dosage
A fentanyl IV bolus is high-potency, short-acting, and takes effect within 15 minutes. If pain is not relieved, the dose is repeated until the pain is controlled. Following pain control, continuous infusion or scheduled doses are administered to manage pain.

Priority Nursing Considerations
Fentanyl is lipid-soluble. It is classified as a short-acting opioid with a short half-life, but this depends on how the medication is administered. When given as an IV bolus, it provides rapid relief of pain, but the analgesic effect wears off quickly. This makes IV fentanyl a good choice to treat breakthrough pain, while a longer-acting opioid is taking effect in the background. If fentanyl is delivered by continuous IV infusion over several days, it can accumulate in the fat tissues over time, and the half-life is prolonged. Fentanyl accumulates in the tissues because it is lipid-soluble. In general the side effects are similar to those of morphine, including risk of respiratory depression and hypotension related to vasodilation in hypovolemic patients. Muscle rigidity is an uncommon side effect associated with fentanyl. As with other opioids, the goal of treatment is to alleviate pain while minimizing or avoiding opioid-related side effects.

Clinical Examples
Fentanyl is frequently used to control postoperative pain either as a continuous infusion or with IV bolus dosing in critical care. This practice follows the recommendations of the SCCM guidelines.[9]

Hydromorphone. Hydromorphone is a semisynthetic opioid that has an onset of action and a duration similar to those of morphine.[57] It is an effective opioid with multiple routes of delivery. It is more potent than morphine. Hydromorphone should be used with caution in renal or hepatic failure patients because its metabolite, hydromorphone-3-glucuronide, accumulates and can cause CNS toxicity. Some side effects (e.g., pruritus, sedation, nausea, vomiting) may occur less with hydromorphone than morphine.[58]

Meperidine. Meperidine (Demerol) is a less potent opioid with agonist effects similar to those of morphine. It is the weakest opioid and must be administered in large doses to be equivalent in action to morphine. Because the duration of action is short, dosing is frequent. A major concern with this medication is the metabolite *normeperidine*, which is a CNS neurotoxic agent. At high doses in patients with kidney failure, liver dysfunction, or in elderly patients, meperidine may induce CNS toxicity, including irritability, muscle spasticity, tremors, agitation, and seizures.[15] Although meperidine is useful in short-term specific conditions (e.g., treating postoperative shivering),[59] it should not be used routinely for analgesia in the critical care unit.[56,60,61]

Codeine. Codeine has limited use in the management of severe pain. It is rarely used in the critical care unit. It provides analgesia for mild to moderate pain. It is usually compounded with a non-opioid (e.g., acetaminophen). To be active, codeine must be metabolized in the liver to morphine.[15] Codeine is available only through oral, intramuscular, and subcutaneous routes, and its absorption can be reduced in the critical care patient by altered gastrointestinal motility and decreased tissue perfusion.

Methadone. Methadone is a synthetic opioid with morphine-like properties but less sedation. It is longer-acting than morphine. The long half-life makes it difficult to titrate in the critically ill patient. Methadone lacks active metabolites, and routes other than the kidney eliminate 60% of the medication. This means that methadone does not accumulate in patients with kidney failure. Prolongation of the QT interval may lead to the ventricular dysrhythmia torsades de pointe.[54]

More potent opioids: remifentanil and sufentanil. Remifentanil and sufentanil are agonist opioids. Remifentanil is 250 times more potent than morphine, and it has a rapid onset and predictable offset of action. For this reason, it allows a rapid emergence from sedation, facilitating the evaluation of the neurologic state of the patient after stopping the infusion.[62,63] As opposed to fentanyl, the use of remifentanil was associated with a lower incidence of post-operative delirium.[64]

Sufentanil is 7 to 13 times more potent than fentanyl and 500 to 1000 times more potent than morphine. It has more pronounced sedation properties than fentanyl and other opioids. Patients under sufentanil require minimal sedative agent doses to achieve an adequate sedation level. It has a rapid distribution and a high clearance rate, preventing accumulation when given for a long period.[65] Sufentanil has a longer emergence from sedation compared with remifentanil, but it allows a longer analgesic effect after stopping its administration.[63]

Preventing and Treating Respiratory Depression

Respiratory depression is the most life-threatening opioid side effect. The risk of respiratory depression increases when other medications with CNS depressant effects (e.g., benzodiazepines, antiemetics, neuroleptics, antihistamines) are concomitantly administered to the patient. While no universal definition of respiratory depression exists, it is usually described in terms of decreased respiratory rate (fewer than 8 or 10 breaths/minute), decreased SpO_2 levels or elevated end-tidal carbon dioxide ($ETCO_2$ levels).[55] A change in the patient's level of consciousness or an increase in sedation normally precedes respiratory depression.

Monitoring. Recent ASPMN monitoring guidelines[55] for patients receiving opioid analgesia recommend evaluation of respirations over 1 minute and assessed according to rate, rhythm, and depth of chest excursion. The use of technology-supported monitoring (e.g., continuous pulse oximetry and capnography) are recommended in high-risk patients.

Opioid reversal. Critical respiratory depression can be readily reversed with the administration of the opioid antagonist *naloxone*.[15] The usual dose is 0.4 mg, which is mixed with 10 mL of normal saline (for a concentration of 0.04 mg/mL). Naloxone is administered intravenously very slowly (0.5 mL over 2 minutes) while the patient is carefully monitored. Naloxone administration is discontinued as soon as the patient is responsive to physical stimulation and able to take deep breaths. However, the medication should be kept nearby. Because the duration of naloxone is shorter than most opioids, another dose of naloxone may be needed as early as 30 minutes after the first dose.

Sedative with Analgesic Properties: Dexmedetomidine

Dexmedetomidine (Precedex) is a short-acting alpha-2 agonist that is indicated for the short-term sedation (<24 hours) of mechanically ventilated patients in the critical care unit. Dexmedetomidine acts in the locus ceruleus section of the brainstem. The analgesic effects of dexmedetomidine are principally due to spinal anti-nociception via binding to non-noradrenergic receptors (heteroreceptors) located on the dorsal horn neurons of the spinal cord. Recently, dexmedetomidine was found to decrease postoperative opioid requirements in both adults and children.[66,67]

Nonopioid Analgesics

In the SCCM guidelines, the use of nonopioids in combination with an opioid is recommended in selected critical care patients.[9] This may reduce the opioid requirement. Pharmacologic information is presented in Table 8-4.

Acetaminophen. Acetaminophen is an analgesic used to treat mild-to-moderate pain. It inhibits the synthesis of neurotransmitter prostaglandins in the CNS.[68] Side effects are rare at therapeutic doses (total daily dose should not exceed 4 g in 24 hours). Nonopioids are rarely used alone in critical care patients. Special care must be taken for patients with liver dysfunction, malnutrition, or a history of excess alcohol consumption.

Nonsteroidal antiinflammatory agents. The use of NSAIDs in combination with opioids is indicated in the patient with acute musculoskeletal and soft tissue inflammation.[15] The mechanism of action of NSAIDs is to block the action of cyclooxygenase (COX, which has two forms: COX-1 and COX-2), the enzyme that converts arachidonic acid to prostaglandins. This inhibits the production of prostaglandins. NSAIDs can be grouped as first-generation (COX-1 and COX-2 inhibitors, such as aspirin, ibuprofen, naproxen, and ketorolac) or second-generation (COX-2 inhibitors, such as celecoxib) agents. The inhibition of COX-1 is thought to be responsible for side effects, such as gastric ulceration, bleeding due to platelet inhibition, and acute kidney failure. In contrast, the inhibition of COX-2 is responsible for the suppression of pain and inflammation.[68]

Ketorolac is commonly used in the critical care setting. Research has shown that it is a safe and effective agent for postoperative pain.[69] Caution is advised for using ketorolac for patients with kidney dysfunction because of slower clearance rates. Prolonged use of ketorolac for more than 5 days was associated with an increase in kidney failure and bleeding.[70,71]

Ketamine. Anesthetics may be used to treat pain in the critical care setting. Ketamine is a dissociative anesthetic agent that has analgesic properties. Compared with opioids, ketamine has the benefit of sparing the respiratory drive, but it has many side effects related to the release of catecholamines and the emergence of delirium. For this reason, ketamine is not recommended for routine therapy in critically ill patients.[57,69] Before administering ketamine, the dissociative state should be explained to the patient. *Dissociative state* refers to the feelings of separateness from the environment, loss of control, hallucinations, and vivid dreams. The use of benzodiazepines (e.g., midazolam) can reduce the incidence of this unpleasant effect.[15]

used for pt-for resp compromised

Lidocaine. Lidocaine is another anesthetic that can be used for procedural pain, neuropathic or non-neuropathic pain conditions.[15] Because lidocaine is metabolized in the liver, it should be used with caution in patients with hepatic dysfunction.

Delivery Methods

The most common routes for medication administration are continuous intravenous infusion, bolus administration, or patient-controlled analgesia (PCA). Traditionally, the choice has been intravenous bolus administration. The benefits of this method are the rapid onset of action and the ease of titration. The major disadvantage is the rise and fall of the serum opioid levels, leading to periods of pain control with periods of breakthrough pain.[68]

Continuous infusion of opioids with an infusion pump provides constant opioid blood levels. This promotes a consistent level of comfort. It is particularly helpful during sleep because the patient awakens with an adequate level of pain relief. It is important that the patient be given the loading dose that relieves the pain and raises the circulating dose of the medication. After the basal rate is established, the patient maintains a steady state of pain control unless there is additional pain from a procedure, an activity, or a change in the patient's condition. In this situation, physician orders to administer additional boluses of opioid need to be available.

Patient-Controlled Analgesia

PCA is an effective method using intravenous route and an infusion pump for medication delivery. It allows the patient to self-administer small doses of analgesics. Different opioids can be used, but the most extensively used is morphine. This method of medication delivery allows the patient to control the level of pain and sedation and to avoid the peaks and valleys of intermittent dosing. The patient can self-administer a bolus of medication the moment the pain begins, acting preemptively. Certain patients are not candidates for PCA. Alterations in the level of consciousness or mentation preclude the patient understanding the use of the equipment. Very elderly patients or patients with kidney failure or liver dysfunction may require careful screening for PCA.

The patient is closely monitored during PCA therapy and after every change in the prescription. If the patient's pain does not respond within the first 2 hours of therapy, a total reassessment of the pain state is essential. The nurse monitors the number of boluses the patient delivers. If the patient is pressing the button to bolus medication more often than the prescription, the dose may be insufficient to maintain pain control. Naloxone must be readily available to reverse adverse opioid respiratory effects. Ideally, the patient undergoing an elective procedure requiring opioid analgesia postoperatively is instructed in the use of PCA during preoperative teaching.

Intraspinal Pain Control

Intraspinal anesthesia uses the concept that the spinal cord is the primary link in nociceptive transmission. The goal is to mimic the body's endogenous opioid pain modification system by interfering with the transmission of pain and

TABLE 8-4 **Equianalgesic Chart: Approximate Equivalent Doses of Opioids for Moderate-to-Severe Pain**

ANALGESIC	PARENTERAL (IM, SC, IV) ROUTE[1,2] (mg)	PO ROUTE[1] (mg)	COMMENTS
Mu Opioid Agonists			
Morphine	10	30	Standard for comparison; multiple routes of administration; available in immediate-release and controlled-release formulations; active metabolite M6G can accumulate with repeated dosing in kidney failure
Codeine	130	200 NR	IM has unpredictable absorption and high side effect profile; used PO for mild-to-moderate pain; usually compounded with nonopioid (e.g., Tylenol No. 3)
Fentanyl	100 mcg/hr parenterally and transdermally ≅ 4 mg/hr morphine parenterally; 1 mcg/hr transdermally ≅ 2 mg/24 hr morphine PO	—	Short half-life, but at steady state, slow elimination from tissues can lead to a prolonged half-life (up to 12 hr); start opioid-naïve patients on no more than 25 mcg/hr transdermally; transdermal fentanyl NR for acute pain management; available by oral transmucosal route
Hydromorphone (Dilaudid)	1.5	7.5	Useful alternative to morphine; no evidence that metabolites are clinically relevant; shorter duration than morphine; available in high-potency parenteral formulation (10 mg/mL) useful for SC infusion; 3 mg rectal ≅ 650 mg aspirin PO; with repeated dosing (e.g., PCA), it is more likely than 2-3 mg parenteral hydromorphone =10 mg parenteral morphine
Levorphanol (Levo-Dromoran)	2	4	Longer-acting than morphine when given repeatedly; long half-life can lead to accumulation within 2-3 days of repeated dosing.
Meperidine	75	300 NR	No longer preferred as a first-line opioid for the management of acute or chronic pain due to potential toxicity from accumulation of metabolite, normeperidine; normeperidine has 15-20 hr half-life and is not reversed by naloxone; NR in elderly or patients with impaired kidney functions; NR by continuous IV infusion
Methadone (Dolophine)	10	20	Longer-acting than morphine when given repeatedly; long half-life can lead to delayed toxicity from accumulation within 3-5 days; start PO dosing on PRN schedule; in opioid-tolerant patients converted to methadone, start with 10%-25% of equianalgesic dose
Oxycodone	—	20	Used for moderate pain when combined with a nonopioid (e.g., Percocet, Tylox); available as single entity in immediate-release and controlled-release formulations (e.g., OxyContin); can be used like PO morphine for severe pain
Oxymorphone (Numorphan)	1	10 rectal	Used for moderate-to-severe pain; no PO formulation
Agonist-Antagonist Opioids: Not recommended for severe, escalating pain. If used in combination with mu agonists, may reverse analgesia and precipitate withdrawal in opioid-dependent patients.			
Buprenorphine (Buprenex)	0.4	—	Not readily reversed by naloxone; NR for laboring patients
Butorphanol (Stadol)	2	—	Available in nasal spray
Dezocine (Dalgan)	10	—	
Nalbuphine (Nubain)	10	—	
Pentazocine (Talwin)	60	180	

[1]Duration of analgesia is dose-dependent; the higher the dose, usually the longer the duration.

[2]IV boluses may be used to produce analgesia that lasts approximately as long as IM or SC doses. However, of all routes of administration, IV produces the highest peak concentration of the medication, and the peak concentration is associated with the highest level of toxicity, e.g., sedation. To decrease the peak effect and lower the level of toxicity, IV boluses may be administered more slowly, e.g., 10 mg of morphine over a 15-minute period, or smaller doses may be administered more often, e.g., 5 mg of morphine every 1-1.5 hours.

FDA, U.S. Food and Drug Administration; IM, intramuscular; IV, intravenous; M6G, morphine-6-glucuronide; MCG, micrograms; MG, milligrams; NR, not recommended; PCA, patient-controlled analgesia; PO, by mouth; PRN, pro re nata (as needed); SC, subcutaneous.

Ref: Pasero C. McCaffery M. *Pain Assessment and Pharmacologic Management.* St Louis, Elsevier, 2011.

providing an opioid receptor binding agent directly into the spinal cord. The hemodynamic status of the patient changes very little.

Intraspinal anesthesia is particularly appropriate for pain in the thorax, upper abdomen, and lower extremities. The two intraspinal routes are intrathecal and epidural. Regardless of the route, the effects of the opioid agonist used is the same, and assessment parameters are the same as those used for other routes.

Intrathecal Analgesia

Intrathecal (subarachnoid) opioids are placed directly into the cerebral spinal fluid and attach to spinal cord receptor sites (Figure 8-5). Opioids introduced at this site act quickly at the dorsal horn. The dural sheath is punctured, eliminating the barrier for pathogens between the environment and the cerebral spinal fluid. This creates the risk of serious infections. The intrathecal route is usually reserved for intraoperative use. Side effects of intrathecal pain control include postdural puncture headache and infection.

Epidural Analgesia

Epidural analgesia is commonly used in the critical care unit after major abdominal surgery, nephrectomy, thoracotomy, and major orthopedic procedures. Certain conditions preclude the use of this pain control method: systemic infection, anticoagulation, and increased intracranial pressure. Epidural delivery of opioids provides longer-lasting pain relief with less dosing of opioids. When delivered into the epidural space (Figure 8-5), 5 mg of morphine may be effective for 6 to 24 hours, compared with 3 to 4 hours when delivered intravenously. Opioids infused in the epidural space are more unpredictable than those administered intrathecally. The epidural space is filled with fatty tissue and is external to the dura mater. The fatty tissue interferes with uptake, and the dura acts as a barrier to diffusion, making diffusion rate difficult to predict.

The type of medication used determines the rapidity of diffusion. Medications are *hydrophilic* or *lipophilic*. Hydrophilic medications, such as morphine, are water-soluble and penetrate the dura slowly, providing a longer onset and duration of action. Lipophilic medications, such as fentanyl, are lipid-soluble and penetrate the dura rapidly with a rapid onset and a shorter duration of action.

The dura acts as a physical barrier and causes delay in medication diffusion. Compared with the intrathecal route, it allows more medication to be absorbed into the systemic circulation, requiring greater doses for pain relief. Medications delivered epidurally may be administered by bolus or continuous infusion. The nurse must assess the patient for respiratory depression. This phenomenon may occur early in the therapy or as late as 24 hours after initiation. The epidural catheter also puts the patient at risk for infection. The efficiency of this pain control method and the increased mobility of the patient does not diminish the nurse's responsibility to monitor and evaluate the outcomes of the pain management protocol in use.

Equianalgesia

When a modification of opioid is considered, the goal is to provide equal analgesic effects with the new agents. This concept is referred to as *equianalgesia*. Morphine is the standard for the conversion of opioids. Prescribed dosages must take into account the patient's age and health status.[15] Because of the variety of agents and routes, the professional pain organizations have developed equianalgesia charts for use by health care professionals. All critical care units need to have a chart posted for easy referral. Table 8-5 provides the equianalgesia dose for the different medications used in

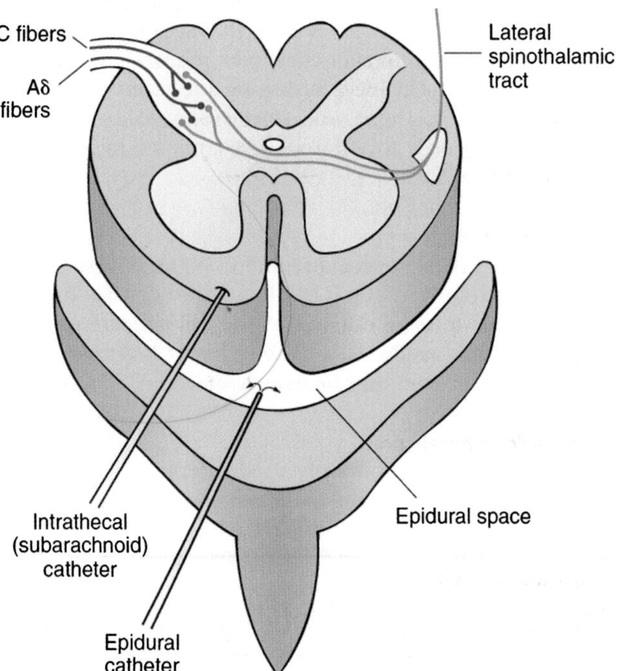

FIG 8-5 Cross section of a section of the spinal cord and vertebrate showing intraspinal catheter placement, intrathecal (subarachnoid) and epidural catheter placement.

TABLE 8-5 Equianalgesic Chart Approximate Equivalent Doses of PO Nonopioids and Opioids for Mild-to-Moderate Pain

ANALGESIC	PO DOSAGE (mg)
Nonopioids	
Acetaminophen	650
Aspirin (ASA)	650
Opioids*	
Codeine	32-60
Hydrocodone†	5
Meperidine (Demerol)	50
Oxycodone‡	3-5
Propoxyphene (Darvon)	65-100

*Often combined with acetaminophen; avoid exceeding maximum total daily dose of acetaminophen (4000 mg/day).
†Combined with acetaminophen (e.g., Vicodin, Lortab).
‡Combined with acetaminophen (e.g., Percocet, Tylox); also available alone as controlled-release OxyContin and immediate-release formulations.
Modified from: Pasero C, McCaffery M. *Pain Assessment and Pharmacologic Management*, St Louis, Elsevier, 2011.

BOX 8-6 A Guide to Using Equianalgesic Charts

- Equianalgesic means approximately the same pain relief.
- The equianalgesic chart is a guideline. Doses and intervals between doses are titrated according to the individual's response.
- The equianalgesic chart is helpful when switching from one medication to another or when switching from one route of administration to another.
- Dosages in the equianalgesic chart for moderate-to-severe pain are not necessarily starting doses. The doses suggest a ratio for comparing the analgesia of one medication with another.
- For elderly patients, initially reduce the recommended adult opioid dose for moderate-to- severe pain by 25% to 50%.
- The longer the patient has been receiving opioids, the more conservative the starting dose of a *new* opioid.

The key to success with any of these therapies is a comprehensive understanding of their mechanism of action so that the therapy matches the needs of the patient. Most of the previously mentioned interventions require the patient's cooperation. There must be some commitment to the treatment on the part of the patient. When handled effectively, nonpharmacologic methods can assist in pain management.

clinical practice. Box 8-6 describes the correct use of an equigesic chart.

Nonpharmacologic Methods of Pain Management

Although numerous methods of pain management other than medications appear in the critical care literature,[72] few studies have been done to provide evidence of their effectiveness in the critical care setting. Nonpharmacologic methods can be used to supplement analgesic treatment, but they are not intended to replace analgesics. In most instances, these therapies may enhance the pharmacologic management of the patient's pain.

Critical care nurses have identifed many barriers to the use of nonpharmacologic methods for pain management, including a lack of knowledge, training, and time.[73] Despite these problems, more than 60% of nurses are willing to use the methods to relieve their patients' pain. It is crucial that critical care nurses be provided with the appropriate training and equipment required to apply nonpharmacologic methods for pain management in the critically ill.

Physical Techniques

Stimulating other non–pain sensory fibers (Aβ) in the periphery modifies pain transmission. These fibers are stimulated by thermal changes as in the application of heat or cold and simple massage.

Cold Application

Ice therapy was found to be helpful to reduce procedural pain in critically ill patients. In a study with 50 post-operative cardiac surgery patients, a significant decrease in pain intensity was obtained after chest tube removal when ice packets were placed around the site for 10 minutes prior to removal.[74] The analgesic property of ice therapy was studied using a 20-minute application of cold packs before chest tube removal.[75] Pain intensity was significantly lower after chest tube removal in patients who received the cold packs and a dose of analgesic compared with a placebo and a control group.

Massage

The effect of massage on pain relief was explored in two studies with postoperative cardiac surgery patients after they have been transferred out of critical care.[76,77] In these two studies with a total of 171 patients, a significant decrease in pain intensity scores was obtained in patients who received a 20-minute massage intervention between postoperative day 2 and day 5 compared to a control group who received standard care and a 20-minute quiet time during the same period.

Cognitive-Behavioral Techniques

Using the cortical interpretation of pain as the foundation, several interventions can reduce the patient's pain report. These modalities include cognitive techniques: patient teaching, relaxation, distraction, guided imagery, music therapy, and hypnosis.

Relaxation

Relaxation is a well-documented method for reducing the distress associated with pain. Although not a substitute for pharmacology, relaxation decreases oxygen consumption and muscle tone, and it can decrease heart rate and blood pressure. Relaxation gives the patient a sense of control over the pain and reduces muscle tension and anxiety. Not all patients are interested in relaxation therapy. For those patients, deep-breathing exercises may be helpful. In a recent study,[3] lower pain scores were found after chest tube removal in 40 critical care patients executing deep breathing and receiving an analgesic compared to those who solely received an analgesic. Excellent references for thorough techniques in relaxation therapy are available.[15]

Guided Imagery

Guided imagery is a technique that uses the imagination to provide control over pain. It can be used to distract or relax. Although this may be difficult in the critical care environment, guiding a patient to a place in his or her imagination that is free from pain may be beneficial.[78]

Music Therapy

Music therapy is a commonly used intervention for relaxation. Music that is pleasing to the patient may have soothing effects, but its effects on reducing pain are controversial.[79] Ideally, the music should be supplied by a small set of headphones. It is important to educate the patient and family regarding the role of music and about other sources of distraction for the patient to assist with relaxation and pain control.

CASE STUDY Patient with Pain

ⓔ Answers to the Case Study Questions can be found on the Evolve website at http://evolve.elsevier.com/Urden/.

Brief Patient History

Ms. X is a woman with type 2 diabetes mellitus and peripheral arterial occlusive disease with neuropathy. Ms. X is disabled because of limited mobility and chronic pain associated with lower extremity claudication and neuropathic pain. She has been admitted for an elective right femoral to distal tibial bypass. Ms. X's chronic pain has been effectively managed with gabapentin (600 mg three times daily) and a 75-mcg fentanyl patch every third day. Ms. X reports that her pain patch is due to be changed the next day. Her diabetes mellitus has been effectively managed with diet and a combination of oral agents. Postoperatively, orders for pain management include her home regimen of gabapentin and fentanyl patch and an order for morphine for breakthrough pain.

Clinical Assessment

Ms. X is admitted to the intensive care unit from the perianesthesia recovery room after an 8-hour surgical revascularization of the right lower extremity. She is awake, alert, and oriented to person, time, place, and situation. Ms. X is breathing through her mouth and taking shallow breaths. She complains of right lower extremity and bilateral foot pain. Her skin is warm and dry. Ms. X is able to move her toes on command, and lower extremity sensation to touch is intact; however, she is complaining of severe burning both feet.

Diagnostic Procedures

Ms. X reports that her pain is a 10 on the Numeric Rating Scale. The Riker Sedation-Agitation Scale score is 5.

Medical Diagnosis

The diagnosis is acute postoperative incisional pain superimposed on chronic neuropathic pain involving both lower extremities. Neuropathic pain is likely worsened because of missed doses of gabapentin.

Questions

1. What major outcomes do you expect to achieve for this patient?
2. What problems or risks must be managed to achieve these outcomes?
3. What interventions must be initiated to monitor, prevent, manage, or eliminate the problems and risks identified?
4. What interventions should be initiated to promote optimal functioning, safety, and well-being of the patient?
5. What possible learning needs do you anticipate for this patient?
6. What cultural and age-related factors may have a bearing on the patient's plan of care?

REFERENCES

1. Chanques G, et al: A prospective study of pain at rest: Incidence and characteristics of an unrecognized symptom in surgical and trauma versus medical intensive care unit patients, *Anesthesiology* 107:858, 2007.
2. Puntillo KA, et al: Patients' perceptions and responses to procedural pain: results from Thunder Project II, *Am J Crit Care* 10:238, 2001.
3. Friesner SA, Curry DM, Moddeman GR: Comparison of two pain-management strategies during chest tube removal: Relaxation exercise with opioids and opioids alone, *Heart Lung* 35:269, 2006.
4. Gélinas C: Management of pain in cardiac surgery ICU patients: have we improved over time? *Intensive Crit Care Nurs* 23:298, 2007.
5. Loeser JD, Treede RD: The Kyoto protocol of IASP basic pain terminology, *Pain* 137:473, 2008.
6. Khalaila R, et al: Communication difficulties and psychoemotional distress in patients receiving mechanical ventilation, *Am J Crit Care* 20:470, 2011.
7. Gélinas C, Johnston C: Pain assessment in the critically ill ventilated adult: validation of the Critical-Care Pain Observation Tool and physiological indicators, *Clin J Pain* 23:497, 2007.
8. Herr K, et al: Pain assessment in the patient unable to self-report: Position statement with clinical practice recommendations, *Pain Manag Nurs* 12:230, 2011.
9. Barr J, et al: Clinical practice guidelines for the management of pain, agitation, and delirium in adult patients in the intensive care unit, *Crit Care Med* 41:263, 2013.
10. International Association for the Study of Pain (IASP): Subcommittee on Taxonomy. Pain terms: a list with definitions and notes on usage, *Pain* 6:249, 1979.
11. McCaffery M: *Nursing management of the patient with pain*, ed 2, Philadelphia, 1979, JB Lippincott.
12. McGuire D: Comprehensive and multidimensional assessment and measurement of pain, *J Pain Symptom Manage* 7:312, 1992.
13. International Association for the Study of Pain (IASP) Task Force on Taxonomy. *Classification of chronic pain*, Seattle, 1994, IASP Press.
14. Melzack R: Pain and stress: A new perspective. In Gatchel RJ, Turk DC, editors: *Psychological factors in pain*, New York, 1999, Guilford Press.
15. Pasero C, McCaffery M: *Pain assessment and pharmacologic management*, St Louis, 2011, Mosby Elsevier.
16. Cervero F, Laird JMA: Visceral Pain, *Lancet* 353:2145, 1999.
17. Kyranou M, Puntillo K: The transition from acute to chronic pain: might intensive care unit patients be at risk? *Ann Intensive Care* 2:36, 2012.
18. Melzack R, Wall PD: *The challenge of pain*, ed 2, London, 1996, Penguin Books.
19. Carr DB, Goudas LC: Acute pain, *Lancet* 353:2051, 1999.
20. Gélinas C, Arbour C: Behavioral and physiological indicators during a nociceptive procedure in conscious and unconscious mechanically ventilated adults: similar or different? *J Crit Care* 24:628.e7, 2009.
21. Rainville P: Brain mechanisms of pain affect and pain modulation, *Curr Opin Neurobiol* 12:195, 2002.
22. Derbyshire SW, Osborn J: Modeling pain circuits: how imaging may modify perception, *Neuroimaging Clin N Am* 17:485, 2007.

23. Marks DM, et al: Serotonin-norepinephrine reuptake inhibitors for pain control: Premise and promise, *Current Neuropharmacology* 7:331, 2009.
24. Lorenz JL, et al: Keeping pain out of mind: The role of the dorsolateral prefrontal cortex in pain modulation, *Brain* 126:5, 2003.
25. Daut RL, Cleeland CS: The prevalence and severity of pain in cancer, *Cancer* 50:1913, 1982.
26. Melzack R: The short form McGill Pain Questionnaire, *Pain* 30:191, 1987.
27. Jarvis C: *Physical examination & health assessment*, ed 6, Philadelphia, 2011, Saunders.
28. Puntillo KA, et al: Pain behaviors observed during six common procedures: results from Thunder Project II, *Crit Care Med* 32:421, 2004.
29. Payen JF, et al: Assessing pain in the critically ill sedated patients by using a behavioral pain scale, *Crit Care Med* 29:2258, 2001.
30. Gélinas C, et al: Validation of the Critical-Care Pain Observation Tool (CPOT) in adult patients, *Am J Crit Care* 15:420, 2006.
31. Gélinas C, et al: The impact of the implementation of the Critical-Care Pain Observation Tool on pain assessment/management nursing practices in the intensive care unit with nonverbal critically ill adults, *Int J Nurs Stud* 48:1495, 2011.
32. Chanques G, et al: Impact of systematic evaluation of pain and agitation in an intensive care unit, *Crit Care Med* 34:1691, 2006.
33. Ahlers S, et al: Comparison of different pain scoring systems in critically ill patients in a general ICU, *Crit Care* 12:1, 2008.
34. Ahlers S, et al: The use of the behavioral pain scale to assess pain in conscious sedated patients, *Anesth Anal* 110:127, 2010.
35. Aïssaoui Y, et al: Validation of a behavioral pain scale in critically ill sedated, and mechanically ventilated patients, *Anesth Analg* 101:1470, 2005.
36. Young J, et al: Use of a Behavioral Pain Scale to assess pain in ventilated, unconscious and/or sedated patients, *Intensive Crit Care Nurs* 22:32, 2006.
37. Marmo L, Fowler S: Pain assessment tool in the critically ill post-open heart surgery patient population, *Pain Manag Nurs* 11:134, 2010.
38. Gélinas C, et al: Item selection and Content validity of the Critical-Care Pain Observation Tool: an instrument to assess pain in critically ill nonverbal adults, *J Adv Nurs* 65:203, 2009.
39. Gélinas C, et al: Sensitivity and specificity of the Critical-Care Pain Observation Tool for the detection of pain in intubated adults following cardiac surgery, *J Pain Symptom Manage* 37:58, 2009.
40. Gelinas C, et al: Nurses' evaluations of the CPOT use at 12-month post-implementation in the intensive care unit, *Nurs Crit Care* 19:272, 2014.
41. Arbour C, Gélinas C: Are vital signs valid indicators for the assessment of pain in cardiac surgery ICU adults? *Int Crit Care Nurs* 26:83, 2010.
42. Gordon DB, et al: American Pain recommendations for improving the quality of acute and cancer pain management, *Arch Intern Med* 165:1574, 2005.
43. Lawrence M: The unconscious experience, *Am J Crit Care* 4:227, 1995.
44. Laureys S, et al: Cortical processing of noxious somatosensory stimuli in the persistent vegetative state, *Neuroimage* 17:732, 2002.
45. Bjoro K, Herr K: Assessment of pain in the nonverbal or cognitively impaired older adult, *Clin Geriatr Med* 24:237, 2008.
46. Hadjistavropoulos T, et al: An interdisciplinary expert consensus statement on assessment of pain in older persons, *Clin J Pain* 23:S1, 2007.
47. Zwakhalen SM, et al: Pain in elderly people with severe dementia: a systematic review of behavioral pain assessment tools, *BMC Geriatr* 6:1, 2006.
48. Fuchs-Labelle S, Hadjistavropoulos T: Development and preliminary validation of the Pain Assessment Checklist for Seniors with Limited Ability to Communicate (PACSLAC), *Pain Manag Nurs* 5:37, 2004.
49. Wary B, Doloplus C: Doloplus-2, a scale for pain measurement, *Soins Gerontol* 19:25, 1999.
50. Warden V, Hurley AC, Volicer L: Development and psychometric evaluation of the Pain Assessment in Advanced Dementia (PAINAD) scale, *J Am Med Dir Assoc* 4:9, 2003.
51. Herr K, et al: Use of pain-behavioral assessment tools in the nursing home: Expert consensus recommendations for practice, *J Gerontol Nurs* 36:18, 2010.
52. Cashman JN, Dolin SJ: Respiratory and haemodynamic effects of acute postoperative pain management: Evidence from published data, *Br J Anaesth* 93:212, 2004.
53. Smith LH: Opioid safety: is your patient at risk for respiratory depression? *Clin J Oncol Nurs* 11:293, 2007.
54. Devlin JW, Mallow-Corbett S, Riker RR: Adverse drug events associated with the use of analgesics, sedatives, and antipsychotics in the intensive care unit, *Crit Care Med* 38:S231, 2010.
55. Jarzyna D, et al: American Society for Pain Management Nursing guidelines on monitoring for opioid-induced sedation and respiratory depression, *Pain Manag Nurs* 12:118, 2011.
56. Brush DR, Kress JP: Sedation and analgesia for the mechanically ventilated patient, *Clin Chest Med* 30:131, 2009.
57. Liu LL, Gropper MA: Postoperative analgesia and sedation in the adult intensive care unit: a guide to drug selection, *Drugs* 63:755, 2003.
58. Sarhill N, et al: Hydromorphone: pharmacology and clinical applications in cancer patients, *Support Care Cancer* 9:84, 2001.
59. Ashley E, Given J: Pain management in the critically ill, *Br J Perioper Nurs* 18:504, 2008.
60. Devlin JW, Roberts RJ: Pharmacology of commonly used analgesics and sedatives in the ICU: Benzodiazepines, propofol, and opioids, *Crit Care Clin* 25:431, 2009.
61. Erstad BL, et al: Pain management principles in the critically ill, *Chest* 135:1075, 2009.
62. Cavalière F, et al: A low-dose remifentanyl infusion is well tolerated for sedation in mechanically ventilated, critically ill patients, *Can J Anaesth* 49:1088, 2002.
63. Soltész S, et al: Recovery after remifentanyl and sufentanyl for analgesia and sedation of mechanically ventilated patients after trauma or major surgery, *Br J Anaesth* 86:763, 2001.
64. Radtke FM, et al: Remifentanyl reduces the incidence of post-operative delirium, *J Int Med Res* 38:1225, 2010.
65. Ethuin F, et al: Pharmacokinetics of long-term sufentanyl infusion for sedation in ICU patients, *Intensive Care Med* 29:1916, 2003.
66. Ohtani N, et al: Perioperative infusion of dexmedetomidine at a high dose reduces postoperative analgesic requirements: A randomized control trial, *J Anesth* 25:872, 2011.

67. Pestieau SR, et al: High-dose dexmedetomidine increases the opioid-free interval and decreases opioid requirement after tonsillectomy in children, *Can J Anaesth* 58:540, 2011.
68. Lehne RA: *Pharmacology for nursing care*, ed 8, Philadelphia, 2012, Elsevier.
69. Summer GJ, Puntillo KA: Management of surgical and procedural pain in a critical care setting, *Crit Care Nurs Clin North Am* 13:233, 2001.
70. Feldman HI, et al: Parenteral ketorolac: the risk for acute renal failure, *Ann Intern Med* 126:193, 1997.
71. Strom BL, et al: Parenteral ketorolac and risk of gastrointestinal and operative site bleeding, *JAMA* 275:376, 1996.
72. Faigeles B, et al: Predictors and use of nonpharmacologic interventions for procedural pain associated with turning among hospitalized adults, *Pain Manag Nurs* 4:85, 2013.
73. Tracy MF, et al: Nurse attitudes towards the use of complementary and alternative therapies in critical care, *Heart Lung* 32:197, 2003.
74. Sauls J: The use of ice for pain associated with chest tube removal, *Pain Manag Nurs* 3:44, 2002.
75. Demir Y, Khorshid L: The effect of cold application in combinaison with standard analgesic administration on pain and anxiety during chest tube removal: a single-blinded, randomized, double-controlled study, *Pain Manag Nurs* 11:186, 2010.
76. Bauer BA, et al: Effect of massage therapy on pain, anxiety, and tension in cardiac surgical patients: a randomized study, *Comp Ther Clin Pract* 16:70, 2010.
77. Cutshall SM, et al: Effect of massage therapy on pain, anxiety, and tension in cardiac surgical patients: a pilot study, *Comp Ther Clin Pract* 16:92, 2010.
78. Good M, et al: Relief of postoperative pain with jaw relaxation, music and their combination, *Pain* 81:163, 1999.
79. Biley FC: The effects on patient well-being of music listening as a nursing intervention: a review of the literature, *J Clin Nurs* 9:668, 2000.

9 CHAPTER

Sedation, Agitation and Delirium Management

Mary E. Lough

Be sure to check out the bonus material, including review questions, on the Evolve website at http://evolve.elsevier.com/Urden/priorities/.

One of the challenges facing clinicians is how to provide a therapeutic healing environment for patients in the alarm-filled, emergency-focused critical care unit. Many critical care patients demonstrate agitation and discomfort caused by painful procedures, invasive tubes, sleep deprivation, fear, anxiety, critical illness, and physiological stress. The goal is to find a balance between providing compassionate patient care and avoiding the perils of excess sedation. Clinical practice guidelines were developed by the Society of Critical Care Medicine (SCCM) to increase awareness of these issues in critical illness. The initial guidelines were published in 2002[1] and substantially revised in 2013.[2]

SEDATION

Pain Assessment Scales: Prior to the assessment of agitation-sedation, the first step is to assess the patient's level of pain. If the patient can communicate, the verbal pain scale of 0 to 10 is optimal. If the patient is intubated and cannot vocalize, pain assessment becomes considerably more complex. The Behavioral Pain Scale (BPS) and the Critical Care Pain Observation (CPOT) scale are the most reliable adult behavioral pain scales. These scales are discussed in detail in Chapter 9. The SCCM guidelines recommend that all critically ill, mechanically ventilated patients have stated goals for administration of analgesia[2] (Figure 9-1). When a patient is nonverbal it can be difficult to determine whether the patient is experiencing pain. After pain medication has been provided, the next step is to perform an assessment to identify levels of agitation-sedation.

Sedation Assessment Scales

The use of a scoring system to assess and record levels of sedation and agitation is strongly encouraged.[2] Because individuals do not metabolize sedative medications at the same rate, use of a standardized scale ensures that sedatives are titrated to a specific behavioral goal rather than a sedative dose. Collaboratively, the critical care team must determine the level of sedation that is most appropriate for each individual patient.[2]

The Richmond Agitation-Sedation Scale (RASS)[3,4] and the Sedation-Agitation Scale (SAS)[5] are recommended for use with critically ill patients.[2] These scales are shown in Table 9-1.

Assessment of agitation-sedation begins by simply observing the patient, as there is a continuum from dangerously agitated to nonresponsive. The level of required sedation varies with the clinical circumstances. Sedation (with analgesia) is appropriately provided during invasive procedures such as bronchoscopy. However, stable mechanical ventilation in the critical care unit is no longer considered a rationale for sedation. In many cases the goal is that the patient feel calm and be sufficiently alert to be able to participate in their care, defined as RASS 0, and SAS 4 (Table 9-1).

Agitation is defined as RASS +1 to +4 and SAS 5 to 7. The higher numbers indicate increased levels of agitation (Table 9-1). Agitation may also be an indicator for pain, for delirium, or for alcohol withdrawal (described later in this chapter). Assessment of the source of the agitation is one of the prerequisites for effective treatment.

Oversedation is recognized as a state of unintended patient unresponsiveness with several levels from drowsy to unarousable. When the patient is drowsy, or difficult to arouse but will respond to verbal stimuli, this is described as a RASS −1 to −3 and SAS 3 to 2 (Table 9-1). Lower numbers indicate deeper levels of sedation. Treatment may be as straightforward as decreasing the amount of sedation that is administered.

When a patient is unarousable, they reside in a state that resembles general anesthesia or coma. Typically this means the patient is responsive only to physical stimulation described as a RASS −4 to −5 and SAS 1 (Table 9-1). It is important to identify the reasons. Examine whether an organic cause, such as liver or kidney encephalopathy, or neurological compromise can be identified from diagnostic tests. Otherwise, if the reason is excess sedation, it is imperative to decrease the dosage to allow normal brain function to resume. Prolonged deep sedation is associated with significant complications of immobility, including pressure ulcers, thromboemboli, gastric ileus, nosocomial pneumonia, and delayed weaning from mechanical ventilation.

Levels of Sedation

In the clinical setting, depth of sedation may also be referred to using general descriptive terms as listed in Box 9-1.

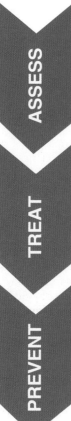

	AGITATION	DELIRIUM
ASSESS	Assess agitation, sedation ≥ 4 times/shift and prn Preferred sedation assessment tools: • RASS(−5 TO +4) or SAS (1 to 7) • NMB → suggest using brain function monitoring Depth of agitation, sedation defined as: • *Agitated* if RASS = +1 to +4, or SAS = 5 to 7 • *Awake and calm* if RASS = 0, or SAS = 4 • *Lightly sedated* if RASS = −1 to −2, or SAS = 3 • *Deeply sedated* if RASS = −3 to −5, or SAS = 1 to 2	Assess delirium every shift and prn Preferred delirium assessment tools: • CAM-ICU (+ or −) • ICDSC (0 to 8) Delirium present if: • CAM-ICU is positive • ICDSC 4
TREAT	Targeted sedation *(Goal: patient purposely follows commands without agitation)*: RASS = −2-0, SAS = 3-4 • If *under sedated* (RASS >0, SAS >4) assess/treat pain → treat with sedatives prn (non-benzodiazepines preferred, unless alcohol withdrawal or benzodiazepine withdrawal is suspected) • If *over sedated* (RASS < −2, SAS <3) hold sedatives until at target, then restart at 50% of previous dose	• Treat pain as needed • Reorient patients; familiarize surroundings; use patient's eyeglasses, hearing aids if needed • Pharmacologic treatment of delirium: – Avoid benzodiazepines unless alcohol withdrawal or benzodiazepine withdrawal is suspected – Avoid rivastigmine – Avoid antipsychotics if increased risk of Torsades de pointes
PREVENT	• Consider daily SBT, early mobility and exercise when patients are at goal sedation level, unless contraindicated	• Identify delirium risk factors: dementia, HTN, alcohol abuse, high severity of illness, coma, benzodiazepine administration • Avoid benzodiazepine use in those at increased risk for delirium • Mobilize and exercise patients early • Promote sleep (control light, noise; cluster patient care activities; decrease nocturnal stimuli) • Restart baseline psychiatric medications, if indicated

FIG 9-1 Agitation and Delirium Care Bundle. *CAM-ICU,* Confusion Assessment Method for the Intensive Care Unit; *HTN,* hypertension; *ICDSC,* Intensive Care Delirium Screening Checklist; *NMB,* neuromuscular blockade; *RASS,* Richmond Agitation-Sedation Scale; *SAS,* Sedation-Agitation Scale; *SBT,* spontaneous breathing trial. (Data from Barr J, et al: Clinical Practice Guidelines for the Management of Pain, Agitation, and Delirium in Adult Patients in the Intensive Care Unit, *Crit Care Med* 2013;41:263-306.)

BOX 9-1 Levels of Sedation

Light Sedation (Minimal Sedation, Anxiolysis)
Medication-induced state during which patients respond normally to verbal commands. Although cognitive function and coordination may be impaired, ventilatory and cardiovascular functions are unaffected.

Moderate Sedation with Analgesia (Conscious Sedation, Procedural Sedation)
Medication-induced depression of consciousness during which patients respond purposefully to verbal commands, alone or accompanied by light tactile stimulation. No interventions are required to maintain a patent airway, and spontaneous ventilation is adequate. Cardiovascular function is usually maintained.

Deep Sedation and Analgesia
Medication-induced depression of consciousness during which patients cannot be easily aroused but respond purposefully after repeated or painful stimulation. The ability to maintain ventilatory function independently is impaired. Patients require assistance in maintaining a patent airway, and spontaneous ventilation may be inadequate. Cardiovascular function is usually maintained.

General Anesthesia
Medication-induced loss of consciousness during which patients are not arousable, even by painful stimulation. The ability to maintain ventilatory function independently is impaired, and assistance to maintain a patent airway is required. Positive-pressure ventilation may be required because of depressed spontaneous ventilation or medication-induced depression of neuromuscular function. Cardiovascular function may be impaired.

Data from Joint Commission on Accreditation of Healthcare Organizations. *Comprehensive Accreditation Manual for Hospitals.* Oakbrook Terrace, IL: The Joint Commission; 2000; Jacobi J, et al. Clinical practice guidelines for the sustained use of sedatives and analgesics in the critically ill adult. *Crit Care Med.* 2002; 30:119.

TABLE 9-1 Sedation Scales

SCORE	DESCRIPTION	DEFINITION
Richmond Agitation-Sedation Scale (RASS)[§,‖]		
Score	**Term**	**Description**
+4	Combative	Overtly combative, violent, immediate danger to staff
+3	Very agitated	Pulls or removes tube(s) or catheter(s); aggressive
+2	Agitated	Frequent nonpurposeful movement; fights ventilator
+1	Restless	Anxious but movements not aggressive vigorous
0	Alert and calm	
−1	Drowsy	Not fully alert, but has sustained awakening (eye-opening/eye contact) to *voice* (≥**10 seconds**)
−2	Light sedation	Briefly awakens with eye contact to *voice* (<**10 seconds**)
−3	Moderate sedation	Movement or eye opening to *voice* (**but no eye contact**)
−4	Deep sedation	No response to voice, but movement or eye opening to *physical* stimulation
−5	Unresponsive	No response to *voice* or *physical* stimulation
Sedation-Agitation Scale (SAS)*		
7	Dangerously agitated	Pulls at endotracheal tube (ETT), tries to remove catheters, climbs over bed rail, strikes at staff, thrashes side to side
6	Very agitated	Does not calm despite frequent verbal reminding of limits, requires physical restraints, bites ETT
5	Agitated	Anxious or mildly agitated, attempts to sit up, calms down to verbal instructions
4	Calm and cooperative	Calm, awakens easily, follows commands
3	Sedated	Difficult to arouse, awakens to verbal stimuli or gentle shaking but drifts off again; follows simple commands
2	Very sedated	Arouses to physical stimuli but does not communicate or follow commands; may move spontaneously
1	Unarousable	Minimal or no response to noxious stimuli; does not communicate or follow commands

Sessler CN, et al. The Richmond Agitation-Sedation Scale: validity and reliability in adult intensive care unit patients. *Am J Respir Crit Care Med* 166: 1338-1344, 2002.
Ely EW, et al. Monitoring sedation status over time in ICU patients: reliability and validity of the Richmond Agitation-Sedation Scale (RASS), *JAMA* 289: 2983-2991, 2003.
Riker RR, et al. Prospective evaluation of the Sedation-Agitation Scale for adult critically ill patients, *Crit Care Med* 27:1325-1329, 1999.

- **Light sedation** refers to pharmacologic relief of anxiety while the patient is alert and communicative (Approximates RASS −1 and SAS 3)
- **Moderate sedation** describes pharmacologic depression of patient consciousness. This is also known as procedural sedation as this is often the target level when tubes or lines are to be inserted (Approximates RASS −3 and SAS 3)
- **Deep Sedation** describes pharmacologic depression of patient consciousness to where the patient cannot maintain an open airway (Approximates RASS −4 and SAS 2).
- **General Anesthesia** describes pharmacologic depression of patient consciousness using multiple medications, administered by a physician anesthesiologist, or a nurse anesthetist. (Approximates RASS −5 and SAS 1).

When the patient has a depressed level of consciousness as a result of sedation (moderate, deep, or general anesthesia), vigilant monitoring of cardiac and respiratory function and vital signs are required. To ensure patient safety, in addition to the person performing the procedure, there must be qualified clinicians present who are able to monitor and recover the patient. Additionally, the person administering the sedative medication must be qualified to manage the patient at whatever level of sedation or anesthesia is achieved.

It is important to be aware that opioids and some antihistamine and antiemetic medications may produce a sedative effect and that the nurse's responsibility to monitor the patient refers to the level of sedation irrespective of the medications that are used.

Pharmacological Management of Sedation

Several categories of sedatives are available. If the patient is experiencing pain, analgesia must be administered in addition to any sedative agents. Sedative agents include the benzodiazepines, sedative-hypnotic agents such as propofol, and the central alpha agonist dexmedotomidine (Table 9-2).[2] Currently, dexmedetomidine-based and propofol-based sedative regimens are recommended for routine sedation of mechanically ventilated adult patients.[2]

Benzodiazepines

Benzodiazepines have powerful amnesic properties that inhibit reception of new sensory information.[1,6] Once a mainstay of sedation, benzodiazepines are no longer recommended for sedation of the mechanically ventilated critically ill adult.[2] This is because benzodiazepine-based sedative regimes are associated with worse patient outcomes, including longer duration of mechanical ventilation and delirium.[7-9]

Benzodiazepines do not confer analgesia. The most frequently used critical care benzodiazepines are diazepam (Valium), midazolam (Versed), and lorazepam (Ativan).

TABLE 9-2 Pharmacologic Management: Sedation

MEDICATION	DOSAGE	ACTION	SPECIAL CONSIDERATIONS
Benzodiazepines			
Diazepam	Loading Dose IV: 5-10 mg slowly Maintenance Dose IV: 0.03-01 mg/kg every 0.5-6.0 hr PRN	Anxiolysis Amnesia Sedation	*Onset:* 2-5 min after IV administration *Side effects:* hypotension, respiratory depression *Half-life:* long (20-120 hr); active metabolites also contribute to prolonged sedative effect *Tolerance:* physical tolerance develops with prolonged use, and higher doses of medication are required to achieve the same effect over time; slow wean required from diazepam after continuous prolonged use Phlebitis occurs with peripheral IV administration.
Lorazepam	Loading Dose IV: 0.02-0.04 mg/kg (≤2 mg) slowly Intermittent maintenance IV every 2-6 hr: 0.02-0.06 mg/kg slowly Continuous IV maintenance infusion: 0.01-0.1 mg/kg/hr (≤10 mg/hr)	Anxiolysis Amnesia Sedation	*Onset:* 15-20 min after IV administration *Side effects:* hypotension, respiratory depression, propylene glycol-related acidosis, nephrotoxicity *Half-life:* relatively long (8-15 hr) *Tolerance:* physical tolerance develops with use, and higher medication dosage is required to achieve the same effect over time; slow wean required from lorazepam after continuous prolonged use Solvent-related acidosis and kidney failure occur at high doses.
Midazolam	Loading Dose IV: 0.01-0.05 mg/kg slowly over several minutes Continuous IV maintenance infusion: 0.02-0.1 mg/kg/hr	Anxiolysis Amnesia Sedation	*Onset:* 2-5 min after IV administration *Side effects:* hypotension, respiratory depression *Half-life:* 3-11 hr; sedative effect is prolonged when midazolam infusion has continued for many days, due to presence of active sedative metabolites; sedative effect is also prolonged in kidney failure. *Tolerance:* physical tolerance develops with prolonged use, and higher medication dosages are required to achieve the same effect over time; slow wean required from midazolam after prolonged use
Sedative-Hypnotics			
Propofol	Loading Dose IV: 5 mcg/kg/min over 5 min Continuous IV maintenance infusion: 5-50 mcg/kg/min	Anxiolysis Amnesia Sedation	*Onset:* very rapid onset (1-2 min) after IV administration *Side effects:* hypotension, respiratory depression (patient must be intubated and mechanically ventilated to eliminate this complication), pain at the injection site if administered via peripheral IV; pancreatitis; hyper triglyceridemia, propofol-related infusion syndrome (PRIS), allergic reactions *Half-life:* 1-2 min when used as a short-term agent *Half-life:* Short term use 3-12 hours. However, with prolonged continuous IV infusion the half life extends to 50 ± 18.6 hours; effective short-term anesthetic agent, useful for rapid "wake-up" of patients for assessment; if continuous infusion is used for many days, emergence from sedation can take hours or days; sedative effect depends on dose administered, depth of sedation, and length of time sedated. Change IV infusion tubing every 12 hr. Requires a dedicated IV catheter and tubing (do not mix with other medications) Monitor serum triglyceride levels.
Central Alpha-Adrenergic Receptor Agonists			
Dexmedetomidine	Loading Dose IV: 1 mcg/kg over 10 min Continuous IV maintenance infusion: 0.2-0.7 mcg/kg/hr	Anxiolysis Analgesia Sedation	*Onset:* 5-10 min *Side effects:* bradycardia, hypotension, loss of airway reflexes *Half life:* 1.8-3.1 hr. No active metabolites Intermittent bolus dosing is not recommended. Maintenance infusion is adjusted to achieve desired level of sedation.

Data from Barr J, et al. Clinical Practice Guidelines for the Management of Pain, Agitation, and Delirium in Adult Patients in the Intensive Care Unit, *Crit Care Med* 2013; 41(1), 276.

hr, hour; *IV*, intravenous; *kg*, kilogram; *mcg*, microgram; *mg*, milligram; *min*, minutes.

Short- acting benzodiazepines (midazolam) are still helpful for control of acute short-term agitation because the intravenous onset of action is rapid. However, when midazolam is administered for longer than 24 hours as a continuous infusion, the sedative effect is prolonged by its active metabolites.[1] One advantage of lorazepam is that it does not have active metabolites that contribute to the overall sedative effect. However, this is outweighed by its long pharmacologic half-life, more days on the ventilator, and an increased risk of delirium.[7,8,9] Another concern with prolonged administration of any benzodiazepine is increasing tolerance, which may be exhibited as increasing agitation as the medication exerts a lessened sedative effect.

Other major unwanted side effects are dose-related respiratory depression and hypotension. If needed, flumazenil (Romazicon) is the antidote used to reverse benzodiazepine overdose in symptomatic patients. Flumazenil should be avoided in patients with benzodiazepine dependence, because rapid withdrawal can induce seizures.[10]

Sedative-Hypnotic Agents

Propofol is a powerful sedative and respiratory depressant used for sedation in mechanically ventilated patients in critical care. It is immediately identifiable by its white milky appearance, always in a glass container. At high doses (>100 to 200 mcg/kg/min), propofol is intended to produce a state of general anesthesia in the operating room.[11] In the critical care unit, propofol is prescribed as a continuous infusion at lower doses (5 to 50 mcg/kg/min) to induce a state of deep sedation.[11] Because propofol is lipid-soluble, it quickly crosses cell membranes, including the cells that comprise the blood–brain barrier. This allows rapid onset of sedation (about 30 seconds), with immediate loss of consciousness. In addition to a rapid onset of action, propofol has very short half-life with initial use (2 to 4 minutes), is rapidly eliminated from the body (30 to 60 minutes), and does not have active metabolites.[11,12] This makes it an ideal sedative for use when a patient needs to be quickly awakened, for a spontaneous awakening trial (SAT), for a spontaneous breathing trial (SBT), or to assess neurological status. This feature makes propofol an ideal medication to manage rapid ventilator weaning post-surgery. Propofol is both clinically effective and cost-effective because it shortens time to extubation. It is important to add an opiate, such as fentanyl, to ensure adequate pain control and amnesia. Propofol is not a reliable amnesic, and patients sedated with only propofol can have vivid recollections of their critical care experience.

Risks of unwanted complications increase when propofol is administered long-term at high doses (>4.00 mg/kg/hour for longer than 48 hours). Propofol is delivered in a fat-based emulsion, and side effects may be related to disruption of fatty acid metabolism, muscle injury, and release of toxic intracellular contents. Complications have been collectively grouped under the term *Propofol Related Infusion Syndrome* (PRIS) including metabolic acidosis, muscular weakness, rhabdomyolysis, myoglobinuria, acute kidney injury, and cardiovascular dysrhythmias. PRIS affects about 1% of all patients who receive propofol; almost one-third of those affected will not survive.[6,12,13] Other secondary side effects related to the fat-emulsion carrier include hyperlipidemia, hypertriglyceridemia, and acute pancreatitis. Vigilance is required to monitor sedation levels and to be alert for the rare but significant risk of propofol- related complications. Serum triglycerides are measured on all patients who receive propofol for longer than 48 hours. For additional information see Table 9-2.

Central Alpha Agonists

Two central α-adrenergic agonists with sedative properties are available. *Clonidine* is typically prescribed as a Catapres patch and *dexmedetomidine* (Precedex) as a continuous infusion. Clonidine may be prescribed for patients experiencing alcohol withdrawal syndrome (see later in chapter).

Dexmedetomidine is an α_2-agonist that is FDA-approved for use as a short-term sedative (<24 hours) in mechanically ventilated patients. Sedation occurs when the medication activates postsynaptic alpha-2 receptors in the central nervous system in the brain. This activation inhibits norepinephrine release and blocks sympathetic nervous system (SNS) fight-or-flight functions, leading to sedation. SNS inhibition may cause hypotension and bradydysrhythmias, both well-known side effects of Dexmedetomidine. Analgesic effects occur because Dexmedetomidine binds to alpha-2 receptors in the spinal cord. These unique mechanisms of action allow patients to be sedated but still arousable, factors that are associated with a shorter time to extubation compared with traditional sedative regimens.

Dexmedetomidine is prescribed with a loading dose of 1.0 mcg/kg over 10 minutes, followed by a continuous infusion of 0.4 mcg/kg (range 0.2 to 0.7 mcg/kg/hr).[14] Dexmedetomidine has a short half-life (6 minutes) and is eliminated from the body in about 2 hours.[14] Elimination from the body is dramatically slowed if the patient has liver failure (see Table 9-2). Complications include bradycardia and hypotension.[15]

Dexmedetomidine confers sedation and analgesic effects without respiratory depression.[14] Consequently, patients can be extubated while still on a Dexmedetomidine infusion. This can be helpful for patients who are anxious during ventilator weaning. Dexmedetomidine has also been used for patients on noninvasive mask ventilation.[16] Because of this favorable pharmacologic profile, many clinicians now use dexmedetomidine as a first-line sedative agent.[17]

Spontaneous Awakening Trial

One strategy to avoid the pitfalls of sedative dependence and withdrawal is a planned strategy to turn off the sedative infusions once each day. This intervention has been given several names, including *sedation vacation* and *spontaneous awakening trial* (SAT). At a scheduled time, all continuously infusing sedatives are stopped. Sometimes analgesics are also stopped, depending on the hospital's protocol, The patient is allowed to regain consciousness for clinical assessment using a standardized instrument such as the RASS or SAS (see Table 9-1).[18,19] The patient is carefully monitored, and when awareness is attained, an assessment of level of consciousness and neurologic function is performed. If the patient becomes agitated, it is essential that a protocol be in place for the nurse to restart the sedatives, plus opiates if applicable. One protocol scheduled the daily interruption of sedatives in the morning and recommended, after a full assessment, restarting the sedative and opiate infusions at 50% of the previous morning dose and adjusting upward until the patient was comfortable.[18]

An important nursing responsibility is to prevent the patient from coming to harm during sedative or analgesic medication withdrawal. If the patient is seriously agitated, it is vital to consult with the physician and pharmacist to establish an effective treatment plan that will allow safe weaning from sedative medications (see Table 9-1).

AGITATION

Agitation describes hyperactive patient movements that range in intensity from slight restless hand and body movements to pulling out lines and tubes, extending to physical aggression and self-harm. Agitation can be caused by pain, anxiety, delirium, hypoxia, ventilator dyssynchrony, neurological injury, uncomfortable position, full bladder, sleep deprivation, alcohol withdrawal, sepsis, a medication reaction or organ failure, to name but a few frequently encountered causes. In the past, when a patient showed physical signs of agitation, a benzodiazepine sedative (lorazepam or midazolam) was quickly administered to reduce the patient's mental awareness. However, because benzodiazepines have been shown to induce delirium, it is now recommended that proactive assessments and interventions be used to treat the causes of agitation.[2] The first step involves systematic assessment using a standardized scale such as the RASS or SAS (Table 9-2).[2] These assessment scales allow clinicians to identify agitation in its milder forms and potentially to ameliorate the patient's symptoms. The goal is to treat the cause of the agitation rather than to overmedicate. Obviously, when a patient is dangerously agitated (RASS +4), is combative (SAS 7), or may endanger themselves or others, immediate sedation is warranted. In these extreme situations, a benzodiazepine is administered.[2]

DELIRIUM

Delirium represents a global impairment of cognitive processes, usually of sudden onset, coupled with disorientation, impaired short-term memory, altered sensory perceptions, such as hallucinations, abnormal thought processes, and inappropriate behavior. Delirium is more prevalent than generally recognized. It is difficult to diagnose in the critically ill patient and represents acute brain dysfunction,[20] caused by sepsis, critical illness, or dysfunction of other vital organs (Box 9-2). Between 60% and 85% of mechanically ventilated patients experience delirium.[21] Delirium increases hospital stay and mortality rates for patients who are mechanically ventilated.[21] The increased mortality remains even after controlling for associated variables, such as coma and administration of sedatives and analgesics.[21]

When patients are agitated, restless, and pulling at tubes and lines, they are often identified as being delirious. In this scenario, delirium may be described as "ICU psychosis" or "sundowner syndrome." However, delirious patients are not always agitated, and it is much more difficult to detect delirium when the patient is physically calm.[1,2,22]

Specific scoring instruments are available to assess delirium, and two have been validated for use with mechanically ventilated critical care patients.[23] They are the *Confusion Assessment Method for the Intensive Care Unit* (CAM-ICU) (Figure 9-2 and Figure 9-3)[24-26] and the *Intensive Care Delirium Screening Checklist* (ICDSC) (Figure 9-4).[27,28] Both instruments are used in tandem with the RASS or SAS to exclude patients in coma (RASS −4 −5; SAS 1) and to identify hyperactive delirium (RASS +4; SAS 7). Both instruments provide a structured format to evaluate delirium both for verbal patients and for nonverbal and mechanically ventilated patients.

Some preexisting conditions increase the likelihood that a patient will experience delirium, including dementia, alcohol use disorder, and prior sedative/opiate dependence.

BOX 9-2 Causes of Delirium in Critically Ill Patients

Metabolic Causes
- Acid-base disturbance
- Electrolyte imbalance
- Hypoglycemia

Intracranial Causes
- Epidural or subdural hematoma
- Intracranial hemorrhage
- Meningitis
- Encephalitis
- Cerebral abscess
- Tumor

Endocrine Causes
- Hyperthyroidism or hypothyroidism
- Addison's disease
- Hyperparathyroidism
- Cushing's syndrome

Organ Failure
- Liver encephalopathy
- Kidney encephalopathy
- Septic shock

Respiratory Causes
- Hypoxemia
- Hypercarbia

Medication-Related Causes
- Alcohol withdrawal syndrome
- Benzodiazepines
- Heavy metal poisoning

Modified from Szokol JW, Vender JS. Anxiety, delirium, and pain in the intensive care unit, *Crit Care Clin* 17(4): 821-842, 2001.

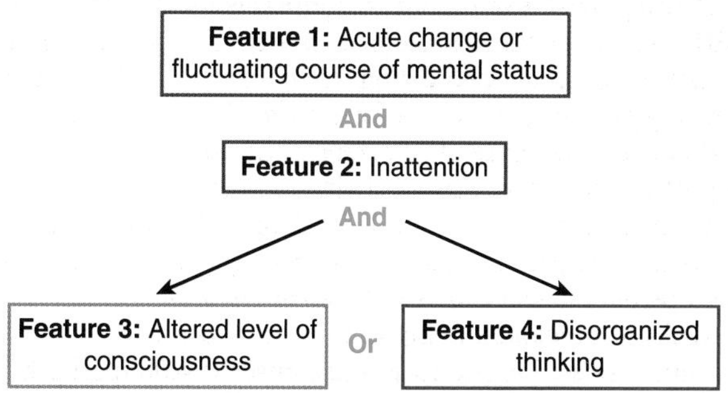

FIG 9-2 The Confusion Assessment Method for the ICU (CAM-ICU). Delirium is defined as positive in feature 1 AND feature 2 and EITHER feature 3 OR feature 4.

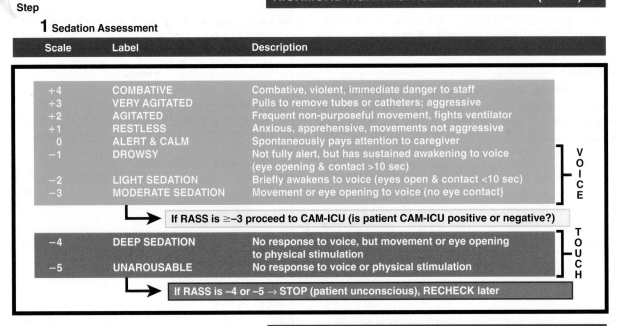

RICHMOND AGITATION-SEDATION SCALE (RASS)

Step

1 **Sedation Assessment**

Scale	Label	Description	
+4	COMBATIVE	Combative, violent, immediate danger to staff	
+3	VERY AGITATED	Pulls to remove tubes or catheters; aggressive	
+2	AGITATED	Frequent non-purposeful movement, fights ventilator	
+1	RESTLESS	Anxious, apprehensive, movements not aggressive	
0	ALERT & CALM	Spontaneously pays attention to caregiver	
−1	DROWSY	Not fully alert, but has sustained awakening to voice (eye opening & contact >10 sec)	VOICE
−2	LIGHT SEDATION	Briefly awakens to voice (eyes open & contact <10 sec)	VOICE
−3	MODERATE SEDATION	Movement or eye opening to voice (no eye contact)	VOICE
−4	DEEP SEDATION	No response to voice, but movement or eye opening to physical stimulation	TOUCH
−5	UNAROUSABLE	No response to voice or physical stimulation	TOUCH

→ **If RASS is ≥−3 proceed to CAM-ICU (is patient CAM-ICU positive or negative?)**

→ **If RASS is −4 or −5 → STOP (patient unconscious), RECHECK later**

Confusion Assessment Method for the ICU (CAM-ICU)

Step

2 **Delirium Assessment**

1. Acute Change or Fluctuating Course of Mental Status:
- **Is there an acute change from mental status baseline? OR**
- **Has the patient's mental status fluctuated during the past 24 hours?**

No → **CAM-ICU negative NO DELIRIUM**

↓ **YES**

2. Inattention:
- ***"Squeeze my hand when I say the letter 'A'."***
  Read the following sequence of letters:
  S A V E A H A A R T or C A S A B L A N C A or A B A D B A D A A Y
  ERRORS: No squeeze with 'A' & Squeeze on letter other than 'A'
- **If unable to complete Letters → Pictures**

0–2 Errors → **CAM-ICU negative NO DELIRIUM**

↓ **> 2 Errors**

3. Altered Level of Consciousness

Current RASS level (think back to sedation assessment in Step 1)

RASS other than zero → **CAM-ICU positive DELIRIUM present**

↓ **RASS = zero**

4. Disorganized thinking:
1. **Will a stone float on water?**
2. **Are there fish in the sea?**
3. **Does one pound weigh more than two?**
4. **Can you use a hammer to pound a nail?**

Command: "Hold up this many fingers" (Hold up 2 fingers)
"Now do the same thing with the other hand" (Do not demonstrate)
OR "Add one more finger" (If patient unable to move both arms)

>1 Error → **CAM-ICU positive DELIRIUM present**

0–1 Error → **CAM-ICU negative NO DELIRIUM**

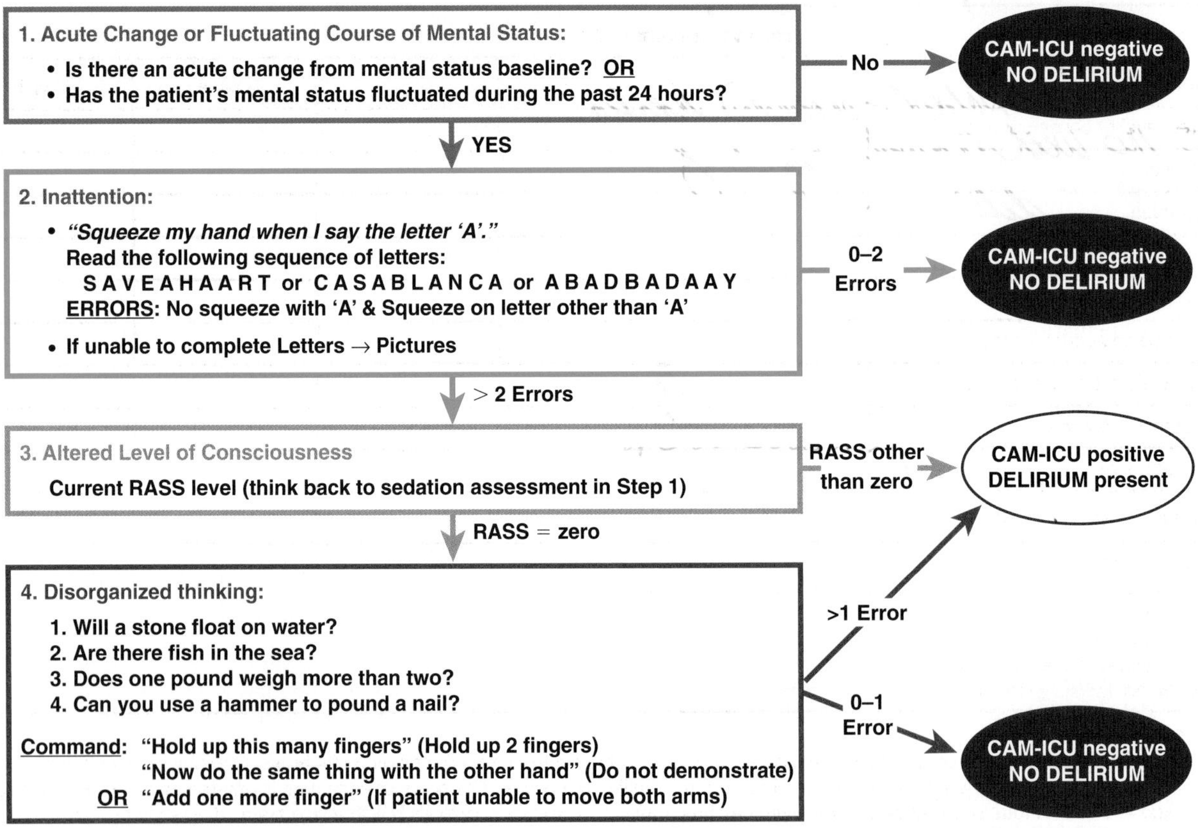

FIG 9-3 The Confusion Assessment for the ICU (CAM-ICU) Delirium Assessment. **A. Step 1**—Sedation Assessment. **B. Step 2**—Delirium Assessment. For detailed information on how to use the CAM-ICU, refer to the CAM-ICU training manual (revised edition March 2014) at www.icudelirium.org.

The Intensive Care Delirium Screening Checklist (ICDSC)

1. Altered level of consciousness

(A) No response or (B) the need for vigorous stimulation in order to obtain any response signified a severe alteration in the level of consciousness precluding evaluation. If there is coma (A) or stupor (B) most of the time period, then a dash (—) is entered and there is no further evaluation for that period.
(C) Drowsiness or response to a mild to moderate stimulation implies an altered level of consciousness and scores 1 point.
(D) Wakefulness or sleeping state that could easily be aroused is considered normal and scores zero points.
(E) Hypervigilance is rated as an abnormal level of consciousness and scores 1 point.

2. Inattention

Difficulty in following a conversation or instruction, easily distracted by external stimuli, or difficulty in shifting focus all score 1 point.

3. Disorientation

Any obvious mistake in time, place or person scores 1 point.

4. Hallucination, delusion or psychosis

The unequivocal clinical manifestation of hallucination or of behaviour probably due to hallucination (e.g., trying to catch a non-existent object) or delusion, or gross impairment in reality testing all score 1 point.

5. Psychomotor agitation or retardation

Hyperactivity requiring the use of additional sedative drugs or restraints in order to control potential danger (e.g., pulling out IV lines, hitting staff), hypoactivity or clinically noticeable psychomotor slowing all score 1 point.

6. Inappropriate speech or mood

Inappropriate, disorganized or incoherent speech, inappropriate mood related to events or situation all score 1 point.

7. Sleep/wake cycle disturbance

Sleeping less than four hours or waking frequently at night (do not consider wakefulness initiated by medical staff or loud environment), or sleeping during most of the day all score 1 point.

8. Symptom fluctuation

Fluctuation of the manifestation of any item or symptom over 24 hours (e.g., from one shift to another) scores 1 point.

How to Calculate a Score for the ICDSC*

Patient Evaluation	Day 1	Day 2	Day 3	Day 4	Day 5
Altered level of consciousness (A-E)*					
Inattention					
Disorientation					
Hallucination, delusion, psychosis					
Psychomotor agitation or retardation					
Inappropriate speech or mood					
Sleep-wake cycle disturbance					
Symptom fluctuation					
Total Score (0-8)					

*Level of Consciousness	Score
A: no response	–
B: response to intense and repeated stimulation (loud voice and pain)	–
C: response to mild or moderate stimulation	1
D: normal wakefulness	0
E: exaggerated response to normal stimulation	1
If **A** or **B**, do not complete patient evaluation for the period.	

Scoring System

The scale is completed based on information collected from each 8-hour shift or from the previous 24 hours. Obvious manifestation of an item = 1 point. No manifestation of an item or no assessment possible = 0 points. The score of each item is entered in the corresponding space and is 0 or 1. A total score of ≥4 on any given day has a 99% sensitivity for correlation with a psychiatric diagnosis of delirium.

*The ICDSC is also used in tandem with the RASS (see Table 9-1) to assess sedation-agitation in addition to delirium.

FIG 9-4 The Intensive Care Delirium Screening Checklist (ICDSC). (From Bergeron N, et al. Intensive Care Delirium Screening Checklist: evaluation of a new screening tool. *Intensive Care Med.* 2001;27:859-864.)

Pharmacologic Management of Delirium

Selecting medications that provide sedation but avoid withdrawal-associated agitation is a priority. The neuroleptic medication haloperidol (Haldol) is administered to treat hyperactive delirium.[29] Haldoperidol stabilizes cerebral function by blocking dopamine-mediated neurotransmission at the cerebral synapses and in the basal ganglia. Because haloperidol prolongs the QTc-interval, it increases the risk of the ventricular dysrhythmia torsade de points. The QTc must be monitored in all patients receiving haloperidol .

Nonpharmacologic Interventions to Prevent Delirium

Several research studies have shown that a "bundle" of interventions may prevent or reduce the duration of delirium in critical illness.[2] In mechanically ventilated patients the interventions include spontaneous awakening trials, early mobility, and daily delirium monitoring.[30,31] Early mobility may also prevent the muscle weakness that accompanies long periods of bed rest during critical illness and may perhaps reduce the cognitive complications associated with prolonged illness that many patients experience.[32] The American Association of Critical Care Nurses (AACN) promotes use of the ABCDE bundle. This is a combination of interventions designed to decrease sedation, reduce delirium and increase mobility in critically ill patients (see the ABCDE bundle implementation link in the Internet Box 9-3). Some critical care units have initiated sleep protocols to increase the opportunity for patients to sleep at night, dimming lights at night, ensuring there are periods of time when tubes are not manipulated and clustering nursing care interventions to provide some uninterrupted rest periods.[33]

ALCOHOL WITHDRAWAL SYNDROME AND DELIRIUM TREMENS

Critically ill patients who are alcohol-dependent, and were drinking prior to hospital admission, are at risk of *alcohol withdrawal syndrome* (AWS).[34] AWS is associated with an increased risk of delirium, hallucinations, seizures, increased need for mechanical ventilation, and death. When hyperactive agitated delirium is caused by alcohol withdrawal, it is termed *delirium tremens*, often verbally described as DTs.[34] Following hospital admission, as the alcohol-dependent patient's blood-alcohol concentration (BAC) falls, about 50% of patients will have AWS-related symptoms.[35] Fewer than 5% will experience severe complications such as delirium tremens or a seizure.[34,35] Screening tools to identify alcohol dependence such as the *Alcohol Use Disorders Identification Test* (AUDIT) shown in the Trauma chapter are very helpful. Management of alcohol withdrawal involves close monitoring of AWS-related agitation and administration of intravenous benzodiazepines, generally diazepam (Valium) or lorazepam (Ativan). Diazepam has the advantage of a longer half-life and high lipid solubility. Lipid-soluble medications quickly cross the blood–brain barrier and enter the central nervous system rapidly to produce a sedative effect.[34,36] Benzodiazepines should be administered in response to increased signs of agitation associated with DTs with dosage guided by a clinical protocol. This is described as an AWS symptom-triggered approach.[34] The severity of alcohol withdrawal can be assessed with a scale such as the Clinical Institute Withdrawal Assessment of Alcohol Scale (revised) (CIWA-Ar).[34,35] Multivitamins, including thiamine (Vitamin B_1), are administered prophylactically to prevent additional neurological sequelae.[34-36] Delirium related to alcohol withdrawal is pharmacologically managed very differently than delirium from other causes. Long-acting benzodiazepines are the medications of choice in AWS.[36] In contrast, benzodiazepines are contraindicated for treatment of delirium from non–alcohol-related causes.[37]

COLLABORATIVE MANAGEMENT

Collaborative management of anxiety, agitation, sedation, and delirium is a responsibility shared by all members of the health care team (see Box 9-4). Recognition of the problem is the first step toward a solution to establish a more effective standard of patient care in management of sedation, agitation, and delirium.

use a Sitter

BOX 9-3 INTERNET RESOURCES

AACN	American Association of Critical Care Nurses	http://www.aacn.org/
	AACN – Implementing the ABCDE Bundle at the bedside	http://www.aacn.org/wd/practice/content/actionpak/withlinks-ABCDE-ToolKit.content?menu=practice
SCCM	Society of Critical Care Medicine	http://www.sccm.org/
	Pain Agitation Delirium guidelines	http://www.learnicu.org/SiteCollectionDocuments/Pain,%20Agitation,%20Delirium.pdf
	ICU Delirium and Cognitive Impairment Study Group Vanderbilt University and Medical Center	http://www.icudelirium.org

BOX 9-4 EVIDENCE-BASED COLLABORATIVE PRACTICE (QSEN)

Summary of Guidelines for Assessment and Treatment of Agitation, Sedation, and Delirium

- Agitation in critically ill patients may result from inadequately treated pain, anxiety, delirium, and/or ventilator dyssynchrony.
- Detection and treatment of pain, agitation, and delirium should be reassessed often in these patients.
- Patients should be awake and able to follow commands purposely in order to participate in their care unless a clinical indication for deeper sedation exists.

Agitation

- Depth and quality of sedation should be routinely assessed in all critical care patients.
- The RASS and SAS are the most valid and reliable scales for assessing quality and depth of sedation in critically ill patients.
- Target the lightest possible level of sedation and/or use daily sedative interruption.
- Use sedation protocols and checklists to facilitate sedation management.
- Suggest using analgesia-first sedation for intubated and mechanically ventilated critically ill patients.
- Suggest using non-benzodiazepines for sedation (either propofol or dexmedetomidine) rather than benzodiazepines (either midazolam or lorazepam) in mechanically ventilated adult critical care patients.

Delirium

- Delirium assessment should be routinely performed in all critically ill patients.
- The CAM-ICU and ICDSC delirium monitoring tools are the most valid and reliable scales to assess delirium in critical care patients.
- Mobilize critical care patients early when feasible to reduce the incidence and duration of delirium and to improve functional outcomes.
- Promote sleep in critically ill patients by controlling light and noise, clustering patient care activities, and decreasing stimuli at night.
- Avoid using rivastigmine to reduce the duration of delirium in critically ill patients.
- Suggest avoiding the use of antipsychotics in patients who are at risk for torsades de pointes.
- Suggest not using benzodiazepines in critically ill patients with delirium unrelated to alcohol/benzodiazepine withdrawal.

CAM-ICU, Confusion Assessment Method for the Intensive Care Unit; ICDSC, Intensive Care Delirium Screening Checklist.
Data from Barr J, et al. Clinical Practice Guidelines for the Management of Pain, Agitation, and Delirium in Adult Patients in the Intensive Care Unit, *Crit Care Med* 2013; 41, 263-306.

CASE STUDY Patient with Delirium

Brief Patient History

Mr. K is a 42-year-old Asian, out-of-town businessman in your city. He is transported to your facility from his hotel because of a witnessed grand mal seizure. Paramedics administered lorazepam in the field. Mr. K's wife reports by phone that he is in good health and that she is not aware that he takes any medications regularly. However, she states that he recently quit drinking alcohol because of pressure from the family. She also comments that she thinks he takes alprazolam to calm his nerves once in a while.

Clinical Assessment

Mr. K is admitted to the intensive care unit from the emergency department with hypertension, restlessness, mental confusion, paranoid ideations with rambling speech, and visual and auditory hallucinations. Mr. K's skin is warm and moist. Intravenous administration of thiamine, folic acid, multivitamins, and magnesium was begun in the emergency department. Physician orders were written for lorazepam every 6 hours and clonidine every 4 hours as needed for delirium-related symptoms.

Diagnostic Procedures

Mr. K's baseline vital signs are as follows: blood pressure of 190/92 mm Hg, heart rate of 130 beats/min (sinus tachycardia), respiratory rate of 26 breaths/min, and temperature of 98.8° F. Pulse oximetry O_2 saturation is 90% on 4 L/min oxygen using a nasal cannula. Confusion Assessment Method indicates presence of acute and fluctuating change in mental status, inattention, and disorganized thinking. The *Riker Sedation-Agitation Scale* score is 5. Serum and urine toxicology studies are negative for ethyl alcohol, cannabis, and opioids; urine is strongly positive for benzodiazepines. The sodium level is 135 mmol/L, potassium level is 4.3 mmol/L, chloride level is 84 mmol/L, carbon dioxide level is 26 mEq/L, calcium level is 8 mg/dL, magnesium level is 2.0 mg/dL, and gamma-glutamyl transpeptidase (GGT) level is 80 IU/L.

Medical Diagnosis

Mr. K is diagnosed with delirium tremens caused by alcohol and benzodiazepine withdrawal.

Questions

1. What major outcomes do you expect to achieve for this patient?
2. What problems or risks must be managed to achieve these outcomes?
3. What interventions must be initiated to monitor, prevent, manage, or eliminate the problems and risks identified?
4. What interventions should be initiated to promote optimal functioning, safety, and well-being of the patient?
5. What possible learning needs do you anticipate for this patient?
6. What cultural and age-related factors may have a bearing on the patient's plan of care?

REFERENCES

1. Jacobi J, et al: Clinical practice guidelines for the sustained use of sedatives and analgesics in the critically ill adult, *Crit Care Med* 30:119–141, 2002.
2. Barr J, et al: Clinical Practice Guidelines for the Management of Pain, Agitation, and Delirium in Adult Patients in the Intensive Care Unit, *Crit Care Med* 41: 263–306, 2013.
3. Ely EW, et al: Monitoring sedation status over time in ICU patients: reliability and validity of the Richmond Agitation-Sedation Scale (RASS), *JAMA* 289:2983–2991, 2003.
4. Sessler CN, et al: The Richmond Agitation-Sedation Scale: validity and reliability in adult intensive care unit patients, *Am J Respir Crit Care Med* 166:1338–1344, 2002.
5. Riker RR, et al: Prospective evaluation of the Sedation-Agitation Scale for adult critically ill patients, *Crit Care Med* 27:1325–1329, 1999.
6. Devlin JW, Roberts RJ: Pharmacology of commonly used analgesics and sedatives in the ICU: benzodiazepines, propofol, and opioids, *Crit Care Clin* 25(3):431–439, 2009.
7. Fong JJ, et al: Propofol associated with a shorter duration of mechanical ventilation than scheduled intermittent lorazepam: a database analysis using Project IMPACT, *Ann Pharmacother* 41:1986–1991, 2007.
8. Pandharipande P, et al: Lorazepam is an independent risk factor for transitioning to delirium in intensive care unit patients, *Anesthesiology* 104:21–26, 2006.
9. Pandharipande PP, et al: Effect of sedation with dexmedetomidine vs lorazepam on acute brain dysfunction in mechanically ventilated patients: the MENDS randomized controlled trial, *JAMA* 298:2644–2653, 2007.
10. Betten DP, et al: Antidote use in the critically ill poisoned patient, *J Intensive Care Med* 21:255–277, 2006.
11. Whitcomb JJ, et al: The use of propofol in the mechanically ventilated medical/surgical intensive care patient: is it the right choice?, *Dimens Crit Care Nurs* 22:60–63, 2003.
12. Zaccheo MM, Bucher DH: Propofol infusion syndrome: a rare complication with potentially fatal results, *Crit Care Nurse* 28:18–26, 2008.
13. Corbett SM, et al: Propofol-related infusion syndrome in intensive care patients, *Pharmacotherapy* 28:250–258, 2008.
14. Lam SW, Alexander E: Dexmedetomidine use in critical care, *AACN Advanced Critical Care* 19:113–120, 2008.
15. Tan JA, Ho KM: Use of dexmedetomidine as a sedative and analgesic agent in critically ill adult patients: a meta-analysis, *Intensive Care Med* 36(6):926–939, 2010.
16. Akada S, et al: The efficacy of dexmedetomidine in patients with noninvasive ventilation: a preliminary study, *Anesth Analg* 107:167–170, 2008.
17. Pichot C, et al: Dexmedetomidine and clonidine: from second- to first-line sedative agents in the critical care setting?, *J Intensive Care Med* 27(4):219–237, 2012.
18. Kress JP, et al: Daily interruption of sedative infusions in critically ill patients undergoing mechanical ventilation, *N Engl J Med* 342:1471–1477, 2000.
19. Girard TD, et al: Efficacy and safety of a paired sedation and ventilator weaning protocol for mechanically ventilated patients in intensive care (Awakening and Breathing Controlled trial): a randomised controlled trial, *Lancet* 371:126–134, 2008.
20. Jackson JC, et al: Depression, post-traumatic stress disorder, and functional disability in survivors of critical illness in the BRAIN-ICU study: a longitudinal cohort study, *Lancet Respir Med* 2(5):369–379, 2014.
21. Ely EW, et al: Delirium as a predictor of mortality in mechanically ventilated patients in the intensive care unit, *JAMA* 291:1753–1762, 2004.
22. Roberts BL, et al: Patients' dreams in ICU: recall at two years post discharge and comparison to delirium status during ICU admission. A multicentre cohort study, *Intensive Crit Care Nurs* 22:264–273, 2006.
23. Plaschke K, et al: Comparison of the confusion assessment method for the intensive care unit (CAM-ICU) with the Intensive Care Delirium Screening Checklist (ICDSC) for delirium in critical care patients gives high agreement rate(s), *Intensive Care Med* 34:431–436, 2008.
24. Ely EW, et al: Evaluation of delirium in critically ill patients: validation of the Confusion Assessment Method for the Intensive Care Unit (CAM-ICU), *Crit Care Med* 29:1370–1379, 2001.
25. Ely EW, et al: Delirium in mechanically ventilated patients: validity and reliability of the confusion assessment method for the intensive care unit (CAM-ICU), *JAMA* 286:2703–2710, 2001.
26. Pun BT, et al: Large-scale implementation of sedation and delirium monitoring in the intensive care unit: a report from two medical centers, *Crit Care Med* 33:1199–1205, 2005.
27. Bergeron N, et al: Intensive Care Delirium Screening Checklist: evaluation of a new screening tool, *Intensive Care Med* 27:859–864, 2001.
28. Ouimet S, et al: Subsyndromal delirium in the ICU: evidence for a disease spectrum, *Intensive Care Med* 33:1007–1013, 2007.
29. Milbrandt EB, et al: Haloperidol use is associated with lower hospital mortality in mechanically ventilated patients, *Crit Care Med* 33:226–229, 2005.
30. Balas MC, et al: Critical care nurses' role in implementing the "ABCDE bundle" into practice, *Crit Care Nurse* 32(2):35–38, 40–48, 2012.
31. Balas MC, et al: Effectiveness and safety of the awakening and breathing *coordination, delirium monitoring/management, and early exercise/mobility bundle, Crit Care Med* 42(5):1024–1036, 2014.
32. Davidson J, et al: Implementation of the Pain, Agitation, and Delirium Clinical Practice Guidelines and promoting patient mobility to prevent post-intensive care syndrome, *Crit Care Med* 41(9 Suppl 1):S136–S145, 2014.
33. Bryczkowski SB, et al: Delirium prevention program in the surgical intensive care unit improved the outcomes of older adults, *J Surg Res* 190(1):280–288, 2013.
34. Sarff M, Gold JA: Alcohol withdrawal syndromes in the intensive care unit, *Crit Care Med* 38(9 Suppl):S494–S501, 2010.
35. Schuckit MA: Alcohol-use disorders, *Lancet* 373:492–501, 2009.
36. Amato L, et al: Benzodiazepines for alcohol withdrawal, *Cochrane Database Syst Rev* 3:CD005063, 2010.
37. Lonergan E, et al: Benzodiazepines for delirium, *Cochrane Database Syst Rev* (4):CD006379, 2009.

CHAPTER 10

End-of-Life Care

Caroline Etland

Be sure to check out the bonus material, including review questions, on the Evolve website at http://evolve.elsevier.com/Urden/priorities/.

End of life has become an important clinical topic in critical care, although requisite improvements in end-of-life care have been slow to follow. Because the primary purpose of admission of patients to a critical care unit is to provide aggressive, life-saving treatment, the death of a patient is generally regarded as a failure. Because the culture emphasizes saving lives, the language that describes the end of life employs negative terms, such as "forgoing life-sustaining treatments," "do not resuscitate (DNR)," and "withdrawal of life support." Sometimes the phrase *withdrawal of care* is used. These words should not be used because families may think there will be no comfort measures or assistance provided after a decision is made to discontinue mechanical ventilation and other life-sustaining treatments. Recently, more accurate language has been proposed to describe end-of-life decision making and medical interventions, such as *allow natural death* instead of "do not resuscitate" and *withholding of non-beneficial treatment* in place of "futile care."[1] This shift toward more realistic descriptors reflects extensive recent research in palliative care and the effectiveness of goals-of-care discussions for people with serious illnesses prior to crisis events. This chapter focuses on the care rendered to the dying critical care patient and his or her family.

PALLIATIVE CARE

The growth of palliative care programs in the United States has demonstrated the importance of this new health care specialty, with a 125% increase from 2000 to 2008.[2] Initiatives such as the IPAL-ICU have demonstrated that a focus on life-saving interventions can be integrated with palliative care concurrently. See the Internet Resources for Palliative Care Box for more information.

Patients who are identified as being critically ill, especially those near the end of life, require aggressive care for their symptom management. Palliative care guidelines have been released by a consortium of organizations concerned with palliative care and end-of-life care, and they may provide guidance when the usual first-line treatments do not promote comfort for critically ill patients who are near death.[3] Strategies that are based on research evidence and expert opinion for specific conditions such as delirium, opioid dose escalation, and dyspnea at the end of life are outlined on the End-of-Life/Palliative Education Resource Center (EPERC) website.[4] (See Box 10-2: Internet Resources for additional information) Palliative care has been thought of as desirable only when the patient nears death or when several interventions have been tried for management of symptoms without success. However, palliative care ideally begins at the time of diagnosis of a life-threatening illness and continues through cure or until death and into the family's bereavement period.

END-OF-LIFE EXPERIENCE IN CRITICAL CARE

Attention to end-of-life care for hospitalized patients has increased since the publication of the Study to Understand Prognoses and Preferences for Outcomes and Risks of Treatment (SUPPORT).[5] In this major report, more than 9000 seriously ill patients in five medical centers were studied. Despite an intervention to improve communication, aggressive treatment was common. Only about half of physicians knew their patients' preferences to avoid cardiopulmonary resuscitation (CPR), more than one-third of patients who died spent at least 10 days in a critical care unit, and for 50% of conscious patients, family members reported moderate-to-severe pain at least one-half of the time.[5]

Following closely after the publication of the SUPPORT study, the Institute of Medicine (IOM) released a report, *Approaching Death: Improving Care at the End of Life*.[6] The group detailed deficiencies in care and gave seven recommendations to improve care:

1. Patients with fatal illnesses and their families should receive reliable, skillful, and supportive care.
2. Health professionals should improve care for the dying.
3. Policymakers and consumers should work with health professionals to improve quality and financing of care.
4. Health profession education should include end-of-life content.
5. Palliative care should be developed, possibly as a medical specialty.
6. Research on end of life should be funded.
7. The public should communicate more about the experience of dying and options available.

Advance Directives

Although advance directives, also known as a *living will* or a *health care power of attorney*, were intended to ensure that patients received the care they desired at the end of their life, their enactment has proven less effective than desired. Like other preventive measures, advance directives are underused, even though they are inexpensive and potentially effective.[7] Completion rates in adults range from 16% to 36% overall with less than one-half of seriously or terminally ill patients having documented their wishes.[8]

Physician Orders for Life-Sustaining Treatment (POLST)

The Physician Orders for Life-Sustaining Treatment (POLST) initiative began in Oregon in the 1990s when medical leaders collaborated to address the problem of patients' advance directives not being honored.[9] Different from an advance directive, POLST forms are medical orders that are honored across all treatment settings and are especially important to emergency responders in the community. Also, they are completed by the patient and physician with the knowledge of a serious chronic illness and should be incorporated into medical orders upon admission to the hospital or skilled nursing facility. Critical care nurses working in states that recognize POLST forms need to know whether state law mandates that health care providers honor wishes documented on POLST forms or if the POLST serves as a guideline only. POLST forms are more easily read than an advance directive in that the format is one of check boxes with specific directions.

Advance Care Planning

Cultural influences in the United States discourage discussion of death. Planning for decisions to be made at a later date if one is deemed incompetent is a difficult process, but this knowledge helps the family members left to make the treatment decisions. Wishes for care should a person become incapacitated may be difficult for a loved one to discuss, but this helps in times of crisis to prevent indecision that could lead to unwanted interventions. When family members hear wishes for end of life care, their actions regarding treatment can be more congruent with their loved one's desires when communicating with healthcare providers. Families and care providers should be informed if patients decline aggressive care, so their families will not be left with difficult decisions in emergency situations. Emotional support for the patient and the family is important as they discuss advance care planning in the critical care setting.[10]

Ethical and Legal Issues

Legal and ethical principles guide many of our decisions in caring for the dying patient and the family. The patient is respected as autonomous and able to make his or her own decisions. When the patient is unable to make decisions, however, the same respect should be accorded to surrogates. These wishes might have been put in writing by the patient as an advance directive and preferably discussed with the surrogate. The Patient Self-Determination Act (PSDA) supports the patient's right to control future treatment in the event the individual cannot communicate.

Comfort Care

The decision to withdraw life-sustaining treatments and switch to comfort care at end of life includes the patient in decision making or a surrogate decision maker if the patient is not able to participate. The patient's intent as understood from discussions or knowledge of the patient should guide the decision about future treatment options. Withholding and withdrawing treatment are considered to be morally and legally equivalent.[11] However, because families experience more stress in withdrawing treatments than in withholding them,[12] interventions should not be started that the patient would not want or that would not provide benefit.

Cardiopulmonary Resuscitation

Cardiopulmonary resuscitation (CPR) was originally developed for those with coronary artery disease, and they are the most likely to survive resuscitation to discharge, as well as those who suffer cardiac arrest in the critical care unit.[13] However, benefits of resuscitation may be overestimated for survival and for return to baseline functional status. Overall survival to discharge after in-hospital CPR is about 13-17%.[14,15] Despite these dismal statistics, CPR is offered as an option without fully informing patients or families of the low possibility of survival and the potential for decline in functional status.

Do Not Resuscitate Orders

A Do Not Resuscitate (DNR) order is intended to prevent the initiation of life-sustaining measures such as endotracheal intubation or CPR. When faced with the decision of whether to withdraw non-beneficial care, families should be assured that patients will continue to receive aggressive pain and symptom management but that aggressive measures to extend life will not be employed. DNR orders should be written before withdrawal of life support is initiated. This documentation ensures that the patient is not subjected to unwanted interventions during the period between initiation of withdrawal and death.

Prognostication and Prognostic Tools

Clinicians' ability to prognosticate the length of time before death is limited,[16,17] and the time to death usually is overestimated. Patients' wishes are often not known, can be vague even when they are known,[18] or change over the course of an illness.[19] Care may not be in accordance with patients' wishes, and this discrepancy is more prevalent when comfort care is desired over aggressive care.[20] Use of prognostic scales can add meaningful information to help patients and families make informed decisions. A summary of commonly used prognostic scales is in Table 10-1.[21]

Despite this information and these tools, uncertainty remains a major issue in decision making for physicians, nurses, patients, and families.[19] Because of uncertain prognosis and anecdotal stories of patients who were never thought likely to survive actually return to visit a critical care unit, professionals are not confident about issues of survivability. Moreover, many families cling to hopes of survival and recovery.

Withdrawal or Withholding of Treatment

Discussions about the potential for impending death are never held early enough. Usually, the first discussion about prognosis occurs in conjunction with the topic of the discontinuation of life support. The late timing of that first discussion is a concern, particularly because some families have

TABLE 10-1 Selected Prognostic Scales

PROGNOSTIC SCALE	DISEASE/CLINICAL CONDITION	PROGNOSTIC SCALE	DISEASE/CLINICAL CONDITION
Palliative Prognostic Scale (PPS)	Any hospice population; palliative care patients	Lung Cancer Prognostic Model (LCPM)	Terminal lung cancer patients
Palliative Prognostic Index (PPI)	Terminal cancer patients	Dementia Prognostic Model (DPM)	Demographic, diagnosis, laboratory, and functional data on dementia residents
Palliative Prognostic Score (PaP)	Terminal cancer patients	Prognostic Index for One-Year Mortality in Older Adults (PIMOA)	Adults >70 years of age with previous stay in hospital
Seattle Heart Failure Model; Heart Failure Risk Scoring System (HFRSS)	Acute heart failure	Cancer Prognostic Scale (CPS)	Terminal cancer patients in Progressive Care Unit
BODE Scale	COPD	Mortality Risk Index Score (MRIS)	New admission to nursing home

Adapted from Lau F, et al. A systematic review of prognostic tools for estimating survival time in palliative care. *J Palliat Care*. 2007; 23(2):93.

arrived at the notion of withdrawal before physicians.[22,23] Equally important is that some family members dread such conversations but are grateful to discuss the uncertainty of their loved one's future. Clinicians should give families time to adjust to this information and make preparations by providing discussions early about prognosis, goals of therapy, and the patient's wishes. After a poor prognosis is established, a period can elapse before end-of-life treatment goals are determined. Proactive palliative care is most helpful when admission diagnoses trigger a consultation instead of after several avenues of treatment have been exhausted.[24]

Steps toward Comfort Care

If a series of interventions is to be withdrawn, dialysis usually is discontinued first, along with diagnostic tests and vasopressors. Next, intravenous fluids, monitoring, laboratory tests, and antibiotics are stopped.[25] Withdrawal of specific treatments may have effects necessitating symptom management. Withdrawal of dialysis may cause dyspnea from volume overload, which may necessitate the use of opioids or benzodiazepines. Efforts to discontinue artificial feeding may be met with concern from the family because offering food has great social significance. It is essential to share information with family and providers regarding the potential benefits of withholding food and fluids in the days immediately prior to death to prevent unnecessary suffering.[26]

Pain Management

Because many critical care patients are not conscious, assessment of pain and other symptoms becomes more difficult.[27] Gélinas and colleagues[28] recommended using signs of body movements, neuromuscular signs, facial expressions, or responses to physical examination for pain assessment in patients with altered consciousness (see Chapter 8).

Nonopioid medications are usually a first-line approach in the general patient population, followed by adding an opioid for additional analgesia when relief is not obtained. However, critically ill patients and those at the end of life usually require stronger analgesics. Because opioids provide sedation, anxiolysis, and analgesia, they are particularly beneficial in the ventilated patient and often are first-line treatment for critical care patients. Morphine is the medication of choice, and there is no upper limit in dosing.

Symptom Management and Promoting Comfort

The nursing interventions at end of life focus on the provision of comfort care as an active, desirable, and important service. Unnecessary checks of vital signs, laboratory work, and any treatment that does not promote comfort should be avoided. Positioning the patient who is actively dying has as its purpose only comfort, not the schedule to promote skin integrity. Coordinating this care with the many members of the critical care team is important to ensure consistency. When symptom management is not successful in ensuring comfort, the services of the pain team or the palliative care service may be required. Provision of comfort and palliation of symptoms at end of life is a major focus of the health care team.

Dyspnea

Dyspnea is best managed with close evaluation of the patient and the use of opioids, sedatives, and nonpharmacologic interventions (oxygen, positioning, and increased ambient air flow).[29] Morphine reduces anxiety and muscle tension and increases pulmonary vasodilatation but is not effective when inhaled. Benzodiazepines may be used in patients who are not able to take opioids or for whom the respiratory effects are minimal. Benzodiazepines and opioids should be titrated to effect. Treatment efforts should be aimed at the patient's expression of dyspnea rather than at respiratory rates or oxygen levels.[30]

Nausea and Vomiting

Nausea and vomiting are common and should be treated with antiemetics. The cause of nausea and vomiting may be intestinal obstruction. Treatment for decompression may be uncomfortable in dying patients, and its use should be weighed using a benefit-to-burden ratio.

Fever

Fever and infection necessitate assessment of the benefits of continuing antibiotics so as not to prolong the dying process. Management of the fever with antipyretics may be appropriate for the patient's comfort, but other methods such as ice or hypothermia blankets should be balanced against the amount of distress the patient may experience.

Edema

Edema may cause discomfort, and diuretics may be effective if kidney function is intact. Dialysis is not warranted at the end of life. The use of fluids may contribute to the edema when kidney function is impaired and the body is slowing its functions.

Delirium

Delirium is commonly observed in the critically ill and in those approaching death. Haloperidol is recommended as useful, and restraints should be avoided.

Metabolic Derangement

Treatments for metabolic derangements, skin problems, anemia, and hemorrhage are tempered with concerns for the patient's comfort. Only interventions promoting comfort should be performed. Patients do not necessarily feel better "when the laboratory values are right."

Withdrawal of Mechanical Ventilation

Standardized withdrawal from life-support order sets are recommended to direct and support nursing judgment in this complex and emotional clinical situation. Recommendations for creating a supportive atmosphere during withdrawal discussions include the following:

- Taking a moment at the beginning of the conversation to inquire about the family's emotional state
- Acknowledging verbal and nonverbal expressions of emotion and using that to support families
- Acknowledging that most family members face a significant emotional burden when a loved one is critically ill or dying

During the family meeting in which a decision to withdraw life support is made, a time to initiate withdrawal is usually established. For example, a distant family member may need to arrive, and then the procedure will occur. When appropriate, the patient should be moved to a separate or special room. It is helpful if other staff members are alerted to the fact that a withdrawal is occurring. A neutral sign hung on the door or use of a special room may caution staff to avoid loud conversations and laughter, which is quite upsetting to grieving families.

After the decision to remove ventilator support is made and the family is gathered, the family should be told what the impending death will be like. When the patient is dependent on ventilator support or vasopressors and that support is removed, death typically follows in minutes. The patient appears as if sleeping, and the usual signs of color and skin temperature changes will not be seen before death. The opposite is true if the patient is not ventilator-dependent. When the patient will be extubated at the beginning of the withdrawal process, the family should be prepared for respiratory noises and gasping respirations. These signs are less likely when the endotracheal tube is removed near the end of the withdrawal process, as is more commonly done.

Pacemakers or implantable cardioverter-defibrillators should be turned off to prevent patient distress from their firing[31] and to avoid interfering with the pronouncement of death.[25] Neuromuscular blocking agents should be discontinued, because paralysis precludes the assessment of the patient's discomfort and the means of the patient to communicate with loved ones. The removal of monitors is usually recommended.[32]

Opioids and Sedatives

Opioids and benzodiazepines are the most commonly administered medications because dyspnea and anxiety are the usual symptoms related to ventilator withdrawal. Medications include an intravenous bolus dose of morphine (2 to 10 mg IV) and a continuous morphine infusion at 50% of the bolus dose per hour. Midazolam (1 to 2 mg IV) is given, followed by an infusion at 1 mg/hr.[33] The intent is to provide effective symptom control so that doses accelerate until the patient's comfort is achieved. Additional medication should be available at the bedside for immediate administration if discomfort is observed in the patient. Opioids or benzodiazepines are used to treat discomfort after the withdrawal of life support and not to hasten death in critically ill patients.[34]

Ventilator Settings

After the patient's comfort is achieved, ventilator settings are reduced. An experienced physician, a respiratory therapist, and a nurse should be present during this time. Ventilator alarms should be turned off. The choice of terminal wean as opposed to extubation is based on considerations of access for suctioning, appearance of the patient for the family, how long the patient will survive off the ventilator, and whether the patient has the ability to communicate with loved ones at the bedside.

If terminal wean is used, positive end-expiratory pressure (PEEP) is reduced to normal, and then the mode is set to patient control. Next, the FiO_2 is reduced to room air (0.21 oxygen). All of these steps are taken slowly while observing the patient for distress or anxiety. If extubation is performed immediately rather than at the end of the terminal wean, the family should be prepared for airway compromise and changes in the appearance of the patient.

ORGAN DONATION

Legal Issues

The Social Security Act Section 1138 requires that hospitals have written protocols for the identification of potential organ donors.[35] The Joint Commission (TJC) has a standard on organ donation, and there is a variety of state legislation to direct health care providers and organ recovery agencies.[36] Although an impending death marks a difficult time for family members, the hospital must notify the organ procurement official to approach the family with a donation request. These individuals have training to make a supportive request and are the ones to decide whether a family may be approached based on the patient's disease. Although organ donation may not be appropriate in some cases, tissue donation remains a consideration.

Brain Death

Death may be pronounced when the patient meets a list of neurologic criteria. However, there are differences among hospital policies for certification of brain death, which may permit differences in the circumstances under which patients are pronounced dead in different U.S. hospitals.[37] Families do not always understand the meaning of brain death, and they are less likely to donate organs when they believe the patient will not be dead until the ventilator is turned off and the heart stops.[38] How these conversations are held will determine families' understanding and positively affect donation. Do not suggest that the organs are alive while the brain is dead, but rather that the organs are functioning as a result of the machines used.[39]

FAMILY CARE

In this chapter, the term *family* means whomever the patient states is the family. An integral part of the patient-family dyad, families expect a cure for any condition the patient may have; they do not expect to receive bad news. They look for the good news in any message received from caregivers and are surprised when told that death is the only outcome possible.[40] Families need assistance in forming their expectations about outcomes. Ongoing communication about the patient's progress is preferable to waiting until the patient is near death and then communicating with the family.

Communication and Decision Making

In critical illness the patients' capacity for decision making is often limited by illness severity or by the therapies or medications used to treat them.[22] When the patient is not able to make health care decisions safely, written documents such as a living will or a health care power of attorney should be obtained if available. Without those documents, the patient's wishes are ascertained from those closest to the patient.

Communication with the patient and family is critical. Families were found to go through a process in their decision making in which they considered the personal domain (rallying support and evaluating quality of life), the critical care unit environment domain (chasing the doctors and relating to the health care team), and the decision domain (arriving at a new belief and making and communicating the decision).[41] Higher levels of shared decision making are associated with greater family satisfaction.

How questions are asked of surrogates is extremely important. The question is not "What do you want to do about (patient's name)?" but rather "What would (patient's name) want if he knew he were in this situation?" These two questions have vastly different meanings and consequences for the patient and the family. Sometimes, this discussion is held during the family meeting, in which goals of care can be discussed.

Family Meetings

Family meetings in the presence of the critical care team have been one method used to arrive at a common understanding of the patient's prognosis and goals for future care.[42,43] An analysis of the amount of time families had to speak in these meetings revealed that when families had greater opportunity to talk, their satisfaction with physician communication increased, and their ratings of conflict with the physician decreased. After the patient's death, greater family satisfaction with withdrawal of life support was associated with the following measures:[44]

- The process of withdrawal of life support being well explained
- Withdrawal of life support proceeding as expected
- Patient appearing comfortable
- Family and friends being prepared
- Appropriate person initiating discussion
- Adequate privacy during withdrawal of life support
- A chance to voice concerns

Waiting for Good News

Patients and families do not come to the critical care unit with the expectation of death. Even those who have had previous admissions expect to be "saved." They tend to listen to imparted information looking for good news; even when bad news is given, they may initially deny it or have great difficulty taking it in.[45] Having this in mind while talking to families may assist professionals in interpreting families' responses.

Preparing families for changes in the patient as the health condition deteriorates helps them make plans. They need to know if other family members should be called, if someone should spend the night, or if financial arrangements should be changed before an impending death (e.g., to enable the widow to have access to funds). Anticipated changes can be described to prepare families. Emotional support and grieving can be facilitated through discussion of the dying patient and their unique qualities and families' memories. Interactive patient education television services provide healing music and videos that help to create a more comfortable environment for families as they wait for the next step in the dying process. Often, families will play the patient's favorite music or movies. Many services also provide access to the Internet through which family pictures or videos can be accessed. Even before the patient dies, provision of these services can be beneficial through visiting a shared past, making the most of the present, and hoping for an end to the patient's suffering and healing for loved ones.

Families may refuse to forgo life-supporting treatments and want "everything done" because of mistrust of health professionals, poor communication, survivor guilt, or religious or cultural reasons.[22] Effective communication throughout the hospitalization and information provided throughout the stay predispose the family to better acceptance of news as the patient deteriorates. Family satisfaction is increased when they feel supported during their decision making[46,47] or hear more empathic statements from physicians.[48]

Visiting Hours

Restricting visiting for dying critical care unit patients is unconscionable. Providing the visiting time to help family members say good-bye is an important function. Family members may have difficulty in seeing the person they knew among all the tubes. Coaching can be provided about how to approach the patient and about how the patient may still be able to hear despite appearing to be nonresponsive. Visitors should be permitted to the extent possible, while not interfering with other patients' privacy or rest. Children, unless they represent a significant source of infection, should be allowed to say good-bye, but they may need adult assistance in understanding the situation. Families may have religious or cultural ceremonies that are important for them to perform before the patient dies or experiences withdrawal of life support. These practices should be encouraged and facilitated as much as possible. Continuity of care by the same nurse is important. As the patient nears death, nurses have sometimes stayed with the family after the end of a shift when death was imminent so that they would not need to adjust to another person at this difficult time.[49]

Family Presence during Resuscitation

Historically, family members were asked to leave the room during resuscitation. The American Association of

Critical-Care Nurses (AACN)[50] and the Emergency Nurses Association (ENA)[51] have issued position statements recommending that families be allowed to be present during CPR and invasive procedures. Family presence is a significant source of support for the patient, and there may be a benefit to the family in observing the resuscitation by knowing that everything possible was done.

Comfort Cart

One intervention used with families at the end of life is the use of a grieving or comfort cart. The cart might have a top drawer with English and Spanish versions of the Bible, Koran, and Book of Mormon and pamphlets about grief and bereavement. The lower portion of the cart holds paper cups, napkins, and condiments. Fresh coffee and tea are brewed and served with muffins and cookies from the cafeteria. Family responses are positive because they do not want to leave the bedside despite their hunger.

Cultural and Spiritual Influences on Communication

Cultural and spiritual influences on attitudes and beliefs about death and dying differ dramatically across cultures and religious communities. These differences may affect how the health care team is viewed, how decisions are made, whether aggressive treatment is preferred, how death is met, and how grieving will occur.[52] Patients who do not follow a particular religion should be assessed for their individual spiritual beliefs or lack thereof. Identifying sources of spiritual comfort strengthens the bond between caregivers, patients, and family. Interpreters are necessary when the patient or the family members do not speak English. A cultural and religious assessment is warranted in all situations because cultural or religious affiliation does not imply that patients or families follow all of the tenets of that group.

Hospice Information

Although hospice care has been available for many years, patients and families often consider this method of care only in the last weeks or months of a patient with end-stage illness, and they frequently view hospice care as "giving up." Health professionals can assist patients and families by providing information about the hospice benefit, particularly regarding the aggressive symptom management and family support. Hospice care is an option that should be considered, especially in end-stage illness.

After Death

After the death, the family may wish to spend time at the bedside. The family members' time with the body should be unhurried and private. They need adequate room to sit and spend time. They can be asked if they need assistance or resources and whether they wish to be alone or have someone nearby. Frequently, the bed is needed for another patient, and juggling is required to ensure that the family has sufficient time even as another patient needs to be admitted. Supporting families after a death involves immediate bereavement support, information on what to do about the death, bereavement support for the future, contact with the family after death, and assessment of the quality of care the patient experienced.[53] Having material already prepared with the necessary after-death information is quite helpful at this time.

PROFESSOINAL ISSUES

Emotional Support for the Nurse

Nurses who care for the dying patient need to have their work as valued as other high-technology functions in the critical care unit. Critical care units usually have several nurses who are looked to by other staff to provide end-of-life care or to assist with withdrawal of life support. When several deaths occur close together, those nurses may be called on frequently. Some consideration in assignment should be given when a nurse has more than one death in a shift or a week. Taking a new admission is also difficult immediately after a death, and it can occur before the family has left the unit. Nurse administrators can provide some additional resources, debriefing, or time off when the burden has been high. Hearing supportive words from colleagues has been reported by critical care nurses as helpful in coping with the death of a patient.[49]

Nurses experience moral distress when aggressive care is offered to patients who are not expected to benefit from it. These levels of distress are high and have implications for retention of highly skilled nurses.[54] Until recently, end-of-life content in nursing school curriculums and textbooks was sparse, and continuing education was limited for licensed nurses on this topic. The Critical Care End of Life Nursing Education Consortium (ELNEC) 2-day course was created in 2006 to provide education for nurses caring for dying patients in critical care units.[55] See the Internet Resources for Palliative Care Box for information about ELNEC.

Collaborative Care

The ability to provide collaborative, compassionate end-of-life care is the responsibility of all clinicians who work with the critically ill. Interdisciplinary collaborative efforts are associated with improvement in care.[56] In 2008, the SCCM published a revised guideline, "Recommendations for End-of-Life Care in the Intensive Care Unit," to provide guidance for end-of-life care for the team.[57] The Evidence-Based Practice feature on end-of-life care provides a summary of the topics included (Box 10-1). The Robert Wood Johnson Foundation (RWJF) Critical Care End-of-Life Peer Workgroup[58] identified seven end-of-life care domains for use in the critical care unit:

1. Patient- and family-centered decision making
2. Communication
3. Continuity of care
4. Emotional and practical support
5. Symptom management and comfort care
6. Spiritual support
7. Emotional and organizational support for ICU clinicians

Internet Resources

Many websites for online tools to improve end-of-life care have been developed. These can provide tools and skills to critical care nurses and physicians to assess the quality of their care at the end of life. Additionally tools and education on the websites may offer guidance on how to become more knowledgeable about assessing perceptions of families and staff, auditing documentation, and making observations of care (see Box 10-2: Internet Resources for additional information).

BOX 10-1 EVIDENCE-BASED PRACTICE GUIDELINE FOR END-OF-LIFE CARE IN THE CRITICAL CARE UNIT QSEN

The key topics of the guidelines for end-of-life care in the critical care unit, based on research and expert panel review, are categorized below.

Patient- and Family-Centered Care and Decision Making: The Comprehensive Ideal for End-of-Life Care
- Use the legal standards for decision making.
- Resolve conflict.
- Communicate with families.

Ethical Principles Related to Withdrawal of Life-Sustaining Treatment
- Withholding versus withdrawing
- Killing versus allowing to die
- Intended versus merely foreseen consequences

Practical Aspects of Withdrawing Life-Sustaining Treatments in the Critical Care Unit
- The procedure
- Specific issues
- Use of paralytics

Symptom Management in End-of-Life Care
- Pain and dyspnea
- Delirium
- Medications used

Considerations at the Time of Death
- Notification of death
- Brain death
- Organ donation
- Bereavement and support
- Needs of the interdisciplinary team

Research, Quality Improvement, and Education
- Develop interventions likely to improve the quality of care.
- Develop education programs.

Data from Truog RD, et al. Recommendations for end-of-life care in the intensive care unit: a consensus statement by the American Academy of Critical Care Medicine. *Crit Care Med.* 2008; 36(3):953.

BOX 10-2 INTERNET RESOURCES FOR PALLIATIVE CARE

AAHPM	American Academy of hospice and Palliative Care Medicine	http://www.aahpm.org
ELNEC	End of Life Nursing Education Consortium	http://www.aacn.nche.edu/elnec
EPERC	End of life/Palliative Education Resource Center:	http://www.eperc.mcw.edu/EPERC
HPNA	Hospice and Palliative Care Nurses Association:	http://www.hpna.org
IPAL-ICU	Improving Palliative Care in the ICU	http://www.capc.org/ipal/ipal-icu/professional-education
Promoting Excellence in End of-Life Care		http://www.promotingexcellence.org.

CASE STUDY Patient at the End of Life

Brief Patient History

Mr. C is a 17-year-old, African American teenager who was involved in a motor vehicle accident. He sustained a cervical fracture at the level of C2 that transected his spinal column and both vertebral arteries. Bystanders began rescue breathing, and he was intubated by paramedics en route to the hospital. Mr. C's parents state that they want everything possible done and that they have faith that God will heal their son.

Clinical Assessment

Mr. C is admitted to the critical care unit from the emergency department. He is ventilator- dependent. His skin is warm and dry. He is unresponsive to verbal or painful stimuli, and there is no physical movement. Mr. C's family remains at the bedside 24 hours each day throughout the week. They converse with Mr. C, speaking about all the things they are going to do when he gets home.

Diagnostic Procedures

Mr. C's vital signs are as follows: blood pressure of 120/72 mm Hg, heart rate of 120 beats/min (sinus tachycardia), no spontaneous respiration, temperature of 97.8° F, and Glasgow Coma Scale score of 3. Computed tomography of the head showed a global ischemic infarct involving both ventricles, and electroencephalography revealed no detectable cortical activity.

Medical Diagnosis

Mr. C is diagnosed with brain death.

Questions

1. What major outcomes do you expect to achieve for this patient?
2. What problems or risks must be managed to achieve these outcomes?
3. What interventions must be initiated to monitor, prevent, manage, or eliminate the problems and risks identified?
4. What interventions should be initiated to promote optimal functioning, safety, and well-being of the patient?
5. What possible learning needs do you anticipate for this patient?
6. What cultural and age-related factors may have a bearing on the patient's plan of care?

REFERENCES

1. Siegel MD: End of life decision making in the ICU, *Clin Chest Med* 30:181, 2009.
2. *Center to Advance Palliative Care*: Palliative care programs continue rapid growth in U.S. hospitals becoming standard practice throughout the country. http://www.capc.org/news-and-events/releases/analysis-of-us-hospital-palliative-care-programs-2010-snapshot.pdf/file_view. Accessed June 28, 2014.
3. National Consensus Project: *Clinical practice guidelines for quality palliative care*, ed 2, 2009. http://www.nationalconsensusproject.org. Accessed June 28, 2014.
4. EPERC: End of Life and Palliative Education Resource Center. Fast Facts. http://www.eperc.mcw.edu/EPERC/FastFactsandConcepts. Accessed June 28, 2014.
5. SUPPORT Investigators: A controlled trial to improve care for seriously ill hospitalized patients. The study to understand prognoses and preferences for outcomes and risks of treatments (SUPPORT), *JAMA* 274(20):1591, 1995.
6. Field MJ, Cassell CK, editors: *Approaching death: improving care at the end of life*, Washington, DC, 1997, National Academy Press.
7. Gillick MR: Advance care planning, *N Engl J Med* 350(1):7, 2004.
8. DHHS. Department of Health and Human Services: *Advance directives and advance care planning: Report to Congress*, August, 2008. http://aspe.hhs.gov/daltcp/reports/2008/adcongrpt.htm. Accessed June 28, 2014.
9. Center for Ethics in Health Care: Oregon Health Sciences University. History of the POLST paradigm initiative, 2008. http://www.ohsu.edu/xd/education/continuing-education/center-for-ethics/ethics-programs/polst.cfm?WT_rank=10. Accessed June 28, 2014.
10. Smith R: A good death, *BMJ* 320:129, 2000.
11. Rubenfeld GD: Principles and practice of withdrawing life-sustaining treatments, *Crit Care Clin* 20(3):435, 2004.
12. Tilden V, et al: Family decision-making to withdraw life-sustaining treatments from hospitalized patients, *Nurs Res* 50(2):105, 2001.
13. Ebell MH, et al: Survival after in-hospital cardiopulmonary resuscitation: a meta-analysis, *J Gen Intern Med* 13(12):805, 1998.
14. Brindley PG, et al: Predictors of survival following in-hospital adult cardiopulmonary resuscitation, *CMAJ* 167(4):343, 2002.
15. Elshove-Bolk J, et al: In-hospital resuscitation of the elderly: characteristics and outcome, *Resuscitation* 74(2):372, 2007.
16. Christakis NA, Lamont EB: Extent and determinants of error in doctors' prognoses in terminally ill patients: prospective cohort study, *BMJ* 320(7233):469, 2004.
17. Lynn J, et al: Prognoses of seriously ill hospitalized patients on the days before death: implications for patient care and public policy, *New Horiz* 5(1):56, 1997.
18. McDonald DD, et al: Communicating end-of-life preferences, *West J Nurs Res* 25(6):652, discussion 667–675, 2003.
19. Fried TR, Bradley EH: What matters to seriously ill older persons making end-of-life treatment decisions? A qualitative study, *J Palliat Med* 6(2):237, 2003.
20. Teno JM, et al: Medical care inconsistent with patients' treatment goals: association with 1-year Medicare resource use and survival, *J Am Geriatr Soc* 50(3):496, 2002.
21. Lau F, et al: A systematic review of prognostic tools for estimating survival time in palliative care, *J Palliat Care* 23(2):93, 2007.
22. Prendergast TJ, Puntillo KA: Withdrawal of life support: intensive caring at the end of life, *JAMA* 288(21):2732, 2002.
23. Breen CM, et al: Conflict associated with decisions to limit life-sustaining treatment in intensive care units, *J Gen Intern Med* 16(5):283, 2001.
24. Campbell ML, Guzman JA: Impact of a proactive approach to improve end-of-life care in a medical ICU, *Chest* 123(1):266, 2003.
25. Faber-Langendoen K, Lanken PN: Dying patients in the intensive care unit: forgoing treatment, maintaining care, *Ann Intern Med* 133(11):886, 2000.
26. *National Hospice and Palliative Care Organization*: HPNA Position Statement: Artificial nutrition and hydration in advanced illness. http://www.hpna.org/pdf/Artifical_Nutrition_and_Hydration_PDF.pdf. Accessed June 28, 2014.
27. Mularski RA: Pain management in the intensive care unit, *Crit Care Clin* 20(3):381, 2004.
28. Gélinas C, et al: Pain assessment and management in critically ill intubated patients: a retrospective study, *Am J Crit Care* 13(2):126, 2004.
29. Campbell ML: Terminal dyspnea and respiratory distress, *Crit Care Clin* 20(3):403, 2004.
30. Fabbro ED, et al: Symptom control in palliative care, part III: dyspnea and delirium, *J Palliat Med* 9(2):422, 2006.
31. Mueller PS, et al: Ethical analysis of withdrawal of pacemaker or implantable cardioverter-defibrillator support at the end of life, *Mayo Clin Proc* 78(8):959, 2003.
32. Rubenfeld GD, Crawford SW: Withdrawal of life-sustaining treatment. In Curtis JR, Rubenfeld GD, editors: *Managing death in the intensive care unit: the transition from cure to comfort*, Oxford, 2001, Oxford University Press.
33. von Gunten C, Weissman DE: Fast fact and concept #034: symptom control for ventilator withdrawal in the dying patient (part II), 2009. http://www.eperc.mcw.edu/EPERC/FastFactsIndex/ff_034.htm. Accessed June 28, 2014.
34. Chan JD, et al: Narcotic and benzodiazepine use after withdrawal of life support: Association with time to death?, *Chest* 126(1):286, 2004.
35. *Social Security Administration*: Hospital protocols for organ procurement and standards for organ procurement agencies, 2004: compilation of the Social Security laws. http://www.ssa.gov/OP_Home/ssact/title11/1138.htm. Accessed June 28, 2014.
36. The Joint Commission: Approved: revisions to Standard LD.3.1.10, Element of Performance 12, for critical access hospitals and hospitals, *Jt Comm Perspect* 27(6):14, 2007.
37. Powner DJ, et al: Variability among hospital policies for determining brain death in adults, *Crit Care Med* 32(6):1284, 2004.
38. Siminoff LA, et al: Families' understanding of brain death, *Prog Transplant* 13(3):218, 2003.
39. Campbell ML: *Forgoing life-sustaining therapy: how to care for the patient who is near death*, Aliso Viejo, CA, 1998, AACN Critical Care.
40. Kirchhoff KT, et al: Preparing ICU families for withdrawal of life support: a pilot study, *Am J Crit Care* 17(2):113, 2008.
41. Limerick MH: The process used by surrogate decision makers to withhold and withdraw life-sustaining measures in an

intensive care environment, *Oncol Nurs Forum* 34(2):331, 2007.

42. Ambuel B, Weissman D: Fast fact and concept #016: conducting a family conference, 2001. http://www.eperc.mcw.edu/EPERC/FastFactsIndex/ff_016.htm. Accessed June 28, 2014.
43. Curtis JR, et al: The family conference as a focus to improve communication about end-of- life care in the intensive care unit: opportunities for improvement, *Crit Care Med* 29(2 Suppl):N26, 2001.
44. Keenan SP, et al: Withdrawal of life support: how the family feels, and why, *J Palliat Care* 16(Suppl):S40, 2000.
45. Kirchhoff KT, et al: The vortex: families' experiences with death in the intensive care unit, *Am J Crit Care* 11(3):200, 2002.
46. Gries CJ, et al: Family member satisfaction with end-of-life decision making in the ICU, *Chest* 133(3):704, 2008.
47. Stapleton RD, et al: Clinician statements and family satisfaction with family conferences in the intensive care unit, *Crit Care Med* 34(6):1679, 2006.
48. Selph RB, et al: Empathy and life support decisions, *J Gen Intern Med* 23(9):1311, 2008.
49. Kirchhoff KT, et al: Intensive care nurses' experiences with end-of-life care, *Am J Crit Care* 9(1):36, 2000.
50. American Association of Critical-Care Nurses: *Family presence during CPR and invasive procedures*, 2004. www.aacn.org/WD/Practice/Docs/Family_Presence_During_CPR_11-2004.pdf. Accessed June 28, 2014.
51. Emergency Nurses Association: *Family presence at the bedside during invasive procedures and cardiopulmonary resuscitation*, 2005. http://www.ena.org/publications/ena/Pages/FamilyPresence.aspx. Accessed June 28, 2014.
52. Degenholtz HB, et al: Race and the intensive care unit: disparities and preferences for end-of-life care, *Crit Care Med* 31(5 Suppl):S373, 2003.
53. Shannon S: Helping families cope with death in the ICU. In Curtis JR, Rubenfeld GD, editors: *Managing death in the intensive care unit: the transition from cure to comfort*, Oxford, 2001, Oxford University Press.
54. Elpern EH, et al: Moral distress of staff nurses in a medical intensive care unit, *Am J Crit Care* 14(6):523, 2005.
55. Ferrell BR, Virani R, Malloy P: Evaluation of the end of life nursing education consortium in the USA, *Int J Palliat Care* 12(6):269, 2006.
56. Baggs JG, et al: The dying patient in the ICU: role of the interdisciplinary team, *Crit Care Clin* 20(3):525, 2004.
57. Truog RD, et al: Recommendations for end-of-life care in the intensive care unit: a consensus statement by the American Academy of Critical Care Medicine, *Crit Care Med* 36(3):953, 2008.
58. Clarke EB, et al: Quality indicators for end-of-life care in the intensive care unit, *Crit Care Med* 31(9):2255, 2003.

11 CHAPTER

Cardiovascular Clinical Assessment and Diagnostic Procedures

Mary E. Lough

Be sure to check out the bonus material, including review questions, on the Evolve website at http://evolve.elsevier.com/Urden/priorities/.

Physical assessment of the cardiovascular patient is a skill that must not be lost amid the technology of the critical care setting.[1] Data collected from a thorough, thoughtful history and examination contribute to both the nursing and the medical decisions for therapeutic interventions.

HISTORY

The patient history is important because it provides data that contribute to the cardiovascular diagnosis and treatment plan. For a patient with chest pain or in acute distress, the history is curtailed to just a few questions about the patient's chief complaint, the precipitating events, and current medications. Acute distress may be symptoms of acute decompensated heart failure, hypertension or hypotension, and any symptoms of chest pain.

For a patient *without* obvious distress, the history focuses on the following four areas:

1. Review of the patient's present illness
2. Overview of the patient's general cardiovascular status, including previous cardiac diagnostic studies, interventional procedures, cardiac surgeries, and current medications including cardiac, noncardiac, and over-the-counter medications
3. Examination of the patient's general health status, including family history of coronary artery disease (CAD), hypertension, diabetes, peripheral arterial disease, or stroke
4. Survey of the patient's lifestyle, including risk factors for CAD

One of the unique challenges in cardiovascular assessment is identifying when "chest pain" is of cardiac origin and when it is not. The following safety information should always be considered:

- If there is any evidence of CAD or risk of heart disease, assume that the chest pain is caused by myocardial ischemia until proven otherwise.[2]
- Questions to elicit the nature of the chest pain cover five basic areas: quality, location, duration of pain, factors that provoke the pain, and factors that relieve the pain.
- There may be little correlation between the severity of chest discomfort and the gravity of its cause. This is a result of the subjective nature of pain and the unique presentation of ischemic disease in women, elderly patients, and individuals with diabetes.
- Subjective descriptors vary greatly among individuals. Not all patients use the word "pain"; some may describe "pressure," heaviness," discomfort," or "indigestion."
- Other symptoms that may signal cardiac dysfunction are dyspnea, palpitations, cough, fatigue, edema, ischemic leg pain, nocturia, syncope, and cyanosis.

A patient's description of chest pain is a powerful bedside predictor of underlying coronary disease, especially when combined with a 12-lead electrocardiogram.[2,3]

PHYSICAL EXAMINATION

A comprehensive physical assessment is fundamental to the achievement of an accurate diagnosis. The nurse who has developed the skills of inspection, palpation, and auscultation can be confident when assessing patients with cardiovascular disease. Percussion is not employed when assessing the cardiovascular system.

Inspection

The priorities for inspection of the patient with cardiovascular dysfunction are 1) assessing the general appearance, 2) examining the extremities, 3) estimating jugular venous distention, and 4) observing the apical impulse.

Assessing General Appearance

The face is observed for the color of the skin (i.e., cyanotic, pale, or jaundiced) and for apprehensive or painful expressions. The skin, lips, tongue, and mucous membranes are inspected for pallor or cyanosis. *Central cyanosis* is a bluish discoloration of the tongue and sublingual area. Multiracial studies indicate that the tongue is the most sensitive site for observation of central cyanosis, which must be recognized and treated as a medical emergency. Pulse oximetry, arterial blood gas analysis, and treatment with 100% oxygen must be instituted immediately.

The anterior thorax and posterior thorax are inspected for skeletal deformities that may displace the heart and cause cardiac compromise. The skin on the chest wall and abdomen is inspected for scars, bruises, wounds, and bulges associated with pacemaker or defibrillator implants. Respiratory rate, pattern, and effort are also observed and recorded. The abdomen is assessed for signs of distention or ascites that may be associated with right-sided heart failure. Abdominal adiposity is a known risk factor for CAD.[4] Body posture can indicate the amount of effort it takes to breathe. For example, sitting upright to breathe may be necessary for the patient with acute decompensated heart failure, and leaning forward may be the least painful position for the patient with pericarditis. The patient is observed for signs of confusion or lethargy that may indicate hypotension, low cardiac output, or hypoxemia.

Examining the Extremities

The nail beds are inspected for signs of discoloration or cyanosis.[5] *Clubbing* in the nail bed is a sign associated with longstanding central cyanotic heart disease or pulmonary disease with hypoxemia.[5,6] Clubbing describes a nail that has lost the normal angle between the finger and the nail root; the nail becomes wide and convex. The terminal phalanx of the finger also becomes bulbous and swollen[7] (Figure 11-1). *Peripheral cyanosis,* a bluish discoloration of the nail bed, is more commonly seen. Peripheral cyanosis results from a reduction in the quantity of oxygen in the peripheral extremities from arterial disease or decreased cardiac output. Clubbing never occurs as a result of peripheral cyanosis.

The legs are inspected for signs of peripheral arterial or venous vascular disease. The visible signs of peripheral arterial vascular disease include pale, shiny legs with sparse hair growth. Research indicates that many individuals, especially women, can have peripheral atherosclerosis without obvious signs or symptoms.[8] Venous disease creates an edematous limb with deep red rubor, brown discoloration, and, frequently, leg ulceration. A comparison of typical assessment findings in arterial and venous disease is presented in Table 11-1.

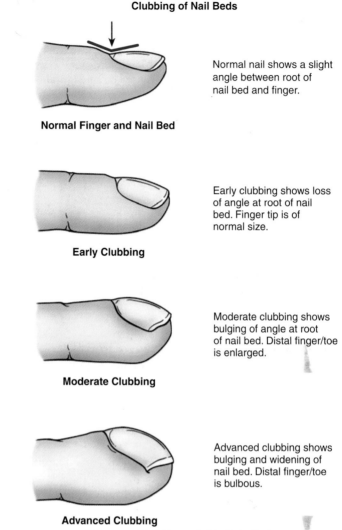

Clubbing of Nail Beds

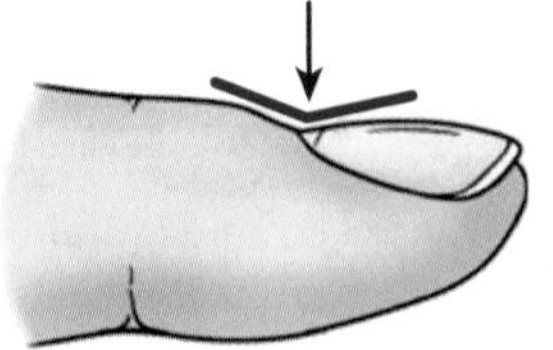

Normal nail shows a slight angle between root of nail bed and finger.
Normal Finger and Nail Bed

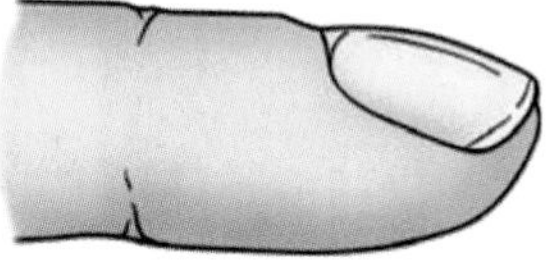

Early clubbing shows loss of angle at root of nail bed. Finger tip is of normal size.
Early Clubbing

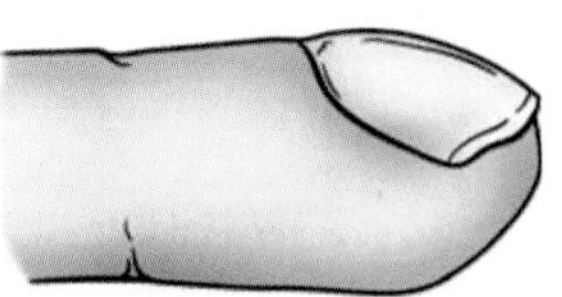

Moderate clubbing shows bulging of angle at root of nail bed. Distal finger/toe is enlarged.
Moderate Clubbing

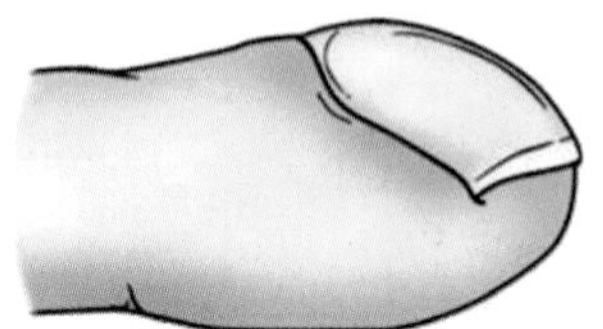

Advanced clubbing shows bulging and widening of nail bed. Distal finger/toe is bulbous.
Advanced Clubbing

FIG 11-1 Clubbing of the Nail Beds.

TABLE 11-1 Inspection and Palpation of Extremities: Comparison of Arterial and Venous Disease

CHARACTERISTIC	ARTERIAL DISEASE	VENOUS DISEASE
Hair loss	Present	Absent
Skin texture	Thin, shiny, dry	Flaking, stasis, dermatitis, mottled
Ulceration	Located at pressure points; painful, pale, dry with little drainage; well-demarcated with eschar or dried; surrounded by fibrous tissue; granulation tissue scant and pale	Usually at the ankle; painless, pink, moist with large amount of drainage; irregular, dry, and scaly; surrounded by dermatitis; granulation tissue healthy
Skin color	Elevational pallor, dependent rubor	Brown patches, rubor, mottled cyanotic color when dependent
Nails	Thick, brittle	Normal
Varicose veins	Absent	Present
Temperature	Cool	Warm
Capillary refill	Greater than 3 seconds	Less than 3 seconds
Edema	None or mild, usually unilateral	Usually present foot to calf, unilateral or bilateral
Pulses	Weak or absent (0 to 1+)	Normal, strong, and symmetric

Estimating Jugular Venous Distention

The jugular veins of the neck are inspected for a noninvasive estimate of intravascular volume and pressure. The external jugular veins are observed for *jugular vein distention* (JVD) (Figure 11-2 and Box 11-1). JVD is caused by an elevation in central venous pressure (CVP). This occurs with fluid volume overload, right ventricular dysfunction, pericardial effusion, or any condition that elevates right atrial pressure.[9,10] The right internal jugular vein can be used for measurement of CVP in centimeters of water (Figure 11-3 and Box 11-2).

The abdominojugular reflux sign can assist with the diagnosis of right ventricular failure. This noninvasive test is used in conjunction with measurement of JVD. The procedure for assessing abdominojugular reflux is described in Box 11-3. A positive abdominojugular reflux sign is an increase in the jugular venous pressure (CVP equivalent) of greater than 3 cm sustained for at least 15 seconds.[11]

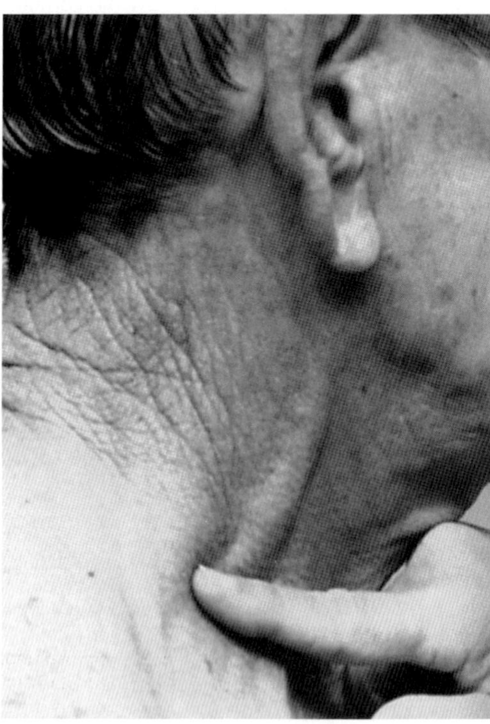

FIG 11-2 Assessment of Jugular Vein Distention (JVD). Applying light finger pressure over the sternocleidomastoid muscle, parallel to the clavicle, helps identify the external jugular vein by occluding flow and distending it. The finger pressure is released, and the patient is observed for true distention. If the patient's trunk is elevated to 30 degrees or more, JVD should not be present.

Observing the Apical Impulse

The thoracic cage is divided with imaginary vertical lines (sternal, midclavicular, axillary, vertebral, and scapular), and the intercostal spaces are divided with horizontal lines to serve as reference points in locating or describing cardiac findings (Figure 11-4). The anterior thorax is inspected for the *apical impulse*, sometimes referred to as the *point of*

BOX 11-1 Procedure for Assessing Jugular Vein Distention

1. Patient reclines at a 30- to 45-degree angle.
2. The examiner stands on the patient's right side and turns the patient's head slightly toward the left.
3. If the jugular vein is not visible, light finger pressure is applied across the sternocleidomastoid muscle just above and parallel to the clavicle. This pressure fills the external jugular vein by obstructing flow (see Fig. 11-2).
4. After the location of the vein has been identified, the pressure is released, and the presence of jugular vein distention (JVD) is assessed.
5. Because inhalation decreases venous pressure, JVD should be assessed at end-exhalation.
6. Any fullness in the vein extending more than 3 cm above the sternal angle is evidence of increased venous pressure. Generally, the higher the sitting angle of the patient when JVD is visualized, the higher the central venous pressure.
7. Documentation: JVD is reported by including the angle of the head of the bed at the time JVD was evaluated (e.g., "presence of JVD with the head of the bed elevated to 45 degrees").

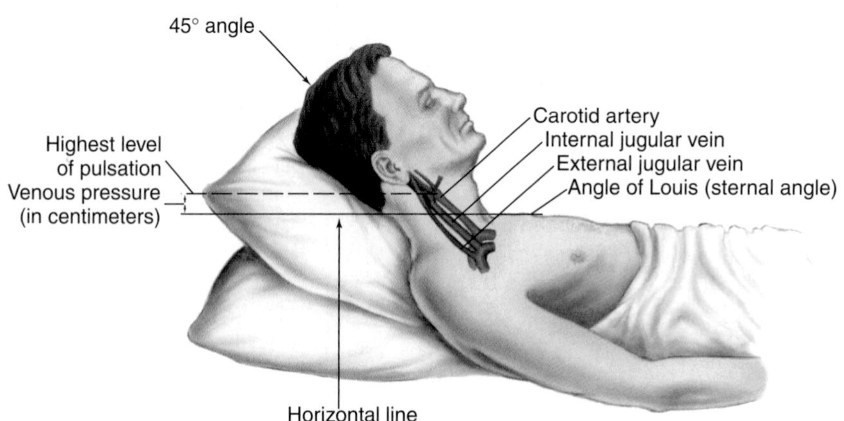

FIG 11-3 Position of Internal and External Jugular Veins. Pulsation in the internal jugular vein can be used to estimate central venous pressure. (Modified from Thompson JM et al: *Mosby's clinical nursing*, ed 5, St Louis, 2002, Mosby.)

BOX 11-2 Procedure for Assessing Central Venous Pressure

1. The patient reclines in the bed. The highest point of pulsation in the internal jugular vein is observed during exhalation.
2. The vertical distance between this pulsation (top of the fluid level) and the sternal angle is estimated or measured in centimeters.
3. This number is then added to 5 cm for an estimation of CVP. The 5 cm is the approximate distance of the sternal angle above the level of the right atrium (see Fig. 11-3).
4. Documentation: The degree of elevation of the patient is included in the report (e.g., "CVP estimated at 13 cm, using internal jugular vein pulsation, with the head of the bed elevated 45 degrees").

BOX 11-3 Procedure for Assessing Abdominojugular Reflux

1. Ask the patient to relax and breathe normally through an open mouth.
2. Measure the jugular vein distention (JVD) in the patient's right internal jugular vein, following the procedure described in Box 11-1.
3. Apply firm pressure of approximately 20 to 35 mm Hg to the patient's midabdomen for 15 to 30 seconds and remeasure the JVD during the compression.
4. Measure the right JVD a third time after the compression is released.
5. Ask the patient not to tense or hold the breath during the test. (Doing so increases venous return to the heart and may produce a falsely positive result.)
6. A positive abdominojugular reflux (AJR) is identified when abdominal compression causes a sustained JVD increase of 4 cm or more. This sign is indicative of right-sided heart failure.
7. A normal AJR is reported if there is no rise in JVD, a transient (<10 seconds) rise in JVD, or a rise in JVD less than or equal to 3 cm sustained throughout compression.

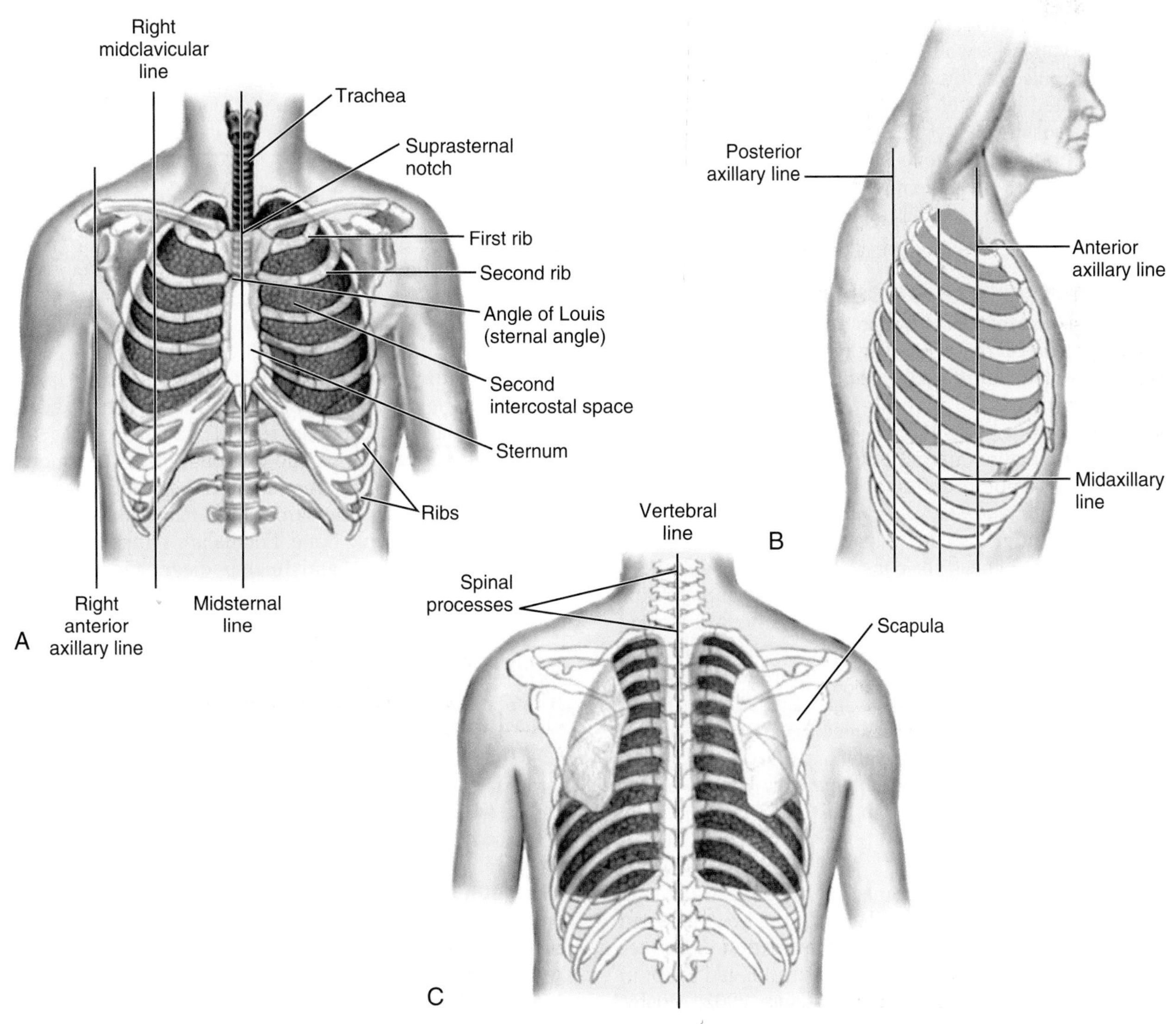

FIG 11-4 Thoracic Landmarks. *A,* Anterior Thorax. *B,* Right Lateral Thorax. *C,* Posterior Thorax.

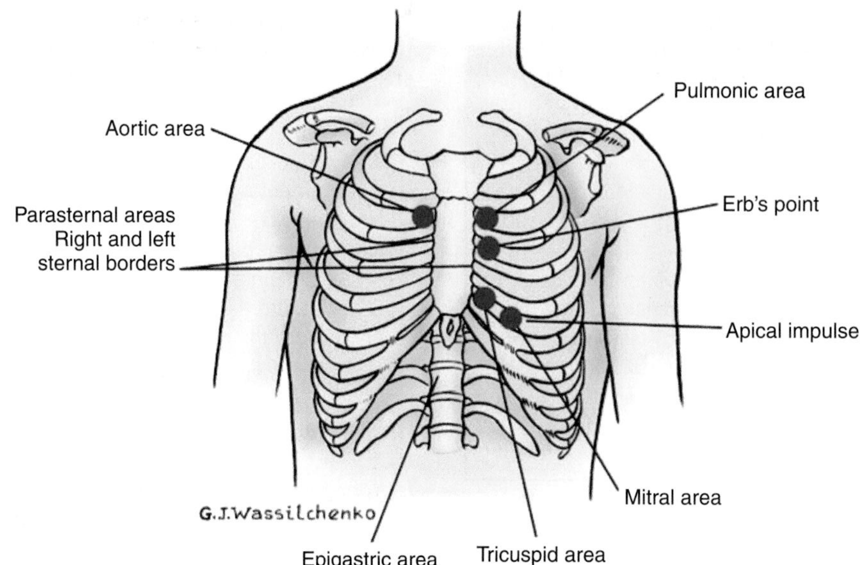

FIG 11-5 Thoracic Palpation and Auscultation Points.

maximal impulse (PMI). The apical impulse occurs as the left ventricle contracts during systole and rotates forward, causing the left ventricular apex of the heart to touch the chest wall. The apical impulse is a quick, localized, outward movement normally located just lateral to the left midclavicular line at the fifth intercostal space in the adult patient (Figure 11-5). The apical impulse is the only normal pulsation visualized on the chest wall. In the patient without cardiac disease, PMI may not be noticeable (see Fig. 11-5).

Palpatation

The priorities for palpation of the patient with cardiovascular dysfunction are 1) assessing arterial pulses, 2) evaluating capillary refill, 3) estimating edema, and 4) assessing for signs of deep vein thrombosis.

Assessing Arterial Pulses

Seven pairs of bilateral arterial pulses may be palpated. The examination incorporates bilateral assessment of the carotid, brachial, radial, ulnar, popliteal, dorsalis pedis, and posterior tibial arteries. The pulses are palpated separately and compared bilaterally to check for consistency.[12] Pulse volume is graded on a scale of 0 to 3+ (Box 11-4). The abdominal aortic pulse can also be palpated. If a distal pulse cannot be palpated using light finger pressure, a Doppler ultrasound stethoscope may increase diagnostic accuracy. It is important to mark the location of the audible signal with an indelible ink marker pen for future evaluation of pulse quality. The radial and ulnar arterial pulses must be evaluated for collateral flow before an arterial line is inserted; this test, known as the modified *Allen Test,* is described in Box 11-5.

Evaluating Capillary Refill

Capillary refill assessment is a maneuver that uses the patient's nail beds to evaluate arterial circulation to the extremity and overall perfusion. The nail bed is compressed to produce blanching, after which release of the pressure should result in a return of blood flow and baseline nail color in less than 2 seconds.[12] The severity of arterial insufficiency is directly proportional to the amount of time required to reestablish flow and color.

BOX 11-4 Pulse Palpation Scale

0	Not palpable
1 +	Faintly palpable (weak and thready)
2+	Palpable (normal pulse)
3+	Bounding (hyperdynamic pulse)

Estimating Edema

Edema is fluid accumulation in the extravascular spaces of the body. The dependent tissues within the legs and sacrum are particularly susceptible. The edema may be dependent, unilateral or bilateral, pitting or nonpitting. The amount of edema is quantified by measuring the circumference of the limb or by pressing the skin of the feet, ankles, and shins against the underlying bone. Edema is a symptom associated with several diseases, and further diagnostic evaluation is required to determine the cause. Typical scales for pitting edema use a 0 to 4+ system (Table 11-2).

Ausculation

The priorities for auscultation of the patient with cardiovascular dysfunction are 1) measuring blood pressure, 2) detecting orthostatic hypotension, 3) measuring pulse pressure, 4) detecting pulsus paradoxus, 5) assessing normal heart sounds, and 6) identifying abnormal heart sounds, murmurs, and pericardial rubs.

Measuring Blood Pressure

Blood pressure measurement is an essential component of every complete physical examination. The most recent blood pressure (BP) management guidelines (JNC8)[13] specify antihypertensive medication treatment targets by age range. For individuals who are 60 years and older, a BP less than 150/90 millimeters of mercury (mm Hg) is the goal. For individuals between 30 and 59 years a BP below 140/90 mm Hg is the target.[13] In patients with chronic kidney disease or diabetes, the goal is a BP below 140/90 mm Hg.[13]

BOX 11-5 Procedure for Assessment of Arterial Blood Supply to the Hand:

The Allen Test

Before a radial artery is punctured or cannulated, the Allen test is performed to assess blood flow to the hand and ensure that it is adequate.

Allen Test by Visual Inspection

1. If the patient is alert and cooperative, he or she is asked to make a tight fist repeatedly to squeeze the blood out of the hand.
2. The radial artery is compressed with firm thumb pressure by the examiner.
3. The patient is requested to open the hand, palm side up, while the radial artery is still occluded.
4. Pressure is released, and the time it takes for the color to return to the hand is noted.

If the ulnar artery is patent, the color will return within 3 seconds. The patient may describe a tingling in the palm as blood flow returns. Delayed color return (a "failed" Allen test) implies that the ulnar artery is inadequate. This means radial artery provides the only reliable source of arterial blood flow to the hand and it must not be punctured or cannulated.

Allen Test with Pulse Oximetry

1. If the patient is unable to cooperate to make a fist, an alternative approach is to use a pulse oximeter that displays a pulse waveform.
2. Place the pulse oximeter on the middle finger and establish an adequate pulse amplitude display on the monitor.
3. Simultaneously compress the radial and ulnar arteries until the waveform clearly decreases or vanishes.
4. Release pressure off the ulnar artery only. If the ulnar artery is patent, the pulse amplitude recovers its normal appearance.
5. Repeat the procedure with the radial artery.
6. Only if there is adequate blood supply to the hand can arterial catheterization of the radial artery be accomplished safely.

In the critical care setting, systemic blood pressure may be measured directly or indirectly. Direct arterial pressure monitoring via an invasive arterial catheter is considered the gold standard in critical care. Accurate use of a stethoscope and sphygmomanometer or electronic measuring device can produce indirect blood pressure values that closely reflect direct measurements.

Detecting Orthostatic Hypotension

When a healthy person stands, 10% to 15% of the blood volume pools in the legs; this reduces venous return to the right side of the heart, which decreases cardiac output and lowers arterial blood pressure.[14] Transient orthostatic intolerance is part of daily life for many people, but acute orthostatic hypotension is a cause of concern.[15] The fall in blood pressure activates baroreceptors; the subsequent reflex increase in sympathetic outflow and parasympathetic inhibition leads to peripheral vasoconstriction, with increased heart rate and contractility.[14] Postural (orthostatic) hypotension occurs when the systolic BP drops 10 to 20 mm Hg after a change from the supine to the upright posture. Postural hypotension is usually accompanied by dizziness, lightheadedness, or syncope. If a patient experiences these symptoms, it is important to complete a full set of postural vital signs before increasing the activity level (Box 11-6). Orthostatic hypotension can have many causes.[15] The three most common causes of orthostatic vital sign changes (i.e., drop in blood pressure and rise in heart rate) observed in critical care are

1. Intravascular volume depletion or fluid loss caused by bleeding, excessive diuresis, or fever
2. Inadequate vascular vasoconstrictor mechanisms to constrict the arterial bed, which can occur in elderly patients after prolonged immobility or as a result of spinal cord injury
3. Autonomic insufficiency caused by administration of medications such as beta-blockers, angiotensin converting enzyme (ACE) inhibitors, and calcium channel blockers.

Measuring Pulse Pressure

Pulse pressure describes the difference between the systolic and diastolic values. The normal pulse pressure is about 40 mm Hg (i.e., the difference between a systolic BP of 120 mm Hg and a diastolic BP of 80 mm Hg). In the critically ill patient, a low blood pressure is frequently associated with a narrow pulse pressure. For example, a patient with a blood pressure of 90/72 mm Hg has a pulse pressure of 18 mm Hg. The narrowed pulse pressure is a temporary compensatory mechanism caused by arterial vasoconstriction resulting from volume depletion or acute decompensated heart failure. The narrow pulse pressure ensures that the mean arterial

TABLE 11-2 Pitting Edema Scale

SCALE	EDEMA	INDENTATION DEPTH: ENGLISH UNITS	INDENTATION DEPTH: METRIC UNITS	TIME TO BASELINE
0	None	0	0	
1 +	Trace	0-0.25 inch	<6.5 mm	Rapid
2+	Mild	0.25-0.5 inch	6.5-12.5 mm	10-15 sec
3+	Moderate	0.5-1 inch	12.5 mm-2.5 cm	1-2 min
4+	Severe	>1 inch	> 2.5 cm	2-5 min

BOX 11-6 Measurement of Postural (Orthostatic) Vital Signs

Guidelines

1. Record blood pressure (BP) and heart rate (HR) in each position.
2. Do not remove cuff between measurements.
3. Record all associated signs and symptoms.
4. Clearly document patient position.

Lying

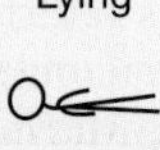

Sitting

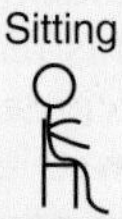

Standing

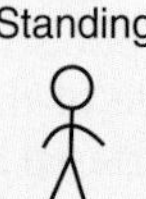

Technique

1. Keep patient as flat as possible for 10 minutes before the initial assessment.
2. Patient supine: Obtain initial BP and HR measurements.
3. Patient sitting with legs hanging: Measure immediately and after 2 minutes.
4. Patient standing: Measure immediately and after 2 minutes. If BP and HR are stable but orthostasis is suspected, BP and HR can be repeated every 2 minutes. Note that this is rarely practical for the critically ill patient.

Results

Normal Changes

HR increases by 5 to 20 beats/min (transiently).
Systolic BP drops 10 mm Hg.
Diastolic BP drops 5 mm Hg.

Positive Orthostasis

Drop in systolic BP by more than 20 mm Hg
Drop in diastolic BP by more than 10 mm Hg within 3 minutes

BOX 11-7 Procedure for Measuring Pulsus Paradoxus

Measurement with a Sphygmomanometer

1. The patient should be lying supine in a comfortable position.
2. The breathing pattern should be of normal depth and rate to avoid excessive respiratory interference.
3. Blood pressure is measured following standard procedures. The sphygmomanometer cuff is inflated to a pressure greater than the systolic blood pressure (SBP), and Korotkoff sounds are auscultated over the brachial artery while the cuff is deflated at rate of approximately 2 to 3 mm Hg per heartbeat.
4. The peak SBP during expiration (i.e., the pressure at which Korotkoff sounds are heard only during expiration) should be identified and then reconfirmed.
5. The cuff is then deflated slowly to establish the SBP at which Korotkoff sounds become audible during both inspiration and expiration.
6. If the auscultated difference between these two SBP values exceeds 10 mm Hg during quiet respiration, a paradoxical pulse is present.

Measurement by Waveform Analysis

1. A pulse oximetry sensor with a visible pulse waveform can be used as an additional measurement device.
2. In the critical care unit, an arterial waveform from an indwelling arterial catheter (if present) can be used to measure the difference in SBP between expiration and inspiration.

pressure (78 mm Hg, in this example) remains in a therapeutic range to provide adequate organ perfusion.

Detecting Pulsus Paradoxus

In normal physiology, the strength of the pulse fluctuates throughout the respiratory cycle. When the "pulse" is measured using the systolic BP, it will decrease slightly during inspiration and rise slightly during respiratory exhalation. The normal difference is 2 to 4 mm Hg. In some clinical conditions, such as cardiac tamponade, the blood pressure decline is abnormally large during inspiration. In general, an inspiratory decline of greater than 10 mm Hg is considered diagnostic for *pulsus paradoxus*.[16-18] The traditional technique for measuring pulsus paradoxus using a sphygmomanometer and a blood pressure cuff and pulse oximetry is described in Box 11-7. If the patient is hypotensive, pulsus paradoxus is more accurately assessed in the critical care unit by monitoring a pulse oximetry waveform or an indwelling arterial catheter waveform.[16-18]

Assessing Normal Heart Sounds

Auscultation of the heart is the most challenging part of the cardiac physical examination, and, in an era of increasing technologic demands, it is daunting to new clinicians. To summarize the advice given by most experts, the examiner must do the following:[19-21]

1. Auscultate systematically across the precordium.
2. Visualize the cardiac anatomy under each point of auscultation, expecting to hear the physiologically associated sounds.
3. Memorize the cardiac cycle to enhance the ability to hear abnormal sounds.
4. Practice, practice, practice.

First and second heart sounds. Normal heart sounds are referred to as the *first heart sound* (S_1) and the *second heart sound* (S_2). S_1 is the sound associated with mitral and tricuspid valve closure and is heard most clearly in the mitral and tricuspid areas. S_2 (aortic and pulmonic closure) can be heard best at the second intercostal space to the right and left of the sternum (see Fig. 11-5). Both sounds are high-pitched and heard best with the diaphragm of the stethoscope (Box 11-8). Each sound is loudest in an auscultation area located downstream from the actual valvular component of the sound, as shown in Figure 11-6.

Pathologic splitting of S_1 and S_2. A variety of abnormalities can alter the intensity and timing of split heart sounds. For example, during auscultation in the pulmonic area, a pathologic split is audible with a stethoscope if the pulmonic valve closure occurs after the aortic valve closure. Pathologic splitting of S_1 and S_2 is associated with specific cardiovascular conditions such as pulmonary hypertension, pulmonic stenosis, and right ventricular failure and with electrical conduction disturbances such as right bundle branch block and premature ventricular contractions.

Identifying Abnormal Heart Sounds, Murmurs, and Pericardial Rubs

Third and fourth heart sounds. The abnormal heart sounds are known as the *third heart sound* (S_3) and the *fourth heart sound* (S_4); they are referred to as *gallops* when auscultated during an episode of tachycardia. These low-pitched sounds occur during diastole and are best heard with the bell of the stethoscope positioned lightly over the apical impulse. The characteristics of S_3 and S_4 are detailed in Box 11-9. The presence of S_3 may be normal in children, young adults, and pregnant women because of rapid filling of the ventricle in a young, healthy heart. However, an S_3 in the presence of cardiac symptoms is an indicator of acute decompensated heart failure in a noncompliant ventricle with fluid overload.[22] Not unexpectedly, the development of an S_3 heart sound is strongly associated with elevated levels of B-type natriuretic peptide (BNP or proBNP).[22]

Auscultation of an S_4 also leads the examiner to suspect an acute exacerbation of heart failure and decreased ventricular compliance.[23] An S_4, also referred to as an atrial gallop, occurs at the end of diastole (just before S_1), when the ventricle is full. It is associated with atrial contraction, also called atrial kick.

Heart murmurs. *Heart valve murmurs* are prolonged extra sounds that occur during systole or diastole. Murmurs are produced by turbulent flood flow through the chambers of the heart, from forward flow through narrowed or irregular valve openings or backward regurgitant flow through an incompetent valve.[24] Murmurs occur in both systole and diastole. Most murmurs are caused by structural cardiac changes. The steps to auscultate for cardiac murmurs effectively and accurately are listed in Box 11-10. Murmurs are characterized by specific criteria:

Timing: place in the cardiac cycle (systole/diastole)
Location: where it is auscultated on the chest wall (mitral/aortic area)
Radiation: how far the sound spreads across chest wall
Quality: whether the murmur is blowing, grating, or harsh
Pitch: whether the tone is high or low
Intensity: the loudness is graded on a scale of 1 through 6; the higher the number, the louder the murmur.

Pericardial friction rub. A *pericardial friction rub* results from pericardial inflammation (*pericarditis*).[25] Classically, a pericardial friction rub is a grating or scratching sound that is both systolic and diastolic, corresponding with cardiac motion within the pericardial sac. It is often associated with chest pain, which can be aggravated by deep inspiration, coughing, and changing position. It is important to differentiate pericarditis from acute myocardial ischemia, and the detection of a pericardial friction rub through

BOX 11-8 Characteristics of the First and Second Heart Sounds

FIRST HEART SOUND (S_1)	SECOND HEART SOUND (S_2)
• High-pitched • Loudest in mitral area (apex)	• High-pitched • Loudest in aortic area (base)
SPLIT S_1	**SPLIT S_2**
• Normal split less than 20 msec • Split heard best in tricuspid area • Important to differentiate between split S_1 and S_4 • Occurs immediately before carotid upstroke	• Normal split less than 30 msec • Split heard best in pulmonic area • ↑ Split with inhalation • ↓ Split with exhalation

↑, increased; ↓, decreased.

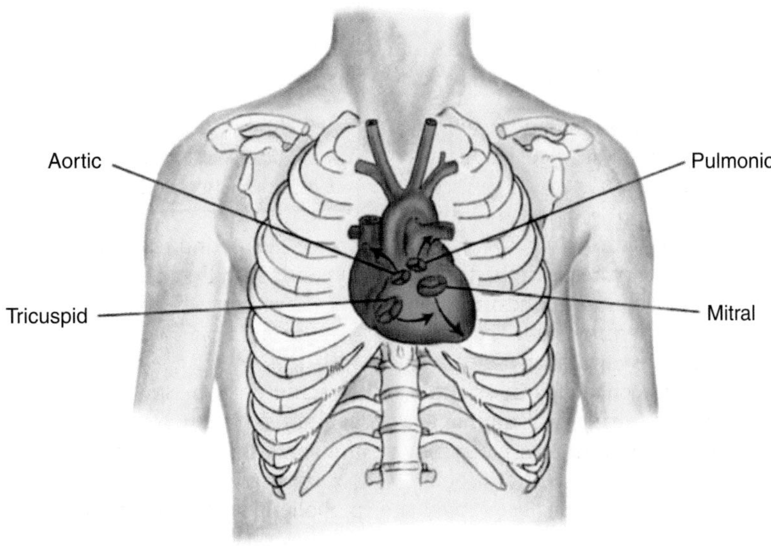

FIG 11-6 Transmission of Heart Sounds to the Thorax and Their Relationship to the Anatomic Position of the Heart Valves.

BOX 11-9 Characteristics of the Third and Fourth Heart Sounds

Third Heart Sound (S_3)

Physiologic Causes
- Related to diastolic motion and rapid filling of ventricles in early diastole
- Can be normal in children and young adults (age <40 years)

Pathologic Causes
- Ventricular dysfunction with an increase in end-systolic volume (MI, heart failure, valvular disease, systemic or pulmonary hypertension)
- Hyperdynamic states (anemia, thyrotoxicosis, mitral ortricuspid regurgitation)

Rhythmic Word Association
- Kentucky: S_1, S_2, S_3

Synonyms
- Ventricular gallop
- Protodiastolic gallop

Fourth Heart Sound (S_4)
- Related to diastolic motion and ventricular dilation with atrial contraction in late diastole
- May occur with or without cardiac decompensation
- Ventricular hypertrophy with a decrease in ventricular compliance (CAD, systemic hypertension, cardiomyopathy, aortic or pulmonary stenosis, increase in intensity with acute MI or angina)
- Hyperkinetic states (anemia, thyrotoxicosis, arteriovenous fistula)
- Acute valvular regurgitation

Rhythmic Word Association
- Tennessee: S_4, S_1, S_2

Synonyms
- Atrial gallop
- Presystolic gallop

CAD, coronary artery disease; MI, myocardial infarction.

BOX 11-10 Technique of Auscultation of Heart Sounds and Murmurs

1. Stethoscope
   - Diaphragm
     Larger surface area
     Brings out higher frequency and filters out low frequency
     Use for listening to S_1/S_2 (split S_1/S_2), loud murmurs, pericardial friction rubs
   - Bell
     Smaller surface area
     Filters out high-frequency sounds and accentuates low-frequency sounds
     Rest lightly on area (or else it becomes a diaphragm)
2. Location: heart sounds auscultated at APTM
   A: aortic area (second right ICS along sternal border)
   P: pulmonic area (second left ICS along sternal border)
   T: tricuspid area (fourth left ICS along sternal border)
   M: mitral area (fifth ICS at MCL)
3. "Know your bases"
   - Base of the heart refers to the right and left second ICS beside the sternum S_2 where the aortic or pulmonic sounds are auscultated
   - Apex or left ventricular area refers to the fifth ICS along the MCL
     Most commonly referred to as the PMI
     Also referred to as the mitral area
     S_1 and mitral sounds are loudest here
   - Erb point: second aortic area (third left ICS along sternal border); pericardial friction rubs are heard best here.
4. Palpation
   - Location
   - Palpate carotid pulse (or observe the ECG to identify S_1 and S_2)
5. Be quiet and patient!
   - Listen for S_1 and S_2 first, ignoring all other sounds.
   - Inching technique
   - After you are sure which is S_1 or S_2, try to determine when the other sound comes in.
   - Is it systolic or diastolic?
   - S_3 and S_4 are best heard with patient in left lateral decubitus position. Notice the location (suggests origin of sound).
   - Notice the timing (S_4 comes just before S_1, and S_3 comes just after S_2).
6. Interpret the sounds based on the clinical condition.

auscultation can assist in this differentiation, leading to effective diagnosis and treatment.

BEDSIDE HEMODYNAMIC MONITORING

Hemodynamic monitoring is at a critical juncture. The technology that launched invasive hemodynamic monitoring is more than 40 years old, and the search to find viable replacement monitoring technologies that are minimal or noninvasive is intense. This has created a new challenge in critical care. Although the use of invasive monitoring is declining, it is still employed for hemodynamically unstable patients. Critical care nurses must be knowledgeable about traditional hemodynamic monitoring methods and also be able to apply established physiologic principles in new situations. As the technology evolves, clinicians will apply the same physiologic principles to the new methods to ensure safety and optimal outcomes for each patient. The following discussion of hemodynamic monitoring describes both established and emerging technologies.

Equipment

A traditional hemodynamic monitoring system has four component parts as shown in Figure 11-7 and described in the following list:

1. An invasive catheter and high-pressure tubing connect the patient to the transducer.
2. The transducer receives the physiologic signal from the catheter and tubing and converts it into electrical energy.
3. The flush system maintains patency of the fluid-filled system and catheter.

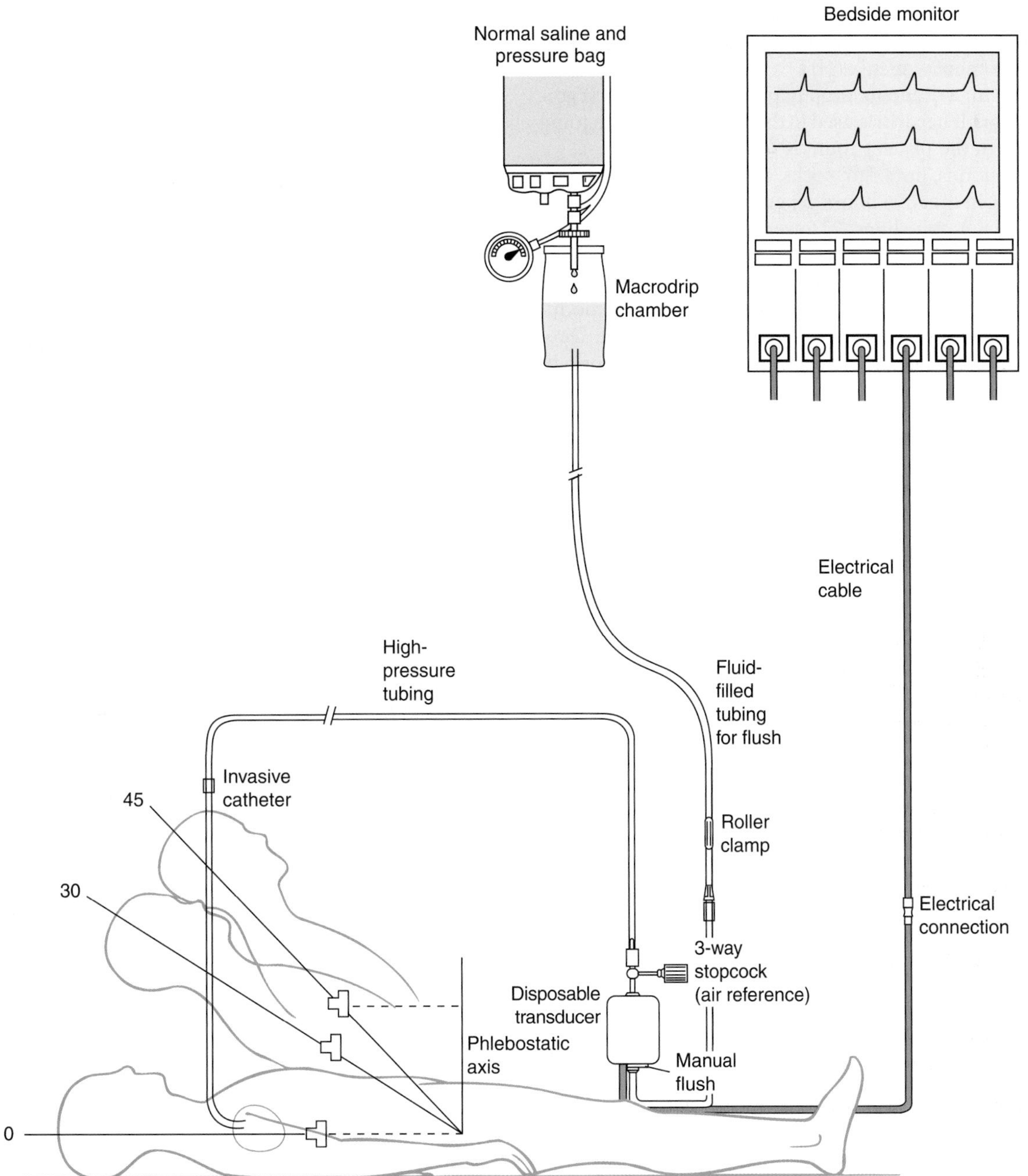

FIG 11-7 The Four Parts of a Hemodynamic Monitoring Include an Invasive Catheter Attached to High-Pressure Tubing to Connect to the Transducer; a Transducer; a Flush System, Including a Manual Flush, and a Bedside Monitor.

4. The bedside monitor contains the amplifier with recorder, which increases the volume of the electrical signal that is displayed as a waveform and numerical value in mm Hg.

Although many different types of invasive catheters can be inserted to monitor hemodynamic pressures, all such catheters are connected to similar equipment (see Figure 11-7). The basic setup consists of the following:

- A bag of 0.9% sodium chloride (normal saline) is used as a flush solution. In some hospitals heparin is added as an anticoagulant. A pressure infusion cuff covers the bag of flush solution and is inflated to 300 mm Hg.
- The system contains intravenous tubing, three-way stopcocks, and an in-line flow device for continuous fluid infusion and manual flush. High-pressure tubing must be used to connect the invasive catheter to the transducer to prevent damping (flattening) of the waveform.
- A disposable pressure transducer.

Heparin

The use of the anticoagulant heparin added to the normal saline (NS) flush setup to maintain catheter patency remains controversial.[26,27] While many units do add heparin to flush solutions, other critical care units avoid heparin because of concern about development of heparin-induced antibodies that can trigger the autoimmune condition known as heparin-induced thrombocytopenia (HIT).[27,28] When present, HIT is associated with a dramatic drop in platelet count and thrombus formation. If heparin is used in the flush infusion, ongoing monitoring of the platelet count is recommended.[27,28]

Flush solutions, lines, stopcocks, and disposable transducers are changed every 96 hours per current Center for Disease Control (CDC) guidelines.[29] However, there is variation in practice between hospitals; some change the flush solutions every 24 hours. For this reason, it is essential to be familiar with the specific written procedures that concern hemodynamic monitoring equipment in each critical care unit. Dextrose solutions are not recommended as flush solutions in monitoring catheters.[29]

Calibrating Hemodynamic Monitoring Equipment

To ensure accuracy of hemodynamic pressure readings, two baseline measurements are necessary:

1. Calibration of the system to atmospheric pressure, also known as *zeroing the transducer*
2. Determination of the phlebostatic axis for transducer height placement, also called *leveling the transducer*[30]

Zeroing the transducer. To calibrate the equipment to atmospheric pressure, referred to as zeroing the transducer, the three-way stopcock nearest to the transducer is turned simultaneously to open the transducer to air (atmospheric pressure) and to close it to the patient and the flush system. The monitor is adjusted so that "0" is displayed, which equals atmospheric pressure. Atmospheric pressure is not zero; it is 760 mm Hg at sea level. Using zero to represent current atmospheric pressure provides a convenient baseline for hemodynamic measurement purposes.

Some monitors also require calibration of the upper scale limit while the system remains open to air. At the end of the calibration procedure, the stopcock is returned to the closed position, and a closed cap is placed over the open port. At this point, the patient's waveform and hemodynamic pressures are displayed.

Disposable transducers are very accurate, and after they are calibrated to atmospheric pressure, drift from the zero baseline is minimal. Although in theory this means that repeated calibration is unnecessary, clinical protocols in most units require the nurse to calibrate the transducer at the beginning of each shift for quality assurance.

Phlebostatic axis. The phlebostatic axis is a physical reference point on the chest that is used as a baseline for consistent transducer height placement. To obtain the axis, a theoretic line is drawn from the fourth intercostal space, where it joins the sternum, half the anterior-posterior diameter of the chest,[30] as shown in Figure 11-7. It is used as the reference mark for central venous pressure (CVP) and pulmonary artery catheter transducers. The level of the transducer "air reference stopcock" approximates the position of the tip of an invasive hemodynamic monitoring catheter within the chest.

Leveling the transducer. Leveling the transducer is different from zeroing. This process aligns the transducer with the level of the atria. The purpose is to line up the *air-fluid interface* with the atria to correct for changes in *hydrostatic pressure* in blood vessels above and below the level of the heart.[30]

A carpenter's level or laser-light level can be used to ensure that the transducer is parallel with the phlebostatic axis reference point. When there is a change in the patient's position, the transducer must be leveled again to ensure accurate hemodynamic pressure measurements are obtained.[30] Errors in measurement can occur if the transducer is placed below the phlebostatic axis because the fluid in the system weighs on the transducer, creating additional hydrostatic pressure, and produces a falsely high reading. For every inch the transducer is below the tip of the catheter, the fluid pressure in the system increases the measurement by 1.87 mm Hg. For example, if the transducer is positioned 6 inches below the tip of the catheter, this falsely elevates the displayed pressure by 11 mm Hg.

If the transducer is placed above this atrial level, gravity and lack of fluid pressure will give an erroneously low reading. For every inch the transducer is positioned above the catheter tip, the measurement is 1.87 mm Hg less than the true value. If several clinicians are taking measurements, the reference point can be marked on the side of the patient's chest to ensure consistent measurements.

Accommodating Changes in Patient Position

Head of bed backrest position. Nurse researchers have determined that the CVP, pulmonary artery pressure (PAP), and pulmonary artery occlusion pressure (PAOP), also known as the *pulmonary artery wedge pressure* can be reliably measured at head-of-bed backrest positions from 0 (flat) to 60 degrees if the patient is lying on his or her back (supine).[30] If the patient is normovolemic and hemodynamically stable, raising the head of the bed usually does not affect hemodynamic pressure measurements. Most patients do not need the head of the bed to be lowered to 0 degrees to obtain accurate CVP, PAP, or PAOP readings.

Lateral position. The landmarks for leveling the transducer are different if the patient is turned to the side. Researchers have evaluated hemodynamic pressure measurement readings with the patients in the 30- and 90-degree lateral positions with the head of the bed flat, and they found the measurements to be reliable.[30]

In the 30-degree angle position, the landmark to use for leveling the transducer is one-half the distance from the surface of the bed to the left sternal border.[30] In the 90-degree right-lateral position, the transducer fluid-air interface is positioned at the fourth ICS at the midsternum. In the 90-degree left-lateral position, the transducer is positioned at the fourth ICS left parasternal border (beside the sternum).[30] It is important to know that measurements can be recorded in nonsupine positions because critically ill patients must be turned to prevent development of pressure ulcers and other complications of immobility.

Solving Hemodynamic Equipment Problems

Typical problems with bedside monitoring equipment and nursing measures to ensure patient safety and troubleshoot equipment problems are addressed in Table 11-3.

Intraarterial Blood Pressure Monitoring

Indications

Arterial pressure monitoring is indicated for any major medical or surgical condition that compromises cardiac output, tissue perfusion, or fluid volume status. The system is designed for continuous measurement of three blood pressure parameters: systole, diastole, and mean arterial blood pressure (MAP). The direct arterial access is helpful in the

TABLE 11-3 Nursing Measures to Ensure Patient Safety and to Troubleshoot Problems with Hemodynamic Monitoring Equipment

PROBLEM	PREVENTION	RATIONALE	TROUBLESHOOTING
Overdamping of waveform	Provide continuous infusion of solution containing heparin through an in-line flush device (1 unit of heparin for each 1 mL of flush solution).	Ensure that recorded pressures and waveform are accurate because a damped waveform gives inaccurate readings.	Before insertion, completely flush the line and/or catheter. In a line attached to a patient, back flush through the system to clear bubbles from tubing or transducer.
Underdamping ("overshoot" or "fling")	Use short lengths of noncompliant tubing. Use fast-flush square wave test to demonstrate optimal system damping. Verify arterial waveform accuracy with the cuff blood pressure.	If the monitoring system is underdamped, the systolic and diastolic values will be overestimated by the waveform and the digital values. False high systolic values may lead to clinical decisions based on erroneous data.	Perform the fast-flush square wave test to verify optimal damping of the monitoring system.
Clot formation at end of the catheter	Provide continuous infusion of solution containing heparin through an in-line flush device (1 unit of heparin for each 1 mL of flush solution).	Any foreign object placed in the body can cause local activation of the patient's coagulation system as a normal defense mechanism. The clots that are formed may be dangerous if they break off and travel to other parts of the body.	If a clot in the catheter is suspected because of a damped waveform or resistance to forward flush of the system, gently aspirate the line using a small syringe inserted into the proximal stopcock. Flush the line again after the clot is removed and inspect the waveform. It should return to a normal pattern.
Hemorrhage	Use luer-lock (screw) connections in line setup. Close and cap stopcocks when not in use. Ensure that the catheter is sutured or securely taped in position.	A loose connection or open stopcock creates a low-pressure sump effect, causing blood to back into the line and into the open air. If a catheter is accidentally removed, the vessel can bleed profusely, especially with an arterial line or if the patient has abnormal coagulation factors (resulting from heparin in the line) or has hypertension.	After a blood leak is recognized, tighten all connections, flush the line, and estimate blood loss. If the catheter has been inadvertently removed, put pressure on the cannulation site. When bleeding has stopped, apply a sterile dressing, estimate blood loss, and inform the physician. If the patient is restless, an armboard may protect lines inserted in the arm.
Air emboli	Ensure that all air bubbles are purged from a new line setup before attachment to an indwelling catheter. Ensure that the drip chamber from the bag of flush solution is more than one-half full before using the in-line, fast-flush system. Some sources recommend removing all air from the bag of flush solution before assembling the system.	Air can be introduced at several times, including when central venous pressure (CVP) tubing comes apart, when a new line setup is attached, or when a new CVP or pulmonary artery (PA) line is inserted. During insertion of a CVP or PA line, the patient may be asked to hold his or her breath at specific times to prevent drawing air into the chest during inhalation. The in-line, fast-flush devices are designed to permit clearing of blood from the line after withdrawal of blood samples. If the chamber of the intravenous tubing is too low or empty, the rapid flow of fluid will create turbulence and cause flushing of air bubbles into the system and into the bloodstream.	Because it is impossible to get the air back after it has been introduced into the bloodstream, prevention is the best cure. If air bubbles occur, they must be vented through the in-line stopcocks, and the drip chamber must be filled. The left atrial pressure (LAP) line setup is the only system that includes an air filter specifically to prevent air emboli.

TABLE 11-3 Nursing Measures to Ensure Patient Safety and to Troubleshoot Problems with Hemodynamic Monitoring Equipment—cont'd

PROBLEM	PREVENTION	RATIONALE	TROUBLESHOOTING
Normal waveform with *low* digital pressure	Ensure that the system is calibrated to atmospheric pressure.	To provide a 0 baseline relative to atmospheric pressure.	Recalibrate the equipment if transducer drift has occurred.
	Ensure that the transducer is placed at the level of the phlebostatic axis.	If the transducer has been placed *higher* than the phlebostatic level, gravity and the lack of hydrostatic pressure will produce a false *low* reading.	Reposition the transducer at the level of the phlebostatic axis. Misplacement can occur if the patient moves from the bed to the chair or if the bed is placed in a Trendelenburg position.
Normal wave form with *high* digital pressure	Ensure that the system is calibrated to atmospheric pressure.	To provide a 0 baseline relative to atmospheric pressure.	Recalibrate the equipment if transducer drift has occurred.
	Ensure that the transducer is placed at the level of the phlebostatic axis.	If the transducer has been placed *lower* than the phlebostatic level, the weight of hydrostatic pressure on the transducer will produce a false *high* reading.	Reposition the transducer at the level of the phlebostatic axis. This situation can occur if the head of the bed was raised and the transducer was not repositioned. Some centers require attachment of the transducer to the patient's chest to avoid this problem.
Loss of waveform	Always have the hemodynamic waveform monitored so that changes or loss can be quickly noted.	The catheter may be kinked, or a stopcock may be turned off.	Check the line setup to ensure that all stopcocks are turned in the correct position and that the tubing is not kinked. Sometimes, the catheter migrates against a vessel wall, and having the patient change position restores the waveform.

management of patients with acute respiratory failure who require frequent arterial blood gas measurements.

Catheters

The size of the catheter used is proportionate to the diameter of the cannulated artery. In small arteries—such as the radial and dorsalis pedis—a 20-gauge, 3.8-cm to 5.1-cm, catheter is used most often. If the larger femoral or axillary arteries are used, a 19- or 20-gauge, 16-cm catheter is inserted.

The catheter insertion is usually percutaneous. Catheters are inserted into smaller arteries, using a "catheter-over-needle" unit in which the needle is used as a temporary guide for catheter placement. With this method, after the unit has been inserted into the artery, the needle is withdrawn, leaving the supple plastic catheter in place. Insertion of a catheter into a larger artery typically uses the Seldinger technique, which involves the following steps:

1. Entry into the artery using a needle
2. Passage of a supple guidewire through the needle into the artery
3. Removal of the needle
4. Passage of the catheter over the guidewire
5. Removal of the guidewire, leaving the catheter in the artery

Insertion and allen test. Several major peripheral arteries are suitable for receiving a catheter and for long-term hemodynamic monitoring. The most frequently used site is the radial artery.[27] The femoral artery is a larger vessel that is frequently cannulated. Other smaller arterials such as the dorsalis-pedis, axillary, or brachial arteries are only used when radial or femoral arterial access is unavailable.

The major advantage of the radial artery is the supply of collateral circulation to the hand provided by the ulnar artery through the palmar arch in most people. Before radial artery cannulation, collateral circulation must be assessed by using Doppler flow, or by the modified Allen test according to institutional protocol.[27] In the Allen test the radial and ulnar arteries are compressed simultaneously. The patient is asked to clench and unclench the hand until it blanches. One of the arteries is then released, and the hand should immediately flush from that side. The same procedure is repeated for the remaining artery (Box 11-5).

Nursing Management

Nursing priorities for the patient with arterial pressure monitoring focus on 1) preventing infection, 2) assessing arterial perfusion pressure, 3) interpreting the arterial pressure waveform, and 4) troubleshooting arterial waveform problems.

Intraarterial blood pressure monitoring is designed for continuous assessment of arterial perfusion to the major organ systems of the body. MAP is the clinical parameter most often used to assess perfusion because MAP represents perfusion pressure throughout the cardiac cycle. Because one-third of the cardiac cycle is spent in systole and two-thirds in diastole, the MAP calculation must reflect the greater amount of time spent in diastole. This MAP formula can be calculated, where

$$\frac{(\text{Diastole} \times 2) + (\text{Systole} \times 1)}{3} = \text{MAP}$$

A blood pressure of 120/60 mm Hg produces a MAP of 80 mm Hg. However, the bedside hemodynamic monitor may show a slightly different digital number because bedside monitoring computers calculate the area under the curve of the arterial line tracing.

Preventing infection in arterial catheters. Infection was once believed to be rare in arterial catheters because of the rapid arterial blood flow. New evidence suggests that arterial catheters are associated with the same risk of bloodstream infections as central venous catheters.[31] This means that infection prevention measures must be just as meticulous for arterial catheters as for central venous catheters.[31]

Assessing arterial perfusion pressure. A MAP greater than 60 mm Hg is necessary to perfuse the coronary arteries. A higher MAP may be required to perfuse the brain and the kidneys. A MAP between 70 and 90 mm Hg is ideal for the cardiac patient to decrease left ventricular (LV) workload. After a carotid endarterectomy or neurosurgery, a MAP of 90 to 110 mm Hg may be more appropriate to increase cerebral perfusion pressure. Systolic and diastolic pressures are monitored in conjunction with the MAP as a further guide to the accuracy of perfusion. If CO decreases, the body compensates by constricting peripheral vessels to maintain the blood pressure. In this situation, the MAP may remain constant, but the pulse pressure (difference between systolic and diastolic pressures) narrows. The following examples explain this point:

Mr. A: BP, 90/70 mm Hg; MAP, 76 mm Hg
Mr. B: BP, 150/40 mm Hg; MAP, 76 mm Hg

Both patients have a perfusion pressure of 76 mm Hg, but they are clinically very different. Mr. A is peripherally vasoconstricted, as is demonstrated by the narrow pulse pressure (90/70 mm Hg). His skin is cool to touch, and he has weak peripheral pulses. Mr. B has a wide pulse pressure (150/40 mm Hg), warm skin, and normally palpable peripheral pulses. Nursing assessment of the patient with an arterial line includes comparison of clinical findings with arterial line readings, including perfusion pressure and MAP.

Interpreting the arterial pressure waveform. As the aortic valve opens, blood is ejected from the left ventricle and is recorded as an increase of pressure in the arterial system. The highest point recorded is called *systole.* After peak ejection (systole), the force decreases, and the pressure drops. A notch (dicrotic notch) may be visible on the downstroke of the arterial waveform, representing closure of the aortic valve. The *dicrotic notch* signifies the beginning of diastole. The remainder of the downstroke represents diastolic runoff of blood flow into the arterial tree. The lowest point recorded is called *diastole.* A normal arterial pressure tracing is shown in Figure 11-8. Notice that electrical stimulation (QRS) is always first and that the arterial pressure tracing follows the initiating QRS. If the arterial line becomes unreliable or dislodged, a cuff pressure can be used as a reserve system.

Troubleshooting arterial pressure monitoring problems. Major complications associated with arterial pressure monitoring are rare. The most life-threatening risk is exsanguination if the Luer-Lock connections are not tight or if an in-line stopcock is inadvertently opened to air. Pressure monitor alarms must always be on, with alarm limits (high and low) set at a safe, audible warning range for each patient. Box 11-11 for the QSEN Patient Safety Alert feature on Clinical Alarm Systems.

When the arterial monitor displays a low blood pressure digital reading, it is a nursing responsibility to determine

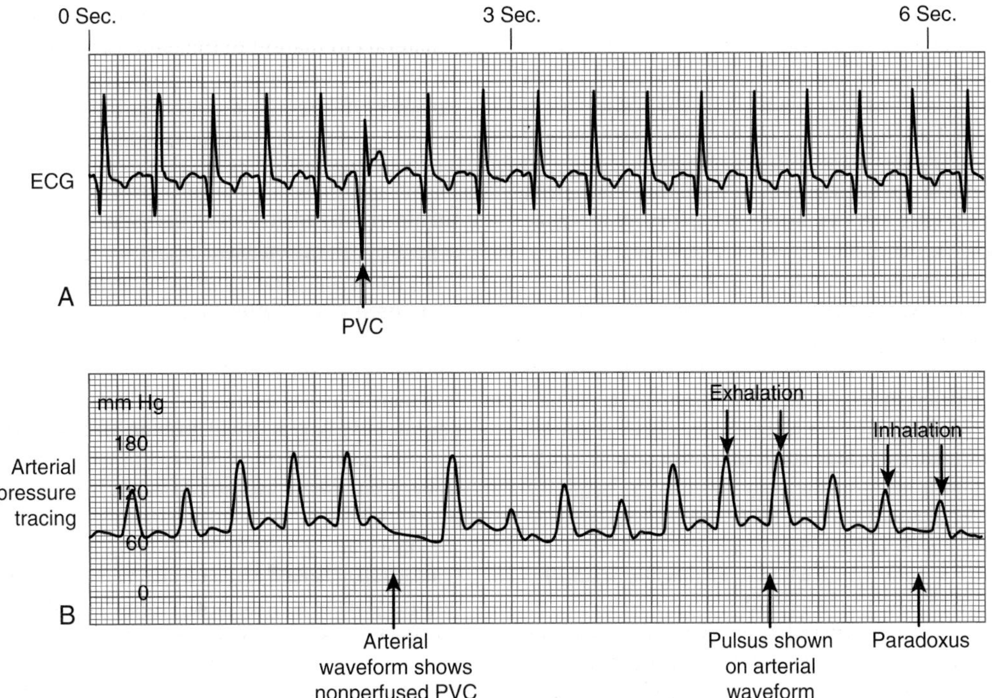

FIG 11-8 Simultaneous ECG and Normal Arterial Pressure Tracing.

BOX 11-11 PATIENT SAFETY QSEN ALERT CLINICAL ALARM SYSTEMS

Clinical Alarm System Effectiveness

1. Implement regular preventive maintenance and testing of alarm systems.
2. Ensure that alarms are activated with appropriate settings and are sufficiently audible with respect to distances and competing noise within the unit.

Clinical Alarm Safety

Alarm Identification

1. Audible and visual indication should be present for any condition that poses a risk to the patient. Indicators should be visible from at least 10 ft (3 m).
2. Cause of the alarm must be easily identifiable by the health care practitioner.
3. Life-threatening conditions should be clearly differentiated from noncritical alarm situations.
4. High-priority alarms should override low-priority alarms.
5. Alarm must be sufficiently loud or distinctive to be heard over the environmental noise of a busy critical care unit.
6. It should never be possible to turn the volume control to "off."

Disabling and Silencing Alarms

1. Alarm silence must have visual indicator to show clearly it is disabled.
2. Critical alarms should not be permanently overridden (turned "off").
3. New, life-threatening alarm conditions should override a silenced alarm.

Power

Battery units should initiate an alarm before a unit stops working effectively.

Alarm Limits

1. Alarm limits can be adjusted to meet the clinical needs of a patient. The system should default to standard settings between patients.
2. Alarm limits should preferably be displayed on the monitor.

Based on data from *The Joint Commission*. http://www.jointcommission.org; and Critical alarms and patient safety. ECRI's guide to developing effective alarm strategies and responding to JCAHO's alarm-safety goal. *Health Devices*. 2002; 31(11):397.

whether this is a true patient problem or a problem with the monitoring equipment. A damped waveform occurs when communication from the artery to the transducer is interrupted and produces false values on the monitor and oscilloscope. Troubleshooting techniques to identify the origin of the problem and to remove the cause of damping are described in Table 11-3.

Another cause of arterial waveform distortion is *underdamping*, also called *overshoot* or *fling*. Underdamping is characterized by a narrow upward systolic peak that produces a falsely high systolic reading. The overshoot is caused by an increase in dynamic response or increased oscillations within the system.

Fast-flush square waveform test. The monitoring system's dynamic response can be verified for accuracy at the bedside by the *fast-flush square waveform test*, also called the *dynamic frequency response test*.[30] The nurse performs this test to ensure that the patient pressures and waveform shown on the bedside monitor are accurate.[30] The test makes use of the manual flush system on the transducer. Normally, the flush device allows only 3 mL of fluid per hour. With the normal waveform displayed, the manual fast-flush procedure is used to generate a rapid increase in pressure, which is displayed on the monitor oscilloscope. As shown in Figure 11-9, the normal dynamic response waveform shows a square pattern with one or two oscillations before the return of the arterial waveform. If the system is overdamped, a sloped (rather than square) pattern is seen. If the system is underdamped, additional oscillations—or vibrations—are observed on the fast-flush square wave test. This test can be performed with any hemodynamic monitoring system. If air bubbles, clots, or kinks are in the system, the waveform becomes damped, or flattened, and this is reflected in the square waveform result.

This is an easy test to perform, and it should be incorporated into nursing care procedures at the bedside when the hemodynamic system is first set up, at least once per shift, after opening the system for any reason, and when there is concern about the accuracy of the waveform.[30] If the pressure waveform is distorted or the digital display is inaccurate, the troubleshooting methods described in Table 11-3 can be implemented. The nurse caring for the patient with an arterial line must be able to assess whether a low MAP or narrowed perfusion pressure represents decreased arterial perfusion or equipment malfunction. Assessment of the arterial waveform on the bedside monitor, in combination with clinical assessment, and use of the square waveform test will yield the answer.

Hemodynamic Equipment and Monitor Alarms

All critically ill patients must have the hemodynamic monitoring alarms on and adjusted to sound an audible alarm if the patient should experience a change in blood pressure, heart rate, respiratory rate, or other significant monitored variable. The key issues concerning monitor alarms are presented in the QSEN Patient Safety Alert feature on Clinical Alarm Systems.

Central Venous Pressure Monitoring

CVP monitoring is indicated when a patient has significant alteration in fluid volume or requires central vein access for administration of vasoactive medications.

Central Vein Insertion Sites

A range of CVC options are available as single-, double-, triple- and quad-lumen infusion catheters, depending on the specific needs of the patient. Many CVCs are antimicrobial-impregnated or heparin-coated to reduce bloodstream infection risk.[29]

The large veins of the upper thorax—subclavian (SC) and internal jugular (IJ)—are most commonly used for percutaneous CVC line insertion.[29] The femoral vein is used when the thoracic veins are not accessible. All three major sites have advantages and disadvantages.

Internal jugular vein. The IJ vein is the most frequently used access site for CVC insertion. Compared with the other

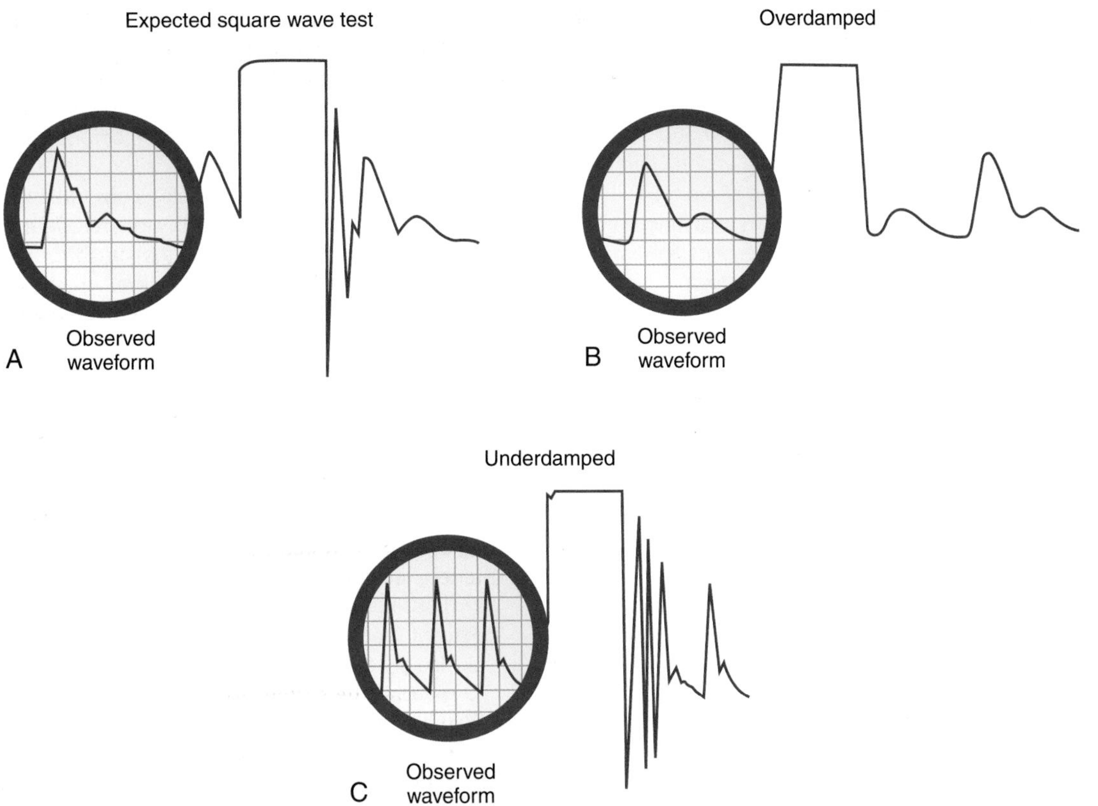

FIG 11-9 Square Wave Test. *A,* Expected square wave test result. *B,* Overdamped. *C,* Underdamped. (From Darovic GO: *Hemodynamic monitoring: invasive and noninvasive clinical application,* ed 3, Philadelphia, 2002, WB Saunders.)

thoracic veins, it is the easiest to cannalize. If the IJ vein is not available, the external jugular (EJ) vein may be accessed. A further advantage of the IJ vein is that the risk of creating an iatrogenic pneumothorax is small. Disadvantages to the IJ vein are patient discomfort from the indwelling catheter when moving the head or neck and contamination of the IJ vein site from oral or tracheal secretions, especially if the patient is intubated or has a tracheostomy.

Subclavian vein. If the anticipated CVC dwelling time is prolonged more than 5 days, the subclavian site is preferred. The subclavian position has the lowest infection rate and produces the least patient discomfort from the catheter. The disadvantages are that the subclavian vein is more difficult to access and carries a higher risk of iatrogenic pneumothorax or hemothorax, although the risk varies greatly, depending on the experience and skill of the physician inserting the catheter.

Femoral vein. The femoral vein is considered the easiest cannulation site because there are no curves in the insertion route. The large diameter of the femoral vein carries a high blood flow that is advantageous for specialized procedures such as continuous renal replacement therapy (CRRT). Because of the higher risk of nosocomial infection with femoral catheters, this site is not recommended as a routine selection.[29]

Insertion

During insertion of a catheter in the subclavian or IJ vein, the patient may be placed in a Trendelenburg position. Placing the head in a dependent position causes the IJ veins in the neck to become more prominent, facilitating line placement. To minimize the risk of air embolus during the procedure, the patient may be asked to "take a deep breath and hold it" any time the needle or catheter is open to air. The tip of the catheter is designed to remain in the vena cava and should not migrate into the right atrium. Because many patients are awake and alert when a CVC is inserted, a brief explanation about the procedure can minimize patient anxiety and result in cooperation during the insertion. This cooperation is important because CVC insertion is a sterile procedure and because the supine or Trendelenburg position may be uncomfortable for many patients. The electrocardiogram (ECG) should be monitored during CVC insertion because of the associated risk of dysrhythmias.

All central catheters are designed for placement by percutaneous injection after skin preparation and administration of a local anesthetic. Visualization of the vein with a bedside utlrasound prior and during insertion is recommended to reduce the number of placement attempts.[29] A prepackaged CVC kit typically is used for the procedure. The standard CVC kit contains sterile towels, chlorhexidine and alcohol for skin preparation, a needle introducer, a syringe, guidewire, and a catheter. The Seldinger technique, in which the vein is located by using a needle and syringe, is the preferred method of placement. A guidewire is passed through the needle, the needle is removed, and the catheter is passed over the guidewire. After the tip of the catheter is correctly placed in the vena cava, the guidewire is removed. A sterile intravenous

BOX 11-12 PATIENT SAFETY ALERT PREVENTION OF CENTRAL VENOUS CATHETER-RELATED BLOODSTREAM INFECTIONS QSEN

1. Education, Training, and Staffing
   a. Nurses and other health care providers should receive education about indications for central venous catheter (CVC) use, maintenance, and infection prevention.
   b. Only trained personnel should insert and maintain CVCs.
   c. Adequate staffing levels in critical care units are associated with fewer catheter-related bloodstream infections (CRBSI).
2. Selection of Catheters and Sites
   a. Use subclavian site rather than jugular or femoral insertion sites to minimize infection risk.
   b. Use ultrasound guidance to place CVCs.
   c. Remove any catheter that is no longer essential.
   d. If a CVC was placed in a medical emergency when aseptic technique was not assured, replace CVC within 48 hours.
3. Hand Hygiene and Aseptic Technique
   a. Perform hand hygiene procedures by washing hands with soap and water or alcohol-based hand rubs (ABHR) before and after palpating the CVC site, dressing the site, or any other intervention.
   b. New sterile gloves must be worn by the professional inserting the CVC.
   c. New sterile gloves must be donned before touching a new catheter for CVC exchange over guidewire.
   d. Wear clean or sterile gloves when changing the catheter dressing.
4. Maximal Sterile Barrier Precautions
   a. For insertion, use maximal sterile barrier precautions including cap, mask, sterile gown, sterile gloves, and a full-body drape.
5. Skin Preparation
   a. Prepare clean skin with greater than 0.5% chlorhexidine preparation with alcohol before CVC insertion.
   b. Antiseptics should be allowed to dry according to the manufacturer's recommendation before CVC insertion.
6. Catheter Site Dressing Regimens
   a. Transparent, semipermeable polyurethane dressings permit continuous visualization of the CVC insertion site.
   b. Replace transparent dressings on CVC sites at least every 7 days.
   c. Monitor the site when changing the dressing or by palpation through an intact dressing.
   d. Replace catheter site dressing whenever the dressing becomes damp, loose, or soiled.
   e. Do not use topical antibiotic ointment or creams on insertion sites (except for dialysis catheters) because of increased fungal infection risk.
   f. Use a chlorhexidine-impregnated sponge dressing at CVC site if CRBSI rate is not decreasing by other means (no recommendation for other types of chlorhexidine dressings).
7. Patient Cleansing
   a. Use 2% chlorhexidine wash for daily skin cleaning to reduce CRBSI.
8. Catheter Securement Device
   a. Use a sutureless catheter securement device to reduce catheter movement, which may reduce infection risk.
9. Antimicrobial Strategies
   a. Use an antimicrobial impregnated CVC when catheters are expected to remain in place for longer than 5 days.
   b. Do not administer systemic antimicrobial prophylaxis to prevent CRBSI.
   c. Do not routinely use anticoagulant therapy to prevent CRBSI.
10. No Routine CVC Replacement
    a. Do not routinely replace CVCs.
    b. Do not replace CVCs on the basis of fever alone.

Data from O'Grady NP, et al. Guidelines for the prevention of intravascular catheter-related infections, *Am J Infect Control* 39(4)suppl 1: S1-S34, 2011.

tubing and solution is attached, and the catheter is sutured in place. Following upper thoracic CVC placement, a chest radiograph is obtained to verify placement and the absence of an iatrogenic hemothorax or pneumothorax, especially if the SC vein was accessed. Box 11-12 for the QSEN Patient Safety Alert feature on Prevention of Central Venous Catheter-related Bloodstream Infections.

Nursing Management

Nursing priorities for the patient with CVP monitoring focus on 1) preventing CVC-associated complications, 2) assessing fluid volume status, 3) accommodating changes in patient position, 4) accurately interpreting the CVP waveforms and pressures, and 5) safely removing the CVC.

Preventing central venous catheter-associated complications. The CVC is an essential tool in care of the critically ill patient, but it is associated with some risks, and it is the responsibility of all clinicians to be informed about these hazards and to follow hospital procedures to avoid iatrogenic complications. CVC complications include air embolus, catheter-associated thrombus formation, and infection.

Air embolus. The risk of air embolus, although uncommon, is always present for the patient with a central venous line in place. Air can enter during insertion[32] through a disconnected or broken catheter by means of an open stopcock, or air can enter along the path of a removed CVC.[33,34] This is more likely if the patient is in an upright position because air can be pulled into the venous system due to negative intrathoracic pressure during inspiration in spontaneous breathing. If a large volume of air is infused rapidly, it may become trapped in the right ventricular outflow tract, stopping blood flow from the right side of the heart to the lungs. Based on animal studies, this volume is approximately 4 mL/kg.[35] If the air embolus is large, the patient will experience respiratory distress and cardiovascular collapse. An auscultatory clinical sign specifically associated with a large venous air embolism is the *mill wheel murmur*.[32-34] A mill wheel murmur is a loud, churning sound heard over the middle chest, caused by the obstruction to right ventricular outflow. Treatment involves immediately occluding the external site where air is entering, administering 100% oxygen, and placing the patient on the left side with the head downward (left lateral Trendelenburg position).[36] This position displaces the air from the right ventricular outflow tract to the apex of the heart, where the air may be aspirated by catheter intervention or gradually absorbed by the bloodstream as the patient remains in the left lateral Trendelenburg position. Precautions to prevent an air embolism in a CVP line include using only screw (Luer-Lock) connections, avoiding long loops of intravenous tubing, and using closed-top screw caps on the three-way stopcock.

Thrombus formation. Clot formation (thrombus) at the CVC site is unfortunately common. Thrombus formation is not uniform; it may involve development of a *fibrin sleeve* around the catheter,[37] or the thrombus may be attached directly to the vessel wall. Other factors that promote clot formation include rupture of vascular endothelium, interruption of laminar blood flow, and physical presence of the catheter, all of which activate the coagulation cascade. The risk of thrombus formation is higher if insertion was difficult or there were multiple needlesticks. Gradual thrombus formation may lead to "sudden" CVC occlusion. Usually, the CVC becomes more difficult to withdraw blood from, or the CVP waveform becomes intermittently damped over a period of hours or days. This situation is caused by the continued lengthening of a fibrin sleeve that extends along the catheter length from the insertion site past the catheter tip.[37] Some catheters are heparin-coated to reduce the risk of thrombus formation, although the risk of HIT does not make this a benign option.[28] Sometimes, CVC complications are additive; for example, the risk of catheter-related infection is increased in the presence of thrombi, where the thrombus likely serves as a culture medium for bacterial growth. Because of concerns over the development of HIT, many hospitals use a saline-only flush to maintain CVC patency.[38, 39]

Central line-associated bloodstream infection (CLABSI). Infection related to the use of CVCs is a major problem. The incidence of CVC-associated infection strongly correlates with the length of time the catherer has been inserted. Longer insertion times are associated with a higher infection rate.[29,40] CVC-related infections are identified at the catheter insertion site or as a bloodstream infection. Systemic manifestations of infection can be present without inflammation at the catheter site. No decrease in bloodstream infections was found when catheters were routinely changed, and this practice is not recommended.[29] When a CVC is infected, it must be removed, and a new catheter inserted in a different site. If a catheter infection is suspected, the CVC should not be changed over a guidewire because of the risk of transferring the infection.[29] Most infections are transmitted from the skin, and infection prevention begins prior to insertion of the CVC. CVC insertion guidelines state that the physician must use effective hand-washing procedures, clean the insertion site with 2% chlorhexidine gluconate in 70% isopropyl, use sterile technique during catheter insertion, and maintain maximal sterile barrier precautions.[29] In many hospitals the bedside nurse is authorized to stop the procedure if these insertion infection control guidelines are not followed. A daily review to determine whether the catheter is still required is recommended to ensure CVCs are removed promptly when no longer needed (see the QSEN Patient Safety Alert feature on Guidelines for Prevention and Management of Central Venous Catheter Infections).[29]

All clinicians must use good hand-washing technique and follow aseptic procedures during site care and any time the CVC system is entered to withdraw blood, give medications, or change tubing.[29] Site dressings impregnated with chlorhexidine are recommended to lower CVC infection rates.[29]

Questioning CVP accuracy for assessment of fluid volume status. The time-honored practice of using the CVP value to assess central volume status has now been challenged.[41] A landmark systematic review of the literature revealed a weak relationship between the CVP measurement and fluid volume responsiveness.[41] In patients with a CVP between 0 and 5 mm Hg, up to 25% do not respond to a fluid challenge as expected.[42] Overall only about half of critically ill patients respond as expected to a fluid challenge.[41] In this situation the clinician must look at other indices of poor tissue perfusion such as an elevated lactate level, low base deficit, or decreased urine output.[42]

Passive leg raise. Another method to assess fluid responsiveness is to raise and support the patient's legs passively, to allow the venous blood from the lower extremities to flow rapidly into the vena cava and return to the right heart. If this maneuver increases the CVP by at least 2 mm Hg, this suggests that the patient will have a positive response to an IV fluid bolus.[43]

Accommodating changes in patient position. To achieve accurate CVP measurements, the phlebostatic axis is used as a reference point on the body, and the transducer must be level with this point. If the phlebostatic axis is used and the transducer is correctly aligned, any head-of-bed position of up to 60 degrees may be used to obtain CVP readings for most patients.[30] Elevating the head of the bed is especially helpful for patients with respiratory or cardiac problems who cannot tolerate a flat position.

Interpreting CVP waveforms and pressures. The normal right atrial (CVP) waveform has three positive deflections—*a*, *c*, and *v* waves—that correspond to specific atrial events in the cardiac cycle (Figure 11-10). The *a* wave reflects atrial contraction and follows the P wave seen on the ECG. The downslope of this wave is called the *x* descent and represents atrial relaxation. The *c* wave reflects the bulging of the closed tricuspid valve into the right atrium during ventricular contraction; this wave is small and not always visible but corresponds to the QRS-T interval on the ECG. The *v* wave represents atrial filling and increased pressure against the closed tricuspid valve in early diastole. The downslope of the *v* wave is named the *y* descent and represents the fall in pressure as the tricuspid valve opens and blood flows from the right atrium to the right ventricle.

Cannon waves. Dysrhythmias can change the pattern of the CVP waveform. In a junctional rhythm or after a PVC, the atria are depolarized after the ventricles if retrograde conduction to the atria occurs. This may be seen as a retrograde P wave on the ECG and as a large combined *ac* or *cannon wave* on the CVP waveform (Figure 11-11). These cannon waves can be easily detected as large pulses in the jugular veins. Other pathologic conditions, such as advanced right ventricular failure or tricuspid valve insufficiency, allow regurgitant backflow of blood from the right ventricle to the right atrium during ventricular contraction, producing large *v* waves on the right atrial waveform.

Fiberoptic central venous catheters. A CVC that incorporates a fiberoptic sensor to measure central venous oxygen saturation ($S_{CV}O_2$) continuously can be used as a traditional CVC and used to follow the trend of venous oxygen

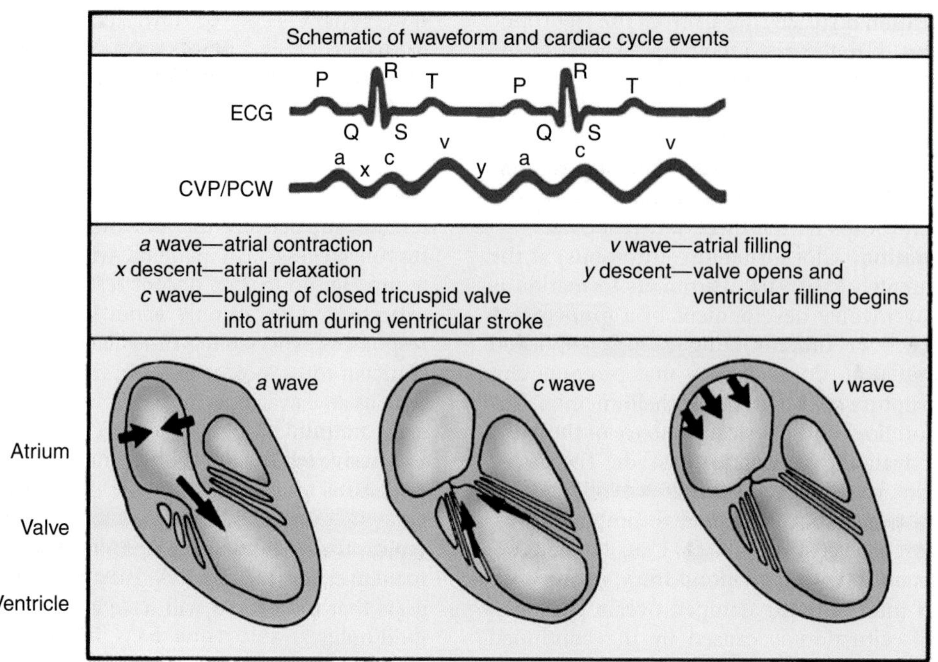

FIG 11-10 Cardiac Events That Produce the CVP Waveform with *a, c,* and *v* Waves. The *a* wave represents atrial contraction. The *x* descent represents atrial relaxation. The *c* wave represents the bulging of the closed tricuspid valve into the right atrium during ventricular systole. The *v* wave represents atrial filling. The *y* descent represents opening of the tricuspid valve and filling of the ventricle.

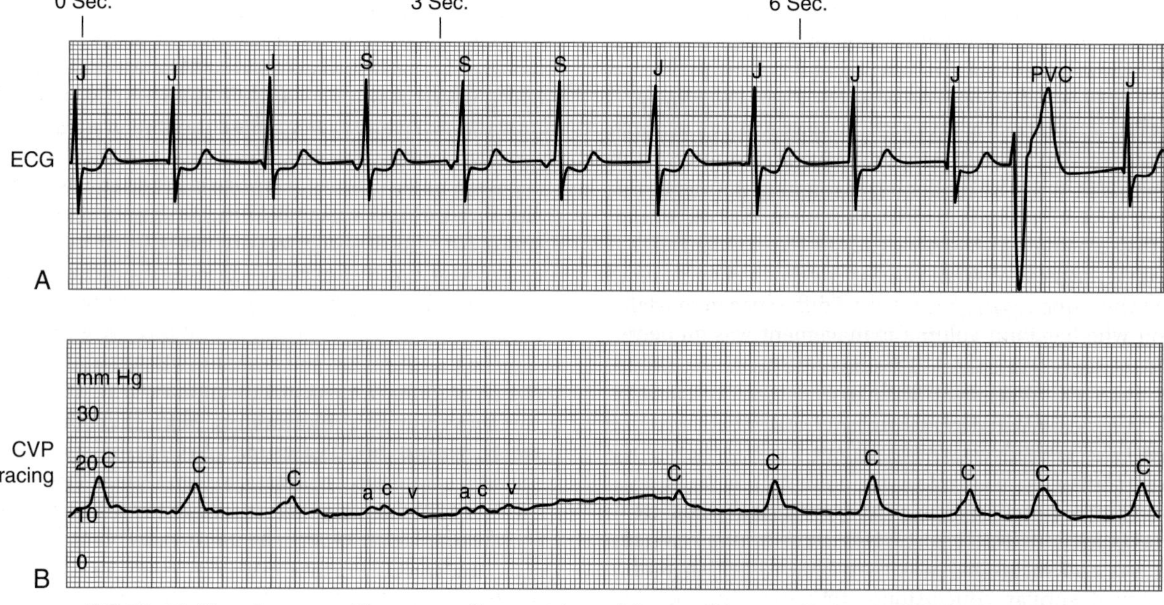

FIG 11-11 Simultaneous Electrocardiographic and Central Venous Pressure (CVP) Tracings. The CVP waveform shows large cannon waves (c waves) corresponding to the junctional beats or premature ventricular contractions (*bottom strip*). As the patient converts to sinus rhythm, the CVP waveform has a normal configuration. ac, normal right atrial pressure tracing; c, cannon waves on CVP tracing; J, junctional rhythm followed by cannon waves on CVP waveform; PVC, premature ventricular contraction followed by cannon wave on CVP; S, sinus rhythm followed by normal CVP tracing with *a, c,* and *v* waves.

saturation.[44] The physiology underlying use of this fiberoptic technology is discussed later in sections on monitoring mixed venous oxygen saturation (SvO_2) and $ScvO_2$.

Safely removing the CVC. Removal of the CVC usually is a nursing responsibility. Complications are infrequent, and the ones to anticipate are bleeding and air embolus. Recommended techniques to avoid air embolus during CVC removal include removing the catheter when the patient is supine in bed (not in a chair) and placing the patient flat or in reverse Trendelenburg position if the patient's clinical condition permits this maneuver. Patients with acute decompensated heart failure, pulmonary disease, and neurologic conditions with raised intracranial pressure (ICP) should not be placed flat. If the patient is alert and able to cooperate, he or she is asked to take a deep breath to raise intrathoracic pressure during removal. After removal, to decrease the risk of air entering by a "track," an occlusive dressing is applied to the site. If bleeding at the site occurs after removal, firm pressure is applied. If a patient has prolonged coagulation times, fresh-frozen plasma or platelets may be prescribed before CVC removal.

Pulmonary Artery Pressure Monitoring

The pulmonary artery (PA) catheter is the most invasive of the critical care monitoring catheters. It is also known as a *right heart catheter* or *Swan-Ganz catheter* (named after the catheter's inventors). The practice of routinely using PA catheters is highly controversial. Several randomized, controlled trials of critically ill patients have not demonstrated a benefit to use of the PA catheter. A randomized, controlled trial of 676 critical care patients with acute respiratory distress syndrome (ARDS) in France reported no difference in mortality rates for patients when treatment was guided by PA catheter and for patients without this information.[45] A randomized, controlled trial of 1000 patients with acute lung injury in the United States found no difference in mortality rates for patients when treatment was guided by a PA catheter and those for whom diagnostic information was obtained from a CVP.[46]

The impact of PA catheterization on mortality rates for patients with acute heart failure has also been examined. A randomized, controlled trial of 433 patients with acute heart failure in the United States reported no difference in mortality based on whether fluid volume management was guided by PA catheter insertion or not.[47] Similar results were reported from a British multicenter trial enrolling more than 1000 critical care patients; there were no differences in mortality or in length of stay.[48] No survival benefit was found in a randomized, controlled trial enrolling older high-risk surgical patients who required critical care monitoring when treatment was guided by PA catheter diagnostics or not.[49] Systematic reviews and meta-analysis of studies of PA catheter use have reached similar conclusions—that insertion of a PA catheter is neutral; it neither conferred a benefit nor increased risk to the patient. There was no increase in mortality or increase in the number of days in the critical care unit or the hospital.[50, 51]

These findings have raised concerns about routine use of PA catheters for critically ill patients. The PA catheter is invasive. It previously seemed intuitive that the diagnostic information provided would confer a survival advantage over less invasive methods, but research has shown this is not the case. Consequently, PA catheter use has decreased dramatically. The number of PA catheters inserted in the USA has declined by 65% over 10 years (1993-2004).[52] In western Canada the decline in PA catheter use was 50% over 5 years (2002-2006).[53]

Although the PA catheter is inserted less frequently in critical care units, right heart catheterization is still used as a diagnostic tool in the cardiac catheterization laboratory. In many critical care units, the PA catheter is reserved for patients who are refractory to conventional treatment,[54] and in many settings, it has been replaced by less invasive technologies such as echocardiography as discussed later in this chapter.

Indications

The thermodilution PA catheter is reserved for the most hemodynamically unstable patients, for the diagnosis and evaluation of heart disease[55] and shock states. The PA catheter can simultaneously assess pulmonary artery systolic and diastolic pressures, pulmonary artery mean pressure, and PAOP (wedge pressure). The PA catheter is used to measure CO, determine mixed-venous oxygen saturation, and calculate additional hemodynamic parameters.

Pulmonary Artery Catheter Lumens

The traditional PA catheter, invented by Swan and Ganz, has four lumens for measurement of right atrial pressure (RAP) or CVP, PA pressures, PAOP, and cardiac output (Figure 11-12A). Multifunction catheters may have additional lumens, which can be used for intravenous infusion (Figure 11-12B) and to measure continuous mixed venous oxygen saturation ($S\bar{v}O_2$), and continuous cardiac output (Figure 11-12C). Other PA catheters include transvenous pacing electrodes to pace the heart if needed.

The PA flow-directed catheter is 110 cm long. The most commonly used sizes are 7.5 or 8.0 Fr, although 5.0 and 7.0 Fr sizes are available. Each of the four lumens exits into the heart or pulmonary artery at a different point, graduated along the catheter length.

Right atrial lumen. The proximal lumen is situated in the right atrium and is used for intravenous infusion, CVP measurement, withdrawal of venous blood samples, and injection of fluid for cardiac output determinations. This port is often described as the *right atrial port*, or *CVP port*.

Pulmonary artery lumen. The distal PA lumen is located at the tip of the PA catheter and is situated in the pulmonary artery. It is used to record pulmonary artery pressures and can be used for withdrawal of blood samples to measure mixed venous blood gases (e.g., SvO_2).

Balloon lumen. The third lumen opens into a balloon at the end of the catheter that can be inflated with 0.8 mL (7 Fr) to 1.5 mL (7.5 Fr) of air. The balloon is inflated during catheter insertion after the catheter reaches the right atrium to assist with forward flow of the catheter and to minimize right ventricular ectopy from the catheter tip. The balloon is also inflated to obtain the PAOP (wedge) measurements when the PA catheter is correctly positioned in the pulmonary artery.

Thermistor lumen. The fourth lumen is a thermistor (temperature sensor) used to measure changes in blood temperature. It is located 4 cm from the catheter tip and is used to measure thermodilution cardiac output. The connector end of the lumen is attached directly to the cardiac output module of the bedside monitor.

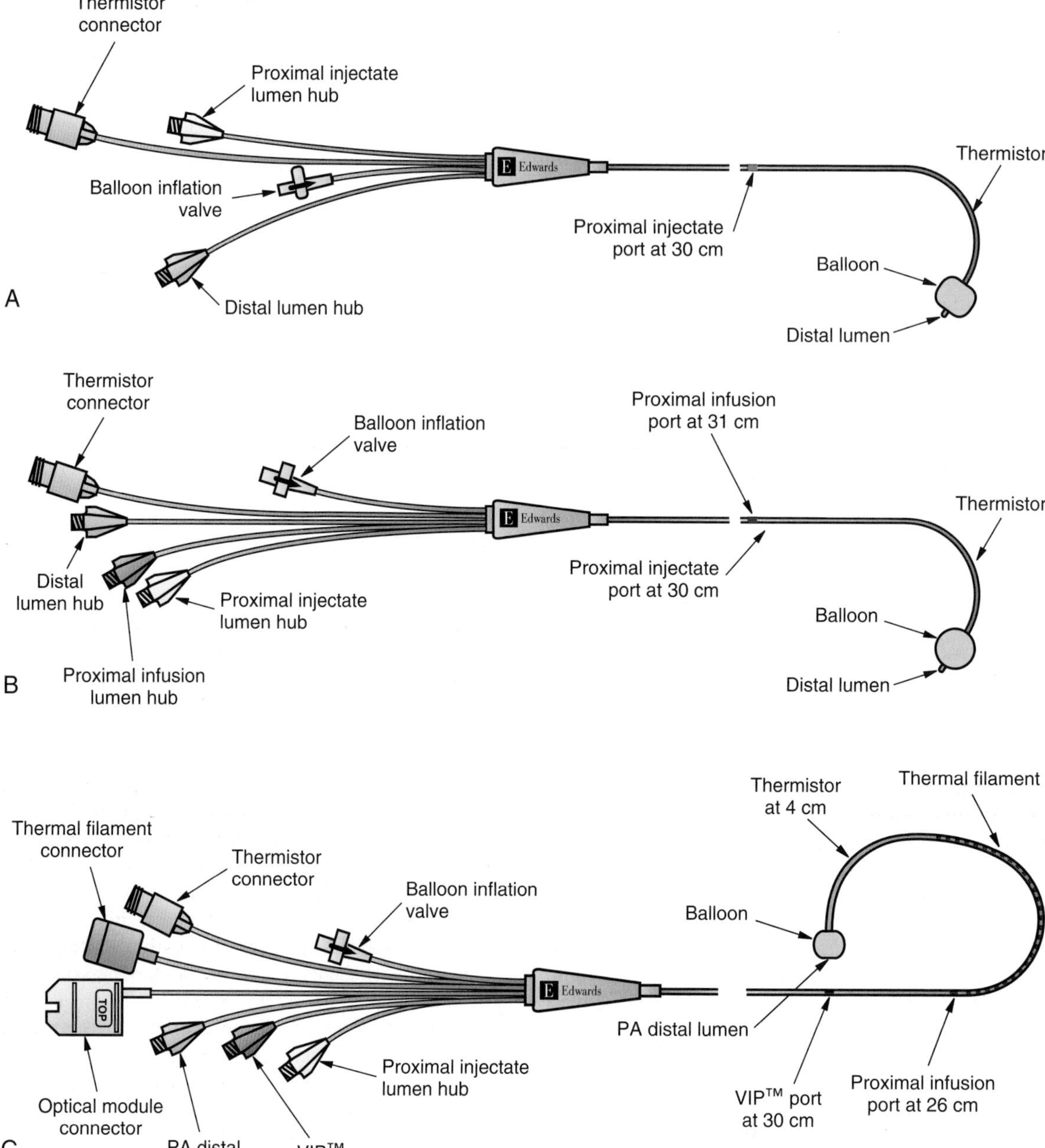

FIG 11-12 Types of Pulmonary Artery Catheters. *A*, Four-lumen catheter. *B*, Five-lumen catheter that includes an additional venous infusion port (VIP) into the right atrium. *C*, Seven-lumen catheter that includes a VIP port and two additional lumens for continuous cardiac output (CCO) and a thermal filament for continuous mixed venous oxygen saturation (SvO_2) monitoring (i.e., optical module connector). An additional option is to combine the use of the CCO filament and the thermistor response time to calculate continuous end-diastolic volume (CEDV). (© 2001 Edwards Lifesciences LLC. All rights reserved. Reprinted with permission of Edwards Lifesciences, Swan-Ganz is a trademark of Edwards Lifesciences Corporation, registered in the US Patent and Trademark Office.)

Fiberoptic lumen. If continuous SvO_2 is measured, the catheter has an additional fiberoptic lumen that exits at the tip of the catheter (see Figure 11-12C).

Insertion

If a PA catheter is to be inserted into a patient who is awake, some brief explanations about the procedure are helpful to ensure that the patient understands what is going to happen. The initial insertion techniques used for placement of a PA catheter are similar to those described for CVC insertion. Because the PA catheter is positioned within the heart chambers and pulmonary artery on the right side of the heart, catheter passage is monitored using fluoroscopy or waveform analysis on the bedside monitor (Figure 11-13).

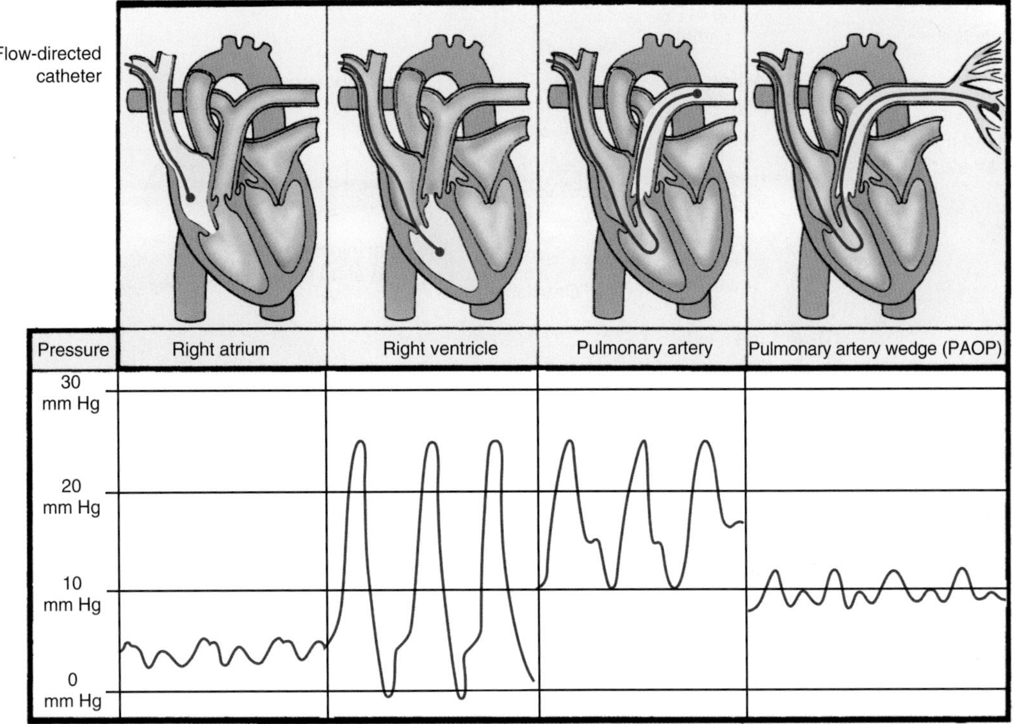

FIG 11-13 Pulmonary Artery (PA) Catheter Insertion with Corresponding Waveforms.

Before inserting the catheter into the vein, the physician—using sterile technique—tests the balloon for inflation and flushes the catheter with normal saline solution to remove any air. The PA catheter is then attached to the bedside hemodynamic line setup and monitor so that the waveforms can be visualized while the catheter is advanced through the right side of the heart (see Fig. 11-13). A larger introducer sheath (8.5 Fr)—with an additional intravenous side-port lumen—is used to cannulate the vein first. This introducer sheath remains in place, and the supple PA catheter is threaded through it into the vena cava and into the right side of the heart.

Nursing Management

Nursing priorities for the patient with PA catheter monitoring focus on 1) accurately interpreting PA waveforms, 2) accommodating changes in patient position, 3) recognizing the effects of respiratory variation, 4) preventing PA catheter-related complications, 5) monitoring cardiac output, and 6) evaluating hemodynamic performance.

Accurately interpreting PA waveforms. Each chamber of the heart has a distinctive waveform with recognizable characteristics. It is the responsibility of the critical care nurse to recognize each waveform displayed on the bedside monitor when the catheter enters the corresponding chamber during insertion and during routine monitoring.

Right atrial waveform. As the PA catheter is advanced into the right atrium during insertion, a right atrial waveform must be visible on the monitor, with recognizable *a*, *c*, and *v* waves (see Fig. 11-13). The normal mean pressure in the right atrium is 2 to 5 mm Hg. Before passage through the tricuspid valve, the balloon at the tip of the catheter is inflated for two reasons. First, it cushions the pointed tip of the PA catheter so that if the tip comes into contact with the right ventricular wall, it will cause less myocardial irritability and, consequently, fewer ventricular dysrhythmias. Second, inflation of the balloon assists the catheter to float with the flow of blood from the right ventricle into the pulmonary artery. It is because of these features and the balloon that PA catheters are described as *flow-directional catheters*.

Right ventricular waveform. The right ventricular waveform is distinctly pulsatile, with distinct systolic and diastolic pressures. Normal right ventricular pressures are 20 to 30 mm Hg systolic and 0 to 5 mm Hg diastolic. Even with the balloon inflated, it is not uncommon for ventricular ectopy to occur during passage through the right ventricle. All patients who have a PA catheter inserted must have simultaneous ECG monitoring, with defibrillator and emergency resuscitation equipment nearby.

Pulmonary artery waveform. As the catheter enters the pulmonary artery, the waveform again changes. The diastolic pressure rises. Normal PA pressures range from 20 to 30 mm Hg systolic over 10 mm Hg diastolic. A dicrotic notch, visible on the downslope of the waveform, represents closure of the pulmonic valve.

Pulmonary artery occlusion waveform (wedge). While the balloon remains inflated, the catheter is advanced into the wedge position. This maneuver produces the PAOP. The waveform decreases in size and is nonpulsatile, reflecting a normal left atrial tracing with *a* and *v* wave deflections. This is often described as a *wedge tracing*, because the balloon is "wedged" into a small pulmonary vessel, but it is technically described as the PAOP (see Fig. 11-13). The balloon occludes the pulmonary vessel so that the PA catheter tip and lumen are exposed only to left atrial pressure. When the balloon is deflated, the catheter should spontaneously float back into the pulmonary artery. When the balloon is reinflated, the wedge tracing should be visible. The normal PAOP ranges from 5 to 12 mm Hg.

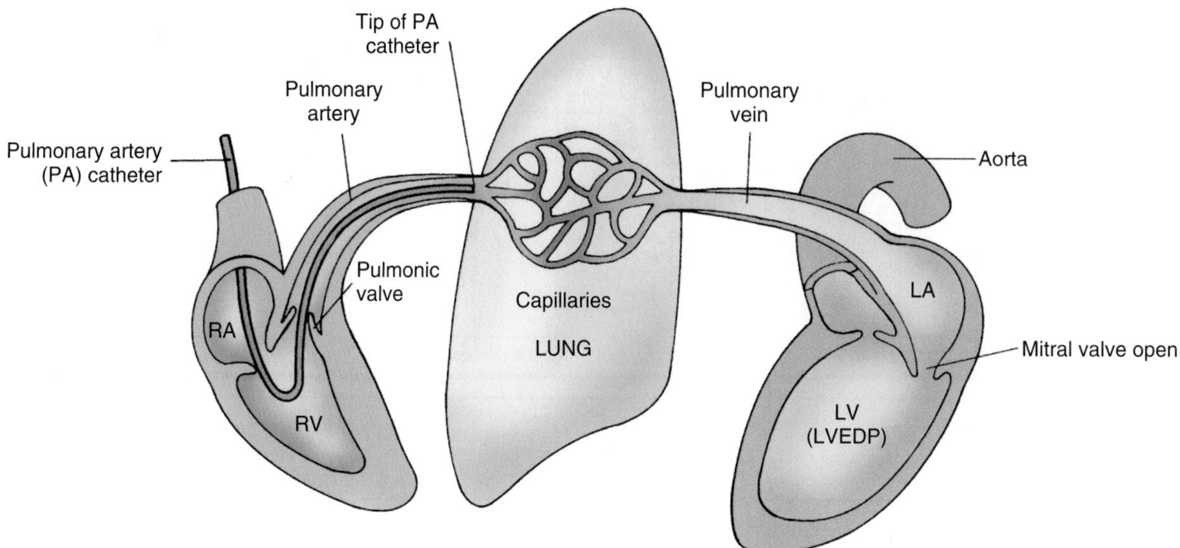

FIG 11-14 Relationship of the Pulmonary Artery Occlusion Pressure (PAOP) (i.e., Wedge Pressure) to the Left Ventricular end Diastolic Pressure (LVEDP) (i.e., Left Ventricular Preload). In most clinical situations the PAOP accurately reflects the LVEDP. During diastole when the mitral valve is open, there are no other valves or obstructions between the tip of the catheter and the left ventricle (LV). The pressure exerted by the volume in the LV is reflected through the left atrium (LA), through the pulmonary veins, and to the pulmonary capillaries. PA, pulmonary artery; RA, right atrium; RV, right ventricle.

During insertion, if the catheter is advanced, or spontaneously floats too far into the pulmonary vascular bed, the patient is at risk for pulmonary infarction.[56] If the PA catheter is not sufficiently advanced into the pulmonary artery, it will not be useful for PAOP readings.

PAD–PAOP relationship. The pulmonary artery diastolic (PAD) pressure may be used as a surrogate for the PAOP in left heart failure, even with an elevated wedge pressure. If the two values (PAD and PAOP) have been shown to be similar, trending the PAD is acceptable. This has the benefit of reducing the number of times the PAC is wedged. The normal difference between the PAOP and the PAD is 1-4 mm Hg with the PAD being the higher value.[56] The relationship from the tip of the PAC to the left ventricle is illustrated in Figure 11-14. It is important to know that the PAD pressure cannot substitute for the PAOP in situations where the PAD is elevated and the PAOP is low, as in patients with acute respiratory distress syndrome (ARDS).

Accommodating changes in patient position. The patient does not need to be flat for accurate pressure readings to be obtained. In the supine position, when the transducer is placed at the level of the phlebostatic axis, a head-of-bed position from flat up to 60 degrees is appropriate for most patients.[30] It is important to know that PAD and PAOP measurements in the lateral position may be significantly different from those taken when the patient is lying supine. If there is concern about the validity of pressure readings in a particular patient, it is more reliable to take measurements with the patient on his or her back, with the head of bed elevated from flat to 60 degrees as tolerated. After a patient changes position, a stabilization period of 5 to 15 minutes is recommended before taking pressure readings.[30] The stabilization period is usually longer if the patient has left ventricular dysfunction or is hemoydynamically unstable.

Recognizing the effects of respiratory variation. All PAD pressure and PAOP tracings are subject to respiratory interference, especially when the patient is on a positive-pressure, volume-cycled ventilator.[30] During the positive-pressure inhalation phase, the increase in intrathoracic pressure may "push up" the pulmonary artery tracing, producing an artificially high reading (Figure 11-15A). During spontaneous breaths, negative intrathoracic pressure "pulls down" the waveform, producing an erroneously low measurement (see Figure 11-15B). To minimize the impact of respiratory variation, the reading is taken at end-expiration, which is the most stable point in the respiratory cycle when intrapleural pressures are close to zero. If the digital number fluctuates with respiration, a printed readout on paper can be obtained to verify the pressure. In some clinical settings, a respiratory waveform or airway pressure waveform are recorded simultaneously with the PAD/PAOP tracing to identify end-expiration accurately.[30]

Positive end expiratory pressure. Some clinical diagnoses, such as acute lung injury, require the use of high levels of positive end-expiratory pressure (PEEP) set with the ventilator to treat refractory hypoxemia. If a PEEP of greater than 10 cm H_2O is used, the PAOP and pulmonary artery pressures will be artificially elevated, and cardiac output may be negatively affected. Because of this impact of PEEP, in the past, patients in some critical care units were taken off the ventilator to record pulmonary artery pressure measurements. It has since been shown that this practice closes alveoli, decreases the patient's oxygenation level, and may result in persistent hypoxemia.

Because patients remain on PEEP for treatment, they remain on it during measurement of pulmonary artery pressures. In this situation, the trend of pulmonary artery readings is more important than one individual measurement.

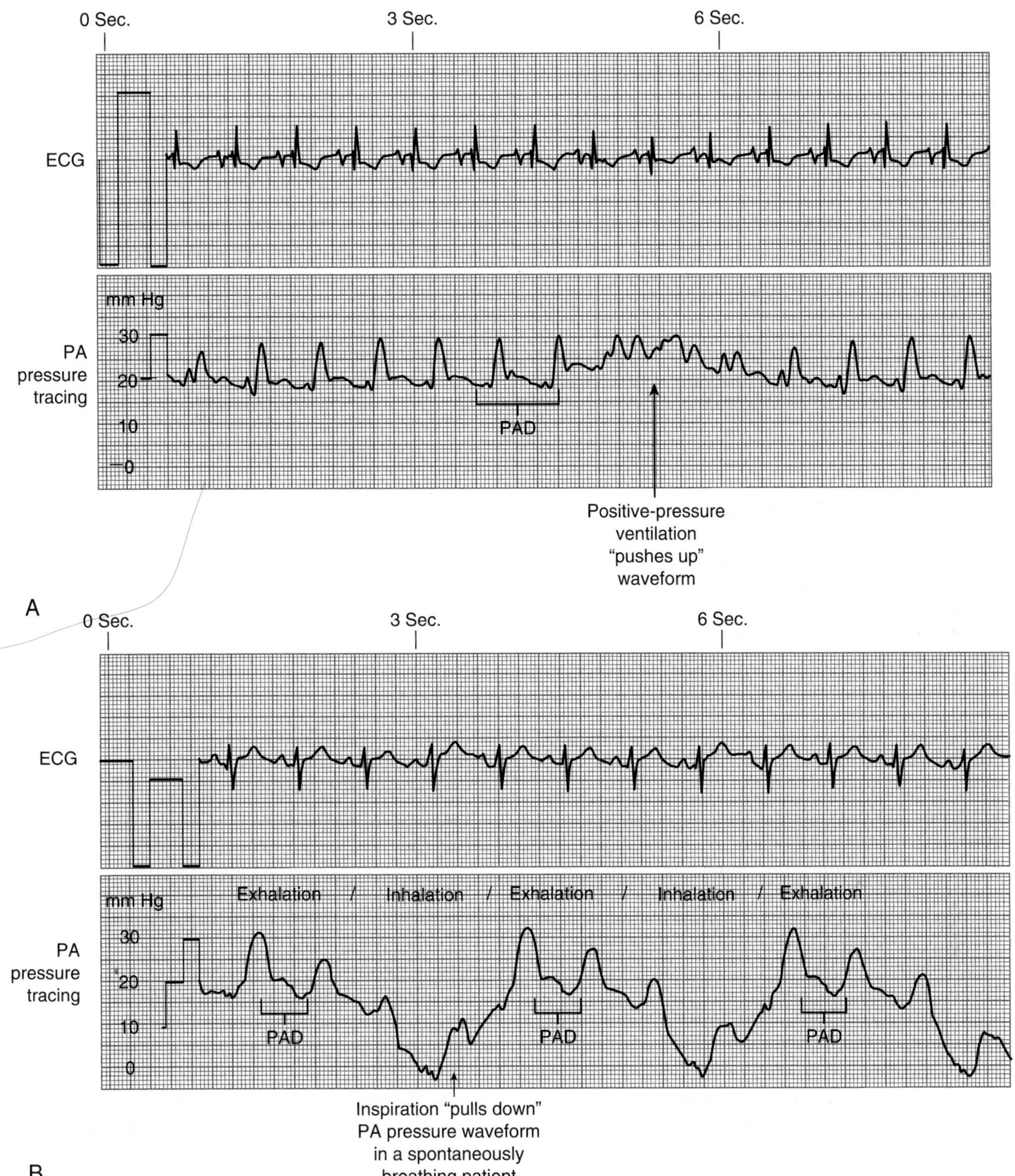

FIG 11-15 Pulmonary Artery (PA) Waveforms That Demonstrate the Impact of Ventilation on PA Pressure Readings. For accuracy, PA pressures are read at the end of exhalation. *A*, In positive-pressure ventilation, the increase in intrathoracic pressure during inhalation "pushes up" the PA pressure waveform, creating a falsely high reading. *B*, In spontaneous breathing, the decrease in intrathoracic pressure during normal inhalation "pulls down" the PA waveform, creating a falsely low reading.

Preventing pulmonary artery catheter-related complications. After insertion of the catheter, the chest radiograph or fluoroscopy is used to verify the PA catheter position to make sure that it is not looped or knotted in the right ventricle and to rule out pneumothorax or hemorrhagic complications.

A thin plastic sleeve is placed on the outside of the catheter when it is inserted to maintain sterility of the part of the PA catheter that exits from the patient. If the PA catheter is not in the desired position or if it migrates out of position, it can be repositioned. Use of this external sleeve on PA catheters has been associated with lower rates of bloodstream infection.[29] Infection is always a risk with a PA catheter. The risks are similar to those discussed in the section on CVCs (see the QSEN Patient Safety Alert feature on

Guidelines for Prevention and Management of Central Venous Catheter Infections).

The PA waveform is continuously monitored to ensure that the catheter does not migrate forward into a spontaneous wedge or PAOP position. A segment of lung can suffer infarction if the wedged catheter occludes an arteriole for a prolonged period. If the catheter is spontaneously wedged, the catheter must be gently pulled back out of the wedge position to prevent pulmonary infarction. Additionally, the PA waveform is monitored to ensure the catheter tip does not migrate back into the right ventricle (see Fig. 11-13).

Pulmonary artery catheter removal. PA catheters can be safely removed from the patient by critical care nurses competent in this procedure.[30] Removal is not usually associated with major complications. Sometimes there are PVCs as the catheter is pulled through the right ventricle.[30]

Monitoring cardiac output. Cardiac output (CO) is the product of heart rate (HR) multiplied by stroke volume (SV). Stroke volume is the volume of blood ejected by the heart during each beat (reported in milliliters).

$$HR \times SV = CO$$

The normal adult stroke volume is 60 to 70 mL. The clinical factors that contribute to the heart's stroke volume are *preload, afterload,* and *contractility* (Figure 11-16). Preload and afterload are calculated with data obtained from the PAC. The PA catheter measures cardiac output using either intermittent (bolus) or continuous methods.

Thermodilution cardiac output bolus method. The bolus thermodilution method is performed at the bedside and results in a cardiac output calculated in liters per minute. Three bolus thermodilution cardiac output values that are within a 10% mean range are obtained at one time and are averaged to provide one number. Typically, 10 mL of room-temperature normal saline solution is injected into the proximal lumen of the PA catheter. The injectate exits into the right atrium and travels with the flow of blood past the thermistor (temperature sensor) located at the distal end of the catheter in the pulmonary artery. The injectate can be delivered by hand injection using individual syringes of saline. Frequently, a closed in-line system attached to a 500-mL bag of normal saline is used as a reservoir to deliver the individual injections.

Cardiac output curve interpretation. The thermodilution CO method uses the indicator-dilution method, in which a known temperature is the indicator. It is based on the principle that the change in temperature over time is inversely proportional to blood flow. Blood flow can be diagrammatically represented as a curve where temperature is plotted against time (Figure 11-17). Most hemodynamic monitors display this curve, which must then be interpreted to determine whether the bolus injection is valid. The normal curve has a smooth upstroke, with a rounded peak and a gradually tapering down-slope. If the curve has an uneven pattern, it may indicate faulty injection technique, and the cardiac output measurement must be repeated. Patient movement or coughing also alters the validity of the measurement.

Injectate temperature. To ensure accurate readings, the difference between injectate temperature and body temperature must be at least 10° Centigrade, and the injectate must be delivered within 4 seconds, with minimal handling of the syringe to prevent warming of the solution. This is particularly important if iced injectate is used. With all delivery systems, the injectate is delivered at the same point in the respiratory cycle, usually end-expiration.

Patient position and cardiac output. In the normovolemic, stable patient, reliable cardiac output measurements can be obtained in a supine position (patient lying on his or her back) with the head of the bed elevated up to 60 degrees.[30] If the patient is hypovolemic or unstable, leaving the head of the bed in a flat position or only slightly elevated may be a more clinically appropriate choice.

Clinical conditions that alter cardiac output. Two clinical conditions that affect the right side of the heart produce errors in the thermodilution cardiac output values: tricuspid valve regurgitation and ventricular septal rupture. If the patient has tricuspid valve regurgitation, the expected flow of blood is disrupted by backflow from the right ventricle to the right atrium. This lowers cardiac output measurement compared with the patient's actual output. If the person has an intracardiac left-to-right shunt, as occurs after ventricular septal rupture, the thermodilution method measures the large pulmonary volume and records a higher cardiac output than the patient's true systemic output.

Continuous cardiac output measurement. The bolus thermodilution method is reliable but performed intermittently. Continuous cardiac output monitoring using a PA catheter is also frequently used in clinical practice. One method employs a thermal filament on the PA catheter to emit small pulses of energy (the indicator) into the bloodstream. These signals are then detected by the thermistor near the tip of the PA catheter. The equivalent of an indicator curve is created, and a cardiac output value is calculated from this data.

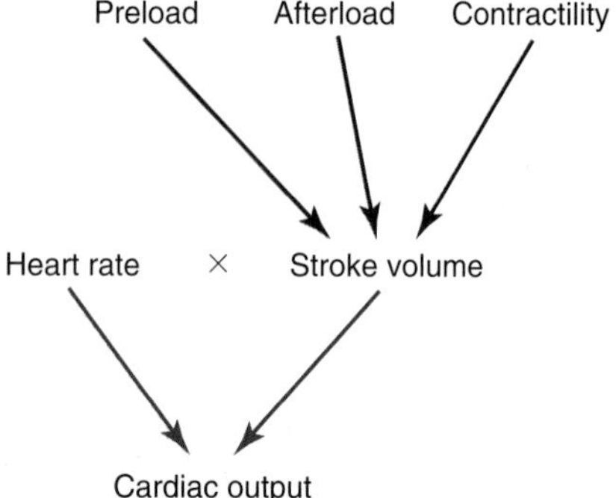

FIG 11-16 Preload, afterload, and contractility contribute to the heart's stroke volume. Stroke volume × Heart rate = Cardiac output.

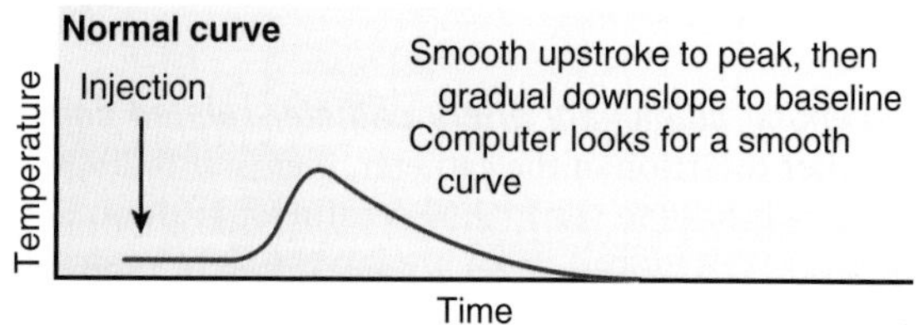

FIG 11-17 Normal Cardiac Thermodilution Bolus Output Curve.

Evaluating hemodynamic profiles. For the patient with a thermodilution PA catheter in place, additional hemodynamic information can be calculated using routine vital signs, cardiac output, and body surface area (BSA). These measurements are calculated using specific formulas that are indexed to individual body size. The BSA is calculated when the patient's height and weight are entered into the bedside monitor.

The calculated values used in the hemodynamic profiles are described in Appendix B.

Noninvasive and minimally invasive measurement of cardiac output. As a result of the perceived risks associated with use of the PA catheter, combined with studies that have not shown improved outcomes with routine monitoring, there is tremendous interest in finding less invasive methods of cardiac output measurement. Bedside echocardiography is the most frequently used noninvasive method. Minimally invasive techniques can involve vascular catheters or esophageal probes as described in Table 11-4. All have been compared with the thermodilution cardiac output method.

TABLE 11-4 Minimally and Non-Invasive Cardiac Output Measurement

DEVICE NAME	PROBE PLACEMENT	METHOD	CARDIAC OUTPUT CALCULATION	CLINICAL ISSUES
Noninvasive Methods				
Bioimpedance	External electrodes placed on the neck and chest	Thoracic electric bioimpedance	1. A small alternating current is applied across the chest by skin electrodes. 2. Pulsatile changes in thoracic blood volume result in changes in electrical impedance. The rate of change of impedance during systole is measured and used to calculate CO.	Noninvasive Less accurate with low body temperature
Transcutaneous Doppler (USCOM, Sydney, Australia)	External probe placed on skin	Ultrasound Continuous wave Doppler	1. Intermittent measurement 2. Measures flow across the aortic and pulmonic valves. 3. Measures real-time stroke volume	Noninvasive Highly accurate
Finger Cuff methods (Edwards Lifesciences, Irvine CA)	Multiple small cuffs on fingers	Arterial pressure monitor	Measures SV, SVV, CO, and SVR	Noninvasive, short-time use
Minimally Invasive Methods				
Pulse Contour Waveform Methods				
LiDCO (LiDCO Ltd., Cambridge, United Kingdom)	Requires a venous access catheter (central or peripheral) and an arterial catheter with a lithium-monitoring sensor attached	Pulse contour waveform analysis method (calibrated)	Independent calibration with a lithium dilution technique is initially required: 1. A small, subtherapeutic dose of isotonic lithium chloride is injected through the venous catheter. 2. The lithium is detected at the arterial sensor (femoral artery), where a fixed flow pump ensures constant flow. 3. A concentration-time curve is produced for lithium before recirculation. 4. CO is calculated based on the lithium dose given and the measurement of area under the curve.	Easy to set up, uses conventional venous and arterial catheters; can measure extravascular lung water for patients in pulmonary edema. CO measurement is affected by artifact on arterial waveform and by irregular and damped arterial waveforms; can be used in conscious and in unresponsive patients. Requires calibration at least every 8 hours to maintain accuracy; cannot be used in patients on lithium therapy because this interferes with the calibration.

Continued

TABLE 11-4 Minimally and Non-Invasive Cardiac Output Measurement—cont'd

DEVICE NAME	PROBE PLACEMENT	METHOD	CARDIAC OUTPUT CALCULATION	CLINICAL ISSUES
PiCCO (Pulsion Medical Systems, Munich, Germany)	Requires a central venous access catheter and uses a specialized arterial thermistor-tipped catheter in the femoral artery	Pulse contour waveform analysis method that uses transpulmonary thermodilution	1. A set volume of cold saline is injected through the central venous catheter. The arterial thermistor-tipped catheter detects the blood temperature change. 2. Continuous CO measurements are achieved by analyzing the systolic component of the arterial waveform.	CO measurement is affected by artifact on arterial waveform and irregular arterial waveforms. Three calibrations are required initially, and frequent recalibration is required to maintain accuracy.
Vigileo (Edward Lifesciences, Irvine, CA)	Requires a functional arterial catheter	Pulse contour waveform analysis method (does not require calibration)	1. Calculates CO by use of the arterial pressure waveform analysis in conjunction with patient data (age, sex, height, weight). 2. Uses an internal proprietary algorithm based on the principle that pulse pressure (difference between systolic and diastolic pressure) is proportional to stroke volume and inversely proportional to aortic compliance. 3. Aortic pressure is sampled at 100 Hz and is updated every 20 seconds.	Does not require external calibration but requires zeroing of the transducer Lack of calibration procedures is controversial.
Esophageal Probe Methods				
Esophageal Doppler	Ultrasound probe placed in the lower esophagus	Stroke volume is calculated by measurement of the aortic blood velocity in the descending thoracic aorta (by continuous wave Doppler) plus calculation of the cross-sectional area of the aorta; these values are used to calculate the CO.	1. Measurement of the aorta cross-sectional area, measured using M-mode ultrasound, and multiplying this value by blood velocity to calculate flow or CO. 2. The value of total CO is derived from a nomogram using aortic blood velocity, height, weight, and age.	Useful in the operating room or with deeply sedated patients. Probe is stiff, and placement is not well-tolerated by conscious patients.
Transesophageal echocardiography (TEE)	Ultrasound probe placed in the esophagus	Probe placement allows imaging of the left ventricular outflow tract. SV measured by Doppler.	1. The left ventricular (LV) outflow tract area is measured; this value is squared and multiplied by the velocity time interval of blood flow and heart rate. 2. LV stroke volume can be measured, as can heart rate to use the SV × HR = CO formula.	Useful in the operating room or with deeply sedated patients Probe is stiff, and placement is not well-tolerated by conscious patients. Requires skill to position probe accurately to visualize the LV outflow tract.

CO, cardiac output; HR, heart rate; LV, left ventricle; SV, stroke volume; SVR, systemic vascular resistance; SVV, stroke volume variation.

Continuous Monitoring of Venous Oxygen Saturation

Indications

Continuous monitoring of venous oxygen saturation is indicated for the critically ill patient who has the potential to develop an imbalance between oxygen supply and metabolic tissue demand. This includes patients after high-risk surgery[57] and in severe sepsis or septic shock.[58]

Continuous venous oxygen monitoring permits a calculation of the balance achieved between arterial oxygen supply (SaO_2) and oxygen demand at the tissue level by sampling venous blood from the distal tip of the PAC. This sample is called mixed venous oxygen saturation (SvO_2) because it is a mixture of all the venous blood drained from upper body and lower body tissues. The same fiberoptic technology has been combined with a fiberoptic triple-lumen CVC. In this situation, the venous blood is sampled from the superior vena cava, just above the right atrium, and the central venous oxygen saturation ($ScvO_2$) is measured.

Under normal conditions, the cardiopulmonary system achieves a balance between oxygen supply and demand. Four factors contribute to this balance:

1. Cardiac output (CO)
2. Hemoglobin (Hgb)
3. Arterial oxygen saturation (SaO_2)
4. Tissue oxygen metabolism (VO_2)

Three of these factors (CO, Hgb, and SaO_2) contribute to the supply of oxygen to the tissues. Tissue metabolism (VO_2) determines oxygen consumption or the quantity of oxygen extracted at tissue level that creates the demand for oxygen. The relationships of these factors are illustrated in Figure 11-18.

In addition to measurement of venous oxygen saturation, it is possible to calculate the quantity of oxygen (in mL/min) that is provided to the tissues by the cardiopulmonary system and to assess the amount of oxygen consumed by the body tissues. These calculations rely on principles of oxygen transport physiology and are the basis for calculation of SvO_2. These formulas are listed in Appendix B.

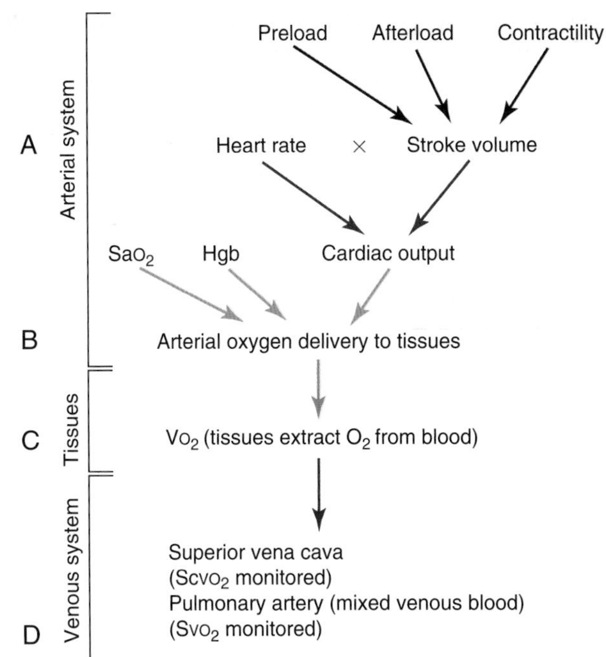

FIG 11-18 Several factors contribute to the mixed venous oxygen saturation ($S\bar{v}O_2$) value. *A*, Cardiac output (CO) is determined by heart rate (HR) × stroke volume (SV). *B*, The oxygen saturation (SaO_2) hemoglobin (Hgb) level, and CO contribute to arterial oxygen delivery at the tissue level. *C*, Tissues extract and use the oxygen carried in the blood. This process of cellular oxygen consumption is VO_2. *D*, Blood returns to the superior vena cava (recorded as $ScvO_2$) and blood from both the superior and inferior vena cavae return to the pulmonary artery, where the mixed venous blood is recorded as SvO_2.

Catheters

The type of catheter used to measure venous oxygen saturation is defined by where the fiberoptic tip is located, either at the tip of a CVC or on the distal tip of a PA catheter.

SvO_2 catheter. The pulmonary arterial S_VO_2 catheter has the traditional four lumens plus a lumen containing two or three optical fibers. The fiberoptics are attached to an optical module that transmits a narrow band of light down one optical fiber. This light is reflected off the hemoglobin in the blood and returns to the optical module through the receiving fiberoptic. The SvO_2 signal is recorded on a continuous display on the bedside monitor.

$ScvO_2$ catheter. The central venous $ScvO_2$ technology is incorporated into a multi-lumen CVC. The fiberoptic catheter tip is positioned in a central vein, such as the superior vena cava. The technology used to measure the venous saturation is identical in both types of catheters, and the same continuous display module is used for both catheters.

The $ScvO_2$ catheter has been recommended to guide resuscitation in patients with sepsis.[58] However, results of the 2014 ProCESS clinical trial indicate that the early identification and treatment of sepsis may be more important for survival than invasive technology including $ScvO_2$.[59]

SvO_2 and $ScvO_2$ relationship. The SvO_2 value (from the pulmonary artery) is normally about 5% higher than the $ScvO_2$ (superior vena cava) value. However, in severe sepsis and septic shock, the trend is reversed, and the SvO_2 value is lower than the $ScvO_2$.

S_VO_2 or $S_{CV}O_2$ catheter calibration. The catheter is calibrated before insertion into the patient through a standardized color reference system, which is part of the catheter package. Insertion technique and sites are identical to those used for placement of conventional PA or CVC catheters. Waveform analysis or venous saturation measurement or both can be used for accurate placement. After the catheter is inserted, recalibration is unnecessary unless the catheter becomes disconnected from the optical module.

To recalibrate the fiberoptic module to verify accuracy when the catheter is already inserted in a patient, a mixed venous blood sample (SvO_2) or central venous sample ($ScvO_2$) must be drawn from the appropriate catheter tip and sent to the laboratory for oxygen saturation analysis. In many critical care units, this is a standard daily procedure to ensure that readings used to guide patient care remain accurate.

Nursing Management

Nursing priorities for the patient with a fiberoptic catheter that monitors venous oxygenation include 1) assessing the

accuracy of the SvO_2/$ScvO_2$ values and 2) incorporating the SvO_2/$ScvO_2$ values into the hemodynamic assessment.

Assessing the accuracy of the SvO_2 or $S_{CV}O_2$ values. SvO_2 monitoring provides a continuous assessment of the balance of oxygen supply and demand for an individual patient. Nursing assessment includes evaluation of the SvO_2 or $ScvO_2$ value and evaluation of the four factors that maintain the oxygen supply-demand balance. These factors are arterial oxygen saturation (SaO_2 or SpO_2), cardiac output (CO), hemoglobin (Hgb), and tissue oxygenation (VO_2) to maintain the oxygen supply-demand balance.

Normal SvO_2 values. Normal SvO_2 is approximately 75% in the healthy individual (range, 60% to 80%). In critically ill patients, an SvO_2 value between 60% and 80% is evidence of adequate balance between oxygen supply and demand.

Normal $ScvO_2$ values. The normal values for the $ScvO_2$ catheter are slightly higher because the reading is taken before the blood enters the right heart chambers, where the cardiac sinus (vein) delivers desaturated venous blood drained from the myocardium into the right atrium. As described above, this situation is reversed in severe sepsis or septic shock.

If SvO_2 or $ScvO_2$ is within the normal range of 60% to 80% and the patient is not clinically compromised, the nurse can assume that oxygen supply and demand are balanced for that individual.

Assessment of ScO_2 or $ScvO_2$. If SvO_2 or $ScvO_2$ falls below 60% and is sustained, the critical care nurse must assume that oxygen supply is not equal to demand. It is helpful to assess the cause of decreased SvO_2 or $ScvO_2$ in a logical sequence that reflects knowledge of the meaning of the venous saturation value. The following is one such assessment sequence:

1. Clinically assess the patient.
2. Assess whether the decreased SvO_2 or $ScvO_2$ is caused by low oxygen supply. Verify the effectiveness of the ventilator or oxygen mask or check arterial oxygen saturation (SaO_2) from arterial blood gas values.
3. Assess cardiac function by performing a cardiac output measurement.
4. Assess the hemoglobin value by checking recent laboratory results or by withdrawing a blood sample for laboratory analysis.
5. Assess whether the decreased SvO_2 or $ScvO_2$ is the result of a recent patient movement or nursing action that may have temporarily increased tissue oxygen consumption.

Incorporating SvO_2 or $ScvO_2$ values into the hemodynamic assessment.

Therapeutic goals for SvO_2 or $ScvO_2$. Therapeutic values for venous oximetry are an SvO_2 of 70% or above and an $ScvO_2$ of 65% or above. Patients with lower values are at greater risk for organ hypoperfusion and increased mortality. The Surviving Sepsis Campaign guidelines recommend that $ScvO_2$ be maintained above 70% during resuscitation.[58]

Low SvO_2 or $ScvO_2$. If SvO_2 or $ScvO_2$ falls below 40% and is maintained at this low value, the imbalance of oxygen supply and demand will not be adequate to meet tissue needs at the cellular level. At some point, the cells change from an aerobic to anaerobic mode of metabolism, which results in the production of lactic acid and is representative of a shock state in which cellular injury or cell death may result. At this point, every attempt must be made to determine the cause of the low SvO_2 or $ScvO_2$ and to correct the oxygen supply-demand imbalance. To avoid the risk of lactic acidosis, it is helpful to monitor the trend of the SvO_2 or $ScvO_2$ and to intervene early with a goal of returning the venous oxygen saturation to above 70%.

High SvO_2 or $ScvO_2$. In certain clinical conditions, SvO_2 or $ScvO_2$ may increase to an above-normal level (>80%). This may occur during times of low oxygen demand, such as during anesthesia or hypothermia. If the SvO_2 PA catheter drifts into a wedged position, the SvO_2 increases because the fiberoptic tip of the catheter comes into contact with newly oxygenated blood (Table 11-5).

ELECTROCARDIOGRAPHY

Nursing Management

Nursing priorities for the patient with bedside ECG monitoring focus on accurate 1) selection of the ECG lead, 2) interpreting the ECG, and 3) initiation of emergency measures to treat dysrhythmias when required.

Selecting ECG Leads

ECG leads. The basic 3-lead ECG system consists of three bipolar electrodes that are applied to the chest wall and labeled right arm (RA), left arm (LA), and left leg (LL) (Figure 11-19A). Three leads are created from this configuration, called simply Lead I, Lead II, and Lead III, plus three augmented vector (aV) leads: aVR, aVL, and aVF calculated from a theoretical triangle (Einthoven's triangle) as shown in Figure 11-20.

A 5-lead ECG system is typically used in critical care. This system incorporates Leads I-III, aVR, aVL, aVF, (see Figure 11-19B) and at least one chest lead (precordial lead), also known as a "V" lead. Leads are color-coded to decrease the risk of misplacement. A multi-select function on the bedside monitor allows clinicians to switch between views and quickly obtain multiple images of the patient's ECG rhythm.

A bipolar lead system means that each displayed ECG lead has a positive and a negative pole. One lead also acts as a ground. The function of the ground electrode is to prevent the appearance of background electrical interference on the ECG tracing. Leads do not transmit any electricity to the patient; they record electrical impulses.

ECG paper. ECG paper records the speed and magnitude of electrical impulses on a grid composed of small and large boxes (Figure 11-21). Every large box has five small boxes in it. At a standard paper speed of 25 mm/sec, on the horizontal axis, one small box (1 mm) is equivalent to 0.04 second, and one large box (5 mm) represents 0.20 second. Distances along the horizontal axis represent speed and are stated in seconds rather than in millimeters or number of boxes. The vertical axis represents the magnitude, or force, of the electrical signal. One small vertical box equals 0.1 mm. The vertical scale is also standardized to a specific calibration, usually a rise of 10 mm (2 large boxes) in response to a 1 mV electrical signal, evident at the beginning of the ECG tracing.

Interpreting the ECG

Waveforms

The analysis of waveforms and intervals provide the basis for ECG interpretation (Figure 11-22).

P wave. The P wave represents atrial depolarization.

TABLE 11-5 Alterations in Oxygen Consumption

CONDITION OR ACTIVITY	% INCREASE OVER RESTING $V\!O_2$	% DECREASE UNDER RESTING $V\!O_2$
Clinical Conditions That Increase $V\!O_2$		
Fever	10% (for each 1°C above normal)	
Skeletal injuries	10%-30%	
Work of breathing	40%	
Severe infection	60%	
Shivering	50%-100%	
Burns	100%	
Routine postoperative procedures	7%	
Nasal intubation	25%-40%	
Endotracheal tube suctioning	27%	
Chest trauma	60%	
Multiple organ dysfunction syndrome	20%-80%	
Sepsis	50%-100%	
Head injury, with patient sedated	89%	
Head injury, with patient not sedated	138%	
Critical illness in emergency department	60%	
Nursing Activities That Increase $V\!O_2$		
Dressing change	10%	
Electrocardiogram	16%	
Agitation	18%	
Physical examination	20%	
Visitor	22%	
Bath	23%	
Chest radiograph examination	25%	
Position change	31%	
Chest physiotherapy	35%	
Weighing on sling scale	36%	
Conditions That Decrease $V\!O_2$		
Anesthesia		25%
Anesthesia in burned patients		50%

$V\!O_2$, Oxygen consumption.
Modified from White KM, et al. The physiologic basis for continuous mixed venous oxygen saturation monitoring. *Heart Lung.* 1990; 19(5 Pt 2):548.

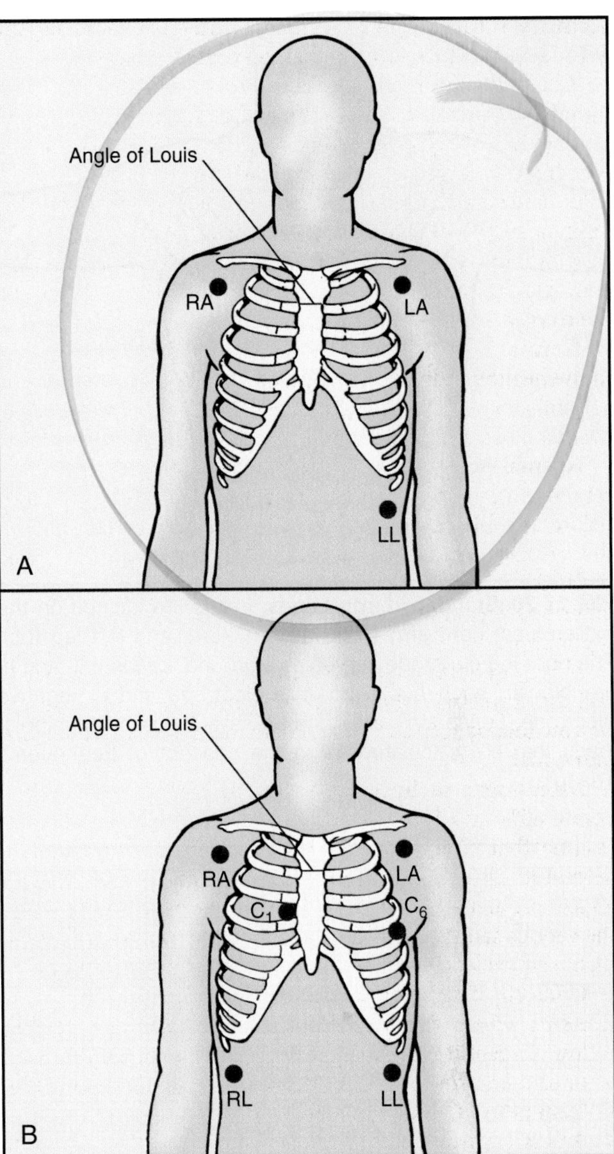

FIG 11-19 *A,* Three electrodes and lead-wire cables allow monitoring of three of the limb leads: I, II, and III. *B,* Five electrodes and lead-wire cables allow monitoring of any of the six standard limb leads (I, II, III, aVR, aVL, or aVF) and any one precordial or chest (C) lead from position V_1 to V_6. The label C_1 indicates the correct position of the chest electrode for monitoring leads V_1, and C_6 indicates the proper position of the chest electrode for monitoring V_6. In a multilead monitoring system, five electrodes and lead-wire cables allow monitoring of any of the six standard limb leads (I, II, III, aVR, aVL, or aVF) and any one precordial lead (V_1 or V_6). C_1 indicates the proper position of the chest electrode for monitoring lead V_1, and C_6 indicates the proper position of the chest electrode for monitoring V_6. Some systems use all six precordial leads for continuous ECG monitoring. Color-coded cable attachments allow quick identification and accurate electrode placement.

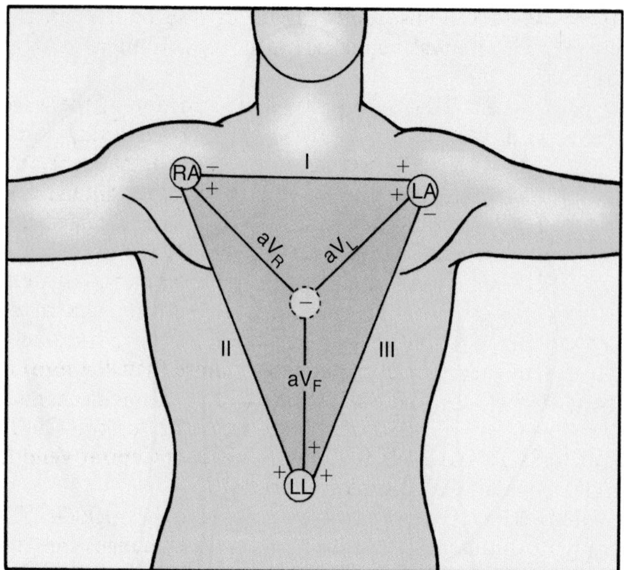

FIG 11-20 Standard Limb Leads. Leads are located on the extremities: right arm (RA), left arm (LA), and left leg (LL). The right leg electrode serves as a ground. Leads I, II, and III are bipolar; each has a positive electrode and a negative electrode. Leads aVR, aVL, and aVF are augmented unipolar leads that are calculated using the concept of Einthoven's Triangle.

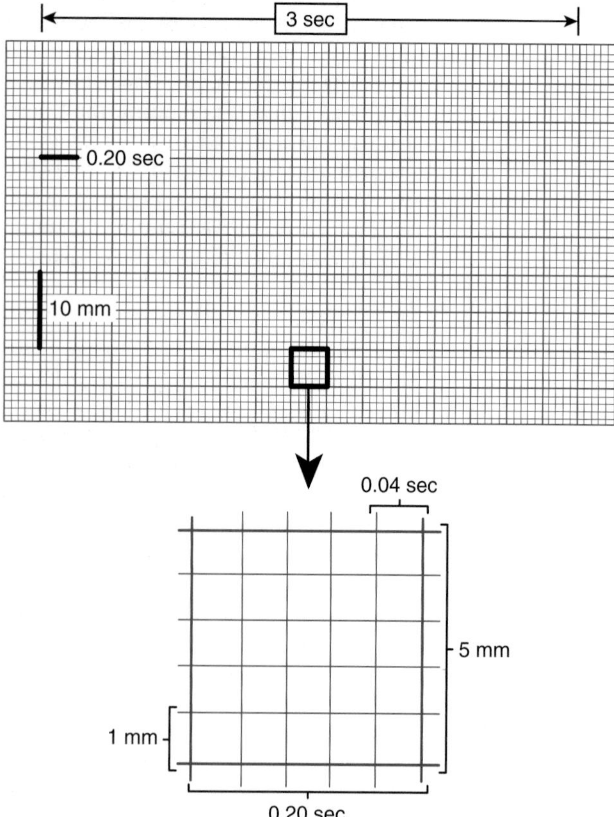

FIG 11-21 ECG Graph Paper. The horizontal axis represents time, and the vertical axis represents the magnitude of voltage. Horizontally, each small box is 0.04 second, and each large box is 0.20 second. Vertically, each large box is 5 mm. Markings are present every 3 seconds at the top of the paper for ease in calculating heart rate.

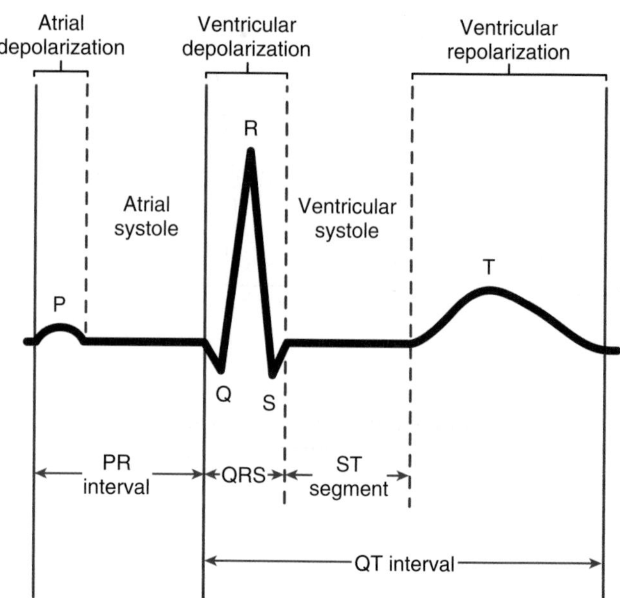

FIG 11-22 Normal ECG Waveforms, Intervals, and Correlation with Events of the Cardiac Cycle. The *P wave* represents atrial depolarization, followed immediately by atrial systole. The *QRS* represents ventricular depolarization, followed immediately by ventricular systole. The *ST segment* corresponds to phase 2 of the action potential, during which time the heart muscle is completely depolarized and contraction normally occurs. The *T wave* represents ventricular repolarization. The *PR interval*, measured from the beginning of the P wave to the beginning of the QRS, corresponds to atrial depolarization and impulse delay in the atrioventricular (AV) node. The *QT interval*, measured from the beginning of the QRS complex to the end of the T wave, represents the time from initial depolarization of the ventricles to the end of ventricular repolarization.

QRS complex. The QRS complex represents ventricular depolarization, corresponding to phase 0 of the ventricular action potential. It is referred to as a *complex* because it consists of several different waves. The letter *Q* is used to describe an initial negative deflection; only if the first deflection from the baseline is negative will it be labeled a Q wave. The letter *R* applies to any positive deflection from baseline. If there are two positive deflections in one QRS complex, the second is labeled R' ("R prime") and is commonly seen in lead V_1 in patients with right bundle branch block. The letter *S* refers to any subsequent negative deflections. Any combination of these deflections can occur and is collectively called the *QRS complex* (Figure 11-23). The QRS duration is normally less than 0.10 second or 2.5 small boxes in a horizontal direction.

T wave. The T wave represents ventricular repolarization, corresponding to phase 3 of the ventricular action potential. The onset of the QRS to approximately the midpoint or peak of the T wave represents an absolute refractory period, during which the heart muscle cannot respond to another stimulus no matter how strong that stimulus may be (Figure 11-24). From the midpoint to the end of the T wave, the heart muscle is in the relative refractory period. The heart muscle has not yet fully recovered, but it can be depolarized again if a strong enough stimulus is received. This can be a particularly

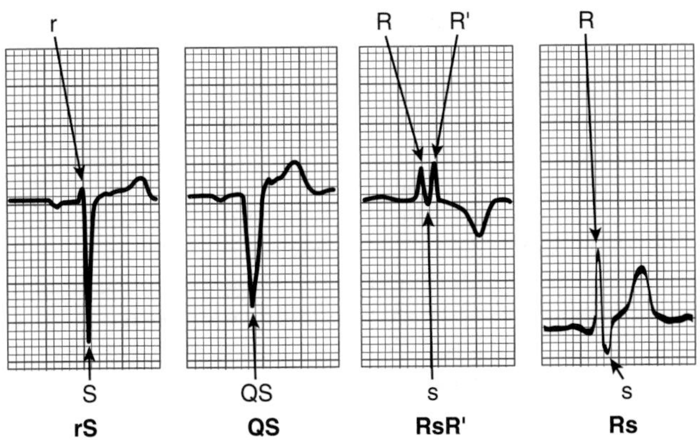

FIG 11-23 Examples of QRS Complexes. Small deflections are labeled with lowercase letters, and uppercase letters are used for larger deflections. A second upward deflection is labeled R′.

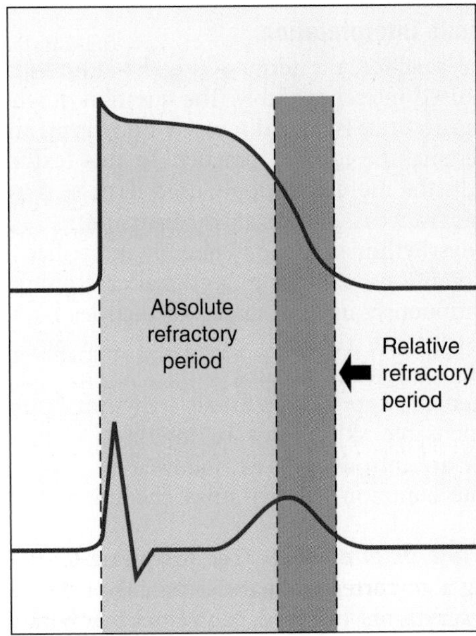

FIG 11-24 Absolute and Relative Refractory Periods are Correlated with the Cardiac Muscle's Action Potential and with an ECG Tracing.

dangerous time for ventricular ectopy to occur, especially if any portion of the myocardium is ischemic, because the ischemic muscle takes even longer to repolarize fully. This sets the stage for the disorganized, self-perpetuating depolarizations of various sections of the myocardium known as *ventricular fibrillation* (VF).

Intervals between waveforms. The intervals between waveforms are evaluated (see Fig. 11-22).

PR interval. The PR interval is measured from the beginning of the P wave to the beginning of the QRS complex. Normally, the PR interval is 0.12 to 0.20 second long and represents the time between sinus node discharge and the beginning of ventricular depolarization. Because most of this period results from delay of the impulse in the AV node, the PR interval is an indicator of AV nodal function.

In the electrophysiology laboratory and in some critical care units, these time values are described in milliseconds. There are 1000 milliseconds (msec) in 1 second. Thus, the normal PR interval value can also be written as 120 to 200 msec.

ST segment. The ST segment is the portion of the wave that extends from the end of the QRS to the beginning of the T wave. Its duration is not measured. Instead, its shape and location are evaluated. The ST segment is normally flat and at the same level as the isoelectric baseline. Any change from baseline is expressed in millimeters and may indicate myocardial ischemia (one small box equals 1 mm). ST-segment elevation (increase of 1-2 mm) is associated with acute myocardial injury, preinfarction, and pericarditis. ST-segment depression (decrease from baseline of more than 1-2 mm) is associated with myocardial ischemia.[60] ST segment changes are shown in Figure 11-25. (See Box 11-12 for the QSEN Patient Safety Alert feature on Prevention of Central Venous Catheter-related Bloodstream Infections.)

Bedside monitoring systems increasingly include ST-segment monitoring software. ST-segment changes may be accompanied by classic symptoms such as chest pain, or they may be silent, without any clinical symptoms except ST-segment depression or elevation as observed on the ECG monitor.[65]

ST-segment deviation is measured as the number of millimeters of ST-segment vertical displacement from the isoelectric line or from the patient's baseline. Because ST segments may slope or arc, the measurement position is typically selected 60 msec to the right of the J point.[60] The J point is chosen to avoid monitoring the upstroke of the T wave. On the bedside monitor, ST-segment elevation is displayed as a positive number, whereas ST-segment depression is indicated as a negative number. To be clinically significant, the J point of the ST segment must be displaced up or down from the isolectric baseline by at least 1 mm or 2 mm (one or two small boxes on ECG paper) depending on the specific ECG lead being monitored.[66] Specific values for recognition of abnormal J-point thresholds in different ECG leads are listed in Box 11-13.

QT interval. The QT interval is measured from the beginning of the QRS complex to the end of the T wave and indicates the total time interval from the onset of depolarization to the completion of repolarization. There is no established bedside monitoring lead recommended for measuring the QT interval.[61] On the 12-lead ECG, the QT interval is usually the longest in precordial leads V_3 and V_4.[61] The important point is that each clinician measures the QT interval using the same ECG lead.[61] At normal heart rates, the QT interval is less than one-half of the R-R interval when measured from one QRS complex to the next. However, the length of a QT interval depends on heart rate and must be adjusted according to the heart rate to be evaluated in a clinically meaningful way.

QTc. Because the QT interval shortens at faster heart rates and lengthens with slower heart rates, it is often written as a "corrected" value (QTc), meaning the QT value was mathematically corrected as if the heart rate were 60 beats/min. The upper limit of normal for the QTc is 0.48 second (480 msec) in women and less than 0.47 second (470 msec) in men.[61] A QTc of 440 msec is described as borderline.[62] A prolonged QT interval is significant because it can predispose the patient to the development of polymorphic VT, known also as *torsade de pointes.* A long QT interval can be

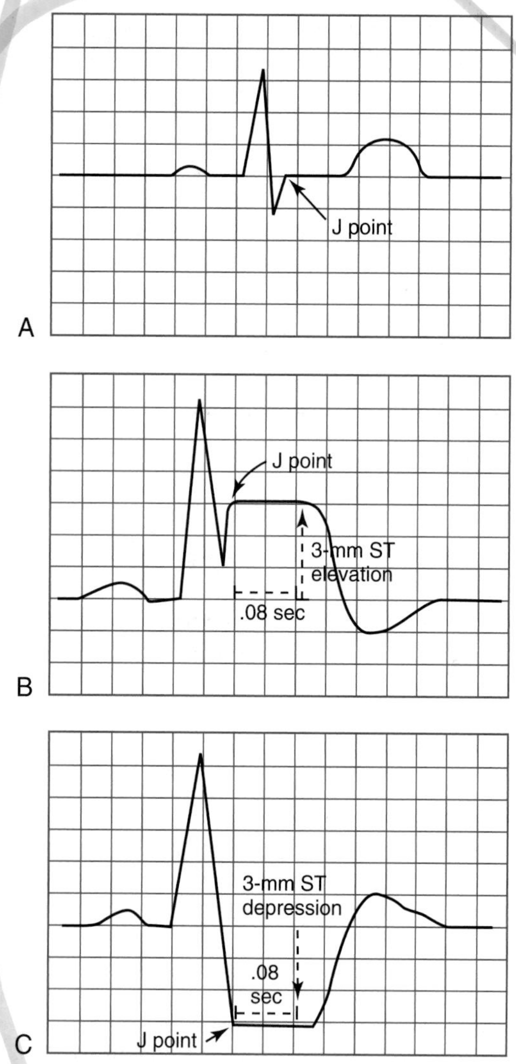

FIG 11-25 *A*, Normal Position of the J Point. *B*, A 3-mm ST-Segment Elevation. *C*, A 3-mm ST-Segment Depression. ST-segment changes are measured 60 to 80 msec (0.06 to 0.08 sec) after the J point.

congenital, as a result of genetic inheritance, or it can be acquired from an electrolyte imbalance or medications.

Many antidysrhythmic medications can prolong the QT interval, notably class Ia antidysrhythmics (quinidine, procainamide, disopyramide) and class III antidysrhythmics (amiodarone, ibutilide, sotalol). Not all high-risk mediations are antidysrhythmics. The U.S. Food and Drug Administration (FDA) has added a "black box" warning and a requirement for QT monitoring for the antipsychotic medication Haloperidol (Haldol), used in critical care for treatment of agitation and delirium.[63] See Table 11-6 for a list of medications used in the critical care unit that can prolong the QT interval.

When medications associated with a high risk of torsade de pointes are started, it is important to record the premedication baseline QTc and to continue to monitor the QTc during treatment. The risk of torsade de pointes is increased with prolongation of the QTc beyond 0.5 second (500 msec), or an increase of 60 msec compared to the baseline QTc.[64]

Dysrhythmia Interpretation

In clinical practice, the terms *dysrhythmia* and *arrhythmia* often are used interchangeably. The question of which word is the more accurate is often discussed. Both terms are correct, and either may be used in practice. In this textbook, dysrhythmia is the more commonly used term. A dysrhythmia is any disturbance in the normal cardiac conduction pathway. Because dysrhythmias occur frequently in cardiac and noncardiac conditions, patients in a critical care unit are monitored continuously using a single- or dual-lead system, and rhythm strips are recorded each shift and any time the patient's heart rhythm changes.

A systematic approach to assess a rhythm disturbance is an indispensable skill. Steps to interpret a rhythm strip accurately are introduced first, followed by specific criteria to evaluate common dysrhythmias encountered in clinical practice.

Heart rate determination. The first thing to assess when evaluating a rhythm strip is the ventricular rate. Regardless of the dysrhythmia involved, the ventricular rate holds the key to whether the patient can tolerate the dysrhythmia by

BOX 11-13 Abnormal J-Point Thresholds Vary with Age, Gender, and ECG Lead

Anterior, Lateral, and Inferior Wall MI—J-Point Threshold

For men older than 40 years, the threshold for abnormal J-point elevation is 0.2 mV (2 mm) in leads V_2 and V_3 and 0.1 mV (1 mm) in all other leads.

For men younger than 40 years, the threshold for abnormal J-point elevation in leads V_2 and V_3 is 0.25 mV (2.5 mm).

For women, the threshold for abnormal J-point elevation is 0.15 mV (1.5 mm) in leads V_2 and V_3 and greater than 0.1 mV (1 mm) in all other leads.

Right Ventricular Wall MI—J-Point Threshold

For men and women, the threshold for abnormal J-point elevation in V_3R and V_4R is 0.05 mV (0.5 mm), except for males less than 30 years of age who have a lower threshold of 0.1 mV (1 mm).

Posterior Wall MI—J-Point Threshold

For men and women, the threshold for abnormal J-point elevation in V_7 through V_9 should be 0.05 mV (0.5 mm).

J-Point Depression

For men and women of all ages, the threshold for abnormal J-point depression should be 0.05 mV (−0.5 mm) in leads V_2 and V_3 and −0.1 mV (−1 mm) in all other leads.

From Wagner GS, Macfarlane P, Wellens H, et al. AHA/ACCF/HRS recommendations for the standardization and interpretation of the electrocardiogram: part VI: acute ischemia/infarction: a scientific statement from the American Heart Association Electrocardiography and Arrhythmias Committee, Council on Clinical Cardiology; the American College of Cardiology Foundation; and the Heart Rhythm Society: endorsed by the International Society for Computerized Electrocardiology. *Circulation.* 2009; 119(10):e262

TABLE 11-6 Medications That May Cause Torsade De Pointes

GENERIC NAME	BRAND NAME	CLINICAL USE	COMMENTS
Arsenic trioxide	Trisenox®	Anticancer for leukemia	
Azithromycin	Zithromax®	Antibiotic	
Bepridil	Vascor®	Antianginal	Females>Males
Chloroquine	Aralen®	Antimalarial	
Chlorpromazine	Thorazine®	Antipsychotic; antiemetic	
Citalopram	Celexa®	Antidepressant	
Clarithromycin	Biaxin®	Antibiotic	
Disopyramide	Norpace®	Antidysrhythmic	Females>Males
Dofetilide	Tikosyn®	Antidysrhythmic	Females>Males
Droperidol	Inapsine®	Sedative; antinausea	
Erythromycin	E.E.S.® Erythrocin®	Antibiotic; increase GI motility	Females>Males
Flecainide	Tambocor®	Antidysrhythmic	
Halofantrine	Halfan®	Antimalarial	Females>Males
Haloperidol	Haldol®	Antipsychotic	TdP risk with IV or excess dosage
Ibutilide	Corvert®	Antidysrhythmic	Females>Males
Mesoridazine	Serentil®	Antipsychotic	
Methadone	Dolophine®	Opiate agonist for pain control	Females>Males
Methadone	Methadose®	Opiate agonist for pain control	Females>Males
Moxifloxacin	Avelox®	Antibiotic	
Pentamidine	NebuPent® Pentam®	Anti-infective for pneumocystis pneumonia	Females>Males
Pimozide	Orap®	Antipsychotic; Tourette's tics	Females>Males
Procainamide	Pronestyl® Procan®	Antidysrhythmic	
Quinidine	Quinaglute® Cardioquin®	Antidysrhythmic	Females>Males
Sotalol	Betapace®	Antidysrhythmic	Females>Males
Thioridazine	Mellaril®	Antipsychotic	
Vandetanib	Caprelsa®	Anticancer for thyroid cancer	

Table only includes medications with a documented risk of torsade de pointes in the United States. Low-risk medications are not included.
Modified from the *Arizona Center for Education and Research on Therapeutics (CERT)*. http://www.qtdrugs.org. Accessed August 27, 2012.

maintaining adequate blood pressure, cardiac output, and mentation. If the ventricular rate is consistently greater than 200 or less than 30, emergency measures must be started to correct the rate. A detailed analysis of the underlying rhythm disturbance can proceed later, when the immediate crisis is over. The three methods for calculating rate (Figure 11-26A) follow:

1. Number of R-R intervals in 6 seconds times 10 (ECG paper is usually marked at the top in 3-second increments, making a 6-second interval easy to identify.)
2. Number of large boxes between QRS complexes divided into 300
3. Number of small boxes between QRS complexes divided into 1500

In the healthy heart, the atrial rate and the ventricular rate are the same. However, in many dysrhythmias, the atrial and ventricular rates are different, and both must be calculated. To find the atrial rate, the PP interval, instead of the R-R interval, is used in one of the three methods listed for determining rate.

When the rhythm is regular, any of the three methods can be used. When the rhythm is irregular, the first method (R-R intervals in 6 seconds × 10) is the only method that can be used (see Figure 11-26B).

Rhythm determination. The term *rhythm* refers to the regularity with which the P waves or R waves occur. Calipers assist in determining rhythm. One point of the calipers is placed on the beginning of one R wave, and the other point is placed on the next R wave. Leaving the calipers "set" at this interval, each succeeding R-R interval is checked to be sure it is the same width as the first one measured.

P-wave evaluation. The P wave is analyzed by answering the following questions. First, is the P wave present or absent? Second, is it related to the QRS? It is hoped that one P wave will be in front of every QRS. Sometimes, two, three, or four P waves may be in front of every QRS. If this pattern is consistent, the P wave and QRS are still related, although not on a 1:1 basis.

PR-interval evaluation. The duration of the PR interval, which normally is 0.12 to 0.20 second (120 to 200 msec), is measured first. This is measured from the start of a visible P wave to the beginning of the next QRS (Fig. 11-22). All PR intervals on the strip are verified to be sure they have the same duration as the original interval.

QRS complex evaluation. The entire ECG strip must be evaluated to ascertain that the QRS complexes are consistently the same shape and width. The normal QRS duration is 0.06 to 0.10 second (60 to 110 msec). Any QRS longer than

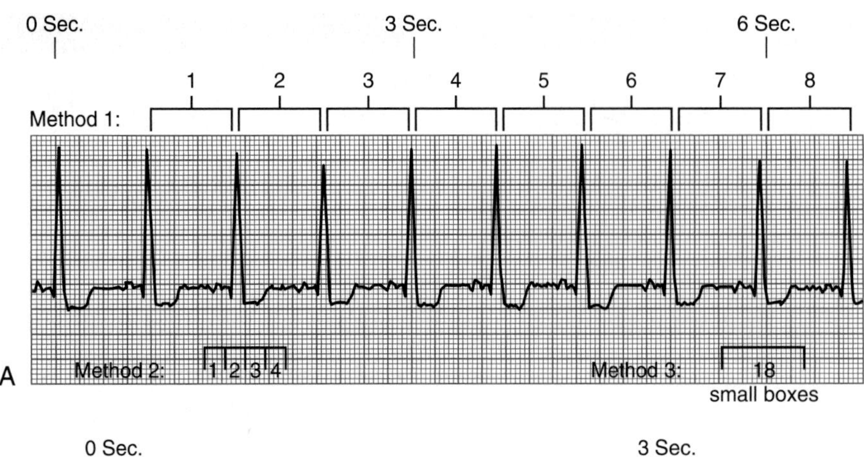

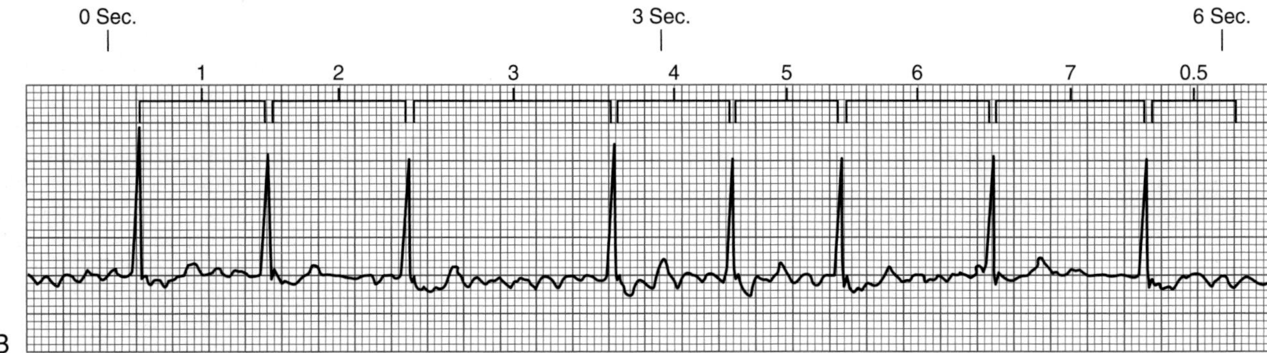

FIG 11-26 *A*, **Calculation of the Heart Rate if the Rhythm is Regular.** Method 1: number of R-R intervals in 6 seconds multiplied by 10 (e.g., 8 × 10 = 80/min). Method 2: number of large boxes between QRS complexes divided into 300 (e.g., 300 ÷ 4 = 75/min). Method 3: number of small boxes between QRS complexes divided into 1500 (e.g., 1500 ÷ 18 = 84/min). *B*, Rate calculation if the rhythm is irregular. Only method 1 can be used (e.g., 7.5 intervals × 10 = 75/min).

0.10 second is considered abnormal.[67] If more than one QRS shape is on the strip, each QRS must be measured. The QRS is measured from where it leaves the baseline to where it returns to the baseline as shown in Figure 11-22.

QT evaluation. The length of the QT interval varies with the heart rate. The QT interval is shorter when the heart rate is faster. A QT interval corrected for heart rate (QTc) that is longer than 0.50 second (500 msec) is of concern, as discussed in the earlier section on QT Interval.

Sinus rhythms. There are four rhythms that begin with the word sinus, indicating that the rhythm originates from within the sinus node. Table 11-7 provides a summary of the major features of this category of rhythms.

Normal sinus rhythm. The following are the criteria for normal sinus rhythm as shown in Figure 11-27.

Rate: 60 to 100 beats/min

Rhythm: Regular (±10%)

P wave: Present, all the same shape, with only one preceding each QRS complex

PR interval: 0.12 to 0.20 second

QRS duration: 0.06 to 0.10 second

QRS complex: Shape and whether deflection is positive or negative vary depending on lead placement and do not provide key diagnostic information.

Sinus bradycardia. Sinus bradycardia meets all of the criteria for normal sinus rhythm except that the rate is fewer than 60 beats/min (see Table 11-9). Sinus bradycardia usually does not require treatment unless the patient displays symptoms of hypoperfusion, such as hypotension, dizziness, chest pain, or changes in level of consciousness.

Sinus tachycardia. Sinus tachycardia meets all the criteria for normal sinus rhythm except that the rate is greater than 100 beats/min (see Table 11-9). Rates may be as high as 180 to 200 beats/min in healthy, young adults during strenuous exercise. However, in the critical care setting, bed rest is prescribed for most patients. It is wise to be skeptical of any "sinus tachycardia" with a rate greater than 150 and to search for a triggering focus other than the sinus node. Many medications used in critical care can cause sinus tachycardia; common culprits are dopamine, hydralazine, atropine, and epinephrine. Tachycardia is detrimental to anyone with ischemic heart disease because it decreases the time for ventricular filling, decreases stroke volume, and compromises cardiac output. Tachycardia increases heart work and myocardial oxygen demand while decreasing oxygen supply by decreasing coronary artery filling time. If the cause of the tachycardia can be determined, such as fever or pain, that symptom is treated rather than trying to treat the heart rate directly.

Sinus dysrhythmia. Sinus dysrhythmia, commonly called sinus arrhythmia in clinical practice, meets all of the criteria for normal sinus rhythm except that the rhythm is irregular (see Table 11-7). This irregularity coincides with the respiratory pattern; heart rate changes with the respiratory cycle, increasing with inspiration and decreasing with expiration[96]

TABLE 11-7 Sinus Rhythms

PARAMETERS	NORMAL SINUS RHYTHM	SINUS BRADYCARDIA	SINUS TACHYCARDIA	SINUS DYSRHYTHMIA
Rate	60-100/min	<60/min	>100/min	Variable
Rhythm	Regular	Regular	Regular	Irregular; respiratory variation
P wave	Present, with one per QRS	Present, with one per QRS	Present, with one per QRS	Present, with one per QRS
PR interval	0.12-0.20 sec and constant	0.12-0.20 sec and constant	0.12-0.20 sec and constant	0.12-0.20 sec and constant
QRS	0.06-0.10 sec	0.06-0.10 sec	0.06-0.10 sec	0.06-0.10 sec

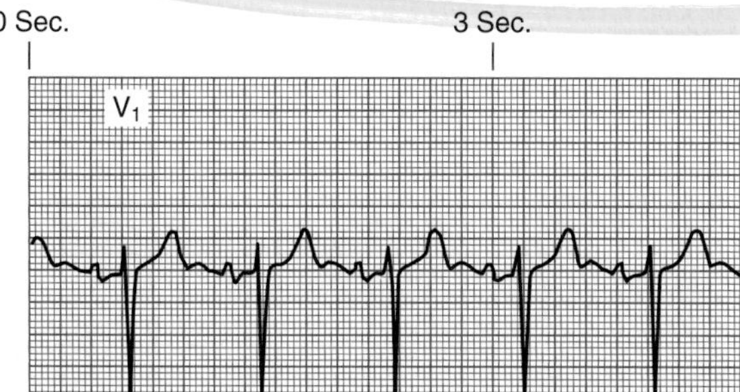

FIG 11-27 Normal Sinus Rhythm. The rate is 70, and the rhythm is regular. One P wave is present before each QRS complex. The PR interval is 0.18 second and does not vary throughout the strip. The QRS duration is 0.08 second. All evaluation criteria are within normal limits.

(Figure 11-28). Sinus dysrhythmia often occurs in children and young adults and decreases with age. No treatment is required. To detect sinus dysrhythmia accurately, look at all P waves closely to verify that they are all the same shape and that the PR intervals are all constant.

Atrial dysrhythmias. Atrial dysrhythmias originate from an ectopic focus in the atria, somewhere other than the sinus node. The ectopic impulse occurs prematurely, before the normal sinus impulse occurs. Table 11-8 provides a summary of the major features of atrial dysrhythmias.

Premature atrial contractions. Premature atrial contractions (PACs) are isolated, early beats from an ectopic focus in the atria. The underlying rhythm is usually sinus. The regular sinus rhythm is interrupted by an early, abnormally shaped atrial P wave. The early atrial wave usually looks different from the sinus P wave and may be inverted. The PR interval may be longer, shorter, or the same as the PR interval of a sinus impulse. The QRS that follows the ectopic atrial P wave can vary in shape depending on the degree of refractoriness of the AV node.

PAC with normal QRS. If the atrial impulse arrives in the AV node after the AV node is fully repolarized, the resultant QRS impulse is of normal width and shape (Figure 11-29A).

PAC with wide QRS. Occasionally, the early ectopic P wave can be conducted through the AV node, but part of the conduction pathway through the ventricular bundle branches is blocked. This produces a QRS that is wider than 0.12 second (120 msec) or wider than three small boxes on the ECG paper (see Figure 11-29B).

Pause with no QRS. Sometimes, the ectopic P wave arrives so early that the AV node is still in its absolute refractory period. In this case, the wave of depolarization does not move past the AV node and no QRS follows. All that is seen on the ECG is an early, abnormal P wave followed by a pause until the next sinus P wave occurs (see Figure 11-29C). This is called a *nonconducted PAC.* Usually, these P waves are so early that they are superimposed on the T wave of the previous beat, making them difficult to find. The pause that follows is still clearly seen.

PACs are not restricted to individuals with heart disease and are accentuated by emotional upheaval, nicotine, and caffeine. Heart failure is associated with PACs. As atrial pressure rises, the atrial walls are stretched, causing irritability of atrial cells and the occurrence of PACs.

Supraventricular tachycardia. The term *supraventricular tachycardia* (SVT) is used clinically to describe a varied group of dysrhythmias that originate above the AV node. SVT is not a specific term; it includes sinus tachycardia, atrial tachycardia, multifocal atrial tachycardia, atrial flutter, atrial fibrillation, and junctional tachycardia. Each of these entities has a distinct pathophysiology, specific therapy, and expected outcome. SVT may also be described as a *narrow-complex tachycardia,* defined as a QRS that is less than 0.12 second (120 milliseconds).[68] After the specific dysrhythmia is identified, it usually is referred to by its specific name, such as atrial fibrillation with a rapid ventricular response. The term SVT is used to describe a rapid, sustained atrial or junctional tachycardia when the exact mechanism is unknown. Women are affected by episodic SVT at about twice the rate of men.[68]

SVT is not always benign. About 15% of people with SVT experience syncope (lose consciousness). Medications are used to limit the SVT rate and prevent "blackouts" or syncope.[68] SVT that is persistent for weeks or months may lead to a tachycardia-mediated cardiomyopathy.[68] A baseline 12-lead ECG is helpful, and when possible, a 12-lead ECG should be obtained during the palpitations.[68]

Paroxysmal supraventricular tachycardia. *Paroxysmal* means starting and stopping abruptly. *Paroxysmal supraventricular tachycardia* (PSVT) refers to the sudden interruption of sinus rhythm by an atrial ectopic focus that depolarizes repetitively at a rate of 150 to 250 beats/min and eventually stops as suddenly as it began (Figure 11-30). PSVT usually responds rapidly to the use of vagal maneuvers that include the following:[68]

Valsalva maneuver. The patient is asked to "bear down," as if going to the bathroom.

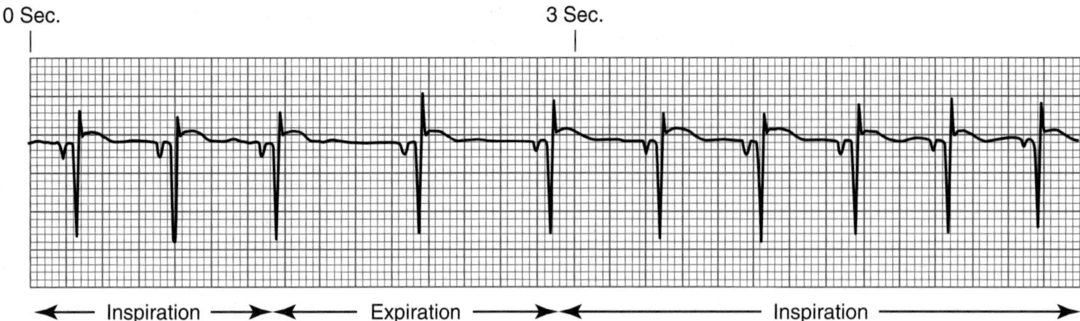

FIG 11-28 **Sinus Dysrhythmia.** Notice the increased heart rate during inspiration and decreased heart rate during expiration.

TABLE 11-8 Atrial Dysrhythmias

PARAMETER	PAROXYSMAL SUPRAVENTRICULAR TACHYCARDIA	MULTIFOCAL ATRIAL TACHYCARDIA	ATRIAL FLUTTER	ATRIAL FIBRILLATION
Rate				
Atrial	150-250/min	100-160/min	250-350/min	>350/min (unable to count it)
Ventricular	Same or less	Same	250-350/min, one half or less	100-180/min (uncontrolled); <100/min (controlled)
Rhythm	Regular	Irregular	Atrial: regular; ventricular: may or may not be regular	Irregularly irregular
P wave	Present; abnormally shaped	Present; three or more different shapes	F waves	Fibrillatory baseline
PR interval	May be normal or prolonged	Variable	Conduction ratio: flutter waves per QRS	Absent
QRS	0.06-0.10 sec	0.06-0.10 sec	0.06-0.10 sec	0.06-0.10 sec

Carotid sinus massage. It is performed on only one side of the neck over the carotid artery by a physician on a patient with a monitored ECG and avoided on older patients who may have atherosclerotic disease of the carotid arteries.

If vagal maneuvers are unsuccessful at terminating the PSVT, the next step usually is the use of intravenous medications if the patient is hemodynamically stable.[68] The intravenous drug of choice to block conduction briefly through the AV node is adenosine (Adenocard). In PSVT, adenosine alone is often sufficient to restore normal sinus rhythm, but if not, it will unmask the ectopic P waves and confirm or provide strong clues to diagnose the SVT.[68] The usual dose is 6 mg given intravenously by rapid push, followed by a normal saline bolus. If this does not create a temporary AV block or restore sinus rhythm, a 12-mg intravenous dose is administered. Potential dysrhythmic side effects of adenosine include a 1% to 15% chance of initiating atrial fibrillation. Adenosine is contraindicated in patients with severe asthma.[68]

Other intravenous medications that may be used to slow the rate in PSVT are amiodarone (Cordarone), a class III antidysrhythmic with a rapid onset and a short half-life.[68] Alternatively, diltiazem, a class IV calcium channel blocker in the nondihydropyridine group, can be administered. The action of these medications is to slow conduction through the AV node.[68] If intravenous medications do not convert the PSVT or sustained SVT or if the patient becomes hemodynamically unstable, the next step is electrical cardioversion.[68]

Atrial flutter. Atrial flutter is recognized on the ECG by the *sawtooth* atrial pattern. These sawtooth-shaped atrial wavelets are not P waves; they are more appropriately called F waves (atrial flutter waves). Fortunately, at a rapid rate the AV node does not allow conduction of all these impulses to the ventricles. The following are the criteria for atrial flutter as shown in Figure 11-31.

Rate: Atrial rate 250 to 350 beats/min

Rhythm: Regular flutter waves. The ventricular QRS complexes may be regular or irregular.

P wave: Replaced by flutter (F) waves

PR interval: No longer applies; instead a conduction ratio of flutter waves to *QRS complexes* (e.g., 2:1, 3:1, 4:1) is used. Both atrial and ventricular rates must be calculated. The atrial rate is always faster.

QRS complex: Shape is usually narrow and normal.

Pathogenesis of atrial flutter. Atrial flutter can be started by any isolated atrial impulse, but to be maintained, the atrial flutter requires a *reentry circular pathway* around macroscopic structures in the atria. Typically, these structures are in the right atrium and involve the vena cava and the tricuspid valve in an area known as the *cavotricuspid isthmus.* The *reentry loop* typically circles counterclockwise around the tricuspid valve[68,69] and can circle the inferior vena cava (IVC) or the IVC and the tricuspid valve. To maintain a viable, self-perpetuating reentry pathway, the loop must avoid the sinoatrial node and be large enough always to meet tissue that is ready to be depolarized (accept a new electrical stimulus). The atrial reentry rate in atrial flutter is typically between 250 to 350 beats/min, producing the classic sawtooth or flutter wave pattern.[68] The atrial flutter wavelet always appears regular, because the circuit is always the same length and requires exactly the same amount of time to complete the reentry loop.

Sometimes, it is difficult to identify the flutter waves, especially if the conduction ratio is 2:1. Vagal maneuvers or adenosine can be useful diagnostic tools to allow better visualization of the flutter waves (see Figure 11-31A). Vagal maneuvers or intravenous adenosine cannot terminate atrial flutter but do create a temporary AV block to permit visualization of the atrial waveform and thereby facilitate accurate diagnosis, as seen in Figure 11-31B.

Atrial flutter management. Antidysrhythmic medications are prescribed for two reasons: to convert the atrial flutter to sinus rhythm and to slow conduction through the AV node.[68] Intravenous medications such as amiodarone, calcium channel blockers (verapamil or diltiazem), or beta blockers may be used prior to electrical cardioversion. See Chapter 13 for additional information on antidysrhythmic medications for the treatment of atrial dysrythmias.

Electrical cardioversion is the most successful treatment, with a 95% to 100% return to sinus rhythm.[68] If atrial flutter has been present for more than 48 hours, up to one-third of patients will have thrombi in the atria, and anticoagulation is mandated before pharmacologic or electrical cardioversion. The risk of systemic emboli after cardioversion ranges from

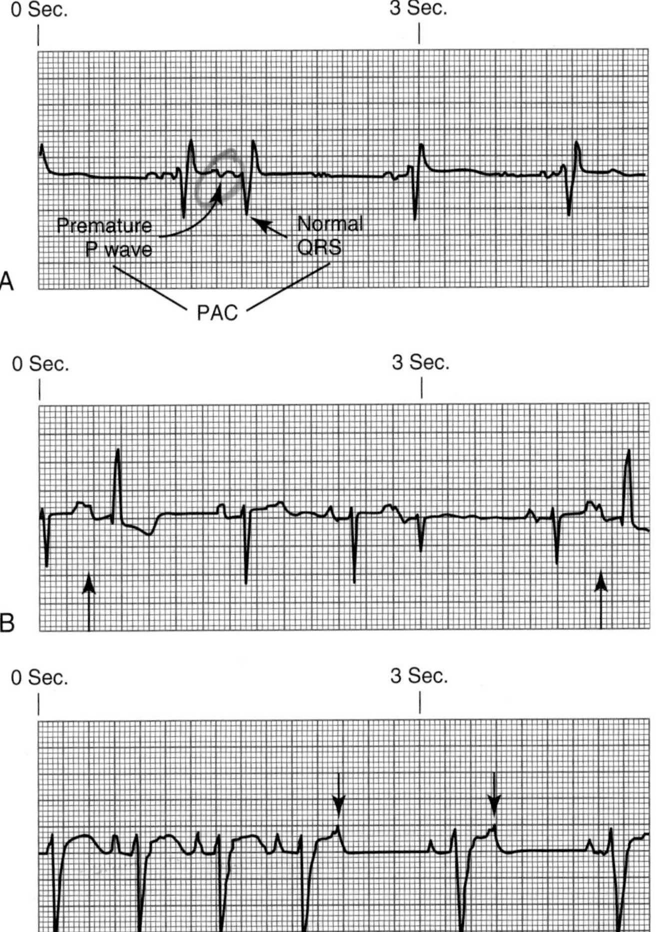

FIG 11-29 Premature Atrial Contractions (PACs). *A,* Normally conducted PAC. The early P wave is indicated by the *arrow,* and the QRS that follows has a normal shape and duration. *B,* Nonconducted (blocked) PACs. The early P waves are indicated by *arrows.* Notice how the early P waves distort the T waves, making the T wave appear peaked compared with the normal T waves seen after the third and fourth QRS complexes. *C,* Right bundle branch block aberration after a PAC.

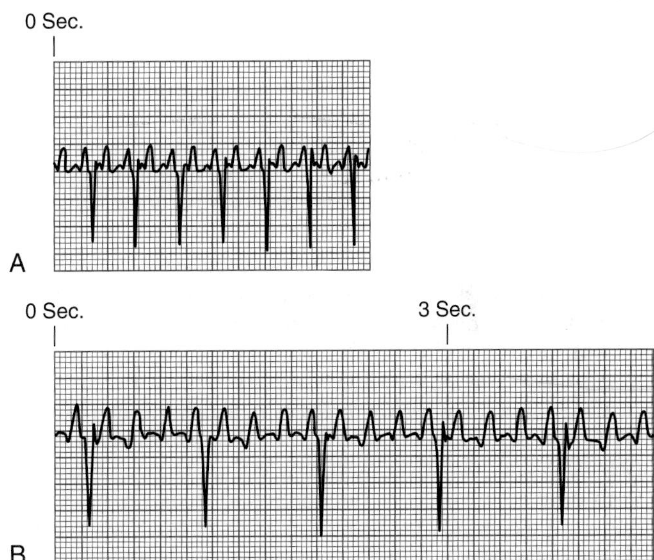

FIG 11-31 *A,* Initial Strip Shows Atrial Flutter with 2:1 Conduction Through the Atrioventricular (AV) Node. *B,* During Carotid Sinus Massage, the AV Conduction Rate is Decreased, More Clearly Revealing the Flutter Waves.

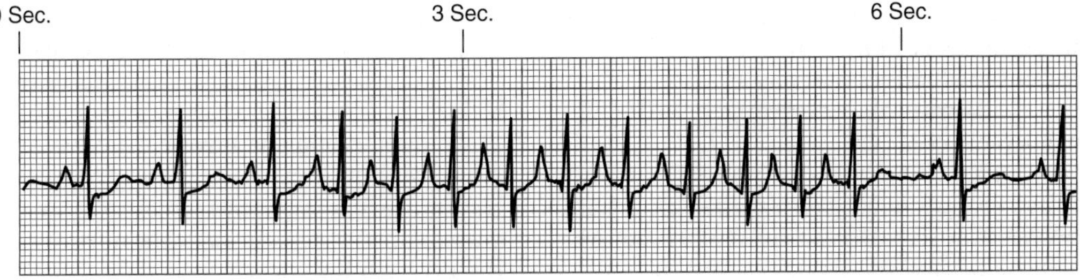

FIG 11-30 Paroxysmal Supraventricular Tachycardia (PSVT). Notice that the atrial rate during tachycardia is 158 beats/min. The run starts and stops abruptly.

2% to 7%.[68] Overdrive atrial pacing may be favored to convert atrial flutter after cardiac surgery. Epicardial wires that are placed at the time of surgery are connected to an external pacemaker with a successful conversion rate between 83% and 100%.[68]

For patients with atrial flutter unrelated to an acute disease process, permanent termination of the atrial flutter circuit can be achieved by *radiofrequency ablation* (RFA).[69] RFA is a catheter procedure used to create a line of conduction block across one of more sections of the reentry pathway. The most frequent location for RFA is a narrow band of tissue between the inferior vena cava and the tricuspid annulus known as the *cavotricuspid isthmus*.[69]

Atrial fibrillation. Atrial fibrillation is the most frequently encountered dysrhythmia in the developed world. The following are the criteria for atrial fibrillation as shown in Figure 11-32.

Rate: Atrial rate 240-300 waves per minute.[70] Ventricular rate 60 to 100 (when controlled by medication), greater than 100 (when uncontrolled by medication).
Rhythm: Irregularly irregular ventricular rhythm
P wave: Replaced by fibrillating baseline or waves.
PR interval: Absent. Replaced by fibrillating baseline.
RR interval: Irregular
QRS duration: 0.06 to 0.10 second
QRS complex: Usually normal because pathway through ventricles is unchanged once impulse leaves AV node

Pathogenesis of atrial fibrillation. Atrial fibrillation is frequently associated with underlying heart disease and may occur as a consequence of atrial remodeling.[70] Ectopic foci may originate the atrial fibrillation, but it is sustained by multiple reentry circuits within the atria that originate in some cases from specific anatomic sites such as ectopic tissues that project from the left atrium into the four pulmonary veins that drain into the left atrium. The risk of developing atrial fibrillation is higher for people with a history of hypertension, heart failure, obesity, or acute coronary syndrome.

Rhythm control in atrial fibrillation. For the hospitalized patient with *new-onset* atrial fibrillation with unstable hemodynamics, the primary focus is generally on rhythm control (conversion to sinus rhythm) using antidysrhythmic medications or electrical cardioversion. Emergency medications used to convert atrial fibrillation to sinus rhythm, also known as a chemical cardioversion, include amiodarone and ibutilide. Antidysrhythmic medications used long-term to maintain sinus rhythm include amiodarone, dronedarone disopyramide, flecainide, propafenone, quinidine, sotalol, and dofetilide.[70] Even with medication therapy, recurrence of atrial fibrillation is likely. Electrical cardioversion may be successful in converting the atria to sinus rhythm if attempted within a few days of the onset of atrial fibrillation. Success is less likely if the atrial fibrillation has existed for a long time.

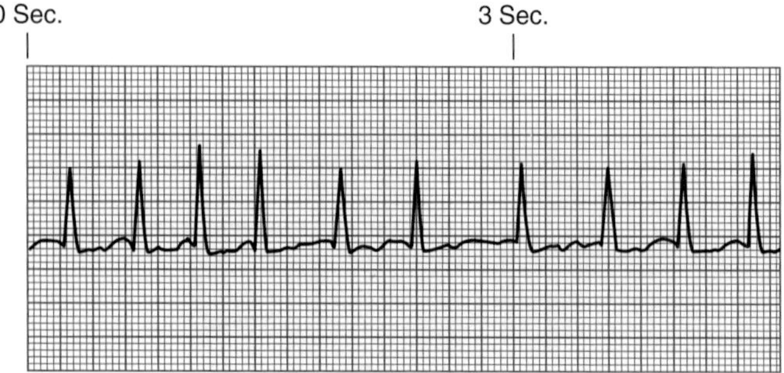

FIG 11-32 Atrial Fibrillation. Notice the irregular ventricular rhythm.

Rate control in atrial fibrillation. The most frequently prescribed medications used to control the ventricular rate in atrial fibrillation include calcium channel blockers and beta-blockers. These medications work to slow conduction through the AV node without impact on the fibrillating atria. In the past, it was assumed that rate control was an inferior strategy because the patient stayed in atrial fibrillation, lost "atrial kick," and was presumed to have an increased risk of embolic stroke. Two multicenter clinical trials have altered that perception: the *A*trial *F*ibrillation *F*ollow-up: *I*nvestigation of *R*hythm *M*anagement (AFFIRM) and the *RA*te *C*ontrol vs. *E*lectrical Cardioversion for Persistent Atrial Fibrillation (RACE). These two trials found similar morbidity, mortality, and quality of life in patients treated with rhythm conversion or rate control. For long-term management of permanent atrial fibrillation, rate control is the recommended approach, and therapeutic anticoagulation to prevent embolic stroke is mandatory.[70] Antidysrhythmic medications used to manage atrial fibrillation are listed in Chapter 13, Table 13-17.

Stroke risk assessment and antithrombotic therapy in atrial fibrillation. Atrial fibrillation, because of the development of thrombi in the atria, greatly increases the risk of embolic stroke. Several scoring mechanisms have been developed to help predict which patients with atrial fibrillation require prophylactic anticoagulation.

CHADS2. The acronym CHADS2 is an easy-to-remember risk assessment tool used to predict stroke risk in atrial fibrillation and to guide antithrombotic therapy (see Box 11-14). The letters stand for **C**ardiac failure, **H**ypertension, **A**ge, **D**iabetes, **S**troke (double points).[70] The score ranges from 0 to 6. For a score of 0, no treatment or aspirin is recommended; for a score of 1, aspirin or warfarin is recommended; for a score between 2 and 6, anticoagulation with warfarin is recommended.[70] There are newer oral anticoagulants: *dabigatran*, a thrombin-inhibitor, and *rivaroxaban* and *apixaban*, factor Xa inhibitors, can be prescribed for atrial fibrillation in patients with higher CHADS2 scores.[71]

BOX 11-14 CHADS2 Score

LETTER	RISK FACTOR	SCORE
C	Chronic heart failure	1
H	Hypertension	1
A	Age >75 years	1
D	Diabetes mellitus	1
S	Stroke or TIA	2

The CHADS2 score is used to predict the risk of having a stroke in atrial fibrillation. A higher score is associated with a higher risk of embolic stroke.

CHADS2 minimum score = 0; CHADS2 maximum score = 6.
A score of 0—no treatment or aspirin
A score of 1—aspirin or warfarin
A score of 2 to 6—warfarin

TIA, Transient ischemic attack.

CHA2DS2-VASc. Other scoring systems, such as the CHA2DS2-VASc have expanded the risk factor profile to include congestive heart failure, hypertension, age 75 years or older (double points), diabetes, stroke (double points), vascular disease, age 65-74 and sex (female).[71]

Electrical and chemical (medication-induced) forms of cardioversion entail the threat of precipitating emboli into the systemic circulation. To prevent embolic stroke, it is important to pay attention to the *48-hour rule.* Patients who have been in atrial fibrillation for 48 hours or longer (how long may not be known) must be adequately anticoagulated with an oral vitamin K antagonist (warfarin) to achieve a target international normalized ration (INR) of 2.0 to 3.0 for at least 3 weeks before elective cardioversion.[72] After successful cardioversion, patients should be anticoagulated for an additional 4 weeks.[72] Advancements in antithrombotic therapies have resulted in several newer oral agents in addition to warfarin. These medications are available specifically for prevention of stroke in non-valvular atrial fibrillation:[72] dabigatran,[73] rivaroxaban,[74] and apixaban.[75] These three antithrombotics do not require routine anticoagulation monitoring.

Transesophageal echocardiography (TEE) is helpful in identifying the presence or absence of thrombi in the fibrillating atria and is recommended as a screening tool before elective cardioversion.[72] It is especially helpful for patients in atrial fibrillation for less than 48 hours who, in the absence of atrial thrombi, may undergo cardioversion without anticoagulation.[72]

Procedures to treat atrial fibrillation. Several catheter interventions to treat atrial fibrillation are being explored, including atrial pacing, cardiac surgery, and catheter isolation of the pulmonary veins.

The Cox-Maze III procedure (typically called the MAZE procedure) is an open-heart surgical operation designed to cure atrial fibrillation permanently by a "cut and sew" insertion of strategic scar lines into the atria. The surgical MAZE procedure is now rarely performed. It has been replaced by catheter interventions that use radiofrequency energy sources to create lines of conduction block (scar) around the pulmonary veins.[69] The success of radiofrequency ablation (RFA), measured as freedom from atrial fibrillation, varies by number of ablation procedures. After one procedure 46%-60% of patients no longer have atrial fibrillation.[76] After multiple procedures 75%-80% of patients are free from atrial fibrillation.[76,77] Number of ablation procedures averages 1.5 per patient.[76]

Junctional dysrhythmias. Only certain areas of the AV node have the property of automaticity. The entire area around the AV node is collectively called the *junction;* impulses generated there are called *junctional.* After an ectopic impulse arises in the junction, it spreads in two directions at once. One wave of depolarization spreads upward into the atria and depolarizes them, causing the recording of a P wave on the ECG. This is called *retrograde (backward) conduction*, and the P wave is inverted when viewed in lead II. At the same time, another wave of depolarization spreads downward into the ventricles through the normal conduction pathway, producing a normal QRS complex. This is called *antegrade (forward) conduction.*

Depending on timing, the P wave 1) may be seen in front of the QRS, with a short PR interval of less than 0.12 second; 2) may be obscured entirely by the QRS, or 3) may immediately follow the QRS.

Table 11-9 provides a summary of the major features of junctional dysrhythmias.

Premature junctional contraction. The following are the criteria for a premature junctional contraction as shown in Figure 11-33.

TABLE 11-9 Junctional Rhythms

PARAMETER	JUNCTIONAL ESCAPE RHYTHM	ACCELERATED JUNCTIONAL RHYTHM	JUNCTIONAL TACHYCARDIA
Rate	40-60/min	60-100/min	>100/min
Rhythm	Regular	Regular	Regular
P waves	May be present or absent; inverted in lead II	May be present or absent; inverted in lead II	May be present or absent; inverted in lead II
PR interval	<0.12 sec	<0.12 sec	<0.12 sec
QRS	0.06-0.10 sec	0.06-0.10 sec	0.06-0.10 sec

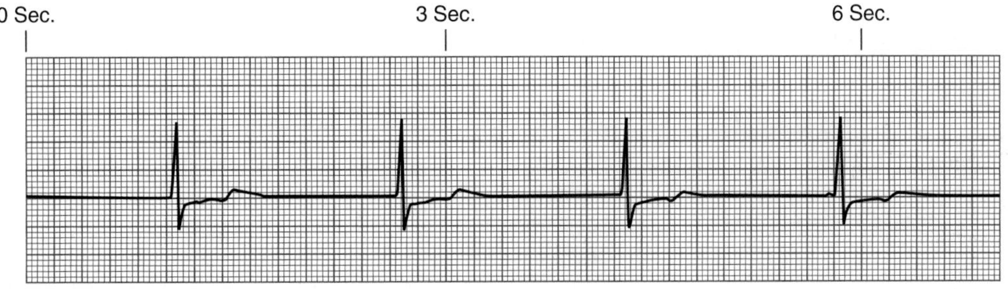

FIG 11-33 Junctional Escape Rhythm. The ventricular rate is 38. P waves are absent, and the QRS has a normal width.

Rate: Depends on underlying rhythm, usually sinus rhythm
Rhythm: The ECG rhythm is regular from sinus node except for early QRS complex (PJC).
P wave: May be entirely absent, may be seen in T wave, or may be inverted
PR interval: Usually absent. Absent or short PR interval is a defining characteristic of junctional rhythms.
QRS duration: 0.06 to 0.10 second
QRS complex: Usually narrow with normal shape

If only a single ectopic impulse originates in the junction, it is simply called a *premature junctional contraction.* On the ECG, the rhythm is regular from the sinus node, except for one early QRS complex of normal shape and duration. The P wave can be entirely absent. If a P wave can be found, it very closely precedes or follows the QRS. In lead II, the P wave appears inverted (having a negative deflection) because the atria are being depolarized from the AV node upward, which is the opposite direction from the wave of depolarization that occurs when triggered by the sinus node. If the P wave appears before the QRS, the PR interval is less than 0.12 second.

Junctional escape rhythm. The following are the criteria for a junctional escape rhythm as shown in Figure 11-33.
Rate: Intrinsic rate of junction is 40 to 60 beats/min if dominant pacemaker of heart.
Rhythm: Regular
P wave: Same as for PJC
PR interval: Usually absent or very short
QRS duration: 0.06 to 0.10 second
QRS complex: Usually narrow and normal because impulse originates above ventricles.

Sometimes, the junction becomes the dominant pacemaker of the heart (Table 11-10). Normally, the intrinsic rate of the junction is 40 to 60 beats/min. The intrinsic rate of the sinus node is 60 to 100 beats/min. Under normal conditions, the junction never has a chance to escape and depolarize the heart because it is overridden by the sinus node. However, if the sinus node fails, the junctional impulses can depolarize completely and pace the heart. This is called a *junctional escape rhythm*, and it is a protective mechanism to prevent asystole in the event of sinus node failure. Generally, a junctional escape rhythm (Figure 11-33) is well-tolerated hemodynamically, although efforts must be directed toward restoring sinus rhythm. Sometimes, a pacemaker is inserted as a protective measure because of concern that the AV junction may also fail.

Junctional tachycardia and accelerated junctional rhythm. A junctional rhythm can also occur at a faster rate (see Table 11-10). As with sinus rhythm, the term *tachycardia* is reserved for rates greater than 100 beats/min; junctional tachycardia is a junctional rhythm, usually regular, at a rate greater than 100 beats/min. When the junctional rate is greater than 60 beats/min and less than 100 beats/min, it is described as an *accelerated junctional rhythm*. Accelerated junctional rhythm is usually well-tolerated by the patient, mainly because the heart rate is within a reasonable range. Junctional tachycardia may not be tolerated as well, depending on the rate and the patient's underlying cardiac reserve.

Ventricular dysrhythmias. Ventricular dysrhythmias result from an ectopic focus in any portion of the ventricular myocardium. The usual conduction pathway through the ventricles is not used, and the wave of depolarization must spread from cell to cell. As a result, the QRS complex is prolonged and is always greater than 0.12 second. It is the width of the QRS not the height that is important in the diagnosis of ventricular ectopy. Table 11-10 provides a summary of the major features of ventricular dysrhythmias.

Premature ventricular contractions. The following are the criteria for a premature ventricular contraction (PVC) is shown in Figures 11-34, 11-35, and 11-36.
Rate: Depends on underlying HR, usually sinus rhythm
Rhythm: Early QRS complexes interrupt underlying rhythm.
PR interval: Absent or retrograde after PVC

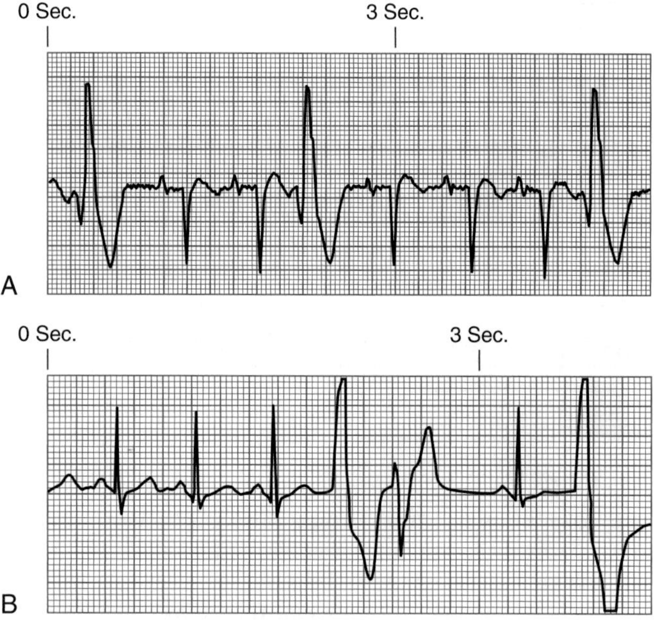

FIG 11-34 *A*, Unifocal Premature Ventricular Contractions (PVCs). *B*, Multifocal PVCs.

TABLE 11-10 Ventricular Rhythms

PARAMETER	IDIOVENTRICULAR RHYTHM	ACCELERATED IDIOVENTRICULAR RHYTHM	VENTRICULAR TACHYCARDIA	VENTRICULAR FIBRILLATION
Rate	20-40/min	40-100/min	>100/min	None
Rhythm	Usually regular	Usually regular	Usually regular	Irregular
P waves	Absent or retrograde	Absent or retrograde	Absent or retrograde	None
PR interval	None	None	None	None
QRS	>0.12 sec	>0.12 sec	>0.12 sec	Fibrillatory waves

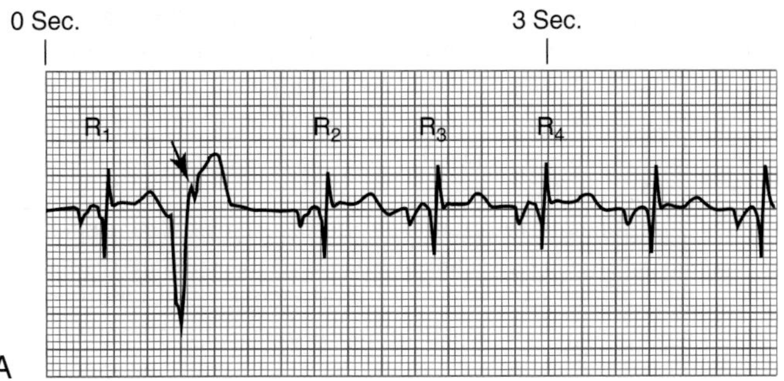

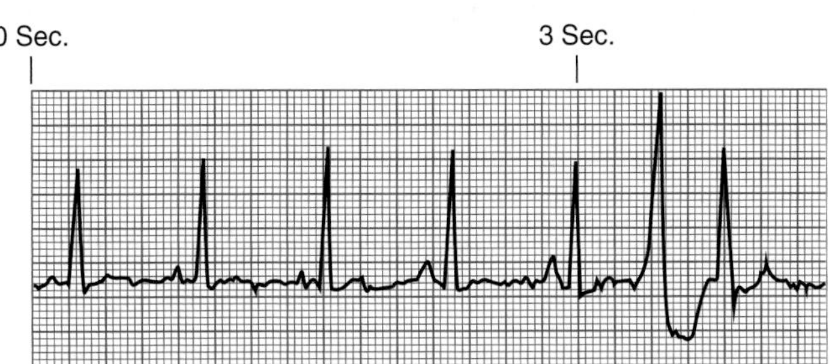

FIG 11-35 *A*, Premature Ventricular Contraction (PVC) with a Fully Compensatory Pause. The interval between the two sinus beats that surround the PVC (R_1 and R_2) is exactly two times the normal interval between sinus beats (R_3 and R_4). The fully compensatory pause occurs because the sinus node continues to pace despite the PVC. Notice the sinus P wave (*arrow*) hidden in the ST segment of the PVC. This P wave did not conduct through to the ventricles because they had just been depolarized and were still in the absolute refractory period. *B*, Interpolated PVC. The PVC falls between two normal QRS complexes without disturbing the rhythm. Notice that the R-R interval between sinus beats remains the same.

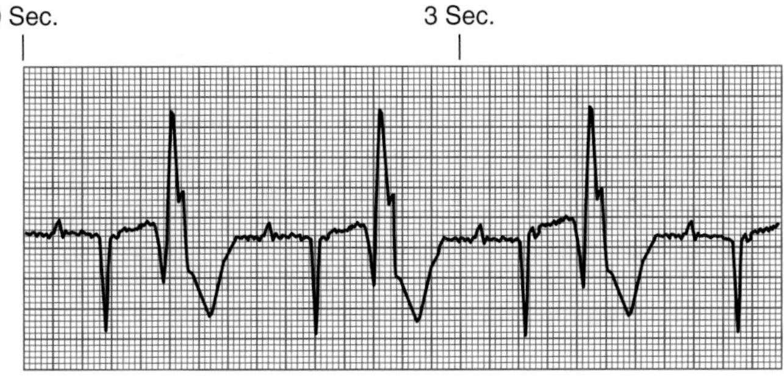

FIG 11-36 Ventricular Bigeminy.

QRS duration: Greater than 0.12 second
QRS complex: Wide, with bizarre shape

A single ectopic impulse originating in the ventricles is called a *premature ventricular contraction* (PVC). Some PVCs are very small in height but remain wider than 0.12 second. If in doubt, a different lead is evaluated. The shape of the QRS depends on the location of the ectopic focus.

Because the ectopic focus may be any cell in the ventricle, the QRS can manifest in an unlimited number of shapes or patterns. If all of the ventricular ectopic beats look the same in a particular lead, they are called *unifocal*, which means that they probably all result from the same irritable focus (Fig. 11-34A). Conversely, if the ventricular ectopics are of various shapes in the same lead, they are called *multifocal* (see Fig. 11-34B). Multifocal ventricular ectopics are more serious than unifocal ventricular ectopics because they indicate a greater area of irritable myocardial tissue and are more likely to deteriorate into VT or fibrillation. In general, ventricular dysrhythmias have more serious implications than do atrial or junctional dysrhythmias and occur only rarely in healthy individuals.

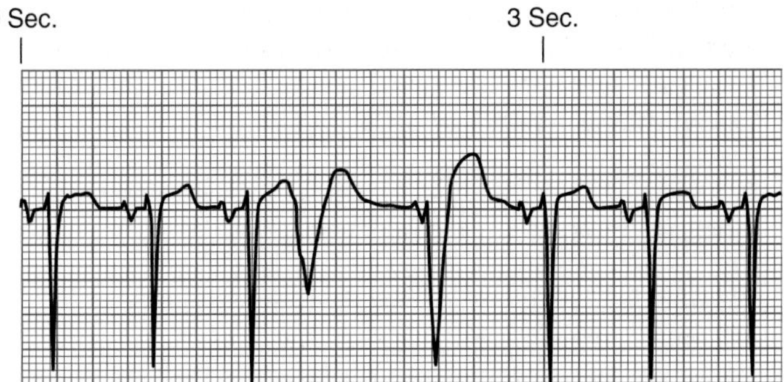

FIG 11-37 R-on-T Phenomenon.

Compensatory pause after a PVC. If the interval from the last normal QRS preceding the PVC to the next one is exactly equal to two complete cardiac cycles (Fig. 11-35A), a compensatory pause is present. Because this does not usually occur in PACs or premature junctional contractions, it is somewhat diagnostic of ventricular ectopy. If the normal sinus P wave that occurs immediately after the PVC finds the ventricles sufficiently recovered to accept another impulse, a normal QRS results, and the PVC is sandwiched between two normal beats (see Fig. 11-35B). This PVC is referred to as *interpolated*, meaning *between*. Interpolated PVCs usually occur when the PVC is very early or the normal sinus rate is relatively slow.

Occasionally, the ventricular impulse spreads backward across the AV node to depolarize the atria. When this occurs, the sinus node is reset, and no full compensatory pause occurs.

If a PVC occurs at this critical point when only a part of the muscle is repolarized, individual segments of muscle can depolarize separately from each other, resulting in VF. This is called the *R-on-T phenomenon* as shown in Figure 11-36. R on T relates to repolarization and absolute and relative refractory periods illustrated in Figure 11-24.

Two consecutive PVCs are described as a *couplet*, and three consecutive PVCs are called a *triplet* or a *three-beat run of ventricular tachycardia*. More than three consecutive PVCs are considered VT, but it is still useful to state how many beats of VT occurred if the run was short, lasting fewer than 20 beats.

Idioventricular rhythms. The following are the criteria for an idioventricular rhythm as shown in Figure 11-37.
Rhythm: Regular
PR interval: Absent
QRS duration: Greater than 0.12 second
P wave: Present, but not associated with QRS complex
QRS complex: Wide and bizarre because the complexes originate in ventricles

Sometimes, an ectopic focus in the ventricle can become the dominant pacemaker of the heart (Table 11-11). If the sinus node and the AV junction fail, the ventricles depolarize

TABLE 11-11 Atrioventricular Block

PARAMETER	FIRST DEGREE	SECOND-DEGREE MOBITZ I (WENCKEBACH)	SECOND-DEGREE MOBITZ II	THIRD DEGREE (COMPLETE)
PR interval	>0.20 sec and constant	Increases with each consecutively conducted P wave	Constant	Varies randomly
P waves	1 P wave for each QRS	Intermittently not conducted, yielding more P waves than QRS complexes	Intermittently not conducted, yielding more P waves than QRS complexes	P waves independent and not related to QRS complexes
QRS	0.06-0.10 sec	0.06-0.10 sec	May be normal, but usually coexists with bundle branch block (>0.12 sec)	0.06-0.10 sec if junctional escape pacemaker activates the ventricles >0.12 sec if ventricular escape pacemaker activates the ventricles

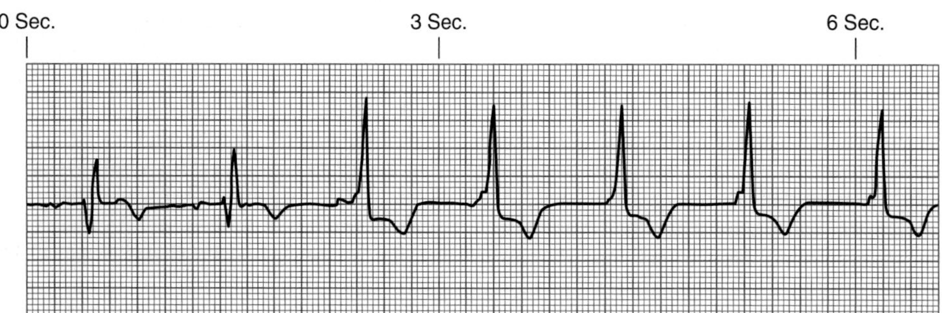

FIG 11-38 Accelerated Idioventricular Rhythm (AIVR). The QRS Duration is 0.14 Second, and the Ventricular Rate is 65.

at their own intrinsic rate of 20 to 40 times per minute. This is called an *idioventricular rhythm* and is a protective mechanism. Rather than trying to abolish the ventricular beats, the aim of treatment is to increase the effective heart rate and reestablish dominance of a higher pacing site such as the sinus node or the AV junction. Usually, a temporary pacemaker is used to increase the heart rate until the underlying problems that caused failure of the other pacing sites can be resolved.

An *accelerated idioventricular rhythm* (AIVR) occurs when a ventricular focus assumes control of the heart at a rate greater than its intrinsic rate of 40 beats/min but less than 100 beats/min (Fig. 11-38). Although relatively benign in and of itself, this rhythm must be closely observed for any increase in rate, and the patient must be observed for hemodynamic deterioration. Usually, AIVR is not treated pharmacologically if well-tolerated with a stable blood pressure, although a transvenous temporary pacemaker should be inserted electively as a precaution against sudden hemodynamic deterioration. Intravenous lidocaine must never be administered to a patient with an idioventricular rhythm because it suppresses the ventricular pacemaker and converts the rhythm to asystole.

Ventricular tachycardia. Ventricular tachycardia (VT) is caused by a ventricular pacing site firing at a rate of 100 times or more per minute, usually maintained by a reentry mechanism within the ventricular tissue. The following are the criteria for ventricular tachycardia as shown in Figure 11-39.

Rate: Greater than 100 beats/min

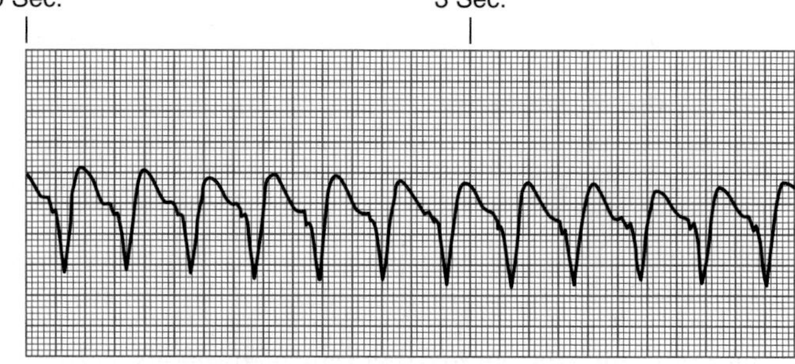

FIG 11-39 Ventricular Tachycardia.

Rhythm: Mostly regular. May have some irregularities.
P wave: Not related to QRS. Sinus node is unaffected and will continue to depolarize the atria, unrelated to the ventricular rate.
PR interval: Absent
QRS duration: Greater than 0.12 second
QRS complex: Wide, with bizarre shape compared with sinus QRS

The complexes are wide, and the rhythm may be slightly irregular, often accelerating as the tachycardia continues (see Table 11-11). In most cases, the sinus node is not affected, and it continues to depolarize the atria on schedule. P waves can sometimes be seen on the ECG tracing. They are not related to the QRS and may even appear to conduct a normal impulse to the ventricles if their timing is just right.

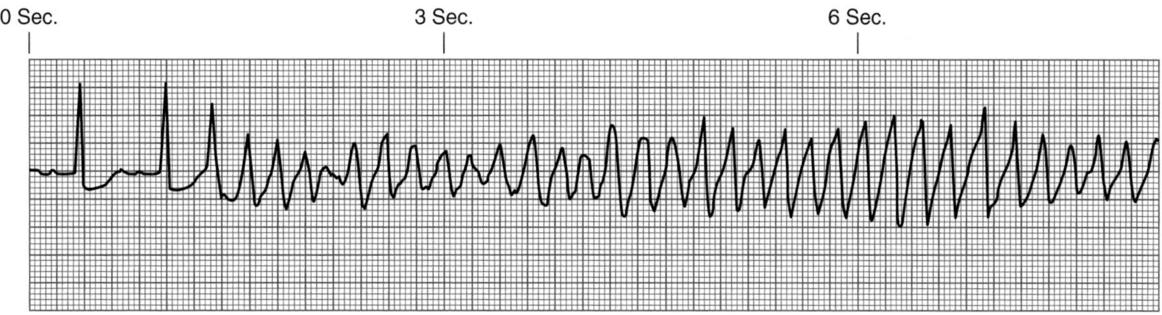

FIG 11-40 Torsade De Pointes.

Most VT occurs in the presence of structural cardiac disease, such as myocardial ischemia, congenital heart disease, valvular dysfunction, and cardiomyopathy. Other triggers include drug toxicities, electrolyte disturbances, and as an adverse reaction to certain antidysrhythmic medications (prodysrhythmia).

VT is a life-threatening dysrhythmia and must be treated quickly. The rapid ventricular rate decreases blood pressure, and the patient may lose consciousness. The loss of the synchronized timing of atrial contraction, which normally adds volume to the ventricles just before contraction and enhances the force of contraction, is lost, greatly reducing cardiac output. If not terminated quickly, VT is likely to degenerate into VF and death.

How VT is clinically managed depends on whether the patient is stable or unstable, as well as whether a pulse and adequate blood pressure are present. Pulseless VT is a life-threatening condition. The patient will lose consciousness and will need immediate cardiopulmonary resuscitation and defibrillation as described in the American Heart Association (AHA) protocols for advanced cardiac life support (ACLS).

After the acute episode is over, patients who have already experienced sustained VT or cardiac arrest continue to be at risk for sudden cardiac death. An extensive clinical evaluation is warranted, including cardiac catheterization and electrophysiologic testing with programmed ventricular stimulation. Treatment is aimed at preventing a recurrence of sustained VT or VF. It may include treating the underlying cause, administering antidysrhythmic medications, performing ablation of the reentrant pathway within the ventricle, or inserting an implantable cardioverter defibrillator (ICD). Chapter 12 provides more detail on sudden cardiac death, and Chapter 13 provides more information on implantable cardioverter defibrillators.

Torsade de pointes. One form of polymorphic VT is termed *torsade de pointes* or "twisting of the points" because of its appearance on the ECG (Figure 11-40). Because torsade de pointes is associated with a lengthening of the QT interval, monitoring this parameter is essential when medications that may prolong the QT interval are administered (see Table 11-6).

Ventricular fibrillation. VF is the result of chaotic electrical activity in the ventricles where the ventricles merely quiver and no forward flow of blood occurs. On the ECG, VF appears as a continuous, undulating pattern without clear P, QRS, or T waves. The following are the criteria for ventricular fibrillation as shown in Figure 11-41.

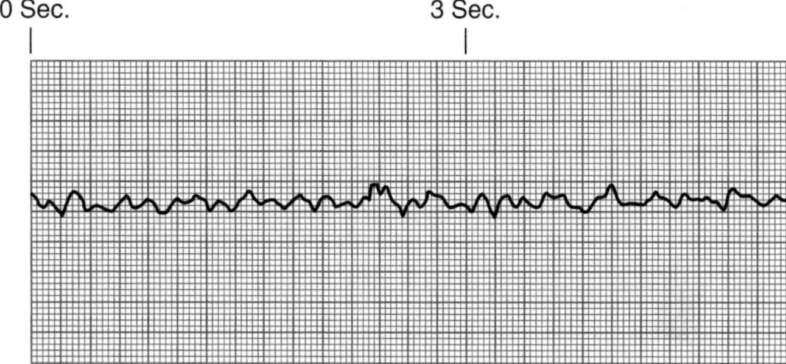

FIG 11-41 Ventricular Fibrillation.

Rate: Indeterminable
Rhythm: Irregular, wavy baseline without recognizable QRS complexes
P wave: Absent. Cannot be distinguished from fibrillating ventricular baseline.
PR interval: Absent
QRS duration: Absent. No QRS complexes present.
QRS complex: Normal P wave and QRS are replaced by a wavy baseline.

When VF occurs in the setting of an acute ischemic event and is accompanied by a significant amount of myocardial damage, the survival rate is poor. Resuscitation is often unsuccessful. VF is seen on the ECG as larger erratic undulations of the baseline (coarse VF) or as a mild tremor (fine VF). In VF, the patient does not have a pulse, no blood is being pumped forward, and defibrillation is the only definitive therapy. As with any cardiac arrest, supportive measures such as cardiopulmonary resuscitation (CPR), intubation, and correction of metabolic abnormalities are performed concurrently with definitive therapy.

Atrioventricular conduction blocks. Normally, the sinoatrial node triggers electrical depolarization in the heart. From there, the impulse travels through the right atrium to the AV node. The left atrium is depolarized by a conduction fiber known as *Bachman's bundle* that connects the right and left atria. The electrical impulse is briefly delayed in the AV node to allow the atria to contract and the mitral and tricuspid valves to close before the impulse is conducted to the bundle of His, the bundle branches, and the Purkinje fibers.

On the ECG, the ability of the AV node to conduct is evaluated by measuring the PR interval and the relationship of P waves to QRS complexes (Table 11-11). The normal PR interval, measured from the beginning of the P wave to the beginning of the QRS complex, ranges from 0.12 to 0.20 second.

First-degree atrioventricular block. When all atrial impulses are conducted to the ventricles, but the PR interval is greater than 0.20 second, a condition known as *first-degree AV block* exists. This represents a delay in conduction as all P waves are conducted. The following are the criteria for first-degree AV block as shown in Figure 11-42.

Rate: Depends on underlying rhythm, usually sinus rhythm
Rhythm: Regular if sinus rhythm
P wave: Present, normal shape
PR interval: Greater than 0.20 second
QRS duration: 0.06 to 0.10 second
QRS complex: Unaffected

First-degree AV block represents slowed conduction through the AV node. If the associated QRS is narrow, it is likely that the only conduction abnormality is in the AV node. However, if the associated QRS complex is widened, it is likely that there is also damage to the bundle branches as a result of fibrosis, ischemia, or infarction.

Second-degree atrioventricular block. Second-degree AV block can be broadly defined as a condition in which some atrial impulses are conducted to the ventricles, but others are "blocked" at the AV node. This description of intermittent AV conduction covers two patterns with markedly different clinical significance: second-degree AV block is divided into Mobitz type I (also known as *Wenckebach block)* and Mobitz type II.

Mobitz Type I. In Mobitz type I block (*Wenckebach*), the AV conduction times progressively lengthen until a P wave is not conducted. This typically occurs in a pattern of *grouped beats* and is observed on the ECG by a gradually lengthening PR interval, until ultimately the final P wave in the group fails to conduct. In Mobitz type I, the QRS complex is generally of normal width and appearance. The following are the criteria for Mobitz type I AV block as shown in Figure 11-43.

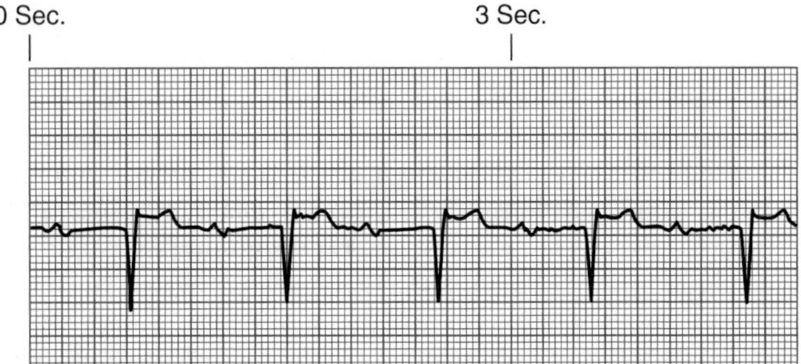

FIG 11-42 First-Degree Atrioventricular (AV) Block. The PR interval is prolonged to 0.44 second.

Rate: Atrial rate depends on underlying sinus rate. Ventricular rate depends on P wave/QRS ratio.
Rhythm: Regular, irregular pattern. P waves are regular. As part of Mobitz I pattern, R-to-R intervals become progressively shorter until sinus P wave is not conducted, resulting in a pause. After the pause, the cycle repeats. The PR interval typically lengthens the most with the second beat of the cycle.
P wave: Normal shape
PR intervals: Progressively lengthen until a P wave is not conducted to ventricles and therefore is not followed by QRS complex
RR intervals: Intervals become progressively shorter until sinus P wave is not conducted, and this results in a longer RR interval, before the cycle starts again.
QRS duration: 0.06 to 0.10 second
QRS complex: Conducted complexes are normal.

Mobitz I block has a specific, repeating pattern that catches the eye. The expected groups are 3 : 2, 4 : 3, or 5 : 4. For example, if four P waves are conducted to the ventricles and the fifth one is not, a 5 : 4 conduction ratio is present (five P waves to four QRS complexes). The nonconducted P ends a *group.* After the pause, the cycle repeats itself. The PR interval typically lengthens the most with the second beat of the cycle.

Mobitz type I does not generally cause significant hemodynamic compromise as long as the ventricular heart rate is maintained. If Mobitz type I occurs in the setting of an acute coronary syndrome, occasionally, placement of a temporary pacemaker as a precautionary measure is warranted.

Mobitz Type II. Mobitz type II block is always anatomically located below the AV node in the bundle of His in the bundle branches. This results in an all-or-nothing situation with respect to AV conduction. Sinus P waves are or are not conducted. When conduction does occur, all PR intervals are the same. Because of the anatomic location of the block, on the ECG the PR interval is seen as constant, and the QRS complexes are usually slightly wider than normal as shown in Figure 11-44, where AV conduction occurs only every other atrial P wave in a 2 : 1 conduction ratio. The following are the criteria for Mobitz type II AV block:

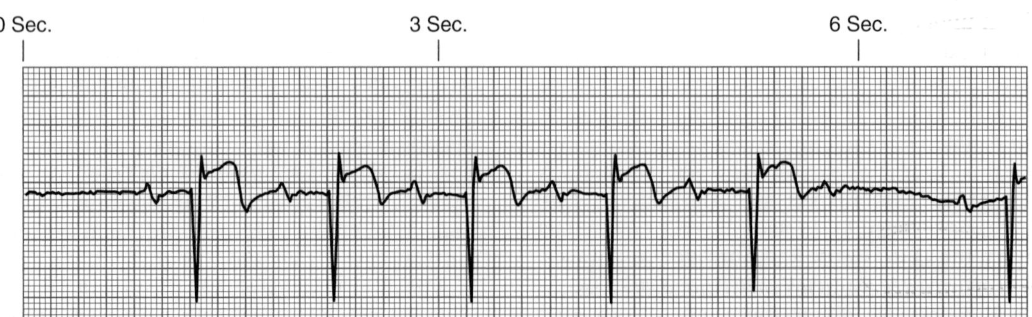

FIG 11-43 Mobitz Type I (Wenckebach) Second-Degree Atrioventricular (AV) Block. Notice that the PR intervals gradually increase from 0.36 to 0.46 second until a P wave is not conducted to the ventricles.

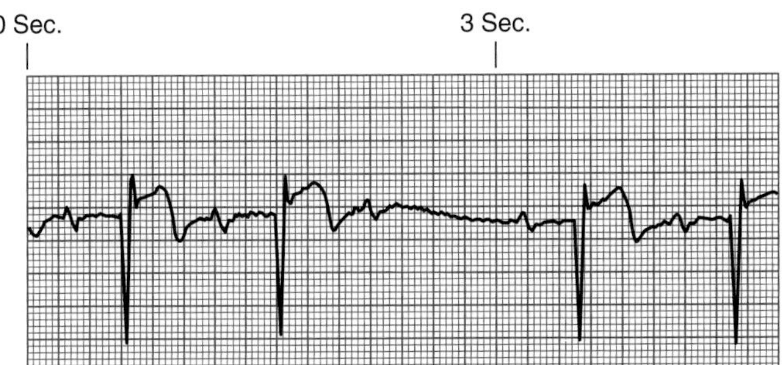

FIG 11-44 Mobitz Type II Second-Degree Atrioventricular (AV) Block. Notice that the PR intervals remain constant.

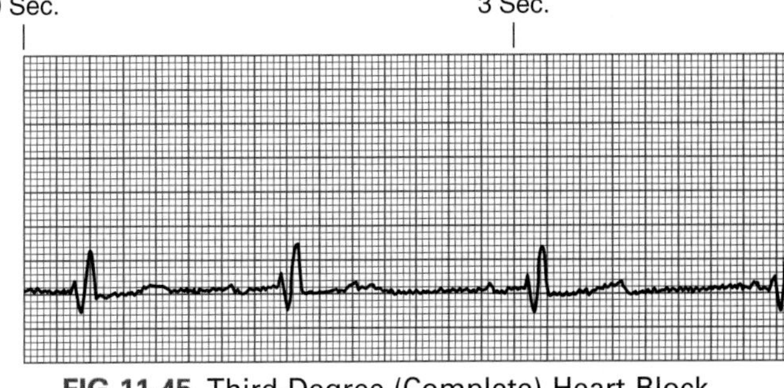

FIG 11-45 Third-Degree (Complete) Heart Block.

Rhythm: Regular if AV node consistently conducts every second or third P wave. Irregular if P waves conducted inconsistently.
P wave: Normal in shape. More P waves than QRS complexes.
PR interval: 0.12 to 0.20 second. Constant interval for P waves that conduct to ventricles.
QRS duration: 0.06 to 0.10 second or wider. The QRS may be wider depending on the location of the block within the bundle branches.
QRS complex: May be normal or widened. Shape may vary depending on location of block within the bundle branches.

Mobitz II block is more ominous clinically than Mobitz I and may progress to complete AV block. For this reason, it is important to prepare for *transcutaneous cardiac pacing* (TCP) by bringing an external pacemaker (often combined with a defibrillator) to the bedside as a precaution. TCP refers to external pacing from outside the chest wall. When pacing is required, two large pacing electrodes are placed on the chest. There is always a diagram on the machine showing where to place the pads on the chest. Consider the possibility that the patient will need a temporary transvenous pacemaker inserted and possibly require a permanent pacemaker before hospital discharge.

Third-degree atrioventricular block. Third-degree, or complete, AV block is a condition in which no atrial impulses can conduct from the atria to the ventricles. This is also described by the terms *complete heart block* or *AV dissociation* to indicate that the atria and the ventricles are controlled by different pacemakers. The block can be located at the level of the AV node or below the node within the bundle of His or the bundle branches. The following are the criteria for third-degree AV block as shown in Figure 11-45.

Rate: Depends on underlying rhythm
Rhythm: Usually regular
P wave: Normal shape
PR interval: P waves are not related to QRS complexes, so there is no PR interval.
QRS duration: Wide, greater than 0.10 second
QRS complex: If a junctional focus is pacing heart, complex is narrow but is not related to P waves. If ventricular focus is pacing heart, the QRS is wide and unrelated to P waves.

Management of third degree atrioventricular block. Complete heart block causes AV dissociation and is associated with a low cardiac output that requires use of a pacemaker. If the patient is hemodynamically unstable, external transcutaneous pacing may be used to maintain an adequate ventricular rate until a transvenous or permanent pacemaker can be inserted.

LABORATORY ASSESSMENT

Nursing Management

The priorities for laboratory assessment for the patient with cardiovascular dysfunction focus on 1) interpreting serum electrolytes and safely replacing electrolyte deficiencies, 2) monitoring cardiac biomarkers, 3) trending hematological studies, 4) assessing coagulation values, and 5) evaluating the serum lipid profile.

Interpreting Serum Electrolyte Levels

Potassium. During depolarization and repolarization of nerve and muscle fiber, potassium and sodium exchange occurs intracellularly and extracellularly. The potassium gradient across the cell membrane determines conduction velocity and helps confine pacing activity to the sinus node. Excess or deficiency of potassium can alter myocardial muscle function. Normal serum potassium levels are 3.5 to 4.5 mEq/L.

Hyperkalemia. Elevated serum potassium, called *hyperkalemia*, can be caused by a variety of conditions that include excess potassium administration, extensive skeletal muscle destruction (rhabdomyolysis), tumor lysis syndrome, and kidney failure. Hyperkalemia can elicit significant changes in the ECG because it decreases AV conduction velocity, slows ventricular depolarization, and accelerates repolarization.[78] As the serum levels of potassium rise, tall, narrow peaked T waves are usually, although not uniquely, associated with early hyperkalemia and are followed by prolongation of the PR interval, loss of the P wave, widening of the QRS complex, heart block, and asystole (Figure 11-46A).[78] Severely elevated serum potassium (greater than 8 mEq/L) causes a wide QRS tachycardia, as shown in the 12-lead ECG in Figure 11-46B. If not corrected, severe hyperkalemia can lead to VF or cardiac standstill. It is important to know that evidence of hyperkalemia is not always visible on the ECG.[79] Furthermore research has shown that ECG waveform changes are not a sensitive indicator of elevated potassium levels.[79] When hyperkalemia is suspected, it is safer to draw serial serum potassium levels than to rely on the ECG waveform alone.[79]

This life-threatening condition can be acutely managed with IV insulin to drive the potassium inside the cell and temporarily out of the plasma. Glucose is usually administered at the same time to avoid hypoglycemia as a secondary complication. Potassium is permanently removed from the

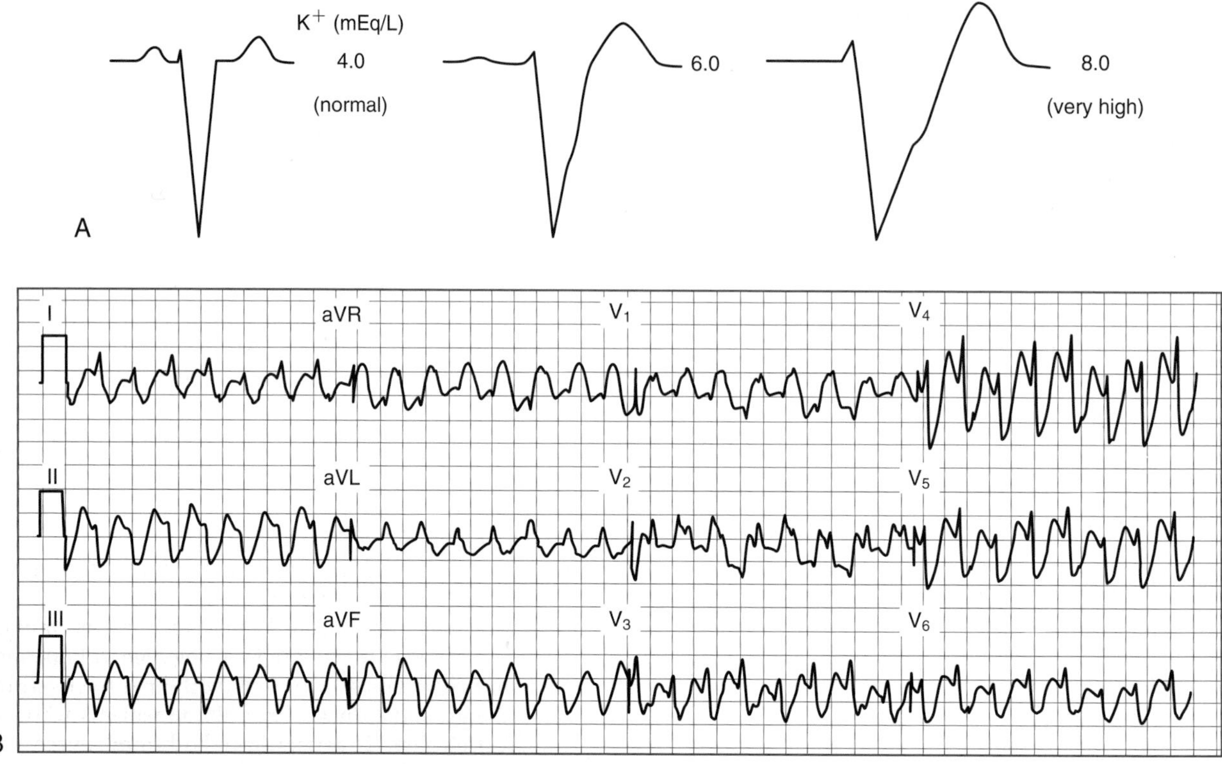

FIG 11-46 Effects of Hyperkalemia on the ECG. *A*, Stages in hyperkalemia from normal potassium levels to plasma levels of 8 mEq/L. At approximately 6 mEq/L, the P wave flattens, the QRS broadens, and the ST segment disappears, with the S wave flowing into the tall, tented T wave. *B*, A 12-lead ECG of a patient with a serum potassium level of 9.1 mEq/L.

bloodstream by cation-exchange resin products, such as Kayexalate, placed into the gastrointestinal tract or removed directly from the blood by hemodialysis.[80] Coexisting low serum sodium, calcium, or pH levels potentiate the cardiac effects of hyperkalemia.

Hypokalemia. A low serum potassium (K^+) level, called *hypokalemia* (<3.5 mEq/L), is commonly caused by gastrointestinal losses, diuretic therapy with insufficient replacement, or chronic steroid therapy. Hypokalemia is also reflected by changes on the ECG (Figure 11-47). The earliest ECG change may be PVCs, which can deteriorate into VT or VF without appropriate potassium replacement.

Hypokalemia impairs myocardial conduction and prolongs ventricular repolarization. This can be seen by a prominent U wave (a positive deflection after the T wave on the ECG).[80] The U wave is not totally unique to hypokalemia, but its presence is a signal for the clinician to check the serum potassium level.[80] In the critical care unit, where patients are receiving diuretics or have gastric tubes to suction, the serum potassium level is checked frequently and replaced to normal levels to prevent dysrhythmias. Great care must be taken when replacing potassium intravenously to ensure it is diluted sufficiently and administered slowly to prevent accidental overdose. Potassium is a high-alert medication, and additional safety procedures are recommended for replacement of this electrolyte (Box 11-15 provides the electrolyte values that impact cardiac contractility. See Box 11-16 for the QSEN Patient Safety Alert feature on Medication Administration.)

Calcium. Calcium (Ca^{2+}) is an important cation in the body. Calcium metabolism is controlled by many factors, including normal parathyroid hormone (PTH) function, calcitonin, and vitamin D acting on target organs such as the kidney, bone, and gastrointestinal tract. Calcium is an important mediator of many cardiovascular functions because of its effect on vascular tone, myocardial contractility, and cardiac excitability.

Serum calcium values are recorded in three possible ways, depending on the hospital laboratory: milliequivalents per liter (mEq/L), milligrams per deciliter (mg/dL), or millimols per liter (mmol/L).

In the bloodstream, about 50% of calcium is biologically active and is known as the *ionized calcium.*[81] The remaining non-active calcium is bound to protein (primarily albumin) and inorganic ions such as sulphate and phosphate.[81] The normal values for total and ionized serum calcium levels are listed in Table 11-12. The normal serum concentration of ionized calcium is maintained within very narrow limits; changes in ionized calcium level are responsible for the clinical effects of hypercalcemia and hypocalcemia. The only accurate way to determine the level of ionized calcium—described as physiologically active, unbound, or free—is to measure the ionized serum value with a laboratory assay.[81] The mathematically calculated values that extrapolate from total calcium and serum albumin levels have been shown to be inaccurate.[81]

Hypercalcemia. Hypercalcemia is defined as increased amounts of ionized calcium (>5.6 mg/dL or 1.40 mmol/L) or increased amounts of total serum calcium (>10.5 mg/dL or 2.60 mmol/L).[82] Serum calcium levels are increased by bone tumors; primary hyperparathyroidism caused by elevated

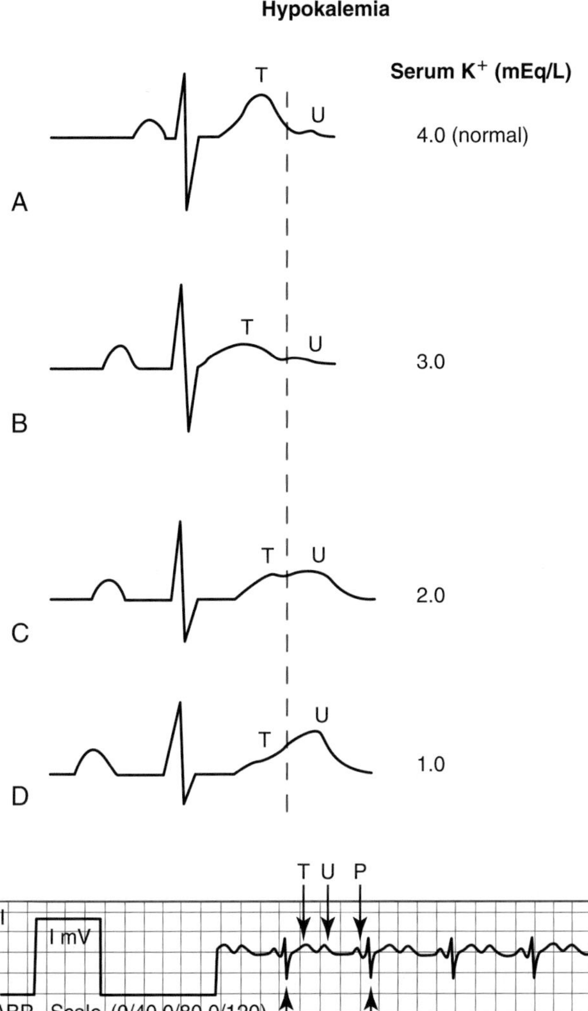

FIG 11-47 Effects of Hypokalemia on the ECG. *A*, At a normal serum concentration of 3.5 to 4.5 mEq/L, the amplitude of the T wave is appreciably greater than that of the U wave. *B*, By the time the serum potassium level has dropped to 3 mEq/L, the amplitudes of the T and U waves are approaching each other. *C* and *D*, With a further drop in the level of potassium, the U wave begins to tower over and fuse with the T wave. *E*, ECG tracing from a patient with a serum potassium of 2.6 mEq/L shows a prominent U wave.

PTH levels; excessive intake of supplemental calcium and vitamin D, usually in oral antacids; hypomagnesemia, and as a complication of kidney failure from decreased excretion of calcium in urine. Hypercalcemia affects many organs, causes smooth muscle relaxation, and can lead to neurologic changes such as lethargy, confusion, and even coma. Elevated serum calcium has the cardiovascular effect of strengthening contractility and shortening ventricular repolarization, demonstrated on the ECG by a shortened QTc interval.[80] Rhythm disturbances may include bradycardia; first-, second-, and third-degree heart block, and bundle branch block. Hypercalcemia can potentiate the effects of digitalis, precipitate digitalis toxicity, and cause hypertension.[81]

BOX 11-15 Chemistry Values That Affect Cardiac Contractility and Conduction

	NORMAL RANGES*		
ELECTROLYTE	**mE₀/L**	**mg/dL**	**mmol/L**
Potassium (K^+)	3.5-4.5		3.50-4.50
Ionized calcium (Ca)		4.0-5.0	1.00-1.30
Total calcium (Ca^{2+})		8.5-10.5	2.00-2.60
Magnesium (Mg^{2+})	1.5-2.0	1.8-2.4	0.70-1.10

*Laboratory values may be reported as mEq/L, mg/dL, or mmol/L. Each measurement parameter used produces a different value. Some electrolytes are reported with more than one reference value. Different clinical laboratories use different reference values, and the cited reference values may vary slightly between hospital laboratories.

Management of hypercalcemia involves promotion of excretion of calcium by diuretics using high-volume intravenous normal saline at 200 to 300 mL/hr if tolerated by the heart, lungs, and kidneys. Critically ill patients who cannot tolerate this clinical regimen may be hemodialyzed using a low-calcium dialysate.

Hypocalcemia. *Hypocalcemia* is defined as an ionized calcium level below normal (<4.5 mg/dL or <1.1 mmol/L) or a low total serum calcium level below 8.5 mg/dL.[82] Hypocalcemia (measured by ionized calcium) is a common finding and is reported to occur in 15% to 20% of critically ill patients, depending on the admitting diagnosis.[83] Transfusions of blood from the blood bank lower serum calcium levels because the citrate used as an anticoagulant in banked blood binds to the calcium.[81] This is called *citrate chelation.* If citrate is used during hemodialysis or plasmapheresis, it will have the same calcium-binding (chelating) effect. Phosphate also binds to calcium and can lower the serum calcium level. Metabolic alkalosis often coexists with hypocalcemia. The cardiovascular effects of hypocalcemia include decreased myocardial contractility, decreased cardiac output, and hypotension. Rhythm disturbances with severe hypocalcemia are variable, ranging from bradycardia to VT and asystole. When the ionized calcium is low, the ECG may show a prolonged QTc interval[80] (Figure 11-48). This predisposes a patient to the life-threatening ventricular dysrhythmia *torsade de pointes* (see Table 11-6 and Figure 11-40).

Management of hypocalcemia, especially when the ionized calcium is low, involves infusion of intravenous calcium chloride or calcium gluconate via a central line.[81,82]

- Calcium chloride provides 27 mg of elemental calcium/mL (272 mg in 10 mls).
- Calcium gluconate provides 9 mg of elemental calcium/mL (90 mg in 10 mls).

Magnesium. Magnesium (Mg^{2+}) is essential for many enzyme, protein, lipid, and carbohydrate functions in the body and is critical for the production and use of energy. The body stores most magnesium in bone (53%), muscle (27%), and soft tissues (19%); only a tiny proportion resides within the bloodstream—red blood cells contain 0.5%, and serum contains 0.3%.[84] As with other electrolytes, the ionized

BOX 11-16 PATIENT SAFETY ALERT MEDICATION ADMINISTRATION QSEN

1. Accurate Patient Identification
   - Use at least two patient identifiers (not the patient's room number) when taking blood samples or administering medications or blood products. Examples include the patient name or date of birth.
2. Effective Communication among Caregivers
   - An organizational method to decrease the number of medication errors is the use of *computerized physician order entry* (CPOE), as advocated by the Leapfrog group (http://www.leapfroggroup.org).
   - Hospitals should have a process for taking verbal or telephone orders that requires a verification "read back" of the complete order by the person receiving the order.
   - The Institute of Safe Medication Practices (ISMP) maintains a list of medications with similar-sounding names as name confusion can lead to medication errors. The list is available on the ISMP website at http://www.ismp.org/Tools/confuseddrugnames.pdf. Medication errors can be reported to the Medication Errors Reporting Program (MERP).
   - Standardize the abbreviations, acronyms, and symbols used throughout the organization, including a list of abbreviations, acronyms, and symbols not to use.
   - Examples of problematic abbreviations include "U" for units and "μg" for micrograms. When handwritten, a capital U can be mistaken for a zero (0); in numerous case reports, an insulin dosage written in U was interpreted as 0. Using the abbreviation "μg" instead of "mcg" for micrograms is also problematic; when handwritten, the Greek letter μ can look like an "m." The error-prone abbreviation is available on the ISMP website at http://www.ismp.org/Tools/errorproneabbreviations.pdf.
   - Use of trailing zeros (e.g., 2.0 versus 2) and using a leading decimal point without a leading zero (e.g., .2 instead of 0.2) are dangerous prescription-writing practices. Misinterpretation has caused 10-fold dosing errors.
3. High-Alert Medication Safety
   - Remove concentrated electrolytes (including but not limited to potassium chloride, potassium phosphate, and hypertonic sodium chloride) from patient care units.
   - Standardize and limit the number of medication concentrations available in the organization.
   - In the first 2 years after enacting a *sentinel event reporting mechanism*, the most common category was medication errors, and the most frequently implicated medication was potassium chloride (KCl). The Joint Commission reviewed 10 incidents of patient death resulting from misadministration of KCl. Eight were the result of direct infusion of concentrated KCl. In six of the eight cases, the KCl was mistaken for another medication, primarily because of similarities in packaging and labeling. Most often, KCl was mistaken for sodium chloride, heparin, or furosemide (Lasix).
   - The Joint Commission suggests that health care organizations *not* make concentrated KCl available outside the pharmacy unless appropriate, specific safeguards are in place.
   - A list of high-alert medications is available on the ISMP website at http://www.ismp.org.
4. Infusion Pump Safety
   - Ensure free-flow protection on all general-use and patient-controlled analgesia (PCA) intravenous (IV) infusion pumps used in the organization.
   - Infusion pumps that do not provide protection from the free flow of IV fluid or medication into the patient are hazardous.
   - *Free flow* occurs when IV solution flows freely under the force of gravity without being controlled by the infusion pump. Free flow typically occurs after the administration set is temporarily removed from the pump to transfer a patient to another area, change a patient's gown, or place a patient on a radiography table. Clinicians can greatly reduce this risk by using administration sets with set-based anti–free-flow mechanisms that prevent gravity free flow by closing off the IV tubing to prohibit flow when the administration set is removed from the pump.
5. Hospital Safety
   - Each year The Joint Commission develops Hospital National Patient Safety Goals that incorporate medication safety requirements. This information is available on The Joint Commission website at http://www.jointcommission.org/standards_information/npsgs.aspx.
   - Medication safety is an important component of hospital safety. Hospitals are graded on the safety of their environment for patients. The "safety score" for each hospital is publicly available at http://www.leapfroggroup.org.

More information can be accessed on the websites of the following three safety organizations:
http://www.jointcommission.org
http://www.usp.org
http://www.leapfroggroup.org

portion of the serum magnesium is the biologically active component that is available for biochemical processes. Serum magnesium is 67% ionized, 19% protein-bound, and 14% complexed.[84] The serum magnesium is what is normally measured in a routine blood test. Serum magnesium can be reported in units of mEq/L, mg/dL, or mmol/L, depending on the laboratory running the analysis. The normal serum range is from 1.5 to 2 mEq/L, 1.8 to 2.4 mg/dL, or 0.7 to 1.1 mmol/L. These represent the same serum level of magnesium despite different units of measurement. It is important to anticipate that normal reference values will vary between hospital laboratories.

Hypermagnesemia. The incidence of hypermagnesemia is rare in comparison with hypomagnesemia. It results from kidney failure, tumor lysis syndrome, or iatrogenic overtreatment. Symptoms do not generally occur until the serum magnesium is above 4.8 mg/dL, and dialysis is the recommended treatment.[82]

Hypomagnesemia. A total serum magnesium concentration below 1.5 mEq/L defines *hypomagnesemia.* It is commonly associated with other electrolyte imbalances, most notably alterations in potassium, calcium, and phosphorus. Low serum magnesium levels can result from many causes. Hypomagnesemia is caused by insufficient intake in the diet or in total parental nutrition (TPN) and is associated with chronic alcohol abuse. In the critical care unit, aggressive diuresis with loop diuretics will lower serum levels.[84] Diarrhea can be a significant cause of magnesium loss because lower gastrointestinal fluids contain up to 15 mEq/L magnesium; vomiting or gastric suction causes less depletion because the upper gastrointestinal fluids contain about 1 mEq/L. Another cause of magnesium depletion is rapid administration of citrated blood products, which causes the citrate to bind to the magnesium, a condition known as *citrate chelation.* In patients with chronic hypomagnesemia, the serum levels are replenished from the bone stores.

Hypomagnesemia can cause hypertension and vasospasm, including coronary artery spasm. Some studies have linked magnesium depletion to sudden cardiac death, to an increased incidence of acute myocardial infarction, and to the occurrence of ventricular dysrhythmias.[84]

TABLE 11-12 Chemistry Values That Affect Cardiac Contractility and Conduction

	NORMAL RANGES*		
ELECTROLYTE	**mE_0/L**	**mg/dL**	**mmol/L**
Potassium (K^+)	3.5-4.5		3.50-4.50
Ionized calcium (Ca)		4.0-5.0	1.00-1.30
Total calcium (Ca^{2+})		8.5-10.5	2.00-2.60
Magnesium (Mg^{2+})	1.5-2.0	1.8-2.4	0.70-1.10

*Laboratory values may be reported as mEq/L, mg/dL, or mmol/L. Each measurement parameter used produces a different value. Some electrolytes are reported with more than one reference value. Different clinical laboratories use different reference values, and the cited reference values may vary slightly between hospital laboratories.

In hypomagnesemia, the ECG changes are similar to those seen with hypokalemia and hypocalcemia: prolonged PR and QT intervals, presence of U waves, T-wave flattening, and a widened QRS complex. Cardiac dysrhythmias may be supraventricular or ventricular and includes the polymorphic ventricular rhythm torsades de pointes. In cardiac arrest with pulseless VT with torsades de pointes, IV magnesium 1-2 grams diluted in 10 mls D5W may be administered over 15 minutes.[85] It is important to evaluate kidney function when administering magnesium to avoid precipitating hypermagnesium states.

Cardiac Biomarker Studies

Cardiac biomarkers in acute coronary syndrome. Cardiac biomarkers are proteins that are released from damaged myocardial cells.[86] When myocardial cells are damaged, they release detectable proteins into the bloodstream so that a rise in biomarkers can be correlated with heart muscle injury. The biomarkers that are routinely measured include cardiac *troponin I* (cTnI), cardiac *troponin T* (cTnT), and *CK-MB*. Table 11-13 summarizes the cardiac biomarkers related to myocardial injury and infarction. Unfortunately, in many hospitals, the laboratory turnaround time for results of quantitative cardiac biomarkers is between 60 and 90 minutes, which limits the usefulness of the biomarkers in an emergency. If point-of-care testing at the bedside is used, the results are available more quickly and may be more helpful in the clinical decision-making process.

Creatine kinase-MB. The creatine kinase (CK) muscle/brain (MB) biomarker (CK-MB) is released as a result of myocardial damage, and serum levels rise 4 to 8 hours after MI, peak at 15 to 24 hours, and remain elevated for 2 to 3 days (see Table 11-13). Serial samples are drawn routinely at 6- or 8-hour intervals, and three samples are usually sufficient to support or rule out the diagnosis of MI. CK-MB is never an isolated test; it is always performed in conjunction with cardiac troponin levels.

Troponin T and troponin I. The *troponins* are biomarkers for myocardial damage. cTnI and cTnT are more sensitive markers of myocardial injury and infarction than CK-MB. As a result, more patients with myocardial damage are now being

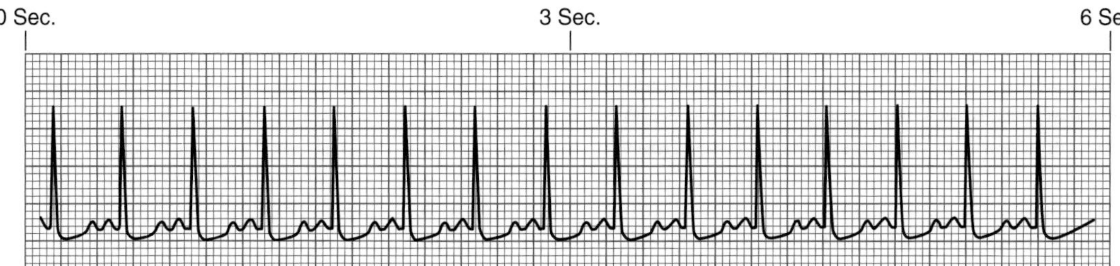

FIG 11-48 Abnormal QT Prolongation in a Hypocalcemic Patient. The patient is a 50-year-old woman admitted to the critical care unit with a diagnosis of alcoholic liver disease and malnourishment. Total calcium concentration is 5.1 mg/dL, and the albumin level is 1.3 mg/dL. The QT interval (0.55 second) is markedly prolonged for the heart rate (100 beats/min). The QT interval varies with the heart rate and can be corrected (QT_c) as if the heart rate were 60 beats/min using the formula $\sqrt{QT/RR} = QT_c$ The QT_c should be 0.44 second or less. The QT_c in the ECG tracing shown is 0.55 second. Hypocalcemia lengthens ventricular repolarization. A quick method for assessing the QT interval is to remember that it is usually less than half of the R-R interval. If it is more than one-half of the R-R interval, it is prolonged. (From Yucha CB, Toto KH: Calcium and phosphorus derangements. Crit Care Nurs Clin North Am 6(4): 747-766, 1994.)

TABLE 11-13 Serum Biomarkers After Acute Myocardial Infarction

SERUM BIOMARKER	TIME TO INITIAL ELEVATION (HOURS)*	PEAK ELEVATION† (HOURS)*	RETURN TO BASELINE (DAYS)*
Cardiac troponin I (cTnI)	3-12	24	5-10
Cardiac troponin T (cTnT)	3-12	12-48	5-14
CK-MB‡	3-12	24	2-3

*Time periods represent average reported values.
†Does not include patients who have had reperfusion therapy.
‡The creatine kinase (CK) enzyme consists of two subunits, the brain type (B) and the muscle type (M).

dectected. Several different methods of laboratory assay are available, which means that normal serum levels will vary between different clinical settings, although cardiac serum cTnI and cTnT levels will be low in the absence of myocardial muscle damage.

The initial elevation of cTnI, cTnT, and CK-MB occurs 3 to 6 hours after the acute myocardial damage. This means that if an individual comes to the emergency department as soon as chest pain is experienced, the biomarkers will not have risen. For this reason, it is clinical practice to diagnose an acute MI by 12-lead ECG and clinical symptoms without waiting for elevation of cardiac biomarkers.

Because cTnI is found only in cardiac muscle, it is a highly specific biomarker for myocardial damage, considerably more specific than CK-MB. As a consequence, patients with a positive cTnI result and a negative CK-MB result usually rule in as an acute MI. A negative cTnI result that remains negative many hours after an episode of chest pain is a strong indicator that the patient is not experiencing an acute MI. Even with a negative cTnI result, symptoms of chest pain still indicate that the patient should have a comprehensive cardiac evaluation to determine if there is underlying CAD present that may later lead to complications.[86]

Cardiac biomarkers and reperfusion. Management of STEMI includes opening the coronary artery obstructed by a thrombus and reperfusing the injured area as rapidly as possible. Individuals who have recent onset of chest pain (within 12 hours) are candidates for reperfusion therapies, including fibrinolytic agents ("clot busters") and cardiac catheterization with catheter interventions such as balloon angioplasty, atherectomy, or stent placement. If successful, these interventions may totally abort or limit the amount of cardiac muscle damage, resulting in an early rise and fall of the cardiac biomarkers as illustrated in Figure 12-11 of Chapter 12. After reperfusion, the serum troponin levels rise dramatically and peak early. Cardiac biomarker samples are drawn at admission, before administration of thrombolytic therapy or PCI, and then at 6-hour or 8-hour intervals for 18 to 24 hours to detect any biomarker rise and assess the return of effective myocardial reperfusion. The advent of newer high sensitivity troponin assays will aid in the detection of injury and infraction in acute coronary syndromes.[87]

Natriuretic peptide biomarkers in acute decompensated heart failure. Natriuretic peptides are biomarkers that provide additional information with which to evaluate the breathless patient accurately.[88] It can be difficult to identify whether a patient who has shortness of breath, has a primary pulmonary problem or is exhibiting symptoms of acute decompensated heart failure with pulmonary edema. Cardiac natriuretic peptides are used to help make the correct diagnosis. In decompensated heart failure, the myocytes in the ventricle release B-type natriuretic peptide (BNP) from the ventricles. Two laboratory assays are commercially available: BNP and a different laboratory test to measure the N-Terminal fragment of pro-BNP (NTpro-BNP). BNP has a half-life of about 20 minutes, whereas NTpro-BNP has a longer half-life of 1 to 2 hours. The choice of test is generally dependent on what is available in the hospital. A BNP point of care test is also available.

The greater the ventricular wall stress, the higher the BNP level rises. The BNP value is combined with the physical examination, the 12-lead ECG, and a chest radiograph to increase the accuracy of heart failure diagnosis (Figure 11-49). A symptomatic patient with a BNP level below 100 pg/mL or an NTpro-BNP below 300 pg/ml is unlikely to be in heart failure, with only a 10% likelihood.[88] Conversely, a patient with a BNP level above 400 pg/dL is almost definitely in decompensated heart failure.[88] BNP is an excellent test to rule out a diagnosis of acute decompensated heart failure.[88] The challenge lies in interpreting the results of patients with a BNP level between 100 and 400 pg/mL, sometimes described as the *gray zone.*[88] This highlights the importance of using a spectrum of clinical and diagnostic tests. As the symptoms of decompensated heart failure are successfully treated, the BNP level usually decreases toward the normal range.

There are some caveats to the use of naturetic peptides as biomarkers, principally because they are not unique to the heart. Naturetic peptides are also released from the endothelium and from the kidney, and this can alter the measured BNP levels. Filtration by the kidney is one of the mechanisms by which BNP is cleared from the bloodstream. BNP levels are higher in patients with kidney failure, especially if the glomerular filtration rate (GFR) is below 60 mL/min/1.7 m^2.[88] BNP levels can also be elevated in septic shock, possibly because of endothelial natriuretic peptide release or myocardial damage.

Conditions such as mitral stenosis that cause pulmonary edema but protect the left ventricle are associated with lower BNP levels than expected from the clinical picture. Even with these caveats, the BNP remains an extremely useful test for the diagnosis of acute decompensated heart failure.

Hematologic Studies

Hematologic laboratory studies that are routinely ordered for the management of patients with altered cardiovascular status are red blood cell (RBC) or erythrocyte level, hemoglobin level, hematocrit level, and white blood cell (WBC) or leukocyte level.

Red blood cells. The normal amount of RBCs in a person varies with age, gender, environmental temperature, altitude, and exercise. Men produce 4.5 to 6 million RBCs/mm^3, whereas the normal level for women is 4 to 5.5 million/mm^3.

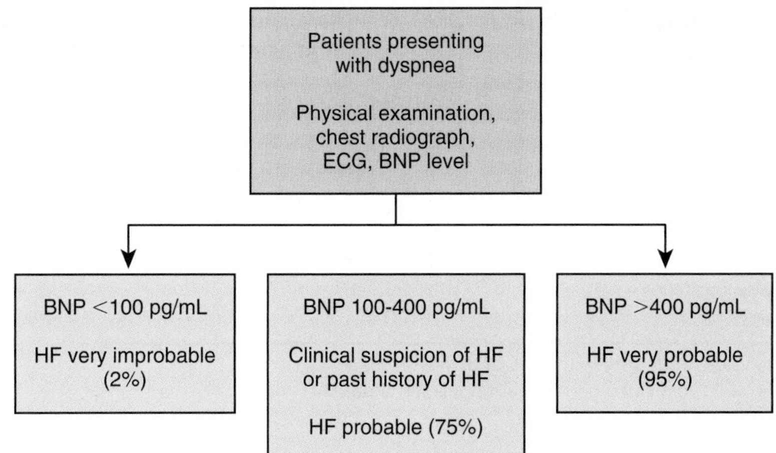

FIG 11-49 The B-Type Natriuretic Peptide (BNP) Algorithm in the Diagnosis of Acute Heart Failure.

Anemia is the clinical condition that occurs when not enough red blood cells are available to carry oxygen to the tissues. *Polycythemia* is the condition that occurs when excess RBCs are produced.

Hemoglobin. Hemoglobin levels normally range from 14 to 18 g/dL in men and from 12 to 16 g/dL in women.

Hematocrit. The hematocrit is the volume percentage of RBCs in whole blood. The value is 40% to 54% for men and 38% to 48% for women.

White blood cells. Most inflammatory processes that produce necrotic tissue within the heart muscle, such as rheumatic fever, endocarditis, and MI, increase the WBC level. WBCs are also known as leukocytes, and a WBC test may be called a serum leukocyte count. The normal WBC level for both men and women is 5000 to 10,000 cells/mm^3. The WBC level also increases in response to infection.

Platelets. The normal platelet count is 150,000 to 400,000 cells/mm^3. Less commonly, the normal platelet count range will be written as 150 to 400 × 10^9/L. Normally, the platelet count is the only laboratory value that is reported. Unfortunately, there is no routine test available for critical care patients that can evaluate platelet functionality. Platelets are important because they are the first cells to be activated when the coagulation system is stimulated. Many medications inhibit platelet function and make the platelets "slippery" so that they do not clump together to activate the clotting process. Sometimes, the anti-platelet action of a medication is its intended role, such as with aspirin used to prevent acute coronary syndrome, and it can be an unintended side effect. A low platelet count is termed *thrombocytopenia.*

Blood Coagulation Studies

Coagulation studies are ordered to determine blood-clotting effectiveness. Anticoagulants—most notably heparin, direct thrombin inhibitors, warfarin, and platelet inhibitory agents—are administered daily in critical care units for many clinical reasons.[89,90] It is essential to understand the laboratory tests that are used to monitor the effectiveness of therapeutic anticoagulation.

Prothrombin time. Most coagulation study results are reported as the length of time in seconds it takes for blood to form a clot in the laboratory test tube. The *prothrombin time* (PT) is no longer directly used to determine the therapeutic dosage of warfarin (Coumadin) necessary to achieve anticoagulation. The PT is not standardized between laboratories, so the result of this test is always reported as a standardized *international normalized ratio* (INR).

International normalized ratio. The INR was developed by the World Health Organization (WHO) in 1982 to standardize PT results among clinical laboratories worldwide. Table 11-14 shows target INR ranges for different cardiovascular conditions that require anticoagulation. A target INR of 2.5 (range 2.0 to 3.0) is desirable.[91,92]

When a patient is first started on warfarin, it is important to know that it can take 72 hours or more to achieve a therapeutic level of anticoagulation. This is because the half-life of prothrombin is between 36 and 42 hours.[91] This delay in anticoagulation effectiveness also occurs if a patient is being converted from heparin-based anticoagulation—monitored by *activated partial thromboplastin* time (aPTT)—to warfarin-based anticoagulation (monitored by INR). To ensure a safe transition, a period of 48 to 72 hours is required in order to obtain a therapeutic INR value before the heparin is discontinued.

Activated partial thromboplastin time. The aPTT is used to measure the effectiveness of intravenous or subcutaneous ultrafractionated heparin (UFH) therapy. Coagulation monitoring is required with UFH, although not with subcutaneous low-molecular-weight heparin (LMWH), because of lower levels of plasma protein binding. In cases of over-anticoagulation with heparin, the antidote is protamine sulfate.

Anti-factor Xa assay of heparin activity. Some critical care units monitor heparin activity directly using the anti-Factor Xa assay. This is currently the only test available to monitor the anticoagulant effects of LMWH and the newer antithrombotic medications.[92,93]

Activated coagulation time. An additional test of heparin effect is the *activated coagulation time* (ACT) also known as the *activated clotting time.* The ACT is a *point of care test* that is performed outside of the laboratory setting in areas such as the cardiac catheterization laboratory, the operating room, or critical care units. Normal and therapeutic values for these coagulation studies are shown in Table 11-14.

TABLE 11-14 Normal and Therapeutic Coagulation Values

TEST	CLINICAL CONDITION	NORMAL VALUE	THERAPEUTIC ANTICOAGULANT TARGET VALUE
INR	Normal coagulation	<1.0	
INR	Atrial fibrillation		2.0-3.0
INR	Treatment of DVT/PE		2.0-3.0
INR	Mechanical heart valves		2.0-3.0
aPTT	Normal coagulation	28-38 sec	1.5-2.5 × normal
PTT	Normal coagulation	60-90 sec	1.5-2.0 × normal
ACT*	Normal coagulation	0-120 sec	150-300 sec

*ACT is normal, but therapeutic values may vary with type of activator used.
ACT, activated coagulation time; aPPT, activated partial thromboplastin time; DVT, deep vein thrombosis; INR, international normalized ratio; PE, pulmonary embolism; PTT, partial thromboplastin time.

Serum Lipid Studies

Four primary blood lipid levels are important in evaluating an individual's risk of developing atherosclerotic cardiovascular disease: total cholesterol, low-density lipoprotein cholesterol (LDL-C), high-density lipoprotein cholesterol (HDLC), and triglycerides. Elevation of LDL-C and triglycerides increases risk. High levels of HDL-C lowers risk of atherosclerotic disease. Risk factor interventions include diet therapy, exercise, and lipid-lowering medications.

Prior clinical guidelines focused on reduction and maintenance of lipid levels below specific thresholds are listed in Table 11-15.[94,95,96] Recently published clinical guidelines focus on the use of statin medications to lower cholesterol levels.[97]

TABLE 11-15 Desirable Lipid Levels

LIPID	DESIRABLE LEVEL
Total cholesterol	<200 mg/dL
	<130 mg/dL without CAD
LDL-C	<100 mg/dL with CAD but not considered high risk
	<70 mg/dL with CAD and considered at high risk for future coronary events
Triglycerides	<150 mg/dL
HDL-C	>40 mg/dL (male)
	>50 mg/dL (female)

Data from the Executive Summary of the Third Report of the National Cholesterol Education Program (NCEP) Expert Panel on Detection, Evaluation, and Treatment of High Blood Cholesterol in Adults (Adult Treatment Panel III), *JAMA* 285(19): 2486-2497, 2001; Grundy SM, et al. Implications of recent clinical trials for the national Cholesterol Education Program (NCEP) Adult Treatment Panel III (ATP III) Guidelines, *Circulation* 110: 227-239, 2004.
CAD, coronary artery disease; HDL-C, high-density lipoprotein cholesterol; LDL-C, low-density lipoprotein cholesterol.

DIAGNOSTIC PROCEDURES

Cardiac Catheterization and Coronary Arteriography

Cardiac catheterization and coronary arteriography are routine diagnostic procedures for patients with known or suspected heart disease. Clinical indications for cardiac catheterization include myocardial ischemia, unstable angina, evolving MI, heart failure with a history that suggests CAD or valvular heart disease, and congenital heart disease. Cardiac catheterization is used to confirm physical findings and to provide a baseline for medical or surgical therapy.[97]

Left-Heart Cardiac Catheterization

During catheterization of the left side of the heart, hemodynamic pressure measurements are taken in the aortic root, the left ventricle, and the left atrium. Radiopaque contrast (dye) is used to visualize the left ventricle (ventriculogram). This information is also used to calculate the LV ejection fraction. The coronary arteries are visualized, and contrast dye is injected directly into each arterial system. The general term for vessel imaging is *angiogram* (veins and arteries), but the more specific term used to describe the visualization of the coronary arteries is *arteriogram.*

Right-Heart Cardiac Catheterization

Catheterization of the right side of the heart is performed using a thermodilution PA catheter. Information obtained includes hemodynamic pressure measurements in the right atrium, the right ventricle, the pulmonary artery, and the pulmonary artery occlusion wedge position, as well as the measurement of cardiac output, calculated hemodynamic values, and oxygen saturations and an angiogram of the right-heart chambers using radiopaque contrast.

Procedure

Before the catheterization, the patient meets with the cardiologist to discuss the purpose, benefit, and risks of the study. For many patients, cardiac catheterization is the first major invasive procedure after a diagnosis of possible heart disease. The patient is often very anxious and has many questions. It is important that nursing and medical staff fully answer patients' questions about the catheterization experience.

The morning of the procedure the patient fasts except for ingesting prescribed cardiac medications. Light premedication is given before the patient goes to the catheterization laboratory. If there is a history of allergy, an antihistamine or corticosteroid may be administered to prevent an anaphylactic reaction to the radiopaque contrast. Throughout the cardiac catheterization, the patient remains awake and alert. He or she is positioned on a hard table with a C-shaped camera arm overhead or to the side. This arm can be positioned to view the heart from several different angles.

Prevention of contrast-induced nephropathy. In patients with an elevated serum creatinine, sodium bicarbonate or normal saline will be administered to protect the kidneys from the damaging effects of the contrast medium.[98] N-acetylcysteine has not been shown to be effective.[98] Up to 10% of acute kidney injury in the hospital occurs as a result of procedures that use IV contrast.[99]

Cardiac catheterization catheters, available in a variety of designs and sizes, are placed in the femoral vein and artery after the patient receives a local anesthetic. The choice of catheters is based on the cardiologist's experience and the diagnostic study required. The femoral artery is used to catheterize the left side of the heart, including the coronary arteries. The femoral vein is frequently used as the access vessel to pass catheters to the right side of the heart. During the study, the patient receives heparin systemically to reduce the risk of emboli. Many patients also receive nitroglycerin to control chest pain, particularly when the coronary arteries are full of contrast material during the coronary arteriographic procedure. At this time, the patient may also experience bradycardia or hypotension. To move the contrast dye more quickly and minimize the vagal effect on heart rate and blood pressure, the patient may be asked to cough. If bradycardia persists, atropine or, occasionally, a transvenous pacemaker may be used. If hypotension continues, IV fluids are administered as a bolus. At the end of the study, the femoral catheters are removed from the vessels. After the catheterization, when the patient is stable, the cardiologist meets with the patient and family to discuss the findings and plan of care.

Nursing Management

Nursing priorities for the patient following a cardiac catheterization focus on 1) assessing the femoral arterial access site, 2) assessing peripheral pulses, 3) monitoring rehydration, 4) assessment of chest pain, and 5) providing patient education.

Assessing the femoral arterial access site. After the diagnostic catheters (and the sheaths through which they are inserted) are removed from the femoral artery and vein, pressure is applied to the femoral vessels until bleeding has stopped. After catheterization, the patient remains flat for up to 6 hours (varies by institutional protocol and catheter size) to allow the femoral arterial puncture site to form a stable clot. Most bleeding occurs within the first 2 to 3 hours after the procedure. During this time, the groin site is checked frequently for evidence of bleeding or hematoma. Three methods may be used to control bleeding at the femoral arterial puncture site after catheter or sheath removal. The most basic method is manual pressure, in which a clinician holds pressure directly on the vein or artery until bleeding stops. The second method uses external mechanical compression over the site (C-clamp or Femstop). The third method is for the cardiologist to use an *arteriotomy closure device* at the end of the catheterization procedure. One closure device is designed to suture the artery closed as the sheath is removed; another option is placement of a collagen plug into the track of the sheath insertion site. All of these methods are effective. After routine diagnostic cardiac catheterization procedures, there is no difference in the rate of femoral arterial site complications for the different methods. The patient is asked to lie still and not to bend at the hip. It usually takes about 40 minutes for a stable clot to form, but it can take longer in some patients, including those with a large body surface area.

Sometimes, when the patient needs to void urine, the movement can dislodge the clot. If the patient cannot void in the supine position, a urinary catheter is usually inserted for women, and a condom catheter is used for men.

Assessing peripheral pulses. The peripheral pulses located distal to the arterial access site are monitored closely by the critical care nurse. If the femoral artery has been used, dorsal pedal and posterior tibial pulses are assessed. If an alternative access site such as the radial artery is used, the radial pulse is assessed. Pulses are assessed every 15 minutes for the first hour after the catheterization and every 30 minutes to 1 hour thereafter. The limb corresponding to the catherization site is assessed for changes in color, temperature, pain, or paresthesia to detect early evidence of acute arterial occlusion.

Monitoring rehydration. The patient is encouraged to drink large amounts of clear liquids, and the intravenous fluid rate is increased to 100 mL/hr. Fluid is given for rehydration because the radiopaque contrast acts as an osmotic diuretic. This is also used to prevent *contrast-induced nephropathy* or damage to the kidney from the contrast dye used to visualize the heart structures. Patients who have elevated blood urea nitrogen (BUN) or creatinine levels before catheterization are at risk for acute renal failure from the dye. For these patients, the quantity of contrast material is consciously limited, and fluid boluses are given to preserve kidney function.

Assessing chest pain. The patient is assessed for chest pain after the procedure. Usually, sublingual nitroglycerin is sufficient to relieve the pain, discomfort, or pressure. Not all patients describe their angina as "pain," and many other descriptors such as "pressure" may be used. Patients are encouraged to use the 0-to-10 pain scale to quantify the angina. A 12-lead ECG must be obtained immediately to identify the coronary arteries involved, and the cardiologist is notified. If the chest pain persists, this may indicate that a clot has formed in a coronary artery, and the patient may need to return to the cardiac catheterization laboratory for an interventional cardiology procedure. More information about PCI is provided under "Catheter Interventions for Coronary Artery Disease" in Chapter 13.

Monitoring dysrhythmias. Dysrhythmias are always a concern after an invasive cardiovascular diagnostic procedure. They result from the underlying cardiac disease and the low potassium levels that can occur after excessive diuresis.

Providing patient education. Because of the invasive nature of cardiac catheterization, many patients express considerable anxiety. Relevant information concerns the sensory details of the procedure, such as lying flat and immobile on a hard table for many hours and sometimes experiencing a feeling of warmth when the dye is injected. Pain is uncommon because opiate analgesics and sedative medications are always provided. Information about possible outcomes—positive and negative—and possible complications must be provided to the patient. Postcatheterization requirements such as lying still and drinking large quantities of fluids are explained. The basic information can be provided using written material or online media, but it is vital to individualize the content and answer any specific concerns or questions. Patients are also asked to report any unusual symptoms, such as chest pain or nausea.

There any many other cardiac diagnostic procedures as listed in Table 11-16. It is important to be familiar with the procedures a patient may have had as part of an elective diagnostic workup or emergently in the hospital. This is because, in addition to clinical presentation, hemodynamic monitoring and ECG information diagnostic procedures contribute significantly to the patient's diagnosis and treatment plan. Clinical practice guidelines that discuss cardiovascular diagnostic procedures can be obtained on the websites of many major professional organizations that are listed in the Internet Resources Box 11-17.

TABLE 11-16 Cardiac Diagnostic Procedures

STUDY	EVALUATES	COMMENTS
Aortography	• Aortic valve insufficiency • Aneurysms or dissection of ascending aorta • Coarctation of the aorta • Injuries to the aorta and major branches	• Contrast medium used: check for allergy to iodine, shellfish, dye; ensure hydration following procedure • Monitor for clinical indications of anaphylaxis (e.g., flushing, urticaria, stridor) • Monitor puncture site
Cardiac biopsy	• Effect of cardiotoxic drugs • Evidence of cardiac transplant rejection • Inflammatory heart disease • Tumors • Cardiomyopathy	• Observe closely for signs of cardiac perforation and/or cardiac tamponade

Cardiac catheterization and coronary angiography	• Severity of coronary artery stenosis
	• Cardiac muscle function
	• Pressures within the heart
	• Cardiac output and ejection fraction
	• Blood gas analysis within chambers
	• Allows angioplasty, atherectomy, intracoronary stents, or lasers to reduce coronary artery obstruction
		• Prior to test:
		  • Check for allergy to iodine, shellfish, dye (contrast medium used)
		• After the test:
		  • Ensure hydration following procedure (contrast medium used)
		  • Keep extremity in which catheter was placed immobilized in a straight position for 6-12 hours.
		  • Monitor arterial puncture point for hemorrhage or hematoma; collagen (e.g., AngioSeal) or stitch device (e.g., Perclose) may be used.
		  • Monitor neurovascular status of affected limb.
		  • Note complaints of back pain and vital sign changes (may indicate retroperitoneal hemorrhage).

Chest x-ray	• Cardiac size and shape and chamber size • Abnormalities of the lungs, ribs, pleura, pulmonary vasculature • Presence of pleural effusions • Presence of thoracic aneurysm or calcification of the aorta • Presence and location of catheters, pacemaker and automatic implantable cardiac defibrillator (AICD) leads	• Inquire about possibility of pregnancy.
Computed tomography (CT) Electron beam computerized tomography (EBCT): high-speed imaging provides improved view of vascular structures including calcification	• Left ventricular wall motion • Cardiac tumors • Myocardial infarction • Pericardial effusion • Aortic aneurysm • Aortic dissection	• May be done with or without contrast medium • If contrast medium used: check for allergy to iodine, shellfish, dye; ensure hydration following procedure.
Digital subtraction angiography	• Vascular disease and degree of occlusion	• Contrast medium used: check for allergy to iodine, shellfish, dye; ensure hydration following procedure. • Monitor for clinical indications of anaphylaxis (e.g., flushing, urticaria, stridor). • Monitor puncture site.

TABLE 11-16 Cardiac Diagnostic Procedures—cont'd

STUDY	EVALUATES	COMMENTS
Doppler ultrasonography Duplex ultrasonography	• Vascular disease and degree of occlusion	

Echocardiography
• M-mode: single ultrasound beam
• 2-D: planar ultrasound beam; wider view of heart and structures
• Doppler: addition of Doppler to demonstrate flow of blood through the heart
• Color flow: Doppler blood flow superimposed on 2-D echocardiogram
• Stress echocardiography: images before, during, and after exercise or pharmacologic stress
• Transesophageal echocardiography (TEE): transducer placed in esophagus
	• Chamber size and wall thickness
	• Valve functioning
	  • Papillary muscle functioning
	  • Prosthetic valve functioning
	• Ventricular wall motion abnormalities
	• Intracardiac masses
	• Presence of pericardial fluid
	• Intracardiac pressures (Doppler)
	• Ejection fraction and cardiac output (Doppler)
	• Valve gradients (Doppler)
	• Intracardiac shunts (Doppler)
	• Thoracic aneurysm (transesophageal)
		• Transesophageal echocardiography is particularly better if patient is obese, has COPD, chest wall deformity, chest trauma, or thick chest dressings.
		• Monitor for methemoglobinemia if local anesthetic (e.g., Cetacaine) is used.
		• If TEE, monitor for clinical indications of esophageal perforation (i.e., sore throat, dysphagia, epigastric or substernal pain).

Electrocardiography (ECG)	• Dysrhythmias • Conduction defects including intraventricular blocks • Electrolyte imbalance • Drug toxicity • Myocardial ischemia, injury, infarction • Chamber hypertrophy	• List what drugs the patient is receiving on ECG request. • Be alert to electrical safety hazards.
Electrophysiologic studies (EPS)	• Dysrhythmias under controlled circumstances • Best therapy for control of dysrhythmia: drug, required dosage of therapy; pacemaker; catheter ablation	• Patients may have near-death experience during EPS; encourage expression of fears, concerns, anxieties. • Monitor puncture site.
Holter monitor	• Suspected dysrhythmias over 24-48 hour period • Pacemaker function • Silent ischemia	• Instruct patient regarding importance of diary-keeping.
Intravascular ultrasound (IVUS)	• Coronary artery size and patency • Structure of vessel wall • Coronary artery stent position and patency • Aorta and presence of aneurysm, aneurysm dissections	• As for cardiac catheterization
Magnetic resonance imaging (MRI)	• Three-dimensional view of the heart • Anatomy and structure of the heart and great vessels including cardiomyopathy, congenital defect, masses, aneurysm • Changes in chemistry of tissues before structural changes occur	• Does not involve radiation or dyes • Cannot be used in patients with any implanted metallic device, including pacemakers, implantable defibrillators, metallic heart valves, intracranial aneurysm clips
Multiple-gated acquisition (MUGA) scan (radionuclide angiography)	• Ventricular size and ventricular wall motion • Cardiac output, cardiac index, end-systolic volume, end-diastolic volume, and ejection fraction • Intracardiac shunts	• Assure patient that amount of radioactive material is minimal.

Continued

TABLE 11-16 Cardiac Diagnostic Procedures—cont'd

STUDY	EVALUATES	COMMENTS
Pericardiocentesis and pericardial fluid analysis	• Presence of blood, pus, pathogens, or malignancy • Also used for emergency relief of cardiac tamponade	• Observe closely for signs of cardiac tamponade.

Peripheral angiography	• Atherosclerotic plaques, occlusion, aneurysms, or traumatic injury	• Prior to test:
		  • Contrast medium used: check for allergy to iodine, shellfish, dye.
		• After the test:
		  • Contrast medium used, ensure hydration postprocedure.
		  • Keep extremity in which catheter was placed immobilized in a straight position for 6-12 hours.
		  • Monitor arterial puncture point for hemorrhage or hematoma.
		  • Monitor neurovascular status of affected limb.
		  • Monitor for indications of systemic emboli.

Plethysmography: arterial or venous	*Arterial*
	  • Patency of peripheral arteries and presence of occlusive vascular disease
	Venous
	  • Patency of peripheral venous system and presence of deep vein thrombosis
		• Requires one normal extremity since one extremity is compared to the other

Positron emission tomography (cardiac PET scan)	• Severity of coronary artery stenosis • Collateral circulation • Patency of bypass grafts • Size and location of infarcted tissue	• Assure patient that amount of radioactive material is minimal.
Sestamibi exercise testing and scan Sestamibi-dipyridamole stress test (for patients with physical limitation preventing exercise)	• Myocardial ischemia during exercise (ischemic areas show increased uptake of radioactivity [hot spots])	• Monitor for myocardial ischemia.
Signal-averaged ECG	• Presence of late electrical potentials which may be responsible for malignant ventricular dysrhythmias; may be performed before and after ablation	• Patient must lie still for 10 minutes.
Stress electrocardiography (also referred to as *Exercise Tolerance Test* [ETT])	• Persons with high risk for CAD, patients with known CAD, or post-CABG patients for ischemia with exercise or pharmacologic agents (e.g., adenosine, dipyridamole, dobutamine) if patient cannot tolerate exercise • Exercise-induced dysrhythmias	• One millimeter or greater transient ST segment depression 80 msec after the J point is suggestive of CAD. • Monitor closely for exercise-induced hypotension or ventricular dysrhythmias. • Adenosine is the preferred agent for pharmacologic stress test because it has a short half-life and does not require reversal agent.
Technetium-99 pyrophosphate scan	• Size, location of acute MI (infarcted areas show increased uptake of radioactivity ["hot spots"] 1-7 days after MI)	• Assure patient that amount of radioactive material is minimal. • Peak accuracy at 12-48 hours after initial symptoms
Thallium stress electrocardiography	• Myocardial ischemia during exercise (ischemic areas show decreased uptake of radioactivity [cold spots])	• Assure patient that amount of radioactive material is minimal.
Thallium-201 scan	• Myocardial ischemia (ischemic areas show decreased uptake of radioactivity [cold spots])	• Assure patient that amount of radioactive material is minimal.

TABLE 11-16 Cardiac Diagnostic Procedures—cont'd

STUDY	EVALUATES	COMMENTS
Vectorcardiography	• Chamber hypertrophy • Bundle branch blocks and hemiblocks • Myocardial ischemia or infarction	
Venography (ascending contrast phlebography)	• Deep leg veins • Presence of deep vein thrombosis (DVT) • Competence of deep vein valves • May be used to locate suitable vein for arterial bypass graft	• Contrast medium used: check for allergy to iodine, shellfish, contrast dye; ensure hydration postprocedure. • Monitor for clinical indications of anaphylaxis (e.g., flushing, urticaria, stridor). • Monitor puncture site.
Ventriculography	• Ventricular wall motion • Wall thickness • Ventricular aneurysm • Mitral valve motion • LV end-diastolic volume, end-systolic volume, stroke volume, ejection fraction • Intracardiac shunt	• Contrast medium used: check for allergy to iodine, shellfish, contrast dye; ensure hydration postprocedure. • Monitor for clinical indications of anaphylaxis (e.g., flushing, urticaria, stridor). • Monitor puncture site.

From Dennison RD. *Pass CCRN!*, ed 4, St Louis, 2013, Mosby.
MI, Myocardial infarction; *2D*, two-dimensional; *TEE*, transesophageal echocardiography; *COPD*, chronic obstructive pulmonary disease; *CAD*, coronary artery disease; *DVT*, deep vein thrombosis.

BOX 11-17 INTERNET RESOURCES FOR CARDIAC ASSESSMENT & DIAGNOSTIC PROCEDURES

AACN	American Association of Critical Care Nurses	http://www.aacn.org/
ACC	American College of Cardiology: AHA/ACC statements and guidelines can be accessed from this page	http://www.cardiosource.org/ACC.aspx
AHA	American Heart Association (for professionals)	http://my.americanheart.org/professional/index.jsp
AHA	American Heart Association (for patients)	http://www.heart.org/HEARTORG/
AHA	American Heart Association (professional journals) AHA/ACC statements and guidelines can be accessed from this page	http://www.ahajournals.org
HFSA	Heart Failure Society of America	http://www.hfsa.org/

REFERENCES

1. Conn RD, O'Keefe JH: Cardiac Physical Diagnosis in the Digital Age: An Important but Increasingly Neglected Skill (from Stethoscopes to Microchips), *Am J Cardiol* 104:590–595, 2009.
2. Amsterdam EA, et al: Testing of low-risk patients presenting to the Emergency Department with chest pain: A scientific statement from the American Heart Association, *Circulation* 122:1756–1776, 2010.
3. Chun AA, McGee SR: Bedside diagnosis of coronary artery disease: a systematic review, *Am J Med* 117(5):334–343, 2004.
4. Cornier MA, et al: Assessing Adiposity: A Scientific Statement From the American Heart Association, *Circulation* 124:1996–2019, 2011.
5. Tully AS, Trayes KP, Suddiford JS: Evaluation of Nail Abnormalities, *Am Fam Physician* 85(8):779–787, 2012.
6. Marrie TJ, Brown N: Clubbing of the digits, *Am J Med* 120(11):940–941, 2007.
7. Spicknall KE, Zirwas MJ, English JC 3rd.: Clubbing: an update on diagnosis, differential diagnosis, pathophysiology, and clinical relevance, *J Am Acad Dermatol* 52(6):1020–1028, 2005.
8. Hirsch AT, et al: A Call to Action: Women and Peripheral Artery Disease: A Scientific Statement From the American Heart Association, *Circulation* 125:1449–1472, 2012.
9. Jolobe O: Disproportionate elevation of jugular venous pressure in pleural effusion, *Br J Hosp Med* 72(10):582–585, 2011.
10. Ferrante G, Pugliese F, Di Mario C: Jugular venous pressure: a cardinal sign, *Lancet* 376(9743):802, 2010.
11. Wiese J: The abdominojugular reflux sign, *Am J Med* 109(1):59–61, 2000.
12. Lewin J, Maconochie I: Capillary refill time in adults, *Emerg Med J* 25(6):325–326, 2008.
13. James PA, et al: 2014 Evidence-based guideline for the management of high blood pressure in adults: report from the panel members appointed to the Eighth Joint National Committee (JNC 8), *JAMA* 311(5):507–520, 2014.
14. Naschitz JE, Rosner I: Orthostatic hypotension: framework of the syndrome, *Postgrad Med J* 83(983):568–574, 2007.
15. Stewart JM: Mechanisms of Sympathetic Regulation in Orthostatic Intolerance, *J Appl Physiol* 113(10):1659–1668, 2012.
16. Swami A, Spodick DH: Pulsus paradoxus in cardiac tamponade: a pathophysiologic continuum, *Clin Cardiol* 26(5):215–217, 2003.

17. Stone MK, Bauch TD, Rubal BJ: Respiratory changes in the pulse-oximetry waveform associated with pericardial tamponade, *Clin Cardiol* 29(9):411–414, 2006.
18. Wu LA, Nishimura RA: Images in clinical medicine. Pulsus paradoxus, *N Engl J Med* 349(7):666, 2003.
19. Treadway K: Heart sounds, *N Engl J Med* 354(11):1112–1113, 2006.
20. Chizner MA: Cardiac auscultation: rediscovering the lost art, *Curr Probl Cardiol* 33(7):326–408, 2008.
21. Barrett MJ, et al: Mastering cardiac murmurs: the power of repetition, *Chest* 126(2):470–475, 2004.
22. Johnston M, Collins SP, Storrow AB: The Third Heart Sound for Diagnosis of Acute Heart Failure, *Curr Heart Fail Rep* 4(3):164–169, 2007.
23. Gupta S, Michaels AD: Relationship Between Accurate Auscultation of the Fourth Heart Sound and the Level of Physician Experience, *Clin Cardiol* 32(2):69–75, 2009.
24. Nishimura RA, et al: 2014 AHA/ACC Guideline for the Management of Patients With Valvular Heart Disease: A Report of the American College of Cardiology/American Heart Association Task Force on Practice Guidelines, *Circulation* 129(23):e521–e643, 2014.
25. Khandaker MH, et al: Pericardial Disease: Diagnosis and Management, *Mayo Clin Proc* 85(6):572–593, 2010.
26. Mitchell MD, et al: Heparin flushing and other interventions to maintain patency of central venous catheters: a systematic review, *J Adv Nurs* 65(10):2007–2021, 2009.
27. Brzezinski M, Luisetti T, London MJ: Radial artery cannulation: a comprehensive review of recent anatomic and physiologic investigations, *Anesth Analg* 109(6):1763–1781, 2009.
28. Linkins LA, et al: Treatment and prevention of heparin-induced thrombocytopenia: Antithrombotic Therapy and Prevention of Thrombosis, 9th ed: American College of Chest Physicians Evidence-Based Clinical Practice Guidelines, *Chest* 141(2 Suppl):e495S–530S, 2012.
29. O'Grady NP, et al: Guidelines for the prevention of intravascular catheter-related infections, *Am J Infect Control* 39(4 Suppl 1):S1–S34, 2011.
30. Pulmonary Artery Pressure Monitoring: AACN Practice Alert. Practice Alerts 12-2009. www.aacn.org. Accessed August 2014.
31. Lucet JC, et al: Infectious risk associated with arterial catheters compared with central venous catheters, *Crit Care Med* 38(4):1030–1035, 2010.
32. Maddukuri P, et al: Echocardiographic diagnosis of air embolism associated with central venous catheter placement: case report and review of the literature, *Echocardiography* 23(4):315–318, 2006.
33. Deceuninck O, et al: Images in cardiovascular medicine. Massive air embolism after central venous catheter removal, *Circulation* 116(19):e516–e518, 2007.
34. Clark DK, Plaizier E: Devastating cerebral air embolism after central line removal, *J Neurosci Nurs* 43(4):193–196, quiz 197–198, 2011.
35. Wang AZ, et al: The Differences Between Venous Air Embolism and Fat Embolism in Routine Intraoperative Monitoring Methods, Transesophageal Echocardiography, and Fatal Volume in Pigs, *J Trauma* 65(2):416–423, 2008.
36. Collyer TC, Yates DR, Bellamy MC: Severe air embolism resulting from a perforated cap on a high-flow three-way stopcock connected to a central venous catheter, *Eur J Anaesthesiol* 24(5):474–475, 2007.
37. Sinno MC, Alam M: Echocardiographically detected fibrinous sheaths associated with central venous catheters, *Echocardiography* 29(3):E56–E59, 2012.
38. Sona C, Prentice D, Schallom L: National survey of central venous catheter flushing in the intensive care unit, *Crit Care Nurse* 32(1):e12–e19, 2012.
39. Schallom ME, et al: Heparin or 0.9% sodium chloride to maintain central venous catheter patency: A randomized trial, *Crit Care Med* 40(6):1820–1826, 2012.
40. Timsit JF, et al: A multicentre analysis of catheter-related infection based on a hierarchical model, *Intensive Care Med* 38(10):1662–1672, 2012.
41. Marik PE, Baram M, Vahid B: Does central venous pressure predict fluid responsiveness? A systematic review of the literature and the tale of seven mares, *Chest* 134(1):172–178, 2008.
42. Kupchik N, Bridges E: Critical analysis, critical care: central venous pressure monitoring: what's the evidence?, *Am J Nurs* 112(1):58–61, 2012.
43. Lakhal K, et al: Central venous pressure measurements improve the accuracy of leg raising-induced change in pulse pressure to predict fluid responsiveness, *Intensive Care Med* 36(6):940–948, 2010.
44. Christensen M: Mixed venous oxygen saturation monitoring revisited: Thoughts for critical care nursing practice, *Aust Crit Care* 25(2):78–90, 2012.
45. Richard C, et al: Early use of the pulmonary artery catheter and outcomes in patients with shock and acute respiratory distress syndrome: a randomized controlled trial, *JAMA* 290(20):2713–2720, 2003.
46. Wheeler AP, et al: Pulmonary-artery versus central venous catheter to guide treatment of acute lung injury, *N Engl J Med* 354(21):2213–2224, 2006.
47. Binanay C, et al: Evaluation study of congestive heart failure and pulmonary artery catheterization effectiveness: the ESCAPE trial, *JAMA* 294(13):1625–1633, 2005.
48. Harvey SE, et al: Post hoc insights from PAC-Man—the U.K. pulmonary artery catheter trial, *Crit Care Med* 36(6):1714–1721, 2008.
49. Sandham JD, et al: A randomized, controlled trial of the use of pulmonary-artery catheters in high-risk surgical patients, *N Engl J Med* 348(1):5–14, 2003.
50. Harvey S, et al: Pulmonary artery catheters for adult patients in intensive care, *Cochrane Database Syst Rev* (3):CD003408, 2006.
51. Shah MR, et al: Impact of the pulmonary artery catheter in critically ill patients: meta-analysis of randomized clinical trials, *JAMA* 294(13):1664–1670, 2005.
52. Wiener RS, Welch HG: Trends in the use of the pulmonary artery catheter in the United States, 1993-2004, *JAMA* 298(4):423–429, 2007.
53. Koo KK, et al: Pulmonary artery catheters: evolving rates and reasons for use, *Crit Care Med* 39(7):1613–1618, 2011.
54. Richard C, Monnet X, Teboul JL: Pulmonary artery catheter monitoring in 2011, *Curr Opin Crit Care* 17(3):296–302, 2011.
55. Kahwash R, Leier CV, Miller L: Role of the pulmonary artery catheter in diagnosis and management of heart failure, *Cardiol Clin* 29(2):281–288, 2011.

56. Headley J: Pulmonary Artery Catheters and Assessment of Pulmonary Artery Wedge Pressure, *Crit Care Nurse* 34:85–86, 2014.
57. Shepherd SJ, Pearse RM: Role of central and mixed venous oxygen saturation measurement in perioperative care, *Anesthesiology* 111(3):649, 2009.
58. Dellinger RP, et al: Surviving sepsis campaign: international guidelines for management of severe sepsis and septic shock: 2012, *Crit Care Med* 41(2):580–637, 2013.
59. ProCESS Investigators, Yealy DM, et al: A randomized trial of protocol-based care for early septic shock, *N Engl J Med* 370(18):1683–1693, 2014.
60. ST segment monitoring: AACN Practice Alert. 5/2009. Accessed August 2014 from: www.aacn.org.
61. Drew BJ, et al: Practice standards for electrocardiographic monitoring in hospital settings: an American Heart Association scientific statement from the Councils on Cardiovascular Nursing, Clinical Cardiology, and Cardiovascular Disease in the Young: endorsed by the International Society of Computerized Electrocardiology and the American Association of Critical-Care Nurses, *Circulation* 110(17):2721–2746, 2004.
62. Drew BJ, Funk M: Practice standards for ECG monitoring in hospital settings: executive summary and guide for implementation, *Crit Care Nurs Clin North Am* 18(2):157–168, 2006.
63. Muzyk AJ, et al: Examination of Baseline Risk Factors for QTc Interval Prolongation in Patients Prescribed Intravenous Haloperidol, *Drug Saf* 35(7):547–553, 2012.
64. Drew BJ, et al: Prevention of torsade de pointes in hospital settings: a scientific statement from the American Heart Association and the American College of Cardiology Foundation, *Circulation* 121(8):1047–1060, 2010.
65. Conti CR, Bavry AA, Petersen JW: Silent ischemia: clinical relevance, *J Am Coll Cardiol* 59(5):435–441, 2012.
66. Wagner GS, et al: AHA/ACCF/HRS recommendations for the standardization and interpretation of the electrocardiogram: part VI: acute ischemia/infarction: a scientific statement from the American Heart Association Electrocardiography and Arrhythmias Committee, Council on Clinical Cardiology; the American College of Cardiology Foundation; and the Heart Rhythm Society: endorsed by the International Society for Computerized Electrocardiology, *Circulation* 119(10):e262–e270, 2009.
67. Surawicz B, et al: AHA/ACCF/HRS recommendations for the standardization and interpretation of the electrocardiogram: part III: intraventricular conduction disturbances: a scientific statement from the American Heart Association Electrocardiography and Arrhythmias Committee, Council on Clinical Cardiology; the American College of Cardiology Foundation; and the Heart Rhythm Society: endorsed by the International Society for Computerized Electrocardiology, *Circulation* 119(10):e235–e240, 2009.
68. Blomstrom-Lundqvist C, et al: ACC/AHA/ESC guidelines for the management of patients with supraventricular arrhythmias–executive summary. a report of the American college of cardiology/American heart association task force on practice guidelines and the European society of cardiology committee for practice guidelines (writing committee to develop guidelines for the management of patients with supraventricular arrhythmias) developed in collaboration with NASPE-Heart Rhythm Society, *J Am Coll Cardiol* 42(8):1493–1531, 2003.
69. January CT, et al: 2014 AHA/ACC/HRS Guideline for the Management of Patients With Atrial Fibrillation: A Report of the American College of Cardiology/American Heart Association Task Force on Practice Guidelines and the Heart Rhythm Society, *Circulation* 129, 2014. [Epub ahead of print].
70. Camm AJ, et al: Guidelines for the management of atrial fibrillation: the Task Force for the Management of Atrial Fibrillation of the European Society of Cardiology (ESC), *Eur Heart J* 31(19):2369–2429, 2010.
71. Schneeweiss S, et al: Comparative efficacy and safety of new oral anticoagulants in patients with atrial fibrillation, *Circ Cardiovasc Qual Outcomes* 5(4):480–486, 2012.
72. You JJ, et al: Antithrombotic therapy for atrial fibrillation: Antithrombotic Therapy and Prevention of Thrombosis, 9th ed: American College of Chest Physicians Evidence-Based Clinical Practice Guidelines, *Chest* 141(2 Suppl):e531S–575S, 2012.
73. Connolly SJ, et al: Dabigatran versus warfarin in patients with atrial fibrillation, *N Eng J Med* 361(12):1139–1151, 2009.
74. Patel MR, et al: Rivaroxaban versus warfarin in nonvalvular atrial fibrillation, *N Eng J Med* 365(10):883–891, 2011.
75. Granger CB, et al: Apixaban versus warfarin in patients with atrial fibrillation, *N Eng J Med* 365(11):981–992, 2011.
76. Ganesan AN, et al: Long-term outcomes of catheter ablation of atrial fibrillation: a systematic review and meta-analysis, *J Am Heart Assoc* 2(2):e004549, 2013.
77. Calkins H: Catheter ablation to maintain sinus rhythm, *Circulation* 125(11):1439–1445, 2012.
78. Freeman K, et al: Effects of presentation and electrocardiogram on time to treatment of hyperkalemia, *Acad Emerg Med* 15(3):239–249, 2008.
79. Montague BT, Ouellette JR, Buller GK: Retrospective Review of the Frequency of ECG Changes in Hyperkalemia, *Clin J Am Soc Nephrol* 3:324–330, 2008.
80. El-Sherif N, Turitto G: Electrolyte disorders and arrhythmogenesis, *Cardiol J* 18(3):233–245, 2011.
81. Kelly A, Levine MA: Hypocalcemia in the Critically Ill patient, *J Intensive Care Med* 28(3):166–177, 2013.
82. Chang WT, Radin B, McCurdy MT: Calcium, magnesium, and phosphate abnormalities in the emergency department, *Emerg Med Clin North Am* 32(2):349–366, 2014.
83. Buckley MS, LeBlanc JM, Cawley MJ: Electrolyte disturbances associated with commonly prescribed medications in the intensive care unit, *Crit Care Med* 38(Suppl):S253–S264, 2010.
84. Noronha JL, Matuschak GM: Magnesium in critical illness: metabolism, assessment, and treatment, *Intensive Care Med* 28(6):667–679, 2002.
85. Neumar RW, et al: Part 8: adult advanced cardiovascular life support: 2010 American Heart Association Guidelines for Cardiopulmonary Resuscitation and Emergency Cardiovascular Care, *Circulation* 122(18 Suppl 3):S729–S767, 2010.
86. Patil H, Vaidya O, Bogart D: A Review of Causes and Systemic Approach to Cardiac Troponin Elevation, *Clin Cardiol* 34(12):723–728, 2011.
87. de Lemos JA: Increasingly sensitive assays for cardiac troponins: a review, *JAMA* 309(21):2262–2269, 2013.
88. Maisel AS, Daniels LB: Breathing Not Properly 10 Years Later: What We Have Learned and What We Still Need to Learn, *J Am Coll Cardiol* 60(4):277–282, 2012.

89. Holbrook A, et al: Evidence-based management of anticoagulant therapy: Antithrombotic Therapy and Prevention of Thrombosis, 9th ed: American College of Chest Physicians Evidence-Based Clinical Practice Guidelines, *Chest* 141(2 Suppl):e152S–184S, 2012.
90. Whitlock RP, et al: Antithrombotic and thrombolytic therapy for valvular disease: Antithrombotic Therapy and Prevention of Thrombosis, 9th ed: American College of Chest Physicians Evidence-Based Clinical Practice Guidelines, *Chest* 141(2 Suppl):e576S–600S, 2012.
91. Douketis JD, et al: Perioperative management of antithrombotic therapy: Antithrombotic Therapy and Prevention of Thrombosis, 9th ed: American College of Chest Physicians Evidence-Based Clinical Practice Guidelines, *Chest* 141(2 Suppl):e326S–350S, 2012.
92. Grundy SM, et al: Implications of recent clinical trials for the National Cholesterol Education Program Adult Treatment Panel III guidelines, *Circulation* 110(2):227–239, 2004.
93. Gehrie E, Laposata M: Test of the month: The chromogenic antifactor Xa assay, *Am J Hematol* 87(2):194–196, 2012.
94. Smith S, et al: AHA/ACCF Secondary Prevention and Risk Reduction Therapy for Patients With Coronary and Other Atherosclerotic Vascular Disease: 2011 Update. A Guideline From the American Heart Association and American College of Cardiology Foundation, *Circulation* 124:2458–2473, 2011.
95. Miller M, et al: Triglycerides and Cardiovascular Disease: A Scientific Statement From the American Heart Association, *Circulation* 123:2292–2333, 2011.
96. Stone NJ, et al: 2013 ACC/AHA guideline on the treatment of blood cholesterol to reduce atherosclerotic cardiovascular risk in adults: a report of the American College of Cardiology/American Heart Association Task Force on Practice Guidelines, *Circulation* 129(25 Suppl 2):S1–S45, 2014.
97. Patel MR, et al: ACCF/SCAI/AATS/AHA/ASE/ASNC/HFSA/HRS/SCCM/SCCT/SCMR/STS 2012 appropriate use criteria for diagnostic catheterization: a report of the American College of Cardiology Foundation Appropriate Use Criteria Task Force, Society for Cardiovascular Angiography and Interventions, American Association for Thoracic Surgery, American Heart Association, American Society of Echocardiography, American Society of Nuclear Cardiology, Heart Failure Society of America, Heart Rhythm Society, Society of Critical Care Medicine, Society of Cardiovascular Computed Tomography, Society for Cardiovascular Magnetic Resonance, and Society of Thoracic Surgeons, *J Am Coll of Cardiol* 59(22):1995–2027, 2012.
98. Stacul F, et al: Contrast induced nephropathy: updated ESUR Contrast Media Safety Committee guidelines, *Eur Radiol* 21(12):2527–2541, 2011.
99. Isaac S: Contrast-induced nephropathy: nursing implications, *Crit Care Nurse* 32(3):41–48, 2012.

CHAPTER 12

Cardiovascular Disorders

Annette Haynes

Cardiovascular disease remains the leading cause of mortality in the United States. In 2010, the overall rate of death attributable to cardiovascular disease (CVD) was 236.6 per 100,000.[1] CVD causes one-third of the deaths in the United States, and 1 in 9 death certificates mentioned heart failure.[1] An understanding of the pathology of CVD processes and clinical management allows the critical care nurse to anticipate and plan interventions accurately. This chapter focuses on cardiac disorders commonly seen in the critical care environment.

CORONARY ARTERY DISEASE

Description and Etiology

The biggest contributor to cardiovascular system–related morbidity and mortality is *coronary artery disease* (CAD). *Atherosclerosis* is a progressive disease that affects arteries throughout the body. In the heart, atherosclerotic changes are clinically known as CAD. This disease process is also known by the term *coronary heart disease* (CHD) because other heart structures ultimately become involved in the disease process. The atherosclerotic vascular changes that lead to CAD may begin in childhood. Research and epidemiologic data collected during the past 50 years have demonstrated a strong association between preventable and nonpreventable risk factors and the development of CAD.[1,2] These risk factors are further delineated as *nonmodifiable* and *modifiable coronary risk factors* (Box 12-1).

Risk Factors for Coronary Artery Disease

Age, Gender, and Race

The severe effects of CAD occur as a person ages. In general, CAD symptoms are seen in persons age 45 years and older.[1] Traditionally, CAD has been regarded as a primarily male disease. Research shows that CAD affects women as well.[1-3] Men typically develop external manifestations of the disease about 5 to 10 years earlier compared with women. The prevalence of cardiovascular disease is higher among women starting at age 75 years.[1-3] CAD rates for postmenopausal women are two to three times higher than those for premenopausal women of the same age.[1]

Family History

A positive family history is one in which a close blood relative has had a myocardial infarction (MI) or stroke before age 60 years. This family history suggests a genetic or lifestyle predisposition to the development of CAD. Individuals with a family history had a 50% greater risk of having an acute MI as demonstrated in the INTERHEART study, a large study that looked at risk factors of patients in 52 countries who experienced an MI.[4]

Hyperlipidemia

Hyperlipidemia is a leading factor responsible for severe atherosclerosis and the development of CAD. Millions of adults above age 20 years have total serum cholesterol levels above 240 milligrams per deciliter (mg/dL). Assessing total serum cholesterol and triglyceride levels is essential to the assessment of cardiovascular risk in patients.[1] A lipid panel blood test will measure the following values:

- High-density lipoprotein (HDL) cholesterol
- Low-density lipoprotein (LDL) cholesterol
- Very-low–density lipoprotein (VLDL) cholesterol
- Triglycerides

New guidelines from the American Heart Association (AHA) and the American College of Cardiology (ACC) focus less on specific lipoprotein target levels and much more on groups of patients known to be at risk, such as those with diabetes.[5] For reference the prior targets for specific serum lipids are listed in Table 12-1.[6]

Total cholesterol. The total cholesterol is the sum of the HDL, LDL, and VLDL cholesterol in the bloodstream. It is used as a starting point for lipid testing. A total cholesterol level higher than 200 mg/dL is an indication to investigate the lipid profile and other risk factors for CAD.[5]

High-density lipoprotein cholesterol. HDL cholesterol is frequently described as the "good cholesterol" because higher serum levels exert a protective effect against acute atherosclerotic events. High HDL cholesterol levels confer antiinflammatory and antioxidant benefits on the arterial wall. HDL cholesterol is generally higher in women, and levels can be raised by physical exercise and by stopping smoking.

Low-density lipoprotein cholesterol. LDL cholesterol is sometimes described as the "bad cholesterol" because high levels are associated with an increased risk of CAD, stroke, and peripheral arterial disease (PAD). High LDL levels in the bloodstream exert an inflammatory effect on the arterial vessel wall. If lifestyle changes are insufficient to reduce the LDL cholesterol level in the bloodstream, the medication category of choice is a statin. Numerous research studies have conclusively demonstrated that lowering the LDL cholesterol with statins for primary or secondary prevention is highly effective in lowering mortality from CAD.[1,3,5,6]

Triglycerides. Triglycerides are serum lipids that constitute an additional atherogenic risk factor. A fasting triglyceride level above 150 mg/dL in adults is considered elevated and is a risk factor for heart disease and stroke. Recent

BOX 12-1 Coronary Artery Disease Risk Factors

Nonmodifiable Risk Factors
- Age
- Gender
- Family history
- Race

Modifiable Risk Factors
- Elevated serum lipids
- Hypertension
- Cigarette smoking
- Prediabetes or diabetes mellitus
- Diet high in saturated fat, cholesterol, and calories
- Elevated homocysteine level
- Metabolic syndrome
- Obesity
- Physical inactivity
- Postmenopause (modification is controversial)

TABLE 12-1 Lipid Guidelines and Risk for Coronary Artery Disease ATP III

Classification of Total, Low-Density Lipoprotein (LDL), and High-Density Lipoprotein (HDL), Cholesterol, and Triglycerides (mg/dL)*

Total Cholesterol	
<200	
200-239	Borderline-high
>240	High
LDL Cholesterol	
<100	Optimal
100-129	Near or above optimal
130-159	Borderline high
160-189	High
>190	Very high
HDL Cholesterol	
<40	Low
>60	High
Triglycerides	
<150	Normal
150-199	Borderline high
200-499	High
>500	Very high

HDL, High-density lipoprotein; *LDL*, low-density lipoprotein; *VLDL*, very–low-density lipoprotein.
*Values outside the target range increase the risk for coronary artery disease.

guidelines suggest that triglyceride levels below 100 mg/dL may be optimal.[7]

Obesity

Obesity is a disease of modern times. A body mass index (BMI) of greater than 30 kilograms per meter squared

BOX 12-2 How to Calculate and Interpret Body Mass Index

Use a Calculator to Determine the Body Mass Index (BMI)

Metric Units: Divide body weight in kilograms by height in meters; divide the result by height in meters:

BMI = $(Weight_{kg}/Height_{m}) \div Height_{m}$

Example: A person weighs 100 kg and is 1.90 m tall:

BMI = 100/1.90 ÷ 1.90 = 27.7

How to Interpret the BMI Result

BMI (KG/M²)	WEIGHT STATUS
<18.5	Underweight
18.5–24.9	Normal weight
25–29.5	Overweight
>30	Obese

(kg/m²) is considered obese. Global estimates are more than 1 billion overweight adults, and at least 300 million of these people are obese. Obesity is often associated with a sedentary lifestyle accompanied by the calories consumed and portion sizes. A high risk of coronary heart disease is among the well-established adverse health effects associated with excess weight. Hypertension, hypercholesterolemia, and diabetes are among the clinical conditions that are important mediators of this association.[1-3] According the Centers for Disease Control and Prevention, 69% of adults in the United States are overweight or obese.[8]

The BMI is a mathematical equation used to assess body weight relative to height. BMI is used to evaluate the threat of excess weight as a risk factor for CAD and permits comparisons of people of different gender, age, height, and body type. BMI is calculated as the weight in kilograms divided by the square of the height in meters (kg/m²), as shown in Box 12-2.

The distribution pattern of body fat is a CAD risk factor. The more fat carried in the abdominal area, indicated by a large waist, the greater is the risk of CAD. Excess abdominal adiposity (apple body shape) indicates additional fat around the abdominal organs compared with individuals who have a smaller waist and larger hips (pear body shape). A waist size greater than 40 inches in men and 35 inches in women increases the risk of CAD.

Physical Activity

Regular vigorous physical activity using large muscle groups promotes physiologic adaptation to aerobic exercise, which can help prevent the development of CAD and reduce symptoms in patients with established cardiovascular disease.[9] Exercise also reduces the incidence of many other diseases, including type 2 diabetes, osteoporosis, obesity, depression, and cancers of the colon and breast.[9] Exercise alters the lipid profile by decreasing cholesterol and triglyceride levels.[9] Exercise reduces insulin resistance at the cellular level, lowering the risk for developing type 2 diabetes, especially if combined with a weight-loss program.[9] Epidemiologic studies indicate that participating in physical athletics in one's youth does not confer protection in later years. A sedentary lifestyle has negative effects, regardless of age, gender, BMI, smoking status, presence or absence of hypertension, or abnormal lipoprotein profile. Lifelong physical activity is necessary to prevent atherosclerotic CAD and stroke.

Hypertension

In the United States, 1 person in 3 has hypertension. Normal blood pressure is described as a systolic blood pressure (SBP) below 120 mm Hg and a diastolic blood pressure (DBP) below 80 mm Hg. Treatment of hypertension is based on the patient's age. Antihypertensive medications are recommended to reduce a SBP greater than 140 mm Hg for patients younger than 40 years of age and to reduce a SBP greater than 150 mm Hg for patients older than 60 years of age. In all ages a DBP below 90 mm Hg is the treatment goal. Patients with kidney failure and/or diabetes should always have a blood pressure below 140/90 mm Hg.[10]

Cigarette Smoking

The greater the number of cigarettes smoked per day, the greater is the risk of developing CAD, acute MI, and stroke.[1] Cigarette smoking unfavorably alters serum lipid levels, decreases HDL cholesterol level, and increases LDL cholesterol and triglyceride levels. Smokers are two to four times more likely to develop CAD compared with nonsmokers.[1]

Diabetes Mellitus

Individuals with diabetes mellitus (types 1 and 2) have a higher incidence of CAD compared with the general population. Elevated blood glucose level is a known risk factor for development of vascular inflammation associated with atherosclerosis. The American Diabetes Association recommends the use of the hemoglobin (Hgb) A_{1C} test and plasma glucose to diagnose diabetes. The A_{1C} threshold is 6.5% or greater.[11] Other diagnostic thresholds are a fasting blood glucose of 126 mg/dL or greater, or 2-hour plasma glucose 200 mg/dL or greater during an oral glucose tolerance test.[11] Or, in a patient with classic symptoms of hyperglycemia, a random plasma glucose above 200 mg/dL signifies diabetes.[11]

A fasting blood glucose concentration between 100 to 125 mg/dL or an A_{1C} of 5.7% to 6.4% represents an increased risk for diabetes (Table 12-2). The upper limit for a normal fasting plasma glucose level is 125 mg/dL.[11] Patients with diabetes have an increased risk of developing CAD.[11]

Chronic Kidney Disease

Chronic kidney disease is considered a risk equivalent for CAD.[1-3,12] This means that patients with chronic kidney disease have as much risk of experiencing a coronary event as if they already had CAD.[1-3,13] The risk of death for the patient with acute MI rises as the serum creatinine level increases.[13]

TABLE 12-2 Fasting Blood Glucose and Risk for Coronary Artery Disease

BLOOD GLUCOSE LEVEL	FASTING PLASMA GLUCOSE LEVEL* (mg/dL)
Normal	70-100
Prediabetes	100-125
Diabetes	126 or higher

CAD, Coronary artery disease.
*Values greater than normal increase the risk for CAD and kidney failure.

Metabolic Syndrome

Metabolic syndrome refers to the clustering of risk factors associated with CVD and type 2 diabetes.[1] About one-third of people in the United States have metabolic syndrome. Any two of the following are risk factors:[1]

- Fasting plasma glucose above 100 mg/dL or taking medications to lower elevated blood glucose
- HDL cholesterol below 40 mg/dL in men and below 50 mg/dL in women or taking medications to raise HDL levels
- Triglycerides above 150 mg/dL or taking medications to lower elevated triglycerides
- Waist circumference above 40 inches (102 cm) in men or above 35 inches (88 cm) in women.
- Blood pressure (BP) above 130 mm Hg systolic or above 85 mm Hg diastolic or taking antihypertensive medications.

Women and Heart Disease

Substantial progress has been made in the awareness, treatment, and prevention of CVD in women[14] Yet, CVD still causes approximately one death per minute among women in the United States.[14] After age 65 years, a higher percentage of women than men have hypertension. Average body weight continues to increase, with nearly 2 out of every 3 women in the United States above age 20 years now being overweight or obese.[14] The incidence of CVD is two to three times higher among postmenopausal women than among women who are premenopausal. Current guidelines do not recommend the use of hormone therapy for primary or secondary prevention of CVD.[14] CVD risk in women is stratified into three categories:

- *At high risk:* documented CAD or CVD risk equivalents, such as the presence of documented CVD, diabetes mellitus, end stage or chronic kidney disease, or 10-year predicted risk for CHD > 20%
- *At risk:* given the presence of subclinical vascular disease or poor exercise tolerance on treadmill testing
- *At optimal risk:* in the setting of a Framingham risk score less than 10%, absence of major CVD risk factors, and engagement in a healthy lifestyle.[1,14]

The American Heart Association (AHA) defined ideal cardiovascular health in women as follows:

- Absence of clinical CVD and the presence of all ideal levels of total cholesterol (<200 mg/dL)
- Blood pressure (<120/80 mm Hg)
- Fasting blood glucose (<100 mg/dL)
- Adherence to healthy behaviors
- Lean body mass index (<25 kg/m^2)
- Participation in physical activity at recommended levels
- Cessation of smoking
- Pursuit of eating pattern as suggested by *Dietary Approaches to Stop Hypertension* (DASH diet)[15]

Cardiovascular disease kills more than 500,000 women annually in the United States. Mortality rates for women after an acute MI are higher than for men: 38% compared with 25%. Risk factors associated with acute MI more strongly in women than in men include hypertension, diabetes mellitus, alcohol intake, and physical inactivity.[14,15] Many reasons contribute to higher mortality from acute MI in women, and these include waiting longer to seek medical care, having smaller coronary arteries, being older when symptoms occur, and experiencing very different symptoms from those of men of the same age.

Vascular Inflammation and C-Reactive Protein

The link between vascular inflammation and atherosclerotic disease is well-established.[16] Research to identify prognostic and sensitive inflammatory markers is ongoing.

The inflammatory marker most frequently cited is *C-reactive protein* (CRP). It is measured as high-sensitivity CRP (hs-CRP).[16] CRP is associated with an increased risk of development of other cardiovascular risk factors including diabetes, hypertension, and weight gain. The higher the hs-CRP value, the greater the risk of a coronary event, especially if all other potential causes of systemic inflammation such as infection can be ruled out. Value ranges for hs-CRP are shown in Table 12-3. If other systemic inflammatory conditions such as bronchitis or urinary tract infection are present, the hs-CRP test loses all predictive value. CRP and other inflammatory markers are used to estimate the probability of future acute coronary events.[16]

Coronary Artery Disease Risk Equivalents

Certain medical conditions are risk equivalents of CAD. A *risk equivalent* means the person has the same risk of having an acute MI as if he or she had coronary heart disease already. Two noncardiac medical conditions considered risk equivalents for CAD: diabetes mellitus and chronic kidney disease.[17] PAD and stroke are atherosclerotic conditions that are also considered CAD risk equivalents.[17]

Multifactorial Risk

CAD has multifactorial causation; the greater the number of risk factors, the greater the risk of developing CAD.[1,3,17] The best time for an individual to make lifestyle changes is *before* the symptoms of CAD occur. Patients with two or more risk factors or with one or more of the CAD risk-equivalent diseases have the greatest potential to benefit from risk factor reduction and lifestyle change.[17] The major risk factors for developing CAD have been extensively documented in large epidemiologic studies: smoking, family history, adverse lipid profile, and elevated blood pressure.

Primary versus Secondary Prevention of Coronary Artery Disease

If a person already has signs and symptoms of CAD and has experienced an acute MI, the goal of any lifestyle change or medication is called *secondary prevention* or preventing another heart attack.[9] If an individual matches the risk profile described previously but does *not* have symptoms of CAD or has *not* had an acute MI, the treatment plan is described as *primary prevention*. The constellation of cardiac risk factors is well-established and can predict development of CAD for most populations in the developed world.[17]

Pathophysiology of Coronary Artery Disease

CAD is a progressive atherosclerotic disorder of the coronary arteries that results in narrowing or complete occlusion. *Atherosclerosis* affects the medium-sized arteries that perfuse the heart and other major organs. Normal arterial walls are composed of three layers: 1) the *intima* (inner lining), 2) the *media* (middle muscular layer), and 3) the *adventitia* (outer coat).

Development of Atherosclerosis

Atherosclerosis is a chronic inflammatory disorder that is characterized by an accumulation of macrophages and T lymphocytes in the arterial intimal wall. A high LDL cholesterol concentration is one of the triggers of vascular inflammation. The inflammation injures the wall, allowing the LDL cholesterol to move into the vessel wall below the endothelial surface. Blood monocytes adhere to endothelial cells and migrate into the vessel wall. Within the artery wall, some monocytes differentiate into macrophages that unite with and then internalize LDL cholesterol. The *foam cells* that result are the marker cells of atherosclerosis.

Atherosclerotic Plaque Rupture

When a mature atherosclerotic plaque develops, it is not uniform in composition. It has a lipid liquid center filled with procoagulant factors. A connective tissue *fibrous cap* covers the top of the fluid lipid center. The abrupt rupture of this cap allows procoagulant lipids to flood into the vessel lumen and rapidly form a coronary thrombosis, as shown in Table 12-4. As the enlarging clot blocks blood flow through the coronary artery, a "heart attack" will occur unless adequate collateral circulation from other coronary vessels occurs. Symptoms and suggested cardiac interventions at appropriate stages in development of CAD are listed in Table 12-4.

Plaques that are likely to rupture are saturated with macrophages and other inflammatory cells. These *vulnerable plaques* are usually not obstructive and are situated at bends or branch points in the arterial tree.[3] It is not known what factors cause the fibrous cap to rupture or erode. As deep fissures in the cap expose the procoagulant factors to the blood plasma, an unstoppable cycle is put into motion. When platelets in the bloodstream are exposed to collagen, necrotic

TABLE 12-3 C-Reactive Protein and Risk for Coronary Artery Disease

CATEGORY	HS-CRP LEVEL* (mg/L)
Low risk (normal)	<1
Moderate risk	1-3
High risk	>3

CAD, Coronary artery disease; *C-reactive*, cross-reactive; *hs-CRP*, high-sensitivity C-reactive protein.

*Values above 1 mg/dL increase the risk for CAD, but test results are not valid in the presence of infection or other inflammatory condition. Normal values may vary slightly between clinical laboratories; however, values below 1 mg/dL are usually considered normal. A test result greater than 10 mg/L suggests a noncoronary source of inflammation or infection.

Based on data from Pearson TA, et al. Markers of inflammation and cardiovascular disease, application to clinical and public health practice: a statement for healthcare professionals from the Centers for Disease Control and Prevention and the American Heart Association. *Circulation*. 2003; 107(3):499.

TABLE 12-4 Timeline of Atherogenesis Development Depicted by Longitudinal Section of An Artery

ATHEROGENESIS OR THROMBOGENESIS	ASSOCIATED SYMPTOMS	CARDIAC INTERVENTION
A. Normal artery, normal vessel wall	No symptoms	Primary prevention of CAD recommended: consume a low-fat diet, take regular physical exercise, avoid smoking, and achieve normal BMI.
B. Lipids in bloodstream	No symptoms	
C. Extracellular lipid accumulates in the intima of the artery (atheroma).	No symptoms	
D. Lipid accumulation evolves to become a fatty-fibrous (atherosclerotic) lesion; some lesions contain a lipid interior covered by a fibrous cap.	Chest pain with exercise that is relieved by rest or NTG (stable angina) or possibly no symptoms until the lesion fills more than 75% of the vessel lumen	PCI if stable angina is present and CAD is diagnosed by cardiac catheterization
E. Rupture of the cap allows lipid in the center to be released into the bloodstream, stimulating clot formation (thrombogenesis).	Chest pain not relieved by rest or NTG (ACS—unstable angina)	Call 911 for immediate transport to a hospital, preferably one with experience treating ACS.
F. Fresh clot blocks the vessel; spasm of the artery may occur near the thrombus.	Chest pain unrelieved by rest or NTG—severity, location of angina, and associated symptoms vary greatly among individuals (ACS—acute MI)	Emergency intervention to open the artery: fibrinolytic or catheter-based procedure (PCI)
G. Vessel is open, but the atherosclerotic lesion remains.	No symptoms	Secondary prevention of CAD to prevent repeat MI; beta-blockers to prevent arrhythmias; ACE-1 medications to prevent ventricular remodeling and heart failure; elective PCI

A B C D E F G

ACE-I, Angiotensin-converting enzyme inhibitor; *ACS*, acute coronary syndrome; *BMI*, body mass index; *CAD*, coronary artery disease; *MI*, myocardial infarction; *NTG*, nitroglycerin; *PCI*, percutaneous coronary intervention.

Illustration modified from Antman EM, et al. ACC/AHA guidelines for the management of patients with ST-elevation myocardial infarction—executive summary. *Circulation*. 2004; 110:588.

debris, von Willebrand factor, and thromboxane, a clot is formed and can occlude the coronary artery. Highly fibrotic plaques do not rupture. The type of atherosclerotic plaque that is prone to rupture has a weak fibrous cap and a large amount of liquid cholesterol within the core (see Table 12-4).

Plaque Regression

A reduction in blood cholesterol decreases atherosclerotic plaque size by decreasing the amount of liquid cholesterol within the plaque core. Lowering cholesterol levels does not change the dimensions of the fibrous or calcified portions of the plaque. However, lower cholesterol levels reduce vascular inflammation and make vulnerable plaque less likely to rupture.

Acute Coronary Syndrome

The term *acute coronary syndrome* (ACS) is used to describe the array of clinical presentations of CAD that range from unstable angina to acute MI (see Table 12-4).[1,2,3] An acute MI is generally described by patients as a "heart attack." The following section discusses stable manifestations of CAD (stable angina) and acute manifestations described as an ACS (unstable angina and acute MI). Figure 12-1 is a concept map of ACS.

Angina

Angina pectoris, or chest pain, caused by myocardial ischemia is not a separate disease, but rather a symptom of CAD. It is

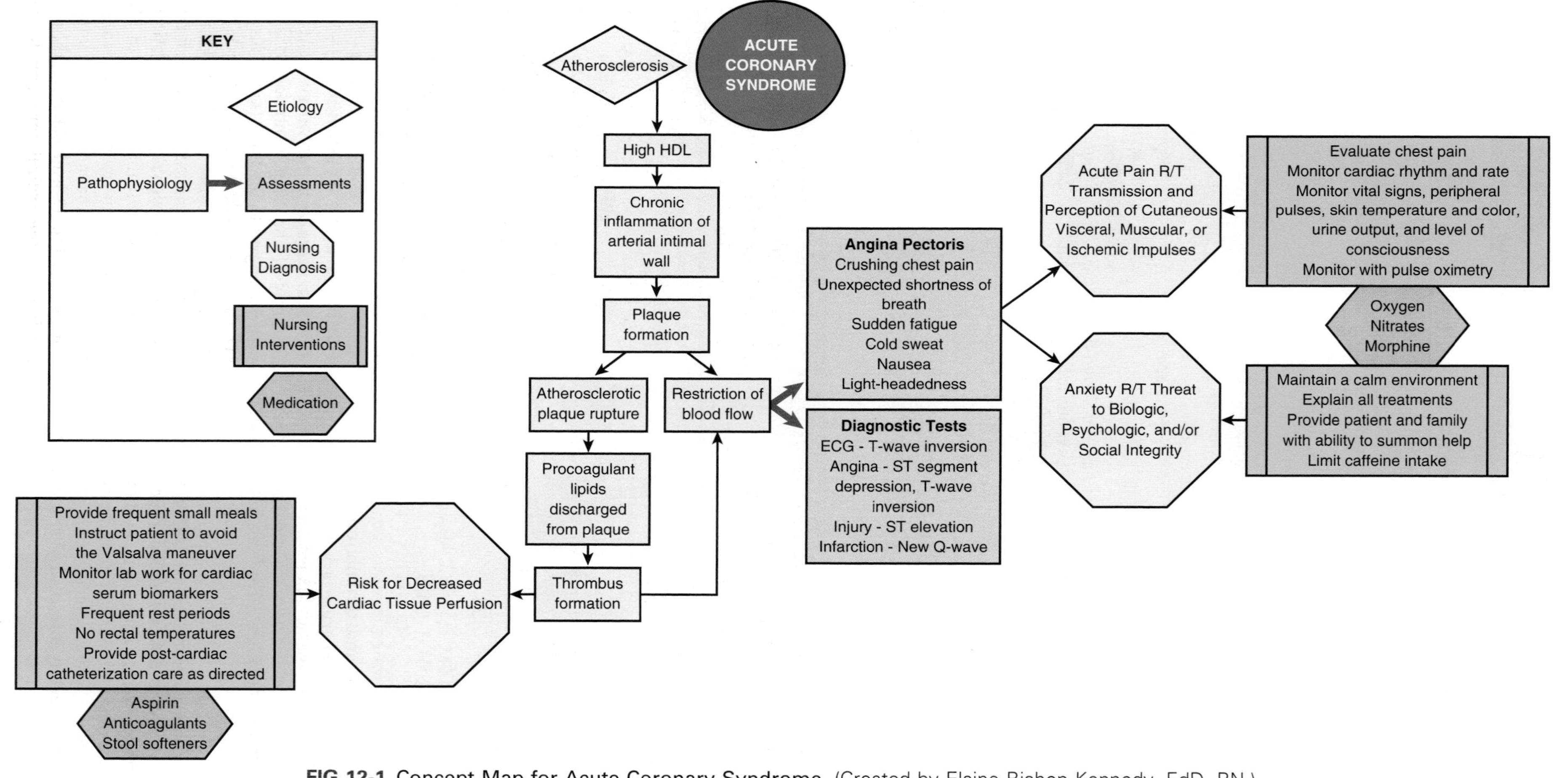

FIG 12-1 Concept Map for Acute Coronary Syndrome. (Created by Elaine Bishop Kennedy, EdD, RN.)

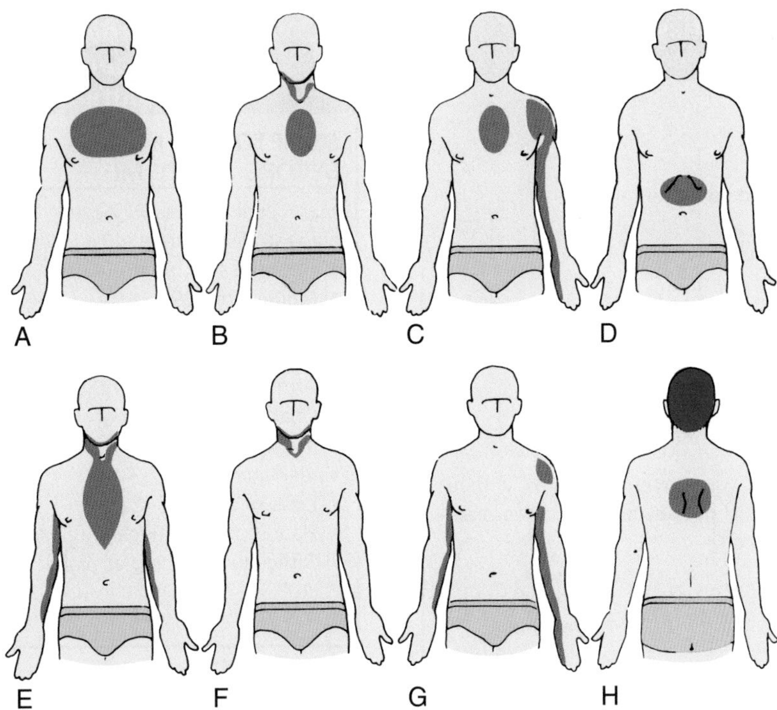

FIG 12-2 Sites for Anginal Pain. *A,* Upper part of chest; *B,* beneath sternum, radiating to neck and jaw; *C,* beneath sternum, radiating down left arm; *D,* epigastric; *E,* epigastric, radiating to neck, jaw, and arms; *F,* neck and jaw; *G,* left shoulder and radiating down both arms; *H,* intrascapular.

caused by a blockage or spasm of a coronary artery, leading to diminished myocardial blood supply. The lack of oxygen causes myocardial ischemia, which is felt as chest discomfort, pressure, or pain. Angina may occur anywhere in the chest, neck, arms, or back, but the most commonly described location is pain or pressure behind the sternum. The pain often radiates to the left arm but can also radiate down both arms and to the back, the shoulder, the jaw, or the neck (Figure 12-2). Angina symptoms are not the same for all individuals, many patients may describe pressure or discomfort rather than pain, and presenting symptoms can be highly individualized, as described in Box 12-3. Patients and families must be taught that angina does not always present in the dramatic heart attack scenario, as often portrayed on television and in movies, in which the person clutches the throat or chest and exhibits extreme distress.[2]

Angina symptom equivalents. Men and women should be made aware of angina symptom equivalents such as unexpected shortness of breath, breaking out in a cold sweat, or sudden fatigue, nausea, or lightheadedness.[18,19]

Women and angina. Many women experience a variety of different symptoms before an acute MI and during the acute event, as shown in Box 12-4.[20] The recognition and publicity about the fact that many women do not experience "crushing chest pain" is important to avoid women's symptoms being trivialized by clinicians. It is important that women are made aware of angina symptom equivalents such as unexplained shortness of breath, breaking out in a cold sweat, or sudden fatigue, nausea, or lightheadedness.[2] More women die every year in the United States of ACS compared with men, a fact that is largely unknown by health care providers.[20]

Stable angina. *Stable angina* is predictable and caused by similar precipitating factors each time; typically, it is exercise-induced. Patients become used to the pattern of this type of angina and may describe it as "my usual chest pain." Pain control should be achieved within 5 minutes of rest and by taking sublingual nitroglycerin. Ischemia and chest pain occur when myocardial demand from exertion exceeds the fixed blood oxygen supply. Additional information on CAD and stable angina is provided in Box 12-5.

Unstable angina. *Unstable angina* is defined as a change in a previously established stable pattern of angina. It is part of the continuum of ACS. Unstable angina usually is more intense than stable angina, may awaken the person from sleep, or may necessitate more than nitrates for pain relief. A change in the level or frequency of symptoms requires immediate medical evaluation. Severe angina that persists for more than 5 minutes, worsens in intensity, and is not relieved by one nitroglycerin tablet is a medical emergency, and the patient or a family member must call 911 immediately.[3] The 911 (Emergency Medical Services [EMS]) system is available to 90% of the population of the United States.[3] Family and friends are discouraged from driving a person experiencing unstable angina to the hospital and instead are urged to call 911. Patients should be instructed never to drive themselves but to contact the EMS by calling 911.

Unstable angina is an indication of atherosclerotic plaque instability. It can signal atherosclerotic plaque rupture and thrombus formation that can lead to MI. The patient who comes to the emergency department with recent-onset unstable angina but who has nonspecific or nonelevated ST-segment changes on the 12-lead electrocardiogram (ECG) may be admitted to the critical care unit to rule out MI. If the

BOX 12-3 Characteristics of Angina Pectoris

Location
- Beneath sternum, radiating to neck and jaw
- Upper chest
- Beneath sternum, radiating down left arm
- Epigastric
- Epigastric, radiating to neck, jaw, and arms
- Neck and jaw
- Left shoulder, inner aspect of both arms
- Intrascapular

Duration
- Less than 5 minutes
- Less than 5 minutes (stable)
- Longer than 5 minutes or worsening symptoms without relief from rest or sublingual nitroglycerin indicates preinfarction symptoms (unstable).

Quality
- Sensation of pressure or heavy weight on the chest
- Feeling of tightness, like a vise
- Visceral quality (deep, heavy, squeezing, aching)
- Burning sensation
- Shortness of breath, with feeling of suffocation
- Most severe pain ever experienced

Radiation
- Medial aspect of left arm
- Jaw
- Left shoulder
- Right arm

Precipitating Factors
- Exertion or exercise
- Cold weather
- Exercising after a large, heavy meal
- Walking against the wind
- Emotional upset
- Fright, anger
- Coitus

Medication Relief
- Usually within 45 seconds to 5 minutes after sublingual nitroglycerin administration

symptoms are typical of an MI, it is important to treat the patient according to the latest published guidelines because not all patients who experience an MI have ST-segment elevation on the 12-lead ECG.[2,18,19]

Variant angina. *Variant angina*, or Prinzmetal angina, is caused by a dynamic obstruction from intense vasoconstriction of a coronary artery.[21] Spasm can occur with or without atherosclerotic lesions. Variant angina commonly occurs when the individual is at rest, and it is often cyclic, occurring at the same time every day. Smoking, alcohol use, and illegal stimulant drug (cocaine) use may precipitate spasm. A definitive diagnosis of variant angina is made during a cardiac catheterization study. Signs of spasm include ST-segment elevation and chest pain. Coronary artery spasm can occur

BOX 12-4 Cardiovascular Symptoms Experienced by Women before Acute Myocardial Infarction

SYMPTOMS 1 MONTH BEFORE ACUTE MI	SYMPTOMS DURING ACUTE MI
• Unusual fatigue (71%)	• Shortness of breath (58%)
• Sleep disturbance (48%)	• Weakness (55%)
• Shortness of breath (42%)	• Unusual fatigue (43%)
• Indigestion (39%)	• Cold sweat (39%)
• Anxiety (36%)	• Dizziness (39%)
• Heart racing (27%)	• Nausea (36%)
• Arms weak or heavy (25%)	• Arm heaviness or weakness (35%)
• Changes in thinking or memory (24%)	• Ache in arms (32%)
• Vision change (23%)	• Heat or flushing (32%)
• Loss of appetite (22%)	• Indigestion (31%)
• Hands or arms tingling (22%)	• Pain centered high in chest (31%)
• Difficulty breathing at night (19%)	• Heart racing (23%)

MI, Myocardial infarction.
From McSweeney JC, et al. Women's early warning symptoms of acute myocardial infarction. *Circulation*. 2003; 108(21):2619.

with or without CAD. The prognosis is excellent when no significant coronary artery stenosis exists. Coronary artery spasm is treated with nitroglycerin or calcium channel blockers to vasodilate the coronary arteries.

Silent ischemia. *Silent ischemia* describes a situation in which objective evidence of ischemia is observed on an ECG monitor but the person does not complain of anginal symptoms. One-third of patients who are having a heart attack do not report chest pain as a symptom.[2] Patients with diabetes are at particular risk for silent ischemia. Many patients who have had type 2 diabetes for more than 10 years have developed autonomic neuropathy, which decreases their ability to experience chest pain. Patients with diabetes may misinterpret angina-equivalent symptoms such as nausea, vomiting, and diaphoresis as signaling a disruption in glucose control rather than a sign of myocardial ischemia.

Medical Management

Accurate assessment of chest pain symptoms is essential if unstable angina is to be recognized and treated effectively. An important reason to ask questions about the chest pain is to differentiate between stable and unstable angina. The change from stable to unstable angina is potentially life-threatening for the patient. If the ST segments are elevated or a newly documented left bundle branch block (LBBB) is seen on the 12-lead ECG, the patient should be treated for acute MI.[2] However, if these classic ECG signs are missing and the chest pain continues, the current pharmacologic treatment of choice is aspirin (If the patient cannot tolerate aspirin, then a thienopyridine such as clopidogrel can be given.). Patients with definite unstable angina or non–ST elevation myocardial infarction (UA or NSTEMI) should receive dual antiplatelet therapy on admission if an invasive strategy is imminent. A glycoprotein (GP) IIb/IIIa inhibitor is administered unless bivalirudin is chosen; and a loading dose of clopidogrel is

BOX 12-5 EVIDENCE-BASED PRACTICE (QSEN)

Coronary Artery Disease and Stable Angina

Strong evidence exists that the following lifestyle interventions help to prevent CAD:

- Diet
  - Diet low in salt and high in fiber, fruit, vegetables, and grains.
  - All dietary fat less than 30% of total calories; saturated fat less than 7%.
  - Limit glucose in diet (simple sugars).
  - Limit calories if overweight.
  - Omega-3 fatty acids included in diet.
- Exercise
  - Start by walking more often and increase physical exercise from there. Refer to cardiac rehabilitation program.
- Obesity
  - Achieve healthy body weight.
- Addiction
  - Stop cigarette smoking. Avoid exposure to environmental (secondhand) tobacco smoke at home and at work.
  - Limit alcohol intake.

Strong evidence exists that the following diagnostic procedures help the patient with angina:

- When a patient presents with chest pain, quickly obtaining a detailed history of symptoms, focused physical examination, and risk factor assessment can help determine whether the probability of CAD is low, intermediate, or high.
- Initial laboratory tests include hemoglobin, fasting blood glucose, lipid panel, cardiac enzymes.
- Obtain a baseline 12-lead ECG at rest, even if chest pain is not present.
- Obtain a 12-lead ECG during an episode of chest pain.
- Obtain a chest radiograph if symptoms of heart failure are present.
- Obtain an exercise 12-lead ECG if the condition is stable and symptoms suggest CAD or if the condition is stable with complete LBBB or RBBB that makes the ECG difficult to interpret for ischemia.
- Obtain cardiac echocardiography for patients with a systolic murmur suggestive of aortic stenosis.
- Use cardiac echocardiography to determine extent of left ventricular (LV) hypertrophy or dysfunction.
- Stress cardiac echocardiography is recommended for patients with greater than 1 mm of ST-segment depression at rest (Stress may be by physical exercise or by pharmacologic stimulation.).
- Coronary angiography (typically as part of a cardiac catheterization procedure) is recommended for patients at high risk for adverse coronary events.

Initial Pharmacologic and Lifestyle Treatment Recommendations

- The goal of treatment is to eliminate chest pain.
- The 10 most important elements of CAD and stable angina management can be remembered using the A-to-E mnemonic:

  A—Aspirin and antianginal medications: Prescribe daily, low-dose (75 to 325 mg) aspirin; oral nitrates; and sublingual nitroglycerin for episodes of angina.

  B—Beta-blockers and blood pressure: Use ACEI and beta-blockers to decrease blood pressure to less than 140/90 mm Hg if no other CAD risk factors are present and to less than 130/80 mm Hg if diabetes or kidney disease is present.

  C—Cholesterol and cigarettes: Obtain a fasting lipid profile. Recommend diet or lipid reduction medication therapy (statin) to lower LDL-C to less than 100 mg/dL (<70 mg/dL if achievable), increase HDL-C to more than 40 mg/dL for men or more than 50 mg/dL for women, and reduce triglycerides to less than 150 mg/dL. Recommend adding plant stanols or sterols (2 g/day) or viscous fiber (>10 g/day), or both, to the diet to lower LDL-C further; add dietary omega-3 fatty acids in the form of fish or capsule (1 g/day). Always ask about tobacco use; strongly recommend smoking cessation; encourage nicotine replacement therapy (nicotine patches or gum) as needed.

  D—Diet and diabetes: Prescribe a low-fat, calorie-appropriate diet and provide nutritional consultation as needed to achieve a fasting blood glucose level of 70 to 100 mg/dL and HbA_{1c} of less than 6.5%.

  E—Education and exercise: Provide education about risk factor modification and the CAD disease process; recommend daily exercise for 30 to 60 minutes (ideal) or at least seven times each week (minimum of 5 days per week). A BMI between 18.5 and 24.9 kg/m^2 and waist less than 40 inches for men or less than 35 inches for women should be recommended. Treat depression, if present. HRT is not recommended as a treatment for symptoms of coronary heart disease. Influenza vaccination is recommended.

Interventional and Surgical Recommendations for Stable High-Risk Patients

Patients are risk-stratified according to their symptoms and the results of cardiac diagnostic tests.

- Percutaneous catheter interventions (PCI)
  - PCI is more frequently performed than open heart surgery for relief of anginal symptoms.
- Coronary artery bypass surgery (CABG)
  - For patients with left main occlusion or multivessel disease
  - For patients with two-vessel disease who have significant proximal LAD stenosis and an LV ejection fraction less than 50%

References

Anderson JL, et al: 2011 ACCF/AHA Focused Update Incorporated into the ACC/AHA 2007 Guidelines for the Management of Patients with Unstable Angina/Non–ST-Elevation Myocardial Infarction: a Report of the American College of Cardiology Foundation/American Heart Association Task Force on Practice Guidelines, *Circulation* 123:e426, 2011.

Fihn SD, et al: 2012 ACCF/AHA/ACP/AATS/PCNA/SCAI/STS Guideline for the Diagnosis and Management of Patients with Stable Ischemic Heart Disease: A Report of the American College of Cardiology Foundation/American Heart Association Task Force on Practice Guidelines, and the American College of Physicians, American Association for Thoracic Surgery, Preventive Cardiovascular Nurses Association, Society for Cardiovascular Angiography and Interventions,

Continued

BOX 12-5 EVIDENCE-BASED PRACTICE—cont'd

Coronary Artery Disease and Stable Angina

and Society of Thoracic Surgeons, *Circulation* 126(25):e354–e471, 2012.

Mosca L, et al: Effectiveness-based guidelines for the prevention of cardiovascular disease prevention in women-2011 update: a guideline from The American Heart Association, *Circulation* 123:1243, 2011.

Wright SR, et al: 2011 ACC/AHA Focused Update of the guidelines for the management of patients with unstable angina/non–ST-elevation myocardial infarction: a report from the American College of Cardiology/American Heart Association Task Force on Practice Guidelines developed in collaboration with the American College of Emergency Physicians, Society for Cardiovascular Angiography and Interventions, and Society for Thoracic Surgeons, *J Am Coll Cardiol* 57:1920, 2011.

ACEI, Angiotensin-converting enzyme inhibitors; *BMI*, body mass index; *CAD*, coronary artery disease; *ECG*, electrocardiogram; *HbA_{1c}*, glycosylated hemoglobin; *HDL-C*, high-density lipoprotein cholesterol; *HRT*, hormone replacement therapy; *LAD*, left anterior descending coronary artery; *LBBB*, left bundle branch block; *LDL-C*, low-density lipoprotein cholesterol; *LV*, left ventricle; *RBBB*, right bundle branch block.

given at least 6 hours prior to the procedure. Patients undergoing noninvasive treatment should receive aspirin and a thienopyridine (clopidgorel, prasugrel, or ticagrelor) for 1 month and ideally up to 1 year. If symptoms persist, a diagnostic angiography is performed. A stress test should be performed on patients who are not undergoing invasive therapy for their UA/NSTEMI, and if negative, the GP IIb/IIIa inhibitor can be discontinued and unfractionated heparin (UFH) administered for 48 hours.

Nursing Management

Nursing management of the patient with CAD and angina incorporates a variety of nursing diagnoses (see Box 12-6 Nursing Diagnosis Priorities: Coronary Artery Disease and Angina). **Nursing priorities focus on 1) recognizing myocardial ischemia, 2) relieving chest pain, 3) maintaining a calm environment, and 4) providing patient education.**

Recognizing Myocardial Ischemia

Complaints of chest discomfort (angina) must be evaluated quickly because angina is an indicator of myocardial ischemia. The patient is asked to rate the intensity of the chest discomfort on a scale of 0 to 10. Pain levels must be assessed with sensitivity to differences in cultural manifestations of pain. The term *chest pain* is not to be used exclusively because some patients describe their angina as "pressure" or "heaviness." It is important to document the characteristics of the pain and the patient's heart rate and rhythm, BP, respirations, temperature, skin color, peripheral pulses, urine output, mentation, and overall tissue perfusion. A 12-lead ECG is used to identify the area of ischemic myocardium. The major concern is that the chest pain may represent preinfarction angina, and early identification is essential so that the patient can be immediately treated. Treatment may include transfer to the cardiac catheterization laboratory for a coronary arteriogram and opening of a blocked artery. If the hospital does not have a cardiac catheterization laboratory, GP IIb/IIIa receptor blockers may be infused to prevent the evolution of the acute MI before transfer.[2,18,19]

Relieving Chest Pain

In the critical care unit, control of angina is achieved by a combination of supplemental oxygen, nitrates, analgesia, and surveillance of the angina and of the effects of pharmacologic therapy.

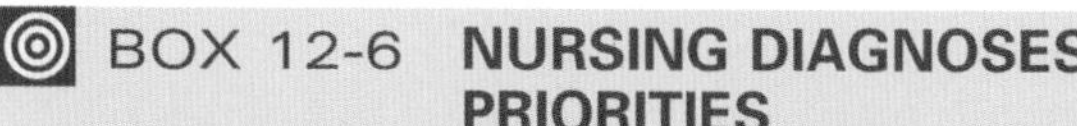

Coronary Artery Disease and Angina

- Acute Pain, related to transmission and perception of cutaneous, visceral, muscular, or ischemic impulses, p. 574
- Risk for Decreased Cardiac Tissue Perfusion, p. 603
- Activity Intolerance, related to cardiopulmonary dysfunction, p. 570
- Powerlessness, related to lack of control over current situation, p. 600
- Anxiety, related to threat to biologic, psychologic, or social integrity, p. 576
- Deficient Knowledge, related to lack of previous exposure to information, p. 585 (see Box 12-7, Patient Education for Coronary Artery Disease and Angina)

- *Oxygen:* All patients with acute ischemic pain are administered supplemental oxygen to increase myocardial oxygenation. Pulse oximetry is used to guide therapy and maintain oxygen saturation above 90% unless patient has a history of chronic obstructive pulmonary disease (COPD) and is a carbon dioxide (CO_2) retainer.
- *Nitrates:* A combination of intravenous and sublingual nitroglycerin is used to vasodilate the coronary arteries and decrease pain. After nitrate administration, the critical care nurse closely observes the patient for relief of chest pain, for return of the ST segment to baseline, and for the potential development of unwanted side effects such as hypotension and headache. Administration of a nitrate is avoided if the SBP is below 90 mm Hg. Medication interactions with nitrates are another potential cause for concern. The phosphodiesterase inhibitor medication *sildenafil* is prescribed for several conditions including pulmonary hypertension (Revatio) and erectile dysfunction (Viagra). Sildenafil and nitrates in combination may contribute to a precipitous fall in blood pressure.[3]
- *Analgesia:* Morphine (2 to 4 mg given intravenously) is the analgesic opiate of choice for preinfarction angina. It relieves pain and decreases fear and anxiety. After administration, the critical care nurse assesses the patient for pain relief and the development of unwanted side effects such as hypotension and respiratory depression.[2,18]

- *Aspirin:* Chewing an oral non–enteric-coated aspirin (162 to 325 mg) at the beginning of chest pain has been shown to reduce mortality. The nonenteric formulation is preferred because it increases absorption in the mouth when chewed, not swallowed.[2,18]

Maintaining a Calm Environment

Patients admitted to a critical care unit with unstable angina experience extreme anxiety and fear of death. The critical care nurse is faced with the challenge of ensuring that the elements of a calm environment that can alleviate the patient's fear and anxiety are maintained, while being ready at all times to respond to an acute emergency such as a cardiac arrest or to assist with emergency intubation or insertion of hemodynamic monitoring catheters.

Providing Patient Education

In the critical care unit, the patient's ability to retain educational information is severely affected by stress and pain. Patient education topics that should be discussed when the clinical condition has stabilized are listed in Box 12-7. It is essential to teach avoidance of the Valsalva maneuver, which is defined as forced expiration against a closed glottis. This can be explained to the patient as "bearing down" during defecation or breath holding when repositioning in bed. The Valsalva maneuver causes an increase in intrathoracic pressure, which decreases venous return to the right side of the heart and can be associated with low blood pressure and symptomatic bradycardia.

After the anginal pain is controlled, longer-term education of the patient and the family can begin. Points to cover include 1) risk factor modification, 2) signs and symptoms of angina, 3) when to call the physician, 4) medications, and 5) dealing with emotions and stress. However, because the acute hospital length of stay for uncomplicated angina is usually less than 3 days, referral to a cardiac rehabilitation program for a controlled exercise program and risk factor modification after discharge may be the most helpful teaching intervention a critical care nurse can provide.

BOX 12-7 PATIENT EDUCATION

Coronary Artery Disease and Angina

- Angina: Describe signs and symptoms such as pain, pressure, and heaviness in chest, arms, or jaw.
- Preinfarction or unstable angina: Any chest pain that is not relieved by a sublingual nitroglycerin (NTG) tablet taken 5 minutes apart times 3 doses provides a reason to call 911 (emergency services).
- Use of the 0-to-10 pain scale: Notify critical care nurse or emergency personnel of any changes in pain intensity.
- Use of sublingual NTG for angina: Pain intensity should decrease on the pain scale after NTG administration. At home, NTG must be kept in a dark, air-tight container, or it loses its potency. To ensure potency, the NTG supply must be replaced about every 6 months. Active NTG has a slight burning sensation when placed under the tongue.
- Avoid Valsalva maneuver.
- Risk factor modification tailored to the patient's individual risk factor profile:
  - Decrease fat intake to 30% of total calories a day.
  - Stop smoking.
  - Reduce salt intake.
  - Control hypertension.
  - Treat diabetes and control blood glucose levels (if patient has diabetes).
  - Increase physical activity; achieve ideal body weight.
- Refer to a cardiac rehabilitation program.
- Medication teaching about indications and side effects
- Follow-up care after discharge
- Symptoms to report to a health care professional
- Discussion of how to handle emotional stress and anger

MYOCARDIAL INFARCTION

Description and Etiology

Myocardial infarction (MI) is the term used to describe irreversible myocardial necrosis (cell death) that results from an abrupt decrease or total cessation of coronary blood flow to a specific area of the myocardium. In the hospital, this is often referred to as an *acute MI*, indicating the sudden onset and the life-threatening nature of the event. Increasingly, an acute MI is described in relation to whether ST-segment elevation is seen on the diagnostic 12-lead ECG. It may be labeled an *acute NSTEMI*[18] or an *acute STEMI.*[2]

Three mechanisms can block the coronary artery and are responsible for the acute reduction in oxygen delivery to the myocardium:

1. Plaque rupture
2. New coronary artery thrombosis
3. Coronary artery spasm close to the ruptured plaque.

Myocardial tissue can best be salvaged within the first 2 hours (120 minutes) after the onset of anginal symptoms, as illustrated in Figure 12-3. The earlier the myocardium is revascularized, the better the chances of survival.[2,18] Unfortunately, many persons do not seek treatment until the acute phase has passed or delay seeking treatment because of denial of symptoms.

Pathophysiology

Ischemia

The outer region of the infarcted myocardial area is the *zone of ischemia*, or penumbra, as illustrated in Figure 12-4. It is composed of viable cells. Priority interventions are targeted to save this viable muscle. Repolarization in this zone is temporarily impaired but eventually will be restored to normal. Repolarization of the cells in this area manifests as T-wave inversion (Figure 12-5B).

Injury

The infarcted zone is surrounded by injured but still potentially viable tissue in an area known as the *zone of injury* (see Figure 12-4). Cells in this area do not fully repolarize because of the deficient blood supply. This is recorded on the ECG as elevation of the ST segment (see Figure 12-5C).

Infarction

The area of dead muscle (necrosis) in the myocardium is known as the *zone of infarction* (see Figure 12-4). On the ECG, evidence of this zone is seen as new pathologic Q waves, which reflect a lack of depolarization from the cardiac surface

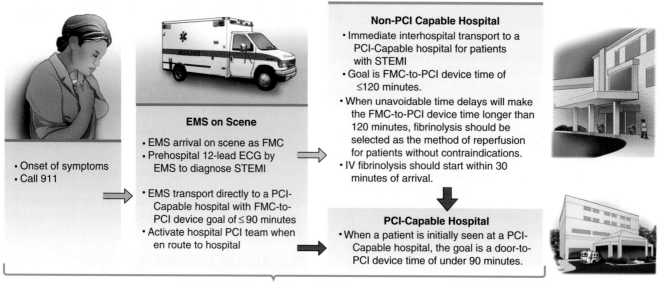

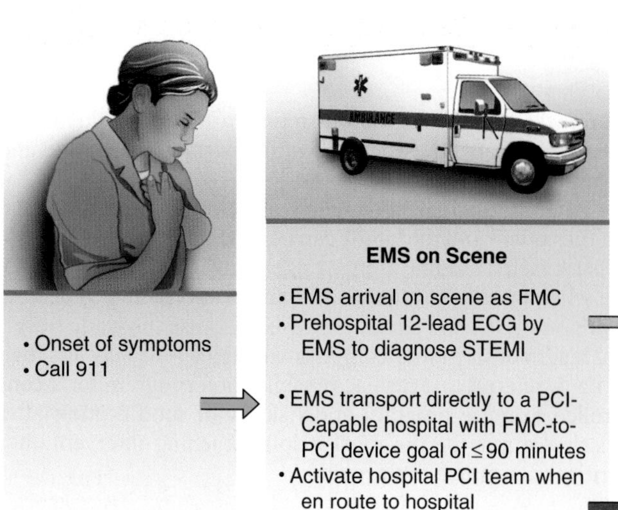

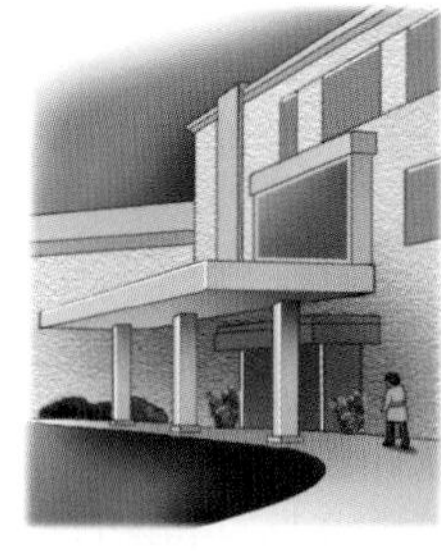

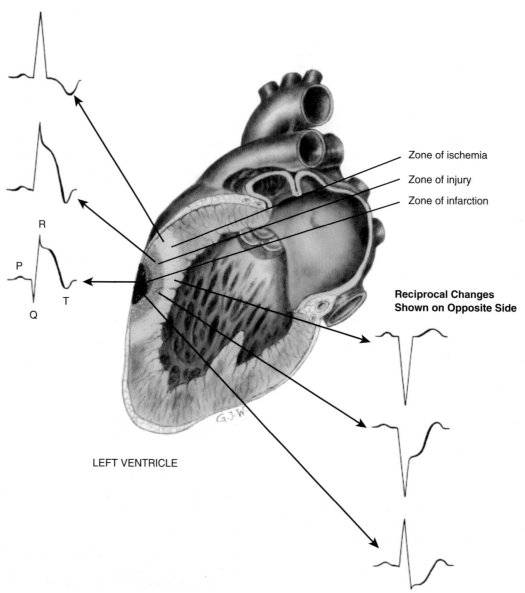

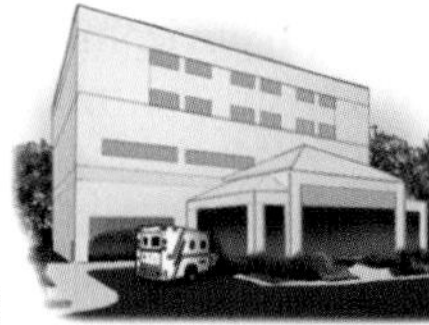

FIG 12-3 Evaluation of Prehospital Chest Pain and Acute Coronary Syndrome and Treatment Options.[2] *ECG,* Electrocardiogram; *EMS,* emergency medical services; *FMC,* first medical contact; *PCI,* percutaneous coronary intervention; *STEMI,* ST-elevation myocardial infarction.

FIG 12-4 Zone of ischemia, zone of injury, and zone of infarction are shown through electrocardiograph waveforms and reciprocal waveforms corresponding to each zone.

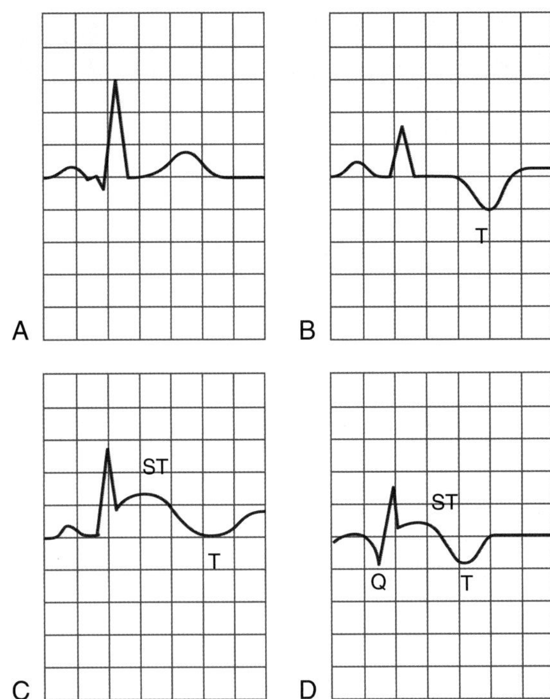

FIG 12-5 Electrocardiograph (ECG) Changes Indicative of Ischemia, Injury, and Infarction (Necrosis) of the Myocardium. *A,* Normal ECG. *B,* Ischemia indicated by inversion of the T wave. *C,* Ischemia and current of injury indicated by T-wave inversion and ST-segment elevation. The ST segment may be elevated above or depressed below the baseline, depending on whether the tracing is from a lead facing toward or away from the infarcted area and depending on whether epicardial or endocardial injury occurs. Epicardial injury causes ST-segment elevation in leads facing the epicardium. *D,* Ischemia, injury, and myocardial necrosis. The Q wave indicates necrosis of the myocardium.

involved in the MI (see Figure 12-5D). As healing takes place, the cells in this area are replaced by scar tissue.

Q-Wave Myocardial Infarction

MIs are classified according to the location on the myocardial surface and the muscle layers affected. Not all infarctions cause necrosis in all layers, as shown in Figure 12-6. A transmural MI involves all three cardiac layers—the *endocardium,* the *myocardium,* and the *epicardium.* A transmural (full-thickness) MI usually provokes significant ECG changes (see Figure 12-5). This is also described as a *Q-wave MI.* Not every acute MI produces a recognizable series of Q waves on the 12-lead ECG. Some patients who had a demonstrated Q wave on a 12-lead ECG as a result of an acute MI lose the Q wave months or years later. The reasons for this are unknown, but it may represent the development of collateral circulation.

12-Lead electrocardiographic changes. The ECG changes produced by an MI demonstrate alteration in myocardial depolarization (QRS complex) and repolarization (ST segment). The changes in repolarization are seen by the presence of new Q waves. These new, pathologic Q waves are deeper and wider than tiny Q waves found on the normal 12-lead ECG.[2]

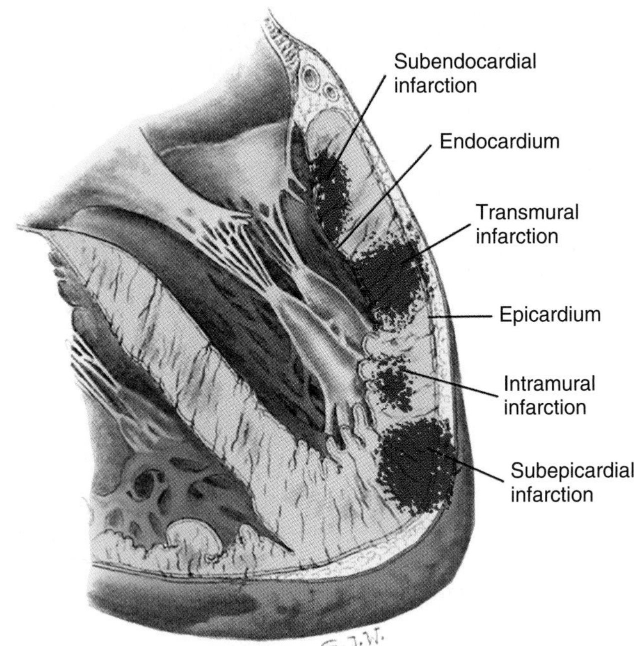

FIG 12-6 Location of Infarctions in Myocardium.

Myocardial Infarction Location

The location of infarction is determined by correlating the ECG leads with Q waves and the ST-segment and T-wave abnormalities (Table 12-5). The ECG manifestations that are used to diagnose an MI and pinpoint the area of damaged ventricle include inverted T waves, ST-segment elevation, and pathologic Q waves in specific lead groupings, as described subsequently.

Anterior wall infarction. Anterior wall infarction results from occlusion of the proximal left anterior descending artery (see Table 12-5). ST-segment elevation is expected in leads V_1 through V_4 on the 12-lead ECG, as shown in Figure 12-7. If the left main coronary artery is occluded, the ECG manifestations will involve almost all of the precordial leads V_1 through V_6 and leads I and aVL (see Table 12-5). These specific groups of ST-segment changes identify the wall of the heart that is infarcting and are called indicative changes. A large anterior wall MI may be associated with left ventricular pump failure, cardiogenic shock, or death.

Left lateral wall infarction. Left lateral wall infarction occurs as a result of occlusion of the circumflex coronary artery. On a 12-lead ECG, new Q waves and ST-segment T-wave changes are seen in leads I, aVL, V_5, and V_6 (Figure 12-8). In reality, few patients present with only lateral wall ECG changes, and some anterior wall leads (V_3 and V_4) may show evidence of injury or infarction.

Inferior wall infarction. Inferior wall infarction occurs with occlusion of the right coronary artery. This infarction manifests by ECG changes in leads II, III, and aV_F (Figure 12-9). Conduction disturbances are expected with an inferior wall MI and are related to the anatomy of the coronary arterial supply. Because the right coronary artery supplies the sinoatrial (SA) node in slightly more than one-half of the population and supplies the proximal bundle of His and the atrioventricular (AV) node in more than 90% of

TABLE 12-5 Correlations Among Ventricular Surfaces, Electrocardiographic Leads, and Coronary Arteries

SURFACE OF LEFT VENTRICLE	ELECTROCARDIOGRAPHIC LEADS	USUALLY INVOLVED
Inferior	II, III, aVF	Right coronary artery
Lateral	V_5-V_6, I, aVL	Left circumflex
Anterior	V_2-V_4	Left anterior descending
Anterior lateral	V_1-V_6, I, aVL	Left main coronary artery
Septal	V_1-V_2	Left anterior descending
Posterior	V_1-V_2	Left circumflex or right coronary artery (reciprocal changes)
	V_7-V_9 (direct)	

I lateral	aVR	V_1 septal	V_4 anterior
II inferior	aVL lateral	V_2 septal	V_5 lateral
III inferior	aVF inferior	V_3 anterior	V_6 lateral

individuals, heart block and other conduction disturbances should be anticipated.

Right ventricular infarction. Infarction of the right ventricle occurs when a blockage occurs in a proximal section of the right coronary artery. This places all of the right ventricle and the inferior wall at risk. Right ventricular ischemia can be demonstrated in up to one-half of inferior wall STEMIs, although only 10% to 15% show the hemodynamic abnormalities associated with classic infarction of the right ventricle. If massive infarction occurs, the patient can suffer cardiogenic shock, which carries a mortality rate of more than 50% in this population.[22]

The ECG leads on the 12-lead ECG also correlate with the coronary arteries. Leads can also be placed on the right side of the chest to assist in the diagnosis of right ventricular infarction and posteriorly to show a posterior infarction. To detect a right ventricular infarction, specific ECG lead placement is used. Electrodes are placed over the right precordium (chest) in a mirror image of the conventional left-sided leads. It is important to write R on the 12-lead ECG (e.g., V_1R-V_6R) in front of the recorded right ventricular chest leads to ensure that the lead location is clear.

Posterior wall infarction. Infarction in the posterior wall can occur because of a blockage in the right coronary artery or in the circumflex artery. This occurs because both arteries supply this section of the heart, although the right coronary artery is generally the dominant vessel. A posterior wall MI is difficult to detect but may be identified by specific leads placed in the left scapular area or by very tall R waves in leads V_1 and V_2.

Non–ST-Segment Elevation Myocardial Infarction

The 12-lead ECG is a highly useful diagnostic tool. For many years, it was considered the gold standard when diagnosing an acute MI. However, the ST segment is not elevated in every acute MI. One reason for the lack of ST-segment elevation may be that the infarction and subsequent necrosis are not full-thickness lesions. Because some of the muscle in the area can still be depolarized, ST-segment elevation may not occur. This type of MI is also less likely to develop Q waves on a subsequent 12-lead ECG after the acute phase has passed. This situation is diagnostically known as an NSTEMI.[18,20] This condition has previously been described by several names, including nontransmural MI, non–Q-wave MI, and subendocardial MI. Because patients who sustain an NSTEMI do have CAD, it is important that they be treated aggressively to minimize the size of the infarcted area. Without the visual clue of the ST-segment elevation on the 12-lead ECG, the patients cannot receive immediate intravenous fibrinolytic agents, but they can be appropriately managed in an interventional catheterization laboratory and receive GP IIb/IIIa inhibitor therapy, as illustrated in the timeline in Figure 12-3. The 12-lead ECG plays a vital role in identifying the treatment plan for an ACS. Visualizing ST-segment elevation is helpful when present. Patients without ST elevation may still be at risk for becoming unstable and should be monitored (Figure 12-10). In this case, the definitive diagnosis may be made in the cardiac catheterization laboratory or by elevation of specific cardiac biomarkers.

Cardiac Biomarkers during Myocardial Infarction

In the presence of damage and necrosis of myocardium, cardiac biomarkers are released.[23] These biomarkers are also called *cardiac enzymes*. To confirm the diagnosis of acute MI, the serum biomarkers creatine kinase–muscle/brain (CK-MB) and troponin I or troponin T are measured. Although CK is still used, the troponins are valuable because the turnaround time is faster. If the coronary artery is opened by fibrinolytic therapy or a percutaneous catheter intervention (PCI), the biomarkers exhibit a more rapid rise and dramatic fall (Figure 12-11). Information on biomarkers is also shown in Table 11-13 in Chapter 11.

Complications of Acute Myocardial Infarction

Many patients experience complications occurring early or late in the postinfarction course. These complications may result from electrical dysfunction or from a decrease in cardiac contractility. Electrical dysfunctions include bradycardia, bundle branch blocks, and various degrees of heart block.[2] Pumping complications can cause heart failure, pulmonary edema, and cardiogenic shock. The presence of a new murmur in a patient with an acute MI warrants special attention, as it may indicate rupture of the papillary muscle or rupture of the intraventricular septum.[2]

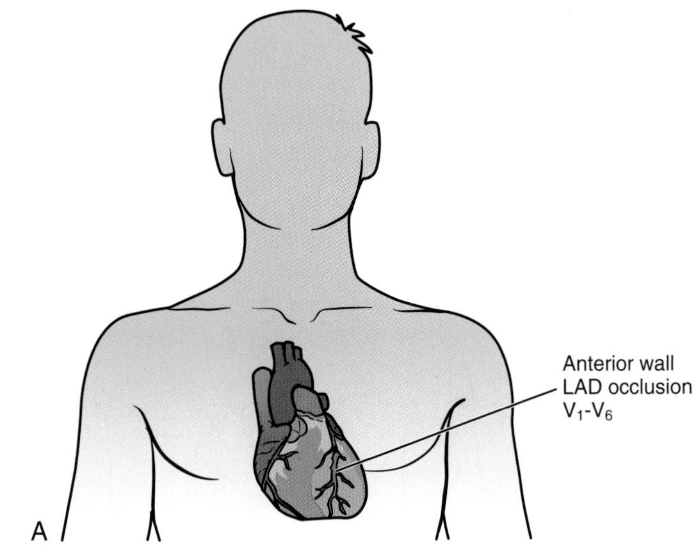

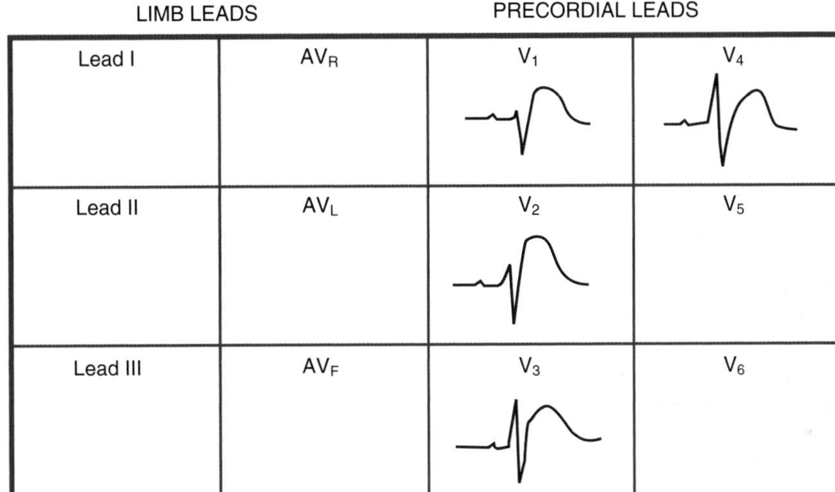

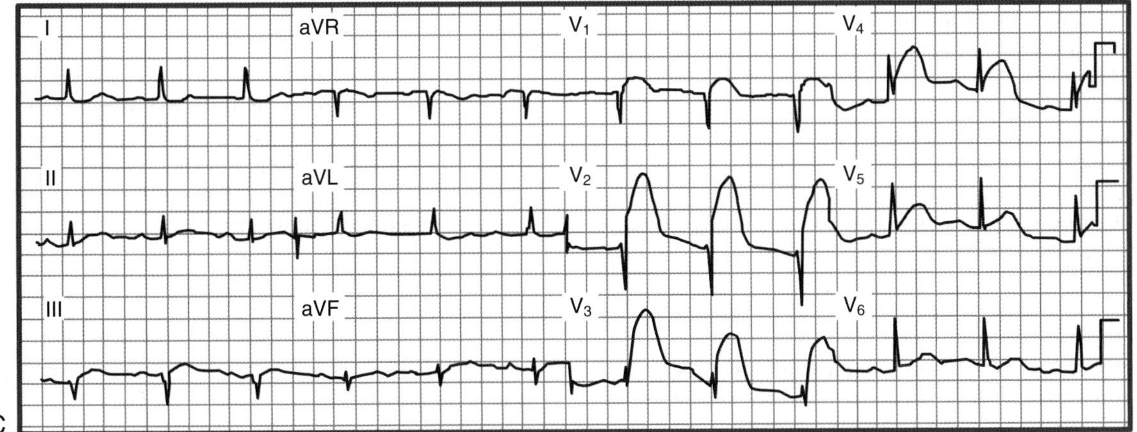

FIG 12-7 Changes Seen on a 12-Lead Electrocardiogram (ECG) with an Anterior Wall Myocardial Infarction (MI). *A,* Infarction location on the cardiac wall; *B,* ECG leads with expected ST-segment elevation; *C,* a 12-lead ECG from a patient experiencing left anterior wall MI. *LAD,* Left anterior descending artery.

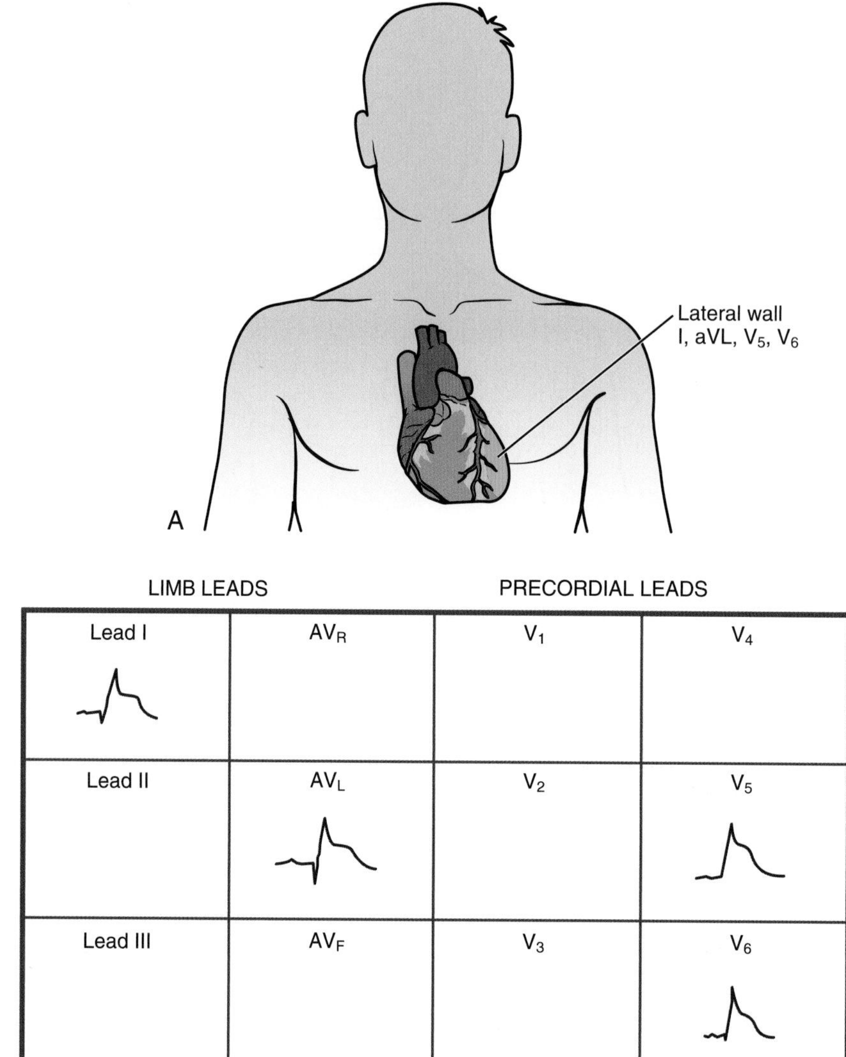

FIG 12-8 **Changes Seen on a 12-Lead Electrocardiogram (ECG) with a Lateral Wall ST-Segment Elevation Myocardial Infarction (STEMI).** *A,* Infarction location on the cardiac wall; *B,* ECG leads with expected ST-segment elevation.

Ventricular aneurysm after myocardial infarction. A left ventricular aneurysm (Figure 12-12) is a noncontractile, thinned left ventricular wall that results from an acute transmural infarction. This complication occurs in less than 5% of patients after an acute MI.

Ventricular septal rupture after myocardial infarction. Postinfarction rupture of the ventricular septal wall is a rare but potentially lethal complication of an acute anterior wall MI (Figure 12-13). This rare complication generally occurs in the first 24 hours after an acute MI. A holosystolic murmur can be auscultated along the left sternal border. Rupture of the septum is a medical and surgical emergency. The patient's condition is stabilized with vasodilators and an intraaortic balloon pump (IABP) to decrease afterload. Most patients with septal rupture also have signs and symptoms of cardiogenic shock. Ventricular septal rupture manifests as severe chest pain, syncope, hypotension, and sudden hemodynamic deterioration caused by shunting of blood from the high-pressure left ventricle into the low-pressure right ventricle through the new septal opening.

Emergency surgical repair is necessary.[2] Surgical mortality is extremely high-ranging from 20%-87%.[2]

Papillary muscle rupture and acute mitral regurgitation after myocardial infarction. Papillary muscle rupture can occur when the infarct involves the area around one of the papillary muscles that support the mitral valve. Infarction of the papillary muscles results in ineffective mitral valve closure, and blood is forced back into the low-pressure left atrium during ventricular systole. The rupture may be partial or complete. Complete rupture is catastrophic and precipitates severe acute mitral regurgitation, cardiogenic shock, and high risk of death.

Partial rupture (Figure 12-14) also results in mitral regurgitation, but the condition can be stabilized with aggressive medical management using the IABP and vasodilators. Urgent surgical intervention is required to replace the mitral valve.[2] Postsurgical mortality is about 20%.[2]

Cardiac wall rupture after myocardial infarction. The incidence of cardiac wall rupture has two peak times. The first occurs within the first 24 hours and the second between

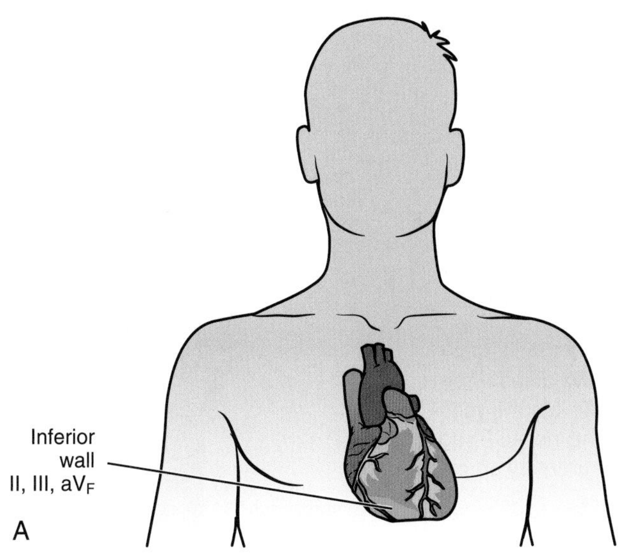

LIMB LEADS		PRECORDIAL LEADS	
Lead I	aV_R	V_1	V_4
Lead II	aV_L	V_2	V_5
Lead III	aV_F	V_3	V_6

B

Example of an Acute Inferior Wall MI

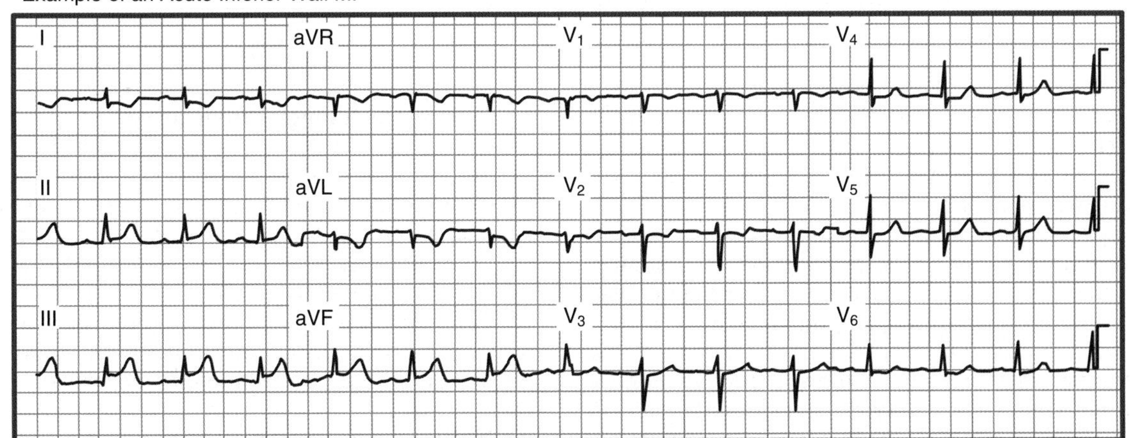

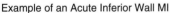

FIG 12-9 Changes Seen on a 12-Lead Electrocardiogram (ECG) with an Inferior Wall Myocardial Infarction (MI). *A,* Infarction location on cardiac wall. *B,* ECG leads with expected ST-segment elevation. *C,* A 12-lead ECG from a patient experiencing inferior wall MI.

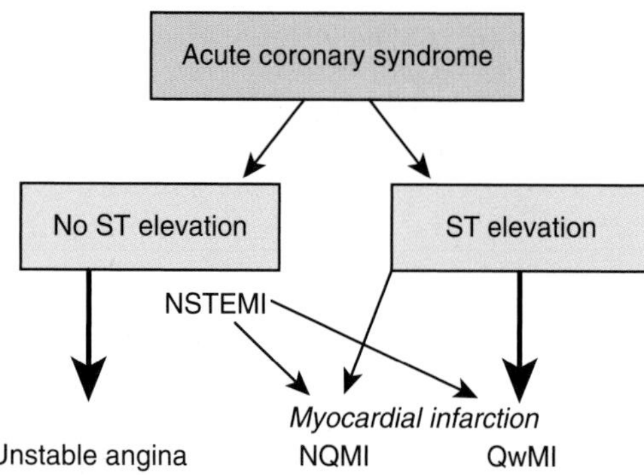

FIG 12-10 Acute Coronary Syndrome. (Modified from Braunwald E, et al. ACC/AHA guideline update for the management of patients with unstable angina and non–ST-segment elevation myocardial infarction—2002: summary article. *Circulation.* 2002; 106[14]:1893.)

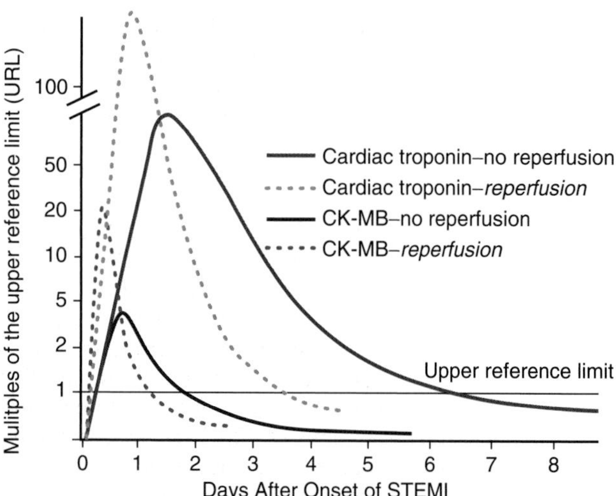

FIG 12-11 Cardiac Biomarkers during Myocardial Infarction (MI). (From Antman EM, et al. ACC/AHA guidelines for the management of patients with ST-elevation myocardial infarction—executive summary: a report of the American College of Cardiology/American Heart Association Task Force on Practice Guidelines [Writing Committee to Revise the 1999 Guidelines for the Management of Patients with Acute Myocardial Infarction]. *Circulation.* 2004; 110[9]:e82.)

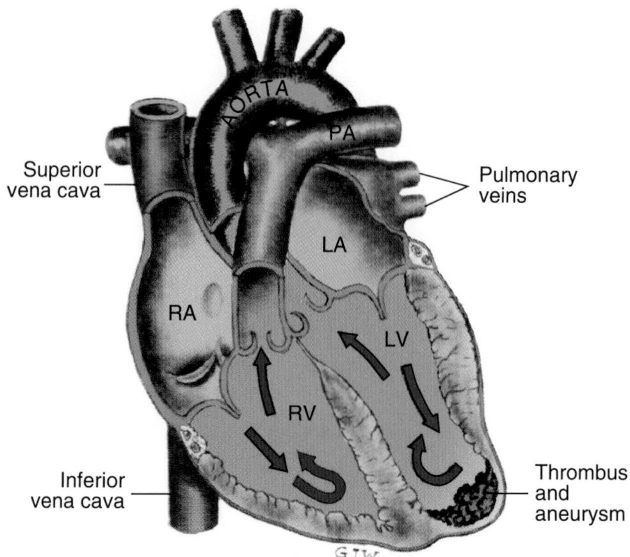

FIG 12-12 Ventricular Aneurysm after Acute Myocardial Infarction. *LA*, Left atrium; *LV*, left ventricle; *PA*, pulmonary artery; *RA*, right atrium; *RV*, right ventricle.

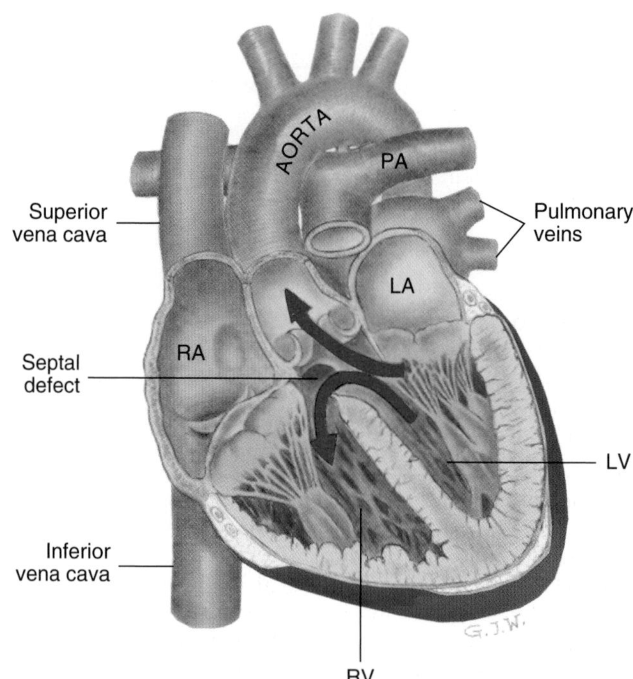

FIG 12-13 Ventricular Septal Rupture after Acute Myocardial Infarction. *LA*, Left atrium; *LV*, left ventricle; *PA*, pulmonary artery; *RA*, right atrium; *RV*, right ventricle.

the third and fifth postinfarction day when leukocyte scavenger cells are removing necrotic debris, thinning the myocardial wall. The onset is sudden and usually catastrophic; bleeding into the pericardial sac results in cardiac tamponade, cardiogenic shock, pulseless electrical activity (PEA), and death. Survival is rare. If rupture occurs in the hospital, emergency pericardiocentesis is required to relieve the tamponade until a surgical repair can be attempted. For the few patients who reach the operating room, postsurgical mortality is about 60%.[2]

Pericarditis after myocardial infarction. Pericarditis is inflammation of the pericardial sac. It can occur during or after an acute MI, although this complication is less frequent because of the aggressive use of reperfusion therapies. Pain is the most common symptom of pericarditis, and a pericardial friction rub is the most common initial sign. The friction rub is best auscultated with a stethoscope at the sternal border and is described as a grating, scraping, or leathery scratching. Pericarditis frequently produces a pericardial effusion. After the effusion occurs, the friction rub may disappear. On the 12-lead ECG, pericarditis may manifest as elevation of the ST segment in all of the typically upright leads. Pericarditis is treated with aspirin, nonsteroidal antiinflammatory medications (NSAIDs), and rest.

Heart failure and acute myocardial infarction. Many patients with acute STEMI also have acute heart failure on

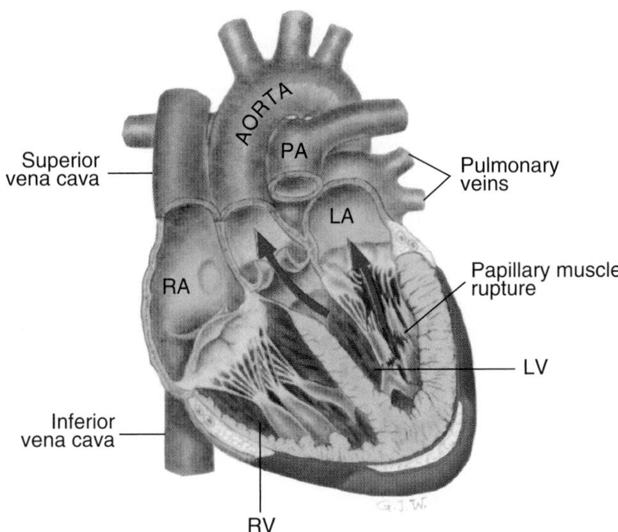

FIG 12-14 Papillary Muscle Rupture after Acute Myocardial Infarction. *LA*, Left atrium; *LV*, left ventricle; *PA*, pulmonary artery; *RA*, right atrium; *RV*, right ventricle.

admission to the hospital. These patients have often waited longer to come to the hospital and are older and more likely to be female. Compared with patients with acute MI but not heart failure, these patients have a higher risk of adverse inhospital events and have longer lengths of stay and higher inhospital mortality rates. More detailed information about heart failure is presented later in this chapter.

Medical Management

Quality outcomes research shows that compliance with the guidelines developed by the American College of Cardiology and the American Heart Association (ACC/AHA) decreases inhospital mortality after acute MI.[24] When the AHA/ACC guidelines for treatment of STEMI or NSTEMI are followed, patients admitted to hospitals have 8% inhospital mortality rate, compared with a 15% mortality rate in patients managed at hospitals where the most recent guidelines are not fully utilized.[24,25] The guidelines are research-based and are designed to improve the outcome of patients admitted to the hospital with an acute MI. Clinical guidelines address the issues of interventions to open the coronary artery, anticoagulation, prevention of dysrhythmias, intensive glucose control, and prevention of ventricular remodeling after STEMI.[2] To facilitate rapid coronary artery revascularization in STEMI, local hospitals are encouraged to develop a coordinated patient transfer strategy between PCI-capable and non–PCI-capable hospitals, as illustrated in Figure 12-3.[2]

Recanalization of the Coronary Artery

The essential immediate interventions are fibrinolytic therapy or PCI to open the occluded artery for the patient with an acute STEMI.[2] All clinical guidelines emphasize the need for patients with symptoms of ACS to be triaged and treated rapidly.[2]

Anticoagulation

In the acute phase after STEMI, heparin is administered in combination with fibrinolytic therapy to recanalize (open) the coronary artery.[2] For patients who will receive fibrinolytic therapy, an initial heparin bolus of 60 units/kg (maximum 5000 units) is given intravenously, followed by a continuous heparin drip at 12 units/kg/hr (maximum 1000 units/hr) to maintain an activated partial thromboplastin time (aPTT) between 50 and 70 seconds (1.5 to 2.0 times) control for 48 hours or until revascularization.[2]

It is also prudent to administer intravenous UFH or subcutaneous low–molecular-weight heparin (LMWH) if the person is at risk for thrombus development. For patients with known heparin-induced thrombocytopenia (HIT), as an alternative to LMWH or UFH, a third class of antithrombotic medications is available—direct antithrombotic agents (e.g., hirudin, bivalirudin, argatroban). Patients at risk for thrombotic emboli include those with an anterior wall infarction, AF, previous embolus, cardiomyopathy, or cardiogenic shock.

Dysrhythmia Prevention

The antidysrhythmic with the best safety record after STEMI is amiodarone. Beta-blockers are another class of antidysrhythmics that are recommended for all patients after STEMI. Beta-blockers prevent ventricular dysrhythmias, lower blood pressure, and prevent reinfarction, especially in patients with left ventricular dysfunction.[2]

Prevention of Ventricular Remodeling

Many patients are at risk for development of heart failure after STEMI. Vasodilating medications (ACEIs or ARBs) can stop or limit the ventricular remodeling that leads to heart failure. Ventricular remodeling is progressive changes in the size, architecture, and shape of the myocardium and occurs because of an injury such as an MI. Ventricular remodeling is modulated by catecholamines and activation of neurohormonal compensatory mechanisms. The heart chamber walls ultimately become dilated, thinned, and poorly contractile. An ACEI is used, or if it is not tolerated, an ARB is indicated for all patients after STEMI.[2] Information about the clinical effects of heart failure is provided later in this chapter.

Nursing Management

Nursing management of the patient with an acute MI incorporates a variety of nursing diagnoses (see Box 12-8 Nursing Diagnoses Priorities: Myocardial Infarction). **Nursing priorities focus on 1) balancing myocardial oxygen supply and demand, 2) preventing complications, and 3) providing patient education.**

Balancing Myocardial Oxygen Supply and Demand

In the acute period, if severe heart muscle damage has occurred, myocardial oxygen supply is increased by the administration of supplemental oxygen to prevent tissue hypoxia. Cardiac medications play an increasingly important role in balancing oxygen supply and demand, and it is the critical care nurse who administers and monitors the effectiveness of these agents. For the patient with a low cardiac output, positive inotropic medications such as dobutamine, dopamine, or both may be administered. Milrinone, a phosphodiesterase inhibitor, which increases contractility by improving sarcolemma calcium uptake and causes positive inotropic effects in the myocardium, may be prescribed. In contrast to dobutamine and dopamine, milrinone does not complete for receptor sites in patients taking beta-blockers.

BOX 12-8 NURSING DIAGNOSES PRIORITIES

Myocardial Infarction

- Acute Pain, related to transmission and perception of cutaneous, visceral, muscular, or ischemic impulses, p. 574
- Decreased Cardiac Output, related to alterations in preload, p. 579
- Decreased Cardiac Output, related to alterations in afterload, p. 580
- Decreased Cardiac Output, related to alterations in contractility, p. 580
- Decreased Cardiac Output, related to alterations in heart rate or rhythm, p. 581
- Activity Intolerance, related to cardiopulmonary dysfunction, p. 570
- Risk for Decreased Cardiac Tissue Perfusion, p. 603
- Disturbed Sleep Pattern, related to fragmented sleep, p. 587
- Anxiety, related to threat to biologic, psychologic, or social integrity, p. 576
- Ineffective Coping, related to situational crisis and personal vulnerability, p. 599
- Powerlessness, related to lack of control over current situation or disease progression, p. 600
- Deficient Knowledge, related to lack of previous exposure to information, p. 585 (see Box 12-9, Patient Education for Myocardial Infarction)

BOX 12-9 PATIENT EDUCATION

Myocardial Infarction

- Pathophysiology of coronary artery disease, angina, and acute myocardial infarction
- Angina: Describe signs and symptoms, such as pain, pressure, or heaviness in chest, arms, or jaw.
- Use of the 0-to-10 pain scale: Notify critical care nurse or emergency personnel of any changes in chest pain intensity.
- Avoid Valsalva maneuver.
- Risk factor modification tailored to the patient's individual risk factor profile:
  - Decrease daily fat intake to less than 30% of total calories.
  - Reduce total serum cholesterol to less than 200 mg/dL.
  - Reduce low-density lipoprotein (LDL) cholesterol to less than 70 mg/dL.
  - Stop smoking.
  - Reduce salt intake.
  - Control hypertension.
  - Control diabetes (if patient has diabetes).
  - Increase physical activity.
  - Achieve ideal body weight, if overweight.
- Refer to cardiac rehabilitation program.
- Medication teaching about indications and side effects
- Follow-up care after discharge
- Symptoms to report to a health care professional
- Discussion of how to handle emotional stress and anger

These inotropic agents are used to increase cardiac contractility in the healthy areas of the heart (increasing oxygen supply) while avoiding damage to the recently infarcted areas. Myocardial oxygen supply can be further enhanced by the use of coronary artery vasodilators. Nitroglycerin is often administered for the first 48 hours to increase vasodilation and prevent myocardial ischemia. Research evidence supports the administration of early beta-blockade therapy to decrease myocardial workload and to prevent dysrhythmias. However, if the patient is in cardiogenic shock, beta-blockers are withheld until the cardiac output has improved.[2] Other interventions to decrease cardiac work and myocardial oxygen consumption include bedrest with bedside commode privileges when the patient is clinically stable.

Preventing Complications

A thorough grasp of the range of potential complications that can occur after STEMI is essential. Cardiac monitoring for early detection of ventricular dysrhythmias is ongoing. Assessment for signs of continued ischemic pain is important because angina is a warning sign of the myocardium being at risk. In response to angina, a 12-lead ECG is obtained to determine if an extension of the infarct exists, and nitroglycerin is administered, and the physician is notified immediately so that interventions may be initiated to limit the size of the MI. Heart failure is a serious complication after STEMI. When the patient's blood pressure is stable, treatment with an ACEI is initiated. These vasodilators are used to prevent left ventricular remodeling and dilation that occurs in many patients after an acute MI. Hypotension is a potential complication of ACEIs, especially with the first dose. It is an important nursing responsibility to monitor blood pressure and patient symptoms after taking this medication. Surveillance to detect obvious and subtle signs of bleeding is also a priority because so many acute MI patients receive antiplatelet, anticoagulant, and fibrinolytic medications.[2,24,25]

In the first 24 hours after a myocardial infarction, diet is progressed as tolerated. Preventing hospital-acquired pneumonia and deep vein thrombosis (DVT) is facilitated by early mobilization and raising the head of the bed 30 degrees or more. An upright position facilitates decrease in venous return, lowering of preload, and decrease in the workload of the myocardium. The patient is taught to avoid increasing intraabdominal pressure (Valsalva maneuver). Stool softeners may be given to the patient to lessen the risk of constipation from analgesics and bedrest and to decrease the risk of straining. Providing a calming and quiet environment that focuses on the well-being of the patient assists in the recovery phase.

Patient Education

It is important to discuss the risk of depression following acute MI.[26] Key symptoms of depression mentioned frequently by cardiac patients are fatigue, change in appetite, and sleep disturbance. Depression is an independent risk factor for increased morbidity and mortality in those with coronary heart disease, and it is a treatable condition.

After the acute phase of an MI, patient and family education becomes a priority. The education focuses on risk factor reduction, manifestations of angina, when to call a physician or emergency services, medications, and resumption of physical and sexual activities (Box 12-9). It is recommended that a referral be made to a cardiac rehabilitation program to reinforce education that was commenced during hospitalization.[2,27] Clinical practice guidelines for multidisciplinary care of the patient with an acute MI are listed in Box 12-10.

CARDIAC ARREST AND SUDDEN CARDIAC DEATH

Description

Sudden cardiac death (SCD) from cardiac arrest accounts for more than 50% of the deaths from CVD.[28] Despite aggressive cardiopulmonary resuscitation (CPR) initiated outside the hospital, few who sustain an out-of-hospital cardiac arrest survive to hospital discharge. Strategies that have been shown to improve resuscitation survival involve huge community-wide programs to teach the public hands-only CPR and how to use an automated external defibrillator (AED).

Etiology

Most SCD incidents occur in patients with preexisting ventricular dysfunction resulting from cardiac disease. Specific SCD risk factors include extensive coronary atherosclerosis with or without a history of an acute MI, dilated or hypertrophic cardiomyopathy, valvular heart disease, autonomic nervous system abnormalities, and electrical system abnormalities such as AV block, Wolff-Parkinson-White (WPW) syndrome, QT syndrome abnormalities, and Brugada syndrome.[28] An ejection fraction less than 30% and a history of

BOX 12-10 EVIDENCE-BASED PRACTICE QSEN

Acute Coronary Syndrome and Acute Myocardial Infarction (Non-STEMI and STEMI)

Prevention of Acute Coronary Syndrome

The term *ACS* is used to define the life-threatening consequences of CAD, notably unstable angina, non-STEMI, and STEMI:

- *Unstable angina* is a term that denotes chest pain that is not relieved by SL nitroglycerin or rest within 5 minutes.
- Non-STEMI is an acute MI *without* ST-segment elevation on the 12-lead ECG.
- STEMI is an acute MI *with* ST-segment elevation on the 12-lead ECG. All of the recommendations are class I, meaning that there is strong research evidence to support these recommendations.

Recommendations that Decrease the Risk of Developing Non-STEMI and STEMI

- Primary care providers should evaluate CAD risk factors for all patients every 3 to 5 years using a validated risk assessment scoring tool.
- The 10-year risk of ACS and acute MI should be assessed for all patients who have more than two major risk factors through the use of evidence-based risk assessment tools.
- An intensive risk factor modification program is recommended for patients with established CAD or high-risk equivalents such as diabetes or chronic kidney disease.

Recommendations about Emergency ACS Symptoms

- A patient who has previously diagnosed CAD should take one SL nitroglycerin dose, and the patient (if alone) or a friend or relative should call 911 if chest pain or discomfort is unrelieved or worsening in 5 minutes.
- The same recommendation applies to a patient without known CAD. If pain is unrelieved with rest or worsening at 5 minutes, the patient (if alone) or a friend or relative should call 911.
- Patients with chest discomfort should be transported to the hospital by ambulance rather than be driven by a friend or relative.
- Family members should be advised to take a CPR course before an ACS emergency occurs. This will teach CPR skills, demonstrate use of an AED, and educate participants about the "chain of survival" concept.

Recommendations for Prehospital EMS-Paramedic First Responders

- First responders such as EMS-paramedics can provide early defibrillation and ACLS for patients in cardiac arrest.
- EMS personnel should administer 162 to 325 mg of nonenteric aspirin (chewed, not swallowed) to patients with chest pain and suspected STEMI.
- A prehospital fibrinolysis protocol is reasonable for patients with STEMI if there are physicians in the ambulance or if there is a well-organized EMS service with full-time paramedics plus 12-lead ECG transmission capability and online medical direction.
- Patients older than 75 years and those with cardiogenic shock should be transported to a hospital with the ability to provide fibrinolytics, emergency PCI, or emergency CABG.
- Patients with STEMI who have a contraindication to fibrinolytic therapy should be brought to a hospital capable of emergency PCI or CABG. At the scene, the door-to-departure time should be *less than 30 minutes.* PCI should be initiated *within 90 minutes* after initial medical contact.

Recommendations for Initial Emergency Clinical Management

- Hospitals should establish multidisciplinary teams to facilitate rapid triage of patients who present to the ED with chest pain.
- Use of written protocols is recommended to standardize care. An immediate cardiology consultation is advised if the patient's symptoms fall outside the written protocol.

STEMI

- *Fibrinolytics for STEMI:* Time from coming into contact with the health care system (paramedics or ED) to receiving fibrinolytics should be *less than 30 minutes*. A brief, focused neurologic examination to determine prior stroke or presence of cognitive defects is necessary before administration of fibrinolytics.
- *PCI for STEMI:* Time from coming into contact with the health care system (paramedics or ED) to balloon inflation PCI should be *less than 90 minutes.*

Continued

BOX 12-10 **EVIDENCE-BASED PRACTICE—cont'd**

Acute Coronary Syndrome and Acute Myocardial Infarction (Non-STEMI and STEMI)

Non-STEMI

- If the level of risk for the patient with non-STEMI is not immediately apparent, a "chest pain unit" within the ED permits close surveillance by competent clinicians without immediate hospital admission.
- Glycoprotein IIb/IIIa inhibitors for non-STEMI, in addition to aspirin and heparin, are indicated if cardiac catheterization or PCI is planned.
- PCI may be indicated for non-STEMI.

Recommendations for Initial Emergency Physical Assessment

Vital Signs

- HR, BP, RR, temperature SpO_2, ECG monitor to detect presence of dysrhythmias

Physical Assessment

- Assess for warm or cool skin, color, capillary refill, peripheral pulses.
- Auscultate heart for cardiac murmur or new S_3 or S_4.
- Auscultate lungs for air entry plus crackles and wheezes.
- Observe for breathlessness and frothy pink sputum (pulmonary edema).
- Ask patient, family, significant others for relevant history.

Recommendations for Emergency Diagnostics

12-Lead ECG

- The 12-lead ECG should be shown to the ED physician within 10 minutes after the patient's arrival in the ED for all patients with chest discomfort or angina-equivalent symptoms.
- If the first ECG is normal but the patient continues to have symptoms of chest pain or discomfort, the 12-lead ECG should be repeated at 5- to 10-minute intervals, *or* continuous 12-lead ECG monitoring can be used.
- In patients with inferior wall infarction, RV infarction must be suspected and right-sided ECG leads recorded. V4R is the diagnostic lead of choice to diagnose ST-segment elevation in the RV.

Laboratory Studies

- Laboratory tests should be performed as part of the general management of STEMI but should not delay the administration of reperfusion therapy.

Cardiac Biomarkers

- Measurement of cardiac-specific troponins is recommended for patients with coexistent skeletal muscle injury. Clinicians are advised not to wait for results of the biomarker assay before initiating reperfusion therapy. Point-of-care (handheld) biomarker assay results can be used for rapid determination of treatment, but subsequent biomarker assays should be done by quantitative laboratory analysis.

Imaging Studies

- *Portable chest radiograph:* Obtaining the chest radiograph must not delay reperfusion therapy unless a major complication such as aortic dissection is suspected.
- *Portable echocardiography (TTE or TEE) or MRI:* A scan should be obtained to distinguish aortic dissection from STEMI, for patients in whom the symptoms are not clear.

Recommendations for Care

Prevent Hypoxia

- Supplemental oxygen administered to maintain oxygen saturation greater than 90%

Coronary Vasodilation

- Nitroglycerin (0.04 mg SL every 5 minutes for three doses) is administered. If chest pain or discomfort is ongoing, start peripheral IV. Administer IV nitroglycerin for relief of chest pain, control of hypertension, or relief of pulmonary congestion.

Pain Control

- Morphine sulfate (2 to 4 mg IV) is administered; can increase to 2- to 8-mg IV increments at 5- to 15-minute intervals for STEMI pain control.

NSAIDs

- Discontinue NSAIDs (except for aspirin), both nonselective and COX-2 selective agents, at time of presentation with STEMI because of increased risk of mortality, reinfarction, hypertension, heart failure, and myocardial rupture associated with NSAID use.

Aspirin

- Aspirin 162 mg to be chewed by patient for rapid buccal absorption.

Beta-Blockers

- Oral beta-blocker therapy is administered to patients with STEMI who do not have contraindications to beta-blockade, regardless of fibrinolytic or primary PCI reperfusion.
- Contraindications for beta-blockade with STEMI include signs of heart failure, low cardiac output, cardiogenic shock risk, heart block or prolonged PR interval (>0.24 second), and active asthma or reactive airway disease.
- While considering the options for reperfusion, beta-blockers are given if the patient has tachycardia or hypertension; otherwise, they are started as soon as possible after STEMI.

Angiotensin-Converting Enzymes Inhibitors

- Oral ACE inhibitors are indicated within the first 24 hours after STEMI unless contraindicated.

Recommendations for Emergency Interventions for STEMI

Fibrinolytic Medications

- Fibrinolytic medications are administered to STEMI patients (if PCI is not available) with ST-segment elevation greater than 0.1 mV (1 mm or one small box) in two contiguous precordial (chest) leads *or* two adjacent limb leads, new LBBB or presumed new LBBB, and onset of symptoms less than 12 hours earlier.
- Before administration of fibrinolytic therapy, rule out neurologic contraindications.
- Rule out facial trauma, uncontrolled hypertension, or ischemic stroke within the last 3 months.
- If contraindications to fibrinolysis are present, PCI is the preferred method of reperfusion.

BOX 12-10 EVIDENCE-BASED PRACTICE—cont'd

Acute Coronary Syndrome and Acute Myocardial Infarction (Non-STEMI and STEMI)

PCI

- Emergency diagnostic coronary angiography should be performed to identify blocked coronary artery before PCI.
- Emergency PCI is recommended over fibrinolytic therapy if symptom onset was longer than 3 hours ago.
- Emergency PCI can be performed within 12 hours after symptom onset for patients with new LBBB or presumed new LBBB.
- Emergency PCI balloon inflation should be done within 90 minutes after arrival at the hospital.

Cardiac Surgery

Emergency CABG surgery is undertaken for specific indications in STEMI:

- Failed PCI with persistent pain or hemodynamic instability
- Recurrent ischemia refractory to medical therapy in patients with suitable anatomy who are not candidates for PCI
- Post-MI VSR or papillary muscle rupture, both of which frequently lead to cardiogenic shock
- Cardiogenic shock less than 36 hours after MI, in patients younger than 75 years with ST-segment elevation, or in patients with new LBBB who have multivessel or left main disease
- Recurrent ventricular dysrhythmias in patients with 50% or greater left main coronary artery lesion or triple-vessel disease or both

Recommendations for Secondary Prevention of Complications

Medications

- ACE inhibitors, to prevent ventricular remodeling
- Beta-blockers, to prevent ventricular dysrhythmias
- Diuretics, if heart failure has developed
- Antihyperlipidemics, if total cholesterol, LDL-C, or triglycerides are elevated

Recommendations for Management of Complications after STEMI Cardiogenic Shock

- IABP for patients with hypotension (BP of 90 mm Hg or SBP of 30 mm Hg below baseline)

Ventricular Arrhythmias

- VF or pulseless VT is managed by standard ACLS criteria.
- Patients with hemodynamically significant VT more than 2 days after STEMI who have ongoing ventricular dysrhythmias are considered for implantation of an ICD.
- Patients with an EF between 30% and 40% at 1 month after STEMI should undergo an EPS; if they are inducible to VT/VF, an ICD is recommended to reduce risk of SCD.
- Patients with an EF of less than 30% at 1 month after STEMI are at high risk for SCD.

AV Block

- Transvenous pacemaker (emergency) or permanent pacemaker (later elective) is inserted for symptomatic second- or third-degree AV block.
- All patients after STEMI who require permanent pacing should also be evaluated for ICD indications.

Provide Relevant Education

Medications

- Written and verbal instructions about medication dosages, administration, and side effects

Emergency Information

- Give patient and family information about calling 911 if pain/angina-equivalent symptoms persist or are worse after 5 minutes.
- Family members of high-risk patients are advised to take a CPR class and learn about AED.

Risk Factors

- Smoking cessation, hypertension control, weight control, normal blood glucose; low-fat diet; normal lipid panel
- Increase physical activity, no new HRT for women

Cardiac Rehabilitation

- Participation in a cardiac rehabilitation program will help the patient continue the process of risk factor and lifestyle modification.

References

Anderson JL, et al: 2011 ACCF/AHA Focused Update Incorporated into the ACC/AHA 2007 Guidelines for the Management of Patients with Unstable Angina/Non–ST-Elevation Myocardial Infarction: a Report of the American College of Cardiology Foundation/American Heart Association Task Force on Practice Guidelines, *Circulation* 123:e426, 2011.

O'Gara PT, et al: 2013 ACCF/AHA Guideline for the Management of ST-Elevation Myocardial Infarction: a Report of the American College of Cardiology Foundation/American Heart Association Task Force on Practice Guidelines, *Circulation* 127(4):e362, 2013.

Wright SR, et al: 2011 ACC/AHA Focused Update of the guidelines for the management of patients with unstable angina/non ST elevation myocardial infarction: a report of the American College of Cardiology/American Heart Association Task Force on Practice Guidelines developed in collaboration with the American College of Emergency Physicians, Society for Cardiovascular Angiography and Interventions, and Society for Thoracic Surgeons, *J Am Coll Cardiol* 57:1920, 2011.

ACE, Angiotensin-converting enzyme; *ACLS*, advanced cardiac life support; *ACS*, acute coronary syndrome; *AED*, automated external defibrillator; *AV*, atrioventricular; *BP*, blood pressure, *CABG*, coronary artery bypass graft surgery; *CAD*, coronary artery disease; *COX-2*, cyclooxygenase 2; *CPR*, cardiopulmonary resuscitation; *ECG*, electrocardiogram; *ED*, emergency department; *EF*, ejection fraction; *EMS*, emergency medical services; *EPS*, electrophysiology study; *HR*, heart rate; *HRT*, hormone replacement therapy; *IABP*, intraaortic balloon pump; *ICD*, implantable cardioverter defibrillator; *IV*, intravenous; *LBBB*, left bundle branch block; *LDL*, low-density lipoprotein cholesterol; *MI*, myocardial infarction; *MRI*, magnetic resonance imaging; *non-STEMI*, non–ST-segment elevation myocardial infarction; *NSAIDs*, nonsteroidal antiinflammatory drugs; *PCI*, percutaneous coronary intervention; *RR*, respiratory rate; *RV*, right ventricle; SaO_2, arterial oxygen saturation; *SCD*, sudden cardiac death; *SL*, sublingual; SpO_2, oxygen saturation from external pulse-oximeter; *STEMI*, ST-segment elevation myocardial infarction; *TEE*, transesophageal echocardiogram; *TTE*, transthoracic echocardiogram; *VF*, ventricular fibrillation; *VSR*, ventricular septal rupture; *VT*, ventricular tachycardia.

BOX 12-11 Causes of Sudden Cardiac Death

Acquired SCD Risk

Most SCD patients are older adults and have a history of CAD, MI, and subsequent heart failure.

- Heart failure
  - Ejection fraction <30%
  - Heart structure is abnormal (systolic or diastolic ventricular dysfunction).
  - CAD and a history of MI that has produced scar tissue is the most common cause of VT/VF leading to SCD.
- Cardiomyopathy (dilated or ischemic)
  - Patients who are inducible for VT/VF in EPS are at highest risk.
  - Risk is decreased by implantation of an ICD and antidysrhythmic medication therapy.

Genetic SCD Risk

Genetic cardiovascular disease accounts for 40% of SCD in young adults.

- Brugada syndrome
  - ECG signs: coved-type ST-segment elevation (>2 mm) in right precordial leads, although ECG variations also occur
  - Heart structure appears normal.
  - High risk of VT or VF in otherwise young healthy adults
  - VT/VF often occurs at night, at rest.
  - Represents 4% of all SCD; average age, 41 years
  - Represents up to 20% of genetic SCD patients
  - Hereditary: autosomal-dominant genetic transmission
  - Five times more common in males
  - Patients who are inducible in EPS are at increased risk.
  - Risk reduced by implantation of an ICD
- Wolff-Parkinson-White syndrome
  - Congenital accessory conduction pathway connects the atria and ventricles.
  - Accessory pathway is *in addition* to the normal conduction system.
  - Accessory pathway allows very rapid transmission of impulses leading to "preexcitation" of the ventricle that can degenerate into VT/VF, especially if atrial dysrhythmias are present.
  - WPW syndrome is usually identified when patient is a teenager or young adult.
  - WPW syndrome is often recognized during exercise by palpitations or breathlessness.
  - It can be cured in many cases by radiofrequency ablation of the accessory pathway.
- Hypertrophic cardiomyopathy
  - Risk of VT/VF with exercise exists.
  - The HOCM form can be cured in many cases by alcohol ablation of the enlarged ventricular septum.
  - For other HCM patients, the risk is reduced by implantation of an ICD.
- Long QT syndrome
  - Risk of VT/VF with exercise exists.
  - The risk is reduced by implantation of an ICD.

CAD, Coronary artery disease; CV, cardiovascular; *ECG*, electrocardiogram; *EPS*, electrophysiology study; *HCM*, hypertrophic cardiomyopathy; *HOCM*, hypertrophic obstructive cardiomyopathy; *ICD*, implantable cardioverter defibrillator; *MI*, myocardial infarction; *SCD*, sudden cardiac death; *VF*, ventricular fibrillation; *VT*, ventricular tachycardia; *WPW*, Wolff-Parkinson-White.

ventricular dysrhythmias are powerful predictors of SCD. Other risk factors are listed in Box 12-11. Unfortunately, many individuals are unaware of their risk or have not considered other risk factors.

Medical Management

Depending on the length of time the patient was unconscious as a result of the cardiac arrest, cognitive defects may be present because of the lack of cerebral blood flow and resultant hypoxia. The cardiac arrest may also have damaged the myocardium and other tissues. Treatment is tailored to the needs of the patient. For comatose patients at high risk for hypoxic brain injury after cardiac arrest, therapeutic hypothermia is initiated to preserve brain function.[28]

HEART FAILURE

Description and Etiology

The number of patients with heart failure is increasing in the United States. Almost 6 million adults (those above the age of 18 years) in the United States have heart failure. It is estimated that by 2030, an additional 3 million more people will be diagnosed with heart failure.[1]

Pathophysiology

Heart failure is a response to cardiac dysfunction, a condition in which the heart cannot pump blood at a volume required to meet the body's needs. Any condition that impairs the ability of the ventricles to fill or eject blood can cause heart failure. Structural heart changes lead to heart failure including acute MI, valvular dysfunction, infection (myocarditis or endocarditis), cardiomyopathy, and uncontrolled hypertension.

Assessment and Diagnosis

Heart failure is typically classified on the basis of the New York Heart Association (NYHA) criteria. Patients are assigned into four groups, I through IV, according to the severity of symptoms and degree of patient activity eliciting symptoms (Table 12-6). Research-based clinical guidelines suggest adding a second level of classification that emphasizes the progressive nature of heart failure through stages identified by increasing distress and intensified clinical interventions.[29] Heart failure can manifest in many different ways, depending on how far ventricular remodeling and dysfunction have advanced. Classic symptoms are dyspnea and fatigue.[29] Heart failure may be discovered because of a known clinical syndrome such as acute MI or because of decreased exercise tolerance, fluid retention, or admission to the critical care unit for an unrelated condition.

The first step in the diagnosis is to determine the underlying structural abnormality creating the ventricular dysfunction and symptoms. Various imaging tests are available to visualize cardiac anatomy, and laboratory tests are used to evaluate the impact of hormonal or electrolyte imbalances. The results of these tests permit the cardiology team to design a treatment plan to control symptoms and possibly correct the underlying cause. All patients do not have the same type of heart failure.

Left Ventricular Failure

Failure of the left ventricle is defined as a disturbance of the contractile function of the left ventricle, resulting in a low cardiac output state. This leads to vasoconstriction of the systemic arterial bed that raises systemic vascular resistance (SVR), a condition also described as "high afterload." A poorly contractile left ventricle will cause congestion in the pulmonary circulation and edema in the alveoli. Clinical manifestations of left ventricular failure include decreased peripheral perfusion with weak or diminished pulses; cool, pale extremities, and, in later stages, peripheral cyanosis (Table 12-7). Over time, with progression of the disease state, the fluid accumulation behind the dysfunctional left ventricle elevates pulmonary pressures, contributes to pulmonary congestion and edema, and produces dysfunction of the right ventricle, resulting in failure of the right side of the heart.

Heart failure with preserved ejection fraction. There has been a change in the descriptors used to define heart failure. Previously the terms "systolic heart failure" and "diastolic heart failure" were used. Recent clinical guidelines focus to a greater extent on whether the ejection fraction is preserved or reduced.[29]

Over one-half of patients with a clinical diagnosis of heart failure have a preserved ejection fraction (HFpEF), meaning they have an ejection fraction greater than 50%.[29,20] This condition was previously referred to as diastolic dysfunction. Most treatments were developed for patients with low ejection fractions, so that research on the optimal treatment regimen for HFpEF is lacking.

Heart failure with reduced ejection fraction. Heart failure with a reduced ejection fraction (HFrEF) was previously named systolic heart failure with an ejection fraction of less than 40%[30] (see Table 12-8).

The patient diagnosed with HFrEF typically experiences the neurohormonal and pulmonary complications of heart failure as described in the following sections.

Neurohormonal Compensatory Mechanisms in Heart Failure

When the heart begins to fail and the cardiac output is no longer sufficient to meet the metabolic needs of tissues, the body activates several major compensatory mechanisms: the sympathetic nervous system, the renin-angiotensin-aldosterone system (RAAS), and, if hypertension is present, the development of ventricular hypertrophy. This process ultimately reshapes the ventricle in a process described as *ventricular remodeling*. These pathophysiologic processes and the pharmacologic measures taken to limit ventricular remodeling are described in this section.

The sympathetic nervous system compensates for low cardiac output by increasing heart rate and blood pressure. As a result, levels of circulating catecholamines are increased, resulting in peripheral vasoconstriction. In addition to raising blood pressure and heart rate, catecholamines cause shunting of blood from nonvital organs such as the skin to vital organs such as the heart and brain. This mechanism, although initially helpful, may become a negative factor if elevation of heart rate increases myocardial oxygen demand while shortening the amount of time for diastolic filling and coronary artery perfusion.

Activation of renin-angiotensin-aldosterone system (RAAS) in heart failure promotes fluid retention. The RAAS is activated by low cardiac output that causes the hormone renin to be secreted by the kidneys. A physiologic chain of events is then set in motion that leads to volume overload. The renin acts on angiotensinogen in the bloodstream and converts it to angiotensin I; when angiotensin passes through the lung tissues, it is activated by angiotensin-converting enzyme (ACE), an enzyme that converts the angiotensin I to

TABLE 12-6 New York Heart Association Functional Classification of Heart Failure

CLASS	DEFINITION
I	Normal daily activity does not initiate symptoms.
II	Normal daily activities initiate onset of symptoms, but symptoms subside with rest.
III	Minimal activity initiates symptoms; patients are usually symptom-free at rest.
IV	Any type of activity initiates symptoms, and symptoms are present at rest.

TABLE 12-7 Clinical Manifestations of Right- and Left-Sided Heart Failure

LEFT VENTRICULAR FAILURE		RIGHT VENTRICULAR FAILURE	
SIGNS	SYMPTOMS	SIGNS	SYMPTOMS
Tachypnea	Fatigue	Peripheral edema	Weakness
Tachycardia	Dyspnea	Hepatomegaly	Anorexia
Cough	Orthopnea	Splenomegaly	Indigestion
Bibasilar crackles	Paroxysmal nocturnal dyspnea	Hepatojugular reflux	Weight gain
Gallop rhythms (S_3 and S_4)	Nocturia	Ascites	Mental changes
Increased pulmonary artery pressures		Jugular venous distention	
Hemoptysis		Increased central venous pressure	
Cyanosis		Pulmonary hypertension	
Pulmonary edema			

TABLE 12-8 Stages in the Development of Heart Failure

AT RISK FOR HEART FAILURE		HEART FAILURE		
STAGE A	**STAGE B**	**STAGE C**		**STAGE D**
At risk for heart failure but without structural heart disease or symptoms of heart failure	Structural heart disease but without symptoms of heart failure	Structural heart disease with prior or current symptoms of heart failure		Refractory heart failure at rest despite optimal guideline-directed therapy
Stage A Risk Factors • Hypertension • Atherosclerotic disease • Diabetes Mellitus • Obesity • Metabolic Syndrome • Using cardiotoxins • Family history of cardiomyopathy	**Stage B Risk Factors** • Previous MI • LV remodeling including LV hypertrophy and low EF% • Asymptomatic valve disease	**Stage C Heart Failure** • Known structural heart disease • Heart failure signs and symptoms • Two presentations of Heart Failure: 1) Heart Failure with preserved Ejection Fraction (HFpEF) 2) Heart Failure with reduced Ejection Fraction (HFrEF)		**Stage D Refractory Heart Failure** • Refractory heart failure symptoms at rest despite optimal therapy • Recurrent hospitalizations for heart failure despite guideline-directed treatment
		HFpEF	**HFrEF**	**LOW EF%**
Stage A Goals of Treatment • Heart-healthy lifestyle • Prevent CAD, stroke, vascular disease • Prevent LV structural abnormalities	**Stage B Goals of Treatment** • Prevent heart failure symptoms • Prevent further cardiac remodeling	**Stage C (HFpEF) Goals of Treatment** • Control symptoms • Health-related quality of life • Prevent hospitalization • Prevent mortality • Identify comorbidities	**Stage C (HFrEF) Goals of Treatment** • Control symptoms • Patient education • Prevent hospitalization • Prevent mortality	**Stage D Goals of Treatment** • Control symptoms • Improve HRQL • Reduce hospital admissions • Establish patients' end-of-life goals
Stage A Medications • ACE inhibitors or ARB blockers for eligible patients with atherosclerotic disease or diabetes mellitus • Statins as appropriate	**Stage B Medications** • ACE inhibitors or ARB blockers as appropriate • Beta-blockers as appropriate (Medications are not required for all patients.)	**Stage C (HFpEF) Medications** Diuretics to relieve symptoms of congestion	**Stage C (HFrEF) Medications for routine use** • Diuretics for fluid retention • ACE Inhibitors • Beta-blockers • Aldosterone antagonists **In selected Patients:** • Hydralazne • Isosorbide dinitrate • ACE Inhibitors and ARBs • Digitalis	**Stage D Medications** As in previous section. Investigational medications
	Stage B Selected Therapies • Implantable cardioverter defibrillator • Revascularization • Valvular surgery	**Stage C (HFpEF)** Follow treatment guidelines for hypertension, atrial fibrillation, coronary artery disease, and diabetes mellitus	**Stage C (HFrEF) Selected Therapies** • CRT • ICD • Revascularization • Valvular surgery	**Stage D Options** • Advanced care measures • Heart transplant • Chronic inotropes • Mechanical circulatory support (temporary or permanent) • Surgery • Palliative care • ICD deactivation
At Risk		Progression of Heart Failure Signs and Symptoms		

ACE, Angiotensin-converting enzyme; *CAD*, coronary artery disease; *CM*, cardiomyopathy; *HF*, heart failure; *IV*, intravenous; *MI*, myocardial infarction.

Modified from Hunt SA, et al. ACC/AHA 2005 guideline update for the diagnosis and management of chronic heart failure in the adult: a report of the American College of Cardiology/American Heart Association Task Force on Practice Guidelines. *Circulation*. 2005; 112(12):e154.

angiotensin II, a powerful vasoconstrictor that increases SVR, raises blood pressure, and increases the workload of the left ventricle; the increased SVR further lowers cardiac output. The mineralocorticoid hormone aldosterone is released from the adrenal glands and stimulates sodium retention by means of the distal tubules of the kidney. In response to the low cardiac output, the renal arterioles constrict, decrease glomerular filtration, and increase reabsorption of sodium from the proximal and distal tubules. To break the RAAS cycle of fluid retention in heart failure, two types of medications are prescribed to interrupt the steps. To inhibit the conversion of angiotensin I to angiotensin II, an ACEI is prescribed (see Table 13-21 (Medications Used for Heart Failure) in Chapter 13). These agents prevent arterial vasoconstriction, decrease blood pressure and SVR, and decrease the amount of ventricular remodeling that often occurs with heart failure. A medication that inhibits angiotensin II directly may be prescribed instead. The medications in this category are ARBs.[31] Aldactone (spirolactone) is a medication from a different category that is also prescribed to break the RAAS cycle. Aldactone is a mineralocorticoid receptor antagonist that inhibits (blocks) the retention of sodium from the distal tubules of the kidney[31] Figure 12-15 depicts the mechanism of action by which these medications act on the RAAS.

Ventricular hypertrophy is the final compensatory mechanism. It is also strongly associated with preexisting hypertension. Because myocardial hypertrophy increases the force of contraction, hypertrophy helps the ventricle overcome an increase in afterload. When this mechanism is no longer efficient for the ventricle, it will remodel by dilation.

Ventricular remodeling occurs as a result of the previously described mechanisms. The shape of the ventricle is changed, or is remodeled, to resemble a round bowl. A dilated ventricle has poor contractility and is enlarged without hypertrophy. Research trial evidence indicates that synergistic use of medications from different categories—ACEI or ARB, aldactone, as well as beta-blockade—can halt or reduce the progression of heart failure remodeling.

Pulmonary Complications of Heart Failure

The clinical manifestations of left-sided heart failure result from tissue hypoperfusion and organ congestion and are progressive. The severity of clinical manifestations progresses as heart failure worsens. Initially, manifestations appear only with exertion, but eventually, they also occur at rest.

Shortness of Breath in Heart Failure

The patient experiences the feeling of shortness of breath first with exertion, but as heart failure worsens, symptoms are also present at rest. A diagnostic blood test is available to assist clinicians in differentiating whether a patient's shortness of breath is caused by cardiac failure or by pulmonary complications. BNP, a cardiac neurohormone released by the ventricles in response to volume expansion and pressure overload, is elevated in heart failure.[29] Heart failure increases left ventricular wall tension because of the excess preload in the ventricles. When the BNP blood level is greater than 100 pg/mL,[32] the dyspnea is most likely related to cardiac failure rather than pulmonary failure. The more severe the heart failure, the higher is the BNP value. If the patient has concomitant kidney disease, the BNP clinical diagnostic point to diagnose heart failure rises to greater than 200 pg/mL[32] There is a newer test, the NT-proBNP, that is used in some settings.[29,32] Breathlessness in heart failure is described by the following terms:

- *Dyspnea:* the patient's sensation of shortness of breath, which derives from pulmonary vascular congestion and decreased lung compliance
- *Orthopnea:* difficulty breathing when lying flat because of an increase in venous return that occurs in the supine position
- *Paroxysmal nocturnal dyspnea:* a severe form of orthopnea in which the patient awakens from sleep gasping for air
- *Cardiac asthma:* dyspnea with wheezing, a nonproductive cough, and pulmonary crackles that progress to the gurgling sounds of pulmonary edema

Pulmonary Edema in Heart Failure

Pulmonary edema, or protein-laden fluid in the alveoli, inhibits gas exchange by impairing the diffusion pathway between the alveolus and the capillary. It is caused by increased left atrial and ventricular pressures and results in an excessive accumulation of serous or serosanguineous fluid in the interstitial spaces and alveoli of the lungs. The normal alveolar-capillary relationship is shown in Figure 12-16A. The formation of pulmonary edema has two stages. The first stage is not as severe and is characterized by interstitial edema, engorgement of the perivascular and peribronchial spaces, and increased lymphatic flow (Figure 12-16B). The later stage is characterized by alveolar edema resulting from fluid moving into the alveoli from the interstitium (see Figure 12-16C). Eventually, blood plasma moves into the alveoli faster than the lymphatic system can clear it, interfering with diffusion of oxygen, depressing the arterial partial pressure of oxygen (PaO_2), and leading to tissue hypoxia (see Figure 12-16D).

Patients experiencing heart failure and pulmonary edema are extremely breathless and anxious and have a sensation of suffocation. They expectorate pink, frothy sputum and feel as if they are drowning. They may sit bolt upright, gasp for breath, or thrash about. The respiratory rate is elevated, and accessory muscles of ventilation are used, with nasal flaring and bulging neck muscles. Respirations are characterized by loud inspiratory and expiratory gurgling sounds. Diaphoresis is profuse, and the skin is cold, ashen, and sometimes cyanotic. This reflects low cardiac output, increased sympathetic stimulation, peripheral vasoconstriction, and desaturation of arterial blood.

Arterial blood gases in pulmonary edema. Arterial blood gas values are variable. In the early stage of pulmonary edema, respiratory alkalosis may be present because of hyperventilation, which eliminates CO_2. As the pulmonary edema progresses and gas exchange becomes impaired, acidosis (pH <7.35) and hypoxemia ensue. A chest radiograph usually confirms an enlarged cardiac silhouette, pulmonary venous congestion, and interstitial edema.

Cardiogenic pulmonary edema versus noncardiogenic pulmonary edema. In the critical care unit, when a patient develops pulmonary edema, it is often a challenge to determine whether the cause is cardiac, known as cardiogenic pulmonary edema, or the origin is pulmonary or systemic in origin. The latter is sometimes referred to as noncardiogenic pulmonary edema or, more commonly, acute respiratory distress syndrome (ARDS). Options to determine the cause of the pulmonary edema include use of the serum BNP

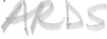

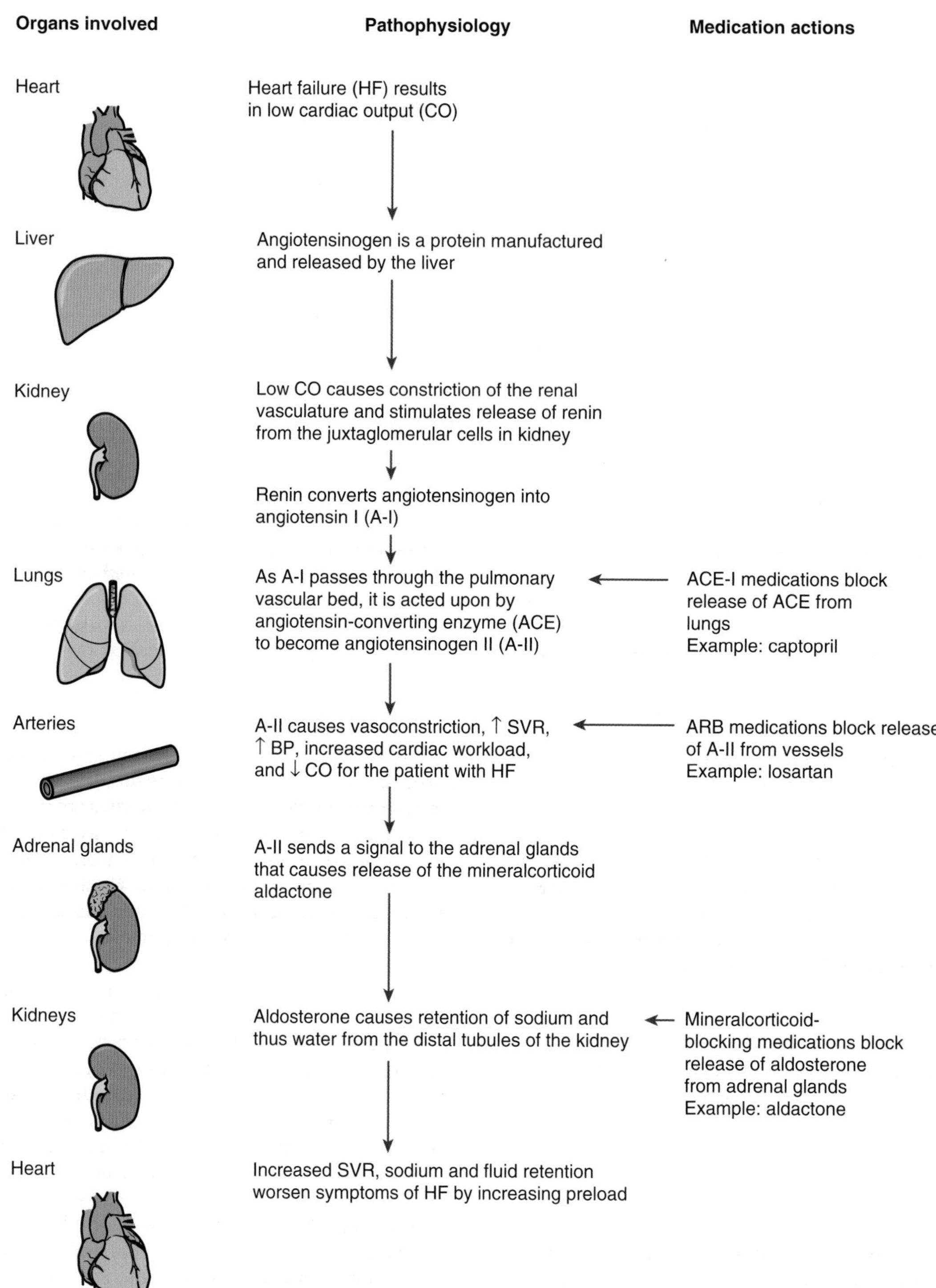

FIG 12-15 Renin-angiotensin-aldosterone system (RAAS), its role in heart failure, and medication actions.

level, diagnostic use of echocardiography, or less frequently insertion of a pulmonary artery catheter. Chapter 20 provides more information on the management of ARDS.

Right Ventricular Failure

Failure of the right side of the heart is defined as ineffective right ventricular contractile function. Pure failure of the right ventricle may result from an acute condition such as a pulmonary embolus or a right ventricular infarction, but it is most commonly caused by failure of the left side of the heart. The common manifestations of right ventricular failure are jugular venous distention, elevated central venous pressure (CVP), weakness, peripheral or sacral edema, hepatomegaly (enlarged liver), jaundice, and liver tenderness.

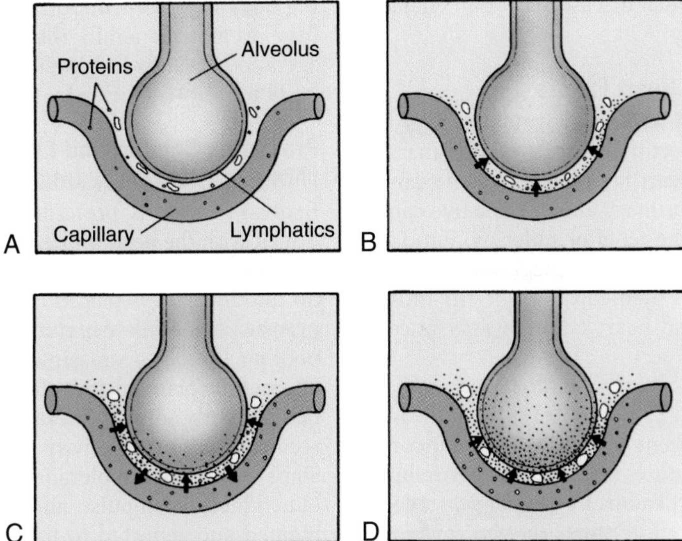

FIG 12-16 As Pulmonary Edema Progresses, Oxygen and Carbon Dioxide Exchange at the Alveolar Capillary Interface are Inhibited. *A,* Normal relationship; *B,* Increased pulmonary capillary hydrostatic pressure causes fluid to move from the vascular space into the pulmonary interstitial space; *C,* Lymphatic flow increases in an attempt to pull fluid back into the vascular or lymphatic space; *D,* Failure of lymphatic flow and worsening of left-sided heart failure results in further movement of fluid into the interstitial space and the alveoli.

Gastrointestinal symptoms include poor appetite, anorexia, nausea, and an uncomfortable feeling of fullness.

Dysrhythmias and Heart Failure

A ventricular ejection fraction below 30% and the presence of NYHA class III or IV heart failure are strongly associated with ventricular dysrhythmias and an increased risk for death. Because sustained VT or VF initiates SCD, high-risk patients with severe heart failure are prescribed antidysrhythmic medications and generally have an ICD inserted.

Medical Management

The goals of the medical management of heart failure are to relieve symptoms, enhance cardiac performance, and correct known precipitating causes.

Relief of Symptoms and Enhancement of Cardiac Performance

In the acute phase of advanced heart failure in the critical care unit, the patient may have a pulmonary artery catheter in place so that left ventricular function can be monitored closely. Control of symptoms involves management of fluid overload and improvement of cardiac output by decreasing SVR and increasing contractility. Diuretics are administered to decrease preload and to eliminate excess fluid from the body. If pulmonary edema develops, additional diuretics are used. Morphine is given to facilitate peripheral dilation and decrease anxiety. Afterload is decreased by vasodilators such as sodium nitroprusside (Nipride) and nitroglycerin. Sodium nitroprusside is a balanced vasodilator medication that relaxes arterial resistance and venous capacitance vessels. By reducing both preload and afterload, it can relieve congestion and also improve cardiac output, particularly in patients with increased SVR. It is useful in favorably redistributing total left ventricular stroke volume in patients with either mitral or aortic insufficiency such that regurgitant flow is reduced while forward flow is increased. Nitrates are used to decrease preload and vasodilate the coronary arteries if CAD is an underlying cause of the acute heart failure. For some patients, an IABP is temporarily required. Contractility is initially increased by continuous infusion of positive inotropic medications (dopamine) or by combination inodilators such as dobutamine or milrinone.

After the acute exacerbation is resolved, the patient is transitioned to oral agents as the intravenous medications are weaned off. Before the transition out of the critical care unit, the patient with heart failure will receive ACEIs to inhibit left ventricular chamber remodeling and slow left ventricular dilation. If the patient does not tolerate ACEIs, ARBs may be substituted. Low-dosage beta-blockers such as carvedilol may also be prescribed, although strict surveillance is required to anticipate and avoid untoward negative inotropic effects. Digoxin may be added to the regimen, especially if the person has concomitant AF. Nonpharmacologic interventions that are increasingly used include *cardiac resynchronization therapy* (CRT).[33] CRT is biventricular pacing, where the right and left ventricles each have a pacing lead in contact with the myocardium. CRT has a beneficial effect on clinical symptoms, exercise capacity, and systolic left ventricular performance in patients with heart failure.[33,34,35]

Correction of Precipitating Causes

After symptoms of heart failure are controlled, diagnostic studies such as cardiac catheterization, echocardiography, and diagnostic imaging tests to determine myocardial perfusion are undertaken to uncover the cause of the heart failure and tailor long-term management to treat the cause. Some structural problems such as valvular disease may be amenable to surgical correction.

Palliative Care for End-Stage Heart Failure

Heart failure is a progressive disease, and patients will not recover.[29] At a point in the trajectory of heart failure, many patients with NYHA class IV heart failure will become candidates for palliative care. The primary aim of palliative care is symptom management and the relief of suffering. Fundamental to all symptom management strategies for heart failure is the relief of symptoms by medications.[29] The most common symptoms of advanced heart failure are dyspnea, pain, and fatigue.

Nursing Management

Nursing management of the patient with heart failure incorporates a variety of nursing diagnoses (see Box 12-12 Nursing Diagnosis Priorities: Acute Heart Failure). **Nursing priorities focus on 1) optimizing cardiopulmonary function, 2) promoting comfort and emotional support, 3) monitoring the effectiveness of pharmacological therapy, 4) providing adequate nutritional intake, and 5) providing patient education.**

Optimizing Cardiopulmonary Function

The patient's ECG is evaluated for dysrhythmias that may be present as a result of medication toxicity or electrolyte imbalance. Patients with heart failure are prone to digoxin toxicity because of decreased renal perfusion and electrolyte imbalances. Breath sounds are auscultated frequently to determine the adequacy of respiratory effort and to assess for onset or worsening of pulmonary congestion. Oxygen is administered through a nasal cannula to relieve dyspnea. Diuretics or vasodilators are used to decrease excessive preload and afterload.[29] If the patient is not hypotensive, morphine may be administered to decrease hyperventilation and anxiety. If the patient's ventilatory status worsens, the nurse must be prepared for endotracheal intubation and mechanical ventilation. Obtaining daily weights is important until the weight stabilizes at a "dry" weight. Generally, the daily weight is used in fluid management, and a weekly weight is optimally used for tracking body weight (e.g., muscle, fat).

Promoting Comfort and Emotional Support

During periods of breathlessness, activity must be restricted. Bedrest usually is prescribed for the patient, who is positioned with the head of the bed elevated to allow for maximal lung expansion. The arms can be supported on pillows so that no undue stress is placed on the shoulder muscles. The legs may be placed in a dependent position to encourage venous pooling, thereby decreasing venous return. Rest periods must be carefully planned and adhered to and independence within the patient's activity prescription fostered. Vital signs are recorded before an activity is begun and after it is completed. Signs of activity intolerance such as dyspnea, fatigue, sustained increase in pulse, and onset of dysrhythmias are documented and reported to the physician. Activity is gradually increased according to the patient's tolerance. Skin breakdown is a risk because of the combination of bedrest, inadequate nutrition, peripheral edema, and decreased perfusion to the skin and subcutaneous tissue. Frequent position changes and mobilization can help to provide comfort and prevent this complication.

Monitoring the Effects of Pharmacologic Therapy

Patients experiencing acute heart failure require aggressive pharmacologic therapy.[36,37] The critical care nurse must know the action, side effects, therapeutic levels, and toxic effects of the diuretics and venodilators used to decrease preload, the positive inotropic agents used to increase ventricular contractility, the vasodilators used to decrease afterload, and any antidysrhythmics used to control heart rate and prevent dysrhythmias. The patient's hemodynamic response to these agents is closely monitored. Fluid intake and output balances are tabulated daily or even hourly in the critical care unit.

Providing Adequate Nutritional Intake

Patients experiencing heart failure often have decreased appetite and nausea, so small, frequent meals may be more appropriate than the standard three large meals. Food must be as tasty as possible; favorite foods and foods from home may be incorporated into the diet as long as the foods are compatible with nutritional restrictions such as low levels of sodium to decrease the risk of fluid retention. Each patient must be assessed for nutritional imbalance individually. Not all patients with heart failure have the same nutritional needs.

Providing Patient Education

The nurse assesses the patient's and family's understanding of the pathophysiology and individual risk factor profile for heart failure.[29] Primary topics of education include the importance of a daily weight, fluid restrictions, and written information about the multiple medications used to control the symptoms of heart failure (Box 12-13).[29] Many patients with a diagnosis of heart failure also require education about lifestyle changes such as smoking cessation, weight loss, energy conservation, and how to incorporate exercise and sodium restriction into their daily lives. Achieving the optimal outcomes for the patient with heart failure requires contributions from a team of educated health care clinicians.

BOX 12-12 NURSING DIAGNOSES

Acute Heart Failure

- Impaired Gas Exchange, related to ventilation/perfusion mismatching or intrapulmonary shunting, p. 594
- Decreased Cardiac Output, related to alterations in preload, p. 579
- Decreased Cardiac Output, related to alterations in contractility, p. 580
- Decreased Cardiac Output, related to alterations in heart rate or rhythm, p. 581
- Activity Intolerance, related to cardiopulmonary dysfunction, p. 570
- Anxiety, related to threat to biologic, psychologic, or social integrity, p. 576
- Ineffective Coping, related to situational crisis and personal vulnerability, p. 599
- Deficient Knowledge, related to lack of previous exposure to information, p. 585 (see Box 12-13, Patient Education for Acute Heart Failure)

CARDIOMYOPATHY

Description and Etiology

Cardiomyopathy is a disease of the heart muscle: *cardio* (heart), *myo-* (muscle), and *-pathy* (pathology). Cardiomyopathies are classified on the basis of structural abnormalities and, if known, genotype. Cardiomyopathies are categorized as *extrinsic*, being caused by external factors such as hypertension, ischemia, inflammation, valvular dysfunction, or as *intrinsic*, which corresponds to myocardial diseases without identifiable external causes.[38,39] The two main forms of primary cardiomyopathies are the hypertrophic and dilated cardiomyopathies. Most of hypertrophic cardiomyopathy and 20% to 50% of dilated cardiomyopathy are familial, showing a genetic disposition.[39] The cardiomyopathy categories are hypertrophic, restrictive, and dilated, as illustrated in Figure 12-17.

BOX 12-13 PATIENT EDUCATION

Acute Heart Failure

- Heart failure: pathophysiology of heart failure
- Fluid balance: low-salt diet to reduce fluid retention; intake and output measurement; signs of fluid overload, such as peripheral edema
- Daily weight: increase or loss of 1 to 2 pounds in a few days is a sign of fluid gain or loss, not true weight gain or loss.
- Breathlessness: increasing shortness of breath, wheezing, and sleeping upright on pillows or in a recliner are symptoms that must be monitored and reported to a health care professional.
- Activity: activity conservation with rest periods as heart failure progresses

Hypertrophic Obstructive Cardiomyopathy

Hypertrophic cardiomyopathy (HCM) is a genetically inherited disease that affects the myocardial sarcomere.[39] As HCM progresses, the left ventricle becomes stiff, noncompliant, and hypertrophied, sometimes in an asymmetric fashion.[38] HCM occurs in two forms. A well-known, but less frequent manifestation is a stiff, noncompliant myocardial muscle, with left ventricular hypertrophy and hypertrophy of the upper ventricular septum. This left ventricular septal hypertrophy obstructs outflow through the aortic valve, especially during exercise (see Figure 12-17A). It also pulls the papillary muscle out of alignment, causing mitral regurgitation. Other patients with HCM have generalized left ventricular hypertrophy, but the septum is not more enlarged than the rest of the myocardium.[38] HCM causes significant diastolic dysfunction because the muscle-bound, stiff, noncompliant heart muscle does not allow adequate filling during diastole.

Two advances in diagnostic medicine have propelled understanding of the differences between these two forms of HCM. *Two-dimensional transthoracic echocardiography* (TTE) is often useful as the first diagnostic test to identify HCM.[38] TTE enables visualization of septal anatomy, septal movement, and ventricular wall thickness and motion. The second advance is *diagnostic genetics*. Genetic testing for HCM usually is performed at a center with expertise in this area.[39] HCM is inherited as an autosomal dominant trait, and

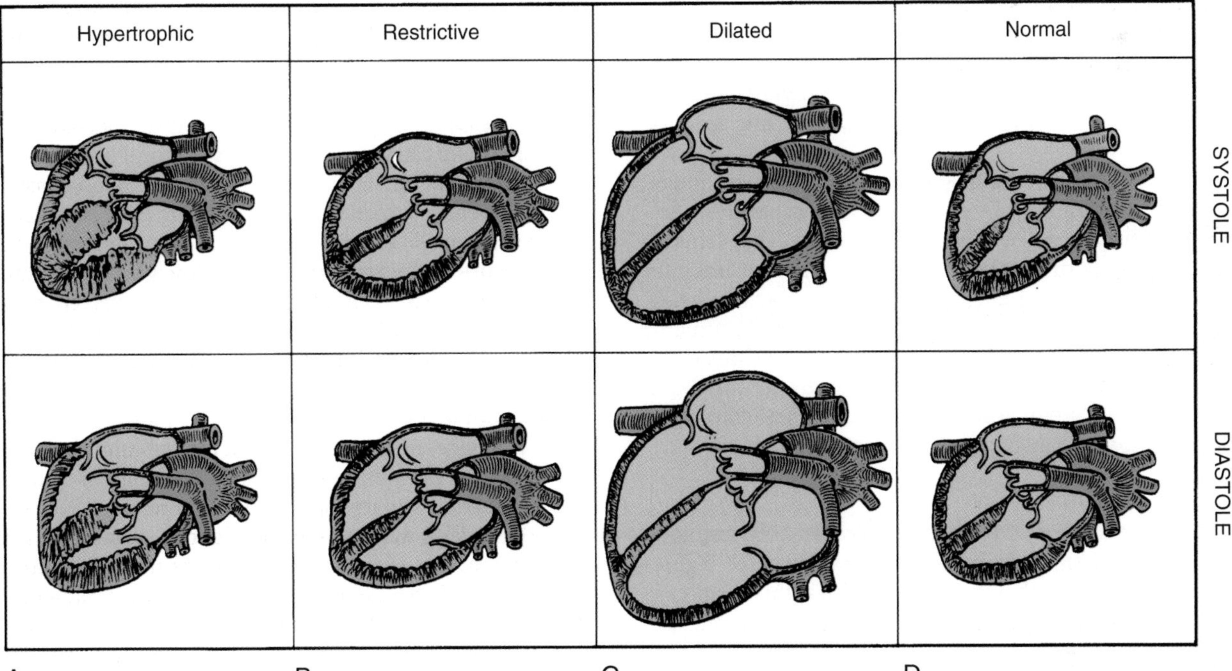

FIG 12-17 Types of Cardiomyopathies and Differences in Ventricular Diameter During Systole and Diastole Compared with a Normal Heart. *A,* Hypertrophic; *B,* restrictive; *C,* dilated; *D,* normal.

the clinical expression is caused by mutations in any of one of 10 genes. Each different gene encodes different protein components of the myocardial sarcomere.[38] Genetic analysis is an area of ongoing research that will undoubtedly help clarify other aspects of this cardiomyopathy within the next decade.

Symptoms are similar to those seen with heart failure, with the addition of myocardial ischemia, supraventricular tachycardia (SVT), VT, syncope, and stroke.[38,39] Symptoms usually are more intense with physical exercise, especially in the obstructive form of HCM, in which the aortic outflow tract is obstructed by the enlarged left ventricular septum. Because a known association exists between HCM and cardiac arrest, limitation of physical activity may be recommended until the patient has an implantable convertor defibrillator (ICD) in situ. Pharmacologic management includes beta-blockers to decrease left ventricular workload, medications to control and prevent atrial and ventricular dysrhythmias, anticoagulation if atrial or left ventricular thrombi are present, and medications to manage heart failure. Interventional procedures include insertion of an ICD to decrease the risk of SCD and percutaneous alcohol ablation of the intraventricular septum to decrease the size of the septal wall.[38,39]

Dilated Cardiomyopathy

Dilated cardiomyopathy is characterized by gross dilation of both ventricles without muscle hypertrophy (see Figure 12-19C). Several distinct causes of dilated cardiomyopathy exist. Dilated cardiomyopathies have both primary and secondary causes and are the most common cause of heart failure, resulting from valvular, ischemic, toxins, metabolic, infectious, and systemic causes.[39]

Ischemic dilated cardiomyopathy results from repeated myocardial infarction that causes ventricular remodeling and a reduced ejection fraction (HFrEF). When the cause of the dilated cardiomyopathy is unknown, it is described as *idiopathic.* Scientific advances in molecular genetics permit detailed studies of affected families. Preliminary research indicates that the genetic picture is highly individual for different family groups, even if the clinical picture appears similar.[40]

In dilated cardiomyopathy, the myocardial muscle fibers contract poorly, resulting in global left ventricular dysfunction, low cardiac output, and atrial and ventricular dysrhythmias. Blood pools tin the heart chambers and that leads to ventricular thrombi and embolic episodes, refractory heart failure, and premature death. The goals of the medical management of dilated cardiomyopathy are similar to those for advanced heart failure: improvement of inotropic function, removal of excess fluid, control of heart failure symptoms, and anticipation and management of complications.

Restrictive Cardiomyopathy

Restrictive cardiomyopathy is the least commonly encountered cardiomyopathy in industrialized countries (see Figure 12-19B). As with the other cardiomyopathies, this form can be idiopathic or can have a known cause. Low cardiac output, dyspnea, orthopnea, and liver engorgement are the most common clinical manifestations of restrictive cardiomyopathy. An elevated jugular venous pressure, S_4 and late S_3, may be present. Both ventricles are typically small with decreased volumes and large atria. The atrial septum and cardiac valves may be thickened, and pericardial effusion may also be present. Medical management is aimed at improving symptoms and preventing tachycardias. Diuretics reduce pulmonary pressure and fluid volume relieving of dyspnea. Nitrates can also provide relief. Patients are advised to reduce sodium intake, weigh daily, and restrict water intake. ACE inhibitors and ARBs improve stroke volume and reduce myocardial oxygen demand.

Nursing Management

Nursing management of the patient with cardiomyopathy incorporates a variety of nursing diagnoses related to the symptoms of heart failure. Nursing interventions are individualized according to the type of cardiomyopathy and are focused on achievement of a stable fluid balance, monitoring the effects of pharmacological therapy, safely increasing mobility, and providing patient and family education. As with heart failure, a collaborative team of compassionate, knowledgeable professionals is required to provide effective care and education for these challenging patients.

ENDOCARDITIS

Description and Etiology

Endocarditis is an inflammation on the endothelial surface of the heart, specifically thrombotic-fibrin vegetations on the cardiac valves. This irritation can be related to infectious or noninfectious sources.[41] Although most commonly associated with valve leaflets, the chordae, chamber walls, paraprosthetic tissue, implanted shunts, conduits, and fistulas may also be affected.[42] The older term of bacterial endocarditis has been replaced by infectious endocarditis (IE) because nonbacterial organisms can be the infective source of the endothelial inflammation. The incidence of IE has not declined over the past 30 years, with 15,000 cases each year and a mortality rate of almost 40%.[43] IE is the fourth most common cause of life-threatening infectious syndromes (after urosepsis, pneumonia, and intraabdominal sepsis). The risk of acquiring IE is higher among patients with congenital heart disease, valvular heart disease, and prosthetic heart valves. Approximately 75% of patients have a preexisting structural abnormality of involved cardiac valve. Increasing incidence of invasive health care interventions such as implantable pacemakers and ICDs, body piercings, intravenous drug abuse (IVDA), and an increase in elderly patients with degenerative valve disease increase the numbers at risk for IE.[41,43] Involvement of right heart valves is highly suspicious for IVDA.[41] Among intravenous drug abusers the incidence of IE is much higher than in the general population.

Development of IE depends on the following events:[44]

- Presence of a nonbacterial thrombotic lesion on a cardiac valve or endothelium
- Bacteremia (bacteria in bloodstream)
- Bacteria attaching to the nonbacterial thrombotic lesion
- Proliferation of bacteria on and within the lesion that may develop into a vegetation.

Research suggests the source of the organism is less likely than previously thought to be related to a specific invasive procedure such as a urogenital procedure or dental work. Instead, IE results from the confluence of multiple daily bacteremic events in the presence of a susceptible cardiac lesion.[44]

Pathophysiology

IE results from a bacterial or fungal organism in the bloodstream that successfully colonizes the cardiac endothelium. It is fatal if not treated. Bacterial organisms, typically streptococci, staphylococci, and enterococci, are the most common pathogens. An increase in multidrug-resistant organisms has led to increased numbers of patients, more serious complications, and higher mortality rates.[44,45] Sites where endocarditis vegetations occur correlate with aberrant intracardiac flow caused by valvular damage or septal defects. After vegetations have colonized, the bacteria multiply at a rapid rate inside a protective platelet-fibrin casing that sequesters the infection.[43]

Assessment and Diagnosis

Diagnosis must be made as soon as possible to initiate treatment and identify patients at high risk for complications. Diagnosis is guided by classic manifestations of bacteremia or fungemia, evidence of active valvulitis, peripheral emboli, and immunologic vascular phenomena.

Modified Duke criteria. The 2008 AHA scientific statement on IE supports use of the modified Duke criteria for diagnosis, early identification, and treatment of IE. This system stratifies patients with suspected IE into three categories: definite cases, possible cases, and rejected cases (Table 12-9). A definite diagnosis of IE requires two major criteria, one major and three minor criteria, or five minor criteria. A possible diagnosis of IE requires one major criteria and one minor criteria or three minor criteria.[44-46]

Blood cultures. Initial symptoms include fever, sometimes accompanied by rigor (shivering), fatigue, malaise, with up to 50% complaining of myalgias and joint pain,[41] Blood cultures are drawn during periods of elevated temperature to detect the infective organism. At least 10 mL of venous blood should be placed in each of the blood culture containers to ensure that the organism will be detected. Culture-negative endocarditis occurs in up to one-third of cases and usually is related to prior antibiotic use or infection by a *fastidious organism* that does not proliferate under conventional laboratory culture conditions.[42] White blood cell (WBC) counts are typically elevated, and the symptoms are identified in the Duke criteria (see Table 12-9).

Chest radiograph. Cough and pleuritic chest pain are present in 40% to 60% of cases. The first noninvasive test is often a chest radiograph to detect nodular infiltrates, cardiomegaly, and enlarged pulmonary vessels.

Echocardiogram. The other essential noninvasive test is an echocardiogram of the heart valves to visualize vegetations. Transthoracic echocardiography (TTE) may be initially performed, but transesophageal echocardiography (TEE) is even more valuable because of the clarity of the heart valve images. TEE is more sensitive in detection of vegetation and abscesses.[45] Color-flow mapping is especially useful to visualize the severity of a valvular regurgitation.[46]

Complications. Heart failure is the most frequent complication of IE and the most frequent cause of death. Embolic complications are the second most common complication, occurring in 22% to 50% of IE cases: 65% of the emboli occur in the central nervous system and can cause a stroke. Pulmonary embolism occurs in 66% to 75% of IVDA cases that involve vegetations on the tricuspid valve. Other organs affected by emboli include liver, spleen, kidney, abdominal mesenteric artery, and peripheral vessels. Septic emboli may be visible on the fingers and toes. Rate of emboli formation rapidly declines with appropriate intravenous antimicrobial administration.[45] Risk of death increases with the development of emboli and decreased arterial perfusion to vital organs.

TABLE 12-9 Modified Duke Criteria

MAJOR CRITERIA*	MINOR CRITERIA*
Blood culture positive for IE Evidence of endocardial involvement	Predisposition: persons with a heart condition or an injectable drug user Fever: temperature >38°C Vascular phenomena: major arterial emboli, septic pulmonary infarcts, mycotic aneurysm, intracranial hemorrhage, conjunctival hemorrhages and Janeway lesions Immunologic phenomena: glomerulonephritis, Osler nodes, Roth spots, and rheumatoid factor Microbial evidence: positive blood culture that does not meet any major criterion or serologic evidence of active infection with organism consistent with IE

*A *definite* diagnosis of infective endocarditis (IE) requires two major criteria, or one major and three minor criteria, or five minor criteria. A *possible* diagnosis of IE requires one major criteria and one minor criteria or three minor criteria.

Based on data from Baddour LM, et al. Infective endocarditis: diagnosis, antimicrobial therapy, and management of complications. A statement for healthcare professionals from the Committee on Rheumatic Fever, Endocarditis, and Kawasaki Disease, Council on Cardiovascular Disease in the Young, and the Councils on Clinical Cardiology, Stroke, and Cardiovascular Surgery and Anesthesia, American Heart Association: endorsed by the Infectious Diseases Society of America. *Circulation.* 2005; 111(23):e394; Wilson W, et al. Prevention of infective endocarditis: guidelines from the American Heart Association. A guideline from the American Heart Association Rheumatic Fever, Endocarditis, and Kawasaki Disease Committee, Council on Cardiovascular Disease in the Young, and the Council on Clinical Cardiology, Council on Cardiovascular Surgery and Anesthesia, and the Quality of Care and Outcomes Research Interdisciplinary Working Group. *Circulation.* 2007; 116(15):1736.

Medical Management

Treatment requires prolonged intravenous therapy with adequate doses of antimicrobial agents tailored to the specific IE microbe and patient circumstances. The antibiotic management of native valve endocarditis (NVE) is frequently different from treatment of prosthetic valve endocarditis (PVE) or IVDA endocarditis. Antibiotic treatment is prolonged, administered in high doses intravenously, and may involve combination therapy.[45] Best outcomes are achieved if therapy is initiated before hemodynamic compromise.

In many cases, antimicrobial drugs are not sufficient to cure the IE. Cardiac surgery to excise the damaged native or prosthetic valve is required for persistent vegetation, valve

BOX 12-14 NURSING DIAGNOSES PRIORITIES

Endocarditis

- Decreased Cardiac Output, related to alterations in preload, p. 579
- Decreased Cardiac Output, related to alterations in afterload, p. 580
- Decreased Cardiac Output, related to alterations in contractility, p. 580
- Decreased Cardiac Output, related to alterations in heart rate or rhythm, p. 581
- Activity Intolerance, related to cardiopulmonary dysfunction, p. 570
- Acute Pain, related to transmission and perception of cutaneous, visceral, muscular, or ischemic impulses, p. 574
- Risk for Infection, related to invasive procedures, p. 607
- Anxiety, related to threat to biologic, psychologic, or social integrity, p. 576
- Deficient Knowledge: Discharge Regimen, related to lack of previous exposure to information, p. 585 (see Box 12-15 Patient Education for Endocarditis)

BOX 12-15 PATIENT EDUCATION

Endocarditis

- Pathophysiology of endocarditis
- Medications: importance of long-term intravenous antibiotics for eradication
- Temperature: daily temperature monitoring
- Infection control: prophylactic antibiotics related to dental work or other invasive procedures after current medical crisis is controlled
- Activity tolerance: Increase activity as tolerated and rest periods as needed.
- Heart failure: If symptoms of heart failure are present, education is given on fluid and sodium restriction, fluid balance, diuretic management, daily weight, and controlling breathlessness.
- Follow-up care after discharge
- Symptoms to report to a health care professional

dysfunction, perivalvular extension, and aggressive fungal- or antibiotic-resistant bacteria. Usually, valve surgery is delayed until the patient is stable. An increasing number of patients with uncomplicated IE are being discharged to home earlier than in the past and are continuing the intravenous antimicrobial therapy by means of a surgically or peripherally implanted long-term central venous catheter at home.[45]

Nursing Management

Nursing management of the patient with IE incorporates a variety of nursing diagnoses priorities (see Nursing Diagnoses Priorities for Management of Endocarditis in Box 12-14). **Nursing priorities are focused on 1) timely antimicrobial administration to resolve the infection, 2) prevention of complications, 3) treatment of pain, and 4) individualizing patient education.**

Resolving the infection. IE requires a long course of intravenous antibiotics, usually for 4 to 6 weeks. This is begun in the hospital and continued at home with an indwelling central catheter after the patient is in stable condition.[45] Nursing assessment includes monitoring for signs of worsening infection, such as persistent temperature elevation, malaise, weakness, easy fatigability, and night sweats, or new emboli on hands or feet (see Box 12-15 Patient Education for Endocarditis).

Preventing complications. Between 20% and 60% of patients with IE experience complications.[43] The nursing assessment is attuned to the early detection of changes such as shortness of breath or chest pain with hemoptysis. As valvular dysfunction accelerates, acute heart failure develops. Cardiac assessment includes auscultation of heart sounds to detect the presence of or change in a cardiac murmur. This can be caused by worsening heart failure or by pulmonary emboli. Changes in level of consciousness, visual changes, or complaints of headache are always reported due to risk of emboli. Evaluation of liver and kidney function is essential to monitor the health of those organs due to embolic risk. With the complex and prolonged antibiotic therapy required for treating IE, adverse drug reactions constitute another important consideration.

Providing Patient Education

The person with IE needs to know the manifestations of infection, how to take an oral temperature, and what medical procedures increase risk of a recurrence of IE. A written list of all medications must be supplied (see the Patient Education feature on Endocarditis). It is essential to reinforce the necessity of the patient providing other health care professionals such as the dentist or podiatrist with a comprehensive endocarditis history.[45,46] The known IVDA has a unique set of challenges to overcome.[47] Multidisciplinary support for the patient to meet the challenge of opiate withdrawal and psychological dependence is essential to prevent a relapse.[47] Many clinicians participate in the care of a patient with IE (Box 12-16).

VALVULAR HEART DISEASE

Description and Etiology

The term *valvular heart disease* describes structural and functional abnormalities of single or multiple cardiac valves. The result is an alteration in blood flow across the valve. The two types of valvular lesions are stenosis (narrowed valve) and insufficiency or regurgitation (backward flow of blood through the valve). These are described with reference to the specific heart valves involved.

Admission of patients with valvular disease to the critical care unit is generally related to surgical replacement or an exacerbation of heart failure. In the past, in the United States, most valvular lesions were rheumatic in origin, and damage was a direct result of group A beta-hemolytic streptococcal pharyngitis. As a result of aggressive treatment of "strep throat," rheumatic valvular disease is rare. Valve lesions are now more commonly related to congenital disorders and

BOX 12-16 EVIDENCE-BASED PRACTICE (QSEN)

Infective Endocarditis and Infective Endocarditis Prophylaxis

Diagnosis of Infective Endocarditis

The Modified Duke Criteria are recommended to guide diagnosis (see Table 12-15). Endocarditis prophylaxis is recommended for patients with the following:

- Prosthetic heart valve with a history of infective endocarditis
- Valve repair
- Complex cyanotic congenital heart disease
- Congenital valve malformation such as bicuspid aortic valve
- HCM with latent or resting obstruction
- MVP with valvular regurgitation and/or thickened valve leaflets

Special considerations apply for patients with prosthetic valve and IE:

- Patients with a risk for IE who have unexplained fever for more than 48 hours should have at least two sets of blood cultures obtained from different sites.
- Surgical valve replacement is indicated for patients with IE of a prosthetic valve who present in heart failure.

Antimicrobial Therapy

Four features mark the antimicrobial therapy administered for IE:

1. It is prolonged.
2. It is bactericidal.
3. It is intravenous.
4. It is high-dosage.

At least two sets of blood cultures are obtained every 24 to 48 hours until the infection is cleared from the bloodstream. IV antimicrobial therapy is continued after hospital discharge in the home setting.

Complications from Infective Endocarditis

- Emboli from infected heart valves occur in 22% to 50% of IE cases, and 65% of embolic events involve the CNS. The rate of embolic events drops significantly during and after 2 to 3 weeks of appropriate antimicrobial therapy.
- Acute heart failure has the greatest impact on overall prognosis.

Complications from Antibiotics

- Toxicity from the high doses of antibiotics may impair kidney function or vestibular function (balance).
- Diarrhea and colitis can be caused by a reaction to the antibiotic therapy or by overgrowth by *Clostridium difficile.*

Indications for Surgery

- Removal of infected device
- Increase in size of valve vegetation despite appropriate antimicrobial therapy
- Mitral or aortic regurgitation with acute heart failure unresponsive to medical therapy
- One or more embolic events during the first 2 weeks of antimicrobial therapy

References

Nishimura RA, et al: ACC/AHA 2008 guideline update on valvular heart disease: focused update on infective endocarditis, *Circulation* 118:887, 2008.

Wilson W, et al: Prevention of infective endocarditis: guidelines from the American Heart Association: a guideline from the American Heart Association Rheumatic Fever, Endocarditis, and Kawasaki Disease Committee, Council on Cardiovascular Disease in the Young, and the Council on Clinical Cardiology, Council on Cardiovascular Surgery and Anesthesia, and the Quality of Care and Outcomes Research Interdisciplinary Working Group, *Circulation* 116(15):1736, 2007.

HCM, Hypertrophic cardiomyopathy; *IE,* infective endocarditis; *MVP,* mitral valve prolapse.

older patients. These patients are more likely to present with symptoms of heart failure and degenerative valve changes.[48]

Pathophysiology

Mitral Valve Stenosis

The term mitral valve stenosis describes a progressive narrowing of the mitral valve orifice. Symptoms occur when the normal valve size is reduced to 2 cm^2 or less. A mitral valve opening less than 1.5 cm^2 is reflective of severe mitral stenosis with a transmitral gradient of 5-10 mm Hg at a normal heart rate.[48] Symptoms occur at rest when the valve area is reduced below 1 cm^2 (Table 12-10A). The diffuse valve leaflets fibrose and fuse, reducing mobility and thickening the chordae tendineae. As a result, the mitral valve can no longer open or close passively in response to left atrial and ventricular pressure changes. Blood flow across the valve is impeded. Mitral stenosis increases the risk of developing AF because of the high pressures in the left atrium that will stimulate left atrial remodeling and enlargement. The valve should be replaced when symptoms develop.

Mitral Valve Regurgitation

Mitral valve regurgitation may result from rheumatic disease, aging of the valve, endocarditis, collagen vascular disease, or papillary muscle dysfunction[48] (see Table 12-10B). In mitral regurgitation, the valve annulus, leaflets, chordae tendineae, and papillary muscles may all be dysfunctional, or the dysfunction may be isolated to just one component of the valve. Mitral valve regurgitation results in retrograde flow of blood into the left atrium with each ventricular contraction. It is always described as chronic or acute because of the very different impact on the left-sided chambers.

In chronic mitral valve regurgitation, the left atrium has dilated to accommodate the additional regurgitant volume, whereas the left ventricle has hypertrophied (increased muscle) to maintain an adequate stroke volume and cardiac output. In contrast, acute mitral valve regurgitation is precipitated by chordae tendineae or papillary muscle rupture resulting from an acute MI or infective endocarditis. This is a medical emergency. The left atrium cannot accommodate

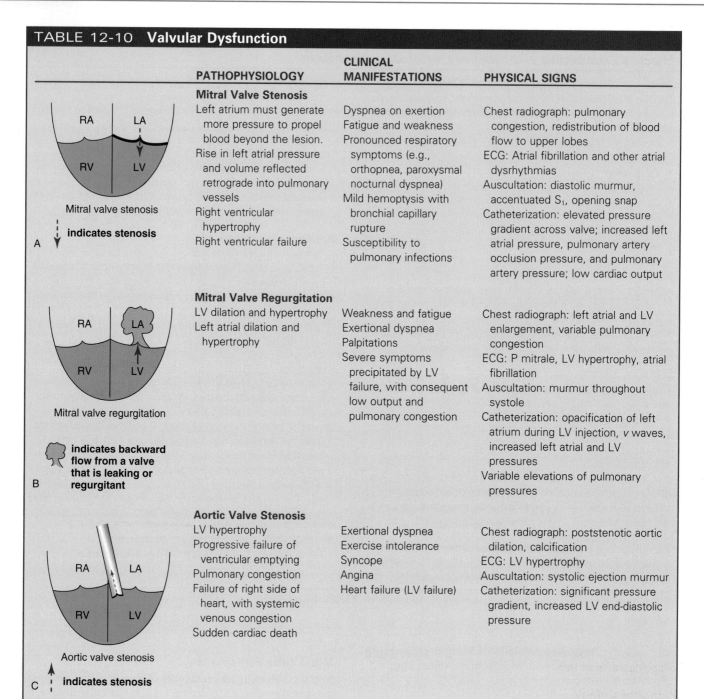

TABLE 12-10 Valvular Dysfunction

	PATHOPHYSIOLOGY	CLINICAL MANIFESTATIONS	PHYSICAL SIGNS
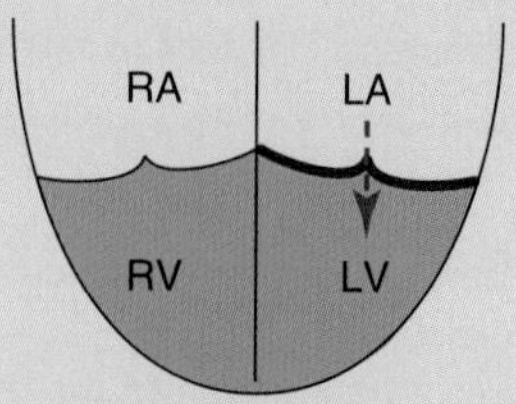 Mitral valve stenosis indicates stenosis A	**Mitral Valve Stenosis** Left atrium must generate more pressure to propel blood beyond the lesion. Rise in left atrial pressure and volume reflected retrograde into pulmonary vessels Right ventricular hypertrophy Right ventricular failure	Dyspnea on exertion Fatigue and weakness Pronounced respiratory symptoms (e.g., orthopnea, paroxysmal nocturnal dyspnea) Mild hemoptysis with bronchial capillary rupture Susceptibility to pulmonary infections	Chest radiograph: pulmonary congestion, redistribution of blood flow to upper lobes ECG: Atrial fibrillation and other atrial dysrhythmias Auscultation: diastolic murmur, accentuated S_1, opening snap Catheterization: elevated pressure gradient across valve; increased left atrial pressure, pulmonary artery occlusion pressure, and pulmonary artery pressure; low cardiac output
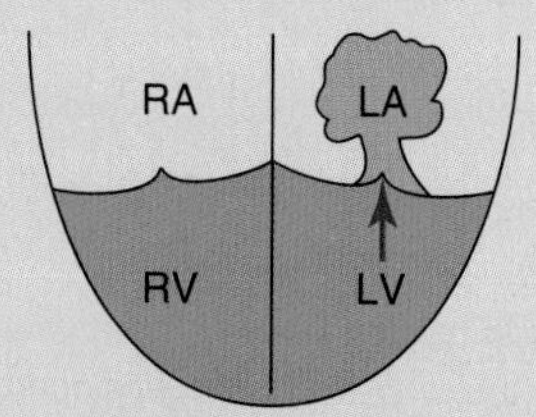 Mitral valve regurgitation indicates backward flow from a valve that is leaking or regurgitant B	**Mitral Valve Regurgitation** LV dilation and hypertrophy Left atrial dilation and hypertrophy	Weakness and fatigue Exertional dyspnea Palpitations Severe symptoms precipitated by LV failure, with consequent low output and pulmonary congestion	Chest radiograph: left atrial and LV enlargement, variable pulmonary congestion ECG: P mitrale, LV hypertrophy, atrial fibrillation Auscultation: murmur throughout systole Catheterization: opacification of left atrium during LV injection, *v* waves, increased left atrial and LV pressures Variable elevations of pulmonary pressures
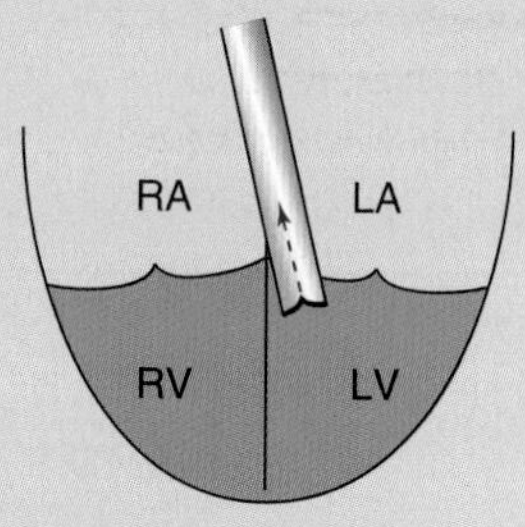 Aortic valve stenosis indicates stenosis C	**Aortic Valve Stenosis** LV hypertrophy Progressive failure of ventricular emptying Pulmonary congestion Failure of right side of heart, with systemic venous congestion Sudden cardiac death	Exertional dyspnea Exercise intolerance Syncope Angina Heart failure (LV failure)	Chest radiograph: poststenotic aortic dilation, calcification ECG: LV hypertrophy Auscultation: systolic ejection murmur Catheterization: significant pressure gradient, increased LV end-diastolic pressure

TABLE 12-10 Valvular Dysfunction—cont'd

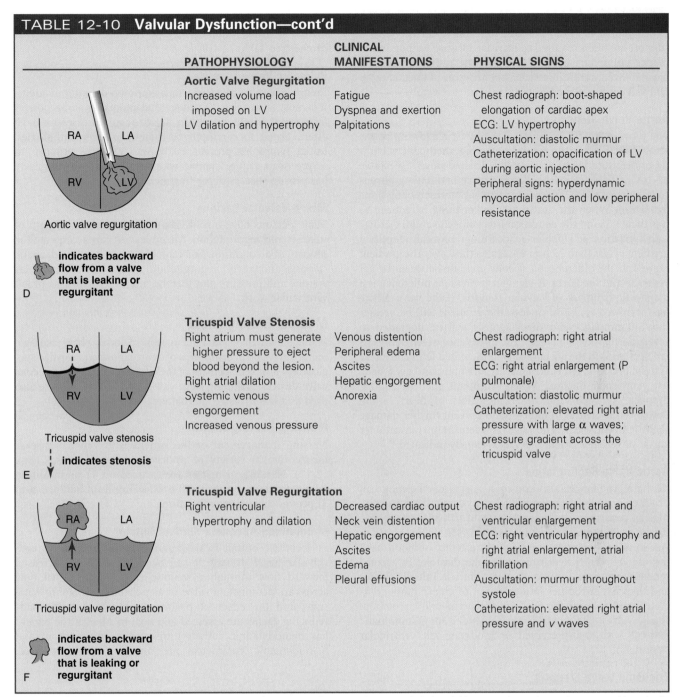

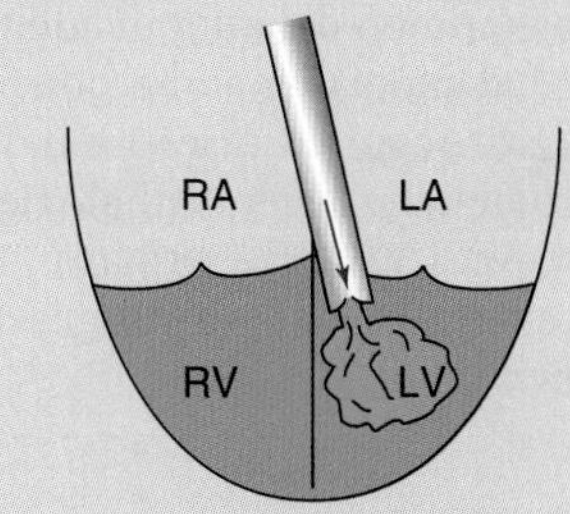

	PATHOPHYSIOLOGY	CLINICAL MANIFESTATIONS	PHYSICAL SIGNS
RA LA RV LV Aortic valve regurgitation indicates backward flow from a valve that is leaking or regurgitant D	**Aortic Valve Regurgitation** Increased volume load imposed on LV LV dilation and hypertrophy	Fatigue Dyspnea and exertion Palpitations	Chest radiograph: boot-shaped elongation of cardiac apex ECG: LV hypertrophy Auscultation: diastolic murmur Catheterization: opacification of LV during aortic injection Peripheral signs: hyperdynamic myocardial action and low peripheral resistance
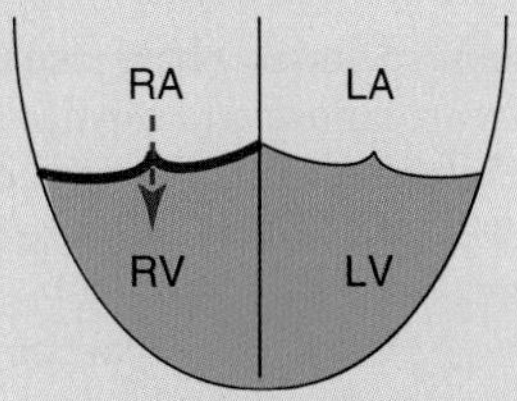 RA LA RV LV Tricuspid valve stenosis indicates stenosis E	**Tricuspid Valve Stenosis** Right atrium must generate higher pressure to eject blood beyond the lesion. Right atrial dilation Systemic venous engorgement Increased venous pressure	Venous distention Peripheral edema Ascites Hepatic engorgement Anorexia	Chest radiograph: right atrial enlargement ECG: right atrial enlargement (P pulmonale) Auscultation: diastolic murmur Catheterization: elevated right atrial pressure with large α waves; pressure gradient across the tricuspid valve
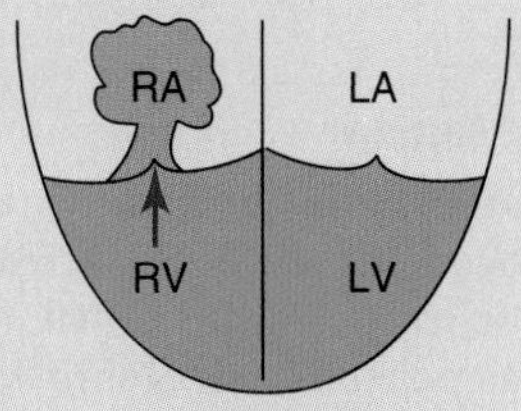 RA LA RV LV Tricuspid valve regurgitation indicates backward flow from a valve that is leaking or regurgitant F	**Tricuspid Valve Regurgitation** Right ventricular hypertrophy and dilation	Decreased cardiac output Neck vein distention Hepatic engorgement Ascites Edema Pleural effusions	Chest radiograph: right atrial and ventricular enlargement ECG: right ventricular hypertrophy and right atrial enlargement, atrial fibrillation Auscultation: murmur throughout systole Catheterization: elevated right atrial pressure and *v* waves

ECG, Electrocardiogram; *LV*, left ventricular; *P mitrale*, m-shaped P waves that occur in left atrial hypertrophy and are often caused by mitral stenosis; *P pulmonale*, tall, peaked P waves that occur in right atrial hypertrophy and are often caused by chronic pulmonary disease.

the sudden increase in volume and pressure, and use of an IABP, inotropic and afterload-reducing pharmacological support are often required to increase forward output and to reduce pulmonary congestion. After the patient's condition has stabilized, surgical replacement or repair of the incompetent valve is performed.[48]

Aortic Valve Stenosis

The term *aortic valve stenosis* describes a narrowing of the aortic valve area. It can result from aging, rheumatic valvulitis, or deterioration of a congenital bicuspid valve[48] (see Table 12-10C). The pathologic hallmarks are inflammation, fibrous valvular thickening, and tissue calcification resembling bone formation. When the aortic valvular opening is reduced to less than 1.5 cm^2, the condition is classified as mild. Cardiac catheterization or Doppler echocardiography can identify a gradient of less than 25 mm Hg across the valve. The gradient represents the difference in systolic pressure between the left ventricle and the aorta. A significant pressure difference is a diagnostic hallmark of valvular stenosis. If the valve orifice has narrowed to 1 cm^2 or less, the gradient will be greater than 40 mm Hg,[48] and the diagnosis will be upgraded to severe aortic valve stenosis.[49] The impedance of left ventricular ejection into the aorta results in increased left ventricular systolic pressure, left ventricular hypertrophy, and eventually left ventricular dilation. When symptoms such as angina, dyspnea, syncope, and other indicators of heart failure develop, it is critical to intervene to prevent further damage to the left ventricle. Aortic valve replacement or transcatheter aortic valve replacement (TAVR) is usually indicated.[49]

Aortic Valve Regurgitation

Aortic regurgitation, also known as aortic insufficiency, can occur as a result of rheumatic fever, systemic hypertension, Marfan syndrome, syphilis, rheumatoid arthritis, aging valve tissue, or discrete subaortic stenosis (see Table 12-10D). Aortic valve incompetence results in a reflux of blood back into the left ventricle during ventricular diastole. To accommodate this extra volume, the left ventricle initially dilates and then hypertrophies in an attempt to empty more completely and to meet the needs of the peripheral circulation. Aortic valve replacement is recommended for symptomatic patients with well-preserved or moderate left ventricular dysfunction.

Tricuspid Valve Stenosis

Tricuspid valve stenosis is rarely an isolated lesion (see Table 12-10E). It often occurs in conjunction with mitral or aortic disease. Its origin most often is rheumatic fever or a complication of IVDA and resultant endocarditis. Tricuspid valve stenosis increases the pressure work of the usually low-pressure right atrium, resulting in right atrial hypertrophy. The right atrium dilates in an attempt to accommodate the residual right atrial volume and the incoming venous return. As a result, systemic venous congestion occurs—the consequences of which include jugular venous congestion, liver failure, hepatomegaly, ascites, and peripheral edema.

Tricuspid Valve Regurgitation

Tricuspid valve regurgitation usually results from advanced failure of the left side of the heart that eventually affects the right side of the heart, severe pulmonary hypertension, or as a complication of IE. Other causes include carcinoid, rheumatoid arthritis, radiation therapy, trauma, and Marfan syndrome (see Table 12-10F).

Pulmonic Valve Disease

Pulmonary valve disease is not a common disorder in adults. It is most often related to congenital anomalies and produces failure of the right side of the heart. Acquired cases are most often related to carcinoid or rheumatic fever pathologies. Initial symptoms present as dyspnea and can progress to severe heart failure symptomatology. Balloon valvuloplasty has proven successful for treatment of these patients.

Mixed Valvular Lesions

Many persons have mixed valvular lesions as an element of stenosis and regurgitation. Mixed lesions can accentuate the severity of a condition. For example, when combined, aortic stenosis and aortic regurgitation increase left ventricular volume and pressure and thereby multiply the degree of left ventricular work.

Medical Management

Management of valvular disorders includes pharmacologic therapy to control symptoms of heart failure and cardiac surgical repair or replacement of the affected valve. Percutaneous valve devices including stent valves and mitral clips are also used as a less invasive alternative.

Nursing Management

Nursing management of the patient with valvular disease incorporates a variety of priority nursing diagnoses (Box 12-17). **Nursing priorities are focused on 1) maintaining adequate cardiac output, 2) optimizing fluid balance, and 3) providing patient education.**

Maintaining Adequate Cardiac Output

Low cardiac output is a common finding in patients with valvular heart disease. It can occur because of decreased forward flow through a stenotic valve, bidirectional flow across an incompetent valve, or associated heart failure. Vital signs and the effect of positive inotropic and afterload-reducing agents are assessed and documented. If the patient has hemodynamic catheters inserted, cardiac output and hemodynamic parameters are measured and evaluated.

BOX 12-17 NURSING DIAGNOSES

Valvular Heart Disease

- Decreased Cardiac Output, related to alterations in preload, p. 579
- Decreased Cardiac Output, related to alterations in afterload, p. 580
- Decreased Cardiac Output, related to alterations in contractility, p. 580
- Decreased Cardiac Output, related to alterations in heart rate or rhythm, p. 581
- Activity Intolerance, related to cardiopulmonary dysfunction, p. 570
- Deficient Knowledge, related to lack of previous exposure to information, p. 585

BOX 12-18 PATIENT EDUCATION

Valvular Heart Disease

- Pathophysiology of valvular disease
- Infection control: prophylactic antibiotics related to dental work or other invasive procedures
- Heart failure: if symptoms of heart failure are present, education is provided on fluid and sodium restriction, fluid balance, diuretic management, daily weight, and controlling breathlessness.
- Surgery: if open-heart surgery was performed, information about postsurgical recovery is provided.
- Medications: medications may be complex, and information must be given in writing and orally.
- Preload: purpose of diuretics, increased urine output, and control of fluid volume
- Afterload: purpose of vasodilators or angiotensin-converting enzyme (ACE) inhibitors in decreasing the workload of the heart
- Heart rate: purpose of digoxin is to control the rate in atrial fibrillation, a frequent dysrhythmia in heart failure.
- Contractility: with the exception of digoxin, no oral contractility medications are approved by the U.S. Food and Drug Administration (FDA).
- Anticoagulation: patients with distended atria, enlarged ventricles, atrial fibrillation, or mechanical valves may be prescribed anticoagulants (Coumadin); risks of bleeding, importance of correct dosages, prothrombin times, international normalized ratio (INR), and nutritional-pharmacologic interactions are emphasized.
- Follow-up care after discharge
- Symptoms to report to a health care professional

Patient care activities are carefully planned to provide adequate rest periods to prevent fatigue.

Optimizing Fluid Balance

Fluid status is evaluated by auscultation of breath sounds for crackles, heart sounds for presence of an S_3, daily weights to trend a "sudden weight gain," and presence of peripheral edema. The appearance of pulmonary crackles or an S_3 heart sound confirms volume overload. The jugular vein is assessed for signs of increased distention. Diuretics and vasodilators are administered to counteract excess fluid retention. The patient is weighed daily, and fluid intake and output are monitored and recorded.

Providing Patient Education

Education for the patient with acute or chronic heart failure caused by valvular dysfunction includes 1) information related to diet, 2) fluid restrictions, 3) the actions and side effects of heart failure medications, 4) the need for prophylactic antibiotics before undergoing any invasive procedures, and 5) when to call the health care provider to report a negative change in cardiac symptoms (Box 12-18).

Many patients also require information about valvular heart surgery. Achieving the optimal outcomes for the patient with valve disease requires contributions from a team of educated health care clinicians. Collaborative multidisciplinary priorities are listed in Box 12-19. The heart valve replacement

BOX 12-19 EVIDENCE-BASED PRACTICE (QSEN)

Valvular Heart Disease

Class I recommendations with strong evidence are provided.

Recommendations for Detection and Surveillance of Valvular Disease by Echocardiography

- Echocardiography is noninvasive and is used for all initial diagnosis and serial follow-up evaluations.

Recommendations for Aortic Stenosis

- Echocardiography is the primary diagnostic tool.
- Coronary arteriography is used before AVR if CAD is suspected.
- AVR recommended for symptomatic patients with severe AS; AVR can be combined with CABG surgery when CAD is present.

Recommendations for Aortic Regurgitation

- Echocardiography is the primary diagnostic tool.
- Cardiac catheterization is used if noninvasive tests are inconclusive.
- AVR is indicated for symptomatic patients with severe AR regardless of LV systolic function.
- AVR is indicated for nonsymptomatic patients with severe AR with LV systolic dysfunction (ejection fraction <0.5 [50%]); AVR can be combined with CABG surgery if CAD is present.

Recommendations for Mitral Stenosis

- Echocardiography is the primary diagnostic tool.
- Anticoagulation is indicated in patients with MS and atrial fibrillation (paroxysmal, persistent, or permanent) and for patients with MS in sinus rhythm with a prior embolic event or left atrial thrombus.
- Cardiac catheterization is used if noninvasive tests are inconclusive.
- Mitral valve repair (preferable) or mitral valve replacement is indicated for symptomatic (NYHA functional class III or IV) moderate or severe MS if percutaneous mitral balloon valvuloplasty is contraindicated.

Recommendations for Mitral Regurgitation

- Echocardiography is the primary diagnostic tool.
- Cardiac catheterization is used if noninvasive tests are inconclusive or if additional hemodynamic measurements are required.
- Mitral valve repair is the operation of choice over valve replacement in most patients with chronic MR.

References

Bonow RO, et al: ACC/AHA 2006 guidelines for the management of patients with valvular heart disease: executive summary, *Circulation* 114:450–527, 2006.

Nishimura RA, et al: ACC/AHA 2008 guideline update on valvular heart disease: focused update on infective endocarditis: a report of the American College of Cardiology/American Heart Association Task Force on Practice Guidelines, *Circulation* 11(8):887–895, 2008.

AR, Aortic regurgitation; *AS*, aortic stenosis; *AVR*, aortic valve replacement; *CABG*, coronary artery bypass graft; *CAD*, coronary artery disease; *IE*, infective endocarditis; *LV*, left ventricular; *MR*, mitral regurgitation; *MS*, mitral stenosis; *NYHA*, New York Heart Association.

BOX 12-20 INTERNET RESOURCES FOR CARDIOVASCULAR DISORDERS

AACN	American Association of Critical Care Nurses	http://www.aacn.org/
ACC	American College of Cardiology: AHA/ACC statements and guidelines can be accessed from this page	http://www.cardiosource.org/ACC.aspx
AHA	American Heart Association (for professionals)	http://my.americanheart.org/professional/index.jsp
AHA	American Heart Association (for patients)	http://www.heart.org/HEARTORG/
AHA	American Heart Association (professional journals) AHA/ACC statements and guidelines can be accessed from this page	http://www.ahajournals.org
HFSA	Heart Failure Society of America	http://www.hfsa.org/

section in Chapter 13 provides more information on the surgical management of valvular heart disease. Clinical practice guidelines that discuss cardiovascular disorders can be obtained on the websites of the professional organizations that are listed in the Internet Resources Box 12-20.

REFERENCES

1. Go AS, et al: American Heart Association. Heart Disease and Stroke Statistics-2014 Update: A Report From the American Heart Association, *Circulation* 129:e28, 2014.
2. O'Gara PT, et al: 2013 ACCF/AHA Guideline for the Management of ST-Elevation Myocardial Infarction: a Report of the American College of Cardiology Foundation/American Heart Association Task Force on Practice Guidelines, *Circulation* 127(4):e362, 2013.
3. Fihn SD, et al: 2012 ACCF/AHA/ACP/AATS/PCNA/SCAI/STS Guideline for the Diagnosis and Management of Patients with Stable Ischemic Heart Disease: a Report of the American College of Cardiology Foundation/American Heart Association Task Force on Practice Guidelines, and the American College of Physicians, American Association for Thoracic Surgery, Preventive Cardiovascular Nurses Association, Society for Cardiovascular Angiography and Interventions, and Society of Thoracic Surgeons, *Circulation* 126(25):e354–e471, 2012.
4. Yusef S, et al: INTERHEART Study Investigators. Effect of potentially modifiable risk factors associated with myocardial infarction in 52 countries (The INTERHEART Study): case-control study, *Lancet* 364(9438):937, 2004.
5. Stone NJ, et al: 2013 AHA/ACC guideline on the treatment of blood cholesterol to reduce atherosclerotic cardiovascular risk in adults: A report of the American College of Cardiology/American Heart Association Task Force on Practice Guidelines, *Circulation* 129:S1–S45, 2014.
6. Adult Treatment Panel: Third Report of the National Cholesterol Education Program (NCP) Expert Panel on Detection, Evaluation, and Treat of High Blood Cholesterol in Adults (Adult Treatment Panel III) final report, *Circulation* 106(25):3143, 2002.
7. Miller M, et al: Triglycerides and Cardiovascular Disease: a Scientific Statement from the American Heart Association, *Circulation* 123:2292, 2011.
8. Centers for Disease Control and Prevention: Obesity and Overweight Data http://www.cdc.gov/nchs/data/hus/hus13.pdf#064. Accessed from: http://www.cdc.gov/nchs/fastats/obesity-overweight.htmon. On July 6, 2014.
9. Smith SC, et al: AHA/ACC Secondary Prevention and Risk Reduction Therapy for Patients with Coronary and Other Atherosclerotic Vascular Disease. 2011 Update: A Guideline from the American Heart Association and American College of Cardiology Foundation, *Circulation* 24:2458, 2011.
10. James PA, et al: 2014 Evidence-Based Guideline for the Management of High Blood Pressure in Adults. Report from the Panel Members Appointed to the Eighth Joint National Committee (JNC 8), *JAMA* 311(5):207, 2014.
11. Standards of Medical Care in Diabetes: American Diabetes Association, *Diabetes Care* 37(Suppl 1):S14–S80, 2014.
12. Smink PA, et al: Albuminuria, Estimated GFR, Traditional Risk Factors, and Incident Cardiovascular Disease: The PREVEND (Prevention of Renal and Vascular Endstage Disease) Study, *Am J Kidney Dis* 60(5):804, 2012.
13. Vassaiwala S, Cannon CR, Foronow GC: Quality of care and outcomes among patients with acute myocardial infarction by level of kidney function at admission: report from the Get with the Guidelines Coronary Artery Disease Program, *Clin Cardiol* 35(9):541, 2012.
14. Mosa L, et al: Effectiveness–Based Guidelines for the Prevention of Cardiovascular Disease in Women-2011 Update: A Guideline from the American Heart Association, *Circulation* 123:1243, 2011.
15. Lloyd-Jones DM, et al: On behalf of the American Heart Association Strategic Planning Task Force and Statistics Committee. Defining and setting national goals for cardiovascular health promotion and disease reduction: the American Heart Association's Strategic Impact Goal through 2020 and beyond, *Circulation* 121:586, 2010.
16. Kavousi M, et al: Evaluation of newer risk markers for coronary heart disease. A cohort study, *Ann Intern Med* 156:438, 2012.
17. Greeland P, et al: 2010 ACCF/AHA Guideline for Cardiovascular Risk in Asymptomatic Adults. A Report of the American College of Cardiology Foundation/American Heart Association Task Force on Practice Guidelines. Writing Committee Members, *Circulation* 122:e584, 2010.
18. Wright SR, et al: 2011 ACC/AHA Focused Update of the guidelines for the management of patients with unstable angina/non–ST-elevation myocardial infarction: a report

of the American College of Cardiology/American Heart Association Task Force on Practice Guidelines developed in collaboration with The American College of Emergency Physicians, Society for Cardiovascular Angiography and Interventions, and Society for Thoracic Surgeons, *J Am Coll Cardiol* 57:1920, 2011.

19. Anderson JL, et al: 2011 ACCF/AHA Focused Update Incorporated into the ACC/AHA 2007 Guidelines for the Management of Patients with Unstable Angina/Non–ST-Elevation Myocardial Infarction: a Report of the American College of Cardiology Foundation/American Heart Association Task Force on Practice Guidelines, *Circulation* 123:e426, 2011.
20. McSweeney JC, et al: Women's early warning symptoms of acute myocardial infarction, *Circulation* 108(21):2619, 2003.
21. Keller KB, Lemberg L: Prinzmetal's angina, *Am J Crit Care* 13(4):350, 2004.
22. Goldstein JA: Acute right ventricular infarction, *Cardiol Clin* 30(2):219, 2012.
23. Newby LK, et al: ACCF 2012 expert consensus document on practical clinical considerations in the interpretation of troponin elevations: a report of the American College of Cardiology Foundation task force on Clinical Expert Consensus Documents, *J Am Coll Cardiol* 60(23):2427–2463, 2012.
24. Krumholz HM, et al: Patterns of hospital performance in acute myocardial infarction and heart failure 30-day mortality and readmission, *Circ Cardiovasc Quality Outcomes* 5(2):407, 2009.
25. Eagle KA, et al: Adherence to evidence-based therapies after discharge for acute coronary syndromes: an ongoing prospective, observational study, *Am J Med* 117(2):73, 2004.
26. Lichtman JL, et al: Depression as a Risk Factor for Poor Prognosis among Patients with Acute Coronary Syndrome: Systematic Review and Recommendations. A Scientific Statement from the American Heart Association, *Circulation* 129:1350, 2014.
27. Balady GJ, et al: Core Components of Cardiac Rehabilitation/Secondary Prevention Programs: 2007 Update A Scientific Statement from the American Heart Association Exercise, Cardiac Rehabilitation, and Prevention Committee, the Council on Clinical Cardiology; the Councils on Cardiovascular Nursing, Epidemiology and Prevention, and Nutrition, Physical Activity, and Metabolism; and the American Association of Cardiovascular and Pulmonary Rehabilitation, *Circulation* 115:2675, 2007.
28. Estes III: NAN Predicting and preventing sudden cardiac death, *Circulation* 124:651, 2011.
29. Yancy CW, et al: 2013 ACCF/AHA Guideline for the management of heart failure: executive summary: A report of the American College of cardiology Foundation/American heart Association Task Force on Practice Guidelines, *Circulation* 128:1810, 2013.
30. Udelson JE: Heart failure with preserved ejection fraction, *Circulation* 124:e540, 2011.
31. Butler J, et al: Update on aldosterone antagonists use in heart failure with reduced left ventricular ejection fraction. Heart Failure Society of America Guidelines Committee, *J Card Fail* 18:265, 2012.
32. Kim HN, Januzzi JL Jr: Naturetic Peptide testing in heart failure, *Circulation* 123:2015, 2011.
33. Sing PJ, Gras D: Biventricular pacing: current trends and future strategies, *Eur Heart J* 33:305, 2012.
34. Arshad A, et al: Cardiac Resynchronization therapy is more effective in women than in men: the MADIT-CRT (Multicenter Automatic Defibrillator Implantation Trial with Cardiac Resynchronization Therapy) trial, *J Am Coll Cardiol* 57:813, 2011.
35. Linde C, Ellenbogen K, McAllister FA: Cardiac resynchronization therapy (CRT): clinical trials, guidelines, and target populations, *Heart Rhythm* 8(Suppl): S3, 2012.
36. Greenberg B: Acute decompensated heart failure: treatment and challenges, *Circulation J* 76(3):532, 2012.
37. Prasad R, Pugh PJ: Drug and device therapy for patients with chronic heart failure, *Expert Rev Cardiovascular Ther* 10(3):313, 2012.
38. Gersh BJ, et al: 2011 AHA/ACC Guideline for the Diagnosis and Treatment of Hypertrophic Cardiomyopathy. A report of the American College of Cardiology Foundation/American Heart Association Task Force on Practice Guidelines, *Circulation* 124:e783, 2011.
39. Friedrich FW, Carrier L: Genetics of hypertrophic and dilated cardiomopathy, *Current Pharm Biotechn* 13(13):2467, 2012.
40. Hershberger RE, Siegfried JD: Update 2011: Clinical and Genetic Issues in Familial Dilated Cardiomyopathy, *JACC* 57(16):1641, 2011.
41. Luttenberger K, DiNapoli M: Subacute bacterial endocarditis: making the diagnosis, *Nurs Prac* 36(3):31–38, 2011.
42. Lester SJ, Wilansky S: Endocarditis and associated complications, *Crit Care Med* 35(8 Suppl):S384, 2007.
43. Bashore M, et al: Update on infective endocarditis, *Curr Probl Cardiol* 31(4):274, 2006.
44. Wilson W, et al: Prevention of infective endocarditis: guidelines from the American Heart Association. A guideline from the American Heart Association Rheumatic Fever, Endocarditis, and Kawasaki Disease Committee, Council on Cardiovascular Disease in the Young, and the Council on Clinical Cardiology, Council on Cardiovascular Surgery and Anesthesia, and the Quality of Care and Outcomes Research Interdisciplinary Working Group, *Circulation* 116(15):1736, 2007.
45. Baddour LM, et al: Infective endocarditis: diagnosis, antimicrobial therapy, and management of complications. A statement for healthcare professionals from the Committee on Rheumatic Fever, Endocarditis, and Kawasaki Disease, Council on Cardiovascular Disease in the Young, and the Councils on Clinical Cardiology, Stroke, and Cardiovascular Surgery and Anesthesia, American Heart Association: endorsed by the Infectious Diseases Society of America, *Circulation* 111(23):e394, 2005.
46. Nishimura RA, et al: ACC/AHA 2008 guideline update on valvular heart disease: focused update on infective endocarditis. A report of the American College of Cardiology/American Heart Association Task Force on Practice Guidelines, *Circulation* 11(8):887, 2008.
47. Broyles LM, Korniewicz DM: The opiate-dependent patient with endocarditis: addressing pain and substance abuse withdrawal, *AACN Clin Issues* 13(3):432, 2002.

48. Bonow RO, et al: ACC/AHA 2006 guidelines for the management of patients with valvular heart disease: a report of the American College of Cardiology/American Heart Association Task Force on Practice Guidelines (Writing Committee to Revise the 1988 Guidelines for the Management of Patients with Valvular Heart Disease) developed in collaboration with the Society of Cardiovascular Anesthesiologists; endorsed by the Society for Cardiovascular Angiography and Interventions and the Society of Thoracic Surgeons, *Circulation* 114(5):e84, 2006.
49. Nishamura RA, et al: 2014 AHA/ACC Guideline for the management of patients with valvular heart disease: A report of the American College of Cardiology/American Heart Association Task Force on Practice Guidelines, *Circulation* 129:e52, 2014.

CHAPTER 13

Cardiovascular Therapeutic Management

Joni L. Dirks, Julie M. Waters

A wide variety of therapeutic interventions are employed in the management of the patient with cardiovascular dysfunction. This chapter focuses on the priority interventions used to manage acute cardiovascular disorders in the critical care setting.

TEMPORARY PACEMAKERS

Pacemakers are electronic devices that can be used to initiate the heartbeat when the heart's intrinsic electrical system cannot effectively generate a rate adequate to support cardiac output. Pacemakers may be used temporarily, either supportively or prophylactically, until the condition responsible for the rate or conduction disturbance resolves. Pacemakers also may be used on a permanent basis if the patient's condition persists despite adequate therapy.[1]

Indications for Temporary Pacing

The clinical indications for instituting temporary pacemaker therapy are similar regardless of the cause of the rhythm disturbance that necessitates the placement of a pacemaker. The causes range from drug toxicities and electrolyte imbalances to sequelae related to acute myocardial infarction (MI) or cardiac surgery.

The Pacemaker System

A pacemaker system is a simple electrical circuit consisting of a pulse generator and a pacing lead (an insulated electrical wire) with one, two, or three electrodes.

Temporary Pacemaker Pulse Generator

The temporary pulse generator is outside the body and generates an electrical current that travels through the pacing lead and exits through an electrode (exposed portion of the wire) that is in direct contact with the heart. This electrical current initiates a myocardial depolarization. The current then seeks to return by one of several pathways to the pulse generator to complete the circuit. The power source for a temporary external pulse generator is a standard 9-volt alkaline battery inserted into the generator.

Temporary Pacing Lead Systems

The pacing lead used for temporary pacing may be bipolar or unipolar. In a bipolar system, two electrodes (positive and negative) are located within the heart, whereas in a unipolar system, only one electrode (negative) is in direct contact with the myocardium. In both systems, the current flows from the negative terminal of the pulse generator, down the pacing lead to the negative electrode, and into the heart. The current is then picked up by the positive electrode (ground) and flows back up the lead to the positive terminal of the pulse generator. Several methods are available for temporary cardiac pacing.

Transcutaneous Pacing

Transcutaneous cardiac pacing involves the use of two large skin electrodes, one placed anteriorly and the other posteriorly on the chest, connected to an external pulse generator. It is a rapid, noninvasive procedure that nurses can perform in the emergency setting and is recommended in the advanced cardiac life support (ACLS) algorithm for the treatment of symptomatic bradycardia that does not respond to atropine.[2] Improved technology related to stimulus delivery and the development of large electrode pads that help disperse the energy have helped reduce the pain associated with cutaneous nerve and muscle stimulation. Discomfort may still be an issue for some patients, particularly when higher energy levels are required to achieve capture. This route is typically used as a short-term therapy until the situation resolves or another route of pacing can be established.

Transvenous Pacing

Temporary transvenous endocardial pacing is accomplished by advancing a pacing electrode wire through a vein, often the subclavian or internal jugular vein, and into the right atrium or right ventricle (RV). Insertion can be guided through direct visualization with fluoroscopy or by the use of the standard ECG. In some cases, the pacing wire is inserted through a special pulmonary artery catheter by means of a port that exits in the right atrium or RV. The bipolar lead used in transvenous pacing has two electrodes on one catheter (Figure 13-1). The distal, or negative, electrode is at the tip of the pacing lead and is in direct contact with the heart, usually inside the right atrium or ventricle. Approximately 1 cm from the negative electrode is a positive electrode. The negative electrode is attached to the negative terminal, and the positive electrode is attached to the positive terminal of the pulse generator, either directly or by means of a bridging cable (see Figure 13-1B).

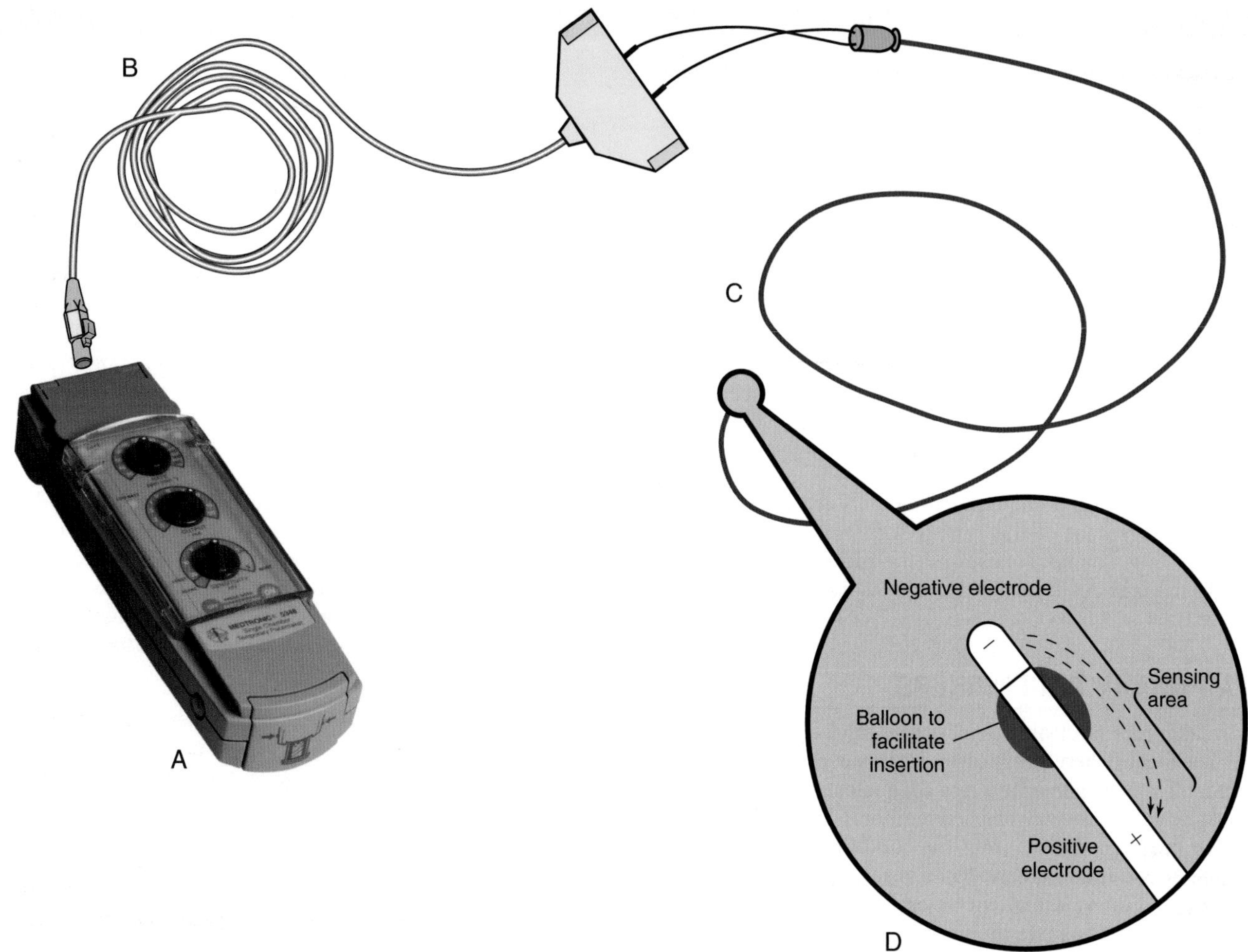

FIG 13-1 The Components of a Temporary Bipolar Transvenous Catheter. *A*, Single-chamber temporary (external) pulse generator. *B*, Bridging cable. *C*, Pacing lead. *D*, Enlarged view of the pacing lead tip. (*A*, Reproduced with permission of Medtronic, Inc.)

TABLE 13-1 NASPE/BPEG Generic Code

POSITION I: CHAMBERS PACED	POSITION II: CHAMBERS SENSED	POSITION III: RESPONSE TO SENSING	POSITION IV: RATE MODULATION	POSITION V: MULTISITE PACING
0 = None	0 = None	0 = None	0 = None	0 = None
A = Atrium	A = Atrium	T = Triggered	R = Rate Modulation	A = Atrium
V = Ventricle	V = Ventricle	I = Inhibited		V = Ventricle
D = Dual (A + V)	D = Dual (A + V)	D = Dual (T + I)		D = Dual (A + V)

BPEG, British Pacing and Electrophysiology Group; *NASPE*, North American Society of Pacing and Electrophysiology.
Modified from Bernstein AD, et al. The Revised NASPE/BPEG generic pacemaker code for antibradycardia, adaptive-rate and multisite pacing. *PACE*. 2002; 25:260.

Epicardial Pacing

The insertion of temporary epicardial pacing wires has become a routine procedure during most cardiac surgical cases. Ventricular and, in many cases, atrial pacing wires are loosely sewn to the epicardium. The terminal pins of these wires are pulled through the skin before the chest is closed. If both chambers have pacing wires attached, the atrial wires exit subcostally to the right of the sternum, and the ventricular wires exit in the same region but to the left of the sternum. These wires can be removed several days after surgery by gentle traction at the skin surface with minimal risk of bleeding.[3]

Pacemaker Codes

The Inter-Society Commission for Heart Disease (ICHD) has a standardized code for describing the various pacing modalities available. This code has five letters as shown in Table 13-1.[4]

The first three letters are used to describe temporary pacemaker function; all five letters refer to permanent pacing modes. In the ICHD code, the first letter refers to the cardiac

TABLE 13-2 Examples of Temporary Pacing Modes

PACING MODE	DESCRIPTION
Asynchronous	
AOO	Atrial pacing, no sensing
VOO	Ventricular pacing, no sensing
DOO	Atrial and ventricular pacing, no sensing
Synchronous	
AAI	Atrial pacing, atrial sensing, inhibited response to sensed P waves
VVI	Ventricular pacing, ventricular sensing, inhibited response to sensed QRS complexes
DVI	Atrial and ventricular pacing, ventricular sensing; both atrial and ventricular pacing are inhibited if a spontaneous ventricular depolarization is sensed
DDD	Both chambers are paced and sensed; inhibited response of the pacing stimuli to sensed events in their respective chambers; triggered response to sensed atrial activity to allow for rate-responsive ventricular pacing

chamber that is paced. The second letter designates which chamber is sensed, and the third letter indicates the pacemaker's response to the sensed event.

Temporary Pacemaker Settings

The controls on all external temporary pulse generators are similar. Their functions must be thoroughly understood so that pacing can be initiated quickly in an emergency situation, and troubleshooting can be facilitated if problems with the pacemaker arise. Examples of temporary pacing modes are listed in Table 13-2.

Rate Control: The *rate control* regulates the number of impulses that can be delivered to the heart per minute. The rate setting depends on the physiologic needs of the patient, but it usually is maintained between 60 and 80 beats/min. Pacing rates for overdrive suppression of tachydysrhythmias may greatly exceed these values. Some generators have special controls for overdrive pacing that allow for rates of up to 800 stimuli per minute. If the pacemaker is operating in a dual-chamber mode, the ventricular rate control also regulates the atrial rate.

Output Dial: The *output dial* regulates the amount of electrical current, measured in milliamperes (mA), that is delivered to the heart to initiate depolarization. The point at which depolarization occurs, called *threshold*, is indicated by a myocardial response to the pacing stimulus (i.e., capture). Threshold can be determined by gradually decreasing the output setting until 1:1 capture is lost. The output setting is then slowly increased until 1:1 capture is re-established; this threshold to pace is less than 1 mA with a properly positioned pacing electrode. The output is set two to three times higher than threshold, because thresholds tend to fluctuate over time. Box 13-1 details the procedure for measuring pacing thresholds. Separate output controls for atrium and ventricle are used with a dual-chamber pulse generator.

BOX 13-1 Determining the Temporary Pacemaker Pacing Threshold

1. Adjust the pacemaker rate setting so that patient is 100% paced. It may be necessary to increase the pacing rate to achieve this setting.
2. Gradually decrease the output (milliampere, mA) setting until 1:1 capture is lost. The pacing threshold is the point at which capture is lost.
3. Slowly increase the output setting until 1:1 capture is re-established. With a properly positioned pacing electrode, the pacing threshold should be less than 1 mA.
4. Set the output setting two to three times higher than measured threshold because thresholds tend to fluctuate over time.
5. If a dual-chamber pulse generator is being used, evaluate pacing thresholds for the atrial and ventricular leads separately.

BOX 13-2 Determining the Temporary Pacemaker Sensitivity Threshold

- Set the sensitivity control to its most sensitive setting.
- Adjust the pulse generator rate to 10 beats/min less than the patient's intrinsic rate (the flash indicator should flash regularly).
- Reduce the generator output to the minimal value to eliminate the risk of competing with the intrinsic rhythm.
- Gradually increase the sensitivity value until the sense indicator stops flashing and the pace indicator starts flashing.
- Decrease sensitivity until the sense indicator begins to flash again; this is the sensitivity threshold.
- Adjust the sensitivity setting on the generator to half of the threshold value; restore the generator output and rate to their original values.

Sensitivity Control: The *sensitivity control* regulates the ability of the pacemaker to detect the heart's intrinsic electrical activity. Sensitivity is measured in millivolts (mV) and determines the size of the intracardiac signal that the generator will recognize. If the sensitivity is adjusted to its most sensitive setting—a setting of 0.5 to 1 mV—the pacemaker can respond even to low-amplitude electrical signals coming from the heart. Turning the sensitivity to its least sensitive setting (i.e., adjusting the dial to a setting of 20 mV or to the area labeled *async)* results in inability of the pacemaker to sense any intrinsic electrical activity and causes the pacemaker to function at a fixed rate. A sense indicator (often a light) on the pulse generator signals each time intrinsic cardiac electrical activity is sensed. A pulse generator may be designed to sense atrial activity or ventricular activity, or both. Box 13-2 describes the procedure for measuring sensitivity.

AV interval: The AV interval control (available only on dual-chamber generators) regulates the time interval between the atrial and ventricular pacing stimuli. This interval is analogous to the PR interval that occurs in the intrinsic ECG. Proper adjustment of this interval to between 150 and 250 milliseconds (msec) preserves AV synchrony and permits maximal ventricular stroke volume and enhanced cardiac output.

Dual Chamber Temporary Pacemaker Settings: Temporary dual chamber pacemakers have other settings that are required in the DDD mode. The lower rate, or base rate, determines the rate at which the generator will pace when intrinsic activity falls below the set rate of the pacemaker. The upper rate determines the fastest ventricular rate the pacemaker will deliver in response to sensed atrial activity. This setting is needed to protect the patient's heart from being paced in response to rapid atrial dysrhythmias.

The *pulse width*, which can be adjusted from 0.05 to 2 msec, controls the length of time that the pacing stimulus is delivered to the heart. There also is an *atrial refractory period*, programmable from 150 to 500 msec, which regulates the length of time, after a sensed or paced ventricular event, during which the pacemaker cannot respond to another atrial stimulus. An emergency button is also available on most models to allow for rapid initiation of asynchronous (DOO) pacing during an emergency.

On all temporary pacemakers, an on/off switch is provided with a safety feature that prevents the accidental termination of pacing. On new generators, there is also a locking feature to prevent unintended changes to the prescribed settings.

Pacing Artifacts

All patients with temporary pacemakers require continuous ECG monitoring. The pacing artifact is the "spike" that is seen on the ECG tracing as the pacing stimulus is delivered to the heart. A *P wave* is visible after the pacing artifact if the atrium is being paced (Figure 13-2A). Similarly, a QRS complex follows a ventricular pacing artifact (see Figure 13-2B). With dual-chamber pacing, a pacing artifact precedes both the P wave and the QRS complex (see Figure 13-2C).

Not all paced beats look alike. For example, the artifact (spike) produced by a unipolar pacing electrode is larger than that produced by a bipolar lead. The QRS complex of paced beats appears different, depending on the location of the pacing electrode. If the pacing electrode is positioned in the RV, a left bundle branch block (LBBB) pattern is displayed on the ECG. A right bundle branch block (RBBB) pattern is visible if the pacing stimulus originates from the left ventricle (LV).

Pacemaker Malfunctions

Most pacemaker malfunctions can be categorized as abnormalities of pacing or of sensing. Problems with pacing can involve failure of the pacemaker to deliver the pacing stimulus, a pacing stimulus that fails to depolarize the heart, or an incorrect number of pacing stimuli per minute.

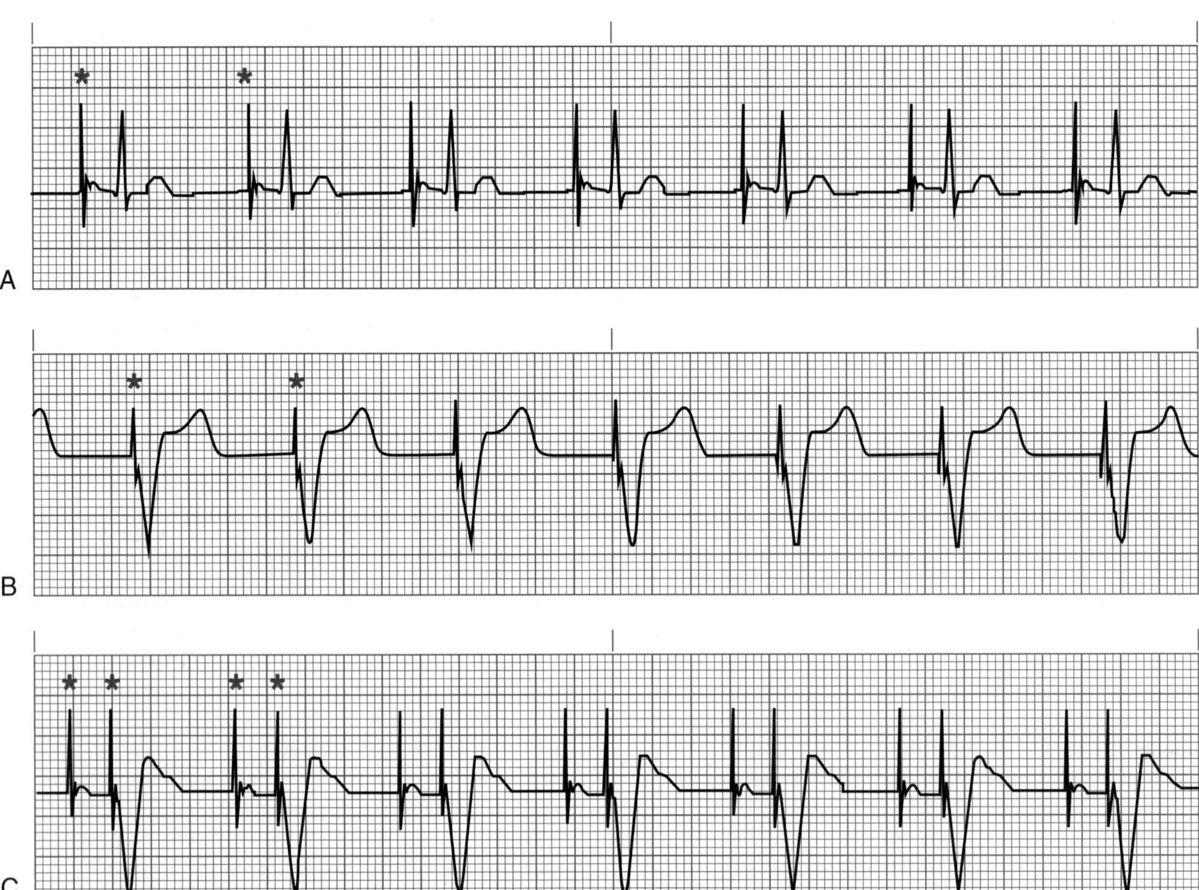

FIG 13-2 Pacing Examples. *A*, Atrial pacing. *B*, Ventricular pacing. *C*, Dual-chamber pacing. Each asterisk represents a pacemaker impulse.

Pacing Abnormalities

No pacing stimulus: Failure of the pacemaker to deliver the pacing stimulus results in disappearance of the pacing artifact, even if the patient's intrinsic rate is less than the set rate on the pacer (Figure 13-3). This can occur intermittently or continuously and can be attributed to failure of the pulse generator or its battery, a loose connection between the various components of the pacemaker system, broken lead wires, or stimulus inhibition as a result of electromagnetic interference (EMI). Tightening connections, replacing the batteries or the pulse generator itself, or removing the source of EMI may restore pacemaker function.

Loss of capture. If the pacing stimulus fires but fails to initiate a myocardial depolarization, a pacing artifact will be present but will not be followed by the expected P wave or QRS complex, depending on the chamber being paced (Figure 13-4). This *loss of capture* most often can be attributed to displacement of the pacing electrode or to an increase in threshold (electrical stimulus necessary to elicit a myocardial depolarization) as a result of medications, metabolic disorders, electrolyte imbalances, or fibrosis or myocardial ischemia at the site of electrode placement. In many cases, increasing the output (mA) elicits capture. For transvenous leads, repositioning the patient onto the left side may improve lead contact and restore capture.

Sensing Abnormalities

Sensing abnormalities include both undersensing and oversensing.

Undersensing. Undersensing is the inability of the pacemaker to sense spontaneous myocardial depolarizations, which results in competition between paced complexes and the heart's intrinsic rhythm. This malfunction is manifested on the ECG by pacing artifacts that occur after or are unrelated to spontaneous complexes (Figure 13-5). Undersensing can result in the delivery of pacing stimuli into a relative refractory period of the cardiac depolarization cycle. A ventricular pacing stimulus delivered into the downslope of the T wave (R-on-T phenomenon) is a real danger with this type of pacer aberration because it may precipitate a lethal dysrhythmia. Quick action to determine the cause and initiate appropriate interventions is essential. Often, the cause can be attributed to inadequate wave amplitude (height of the P or R wave). If this is the case, the situation can be promptly

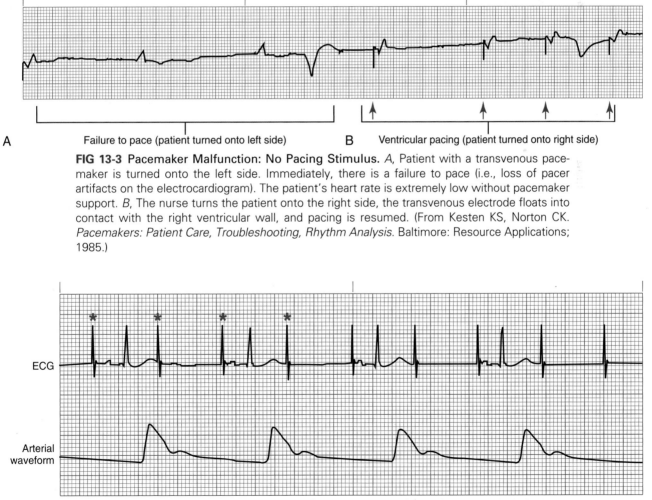

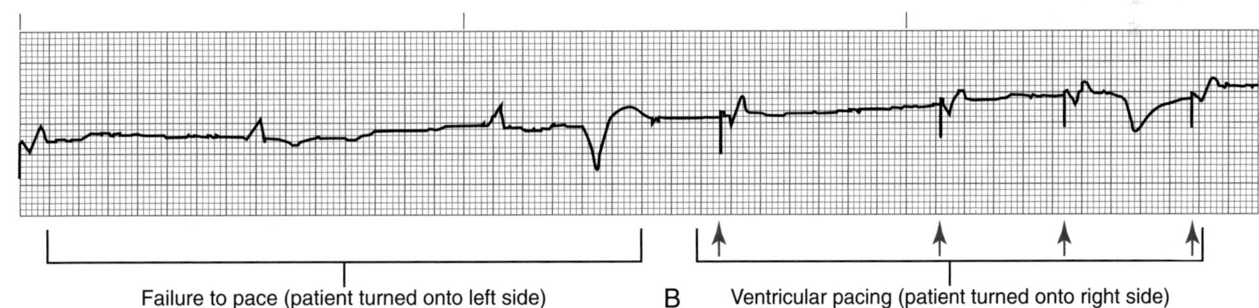

FIG 13-3 Pacemaker Malfunction: No Pacing Stimulus. *A,* Patient with a transvenous pacemaker is turned onto the left side. Immediately, there is a failure to pace (i.e., loss of pacer artifacts on the electrocardiogram). The patient's heart rate is extremely low without pacemaker support. *B,* The nurse turns the patient onto the right side, the transvenous electrode floats into contact with the right ventricular wall, and pacing is resumed. (From Kesten KS, Norton CK. *Pacemakers: Patient Care, Troubleshooting, Rhythm Analysis.* Baltimore: Resource Applications; 1985.)

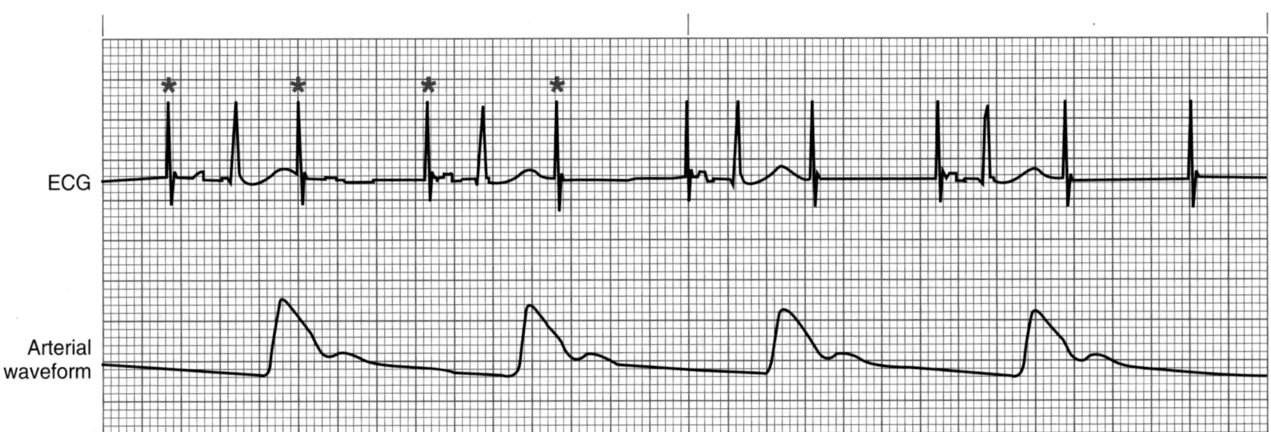

FIG 13-4 Pacemaker Malfunction: Loss of Capture. Atrial pacing and capture occur after pacer spikes 1, 3, 5, and 7. The remaining pacer spikes fail to capture the tissue, resulting in loss of the P wave, no conduction to the ventricles, and no arterial waveform. Each asterisk represents a pacemaker impulse.

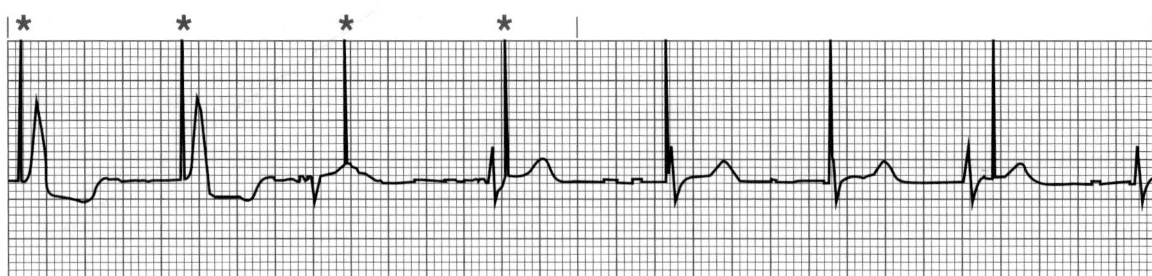

FIG 13-5 Pacemaker Malfunction: Undersensing. After the first two paced beats, a series of intrinsic beats occur; the pacemaker unit fails to sense these intrinsic QRS complexes. These spikes do not capture the ventricle because they occur during the refractory period of the cardiac cycle. Each *asterisk* represents a pacemaker impulse.

remedied by increasing the sensitivity by moving the sensitivity dial toward its lowest setting. Other possible causes include inappropriate (asynchronous) mode selection, lead displacement or fracture, loose cable connections, and pulse generator failure.

Oversensing. Oversensing occurs as a result of inappropriate sensing of extraneous electrical signals that leads to unnecessary triggering or inhibition of stimulus output, depending on the pacer mode. The source of these electrical signals can range from tall peaked T waves to EMI in the critical care environment. Because most temporary pulse generators are programmed in demand modes, oversensing results in unexplained pauses in the ECG tracing as the extraneous signals are sensed and inhibit pacing. Often, moving the sensitivity dial toward 20 mV (less sensitive) stops the pauses.

Medical Management

The physician determines the pacing route based on the patient's clinical situation. Transcutaneous pacing typically is used in emergent situations until a transvenous lead can be secured. If the patient is undergoing heart surgery, epicardial leads may be electively placed at the end of the operation. The physician places the transvenous or epicardial pacing lead(s), repositioning them as needed to obtain adequate pacing and sensing thresholds. Decisions regarding lead placement may later limit the pacing modes available to the clinician. For example, to perform dual-chamber pacing, both atrial and ventricular leads must be placed. In an emergency, however, interventions are focused on establishing ventricular pacing, and atrial lead placement may not be feasible. After lead placement, the initial settings for output and sensitivity are determined, the pacing rate and mode are selected, and the patient's response to pacing is evaluated.

Nursing Management

Nursing priorities in the care of a patient with a temporary pacemaker are directed toward four primary areas: 1) preventing pacemaker malfunction, 2) protecting against microshock, 3) preventing complications, and 4) providing patient education.

Preventing Pacemaker Malfunction

Continuous ECG monitoring is essential to facilitate prompt recognition of and appropriate intervention for pacemaker malfunction. Proper care of the pacing system can prevent pacing abnormalities.

The temporary pacing lead and bridging cable must be properly secured to the body with tape to prevent accidental displacement of the electrode, which can result in failure to pace or sense. The external pulse generator can be secured to the patient's waist with a strap or placed in a telemetry bag for the mobile patient. If the patient is on a regimen of bed rest, the pulse generator can be suspended with twill tape from an IV pole mounted overhead on the ceiling. This prevents tension on the lead while the patient is moved (given adequate length of bridging cable) and alleviates the possibility of accidental dropping of the pulse generator.

The nurse inspects for loose connections between the leads and pulse generator on a regular basis. Replacement batteries and pulse generators must always be available on the unit. Although the battery has an anticipated life span of 1 month, it probably is sound practice to change the battery if the pacemaker has been operating continually for several days. Newer generators provide a low-battery signal 24 hours before complete loss of battery function occurs to prevent inadvertent interruptions in pacing. The pulse generator must always be labeled with the date on which the battery was replaced.

It is important to be aware of all sources of EMI within the critical care environment that may interfere with the pacemaker's function. Sources of EMI in the clinical area include electrocautery, defibrillation current, radiation therapy, magnetic resonance imaging devices, and transcutaneous electrical nerve stimulation (TENS) units.[5] In most cases, if EMI is suspected of precipitating pacemaker malfunction, conversion to the asynchronous mode (fixed rate) can maintain pacing until the cause of the EMI is removed.

Protecting against Microshock

Because the pacing electrode provides a direct, low-resistance path to the heart, the nurse takes special care while handling the external components of the pacing system to avoid conducting stray electrical current from other equipment. Even a small amount of stray current transmitted through the pacing lead could precipitate a lethal dysrhythmia. The possibility of microshock can be minimized by wearing gloves when handling the pacing wires and by proper insulation of terminal pins of pacing wires when they are not in use. The latter precaution can be accomplished by the use of caps provided by the manufacturer or by improvising with a plastic syringe or section of disposable rubber glove. The wires are taped securely to the patient's chest to prevent accidental electrode displacement.

Preventing Complications

Infection at the lead insertion site is a rare but serious complication associated with temporary pacemakers. The site is carefully inspected for purulent drainage, erythema, and edema, and the patient is observed for signs of systemic infection. Site care is performed according to the institution's policies and procedures. Although most infections remain localized, endocarditis can occur in patients with endocardial pacing leads. A less common complication associated with transvenous pacing is myocardial perforation, which can result in rhythmic hiccoughs or cardiac tamponade.

Providing Patient Education

Patient teaching for the person with a temporary pacemaker emphasizes the prevention of complications. The patient is instructed not to handle any exposed portion of the lead wire and to notify the nurse if the dressing over the insertion site becomes soiled, wet, or dislodged. The patient also is advised not to use any electrical devices brought in from home that could interfere with pacemaker functioning. Patients with temporary transvenous pacemakers need to be taught to restrict movement of the affected extremity to prevent lead displacement.

PERMANENT PACEMAKERS

Almost 400,000 permanent pacemakers are implanted annually in the United States, and critical care nurses are likely to encounter these devices in their clinical practice.[6] These pacemakers were originally designed to provide an adequate ventricular rate in patients with symptomatic bradycardia. Today, the goal of pacemaker therapy is to simulate, as much as possible, normal physiologic cardiac depolarization and conduction.

Sophisticated generators permit rate-responsive pacing, effecting responses to sensed atrial activity (DDD) or to a variety of physiologic sensors (body motion or minute ventilation). For patients who do not have a functional sinus node that can increase their heart rate, rate-responsive pacemakers may improve exercise capacity and quality of life.[7] Table 13-3 describes the types of rate-responsive pacing generators in clinical use.

The concept of physiologic pacing continues to evolve because studies have indicated that pacing initiated from the RV apex—even in a dual-chamber mode—may promote heart failure in patients with permanent pacemakers.[8] This has prompted further research to identify alternative sites for pacing and modes that can maximize intrinsic AV conduction and minimize ventricular pacing.[8]

The patient who undergoes implantation of a permanent pacemaker is usually in the hospital for less than 24 hours. Longer lengths of stay are expected for patients with serious complications such as MI or cardiogenic shock. Current generators are smaller, more energy-efficient, and more reliable than previous models. The most recent enhancement has been the release of a pacemaker that is compatible with magnetic resonance imaging (MRI).[9] A rapidly expanding role for permanent pacemakers has been the use of these devices as a type of nonpharmacologic therapy for adjunctive treatment of conditions such as heart failure and atrial fibrillation.

TABLE 13-3 Permanent Pacemaker Rate-Response Pacing Modes

PULSE GENERATOR	DESCRIPTION
AAIR	AAI features plus rate-responsive pacing; used for patients with a symptomatic bradycardia who have a paceable atrium and intact atrioventricular conduction
VVIR	VVI features plus rate-responsive pacing; used for patients with an atrium that is unpaceable as a result of chronic atrial fibrillation or other atrial dysrhythmia
DDDR	DDD features plus rate-responsive pacing; used for patients with a symptomatic bradycardia in which the atrium is paceable but atrioventricular conduction is, or may become, unreliable

Cardiac Resynchronization Therapy

About one-third of patients with severe heart failure have ventricular conduction delays (prolonged QRS duration or bundle branch block). These conduction delays create a lack of synchrony between the contractions of the LV and RV.[10] The hemodynamic consequences of this dyssynchrony includes impaired ventricular filling with decreased ejection fraction, cardiac output, and mean arterial pressure.[11] Cardiac resynchronization therapy (CRT) uses atrial pacing plus stimulation of both the LV and RV (biventricular pacing) to optimize atrial and ventricular mechanical activity. The CRT device uses three pacing leads, one in the right atrium, one in the RV, and a specially designed transvenous lead that is inserted through the coronary sinus to pace the LV.[12] Because many patients with heart failure are also at risk for sudden cardiac death, biventricular pacing is available on most implantable cardioverter defibrillators (ICDs). A number of clinical trials have shown that CRT improves symptoms, functional status, and mortality in patients with moderate-to-advanced heart failure.[12] Research indicates that CRT may also be beneficial in preventing the progression of heart failure in less symptomatic patients.[13]

Atrial Fibrillation Suppression

There is a growing incidence of atrial fibrillation, and atrial pacing has been proposed as a possible preventive therapy for this dysrhythmia in selected patients. Atrial pacing in patients with bradycardia has been shown to lower the recurrence of atrial fibrillation, especially compared with ventricular pacing. Atrial-based modes that promote intrinsic conduction and minimize episodes of ventricular pacing are most effective. Attempts to prevent episodes of atrial fibrillation by overdrive pacing in response to ectopic atrial activity have not proven successful.[1] Most pacemakers can be programmed to *mode switch* to a non–P-wave tracking mode, if rapid atrial rates are sensed, to limit the rate of response for ventricular pacing.

Medical Management

Permanent pacemakers may be implanted with the patient under local anesthesia in the operating room or in the cardiac catheterization laboratory. Transvenous leads usually are inserted through the cephalic or subclavian vein and positioned in the right atrium or RV, or both, with fluoroscopic guidance. Satisfactory lead placement is determined by testing the stimulation and sensitivity thresholds with a pacing system analyzer. The leads are then attached to the generator, which is inserted into a surgically created pocket in the subcutaneous tissue below the clavicle.

Nursing Management

Nursing management for patients after permanent pacemaker implantation includes monitoring for complications related to insertion and for pacemaker malfunction. Postoperative complications are rare but include cardiac perforation and tamponade, pneumothorax, hematoma, lead displacement, and infection.[14]

Identification of permanent pacemaker malfunction is the same as that described previously for temporary pacemakers. To evaluate pacemaker function, the nurse must know at least the pacemaker's programmed mode of pacing and the lower rate setting. With permanent pacemakers, settings are adjusted noninvasively through a specialized programmer that uses pulsed magnetic fields or a radiofrequency signal. If a pacemaker problem is suspected, ECG strips are obtained, and the physician is notified so that the pacemaker settings can be reprogrammed as needed. When oversensing is suspected with permanent pacemakers, a magnet may be placed over the generator to restore pacing in an asynchronous mode until appropriate changes in the generator settings can be programmed. If the patient experiences symptoms of decreased cardiac output, he or she may require support with temporary transcutaneous pacing until the problem is corrected.

The foregoing discussion provides an introduction to the basic concepts of pacemaker therapy. However, the nurse who cares for patients with permanent or temporary pacemakers must be familiar with ever more sophisticated modes of pacemaker function. Only by keeping pace with current technology can the nurse accurately interpret pacer function and thereby safely and effectively care for patients with pacemakers.

IMPLANTABLE CARDIOVERTER DEFIBRILLATORS

An implantable cardioverter defibrillator (ICD) is an electronic device that is used in the treatment of life-threatening tachydysrhythmias. Initially, an ICD was recommended only for patients who had survived an episode of cardiac arrest caused by ventricular fibrillation (VF) or ventricular tachycardia (VT). As clinical trials found improved survival with ICD therapy when compared to treatment with antidysrhythmic medications, ICD use was expanded to include primary prevention of sudden cardiac death. Current heart failure guidelines recommend ICD implantation in high-risk patients with a left ventricular ejection fraction less than 35%, even without evidence of VT or VF on an electrophysiology study (EPS).[15] These expanded ICD indications have resulted in over 100,000 implants per year in the United States.[6]

The ICD System

The ICD system consists of leads and a generator and is similar to a pacemaker but with some key differences. The leads contain not only electrodes for sensing and pacing but also integrated defibrillator coils capable of delivering a shock. The generator is larger to accommodate a more powerful battery and a high-voltage capacitor along with the microprocessor.[16] It is surgically placed in the subcutaneous tissue of the pectoral region in the upper chest (Figure 13-6). The current generation of devices delivers a tiered therapy, with options for programmable antitachycardia pacing, bradycardia backup pacing, low-energy cardioversion, and high-energy defibrillation. With tiered therapy, antitachycardia pacing is used as the first line of treatment in some cases of VT. If the VT can be pace-terminated successfully, the patient will not receive a shock from the generator and may not even realize that the ICD terminated the dysrhythmia. If programmed bursts of pacing do not terminate the VT, the ICD will cardiovert the rhythm. If the dysrhythmia deteriorates into VF, the ICD is programmed to defibrillate at a higher energy. If the dysrhythmia terminates spontaneously, the device will not discharge. Occasionally, the electrical rhythm may deteriorate to asystole or a slow idioventricular rhythm; in such cases, the bradycardia backup pacing function is activated.

ICDs also incorporate dual-chamber pacemakers with leads in both atria and ventricles. This allows dual-chamber pacing to optimize hemodynamic performance and atrial sensing to discriminate more accurately between atrial and ventricular tachycardias and decrease the incidence of inappropriate shocks. Many ICDs also incorporate triple-lead systems (leads in one atrium and both ventricles) to allow for CRT and defibrillation. Other developments in ICD technology include improved diagnostic and telemetry functions, such as the ability to provide real-time electrograms obtained from the ICD electrodes or the ability to perform remote device interrogation by telephone or Internet.[16]

ICD Insertion

Transvenous ICD leads are inserted into the subclavian vein and advanced into the right side of the heart, where contact with the endocardium is achieved. The endocardial leads are connected to the generator by tunneling through the subcutaneous tissue, and thoracotomy is avoided. Procedural complications are infrequent but may include hematoma, pneumothorax, or lead dislodgement.

Medical Management

An electrophysiologist performs the initial programming of the device at the time of implantation. During implantation, defibrillation threshold testing is performed to test device integrity. This involves inducing the dysrhythmia and then evaluating the device's ability to terminate it. After it has been determined that the ICD functions appropriately, further follow-up is conducted on an outpatient basis to monitor the number of discharges and the battery life of the device.

Nursing Management

The nursing management of the patient with an ICD includes assessing for dysrhythmias and monitoring for complications related to insertion. In the case of a ventricular dysrhythmia, it is important to know the type of ICD implanted, how the

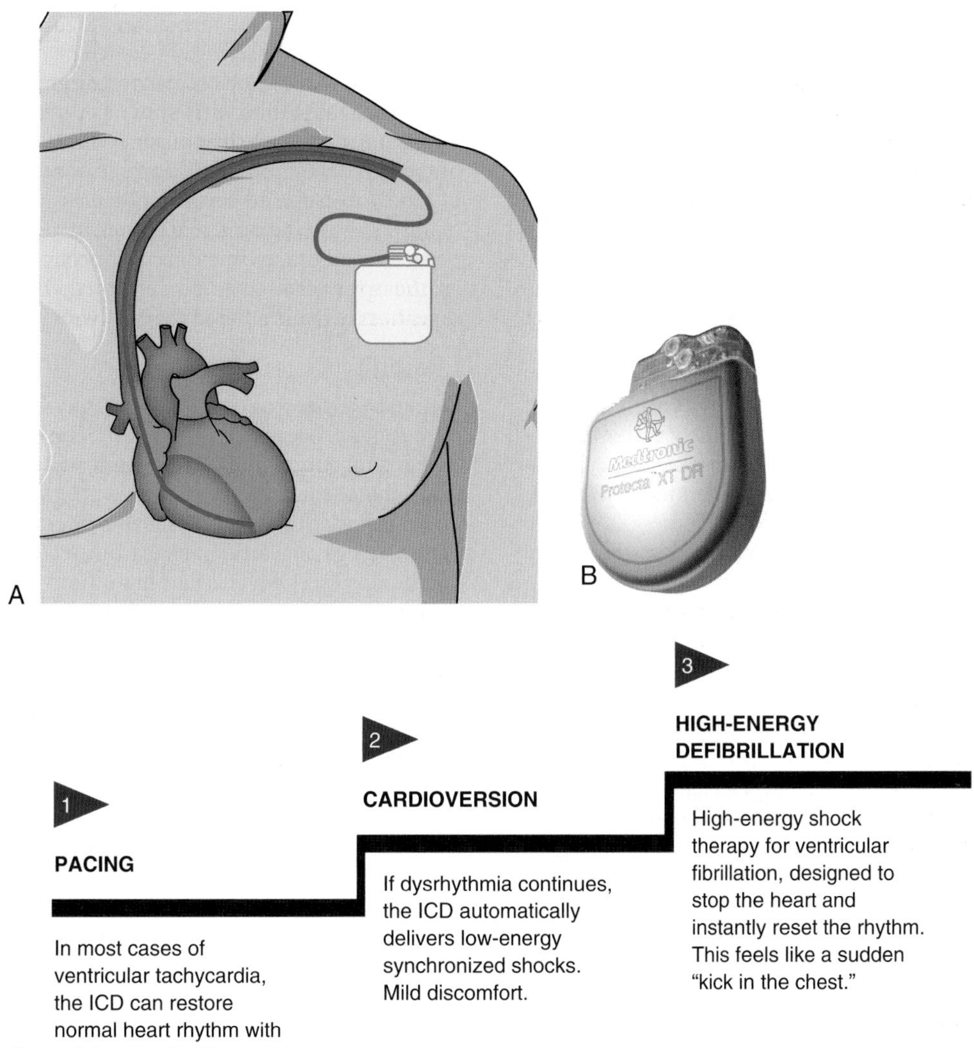

A
B
Medtronic
Protecta XT DR
C
1
PACING
In most cases of ventricular tachycardia, the ICD can restore normal heart rhythm with painless pacing therapy.
2
CARDIOVERSION
If dysrhythmia continues, the ICD automatically delivers low-energy synchronized shocks. Mild discomfort.
3
HIGH-ENERGY DEFIBRILLATION
High-energy shock therapy for ventricular fibrillation, designed to stop the heart and instantly reset the rhythm. This feels like a sudden "kick in the chest."

FIG 13-6 Placement of an Implantable Cardioverter Defibrillator (ICD) with a Transvenous Lead System. *A*, The generator is placed in a subcutaneous "pocket" in the pectoral region. The pacing, cardioversion, and defibrillation functions are all contained in a lead (or leads) inserted into the right atrium and ventricle. *B*, An example of a dual-chamber ICD (Medtronic Protecta XT DR, ICD (approximate dimensions 2.5 × 2.0 × 0.6 inches), with tiered therapy and pacing capabilities. *C*, Tiered therapy is designed to use increasing levels of intensity to terminate ventricular dysrhythmias. (*B*, Reproduced with permission of Medtronic, Inc.)

device functions, and whether it is activated (i.e., on). If the patient experiences a shockable rhythm, the nurse should be prepared to defibrillate in the event that the device fails. During external defibrillation, the paddles or patches should not be placed directly over the ICD generator, as long as this can be accomplished without delay of defibrillation.[17] For recurring shocks, patients should be assessed for underlying causes, such as electrolyte imbalance, ischemia, or worsening heart failure.[16] Most patients continue to take some antidysrhythmic medications to decrease the number of shocks required and to slow the rate of the tachycardia. Complications associated with the permanent ICD include infection from the implanted system, broken leads, and sensing of supraventricular tachydysrhythmias resulting in unneeded discharges.

Patient Education

To facilitate a positive psychologic adjustment to the ICD, education of the patient and family about the device is vital. Preoperative teaching for the ICD patient includes information about how the device works and what to expect during the implantation procedure. After implantation, education is focused on aspects of living with an ICD. Patients need information pertaining to scheduled device follow-up and instructions about what to do if they experience a shock. Many institutions have successfully used family support groups for this patient population. Finally, since the ICD is an adjunctive treatment rather than a cure for heart failure, education must focus on the importance of continued risk-factor modification and role of prescribed medications.

FIBRINOLYTIC THERAPY

Fibrinolytic therapy is an important clinical intervention for the patient experiencing acute ST-elevation myocardial infarction (STEMI). Before the introduction of fibrinolytic agents, medical management of acute MI was focused on decreasing myocardial oxygen demands to minimize myocardial necrosis and preserve ventricular function. Today, efforts to limit the size of the infarction are directed toward timely reperfusion of the jeopardized myocardium through restoration of blood flow in the culprit vessel (the open artery theory). Two options are available for opening the artery—fibrinolytics and mechanical intervention. Although mechanical catheter-based intervention has been proven to yield better outcomes when performed in a timely fashion, only one-third of U.S. hospitals are estimated to have this capability.[18] For this reason, fibrinolytic therapy continues to play a major role in the treatment of acute MI.

The use of fibrinolytic therapy is predicated on the theory that the significant event in acute coronary syndromes (e.g., unstable angina, acute MI) is the rupture of an atherosclerotic plaque with thrombus formation (Figure 13-7). The thrombus, which is composed of aggregated platelets bound together with fibrin strands, occludes the coronary artery, depriving the myocardium of oxygen previously supplied by that artery. The administration of a fibrinolytic agent results in lysis of the acute thrombus, resulting in recanalization, or opening, of the obstructed coronary artery and restoration of blood flow to the affected tissue. In addition to restoring perfusion, adjunctive measures (anticoagulants and antiplatelet therapy) are used to prevent further clot formation and repeat occlusion.

Eligibility Criteria

Patients with recent onset of chest pain (less than 12 hours' duration) and persistent ST elevation (greater than 0.1 mV in two or more contiguous leads) are considered candidates for fibrinolytic therapy.[19] Patients who present with bundle branch blocks that may obscure ST-segment analysis and a history suggesting an acute MI are also considered candidates for therapy (see "Myocardial Infarction" in Chapter 12). The goal is to administer fibrinolytic therapy within 30 minutes

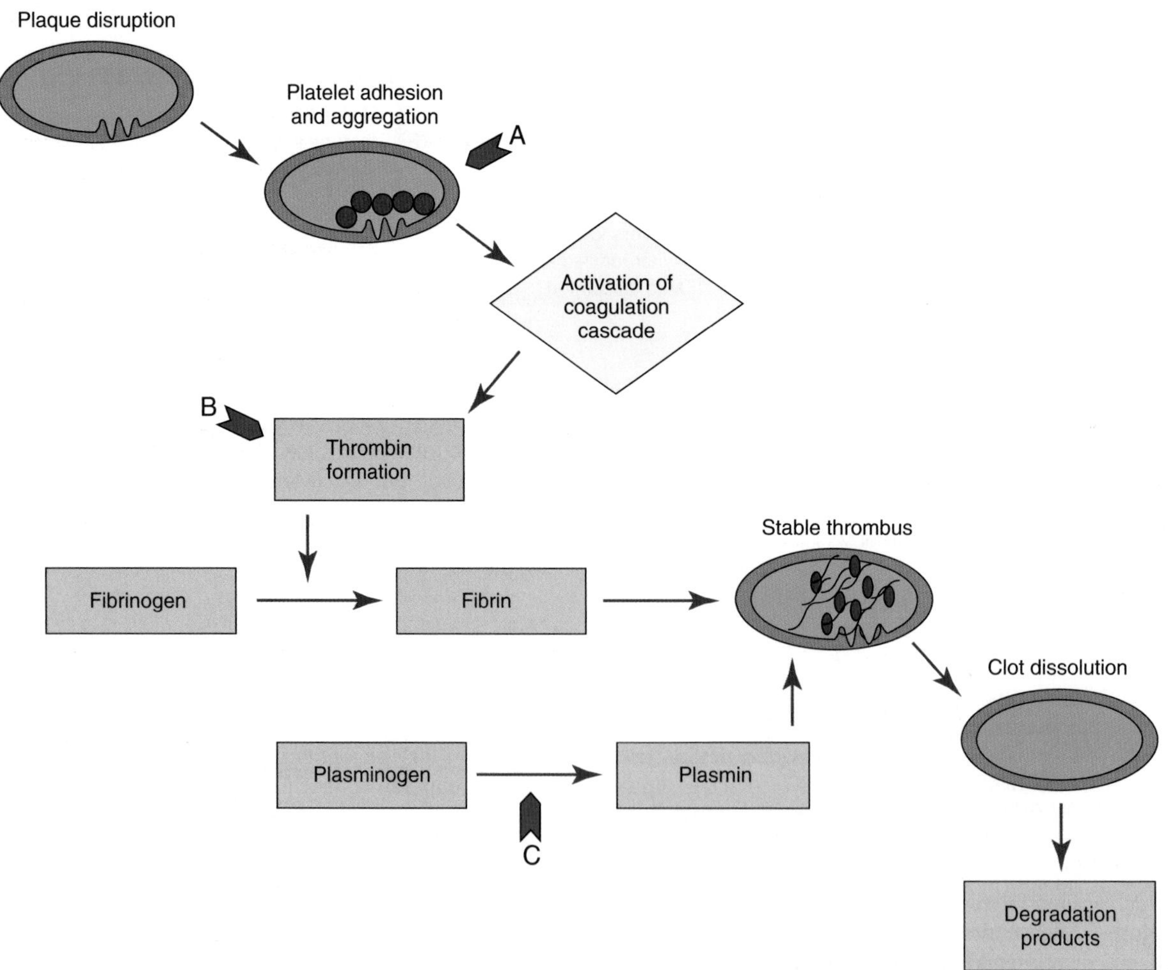

FIG 13-7 Thrombus Formation and Site of Action of Medications used in the Treatment of Acute Myocardial Infarction. *A*, Site of action of antiplatelet agents such as aspirin, thienopyridines, and glycoprotein IIb/IIIa inhibitors. *B*, Heparin bonds with antithrombin III and thrombin to create an inactive complex. *C*, Fibrinolytic agents convert plasminogen to plasmin, an enzyme responsible for degradation of fibrin clots.

after presentation ("door to needle") because early reperfusion yields the greatest benefit.[20]

Exclusion criteria are usually based on the increased risk of bleeding. Patients who have stable clots that might be disrupted by fibrinolytic therapy (recent surgery, facial or head trauma) usually are not considered candidates. Other common criteria for the use of fibrinolytic therapy are presented in Box 13-3.

Currently, fibrinolytic therapy is not indicated for patients with unstable angina or non–ST-elevation myocardial infarction (NSTEMIs).[21] Instead, these patients are treated with antiplatelet agents (e.g., aspirin, clopidogrel, glycoprotein IIb/IIIa inhibitors) and antithrombin medications (e.g., heparin). NSTEMI treatment is discussed in detail in Chapter 12.

Fibrinolytic Agents

A comparison of FDA-approved fibrinolytic agents is provided in Table 13-4. Because patients with an area of plaque disruption are still at risk for clot formation and reocclusion, fibrinolytic therapy is used in conjunction with anticoagulants and antiplatelet agents. Current guidelines recommend that anticoagulant therapy be administered for a minimum of 48 hours after reperfusion. Unfractionated heparin (UFH) has been used traditionally, but low–molecular-weight heparin (LMWH) and fondaparinux are also acceptable options[20] (Table 13-5). Antiplatelet therapy with clopidogrel is recommended for 14 days, and aspirin should be continued indefinitely[20] (Table 13-6).

Outcomes of Fibrinolytic Therapy

The benefit of fibrinolytic therapy correlates with the degree of restoration of normal blood flow in the infarct-related artery. Coronary artery patency is defined by angiographic perfusion grades developed by the Thrombolysis in Myocardial Infarction (TIMI) study group in 1985 (Box 13-4).[22] Achievement of TIMI grade 3 flow is associated with the best long-term survival. Studies also indicate that rapid

BOX 13-3 Fibrinolytic Therapy Selection Criteria

- No more than 12 hours from onset of chest pain and preferably within 30 minutes of STEMI diagnosis
- ST-segment elevation on electrocardiogram or new-onset left bundle branch block
- Ischemic chest pain unresponsive to sublingual nitroglycerin
- No conditions that might cause a predisposition to hemorrhage

BOX 13-4 Flow in the Infarct-Related Artery as Described in the Thrombolysis in Myocardial Infarction Trial

PERFUSION GRADES	FLOW IN THE INFARCT-RELATED ARTERY
TIMI 3	Normal or brisk flow through the coronary artery
TIMI 2	Partial flow, slower than in normal vessels
TIMI 1	Sluggish flow with incomplete distal filling
TIMI 0	No flow beyond the point of occlusion

TIMI, Thrombolysis in Myocardial Infarction Trial.
Modified from The TIMI Study Group. The thrombolysis in myocardial infarction (TIMI) trial: phase I findings. *N Engl J Med.* 1985; 312:932.

TABLE 13-4 Pharmacologic Management

Fibrinolytic Agents for Use in Acute Myocardial Infarction

MEDICATION	DOSAGE	ACTIONS	SPECIAL CONSIDERATIONS
Clot-Specific			
tPA (alteplase)	IV: 100 mg over 90 min with the first 15 mg given as a bolus over 2 minutes (dose is adjusted based on weight for patients ≤67 kg)	Binds to fibrin at the clot and promotes activation of plasminogen to plasmin	Anticoagulants are given concurrently. Aspirin and clopidogrel are begun with administration and continued daily.
rPA (reteplase)	IV: 10 units given as a bolus over 2 minutes, repeated in 30 min	Binds to fibrin at the clot and promotes activation of plasminogen to plasmin	Anticoagulants are given concurrently. Aspirin and clopidogrel are begun with administration and continued daily.
TNKase (tenecteplase)	IV: 30-50 mg based on body weight, given as a single bolus	Binds to fibrin at the clot and promotes activation of plasminogen to plasmin	Anticoagulants are given concurrently. Aspirin and clopidogrel are begun with administration and continued daily.
Non–Clot-Specific			
SK (streptokinase)	IV: 1.5 million units given over 60 min	Catalyzes the conversion of plasminogen to plasmin, which causes lysis of fibrin; has systemic lytic effects	May cause allergic reactions and hypotension. Anticoagulants are given concurrently. Aspirin and clopidogrel are begun with administration and continued daily.

IV, Intravenous; *rPA*, recombinant plasminogen activator; *tPA*, tissue plasminogen activator.

TABLE 13-5 Pharmacologic Management Anticoagulants

MEDICATION	DOSAGE	ACTION	SPECIAL CONSIDERATIONS
Unfractionated Heparin			
Heparin sodium	Initial bolus 60 units/kg (max dose 4000 units), followed by 12 units/kg/hr infusion	Enhances activity of antithrombin III, a natural anticoagulant to prevent clot formation	Effectiveness of treatment may be monitored by aPTT or ACT. Response is variable because of binding with plasma proteins. Effects may be reversed with protamine sulfate. Risk of developing HIT Should not be given to patients already receiving therapeutic SC enoxaparin.
Low Molecular Weight Heparin			
Enoxaparin (Lovenox)	30 mg IV bolus, followed by 1 mg/kg SC every 12 hrs For patients already on SC dosing, an additional bolus of 0.3 mg/kg is given if last dose was >8 hrs prior to PCI.	Enhances activity of antithrombin III	More predictable response than heparin because enoxaparin is not largely bound to protein No need for aPTT or ACT monitoring Lower risk of HIT than with UFH Administer within 30 minutes of initiation of fibrinolytic therapy.
Direct Thrombin Inhibitors			
Bivalirudin (Angiomax)	0.75 mg/kg IV bolus, followed by infusion at 1.75 mg/kg/hr during PCI If infusion continued >4 hrs, rate is decreased to 0.2 mg/kg/hr.	Directly inhibits thrombin	May be administered alone or in combination with glycoprotein IIb/IIIa inhibitors Produces a dose-dependent increase in aPTT and ACT Coagulation times return to baseline within one hour after stopping infusion. Dose should be reduced for patients with kidney dysfunction. No reversal agent is available. May be used instead of UFH for patients with HIT
Argatroban (Argatroban)	Loading dose of 100 mcg/kg IV bolus over 1 minute, followed by infusion of 1 mcg/kg/min (low-dose) or 3 mcg/kg/min (high-dose)	Directly inhibits thrombin	May be used instead of UFH for patients with HIT ACT is monitored during PCI, while aPTT is used during prolonged infusion. Abrupt discontinuation may lead to a rebound hypercoagulable state.
Factor Xa Inhibitor			
Fondaparinux (Arixtra)	2.5 mg IV, followed by 2.5 mg SC once daily	Selective inhibitor of factor Xa	May be used in conjunction with fibrinolytics For PCI, must be administered with another anticoagulant (i.e., UFH) to prevent catheter thrombosis Long half-life (>17 hrs) Contraindicated in patients with kidney failure

ACT, Activated clotting time; *aPTT*, activated partial thromboplastin time; *HIT*, heparin-induced thrombocytopenia; *MI*, myocardial infarction; *PCI*, percutaneous coronary intervention; *SC*, subcutaneous; *UFH*, unfractionated Heparin.

restoration of normal blood flow, within 90 minutes after treatment, results in improved LV function and reduced mortality.

Residual Coronary Artery Stenosis

Fibrinolytic therapy has been determined to be a successful strategy for reopening occluded coronary arteries in the setting of acute STEMI. It limits infarct size, salvaging myocardium and significantly reducing morbidity and mortality associated with cardiogenic shock and VF. However, residual coronary artery stenosis resulting from the atherosclerotic process remains, even after successful fibrinolysis. Subsequent prevention of reocclusion is critical to preserving myocardial function and preventing the risk of late complications. Fibrinolytic therapy is therefore recognized as an emergency procedure to restore patency until more definitive therapy can be initiated to reduce the degree of stenosis effectively (an interventional catheter procedure or surgical coronary artery bypass graft).

Nursing Management

Nursing priorities for the patient receiving fibrinolytic therapy are directed toward 1) identifying candidates for reperfusion therapy, 2) observing for signs of reperfusion,

TABLE 13-6 **Pharmacologic Management Oral Antiplatelet Agents**

MEDICATION	DOSAGE	ACTION	SPECIAL CONSIDERATIONS
Aspirin	81-325 mg	Inhibits synthesis of thromboxane A_2 resulting in irreversible inhibition of platelet activation	Lower doses are recommended when given with other antithrombotics.
Clopidogrel (Plavix)	300-600 mg loading dose 75-150 mg maintenance	Irreversibly inhibits the ADP $P2Y_{12}$ platelet receptor to block platelet activation	Onset of action 2-4 hr Should be held 5-7 days before elective surgery to decrease risk of bleeding Some patients may have a genetic resistance to clopidogrel, resulting in inadequate platelet inhibition.
Prasugrel (Effient)	60 mg loading dose 10 mg daily maintenance	Irreversibly inhibits the ADP $P2Y_{12}$ platelet receptor to block platelet activation	Onset of action 15-30 minutes Should be held 5-7 days before elective surgery to decrease risk of bleeding Contraindicated in patients with prior TIA or stroke; not recommended in patients >75 years of age
Ticagrelor (Brilinta)	180 mg loading dose 90 mg twice daily maintenance	Reversibly inhibits the ADP $P2Y_{12}$ platelet receptor to block platelet activation	Onset of action 30 minutes Should be held 5 days before elective surgery to decrease risk of bleeding Contraindicated in patients with a history of ICH or severe hepatic impairment Maintenance aspirin dose above 100 mg reduces effectiveness.

ADP, Adenosine diphosphate; *ICH*, intracranial hemorrhage; *TIA*, transient ischemic attack.

3) monitoring for signs of bleeding, and 4) providing patient education.

Identifying Candidates for Reperfusion Therapy

Nursing management of the patient undergoing fibrinolytic therapy begins with identifying potential candidates. In many institutions, checklists are used to facilitate the rapid identification of patients who are candidates for fibrinolytics. Baseline laboratory values and vital signs are obtained. Intravenous lines are placed before lytic therapy is administered, and a heparin lock may be used for obtaining laboratory specimens during treatment. Throughout the administration of the fibrinolytic agent, assessment of the patient continues for clinical indicators of reperfusion and complications related to therapy.

Observing for Signs of Reperfusion

Several phenomena may be observed after the reperfusion of an artery that has been completely occluded by a thrombus. While recognition of these noninvasive markers of recanalization is important for assessing the patient's response to fibrinolytic therapy, they are less reliable than angiography in determining whether reperfusion has been successful.

Pain and Reperfusion Dysrhythmias

One possible sign of reperfusion is the abrupt cessation of chest pain as blood flow is restored to the ischemic myocardium. Another potential indicator of reperfusion is the appearance of various "reperfusion dysrhythmias." A variety of dysrhythmias can occur—premature ventricular contractions (PVCs), bradycardias, heart block, VT—but accelerated idioventricular rhythms have shown the best correlation with reperfusion.[23] Reperfusion dysrhythmias are usually self-limiting or nonsustained, and aggressive antidysrhythmic therapy is not required. However, vigilant monitoring of the patient's ECG is essential because a stable condition can deteriorate rapidly, and the dysrhythmias may necessitate emergency treatment.

ST Segment Return to Baseline

Another noninvasive marker of recanalization is rapid return to baseline of the elevated ST segments, which indicates restoration of blood flow to previously ischemic myocardial tissue. A monitoring lead should be chosen that clearly demonstrates ST elevation before initiation of therapy.[24] The inability to achieve 50% resolution of the ST elevation within 60 minutes of administering the medication is generally considered criteria for failure of fibrinolytic therapy.[23]

Cardiac Biomarkers

Serial measurement of serum biomarkers may serve as further evidence of successful reperfusion following fibrinolytics. Cardiac-specific creatine kinase and troponin rise rapidly and then decrease markedly after reperfusion of the ischemic myocardium. This phenomenon is called *washout* because it is thought to result from the rapid readmission of substances released by damaged myocardial cells into the circulation after restoration of blood flow (see "Cardiac Biomarkers" in Chapter 11).

Monitoring for Bleeding

The most common complication related to thrombolysis is bleeding, from the fibrinolytic therapy itself and also because patients routinely receive anticoagulation therapy to minimize the possibility of rethrombosis. Monitoring for clinical manifestations of bleeding is essential. Mild gingival bleeding and oozing around venipuncture sites is common and not a cause of concern. Should serious bleeding occur, such as intracranial or internal bleeding, all fibrinolytic and antithrombotic therapies are discontinued, and volume expanders or coagulation factors, or both, are administered.

In addition to accurate assessment of the patient for evidence of bleeding, nursing management includes preventive measures to minimize the potential for bleeding. For example, patient-handling is limited, injections are avoided, and additional pressure is applied at the catheter insertion site to ensure hemostasis.

Patient Education

Education for the patient receiving fibrinolytic therapy includes information regarding the actions of fibrinolytic agents, with emphasis on precautions to minimize bleeding. For example, the patient is cautioned against vigorous tooth brushing and told to refrain from using straight-edge razors. Information is provided regarding ongoing risk-factor management in the prevention of atherosclerotic CAD.

CATHETER INTERVENTIONS FOR CORONARY ARTERY DISEASE

During the past 3 decades, the use of catheter procedures to open coronary arteries blocked or narrowed by CAD has expanded dramatically. These procedures are collectively referred to as *percutaneous coronary intervention* (PCI). Today, PCI includes balloon angioplasty, atherectomy, and stent implantation. Advances in device technology, along with more effective anticoagulant and antiplatelet regimens, have reduced complication rates and improved procedural outcomes.[25] Patients undergoing scheduled PCI-based interventions generally remain in the hospital overnight and then go home. In the setting of emergency PCI, associated with an MI, the hospital stay lasts a few days, depending on the cardiovascular work-up that is required.

Indications for Catheter-Based Interventions

PCI is preferred as the initial method of treatment for acute MI (primary PCI). Elective PCI is used to treat patients with symptomatic coronary artery disease to address blockages in both native vessels and bypass grafts. Improvements in technology and operator experience have expanded the use of catheter-based interventions to more complex types of lesions, including total occlusions, bifurcation stenoses, and left main coronary artery lesions.[26] Lesion morphology related to shape, size, location, and amount of calcification are used to guide the selection of each catheter-based intervention (see "Coronary Artery Disease" in Chapter 12).

Percutaneous Transluminal Coronary Angioplasty

Percutaneous transluminal coronary angioplasty (PTCA), also known as balloon angioplasty, involves the use of a balloon-tipped catheter that, when advanced through an atherosclerotic lesion (atheroma), can be inflated intermittently to dilate the stenotic area and improve blood flow through the coronary artery (Figure 13-8). After balloon deflation, the vessel exhibits some degree of elastic recoil, resulting in a residual stenosis of approximately 30%. A successful angioplasty procedure is one in which the stenosis is reduced to less than 50% of the vessel lumen diameter.[26]

In recent years, design enhancements have led to low-profile angioplasty catheters that are able to traverse tortuous anatomy and development of noncompliant balloons to prevent overdistention of the vessel.[27] Another modification is the cutting balloon—a device that produces incisions in the plaque before the balloon is inflated. Even with these improvements PTCA is rarely used alone, except to treat lesions in very small coronary arteries.[27]

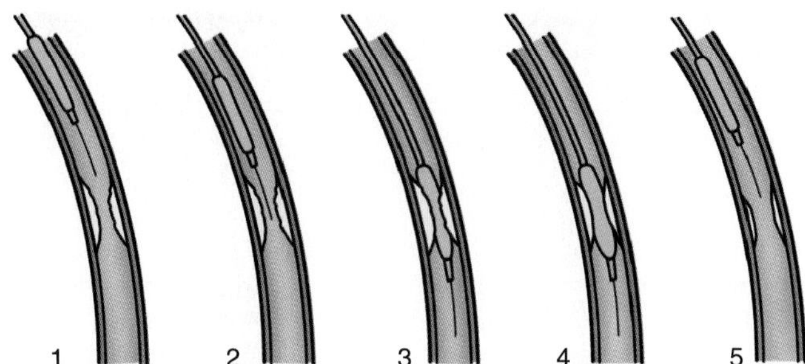

FIG 13-8 Percutaneous Transluminal Coronary Angioplasty (PTCA) is used to open a stenotic vessel occluded by atherosclerosis.

Atherectomy

Atherectomy is the excision and removal of the atherosclerotic plaque by cutting, shaving, or grinding. Two specialized coronary catheters are used in coronary intervention: directional coronary atherectomy (DCA) shown in Figure 13-9A and rotational ablation (Rotablator) shown in Figure 13-9B. Atherectomy is useful for removing plaque in calcified or fibrotic lesions, which helps increase wall compliance and facilitate angioplasty and stent placement. In the current era, atherectomy devices are used in less than 5% of PCI procedures.[27]

Coronary Stents

A stent is a metal structure that is introduced into the coronary artery over a guidewire and expanded into the vessel wall at the site of the lesion. Bare metal stents were first used to treat acute or threatened vessel closure after failed PTCA. The stent acted as a scaffold to tack dissection flaps against the vessel wall and provided mechanical support to minimize elastic recoil. Subsequent studies confirmed the clinical benefits of stents, which led to elective coronary stenting as a primary procedure. Stent implantation was initially limited to large vessels (greater than 3 mm) with proximal, discrete lesions. Improvements in stent design and operator technique allow for their deployment in smaller vessels with diffuse disease, vessels with lesions at bifurcations, and vessels with thrombus. Multiple stents may be implanted sequentially within a vessel to cover the area of the lesion fully. Stents are currently the predominant form of PCI and are used in more than 90% of all interventional procedures.[27]

Numerous stents are available. They are composed of various types of metal (stainless steel, titanium, cobalt chromium) and come in a variety of configurations (e.g., mesh, coil). Most stents are balloon-expandable (Figure 13-10).

Drug-Eluting Stents

In an effort to minimize restenosis, drug-eluting stents (DES) were developed. These stents have polymer coatings impregnated with medications that are released slowly into the endothelium at the site of stent placement to inhibit cellular

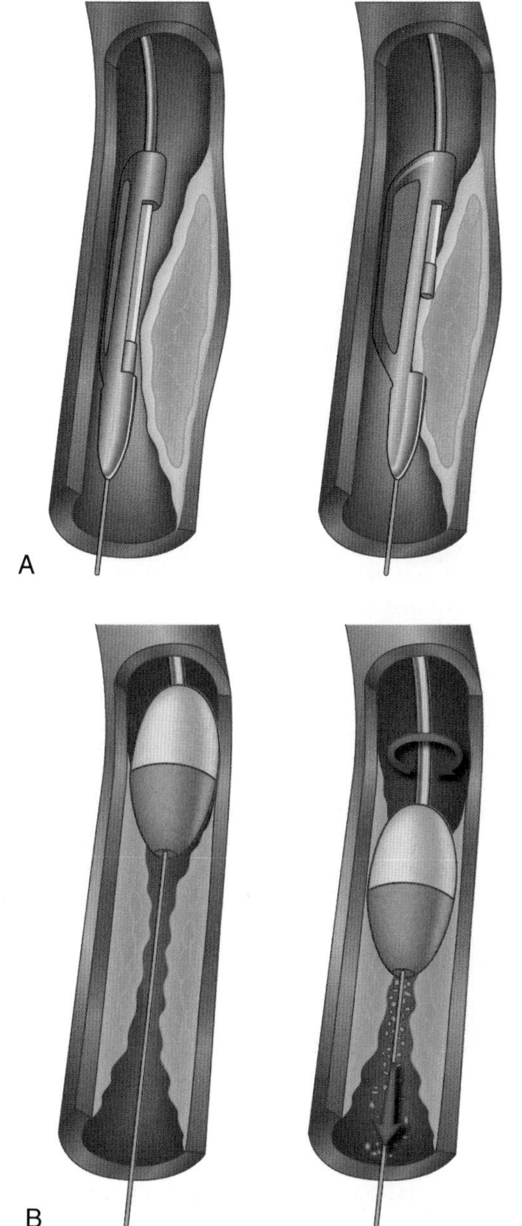

FIG 13-9 Atherectomy Devices. *A*, Directional coronary atherectomy catheter. *B*, Rotational atherectomy catheter.

proliferation. DES coated with sirolimus (an immunosuppressive medication used to prevent organ transplant rejection) and paclitaxel (an anticancer agent) have been approved by the FDA.[28] In initial trials, DES were found to decrease the 6-month restenosis rate to less than 10%, and they soon became the predominant stent, implanted in 90% of patients. Later trials demonstrated similar efficacy between bare metal stents and DES in long-term outcomes (stent thrombosis, MI, or death) and raised concerns regarding the possibility of late stent thrombosis (greater than 1 year) in DES.[25] As a result, DES usage has decreased somewhat to around 75% of patients.[28] Because a DES delays endothelialization, dual antiplatelet therapy must be continued for a longer period to prevent stent thrombosis. A DES is also considerably more expensive than a bare metal stent. A comparison of bare metal stents and DES is provided in Table 13-7.

TABLE 13-7 Comparison of Bare Metal and Drug-Eluting Stents

CHARACTERISTICS	BARE METAL STENT	DRUG-ELUTING STENT
Restenosis rate (at 6 months)	15%-20%	5%-10%
Cost	$	$$$
Duration of dual antiplatelet therapy	Minimum of 1 month for non-ACS patients, at least 12 months for stents implanted for ACS	Minimum of 12 months for either non-ACS or ACS patients, and longer if tolerated
Recommended lesion features	Short lesions <20 mm Large vessel diameter >3 mm	Longer lesions >20 mm Small vessel diameter <3.5 mm

ACS, Acute coronary syndrome.

Stent Thrombosis and Antiplatelet Therapy

Specific interventions are used to prevent subacute stent thrombosis. High-pressure balloon inflations within the stent are employed to open the stent fully, so less anticoagulation is needed to maintain stent patency. Dual antiplatelet therapy (aspirin and a thienopyridine) has been shown to be more important than anticoagulation in preventing stent thrombosis.[25] These agents are administered before the procedure and continued at discharge.[29] A description of oral antiplatelet agents is provided in Table 13-6.

More potent intravenous antiplatelet agents—glycoprotein IIb/IIIa inhibitors—may also be used during PCI procedures, especially in high-risk patients[29] (Table 13-8). These medications act on specific receptors on the platelet membrane to inhibit the final phase of platelet aggregation and prevent platelets from binding with fibrinogen. Indications and dosages for glycoprotein IIb/IIIa medications are listed in Table 13-8.

PCI Procedure

PCI is performed in the cardiac catheterization laboratory under fluoroscopy. An introducer catheter, or sheath, is inserted percutaneously into the femoral, radial, or brachial artery. In some cases, a venous sheath is inserted and used to perform a right-heart catheterization or to insert a pacing catheter, or both. Nitroglycerin or calcium channel blockers may be administered to prevent coronary artery spasm and to maximize coronary vasodilation during the procedure.

Anticoagulation and Antiplatelet Therapy. The patient is systemically anticoagulated to prevent clots from forming on or in any of the catheters. Unfractionated heparin has been used traditionally, initiated with a weight-based bolus and then titrated to achieve a target activated clotting time. Other anticoagulants may be selected based on physician preference or if the patient cannot tolerate heparin.[30] Options for anticoagulant agents are described in Table 13-9.

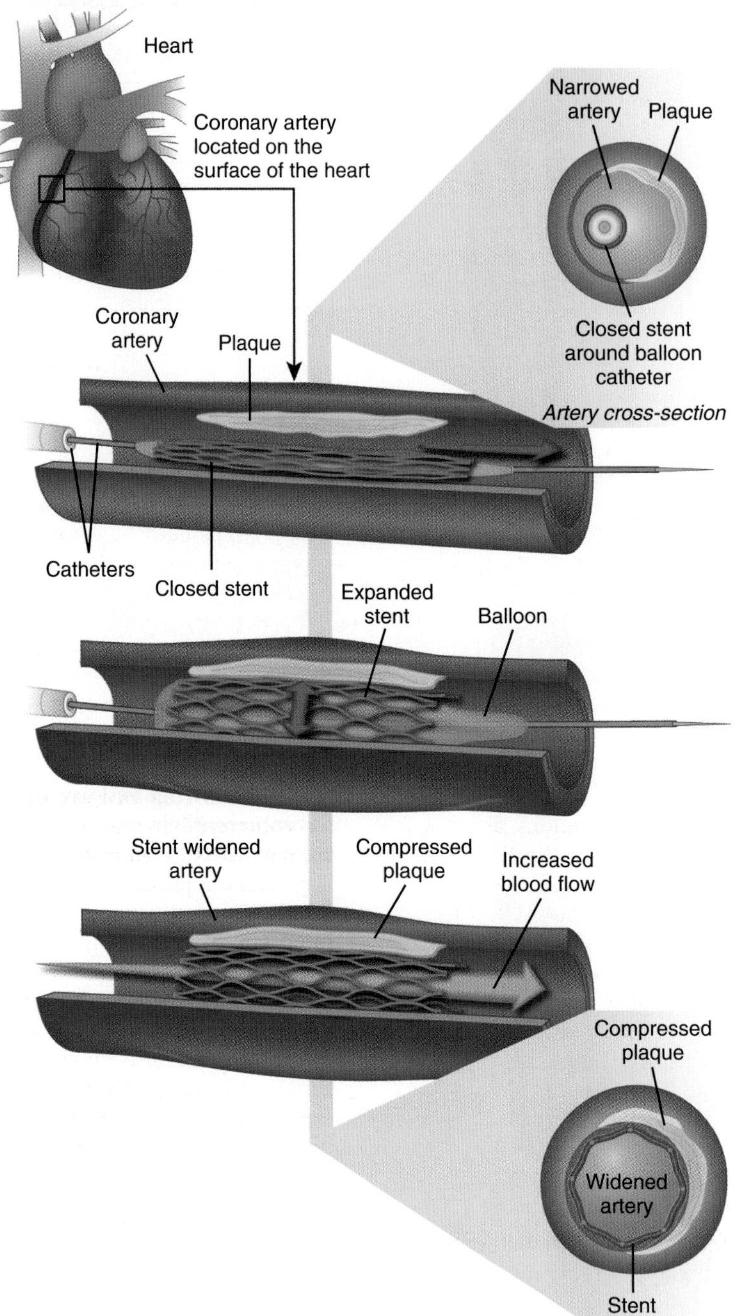

FIG 13-10 The intracoronary stent is a balloon-expandable stent.

In most procedures, vessel dilation is followed by deployment of an intracoronary stent. A stent is positioned at the target site, the stent is expanded, and the catheter is removed, leaving the stent in place.

Intravascular Ultrasound. Intravascular ultrasound is used to evaluate the vessel lumen diameter after stent deployment to ensure optimal expansion.[31] Information obtained by ultrasonography provides a better estimate of residual plaque than that provided by angiography because contrast material may surround the lattice-work of the stent, giving the appearance of a large lumen even when the stent is not fully open.

Post-procedure Care. The patient is transferred to the coronary care or angioplasty unit after the procedure for care and observation. Heparin or other anticoagulants are usually discontinued immediately after the procedure to facilitate early sheath removal. Sheaths are removed when the activated clotting time (ACT) returns to normal in heparinized patients, or sooner if other anticoagulants or a vascular closure device is used. If glycoprotein IIb/IIIa inhibitors were initiated during the procedure, they may be continued for 12 to 24 hours, depending on the agent used. Dual antiplatelet therapy with aspirin and a thienopyridine (clopidogrel, prasugrel or ticagrelor) is routinely prescribed at discharge. Recommendations for antiplatelet medication vary based on the type of stent used (see Table 13-7), whereas aspirin is continued indefinitely.

TABLE 13-8 Pharmacologic Management Intravenous Antiplatelet Agents

MEDICATION	DOSAGE	ACTION	SPECIAL CONSIDERATIONS
Abciximab (ReoPro)	ACS: 0.25 mg/kg IVP, then 10 mcg/min until PCI (continue infusion for a minimum of 18 hrs to a maximum of 26 hrs) PCI: 0.25 mg/kg IVP, then 0.125 mcg/kg/min × 12 hrs	Inhibits the GP IIb/IIIa receptors responsible for platelet aggregation	Used concomitantly with aspirin and anticoagulants May affect platelet function for up to 48 hrs after infusion
Eptifibatide (Integrilin)	ACS: 180 mcg/kg IV bolus, followed by continuous infusion of 2 mcg/kg/min up to 72 hrs PCI: 180 mcg/kg IV bolus immediately before PCI (repeat after 10 minutes) followed by continuous infusion of 2 mcg/kg/min for 12-24 hrs	Reversibly binds to the glycoprotein GP IIb/IIIa platelet receptor and inhibits platelet aggregation	Concomitant aspirin and anticoagulants may be administered. Platelet function returns to baseline within 6-8 hrs. Contraindicated in patients with significant kidney dysfunction
Tirofiban (Aggrastat)	ACS: 0.4 mcg/kg/min for 30 min, then continued at 0.1 mcg/kg/min for 48-108 hrs PCI: 25 mcg/kg bolus followed by an infusion of 0.15 mcg/kg/min for up to 18 hrs	Reversibly binds to the glycoprotein GP IIb/IIIa platelet receptor and inhibits platelet aggregation	Administered in combination with heparin for patients undergoing PCI Platelet function returns to baseline within 4-8 hrs. Dosage should be reduced in patients with kidney dysfunction.

ACS, Acute coronary syndrome; *IV*, intravenous; *IVP*, intravenous push; *PCI*, percutaneous coronary intervention.

Acute Complications

The incidence of serious cardiac complications after PCI, including coronary spasm, coronary artery dissection, and acute coronary thrombosis, has decreased significantly with improvements in technology. Stents have proved efficacious in the repair of coronary dissections, decreasing the need for emergency bypass surgery. Acute thrombosis has decreased with the established use of dual antiplatelet agents. Bleeding and hematoma formation at the site of vascular cannulation, compromised blood flow to the involved extremity, and retroperitoneal bleeding with femoral access occur infrequently but are associated with increased morbidity and lengthened hospitalization.[32] Other complications that can occur in the period immediately after PCI include contrast-induced kidney failure, dysrhythmias, and vasovagal response (hypotension, bradycardia, and diaphoresis) during manipulation or removal of introducer sheaths.

Late Complications

Restenosis after PCI continues to be a problem, although rates are much lower with drug-eluting stents than with angioplasty alone. Patients at greatest risk are those with complex lesions, multivessel disease, or diabetes.[28] Treatment options for in-stent restenosis include balloon dilation, debulking with an atherectomy device, implantation of another stent or brachytherapy—the localized delivery of intracoronary radiation through specialized catheters. Late thrombosis, although rare, is associated with a 45% mortality rate. Premature discontinuation of antiplatelet therapy is the strongest predictor of late stent thrombosis.[28]

Nursing Management

Nursing management and nursing diagnoses after PCI focus on accurate assessment of the patient's condition and prompt intervention. **Nursing priorities in the care of a patient following PCI are directed toward 1) monitoring for recurrent angina, 2) prevention of contrast-induced kidney injury, 3) monitoring the vascular access site, and 4) providing patient education about PCI follow-up and medications.**

Monitoring for Recurrent Angina

It is essential that the nurse observe the patient for recurrent angina or ST elevation, which are clinical indicators of myocardial ischemia. Select monitoring leads that will reflect ischemia in the vessels that were treated during the PCI. Angina during interventional cardiology procedures is an expected occurrence at the time of balloon inflation or when manipulation within the coronary artery occurs. Post-procedure angina may be caused by transient coronary vasospasm, or it may signal a more serious complication—acute thrombosis. Intravenous nitroglycerin is typically infused and may be titrated to alleviate chest pain. Continued angina despite maximal vasodilator therapy usually rules out transient coronary vasospasm as the source of ischemic pain, and a return to the cardiac catheterization laboratory must be considered.

Prevention of Contrast-Induced Acute Kidney Injury

Patients undergoing PCI are exposed to significant amounts of contrast dye, with its associated risk of nephrotoxicity. Protective strategies may be implemented before the procedure, especially for patients with evidence of baseline kidney impairment. This may include preprocedural hydration and infusion of sodium bicarbonate.[33] While an early study indicated that administration of *N*-acetylcysteine (Mucomyst) might be beneficial, current guidelines do not recommend it for prevention of contrast-induced acute kidney injury.[31] After PCI, hydration is important to maintain adequate flow through the kidneys. Intravenous fluids are administered, and patients are encouraged to take oral fluids as tolerated.

TABLE 13-9 Pharmacologic Management Anticoagulants

MEDICATION	DOSAGE	ACTION	SPECIAL CONSIDERATIONS
Unfractionated Heparin			
Heparin sodium	Initial bolus 60 units/kg (max dose 4000 units), followed by 12 units/kg/hr infusion	Enhances activity of antithrombin III, a natural anticoagulant to prevent clot formation	Effectiveness of treatment may be monitored by aPTT or ACT. Response is variable because of binding with plasma proteins. Effects may be reversed with protamine sulfate. Risk of developing HIT Should not be given to patients already receiving therapeutic SQ enoxaparin
Low-Molecular-Weight Heparin			
Enoxaparin (Lovenox)	30 mg IV bolus, followed by 1 mg/kg SC every 12 hrs For patients already on SC dosing, an additional bolus of 0.3 mg/kg is given if last dose was >8 hrs prior to PCI.	Enhances activity of antithrombin III	More predictable response than heparin, because enoxaparin is not largely bound to protein No need for aPTT or ACT monitoring Lower risk of HIT than with UFH Administer within 30 minutes of initiation of fibrinolytic therapy.
Direct Thrombin Inhibitors			
Bivalirudin (Angiomax)	0.75 mg/kg IV bolus, followed by infusion at 1.75 mg/kg/hr during PCI If infusion continued >4 hrs, rate is decreased to 0.2 mg/kg/hr.	Directly inhibits thrombin	May be administered alone or in combination with glycoprotein IIb/IIIa inhibitors Produces a dose-dependent increase in aPTT and ACT Coagulation times return to baseline within 1 hour after stopping infusion. Dose should be reduced for patients with kidney dysfunction. No reversal agent is available. May be used instead of UFH for patients with HIT
Argatroban (Argatroban)	Loading dose of 100 mcg/kg IV bolus over 1 minute, followed by infusion of 1 mcg/kg/min (low-dose) or 3 mcg/kg/min (high-dose)	Directly inhibits thrombin	May be used instead of UFH for patients with HIT ACT is monitored during PCI, while aPTT is used during prolonged infusion. Abrupt discontinuation may lead to a rebound hypercoagulable state.
Factor Xa Inhibitor			
Fondaparinux (Arixtra)	2.5 mg IV, followed by 2.5 mg SC once daily	Selective inhibitor of factor Xa	May be used in conjunction with fibrinolytics For PCI, must be administered with another anticoagulant (i.e., UFH) to prevent catheter thrombosis Long half-life (>17 hrs) Contraindicated in patients with kidney failure

ACT, Activated clotting time; *aPTT*, activated partial thromboplastin time; *HIT*, heparin-induced thrombocytopenia; *MI*, myocardial infarction; *PCI*, percutaneous coronary intervention; *SC*, subcutaneous.

Monitoring the Vascular Access Site

While the sheath is in place or after its removal, bleeding or hematoma at the insertion site may occur due to the effects of anticoagulation. The nurse observes the patient for bleeding or swelling at the puncture site and for changes in vital signs (hypotension, tachycardia) that could indicate hemorrhage. If a femoral approach was used, the nurse also assesses the patient for back pain, which can indicate retroperitoneal bleeding from the internal arterial puncture site.

Limb Ischemia. Peripheral ischemia can occur secondary to cannulation of the artery, so frequent assessment of the adequacy of circulation to the involved extremity is important. The patient is instructed to keep the limb straight and minimize movement. Additional activity restrictions vary, depending on the size and location of the sheath, type of anticoagulation prescribed, methods used to achieve hemostasis, and institutional protocols. For femoral access, the head of the bed is not elevated more than 30 degrees while the sheath is in place (to prevent dislodgment) and for a period of time after its removal (to prevent bleeding). For brachial or radial access, a splint may be used to prevent flexion of the arm or wrist. After sheath removal, direct

TABLE 13-10 **Vascular Closure Devices**

TECHNOLOGY AND EXAMPLES	DESCRIPTION	COMMENTS
Patch		
Chito-Seal Clo-Sur P.A.D. D-Stat Syvek Patch	Patches that contain materials to promote clotting are applied directly to the puncture site, along with manual compression.	Less expensive than active closure devices No foreign material is left in the patient.
Suture		
Perclose A-T ProGlide	Sutures deployed through the sheath are used to close the arteriotomy site.	Allows for immediate reaccess through the site if needed Device failure may require surgical repair.
Plug or Sealant		
Angio-Seal Duett Mynx	Placement of a procoagulant sealant such as collagen or thrombin is used to close the artery. Angio-Seal also includes an intravascular suture to anchor the collagen plug in place. The Mynx system uses a balloon catheter to inject sealant into the puncture site tract.	Reaccess must be done 1 cm above the previous arterial access site to avoid dislodging the sealant. Extrusion of the sealant into the vessel may compromise the arterial lumen. Components are absorbed within 30-90 days, depending on the sealant used.
Clip or Staple		
EVS-Angiolink StarClose	Circumferential staples or clips are deployed at the site of the arteriotomy to close the vessel.	Extravascular clip does not compromise the artery lumen.

pressure is applied to the puncture site for 15 to 30 minutes until hemostasis is achieved.

If direct pressure is inadequate or the patient is at higher risk for bleeding, a C-clamp or other compression device may be used to apply continuous pressure for 1 to 2 hours to ensure adequate hemostasis. Patients usually are allowed to resume ambulation 2 to 6 hours after the procedure, or sooner if a vascular closure device is employed.[34]

Vascular Closure Devices. In the last decade, a number of products have been introduced to facilitate adequate hemostasis at the femoral access site after sheath removal. Active closure devices utilize mechanical sutures, collagen plugs, or metal clips to close the vessel when the sheath is removed. Advantages of these devices include a reduced time to hemostasis (under 5 minutes) regardless of the patient's level of anticoagulation, earlier ambulation, and increased patient comfort.[32]

The Perclose closure device contains needles and sutures that are used to suture the artery closed after the interventional procedure. Angio-Seal is a vascular hemostatic device that uses a collagen plug to seal the arterial puncture site. Gentle pressure is maintained over the puncture site for approximately 5 minutes, until hemostasis is achieved. The StarClose vascular closure device consists of a tiny circumferential nitinol (nickel and titanium) clip that is applied to the surface of the vessel to close the femoral artery at the end of the procedure.

Reports of complications and increased cost have limited the use of active closure devices.[32,35] To avoid these complications, a number of products have been developed to enhance manual compression and shorten the time required to achieve hemostasis. Some of these devices rely on the delivery of prothrombotic materials by a patch, whereas others increase local pressure over the puncture site. These devices do not offer immediate closure but may decrease the time to ambulation.[32] A comparison of vascular closure systems is provided in Table 13-10.

Patient Education

In most cases, patients undergoing elective angioplasty, atherectomy, or stent procedures are hospitalized for approximately 24 hours. All patients require education about their medication regimen and about risk-factor modification. Because of the abbreviated hospital stay, the nurse often has time to do little more than identify the major risk factors and initiate basic instruction. Patients are referred to local cardiac rehabilitation centers for more extensive teaching and follow-up to facilitate understanding and compliance with risk-factor modification.

Another point of instruction that must be addressed is the patient's knowledge deficit related to discharge medications. Patients are sent home on a regimen of antiplatelet medications and medications for secondary prevention, such as lipid-lowering agents and blood pressure medications. A nitrate such as isosorbide may be prescribed to promote vasodilation, or, if the patient has demonstrated evidence of a vasospastic component to the disease, calcium channel blockers may be used. It is essential that the patient clearly understands the rationale for therapy and the potential side effects of each medication. Patients also need to understand the importance of not discontinuing their antiplatelet therapy.[36] Patients should be provided with written information and a number to call if problems occur.

CATHETER INTERVENTIONS FOR VALVE REPAIR

Balloon Valvuloplasty

Percutaneous catheter technology has also been adapted to allow for nonsurgical interventions for valvular heart disease. Balloon valvuloplasty, also known as balloon comissurotomy, is an accepted alternative to surgical repair for patients with mitral valve stenosis. This procedure has a limited role in aortic stenosis because it provides only short-term improvement and is associated with high morbidity and mortality. Current guidelines recommend balloon valvuloplasty for aortic stenosis only as a bridge to surgery or transcatheter valve replacement (discussed below) in severely symptomatic patients (Box 13-5).[37]

Balloon valvuloplasty is performed in the cardiac catheterization laboratory by placing a balloon across the stenotic valve and inflating it to reduce stenosis. Regurgitant flow can result, particularly after mitral valvuloplasty, and may result in the need for emergent valve replacement if severe. The risks of balloon valvuloplasty are similar to those inherent in most catheterization procedures and include cardiac perforation, thromboembolic events, dysrhythmias, and vascular complications caused by the sheath. Postprocedural nursing management is similar to that for other percutaneous cardiac catheter procedures.

Transcatheter Aortic Valve Replacement

Transcatheter aortic valve replacement (TAVR) is a transformational therapy for patients who have severe aortic stenosis but are deemed high-risk surgical candidates or are considered inoperable by virtue of associated comorbidities.[38] TAVR can be performed with spinal or general anesthesia in a cardiac catheterization laboratory or in a hybrid operating room. The procedure consists of positioning a bioprosthetic valve that has been loaded on a stent within the native aortic valve and then expanding the stent to anchor the valve within the aortic annulus.[39] Different approaches are used to deploy the device, but once it is in place, contrast medium is used to ensure correct positioning of the catheter valve across the aortic annulus.[39] Post-procedure patient assessments include monitoring patient rhythm, hemodynamics and fluid balance, and observing for signs of stroke or kidney injury that may require additional medical interventions.

BOX 13-5 Indications for Percutaneous Valve Repair

Aortic Stenosis
- Transcatheter repair recommended for inoperable patients with predicted survival >12 months
- Transcatheter repair reasonable as an alternative to surgery for patients with high surgical risk
- Percutaneous dilation may be considered as a bridge to surgery or TAVR in severely symptomatic patients.

Mitral Stenosis
- Balloon commissurotomy recommended for patients with severe MS and favorable valve morphology
- Balloon commissurotomy reasonable for patients with suboptimal valve if high surgical risk or inoperable

CARDIAC SURGERY

Nursing management of the patient undergoing cardiac surgery is demanding but exciting work that requires the talents of an experienced team of critical care nurses. The following discussion introduces basic cardiac surgical techniques and principles of cardiopulmonary bypass and highlights the key points about postoperative care of the adult patient who requires valve replacement or coronary artery revascularization.

Coronary Artery Bypass Surgery

Since its introduction almost 50 years ago, CABG has proved to be safe and effective in relieving angina symptoms and improving survival in most patients. Although treatment of coronary artery disease has evolved, offering less invasive techniques, improved pharmacologic therapy, and expanded education regarding lifestyle modifications, CABG surgery continues to have an important role in the treatment of coronary artery disease. Information on "Coronary Artery Disease" is presented in Chapter 12 and "Catheter Interventions for Coronary Artery Disease" are discussed earlier in this chapter.

Bypass Conduit. Myocardial revascularization involves the use of a conduit, or channel, designed to bypass an occluded coronary artery. Surgeons must evaluate which conduits will provide the best graft patency and long-term outcomes for the patient. The saphenous vein graft (SVG) is the most frequently utilized conduit for CABG surgery. Saphenous vein grafting involves the anastomosis of an excised portion of the saphenous vein proximal to the aorta and distal to the coronary artery below the obstruction (Figure 13-11). Endoscopic vein harvesting has decreased length of stay and increased patient satisfaction but has also been linked to a possible risk of early graft failure and so requires further research.[40] Vein grafts have traditionally had a high rate of arteriosclerosis, which has limited their long-term patency. Recent studies suggest that SVGs can achieve 5-year patency rates of over 80% through improved harvesting techniques, adjunctive medication strategies (statins and antiplatelet agents), and aggressive risk factor modification such as smoking cessation.[41,42]

The internal mammary artery (IMA), which usually remains attached to its origin at the subclavian artery, is swung down and anastomosed distal to the coronary artery (Figure 13-12). Either the right IMA or the left IMA may be used as a conduit. The IMA is currently recommended as the conduit of choice for CABG, with a standard practice of attaching the LIMA to the artery that supplies the largest myocardial territory, most often the left anterior descending artery.[43] The IMA has continued to demonstrate excellent long-term patency with estimated rates of 85% to 92% at 15 years.[43] A comparison of conduits used for surgical myocardial revascularization is provided in Table 13-11.

Valvular Surgery

Valvular disease results in various hemodynamic dysfunctions that can usually be managed medically as long as the patient remains symptom-free. There is reluctance to

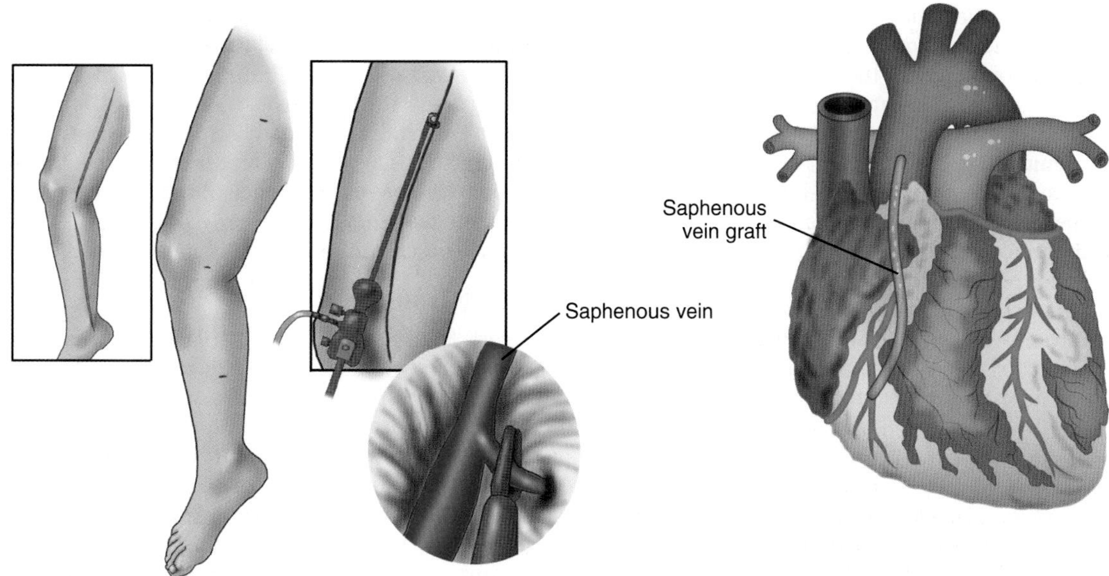

FIG 13-11 Saphenous Vein Graft. (Leg illustration from Moser D, Riegel B. *Cardiac Nursing: A Companion to Braunwald's Heart Disease*. Philadelphia: Saunders; 2007.)

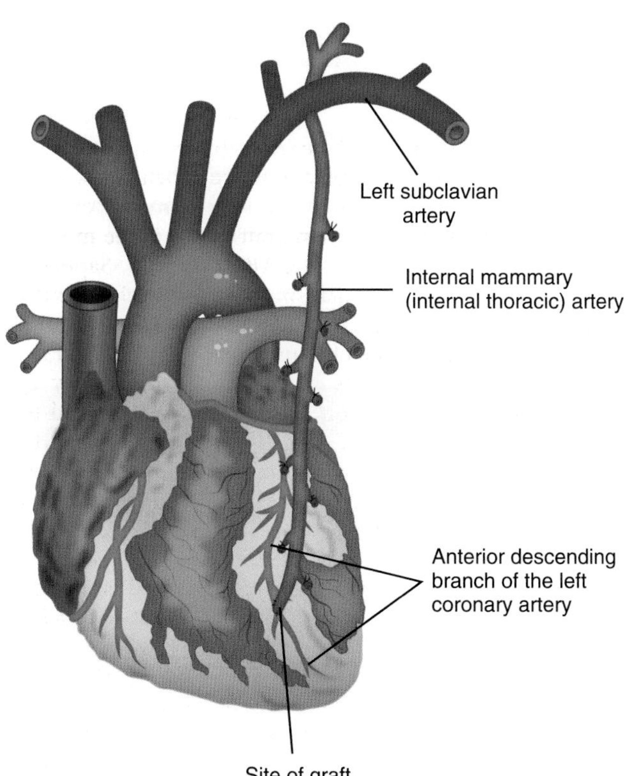

FIG 13-12 Internal mammary artery graft.

TABLE 13-11 Conduits Used for Coronary Artery Bypass Grafts

TYPE OF GRAFT	ADVANTAGES	DISADVANTAGES
Saphenous vein	Easily harvested Length allows for multiple grafts No anatomic limitations to graft sites	Long-term patency still to be determined Requires at least two anastomosis sites
Internal mammary artery	Proven patency rates Requires only one anastomosis	Requires extensive dissection Not accessible for emergency bypass Associated with increased chest wall discomfort postoperatively Anatomic limitations to bypassing some areas of the heart
Radial artery	Improved patency rates Easily harvested	Requires adequate collateral flow to the hand through the ulnar artery May be associated with higher rates of vasospasm Requires two anastomosis sites

intervene surgically early in the course of this disease because of the surgical risks and long-term complications associated with prosthetic valve replacement. These consequences, however, must be weighed against the possibility of irreversible deterioration in LV function that may develop during the compensated asymptomatic phase (see "Valvular Heart Disease" in Chapter 12).

Surgical therapy for aortic valve disease consists primarily of aortic valve replacement, although repairs may be done for selected regurgitant valves.[37] Three surgical procedures are available to treat mitral valve disease: commissurotomy, valve repair, and valve replacement. Commissurotomy is performed for mitral stenosis; the fused leaflets are incised, and calcium deposits are debrided to increase valve mobility.

Repair of damaged leaflets may be accomplished with pericardial patches. In the setting of mitral regurgitation, valve repair may include reshaping of the leaflets and the use of a ring to reduce the size of the dilated mitral annulus, enhancing leaflet coaptation (annuloplasty). Although it is technically more demanding, valve repair is preferred over replacement to avoid the complications inherent with a prosthetic valve: the risk of thromboembolic events and the need for long-term anticoagulation.[44] If reconstruction of the mitral valve is not possible, it is replaced.

The two categories of prosthetic valves are mechanical valves and biologic valves, or tissue valves. *Mechanical valves* are made from combinations of metal alloys, pyrolytic carbon, Dacron, and Teflon and have rigid occluding devices (Figure 13-13).

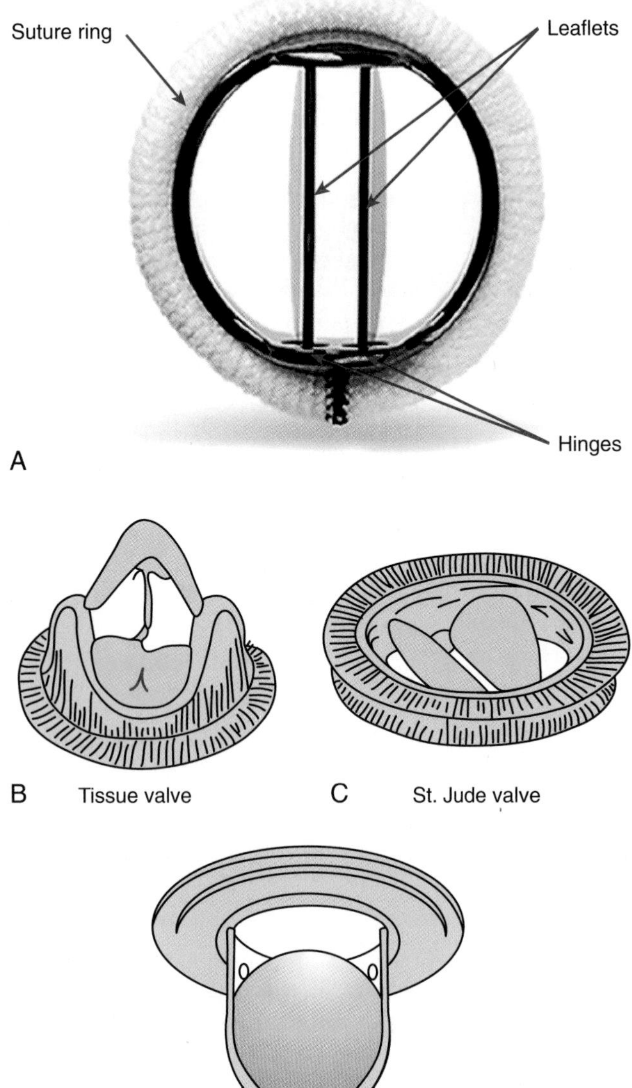

FIG 13-13 *A*, Mechanical bileaflet valve. *B*, Prosthetic tissue valve. *C*, Mechanical bileaflet valve (St. Jude). *D*, Starr-Edwards ball-and-cage valve. *A, B,* and *C* depict valves currently in use; ball-and-cage valve *(D)* is no longer in clinical use. (Courtesy St. Jude Medical.)

Their construction renders them highly durable, but all patients with mechanical valves require anticoagulation to reduce the incidence of thromboembolism. *Biologic valves* are constructed from animal or human cardiac tissue and have flexible occluding mechanisms. Because of their low thrombogenicity, tissue valves offer the patient freedom from therapeutic anticoagulation. Their durability, however, is limited by their tendency toward early calcification. Box 13-6 provides a description of various valvular prostheses.

Heart Transplant

Heart transplant is performed for selected patients with refractory end-stage heart failure.[45] A median incision and sternotomy is performed for visualization of the thorax. All of the diseased heart is removed except the posterior walls of the atria that contain the openings of the pulmonary veins and the vena cava. There are four main anastomoses to connect the donor heart: the right atria, left atria, aorta, and pulmonary artery are connected in that order (Figure 13-14). Immediate postoperative management is similar to other cardiac surgical procedures. For the rest of their lives, recipients must take immunosuppressive drugs to prevent rejection of the new heart.[46] Surveillance for rejection, prevention of infection, and comprehensive education about transplant self-care are essential to ensure long-term success.

Cardiopulmonary Bypass

Cardiopulmonary bypass (CPB) is a mechanical means of circulating and oxygenating the patient's blood while diverting most of the circulation from the heart and lungs during cardiac surgical procedures. The extracorporeal circuit consists of cannulas that drain off venous blood, an oxygenator that oxygenates the blood, and a pump head that propels the

BOX 13-6 Classification of Prosthetic Cardiac Valves

Mechanical Valves

Tilting-disc: a free-floating, lens-shaped disk mounted on a circular sewing ring

- Medtronic Hall
- Omniscience
- Monostrut

Bi-leaflet: two semicircular leaflets, mounted on a circular sewing ring that opens centrally

- St. Jude Medical
- Duromedics
- CarboMedics
- On-X/ATS

Biologic or Tissue Valves (Bioprostheses)

Porcine heterograft: a porcine aortic valve mounted on a semiflexible stent and preserved in glutaraldehyde

- Hancock
- Carpentier-Edwards
- Toronto Stentless (St. Jude)
- Free Style Stentless (Medtronic)

Homograft: a human heart valve (aortic or pulmonic) harvested from a donated heart and cryopreserved; may or may not be mounted on a support ring

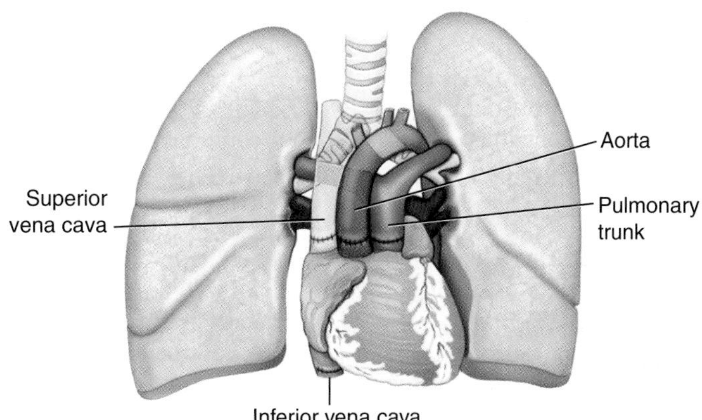

FIG 13-14 Heart Transplant Surgical Procedure.

TABLE 13-12 Physiologic Effects of Cardiopulmonary Bypass

EFFECTS	CAUSES
Intravascular fluid deficit (hypotension)	Third-spacing Postoperative diuresis Sudden vasodilation (medications, rewarming)
Third-spacing (weight gain, edema)	Decreased plasma protein concentration Increased capillary permeability
Myocardial depression (decreased cardiac output)	Hypothermia Increased systemic vascular resistance Prolonged cardiopulmonary bypass pump run Pre-existing heart disease Inadequate myocardial protection
Coagulopathy (bleeding)	Systemic heparinization Mechanical trauma to platelets Depressed release of clotting factors from liver as a result of hypothermia
Pulmonary dysfunction (decreased lung mechanics and impaired gas exchange)	Decreased surfactant production Pulmonary microemboli Interstitial fluid accumulation in lungs
Hemolysis (hemoglobinuria)	Red blood cells damaged in pump circuit
Hyperglycemia (rise in serum glucose concentration)	Decreased insulin release Stimulation of glycogenolysis
Hypokalemia (low serum potassium concentration)	Intracellular shifts during bypass and postoperative diuresis
Hypomagnesemia (low serum magnesium concentration)	Postoperative diuresis resulting from hemodilution
Neurologic dysfunction (decreased level of consciousness, motor/sensory deficits)	Inadequate cerebral perfusion Microemboli to brain (air, plaque fragments, fat globules)
Hypertension (transient rise in blood pressure)	Catecholamine release and systemic hypothermia causing vasoconstriction

arterialized blood back to the ascending aorta—which has been cross-clamped to prevent the back flow of blood into the heart.

Several adjunctive strategies are used to facilitate circulation and oxygenation while the patient is on bypass ("on-pump"). Heparin is administered systemically to prevent clotting within the bypass circuit. Hypothermia is induced through a heat exchanger in the pump to reduce tissue oxygen requirements by approximately 50%. The patient's blood is diluted with the crystalloid solution that is used to prime the bypass circuit. This hemodilution enhances capillary perfusion by reducing blood viscosity (stickiness) and decreases the risk of microthrombi formation. Numerous clinical sequelae can result from cardiopulmonary bypass (Table 13-12). Knowledge of these physiologic effects allows the nurse to anticipate problems and intervene effectively in the postoperative period.

OPCAB. Some surgeons may elect to perform CABG surgery without CPB, referred to as "off-pump" coronary artery bypass (OPCAB), in order to avoid the potential complications associated with CPB and cross-clamping of the aorta. Several techniques are used to stabilize the operative area during an OPCAB procedure. Immobilization devices that use compression or suction have been developed to restrict movement of the heart wall at the site of the anastomosis. Medications that temporarily decrease the heart rate (e.g., esmolol, diltiazem) or cause transient cardiac asystole (e.g., adenosine) may also be used to limit cardiac motion further. Patients still receive heparin but in lower doses than with CPB. OPCAB may be most beneficial in patients with significant comorbid conditions and in those with contraindications to cardiopulmonary bypass.[47]

Nursing Management

Nursing priorities are directed toward 1) optimizing cardiac output, 2) regulating temperature, 3) controlling bleeding, 4) maintaining chest tube patency, 5) recognizing cardiac tamponade, 6) promoting early extubation, 7) assessing for neurological complications, 8) preventing infection, 9) preserving kidney function, and 10) providing patient education.

Optimizing Cardiac Output

Postoperative cardiovascular support often is indicated because of a low output state resulting from pre-existing heart disease, a prolonged cardiopulmonary bypass pump run, inadequate myocardial protection, or some combination of these factors. Cardiac output can be maximized by adjustments in heart rate, preload, afterload, and contractility.

Heart rate. In the presence of low cardiac output, the heart rate can be appropriately regulated by means of temporary pacing or medication therapy. Temporary atrial and/or ventricular epicardial pacing usually is instituted when the heart rate drops to less than 60 beats/min and the patient is hypotensive, requiring a supportive rate of 80 to 100 beats/min. In the case of tachycardia, intravenous beta-blockers (esmolol) or calcium channel blockers (diltiazem) may be used in the acute postoperative period to slow supraventricular rhythms. Electrolyte disturbances such as hypokalemia, hypomagnesemia, hypocalcemia, and hypercalcemia must be quickly identified and corrected to prevent postoperative dysrhythmias.

Atrial fibrillation occurs in roughly one-third of patients after cardiac surgery, with a peak occurrence in the first 2 to 3 days after surgery. This rhythm may induce hemodynamic compromise, prolong hospitalization, and increase the patient's risk of stroke. Prophylactic administration of beta-blockers is recommended to decrease the incidence of atrial fibrillation and its clinical sequelae, or amiodarone as an alternative for those who have contraindications to beta-blockers.[48]

Preload. In most patients, reduced preload is the cause of low postoperative cardiac output. The most common causes of decreased preload are due to hypovolemia from bleeding and fluid shifts caused by the systemic inflammatory response. To enhance preload, volume may be administered in the form of crystalloid, colloid, or packed red cells. Traditionally, preload has been evaluated by intermittent measurements of central venous pressure (CVP) and pulmonary artery occlusion pressure (PAOP) obtained from catheters placed in the right atrium or pulmonary artery. A growing body of research suggests that dynamic measures of preload responsiveness, such as pulse pressure variation (PPV) and systolic pressure variation (SPV), may more accurately predict an increase in cardiac output in response to a volume challenge in post-cardiac surgery patients.[49,50]

Afterload. Many patients who have had cardiac surgery demonstrate postoperative hypertension. Although it is transient, postoperative hypertension can precipitate or exacerbate bleeding from the mediastinal chest tubes. The high SVR (afterload) resulting from the intense vasoconstriction can increase LV workload. Vasodilator therapy with intravenous sodium nitroprusside or nitroglycerin often is used to reduce afterload, control hypertension, and improve cardiac output. Increased afterload may be partially due to the peripheral vasoconstrictive effects of hypothermia, which can be managed with careful rewarming.

Contractility. If the adjustments in heart rate, preload, and afterload fail to produce significant improvement in cardiac output, contractility can be enhanced with positive inotropic support or intra-aortic balloon pumping (IABP) to augment circulation as discussed later in the chapter.

Temperature Regulation

Hypothermia can contribute to depressed myocardial contractility, vasoconstriction, and ventricular dysrhythmias following cardiac surgery. Hypothermia may also contribute to postoperative bleeding because clotting factors are depressed at lower temperatures. After surgery, patients may be rewarmed with the use of warm blankets or forced-air warming devices. Excessive temperature elevations must be avoided, with the goal of maintaining a target body temperature of 36° C to 37° C (96.8° F to 98.6° F).

Controlling Bleeding

Postoperative bleeding from the mediastinal chest tubes can be caused by inadequate hemostasis, disruption of suture lines, or coagulopathy associated with cardiopulmonary bypass or hypothermia. Bleeding is more likely to occur with IMA grafts as a result of the extensive chest wall dissection required to free the IMA. If bleeding in excess of 150 mL/hr occurs early in the postoperative period, clotting factors (fresh-frozen plasma, fibrinogen, and platelets), protamine, or desmopressin may be administered. Medications used in the treatment of postoperative bleeding are described in Table 13-13. Thromboelastography (TEG) is now also being used to determine which part of the clotting cycle is deficient in order to help guide the selection of appropriate factors or medications.

Autotransfusion devices, which facilitate the collection and reinfusion of shed mediastinal blood, previously were used in some institutions. Routine autotransfusion of shed mediastinal blood is no longer recommended because it may further exacerbate bleeding by activating the extrinsic clotting pathway and increase the risk of infection. The use of positive end-expiratory pressure (PEEP) in conjunction with mechanical ventilation may be helpful in controlling excessive bleeding in some cases by increasing the intrathoracic pressure enough to effect tamponade of oozing mediastinal blood vessels.[51,52] Rewarming the patient reverses the depressed manufacture and release of clotting factors that results from hypothermia. However, persistent mediastinal bleeding—usually in excess of 500 mL in 1 hour or 300 mL/hr for 2 consecutive hours despite normalization of clotting studies—is an indication for re-exploration of the surgical site.

Maintaining Chest Tube Patency

Chest tube stripping to maintain patency of the tubes is controversial because of the high negative pressure generated by routine methods of stripping. It is believed to result in tissue

TABLE 13-13 Medications Used to Treat Postoperative Bleeding

MEDICATION	DOSE	ACTION AND SIDE EFFECTS
Aminocaproic acid (Amicar)	Loading dose: 4-5 g over 1 hr, followed by continuous infusion of 1 g/hr for 8 hrs or until bleeding is controlled	Inhibits conversion of plasminogen to plasmin to prevent fibrinolysis, helping to stabilize clots
Desmopressin acetate (DDAVP)	0.3 mcg/kg IV over 20-30 min	Improves platelet function by increasing levels of factor VIII Side effects include facial flushing, tachycardia, headache, and hypotension.
Protamine sulfate	25-50 mg IV slowly over 10 min	Neutralizes the anticoagulant effect of heparin Can cause hypotension, bradycardia, and allergic reactions

damage that can contribute to bleeding. This risk must be carefully weighed against the real danger of cardiac tamponade if blood is not effectively drained from around the heart. Chest tube stripping often is advocated in instances of excessive postoperative bleeding. However, the technique of "milking" the chest tubes is advisable for routine postoperative care because this technique generates less negative pressure and decreases the risk of bleeding.

Recognizing Cardiac Tamponade

A potentially lethal complication, cardiac tamponade may occur after surgery if blood accumulates in the mediastinal space, impairing the heart's ability to pump. Signs of tamponade include elevated and equalized filling pressures (e.g., CVP, PAD, PAOP), decreased cardiac output, decreased blood pressure, jugular venous distention, pulsus paradoxus, muffled heart sounds, sudden cessation of chest tube drainage, and a widened cardiac silhouette on radiographs. A bedside echocardiogram may confirm tamponade. Interventions for tamponade include emergency sternotomy in the critical care unit or a return to the operating room for surgical evacuation of the clot.

Promoting Early Extubation

Mechanical ventilation is utilized initially to provide adequate alveolar oxygenation and ventilation in the postoperative period. Protocols that facilitate early extubation (less than 6 hours after surgery) have been implemented in most institutions to decrease pulmonary complications after cardiac surgery.[53] Early extubation requires a multidisciplinary approach that incorporates anesthesiologists, surgeons, nurses, and respiratory therapists. Potential candidates must be identified before surgery so that the anesthetic regimen supports early extubation.

After surgery, patients are evaluated for hemodynamic stability, adequate control of bleeding, normothermia, and the ability to follow commands. Patients who exhibit hemodynamic instability or intraoperative complications or who have underlying pulmonary disease may require longer periods of mechanical ventilation. After extubation, supplemental oxygen is administered, and patients are medicated for incisional pain to facilitate aggressive pulmonary toilet and early mobility, which is essential to helping prevent postoperative complications.

Assessing for Neurologic Complications

The neurologic dysfunction often seen in patients who have had cardiac surgery has been attributed to decreased cerebral perfusion, cerebral microemboli, hypoxia, and the systemic inflammatory response. The dysfunction can range from subtle cognitive changes to signs of acute stroke. Neurologic dysfunction was thought to be primarily caused by CPB, but newer evidence demonstrates no difference in neuropsychologic outcomes between on-pump and off-pump and indicates that cognitive decline may be influenced more by patient-related factors such as the degree of pre-existing cerebral vascular disease or diabetes.[54]

The risk of delirium is increased in cardiac surgery patients, especially older adults, and is associated with increased mortality and reduced quality of life and cognitive function.[55] Nursing staff can play a critical role in the prevention and recognition of delirium. Nonpharmacologic interventions involve reorienting patients, providing visual and hearing aids, early mobilization, sleep promotion, and the judicious use of medications known to potentiate delirium.[56] Treatment of delirium may require the use of medications such as haloperidol (Haldol). Liberalization of visitation policies to allow family members a prolonged presence at the bedside is also highly desirable.

Preventing Infection

Postoperative fever is fairly common after cardiopulmonary bypass. However, persistent temperature elevation to greater than 101°F (38.3°C) must be investigated. Sternal wound infections and infective endocarditis are the most devastating infectious complications, but leg wound infections, pneumonia, and urinary tract infections also can occur. Infection rates are greater in patients with diabetes, malnutrition, chronic diseases, obesity, and those requiring emergent or prolonged surgery. Using a continuous insulin infusion to maintain blood glucose concentrations less than or equal to 180 mg/dL while avoiding hypoglycemia may reduce the incidence of adverse events, including deep sternal wound infections.[57]

Preserving Kidney Function

Almost one-third of patients develop acute kidney injury after cardiac surgery, owing often to a combination of ischemic processes.[58] Kidney dysfunction in the postoperative period requires frequent monitoring of urine output and serum creatinine levels. Because of fluid retention, diuresis is often required to help mobilize fluids from the interstitial to the intravascular space. The patient's potassium levels may be depleted with the diuresis, requiring that levels be closely monitored and replaced.

Guidelines for Coronary Artery Bypass Grafting

The American College of Cardiology and the American Heart Association have developed a set of clinical practice guidelines for care of the patient undergoing CABG.[57] These guidelines are designed to support clinical decision making with research evidence (Box 13-7).

Patient Education

Patient education includes information related to the surgical procedure, risk-factor management, and prevention of atherosclerosis. Patients who have undergone valve surgery may also require information regarding the need for antibiotic prophylaxis before invasive procedures and specific instructions pertaining to their anticoagulation regimen.

Minimally Invasive Cardiac Surgery

Continuously evolving techniques have expanded the options for patients undergoing cardiac surgery, with a general transition from surgical to minimally invasive (minithoracotomy and small port) therapies along with percutaneous approaches. In minimally invasive direct coronary artery bypass graft (MIDCABG) surgery, a small left anterior thoracotomy incision is used to harvest the left IMA directly, which is then anastomosed to the LAD. Mitral valve repair procedures are also increasingly accomplished via a minimally invasive approach, performed either directly or with robotic assistance.

Robotic-assisted surgery allows the surgeon to view a computer-enhanced image while using robotic arms to

BOX 13-7 EVIDENCE-BASED PRACTICE CORONARY ARTERY BYPASS GRAFT SURGERY (QSEN)

A summary is provided of evidence and evidence-based review recommendations for management of the coronary artery bypass graft (CABG) surgery patient.

Strong Evidence to Support the Following

CABG for Patients

- Emergency CABG for patients with acute MI when primary PCI has failed or cannot be performed, coronary anatomy is suitable for CABG, and persistent ischemia and/or hemodynamic instability refractory to nonsurgical therapy is present
- Emergency CABG for patients undergoing surgical repair of postinfarction mechanical complications of MI, those with cardiogenic shock, or those with life-threatening ventricular dysrhythmias in the presence of left main stenosis or 3-vessel CAD
- Undergoing noncoronary cardiac surgery if ≥50% stenosis of left main or ≥70% stenosis of other major coronary arteries
- Significant (≥50%) stenosis of left main
- Significant (≥70%) stenosis in 3 major coronary arteries or in the proximal LAD plus 1 other major coronary artery
- CABG or PCI in patients with 1 or more significant (≥70%) coronary artery stenosis with unacceptable angina despite guideline-directed medical therapy
- Patients undergoing CABG who have at least moderate aortic stenosis should undergo an aortic valve replacement (AVR).
- Patients undergoing CABG who have severe ischemic mitral valve regurgitation not likely to resolve with revascularization should undergo a mitral valve repair or replacement.

Anesthetic Considerations

- Anesthetic management should be directed toward early postoperative extubation and accelerated recovery of low- to medium-risk patients.

Bypass Graft Conduits

- If possible, the left internal mammary artery (LIMA) should be used to bypass the left anterior descending artery (LAD).

Antiplatelet Therapy

- Aspirin should be administered preoperatively; if not done, initiated within 6 hours postoperatively and continued indefinitely.
- In elective cases, clopidogrel and ticagrelor should be discontinued 5 days before surgery and prasugrel for at least 7 days.

Management of Hyperlipidemia

- All patients should receive statin therapy unless contraindicated.

Blood Glucose Management

- Continuous IV insulin to maintain an early postoperative blood glucose concentration ≤180 mg/dL while avoiding hypoglycemia to reduce adverse events

Dysrhythmia Management

- Beta-blockers should be administered for at least 24 hours before CABG, reinstituted as soon as possible after surgery, and prescribed at discharge unless contraindicated in order to reduce the incidence and clinical sequelae of atrial fibrillation.

Angiotensin-Converting Enzyme (ACE) Inhibitors and Angiotensin-Receptor Blockers (ARBs)

- ACE inhibitors and ARBs should be instituted or restarted postoperatively and continued indefinitely for patients with LVEF ≤40%, hypertension, diabetes, or chronic kidney disease.

Smoking Cessation

- All smokers should receive educational counseling and be offered smoking cessation therapy during CABG hospitalization.

Cardiac Rehabilitation

- Cardiac rehabilitation should be offered to all eligible patients after CABG.

BOX 13-7 EVIDENCE-BASED PRACTICE CORONARY ARTERY BYPASS GRAFT SURGERY—cont'd

Reduction in Risk of Infection

- Preoperative antibiotic administration should be used in all patients to reduce the risk of postoperative infection.

Bleeding/Transfusions

- Aggressive attempts at blood conservation are indicated to reduce the need for RBC transfusions.

Moderate Evidence to Support the Following

CABG for Patients

- In patients with multivessel CAD with recurrent angina or MI within the first 48 hours of STEMI presentation as an alternative to a more delayed strategy
- CABG or PCI for selected patients ≥75 years of age with ST-segment elevation or left bundle branch block who are suitable for revascularization regardless of the time interval from MI to the onset of shock
- Emergency CABG after failed PCI to retrieve a foreign body in a crucial anatomic location or for hemodynamic compromise in patients with impairment of the coagulation system and without previous sternotomy
- Significant (≥70%) stenosis in 2 major coronary arteries with extensive myocardial ischemia or target vessels supplying a large area of viable myocardium
- Mild-moderate LV systolic dysfunction (EF 35%-50%) and significant (≥70% stenosis) multivessel CAD or proximal LAD stenosis with viable myocardium present
- Complex 3-vessel CAD (SYNTAX score >22) with or without involvement of the proximal LAD who are good candidates for CABG
- CABG over PCI to improve survival in patients with multivessel CAD and diabetes mellitus, particularly if a LIMA graft can be anastomosed to the LAD
- Patients undergoing CABG who have moderate ischemic mitral valve regurgitation not likely to resolve with revascularization should undergo a mitral valve repair or replacement.

Hybrid Coronary Revascularization

- The planned combination of LIMA-to-LAD artery grafting and PCI of ≥1 non-LAD coronary arteries is reasonable for 1) limitations to CABG such as heavily calcified proximal aorta or poor target vessels for CABG, 2) lack of suitable graft conduits, 3) unfavorable LAD artery for PCI.

Antiplatelet Therapy

- Clopidogrel 75 mg daily is a reasonable alternative in patients who cannot take aspirin.

Beta-Blockers

- Preoperative beta-blockers, particularly in patients with an EF >30%, can reduce the risk of in-hospital mortality.
- Can reduce the incidence of perioperative myocardial ischemia

Emotional Dysfunction and Psychosocial Considerations

- Cognitive behavior therapy or collaborative care for patients with clinical depression after CABG can be beneficial to reduce objective measures of depression.

Carotid Artery Disease

- For patients with a previous transient ischemic attack or stroke and a significant (50%-99%) carotid artery stenosis, consider carotid revascularization in conjunction with CABG. Sequence and timing (staged or simultaneous) should be determined by the relative magnitude of cerebral and myocardial dysfunction.

Infection Prevention

- Leukocyte-filtered blood can be useful to reduce the rate of overall perioperative infection and in-hospital death.

Adjuncts to Myocardial Protection

- Insertion of an intra-aortic balloon pump (IABP) is reasonable to reduce the mortality rate in CABG patients who are considered to be at high risk (e.g., LVEF <30% or left main CAD).
- Assessment of cardiac biomarkers in the first 24 hours after CABG may be considered.

Dysrhythmia Management

- For patients who cannot take beta-blockers, amiodarone is an alternative to reduce the incidence of postoperative atrial fibrillation.
- Digoxin and nondihydropyridine calcium channel blockers can be useful to control the ventricular rate in the setting of atrial fibrillation but are not indicated for prophylaxis.
- Information regarding prescribed medications (including prescribed pain medication)

Reference

Hillis LD, et al. 2011 ACCF/AHA guideline for coronary artery bypass graft surgery: executive summary: a report of the American College of Cardiology Foundation/American Heart Association Task Force on Practice Guidelines, *Circulation* 124(23):2610, 2011.

manipulate instruments positioned through small (endoscopic) ports in the patient's chest. Total endoscopic coronary artery bypass can either be done on an arrested heart or on a beating heart. Robotically assisted CABG is demonstrating acceptable safety standards with patients experiencing a rapid return to normal activities.[59] Significant surgeon and team learning curves limit these procedures to dedicated centers and highly specialized cardiac surgeons at this time.

Hybrid coronary revascularization combines catheter-based procedures along with surgical interventions to treat CAD, with the idea of capitalizing on the benefits of each. Most commonly, a LIMA bypass graft to the LAD is done surgically with PCI to one or two additional target vessels.[60] Patients who are hemodynamically unstable or with cardiogenic shock would generally be excluded from this procedure.[60] With the increasing availability of hybrid operating rooms, there will be more of these approaches done simultaneously instead of the surgical team trying to decide whether to complete the surgery or percutaneous intervention first.

INTRA-AORTIC BALLOON PUMP

Intra-aortic balloon pump (IABP) is the most commonly used temporary mechanical circulatory- assist device for supporting failing circulation (Box 13-8). The intra-aortic balloon (IAB) catheter consists of a single, sausage-shaped polyurethane balloon that is wrapped around the distal end of a vascular catheter and positioned in the descending thoracic aorta just distal to the takeoff of the left subclavian artery. When attached to a bedside pumping console and properly synchronized to the patient's cardiac cycle, the IAB inflates during diastole and deflates just before systole. Its therapeutic effects are based on the hemodynamic principles of diastolic augmentation and afterload reduction.

Initially, as the balloon is inflated in diastole concurrent with aortic valve closure, the blood in the aortic arch above the level of the balloon is displaced retrograde (backward) toward the aortic root, augmenting diastolic coronary arterial blood flow and increasing myocardial oxygen supply (Figure 13-15A). The blood volume in the aorta below the level of the balloon is propelled forward toward the peripheral vascular system, which may enhance systemic perfusion. Subsequently, the deflation of the balloon just before the opening of the aortic valve creates a potential space or vacuum in the aorta, toward which blood flows unimpeded during ventricular ejection (see Figure 13-15B). This decreased resistance to LV ejection, or decreased afterload, facilitates ventricular emptying and reduces myocardial oxygen demands. The overall physiologic effect of IABP therapy is an improvement in the balance between myocardial oxygen supply and demand. Contraindications to IABP include aortic aneurysm, significant aortic valve insufficiency, and severe peripheral vascular disease.[61]

BOX 13-8 Indications for Use of the Intra-Aortic Balloon Pump

- Failure to wean from cardiopulmonary bypass
- Unstable angina refractory to medications
- Recurrent angina after acute MI
- Hemodynamic support for high-risk PCI and CABG
- Complications of acute MI
  - Cardiogenic shock
  - Papillary muscle dysfunction or rupture with mitral regurgitation
  - Ventricular septal rupture
- Refractory ventricular dysrhythmias
- Septic shock
- Bridge to definitive therapy: cardiac transplantation or ventricular assist device

IAB Catheter Insertion

The IAB catheter may be inserted in the operating room, the cardiac catheterization laboratory, or the critical care unit. The IAB catheter is usually inserted percutaneously through the femoral artery and advanced to the correct position in the descending thoracic aorta. The physician may insert the balloon through an introducer sheath or perform a sheathless insertion to minimize the degree of vessel occlusion created by the catheter. After insertion, the balloon is attached to the console, filled with the prescribed volume of helium, and pumping is then initiated.

IAB Catheter Position

The balloon catheter must be maintained in the correct position, below the left subclavian artery and above the renal arteries to optimize effectiveness and minimize complications. The balloon may migrate proximally and occlude the left subclavian artery or the carotid arteries, or it may move distally, compromising renal and mesenteric circulation. Careful assessment of the left radial pulse, level of consciousness, urinary output, and gastrointestinal symptoms is essential. Measures to prevent accidental displacement of the balloon catheter include ensuring that the IAB is carefully secured and the head of the bed elevated no more than 30 degrees and avoiding any flexion of the involved hip.

IABP Timing

The IABP is dependent upon proper timing to ensure optimal hemodynamic benefits.[62] Although systems now adjust the timing automatically, clinicians must still be aware of how to set the timing, understand the method utilized, and evaluate its effects. The ECG and arterial pressure tracings are constantly monitored to verify the timing and effect of balloon counterpulsation.

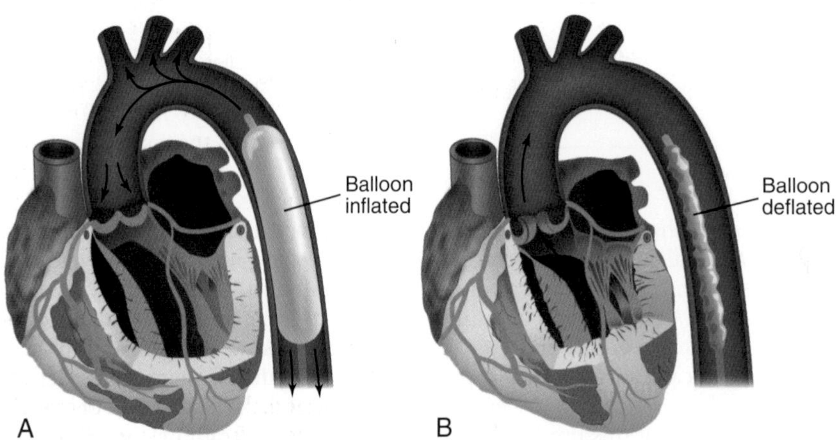

FIG 13-15 Mechanisms of Action of the Intra-Aortic Balloon Pump. *A,* Diastolic balloon inflation augments coronary blood flow. *B,* Systolic balloon deflation decreases afterload.

For counterpulsation to occur, the pump must receive a trigger signal to identify the beginning and end of the cardiac cycle. The trigger can be the R wave of the ECG, the upstroke of the arterial pressure waveform, or a pacemaker spike.[61]

Dysrhythmias

The timing of balloon inflation and deflation depends on a regular heart rhythm, such as sinus rhythm, so dysrhythmias must be detected and treated promptly. Current IABPs have automatic timing features that use internal algorithms to adjust inflation and deflation in response to changes in the patient's heart rate or rhythm. There are also catheters that incorporate a fiberoptic sensor to enhance the quality of the arterial waveform, which allows beat-to-beat adjustments to improve timing accuracy.[62]

Vascular Complications

One complication of IABP support is lower extremity ischemia resulting from occlusion of the femoral artery by the catheter itself or by emboli from thrombus formation on the balloon (see Box 13-9, Patient Safety for Peripheral Ischemia). Although ischemic complications have decreased with sheathless insertion techniques and the introduction of smaller balloon catheters (7 versus 9.5 Fr), evaluation of peripheral circulation remains an important nursing assessment. The presence and quality of peripheral pulses distal to the catheter insertion site are assessed frequently, along with color, temperature, and capillary refill of the involved extremity. Signs of diminished perfusion must be reported immediately. Anticoagulation (e.g., heparin infusion) may be prescribed to decrease the incidence of thrombosis. Other vascular complications associated with IABP include acute aortic dissection and the development of pseudoaneurysms at the catheter insertion site.

Balloon Perforation

Another potential complication of IABP therapy is balloon perforation. Perforation occurs because of repeated contact of the balloon membrane with calcified plaque in the aorta as the balloon inflates and deflates. The patient is monitored for evidence of a balloon leak, such as a gas leak alarm from the pump console or the presence of blood in the IAB tubing. If a balloon leak is detected, pumping is stopped, and the physician is immediately notified so that the balloon can be removed. If the balloon is not promptly removed or pumping is attempted after the perforation, the IAB may become entrapped as the blood hardens within the catheter, creating a mass. If this occurs, the balloon must be surgically removed.

BOX 13-9 PATIENT SAFETY (QSEN) ALERT PERIPHERAL ISCHEMIA

- Maintain head of bed ≤30 degrees.
- Keep cannulated extremity straight (use immobilizer or splint as needed).
- Monitor distal perfusion (pulse strength, capillary refill) frequently.
- Assess color, sensation, and temperature in involved extremity.

Preventing Further Complications

Log rolling, in which the patient is moved from side to side every 2 hours, is used to maintain skin integrity and to prevent pulmonary atelectasis. Because thrombocytopenia may occur as a result of mechanical destruction of the platelets by the pumping action of the balloon, platelet counts are closely monitored, and the patient is observed for evidence of bleeding. Since infection of the insertion site is a potential complication, the dressing is changed in accordance with the hospital policy for other invasive lines.

Psychological Support

The psychological needs of the patient must be considered while on IABP therapy. Sleep deprivation is common and is related in part to the continuous nursing management requirements for the patient and the noise level in the unit, including the sounds made by the balloon pumping device. Anxiety related to fear of nonrecovery and loss of control because of forced immobility is a common occurrence.

Weaning the IABP

Weaning from the IABP is considered after hemodynamic stability has been achieved with no—or only minimal—pharmacologic support. One weaning procedure consists of slowly decreasing the pumping frequency from every beat to every fourth beat, as tolerated. Another, less common, weaning method involves a gradual decrease in balloon volume. To prevent thrombus formation on the balloon surface, the IABP must remain at a minimal pumping ratio (or volume) until its removal.

Patient Education

Patient education for the patient with an IAB should include a description of the device and how it works as well as the need to minimize movement of the affected extremity. The patient should also be instructed to report symptoms that could indicate complications, such as pain in the back, leg or chest. Many of the IABP manufacturers provide helpful educational booklets designed for patients and families.

PHARMACOLOGIC MANAGEMENT

Antidysrhythmic Medications

Antidysrhythmic medications comprise a diverse category of pharmacologic agents used to terminate or prevent an array of abnormal cardiac rhythms. These commonly are classified according to their primary effect on the action potential of cardiac cells (Figure 13-16). The classification scheme shown in Table 13-14 is the most commonly used system. Classification of newer agents is more difficult because some of these agents have characteristics of more than one class and others have no characteristics of the current system.

Class I

Class I agents are sodium channel blockers that decrease the influx of sodium ions through "fast" channels during phase 0 depolarization. This prolongs the absolute (effective) refractory period, thereby decreasing the risk of premature impulses from ectopic foci. These medications also depress automaticity by slowing the rate of spontaneous depolarization of pacemaker cells during the resting phase (phase 4).

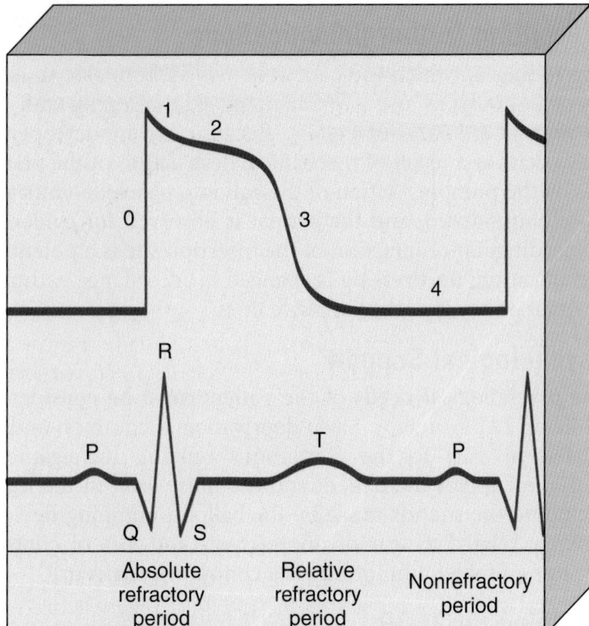

FIG 13-16 The Phases of the Cardiac Action Potential and their Relationship to the Heart's Refractory Periods. *Phase 0,* Depolarization with rapid influx of sodium. *Phase 1,* Rapid repolarization with rapid efflux of potassium ions and decreased sodium conductance. *Phase 2,* Plateau with slow influx of sodium and calcium ions. *Phase 3,* Repolarization with continued efflux of potassium ions. *Phase 4,* Resting phase with restoration of ionic balance by sodium and potassium pumps.

TABLE 13-14 Classification of Antidysrhythmic Agents

CLASS	ACTION	MEDICATIONS
I	Blocks sodium channels (stabilizes cell membrane)	
IA	Blocks sodium channels and delays repolarization, lengthening the duration of the action potential	Quinidine Procainamide Disopyramide
IB	Blocks sodium channels and accelerates repolarization, shortening the duration of the action potential	Lidocaine Mexiletine Tocainide
IC	Blocks sodium channels and slows conduction through the His-Purkinje system, prolonging the QRS duration	Flecainide Encainide Propafenone
II	Blocks beta-receptors	Esmolol Metoprolol Propranolol
III	Slows repolarization and prolongs the duration of the action potential	Amiodarone Ibutilide Sotalol Dofetilide Dronedarone
IV	Blocks calcium channels	Diltiazem Verapamil

TABLE 13-15 Effects of Adrenergic Receptors

RECEPTOR	LOCATION	RESPONSE TO STIMULATION
Alpha (α)	Vessels of skin, muscles, kidneys, and intestines	Vasoconstriction of peripheral arterioles
Beta$_1$ (β_1)	Cardiac tissue	Increased heart rate Increased conduction Increased contractility
Beta$_2$ (β_2)	Vascular and bronchial smooth muscle	Vasodilation of peripheral arterioles Bronchodilation

Class II

Class II agents are beta-adrenergic blockers (beta-blockers). They inhibit dysrhythmias mediated by the sympathetic nervous system by competing with endogenous catecholamines for available receptor sites. As a result, spontaneous depolarization during the resting phase (phase 4) is depressed, and AV conduction is slowed. Antidysrhythmic medications in this class can be further subdivided into cardioselective agents (those that block only beta$_1$-receptors) and noncardioselective agents (those that block both beta$_1$- and beta$_2$-receptors). Knowledge of the effects of adrenergic-receptor stimulation allows for anticipation of both the therapeutic responses brought about by beta-blockade and the potential adverse effects of these agents (Table 13-15). For example, bronchospasm can be precipitated by noncardioselective beta-blockers in a patient with chronic obstructive pulmonary disease (COPD) caused by blockade of the effects of beta$_2$-receptors in the lungs. Beta-blockers also are negative inotropes and must be used cautiously in patients with LV dysfunction. Although numerous beta-blockers are marketed, only esmolol, metoprolol, and propranolol are available as intravenous agents for the treatment of acute dysrhythmias. Of these, esmolol (Brevibloc) offers significant advantages for the critically ill patient because of its short half-life (approximately 9 minutes). It is used in the treatment of supraventricular tachycardias, such as atrial fibrillation and atrial flutter.

Class III

Class III agents include amiodarone, dofetilide, dronedarone, ibutilide, and sotalol. These agents markedly slow the rate of phase 3 repolarization, increasing the effective refractory period and the action potential duration. Although their effects on the action potential are similar, these medications differ greatly in their mechanism of action and their side effects. At this time, sotalol is approved only for oral use. Intravenous amiodarone was originally approved for the treatment of serious ventricular dysrhythmias refractory to other medications. Because of its effectiveness, it is now used for both atrial and ventricular dysrhythmias.[63] Dofetilide (Tikosyn) is a new class III antidysrhythmic agent used for the conversion to and maintenance of normal sinus rhythm in patients with highly symptomatic atrial fibrillation or atrial flutter. Because dofetilide prolongs the refractoriness of both atrial and ventricular tissue, prolongation of the QT interval can occur and is associated with an increased risk of torsades de pointes.[64] Therapy with dofetilide is initiated in a hospital setting under close monitoring. Ibutilide (Covert) is a short-term antidysrhythmic agent used for the rapid conversion of acute atrial fibrillation or atrial flutter to sinus rhythm. Ibutilide is administered as a 10-minute infusion in a carefully monitored clinical setting. The most serious side effect of ibutilide is its potential for inducing life-threatening dysrhythmias, especially torsades de pointes.[65]

Class IV

Class IV agents are calcium channel blockers that inhibit the influx of calcium through slow calcium channels during the plateau phase (phase 2). This effect occurs primarily in tissue in which slow calcium channels predominate, primarily the sinus and AV nodes and the atrial tissue. Verapamil was the first medication in this category available as an intravenous antidysrhythmic. It depresses sinus and AV node conduction and is effective in terminating supraventricular tachycardias caused by AV nodal re-entry. Diltiazem (Cardizem) has become available in intravenous form and is thought to be as effective as verapamil in treating supraventricular dysrhythmias, with fewer hypotensive side effects. Because accessory pathways are not affected by calcium channel blockade, both of these agents must be avoided when treating atrial fibrillation or atrial flutter in patients with Wolff-Parkinson-White syndrome.[2]

Unclassified Antidysrhythmics

Adenosine (Adenocard) is an antidysrhythmic agent that remains unclassified under the current system. Adenosine occurs endogenously in the body as a building block of adenosine triphosphate (ATP). Given in intravenous boluses, adenosine slows conduction through the AV node, causing transient AV block. It is used clinically to convert supraventricular tachycardias and to facilitate differential diagnosis of rapid dysrhythmias. Because of its short half-life, adenosine is administered intravenously as a rapid bolus, followed by a saline flush. The bolus is delivered as centrally as possible, so that the medication reaches the heart before it is metabolized.[2] Side effects are transient because adenosine is rapidly taken up by the cells and is cleared from the body within 10 seconds.

Magnesium is also unclassified under the present system. Although its action as an antidysrhythmic agent is not entirely understood, clinical studies suggest that it may reduce the incidence of both ventricular and supraventricular dysrhythmias in selected patient populations. It is considered the treatment of choice in patients with torsade de pointes. For acute treatment, 1 to 2 g of magnesium is administered over 1 to 2 minutes. In patients with confirmed hypomagnesemia, this bolus may be followed with a 24-hour infusion.[2]

Side Effects

Antidysrhythmic medications carry the risk of serious side effects, some of which can be life- threatening. Selected intravenous antidysrythmic medications with their major side effects are listed in Table 13-16. The most severe complication is the potential for a prodysrhythmic effect. This may result in worsening of the underlying dysrhythmia, the occurrence of a new dysrhythmia, or the development of a bradydysrhythmia. For example, torsades de pointes is a prodysrhythmia caused by a number of medications that prolong the QT interval on the ECG. Because the development of a prodysrhythmia is unpredictable, the nurse plays an important role in evaluating ECG changes, monitoring serum medication levels, and assessing patient symptoms. Antidysrhythmic agents may also alter the amount of energy required for defibrillation and pacing. For example, increases in the dose of an antidysrhythmic medication may increase the amount of output (mA) required to depolarize the myocardium.

Treatment of Atrial Fibrillation

More than 2 million people in the United States have atrial fibrillation, and extensive research has been done on the treatment of this disorder. The goals of pharmacologic therapy for atrial fibrillation include re-establishing and maintaining sinus rhythm, decreasing the rapid ventricular response during episodes of atrial fibrillation, and preventing the risk of thromboembolism. Table 13-17 reviews current medications used in the treatment of atrial fibrillation. Results of some clinical trials suggest that rate control is equivalent to restoration of sinus rhythm in terms of mortality, with a lower incidence of adverse medication effects.[65] In 2010, the FDA approved two new anticoagulant agents for embolism prophylaxis in patients with non-valvular atrial fibrillation. Dabigatrin (Pradaxa) is a direct thrombin inhibitor, and Rivaroxaban is a factor Xa inhibitor. These agents have advantages over warfarin in that they have fewer medication interactions and do not require routine monitoring.[66] Concerns have been raised, however, over possible risks of life-threatening hemorrhage because neither of these medications has an antidote. A recent meta-analysis found that Dabigatrin use was associated with an increased incidence of myocardial infarction.[67]

Inotropic Medications

Critically ill patients with compromised cardiac function often require the use of medications to enhance myocardial contractility (positive inotropes). Clinically available inotropes include cardiac glycosides, sympathomimetics, and phosphodiesterase inhibitors. These agents increase myocardial contractility, resulting in improved cardiac output, more complete emptying of the ventricles, and decreased filling pressures.

Cardiac Glycosides

Cardiac glycosides include digitalis and its derivatives. Although these medications have been used for centuries, their slow onset of action and risk of toxicity make them more appropriate for management of chronic heart failure. Because digoxin also causes slowing of the sinus rate and a decrease in AV conduction, it may be administered intravenously in the acute care setting to control supraventricular dysrhythmias.

Sympathomimetic Agents

Sympathomimetic agents stimulate adrenergic receptors, thereby simulating the effects of sympathetic nerve stimulation. Included in this category are naturally occurring catecholamines (epinephrine, dopamine, and norepinephrine) and synthetic catecholamines (dobutamine and isoproterenol). The cardiovascular effects of these medications, which vary according to their selectivity for specific receptor sites, are often dose-dependent as well. Table 13-18 describes the cardiovascular effects of sympathomimetic agents at various dosages.

TABLE 13-16 Pharmacologic Management

Selected Antidysrhythmic Agents

MEDICATION	DOSAGE	ACTIONS	SPECIAL CONSIDERATIONS
Adenosine	6 mg IV rapid push; if unsuccessful, repeat with 12 mg over 1-2 sec; follow with IV fluid 10 mL flush (NS or D_5W)	Blocks the AV node to terminate SVT, PSVT	Transient; flushing, dyspnea, hypotension
Digoxin	0.5-1 mg loading dose in divided doses; maintenance dose of 0.0625-0.375 mg daily	Conversion and/or rate control in SVT, AFib, AF	Bradycardia, heart block Toxicity: CNS and GI symptoms
Diltiazem	Bolus dose of 0.25 mg/kg IV over 2 min, followed by an infusion of 5-15 mg/hr	Conversion and/or rate control in SVT, AFib, AF	Bradycardia, hypotension, AV block
Esmolol	Loading dose of 500 mcg/kg over 1 min, followed by an infusion of 50 mcg/kg/min for 4 min; repeat procedure every 5 min, increasing infusion by 25-50 mcg/kg/min to maximum of 200 mcg/kg/min	Conversion and/or rate control in SVT, AFib, AF Also used to decrease rate of sinus tachycardia	Hypotension, bradycardia, heart failure
Ibutilide	0.010-0.025 mg/kg infused over 10 min (may repeat once) or 1 mg diluted in 50 mL infused over 10 min (may repeat once)	Conversion of AFib, AF	Minimal side effects except for rare polymorphic VT (torsades de pointes)
Propranolol	1-3 mg IV every 5 min, not to exceed 0.1 mg/kg	Conversion and/or rate control in SVT	Bradycardia, heart block, heart failure
Verapamil	5-10 mg IV, may repeat in 15-30 min	Conversion and/or rate control in SVT	Hypotension, bradycardia, heart failure
Lidocaine	1-1.5 mg/kg bolus, followed by continuous infusion of 1-4 mg/min	Treatment of ventricular dysrhythmias (PVCs, VT, VF)	CNS toxicity, nausea, vomiting with repeated doses
Amiodarone	*VT/VF arrest*: 300 mg IV push; may repeat with 150 mg in 3-5 min (maximum dose, 2.2 g/24 hr) *Pulsatile VT, AFib, AF*: 150 mg IV over 10 min, followed by 360 mg over 6 hrs (1 mg/min); maintenance infusion of 0.5 mg/min	Treatment of atrial (AFib, AF, SVT) and ventricular (PVCs, VT, VF) dysrhythmias	Hypotension, abnormal liver function tests
Procainamide	Loading dose of 12-17 mg/kg at a rate of 20 mg/min, followed by infusion of 1-4 mg/min	Treatment of atrial (AF, SVT) and ventricular (PVCs, VT) dysrhythmias	Hypotension, GI effects Widening of QRS and QT lengthening

AF, Atrial flutter; *AFib*, atrial fibrillation; *AV*, atrioventricular; *CNS*, central nervous system; *D_5W*, 5% dextrose in water; *GI*, gastrointestinal; *IV*, intravenous; *NS*, normal saline; *PSVT*, paroxysmal supraventricular tachycardia; *PVCs*, premature ventricular contractions; *ST*, sinus tachycardia; *SVT*, supraventricular tachycardia; *VF*, ventricular fibrillation; *VT*, ventricular tachycardia.

Dopamine (Intropin) is one of the most widely used medications in the critical care setting. It is a chemical precursor of norepinephrine, which, in addition to both alpha- and beta-receptor stimulation, can activate dopaminergic receptors in the renal and mesenteric blood vessels. The actions of dopamine are dose-related, although there is some overlap in effect.[68] At low dosages of 1 to 2 mcg/kg/min, dopamine stimulates dopaminergic receptors, causing renal and mesenteric vasodilation. The resultant increase in kidney perfusion increases urinary output. However, it is clear that this increase in urine output does not confer protection against the development of acute kidney injury. Moderate dosages result in stimulation of $beta_1$-receptors to increase myocardial contractility and improve cardiac output. At dosages greater than 10 mcg/kg/min, dopamine predominantly stimulates alpha-receptors, resulting in vasoconstriction that often negates both the beta-adrenergic and the dopaminergic effects.

Dobutamine (Dobutrex) is a synthetic catecholamine with predominantly $beta_1$-adrenergic effects. It also produces some $beta_2$ stimulation, resulting in a mild vasodilation. Dobutamine is as effective as dopamine in increasing myocardial contractility and is useful in the treatment of heart failure, especially in hypotensive patients who cannot tolerate vasodilator therapy. The usual dosage range is 2.5 to 20 mcg/kg/min, titrated on the basis of hemodynamic parameters.

Epinephrine (Adrenalin) is produced by the adrenal gland as part of the body's response to stress. This agent has the ability to stimulate both alpha- and beta-receptors, depending on the dose administered (see Table 13-18). At doses of 1 to 2 mcg/min, epinephrine binds with beta-receptors to increase heart rate, cardiac conduction, contractility, and vasodilation, thereby increasing cardiac output. As the dosage is increased, alpha-receptors are stimulated, resulting in increased vascular resistance and increased blood pressure. At these doses, epinephrine's impact on cardiac output depends on the heart's ability to pump against the increased afterload. Epinephrine accelerates the sinus rate and may precipitate ventricular dysrhythmias in the ischemic heart. Other side effects include restlessness, angina, and headache.

Norepinephrine (Levophed) is similar to epinephrine in its ability to stimulate beta- and alpha-receptors, but it lacks the $beta_2$ effects of epinephrine. At low infusion rates,

TABLE 13-17 Medications Used for Atrial Fibrillation

TREATMENT GOAL	CLASSIFICATION AND MEDICATIONS	SPECIAL CONSIDERATIONS
Conversion or maintenance of sinus rhythm	Class IA Quinidine Procainamide (Pronestyl) Disopyramide (Norpace)	Class IA agents prolong QT intervals and may cause torsades de pointes. Rate control should be achieved before initiation of therapy.
	Class IC Flecainide (Tambocor) Propafenone (Rythmol)	Class IC agents are prodysrhythmic in patients with CAD or previous MI and should be avoided in these patients.
	Class III Amiodarone (Cordarone) Dofetilide (Tikosyn) Dronedarone (Multaq) Ibutilide (Corvert) Sotalol (Betapace)	Amiodarone and sotalol also have beta-blocking properties and may help with rate control. Treatment with dofetilide requires careful monitoring for prodysrhythmic effects. Ibutilide is an IV agent and is used for conversion only.
Control of ventricular rate	Beta-blockers Esmolol (Brevibloc) Metoprolol (Lopressor) Propranolol (Inderal)	IV esmolol may be used in acute settings to control ventricular rate. Oral agents are used for maintenance therapy. Beta-blockers provide good rate control during exercise.
	Calcium channel blockers Diltiazem (Cardizem) Verapamil (Isoptin)	Intravenous calcium channel blockers may be used in emergency situations, followed by oral agents for maintenance therapy.
	Digitalis compounds Digoxin (Lanoxin)	Digoxin does not effectively control rate with exercise, so it may be used in combination with other medications.
Prevention of thromboembolism	Anticoagulants Heparin Warfarin (Coumadin) Dabigatran (Pradaxa) Rivaroxaban (Xarelto)	Heparin may be used in emergency situations, before cardioversion. Warfarin is used long term, with monitoring to achieve an INR of 2-3. Dabigatran is an oral direct thrombin inhibitor approved to reduce the risk of thromboembolism in patients with nonvalvular AFib. This medication does not require routine anticoagulant monitoring. Rivaroxaban is a Factor Xa inhibitor approved to reduce the risk of thromboembolism in patients with non-valvular Afib. This medication does not require routine anticoagulant monitoring.
	Antiplatelet agents Aspirin	Aspirin may be used in patients with contraindications to warfarin or in low-risk patients younger than 65 years.

AFib, Atrial fibrillation; *CAD*, coronary artery disease; *INR*, international normalized ratio; *IV*, intravenous; *MI*, myocardial infarction.

TABLE 13-18 Physiologic Effects of Sympathomimetic Agents

		RECEPTOR ACTIVATED*				CARDIOVASCULAR EFFECTS		
MEDICATIONS	DOSAGE	ALPHA	$BETA_1$	$BETA_2$	DOPA	CO	HR	SVR
Dobutamine	<5 mcg/kg/min	0	↑↑↑	↑	0	↑↑	↑	↓↓
	5-20 mcg/kg/min	0	↑↑↑	↑↑	0	↑↑↑	↑↑	↓↓
Dopamine	<3 mcg/kg/min	0	↑	↑	↑↑↑	0/↑	0/↑	0
	3-10 mcg/kg/min	↑↑	↑↑↑	↑	↑↑↑	↑↑↑	↑	↑
	11-20 mcg/kg/min	↑↑↑	↑↑↑	↑	↑↑	↑↑	↑↑	↑↑↑
Epinephrine	<2 mcg/min	0	↑	↑↑	0	0/↑	0/↑	↓
	2-8 mcg/min	↑↑	↑↑↑	↑↑	0	↑↑↑	↑↑	↑
	9-20 mcg/min	↑↑↑	↑↑↑	↑↑	0	↑↑	↑↑	↑↑↑
Isoproterenol	1-7 mcg/min	0	↑↑↑	↑↑↑	0	↑↑↑	↑↑↑	↓↓↓
Norepinephrine	<2 mcg/min	↑↑↑	↑↑	0	0	↑	0/↑	↑↑↑
	2-16 mcg/min	↑↑↑↑	↑↑	0	0	↓	↑	↑↑↑↑
Phenylephrine	10-100 mcg/min	↑↑↑↑	0	0	0	0	↓	↑↑↑

*See Table 13-15 for actions of receptors.
0, No effect; ↑, increased (number of arrows indicates degree of effect); ↓, decreased (number of arrows indicates degree of effect); *CO*, cardiac output; *HR*, heart rate; *SVR*, systemic vascular resistance.

$beta_1$-receptors are activated to produce increased contractility, augmenting cardiac output. At higher doses, the inotropic effects are limited by marked vasoconstriction mediated by alpha-receptors. Clinically, norepinephrine is used most often as a vasopressor to elevate blood pressure in shock states.

Isoproterenol (Isuprel) is a pure beta-receptor stimulant with no alpha-adrenergic effects. It produces dramatic increases in heart rate, conduction, and contractility through $beta_1$ stimulation and vasodilation through $beta_2$ stimulation. Isoproterenol also produces vasodilation of the pulmonary arteries and bronchodilation. It greatly increases the automaticity of cardiac cells and frequently precipitates dysrhythmias, such as PVCs and even ventricular tachycardia. These effects limit its usefulness in most patients, and it is rarely used.

Phosphodiesterase Inhibitors

Phosphodiesterase inhibitors are inotropic agents that also are potent vasodilators (inodilators). Medications in this classification inhibit the enzyme phosphodiesterase, resulting in increased levels of cyclic adenosine monophosphate (AMP) and intracellular calcium. Amrinone (Inocor) and milrinone (Primacor) were the first of these agents approved for use in the United States. Increases in cardiac output occur as a result of increased contractility (inotropic effects) and decreased afterload (vasodilative effects). Amrinone may cause thrombocytopenia, so use of this medication has decreased. Milrinone is associated with a lower rate of thrombocytopenia but can induce atrial and ventricular dysrhythmias (PVCs, VT) in a significant number of patients.[69]

Vasodilator Medications

Vasodilators are pharmacologic agents that improve cardiac performance by various degrees of arterial or venous dilation, or both. The goal of vasodilator therapy may be reduction of preload or of afterload, or both. Afterload reduction is accomplished by vasodilation of arterial vessels. This results in decreased resistance to LV ejection and may improve cardiac output without increasing myocardial oxygen demands. Reduction of preload is accomplished by dilation of venous vessels to increase capacitance. This results in decreased filling pressures for a failing heart. These medications may be classified into four groups on the basis of mechanism of action (Table 13-19).

Direct Smooth Muscle Relaxants

Direct-acting vasodilators include sodium nitroprusside, nitroglycerin, and hydralazine. These medications produce relaxation of vascular smooth muscle through the activation of nitric oxide, which results in decreased systemic vascular resistance (SVR). Hypotension may occur as a result of peripheral vasodilation, and headaches may be caused by cerebral vasodilation. Compensatory mechanisms can occur in response to the drop in blood pressure. These include baroreceptor activation that causes reflex tachycardia and activation of the renin-angiotensin-aldosterone system (RAAS) (see Fig. 12-18 in Chapter 12), with resultant sodium and water retention.

Sodium nitroprusside (Nipride) is a potent, rapidly acting venous and arterial vasodilator that is particularly suitable for rapid reduction of blood pressure in hypertensive emergencies and perioperatively. It also is effective for afterload reduction in the setting of severe heart failure. Sodium nitroprusside is administered by continuous intravenous infusion, with the dosage titrated to maintain the desired blood pressure and SVR. Prolonged administration can result in thiocyanate toxicity, manifested by nausea, confusion, and tinnitus.[70]

TABLE 13-19 Pharmacologic Management Selected Vasodilator Agents

MEDICATION	DOSAGE	ACTION	SPECIAL CONSIDERATIONS
Sodium nitroprusside (Nipride)	0.25-6 mcg/kg/min IV infusion	Potent arterial and moderate venous dilation	May cause hypotension and reflex tachycardia, thiocyanate toxicity with prolonged infusions or kidney dysfunction
Nitroglycerin (Tridil)	5-300 mcg/min IV infusion	Potent venodilator, with arterial effects at higher doses	May cause headache, reflex tachycardia, hypotension
Calcium Channel Blockers			
Clevidipine (Cleviprex)	1-2 mg/hr IV infusion, titrated to 32 mg/hr (500 mg/24 hr)	Potent arterial dilator, with no effect on venous capacitance (preload)	Hypotension, reflex tachycardia, nausea, vomiting, rebound hypertension
Nicardipine (Cardene)	5 mg/hr IV, titrated to 15 mg/hr	Potent arterial dilator, no effect on preload	Hypotension, headache, reflex tachycardia
ACE Inhibitors			
Enalaprilat (Vasotec)	0.625 mg IV over 5 min, then every 6 hr	Moderate dilation of both arteries and veins	Hypotension, elevation of liver enzymes, increase in serum potassium level
α-Adrenergic Blockers			
Labetalol (Normodyne)	20-80 mg IV bolus every 10 min, then 1-2 mg/min infusion	Moderate dilation of both arteries and veins	Orthostatic hypotension, bronchospasm, AV block
Phentolamine (Regitine)	1-5 mg IV slowly every 6 hr	Moderate dilation of both arteries and veins	Hypotension, tachycardia

AV, Atrioventricular; *IV*, intravenous; *PO*, by mouth.

Intravenous nitroglycerin (Tridil) causes both arterial and venous vasodilation, but its venous effect is more pronounced. It is used in the critical care setting for the treatment of acute heart failure because it reduces cardiac filling pressures, relieves pulmonary congestion, and decreases cardiac workload and oxygen consumption. Nitroglycerin dilates the coronary arteries and is a useful adjunct in the treatment of unstable angina and acute MI. The initial dosage is 10 mcg/min, and the infusion is titrated upward to achieve the desired clinical effect: a reduction or elimination of chest pain, decreased PAOP (wedge pressure), or a decrease in blood pressure. The most common side effects of this medication are hypotension, reflex tachycardia, and headache. Nitroglycerin becomes less effective with prolonged infusions, as tolerance develops within 24 to 48 hours.[70]

Hydralazine (Apresoline) is a potent arterial vasodilator. It is not given as a continuous infusion; rather, it is administered in slow intravenous doses of 5 to 10 mg every 4 to 8 hours. Occasionally, hydralazine is given as an intermediate agent during the transition between weaning of a continuous infusion and initiation of oral antihypertensive medications. The major side effect is reflex tachycardia mediated by the sympathetic nervous system. Hydralazine is preferred for treatment of eclampsia or pre-eclampsia because only minimal amounts cross the placenta.[70]

Calcium Channel Blockers

Calcium channel blockers are a chemically diverse group of medications with differing pharmacologic effects (Table 13-20).

Nifedipine (Procardia), nicardipine (Cardene), and clevidipine (Cleviprex) are dihydropyridines. Medications in this group of calcium channel blockers (with the suffix *-pine*) are used primarily as arterial vasodilators. These agents reduce the influx of calcium in the arterial resistance vessels. Both coronary and peripheral arteries are affected. They are used in the critical care setting to treat hypertension. Nifedipine is available only in an oral form, but in the past it was prescribed sublingually during hypertensive emergencies. Reports of adverse events associated with sublingual nifedipine prompted the FDA to issue a warning against using this administration route.[71] Nicardipine was the first available intravenous calcium channel blocker and as such could be more easily titrated to control blood pressure. Because this medication has vasodilatory effects on coronary and cerebral vessels, it has proven beneficial in treating hypertension in patients with coronary artery disease or ischemic stroke. Side effects of nicardipine are related to vasodilation and include hypotension, reflex tachycardia, flushing, headache, and ankle edema.

Clevidipine is a new short-acting calcium channel blocker that allows for even more precise titration of blood pressure in the management of acute hypertension. Advantages of this agent include its short half-life (about 1 minute), rapid onset of action, predictable dose response, and minimal effect on heart rate.[72] Because Clevidipine is mixed in a phospholipid emulsion, it can cause allergic reactions in patients with allergies to soybeans or eggs.[70]

Diltiazem (Cardizem) is from the benzothiazine group of calcium channel blockers. Verapamil (Calan, Isoptin) is part of the phenylalkylamine group. The different classifications account for the differing actions of these calcium channel blockers. These medications dilate coronary arteries but have little effect on the peripheral vasculature. They are used in the treatment of angina, especially that which has a vasospastic component, and as antidysrhythmics in the treatment of supraventricular tachycardias.

Angiotensin-Converting Enzyme Inhibitors

Angiotensin-converting enzyme (ACE) inhibitors produce vasodilation by blocking the conversion of angiotensin I to angiotensin II. Because angiotensin is a potent vasoconstrictor, limiting its production decreases SVR. In contrast to the direct vasodilators and nifedipine, ACE inhibitors do not cause reflex tachycardia or induce sodium and water retention. However, these medications may cause a profound fall in blood pressure, especially in patients who are volume-depleted. Blood pressure must be monitored carefully, especially at the initiation of therapy.

TABLE 13-20 Pharmacologic Management Classification of Calcium Channel Blockers

MEDICATION	DOSAGE	ACTIONS	SPECIAL CONSIDERATIONS
Dihydropyridines			
Nicardipine (Cardene)	5 mg/hr IV, titrated to 15 mg/hr	Short-term control of hypertension	Hypotension, headache, nausea
Nifedipine (Procardia)	10-30 mg PO	Hypertension	Hypotension, headache, reflex tachycardia
Clevidipine (Cleviprex)	1-2 mg/hr IV infusion, titrated to 32 mg/hr	Short-term control of hypertension	Hypotension, reflex tachycardia, nausea, vomiting, rebound hypertension
Benzothiazepines			
Diltiazem (Cardizem)	Bolus dose of 0.25 mg/kg IV over 2 min, followed by an infusion of 5-15 mg/hr	Treatment of SVT, AFib, AF, angina	Bradycardia, hypotension, atrioventricular block
Phenylalkylamines			
Verapamil (Calan, Isoptin)	5-10 mg IV, may repeat in 15-30 min	Treatment of AF, PSVT	Hypotension, bradycardia, heart failure

AF, Atrial flutter; *AFib*, atrial fibrillation; *IV*, intravenous; *PO*, by mouth; *PSVT*, paroxysmal supraventricular tachycardia; *SVT*, supraventricular tachycardia.

ACE inhibitors are used in patients with heart failure to decrease SVR (afterload) and PAOP (preload). Most of these agents are only available in an oral form. Enalaprilat is available in an intravenous form and may be used to decrease afterload in more emergent situations.

B-Type Natriuretic Peptide

Nesiritide (Natrecor) is a vasodilator used in the treatment of acute heart failure. This agent is a recombinant form of human brain natriuretic peptide (BNP), the hormone released by cardiac cells in response to ventricular distention. The primary effects of nesiritide include decreased filling pressures (PAOP, CVP), reduced vascular resistance (SVR, PVR), and increased urine output. Compared with traditional vasodilator therapy for acute heart failure, nesiritide reportedly is as effective as the traditional agents and has fewer side effects (e.g., headache, tachycardia).[73] The recommended dose is an intravenous bolus of 2 mcg/kg, followed by a continuous infusion of 0.01 mcg/kg/min. The primary side effect is hypotension. If this occurs, nesiritide may need to be discontinued for a time and then restarted at a lower dose after the patient has stabilized.[74] Analysis of early clinical studies indicated that this medication may be associated with an increased risk of worsening kidney function (elevated serum creatinine) and short-term mortality compared with traditional treatment of acute decompensated heart failure. More recent studies offered conflicting results, demonstrating no impact on kidney function but increased rates of hypotension.[73]

Alpha-Adrenergic Blockers

Peripheral adrenergic blockers block alpha-receptors in arteries and veins, resulting in vasodilation. Orthostatic hypotension is a common side effect and may result in syncope. Long-term therapy also may be complicated by fluid and water retention.

Labetalol (Normodyne), a combined peripheral alpha-blocker and cardioselective beta-blocker, is used in the treatment of acute stroke and hypertensive emergencies.[75] Because the blockade of $beta_1$-receptors permits the decrease of blood pressure without the risk of reflexive tachycardia and increased cardiac output, Labetalol also is useful in the treatment of acute aortic dissection.[71]

Phentolamine (Regitine) is a nonselective peripheral alpha-blocker that deceases blood pressure through arterial vasodilation. It is administered by slow IV push, 1 to 5 mg every 6 hours to reduce blood pressure. Phentolamine is used only in very specific circumstances for catecholamine-induced hypertension or illegal-drug related toxicities (e.g., cocaine). Phentolamine is the medication of choice to control blood pressure and sweating caused by *pheochromocytoma*, an epinephrine (adrenalin)-secreting tumor that can arise from the adrenal medulla.[70]

Phentolamine also is used to treat the *extravasation of dopamine* or other vasopressors into peripheral tissues. If this occurs, 5 to 10 mg is diluted in 10 mL normal saline and administered intradermally into the infiltrated area as soon as possible following the extravasation.

Dopamine Receptor Agonists

Fenoldopam (Corlopam) is a unique type of vasodilator, a selective, specific dopamine (D_1) receptor agonist.[70] Fenoldopam is a potent vasodilator that affects peripheral, renal, and mesenteric arteries. It is administered by continuous intravenous infusion beginning at 0.1 mcg/kg/min and titrated up to the desired blood pressure effect, with a maximum recommended dose of 0.5 mcg/kg/min. It can be administered as an alternative to sodium nitroprusside or other antihypertensives in the treatment of hypertensive emergencies. Fenoldopam can be used safely in patients with kidney dysfunction.[70]

Vasopressors

Vasopressors are sympathomimetic agents that mediate peripheral vasoconstriction through stimulation of alpha-receptors (see Table 13-17). This results in increased SVR and elevates blood pressure. Some of these medications (epinephrine and norepinephrine) also have the ability to stimulate beta-receptors. Vasopressors are not widely used in the treatment of critically ill cardiac patients because the dramatic increase in afterload is taxing to a damaged heart. Occasionally, vasopressors may be used to maintain organ perfusion in shock states. For example, phenylephrine (Neo-Synephrine) or norepinephrine (Levophed) may be administered as a continuous intravenous infusion to maintain organ perfusion by increasing SVR in cases of severe sepsis or septic shock.

Vasopressin, also known as antidiuretic hormone (ADH), has become popular in the critical care setting for its vasoconstrictive effects. At higher doses, vasopressin directly stimulates V1 receptors in vascular smooth muscle, resulting in vasoconstriction of capillaries and small arterioles. A one-time dose of 40 units intravenously is recommended in the ACLS guidelines as first-line therapy for VF, pulseless VT asystole, or pulseless electrical activity (PEA).[2] In septic shock vasopressin levels have been reported to be lower than anticipated for a shock state. Vasopressin continuous infusion of 0.03 unit/min may be added to the norepinephrine infusion in refractory shock per sepsis guidelines.[68] Patients must be assessed for side effects, such as heart failure caused by the antidiuretic effects, and monitored for increased risk of ischemia in the myocardium, spleen, and periphery. Vasopressin should be infused through a central line to avoid the risk of peripheral extravasation and resultant tissue necrosis. Placement of an arterial line in shock states to monitor blood pressure and SVR is recommended.

Medication Treatment of Heart Failure

Over 6 million Americans have heart failure, making it a major chronic health issue.[6] The goals of treatment in heart failure include alleviating symptoms, slowing the progression of the disease, and improving survival. Findings from a number of randomly controlled clinical trials have resulted in guidelines for the pharmacologic treatment of heart failure.[11] More information about heart failure is available in Chapter 12, (see Table 12-8 for stages and development of heart failure). For an overview of the management of acute decompensated heart failure (ADHF) see Figure 13-17.

Table 13-21 reviews the medications currently recommended for the treatment of heart failure. Types of medications that have been found to worsen heart failure should be avoided, including most antidysrhythmics, calcium channel blockers, and nonsteroidal anti-inflammatory medications.[11]

Clinical practice guidelines that discuss cardiovascular therapeutic interventions can be obtained on the websites of the professional organizations that are listed in the Internet Resources Box 13-10.

TABLE 13-21 Medications Used for Heart Failure

CLASSIFICATION AND MEDICATIONS	MECHANISM OF ACTION	EFFECTS	SPECIAL CONSIDERATIONS
ACE Inhibitors			
Captopril (Capoten) Enalapril (Vasotec) Lisinopril (Prinivil)	Interferes with the renin-angiotensin-aldosterone system by preventing conversion of angiotensin I to angiotensin II	Decreases afterload Decreases preload Reverses ventricular remodeling	Agents appear equivalent in treatment of heart failure. Monitor closely for hypotension when initiating therapy. May be contraindicated in patients with elevated creatinine, indicating kidney failure Monitor serum potassium levels
Angiotensin Receptor Blockers			
Candesartan (Atacand) Valsartan (Diovan) Losartan (Cozaar)	Interferes with the renin-angiotensin-aldosterone system by blocking the effect of angiotensin II at the angiotensin II receptor site	Decreases afterload Decreases preload Reverses ventricular remodeling	Used as primary therapy or as an alternative for patients who can't tolerate ACE inhibitors due to side effects such as severe cough Can also be used in combination with an ACE inhibitor for systolic dysfunction; monitor renal function and serum potassium levels
Beta-Blockers			
Metoprolol Succinate (Toprol XL) Bisoprolol (Zebeta) Carvedilol (Coreg)	Counteracts the SNS response activated in heart failure by blocking receptor sites Metoprolol and bisoprolol are cardioselective beta-blockers, whereas carvedilol blocks alpha- and beta-receptor sites	Slows heart rate Prevents dysrhythmias Decreases blood pressure Reverses ventricular remodeling	Not initiated during decompensated stage of heart failure Use cautiously in patients with reactive airway disease, poorly controlled diabetes, bradydysrhythmias, or heart block Carvedilol dose is increased slowly, while monitoring for symptoms caused by vasodilation, such as dizziness or hypotension.
Aldosterone Antagonists			
Spironolactone (Aldactone) Eplerenone (Inspra)	Counteracts the effects of aldosterone, which include sodium and water retention	Decreases preload Decreases myocardial hypertrophy	May increase serum potassium
Inotropes			
Digoxin (Lanoxin)	Affects the Na^+, K^+-ATPase pump in myocardial cells to increase the strength of contraction	Increases contractility Increases cardiac output Prevents atrial dysrhythmias	Risk of toxicity is increased with hypokalemia.

ACE, Angiotensin-converting enzyme; *Na^+/K^+-ATPase*, sodium-potassium adenosine triphosphatase; *SNS*, sympathetic nervous system.

BOX 13-10 INTERNET RESOURCES

AACN	American Association of Critical Care Nurses	http://www.aacn.org/
ACC	American College of Cardiology: AHA/ACC statements and guidelines can be accessed from this page	http://www.cardiosource.org/ACC.aspx
AHA	American Heart Association (for professionals)	http://my.americanheart.org/professional/index.jsp
AHA	American Heart Association (for patients)	http://www.heart.org/HEARTORG/
AHA	American Heart Association (professional journals) AHA/ACC statements and guidelines can be accessed from this page	http://www.ahajournals.org
HFSA	Heart Failure Society of America	http://www.hfsa.org/

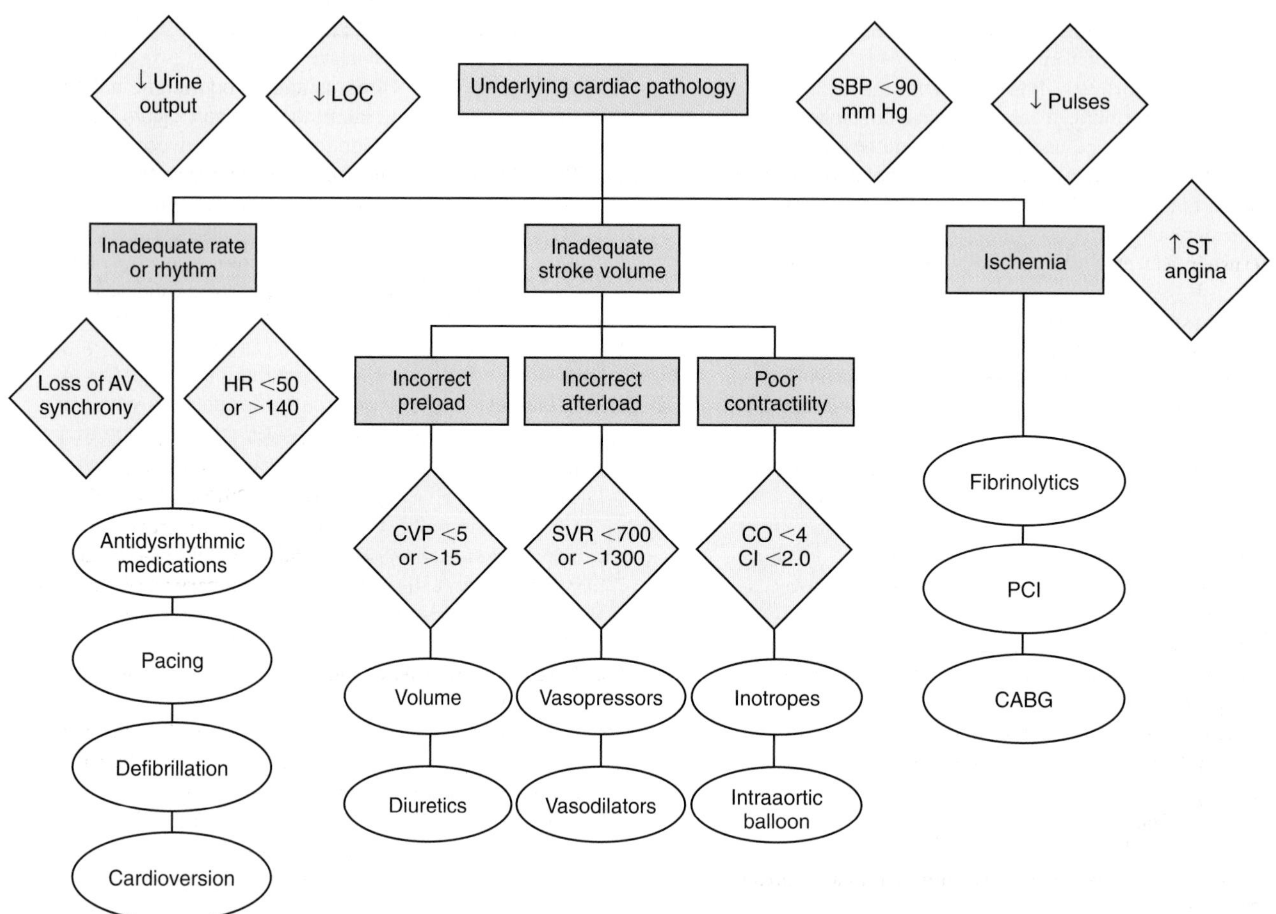

FIG 13-17 Management of acute decompensated heart failure (ADHF). *AV*, Atrial-Ventricular; *CABG*, Coronary artery bypass graft; *CI*, Cardiac index; *CO*, Cardiac output; *CVP*, Central venous pressure; *HR*, Heart rate; *LOC*, Level of consciousness; *PCI*, Percutaneous coronary intervention; *SBP*, Systolic blood pressure; *ST*, Increased ST segment elevation; *SVR*, Systemic vascular resistance; ↑, Increased; ↓, Decreased; >, Indicates greater than; <, Indicates less than.

CASE STUDY Patient with a Cardiac Problem

Brief Patient History

Mrs. G is a 54-year-old African American woman who has been having intermittent indigestion for the past month. She has a history of hypertension and hyperlipidemia. She was admitted as an in-patient on a medical floor for management of her blood pressure and is scheduled to undergo endoscopy tomorrow. Mrs. G suddenly becomes diaphoretic and complains of nausea and epigastric pain.

Clinical Assessment

The rapid response team is called to evaluate Mrs. G. When the team arrives at her bedside, she continues to complain of pain, which now radiates to her neck and back. She has some slight shortness of breath and is vomiting.

Diagnostic Procedures

The admission electrocardiogram (ECG) shows ST-segment elevation in II, III, and AVF.

Baseline vital signs include the following: blood pressure of 160/90 mm Hg, heart rate of 98 beats/min (sinus rhythm), respiratory rate of 18 breaths/min, temperature of 99°F, and O_2 saturation of 94%.

Medical Diagnosis

Mrs. G is diagnosed with an inferior myocardial infarction.

Questions

1. What major outcomes do you expect to achieve for this patient?
2. What problems or risks must be managed to achieve these outcomes?
3. What interventions must be initiated to monitor, prevent, manage, or eliminate the problems and risks identified?
4. What interventions should be initiated to promote optimal functioning, safety, and well-being of the patient?
5. What possible learning needs do you anticipate for this patient?
6. What cultural and age-related factors may have a bearing on the patient's plan of care?

REFERENCES

1. January CT, et al: 2014 AHA/ACC/HRS guideline for the management of patients with atrial fibrillation, *Circulation* 129:000, 2014. [Epub: April 10, 2014].
2. Neumar RW, et al: Part 8: adult advanced cardiovascular life support: 2010 American Heart Association Guidelines for Cardiopulmonary Resuscitation and Emergency Cardiovascular Care, *Circulation* 122(Suppl 3):S729, 2010.
3. Mahon L, et al: Cardiac tamponade after removal of temporary pacer wires, *Am J Crit Care* 21:432–440, 2012.
4. Bernstein AD, et al: The revised NASPE/BPEG generic pacemaker code for antibradycardia, adaptive-rate and multi-site pacing, *Pacing Clin Electrophysiol* 25:260, 2002.
5. Beinart R, Nazarian S: Effects of external electrical and magnetic fields on pacemakers and defibrillators: From engineering principles to clinical practice, *Circulation* 128:2799, 2013.
6. Go AS, et al: Heart disease and stroke statistics—2014 update: a report from the American Heart Association, *Circulation* 129:e28, 2014.
7. Kaszala K, Ellenbogen KA: Device sensing: sensors and algorithms for pacemakers and implantable cardioverter defibrillators, *Circulation* 122(1):1328, 2010.
8. Tops LF, et al: The effects of right ventricular apical pacing on ventricular function and dyssynchrony: implications for therapy, *J Am Coll Cardiol* 54:764, 2009.
9. Mitka M, First MRI: safe pacemaker receives conditional approval from FDA, *JAMA* 305(10):985, 2011.
10. Vernooy K, et al: Strategies to improve cardiac resynchronization therapy, *Nat Rev Cardiol* 11(8):481, 2014.
11. Yancy CW, et al: 2013 ACCF/AHA guideline for the management of heart failure: executive summary, *Circulation* 128:1810–1852, 2013.
12. Ho JK, Mahajam A: Cardiac resynchronization therapy for treatment of heart failure, *Anesth Analg* 111:1353, 2010.
13. Al-Majed NS, et al: Meta-analysis: cardiac resynchronization therapy for patients with less symptomatic heart failure, *Ann Intern Med* 154:401, 2011.
14. Baddour LM, et al: Update on cardiovascular implantable electronic device infections and their management: a scientific statement from the American Heart Association, *Circulation* 121(3):458, 2010.
15. Aronow WS: Implantable cardioverter-defibrillators, *Am J Therapeut* 17:e208, 2010.
16. Turakhia MP: Sudden cardiac death and implantable cardioverter-defibrillators, *Am Fam Physician* 82(11):1357, 2010.
17. Link MS, et al: Part 6: electrical therapies-automated external defibrillators, defibrillation, cardioversion, and pacing: 2010 American Heart Association Guidelines for Cardiopulmonary Resuscitation and Emergency Cardiovascular Care, *Circulation* 122(Suppl 3):S706, 2010.
18. Concannon TW, et al: A percutaneous coronary intervention lab in every hospital?, *Circ Cardiovasc Qual Outcomes* 5:14, 2012.
19. O'Connor RE, et al: Part 10: acute coronary syndromes: 2010 American Heart Association Guidelines for Cardiopulmonary Resuscitation and Emergency Cardiovascular Care, *Circulation* 122(Suppl 3):S787, 2010.
20. O'Gara PT, et al: 2013 ACCF/AHA Guideline for the Management of ST-Elevation Myocardial Infarction: a report of the American College of Cardiology Foundation/American Heart Association Task Force on Practice Guidelines, *Circulation* 127(4):e362, 2013.
21. Jneid H, Anderson JL, et al: 2012 ACCF/AHA Focused update of the guideline for the management of patients with unstable angina/non–ST-elevation myocardial infarction (updating the 2007 guideline and replacing the 2011 focused update), *Circulation* 126:875, 2012.
22. The TIMI Study Group: The Thrombolysis in Myocardial Infarction (TIMI) trial: phase I findings, *N Engl J Med* 312:932, 1985.
23. Antman EM, Morrow DA: ST Elevation myocardial infarction management. In Bonow RO, et al, editors: *Braunwald's Heart Disease*, ed 9, Philadelphia, 2011, Saunders, p 1111.
24. American Association of Critical Care Nurses: *AACN practice alert: ST segment monitoring*, 2009. http://www.AACN.org. Accessed August 15, 2014.
25. St. Laurent PS: Acute coronary syndromes: new and evolving therapies, *Crit Care Nurs Clin N Am* 23:559, 2011.
26. Harold JG, et al: ACCF/AHA/SCAI 2013 update of the clinical competence statement on coronary artery interventional procedures, *Circulation* 128:436–447, 2013.
27. Pompa JJ, Bhatt DL: Percutaneous coronary intervention. In Bonow RO, et al, editors: *Braunwald's Heart Disease*, ed 9, Philadelphia, 2011, Saunders, pp 1270–1300.
28. Garg S, Serruys PW: Coronary stents: current status, *JACC* 56(10 Suppl):S1, 2010.
29. Kim SJ, Giugliano RP, Jang IK: Adjunctive pharmacologic therapy in percutaneous coronary intervention: Part I antiplatelet therapy, *Coron Artery Dis* 22:100, 2011.
30. Fletcher B, Thalinger KK: Prasugrel as antiplatelet therapy in patients with acute coronary syndromes or undergoing percutaneous coronary intervention, *Crit Care Nurse* 30(5):45–54, 2010.
31. Levine GN, et al: 2011 ACCF/AHA/SCAI guideline for percutaneous coronary intervention and executive summary, *Circulation* 124:2574, 2011.
32. Dauerman HL, et al: Bleeding avoidance strategies: consensus and controversy, *JACC Cardiovasc Interv* 58(1):1, 2011.
33. Dirkes S: Acute kidney injury: not just acute renal failure anymore?, *Crit Care Nurse* 31(1):37, 2011.
34. Merriweather N, Sulzbach-Hokes L: Managing risk of complications at femoral vascular access sites in percutaneous coronary intervention, *Crit Care Nurse* 32(5):316, 2012.
35. Biancari F, et al: Meta-analysis of randomized trials on the efficacy of vascular closure devices after diagnostic angiography and angioplasty, *Am Heart J* 159(4):518, 2010.
36. Devabhakthuni S, Seybert AL: Oral antiplatelet therapy for the management of acute coronary syndromes: defining the role of prasugrel, *Crit Care Nurse* 31(1):51–63, 2011.
37. Nishimura RA, et al: 2014 AHA/ACC guideline for the management of patients with valvular heart disease: executive summary, *Circulation* 129:2440–2492, 2014.
38. Holmes DR, et al: 2012 ACCF/AATS/SCAI/STS Expert Consensus Document on Transcatheter Aortic Valve Replacement, *Ann Thorac Surg* 93:1340, 2012.
39. McRae ME, Rodger M: Transcatheter aortic valve implantation outcomes implications for practice, *J Cardiovasc Nurs* 27(3):270, 2012.
40. Kempfert J, et al: Current perspectives in endoscopic vessel harvesting for coronary artery bypass grafting, *Expert Rev of Cardiovasc Therapy* 9(11):1481, 2011.

41. Hayward P, et al: Comparable patencies of the radial artery and right internal thoracic artery or saphenous vein beyond 5 years: results from the Radial Artery Patency and Clinical Outcomes trial, *J Thorac Cardiovasc Surg* 139:60, 2010.
42. Kim FY, et al: Saphenous vein graft disease: Review of pathophysiology, prevention and treatment, *Cardiology Rev* 21:101, 2013.
43. Bello S, et al: Conduits for coronary artery bypass surgery: the quest for the second best, *J Cardiovasc Med* 12(6):411, 2011.
44. Piaschyk M, et al: A journey through heart valve surgery, *Crit Care Nurse* 23:587, 2011.
45. DePasquale EC, Schweiger M, Ross HJ: A contemporary review of adult heart transplantation: 2012 to 2013, *J Heart Lung Transplant* 33(8):775, 2014.
46. Costanzo MR, et al: The International Society of Heart and Lung Transplantation Guidelines for the care of heart transplant recipients, *J Heart Lung Transplant* 29(8):914, 2010.
47. Moller CH, et al: Off-pump versus on-pump coronary artery bypass grafting for ischaemic heart disease, *Cochrane Database Syst Rev* (3):CD007224, 2012.
48. Hillis LD, et al: 2011 ACCF/AHA Guideline for coronary artery bypass surgery: a report of the American College of Cardiology Foundation/American Heart Association task force on practice guidelines, *Circulation* 124(23):e652, 2011.
49. Kupchik N, Bridges E: Central venous pressure monitoring: what's the evidence?, *Am J Nurs* 112(2):58, 2012.
50. Bridges EJ: Arterial pressure based stroke volume and functional hemodynamic monitoring, *J Cardiovasc Nurs* 23(2):105, 2008.
51. Ferraris VA, et al: 2011 Update to the society of thoracic surgeons and the society of cardiovascular anesthesiologists Blood Conservation Clinical Practice Guidelines, *Ann Thorac Surg* 91:944, 2011.
52. Collins TA: Packed red blood cell transfusions in critically ill patients, *Crit Care Nurse* 31(1):25, 2011.
53. Lee ZF, Chee YE: Fast-track cardiac care for adult cardiac surgical patients, *Cochrane Database Syst Rev* (10):CD003587, 2012.
54. South T: Coronary artery bypass surgery, *Crit Care Nurs Clin N Am* 23:573, 2011.
55. Koster S: Consequences of delirium after cardiac operations, *Ann Thorac Surg* 93:705, 2012.
56. Allen J, Alexander E: Prevention, recognition, and management of delirium in the intensive care unit, *AACN Adv Crit Care* 23(1):5, 2012.
57. Hillis LD, et al: 2011 ACCF/AHA guideline for coronary artery bypass graft surgery: executive summary: a report of the American College of Cardiology Foundation/American Heart Association Task Force on Practice Guidelines, *J Thorac Cardiovasc Surg* 143(1):4–34, 2012.
58. Karkouti K, et al: Acute kidney injury after cardiac surgery: focus on modifiable risk factors, *Circulation* 119:495, 2009.
59. Bonatti J, et al: Robotically assisted totally endoscopic coronary bypass surgery, *Circulation* 124:236, 2011.
60. Bonatti J, et al: Hybrid coronary revascularization: which patients? when? how?, *Curr Opin Cardiol* 25:568, 2010.
61. Peura JL, et al: Recommendations for the use of mechanical circulatory support: device strategies and patient selection: a scientific statement from the American Heart Association, *Circulation* 126:2648, 2012.
62. Hanlon-Pena PM, Quaal S: Resource document: evidence supporting current practice in timing assessment, *Am J Crit Care* 20(4):e99, 2011.
63. Roberts M: Clinical utility and adverse effects of amiodarone therapy, *AACN Adv Crit Care* 21(4):333, 2010.
64. Simmons S: Critical care drugs: dofetilide. Nursing 2011, *Crit Care* 6(2):8, 2011.
65. Gutierrez C, Blanchard DG: Atrial fibrillation: diagnosis and treatment, *Am Fam Physician* 83(1):61, 2011.
66. Furie K, et al: Oral antithrombotic agents for the prevention of stroke in nonvalvular atrial fibrillation: a science advisory for healthcare professionals from the American Heart Association/American Stroke Association, *Stroke* 43:3442, 2012.
67. Uchino K, Hernandez AV: Dabigatran association with higher risk of acute coronary events: meta-analysis of noninferiority randomized controlled trials, *Arch Intern Med* 172(5):397, 2012.
68. Hollenberg SM: Inotrope and vasopressor therapy in septic shock, *Crit Care Nurs Clin N Am* 23:127, 2011.
69. Coons JC, McGraw M, Murali S: Pharmacotherapy for acute heart failure syndromes, *Am J Health Syst Pharm* 68:21, 2011.
70. Hays AJ, Wilkerson TD: Management of hypertensive emergencies: a drug therapy perspective for nurses, *AACN Adv Crit Care* 21(1):5, 2010.
71. Rodriguez MA, Kumar SK, DeCaro M: Hypertensive crisis, *Cardiol Rev* 18:102, 2010.
72. Pollack CV, et al: Clevidipine, an intravenous dihydropyridine calcium channel blocker, is safe and effective for the treatment of patients with acute severe hypertension, *Ann Emerg Med* 53:329, 2009.
73. O'Connor CM, et al: effect of nesiritide in patients with acute decompensated heart failure, *N Engl J Med* 365(1):32, 2011.
74. Falk SA: Anesthetic considerations for the patient undergoing therapy for advanced heart failure, *Curr Opin Anesthesiol* 24:314, 2011.
75. Smithburger PL, et al: Recent advances in the treatment of hypertensive emergencies, *Crit Care Nurse* 30(5):24, 2010.

CHAPTER 14

Pulmonary Clinical Assessment and Diagnostic Procedures

Kathleen M. Stacy, Jeanne M. Maiden

Be sure to check out the bonus material, including review questions, on the Evolve website at http://evolve.elsevier.com/Urden/priorities/.

HISTORY

Taking a thorough and accurate history is an essential part of the assessment process. The patient's history provides the foundation and direction for the rest of the assessment. The overall goal of the patient interview is to expose key clinical manifestations that will facilitate the identification of the underlying cause of the illness. This information then assists in the development of an appropriate management plan.[1]

The initial presentation of the patient determines the rapidity and direction of the interview. For a patient in acute distress, the history should be curtailed to just a few questions about the patient's chief complaint and precipitating events. For a patient in no obvious distress, the history should focus on five areas: 1) review of the patient's present illness, 2) overview of the patient's general respiratory status, 3) examination of the patient's general health status, 4) survey of the patient's family and social background, and 5) description of the patient's current symptoms.[1] Specific items regarding each of these areas are outlined in Box 14-1.[1-5]

FOCUSED CLINICAL ASSESSMENT

Inspection

Inspection of the patient focuses on three priorities: 1) observation of the tongue and sublingual area, 2) assessment of chest wall configuration, and 3) evaluation of respiratory effort. If possible, patients should be positioned upright, with their arms resting at their sides.[3]

Observation of the Tongue and Sublingual Area

The patient's tongue and sublingual area should be observed for a blue, gray, or dark purple tint or discoloration indicating the presence of central cyanosis. *Central cyanosis* is a sign of hypoxemia, or inadequate oxygenation of the blood, and it is considered to be a life-threatening condition. It occurs when the amount of reduced hemoglobin (unsaturated hemoglobin) exceeds 5 g/dL. The fingers and toes may also appear discolored, an indication of the presence of peripheral cyanosis.[6]

Assessment of Chest Wall Configuration

The size and shape of the patient's chest wall are assessed for an increase in the anteroposterior (AP) diameter and for structural deviations. Normally, the ratio of anteroposterior diameter to lateral diameter ranges from 1:2 to 5:7.[2,4,5] An increase in the anteroposterior diameter is suggestive of chronic obstructive pulmonary disease (COPD).[2,4,5] The shape of the chest should be inspected for any structural deviations. Some of the more frequently seen abnormalities are pectus excavatum, pectus carinatum, barrel chest, and spinal deformities. In *pectus excavatum* (funnel chest), the sternum and lower ribs are displaced posteriorly, creating a funnel or pit-shaped depression in the chest. This causes a decrease in the anteroposterior diameter of the chest and may interfere with respiratory function. In *pectus carinatum* (pigeon breast), the sternum projects forward, causing an increase in the anteroposterior diameter of the chest. The *barrel chest* also results in an increase in anteroposterior diameter of the chest and is characterized by displacement of the sternum forward and the ribs outward. Spinal deformities such as *kyphosis, lordosis,* and *scoliosis* also may be present and can interfere with respiratory function.[7]

Evaluation of Respiratory Effort

The patient's respiratory effort is evaluated for rate, rhythm, symmetry, and quality of ventilatory movements.[2] Normal breathing at rest is effortless and regular and occurs at a rate of 12 to 20 breaths per minute.[3] There are a number of abnormal respiratory patterns (Figure 14-1). Some of the more commonly seen patterns in patients with pulmonary dysfunction are tachypnea, hyperventilation, and air trapping. *Tachypnea* is manifested by an increase in the rate and decrease in the depth of ventilation. *Hyperventilation* is manifested by an increase in the rate and depth of ventilation. Patients with COPD often experience obstructive breathing, or *air trapping.* As the patient breathes, air becomes trapped in the lungs, and ventilations become progressively shallower until the patient actively and forcefully exhales.[8]

BOX 14-1 Data Collection

Pulmonary History

Common Pulmonary Symptoms

Cough

- Onset and duration:
  Sudden or gradual
  Episodic or continuous
- Characteristics:
  Dry or wet
  Hacking, hoarse, barking, or congested
  Productive or nonproductive
- Sputum:
  Present or absent
  Frequency of production
  Appearance—color (e.g., clear, mucoid, purulent, blood-tinged, mostly bloody), foul odor, frothy
  Amount
- Pattern:
  Paroxysmal
  Related to time of day, weather, activities, talking, or deep breathing
  Change over time
- Severity:
  Causes fatigue
  Disrupts sleep or conversation
  Produces chest pain
- Associated symptoms:
  Shortness of breath
  Chest pain or tightness with breathing
  Fever
  Upper respiratory tract signs (sore throat, congestion, increased mucus production)
  Noisy respirations or hoarseness
  Gagging or choking
  Anxiety, stress, or panic reactions
- Efforts made to treat:
  Prescription or nonprescription medications
  Vaporizers
  Effective or ineffective

Shortness of Breath or Dyspnea on Exertion

- Onset and duration:
  Sudden or gradual
  Gagging or choking episode a few days before onset
- Pattern:
  Related to position—improves when sitting up or with head elevated; number of pillows used to alleviate problems
  Related to activity—exercise or eating; extent of activity that produces dyspnea
  Related to other factors—time of day, season, or exposure to something in the environment
  Harder to inhale or harder to exhale
- Severity:
  Extent activity is limited
  Breathing itself causes fatigue
  Anxiety about getting enough air
- Associated symptoms:
  Pain or discomfort—exact location in respiratory tree
  Cough, diaphoresis, swelling of ankles, or cyanosis
- Efforts made to treat:
  Prescription or nonprescription medications
  Oxygen
  Effective or ineffective

Chest Pain

- Onset and duration:
  Gradual or sudden
  Associated with trauma, coughing, or lower respiratory tract infection
- Associated symptoms:
  Shallow breathing
  Uneven chest expansion
  Fever
  Cough
  Radiation of pain to neck or arms
  Anxiety about getting enough air
- Efforts made to treat:
  Heat, splinting, or pain medication
  Effective or ineffective

Pulmonary Risk Factors

- Tobacco use—current and past:
  Type of tobacco—cigarettes, cigars, pipes, or smokeless
  Duration and amount—age started, inhale when smoking, amount used in the past and present
  Pack years—number of packs per day multiplied by number of years patient has smoked
  Efforts to quit—previous attempts and current interest
- Work environment:
  Nature of work
  Environmental hazards: chemicals, vapors, dust, pulmonary irritants, or allergens
  Use of protective devices
- Home environment:
  Location
  Possible allergens—pets, house plants, plants and trees outside the home, or other environmental hazards
  Type of heating
  Use of air conditioning or humidifier
  Ventilation
  Stairs to climb

Medical History

Child

- Infectious respiratory diseases:
  Strep throat
  Mumps
  Tonsillitis
- Asthma
- Cystic fibrosis
- Immunizations

BOX 14-1 Data Collection—cont'd

Adult
- Previous diagnosis of pulmonary disorders—dates of hospitalization
- Chronic pulmonary disease—date, treatment, and compliance with therapy:
  Tuberculosis
  Bronchitis
  Emphysema
  Bronchiectasis
  Asthma
  Sinus infection
- Other chronic disorders—cardiovascular, cancer, musculoskeletal, neurologic, immune:
  Obstruction of one or both nares
  Mouth breathing often necessary (especially at night)
  History of nasal discharge
  Compromised immune system function
- Nosebleed
- Sleep apnea:
  Obstructive
  Central
- Previous tests:
  Allergy testing
  Pulmonary function tests
  Tuberculin and fungal skin tests
  Chest radiographs

Surgical
- Thoracic trauma
- Thoracic surgery
- Nasal surgery or injury

Family History
- Tuberculosis
- Cystic fibrosis
- Emphysema
- Allergies
- Asthma
- Atopic dermatitis
- Smoking by household members
- Malignancy

Current Medication Use
- Inhalators
- Steroids
- Antibiotics
- Immunizations
  Pneumococcal (Pneumovax)

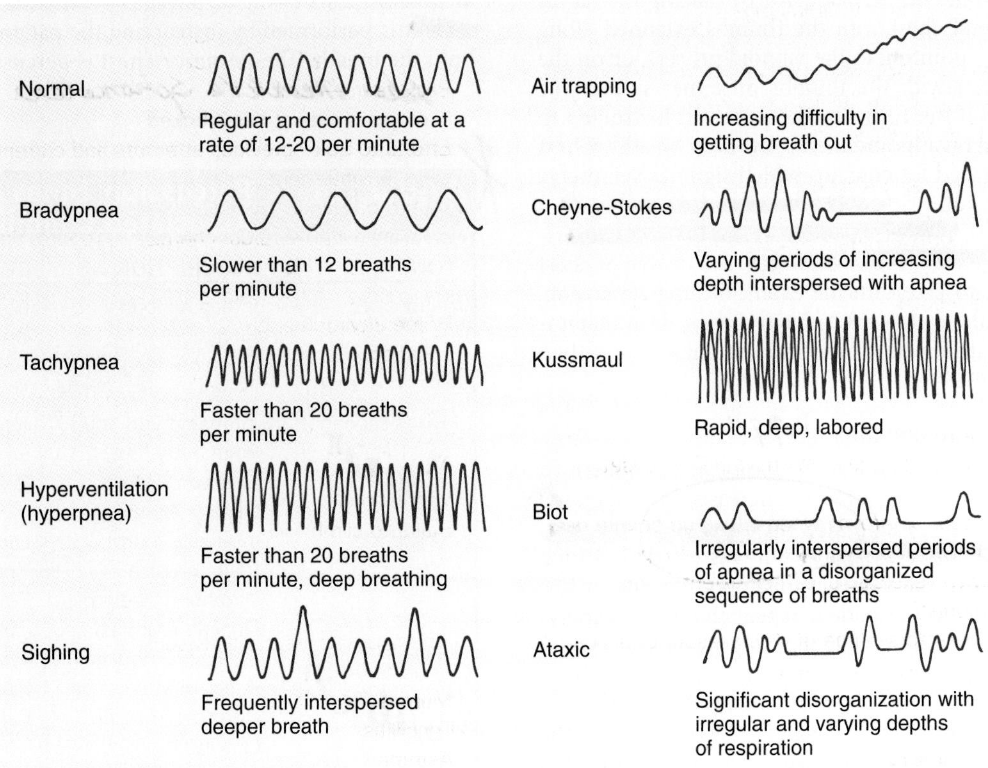

FIG 14-1 Patterns of Respiration. (From Ball JW et al: *Seidel's guide to physical examination*, ed 8, St Louis, 2015, Elsevier.)

Additional Assessment Areas

Other areas assessed are patient position, active effort to breathe, use of accessory muscles, presence of intercostal retractions, unequal movement of the chest wall, flaring of nares, and pausing midsentence to take a breath.[2,4,5] The presence of other iatrogenic features, such as chest tubes, central venous lines, artificial airways, and nasogastric tubes, should be identified because they may affect assessment findings.

Palpation

Palpation of the patient focuses on three priorities: 1) confirmation of the position of the trachea, 2) assessment of thoracic expansion, and 3) evaluation of fremitus. The thorax should be assessed for any areas of tenderness, lumps, or bony deformities. The anterior, posterior, and lateral areas of the chest should be evaluated in a systematic fashion.[2]

Confirmation of Position of the Trachea

The patient's tracheal position is confirmed at midline. It is assessed by placing the fingers in the suprasternal notch and moving upward.[8] Deviation of the trachea to either side may indicate a pneumothorax, unilateral pneumonia, diffuse pulmonary fibrosis, a large pleural effusion, or severe atelectasis. With atelectasis, the trachea shifts to the same side as the problem, and with pneumothorax, the trachea shifts to the opposite side of the problem.[7]

Assessment of Thoracic Expansion

The patient's thoracic expansion is assessed for the degree and symmetry of movement. It is assessed by placing the hands on the anterolateral chest with the thumbs extended along the costal margin, pointing to the xiphoid process, or on the posterolateral chest with the thumbs on either side of the spine at the level of the 10th rib. The patient is instructed to take a few normal breaths and then a few deep breaths. Chest movement is assessed for equality, which signifies symmetry of thoracic expansion.[3,7,8] Asymmetry is an abnormal finding that can occur with pneumothorax, pneumonia, or other disorders that interfere with lung inflation. The degree of chest movement is felt to ascertain the extent of lung expansion. The thumbs should separate 3 to 5 cm during deep inspiration.[5,8] Lung expansion of a hyperinflated chest is less than that of a normal one.[5,8]

Evaluation of Tactile Fremitus

Assessment of tactile fremitus is performed to identify, describe, and localize any areas of increased or decreased fremitus. Fremitus refers to the palpable vibrations felt through the chest wall when the patient speaks. It is assessed by placing the palmar surface of the hands against opposite sides of the chest wall and having the patient repeat the word "ninety-nine". The hands are moved systematically around the thorax until the anterior, posterior, and both lateral areas have been assessed.[7,8] If only one hand is used, it is moved from one side of the chest to the corresponding area on the other side of the chest until all areas have been assessed.[8] Fremitus varies from patient to patient and depends on the pitch and intensity of the voice. Fremitus is described as normal, decreased, or increased. With normal fremitus, vibrations can be felt over the trachea but are barely palpable over the periphery.[2] With decreased fremitus, there is interference with the transmission of vibrations. Examples of disorders that decrease fremitus include pleural effusion, pneumothorax, bronchial obstruction, pleural thickening, and emphysema. With increased fremitus, there is an increase in the transmission of vibrations. Examples of disorders that increase fremitus include pneumonia, lung cancer, and pulmonary fibrosis.[5]

Percussion

Percussion of the patient focuses on two priorities: 1) evaluation of the underlying lung structure and 2) assessment of diaphragmatic excursion. Although the technique is not used often, percussion is a useful method for confirming suspected abnormalities.

Evaluation of Underlying Lung Structure

The patient's underlying lung structure is evaluated to estimate the amounts of air, liquid, or solid material present. It is performed by placing the middle finger of the nondominant hand on the chest wall. The distal portion, between the last joint and the nail bed, is then struck with the middle finger of the dominant hand. The hands are moved systematically and side to side around the thorax to compare similar areas until the anterior, posterior, and both lateral areas have been assessed. Five tones can be elicited: resonance, hyperresonance, tympany, dullness, and flatness. These tones are distinguished by differences in intensity, pitch, duration, and quality. Table 14-1 describes the different percussion tones and their associated conditions.[3,7]

Assessment of Diaphragmatic Excursion

Diaphragmatic excursion is assessed by measuring the difference in the level of the diaphragm on inspiration and expiration. It is performed by instructing the patient to inhale and hold the breath. The posterior chest is percussed downward,

TABLE 14-1 Percussion Tones and Their Associated Conditions

TONE	DESCRIPTION	CONDITION
Resonance	Intensity: loud Pitch: low Duration: long Quality: hollow	Normal lung Bronchitis
Hyperresonance	Intensity: very loud Pitch: very low Duration: long Quality: booming	Asthma Emphysema Pneumothorax
Tympany	Intensity: loud Pitch: musical Duration: medium Quality: drumlike	Large pneumothorax Emphysematous blebs
Dullness	Intensity: medium Pitch: medium-high Duration: medium Quality: thudlike	Atelectasis Pleural effusion Pulmonary edema Pneumonia Lung mass
Flatness	Intensity: soft Pitch: high Duration: short Quality: extremely dull	Massive atelectasis Pneumonectomy

over the intercostal spaces, until the dull sound produced by the diaphragm is heard. The spot is marked. The patient is then instructed to take a few breaths in and out, exhale completely, and then hold his or her breath. The posterior chest is percussed again, and the new area of dullness over the diaphragm is located and marked. The difference between the two spots is identified and measured. Normal diaphragmatic excursion is 3 to 5 cm.[10] It is decreased in disorders or conditions such as ascites, pregnancy, hepatomegaly, and emphysema. It is increased in pleural effusion or disorders that elevate the diaphragm, such as atelectasis or paralysis.[7]

Auscultation

Auscultation of the patient focuses on three priorities: 1) evaluation of normal breath sounds, 2) identification of abnormal breath sounds, and 3) assessment of voice sounds. Auscultation requires a quiet environment, proper positioning of the patient, and a bare chest.[9] Breath sounds are best heard with the patient in the upright position.[5]

Evaluation of Normal Breath Sounds

The patient's breath sounds are auscultated to evaluate the quality of air movement through the pulmonary system and to identify the presence of abnormal sounds. It is performed by placing the diaphragm of the stethoscope against the chest wall and instructing the patient to breathe in and out slowly with his or her mouth open.[2] The inspiratory and expiratory phases should be assessed. Auscultation should be done in a systematic sequence: side-to-side, top-to-bottom, posteriorly, laterally, and anteriorly (Figure 14-2).[5] Normal breath sounds are different, depending on their location. There are three categories: vesicular, bronchovesicular, and bronchial. Figure 14-3 describes the characteristics of normal breath sounds and their associated conditions.[2,5,9]

Identification of Abnormal Breath Sounds

Abnormal breath sounds are identified once the normal breath sounds have been clearly delineated. There are three categories of abnormal breath sounds: absent or diminished

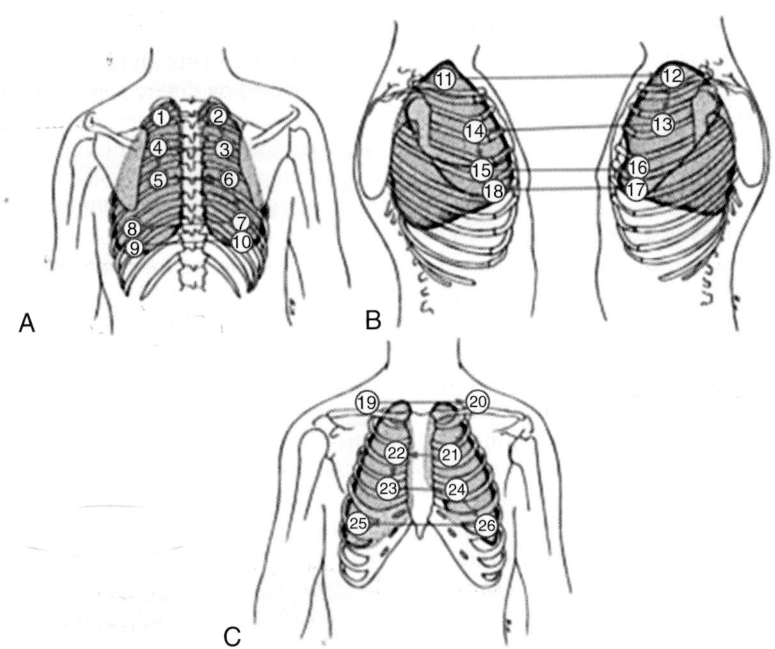

FIG 14-2 Auscultation Sequence. *A*, Posterior. *B*, Lateral. *C*, Anterior. (From Perry AG et al. *Clinical Nursing Skills and Techniques.* 8th ed. St. Louis: Elsevier; 2014.)

BREATH SOUND	PITCH	INTENSITY	LOCATION	DIAGRAM OF SOUND
Vesicular or normal breath sounds	Low	Soft	Peripheral lung areas	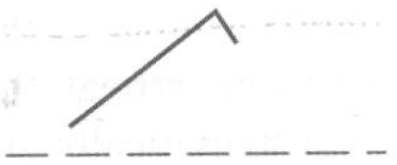
Bronchovesicular	Moderate	Moderate	Around upper part of sternum, between scapulae	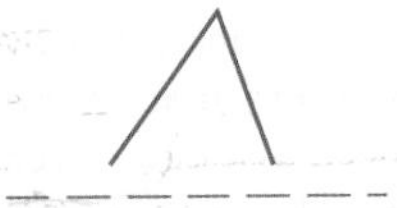
Bronchial	High	Loud	Over trachea	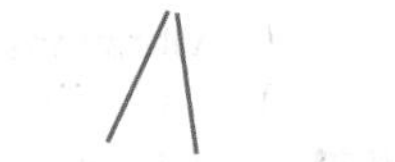

FIG 14-3 Characteristics of Normal Breath Sounds. (From Kacmarek RM, Diamas S. *The Essentials of Respiratory Care.* 4th ed. St. Louis: Elsevier; 2005.)

TABLE 14-2 Abnormal Breath Sounds and Their Associated Conditions

ABNORMAL SOUND	DESCRIPTION	CONDITION
Absent breath sounds	No airflow to particular portion of lung	Pneumothorax Pneumonectomy Emphysematous blebs Pleural effusion Lung mass Massive atelectasis Complete airway obstruction
Diminished breath sounds	Little airflow to particular portion of lung	Emphysema Pleural effusion Pleurisy Atelectasis Pulmonary fibrosis
Displaced bronchial sounds	Bronchial sounds heard in peripheral lung fields	Atelectasis with secretions Lung mass with exudates Pneumonia Pleural effusion Pulmonary edema
Crackles (rales)	Short, discrete popping or crackling sounds	Pulmonary edema Pneumonia Pulmonary fibrosis Atelectasis Bronchiectasis
Rhonchi	Coarse, rumbling, low-pitched sounds	Pneumonia Asthma Bronchitis Bronchospasm
Wheezes	High-pitched, squeaking, whistling sounds	Asthma Bronchospasm
Pleural friction rub	Creaking, leathery, loud, dry, coarse sounds	Pleural effusion Pleurisy

breath sounds, displaced bronchial breath sounds, and adventitious breath sounds. Table 14-2 describes the various abnormal breath sounds and their associated conditions.[2,5,9]

An *absent or diminished breath sound* indicates that there is little or no airflow to a particular portion of the lung (a small segment or an entire lung).[9] *Displaced bronchial breath sounds* are normal bronchial sounds heard in the peripheral lung fields instead of over the trachea. This condition is usually indicative of fluid or exudate in the alveoli.[9] *Adventitious breath sounds* are extra or added sounds heard in addition to the other sounds previously discussed. They are classified as crackles, rhonchi, wheezes, and friction rubs.[9]

Crackles, also called *rales*, are short, discrete popping or crackling sounds produced by fluid in the small airways or alveoli or by the snapping open of collapsed airways during inspiration. They can be heard on inspiration and expiration and may clear with coughing.[2,5,9] Crackles can be further classified as fine, medium, or coarse, depending on pitch.[2,5] *Rhonchi* are coarse, rumbling, low-pitched sounds produced by airflow over secretions in the larger airways or narrowing of the large airways. They are heard mainly on expiration and sometimes can be cleared with coughing. Rhonchi can be further classified as bubbling, gurgling, or sonorous, depending on the characteristics of the sound.[9] *Wheezes* are high-pitched, squeaking, whistling sounds produced by airflow through narrowed small airways. They are heard mainly on expiration but may be heard throughout the ventilatory cycle. Depending on their severity, wheezes can be further classified as mild, moderate, or severe.[9] A *pleural friction rub* is a creaking, leathery, loud, dry, coarse sound produced by irritated pleural surfaces rubbing together. It is usually heard best in the lower anterolateral chest area during inspiration and expiration. Pleural friction rubs are caused by inflammation of the pleura.[2,5]

Assessment of Voice Sounds

Assessment of voice sounds is particularly useful in detecting lung consolidation or lung compression. Three abnormal types of voice sounds are bronchophony, whispering pectoriloquy, and egophony. *Bronchophony* describes a condition in which the spoken voice is heard on auscultation with higher intensity and clarity than usual. Normally, the spoken word is muffled when heard through the stethoscope. It is assessed by placing the diaphragm of the stethoscope against the posterior side of the patient's chest and instructing the patient to say "ninety-nine." Bronchophony is present when the sound heard is clear, distinct, and loud. *Whispering pectoriloquy* describes a condition of unusually clear transmission of the whispered voice on auscultation. Normally, the whispered word is unintelligible when heard through the stethoscope. It is assessed by placing the stethoscope against the posterior side of the patient's chest and instructing the patient to whisper "one, two, three." Whispering pectoriloquy is present when the sound heard is clear and distinct. *Egophony* describes a condition in which the voice sounds increase in intensity and develop a nasal bleating quality on auscultation. It is assessed by placing the stethoscope against the posterior side of the patient's chest and instructing the patient to say "e-e-e." Egophony is present when the "e" sound changes to an "a" sound.[2,4,9]

LABORATORY STUDIES

Arterial Blood Gases

Interpretation of arterial blood gas (ABG) levels can be difficult, especially if the nurse is under pressure to do it quickly and accurately. One method that can help ensure accuracy when analyzing ABG levels is to follow the same steps of interpretation each time. A specific method to be used each time that blood gas values must be interpreted is presented here (Box 14-2).

Steps for Interpretation of Blood Gas Levels

Step 1. Look at the PaO_2 level and answer this question: Does the PaO_2 show hypoxemia? The PaO_2 is a measure of the partial pressure (P) of oxygen dissolved in arterial (a)

BOX 14-2 Steps for Interpretation of Blood Gas Levels

Step 1
Look at the PaO_2 level and answer this question: Does the PaO_2 level show hypoxemia?

Step 2
Look at the pH level and answer this question: Is the pH level on the acid or alkaline side of 7.40?

Step 3
Look at the $PaCO_2$ level and answer this question: Does the $PaCO_2$ level show respiratory acidosis, alkalosis, or normalcy?

Step 4
Look at the HCO_3^- level and answer this question: Does the HCO_3^- level show metabolic acidosis, alkalosis, or normalcy?

Step 5
Look again at the pH level and answer this question: Does the pH show a compensated or an uncompensated condition?

blood plasma. Sometimes, PaO_2 is shortened to PO_2. It is reported in millimeters of mercury (mm Hg). PaO_2 reflects 3% of total oxygen in the blood.[10]

The normal range of PaO_2 values for persons breathing room air at sea level is 80 to 100 mm Hg. However, the normal range is age-dependent for infants and for persons 60 years old or older. The normal level for infants breathing room air is between 50 and 70 mm Hg.[11] The normal level for persons 60 years old or older decreases with age as changes occur in the ventilation/perfusion (V/Q) matching in the aging lung.[10,12] The correct PaO_2 for older persons can be ascertained as follows: 80 mm Hg (the lowest normal value) minus 1 mm Hg for every year of age above 60 years. Using this formula, a 65-year-old individual can have a PaO_2 as low as 75 mm Hg (80 mm Hg − 5 mm Hg = 75 mm Hg) and still be within the normal range. An acceptable range for an 80-year-old person (20 years older than 60 years) is 60 mm Hg (80 mm Hg − 20 mm Hg = 60 mm Hg). At any age, a PaO_2 lower than 40 mm Hg represents a life-threatening situation that necessitates immediate action.[10] A PaO_2 value less than the predicted lowest value indicates hypoxemia, which means that a lower-than-normal amount of oxygen is dissolved in plasma.[10]

Step 2. Look at the pH level and answer this question: Is the pH on the acid or alkaline side of 7.40? The pH is the hydrogen ion (H^+) concentration of plasma. Calculation of pH is accomplished by using the partial pressure of carbon dioxide ($PaCO_2$) and the plasma bicarbonate level (HCO_3^-). The formula used is the Henderson-Hasselbalch equation (see Appendix B).[13]

The normal pH of arterial blood is 7.35 to 7.45, and the mean is 7.40. If the pH level is less than 7.40, it is on the acid side of the mean. A pH level less than 7.35 is known as acidemia, and the overall condition is called acidosis. If the pH level is greater than 7.40, it is on the alkaline side of the mean. A pH level greater than 7.45 is known as alkalemia, and the overall condition is called alkalosis.[10,13,14]

BOX 14-3 Uncompensated Arterial Blood Gas Values

Example 1
PaO_2: 90 mm Hg
pH: 7.25
$PaCO_2$: 50 mm Hg
HCO_3^-: 22 mEq/L
Interpretation: Uncompensated respiratory acidosis

Example 2
PaO_2: 90 mm Hg
pH: 7.25
$PaCO_2$: 40 mm Hg
HCO_3^-: 17 mEq/L
Interpretation: Uncompensated metabolic acidosis

Step 3. Look at the $PaCO_2$ level and answer this question: Does the $PaCO_2$ show respiratory acidosis, alkalosis, or normalcy? The $PaCO_2$ is a measure of the partial pressure of carbon dioxide dissolved in arterial blood plasma, and it is reported in millimeters of mercury (mm Hg). It is the acid–base component that reflects the effectiveness of ventilation in relation to the metabolic rate.[13] In other words, the $PaCO_2$ value indicates whether the patient can ventilate well enough to rid the body of the carbon dioxide produced as a consequence of metabolism.

The normal range for $PaCO_2$ is 35 to 45 mm Hg. This range does not change as a person ages. A $PaCO_2$ value greater than 45 mm Hg defines *respiratory acidosis*, which is caused by alveolar hypoventilation. Hypoventilation can result from chronic obstructive pulmonary disease (COPD), oversedation, head trauma, anesthesia, drug overdose, neuromuscular disease, or hypoventilation with mechanical ventilation.[15] A $PaCO_2$ value that is less than 35 mm Hg defines *respiratory alkalosis*, which is caused by alveolar hyperventilation. Hyperventilation can result from hypoxia, anxiety, pulmonary embolism, pregnancy, and hyperventilation with mechanical ventilation, or as a compensatory mechanism for metabolic acidosis.[13]

Step 4. Look at the HCO_3^- level and answer this question: Does the HCO_3^- show metabolic acidosis, alkalosis, or normalcy? Bicarbonate (HCO_3^-) is the acid–base component that reflects kidney function. The bicarbonate level is reduced or increased in the plasma by renal mechanisms.

The normal range is 22 to 26 mEq/L.[13,14] A bicarbonate level of less than 22 mEq/L defines metabolic acidosis, which can result from ketoacidosis, lactic acidosis, renal failure, or diarrhea. The cumulative effect is a gain of acids or a loss of base. A bicarbonate level that is greater than 26 mEq/L defines metabolic alkalosis, which can result from fluid loss from the upper gastrointestinal tract (vomiting or nasogastric suction), diuretic therapy, severe hypokalemia, alkali administration, or steroid therapy.[13-15]

Step 5. Look again at the pH level and answer this question: Does the pH show a compensated or an uncompensated condition? If the pH level is abnormal (less than 7.35 or greater than 7.45), the $PaCO_2$ value or the HCO_3^- level, or both, will also be abnormal. This is an uncompensated condition because the body has not had enough time to return the pH to its normal range (Box 14-3).[13-16] If the pH level is within normal limits and the $PaCO_2$ value and the HCO_3^- level are abnormal, the condition is compensated because the body has had enough time to restore the pH to within its normal range.[13-16] Differentiating the primary disorder from the compensatory response can be difficult. The primary disorder is the abnormality that caused the pH level to shift initially. It is determined according to the pH level; the primary disorder is considered to be the one on whichever side of 7.40 the pH level occurs (Box 14-4).[13,16] Partial compensation may be present and is evidenced by abnormal pH, $PaCO_2$, and HCO_3^- levels, indications that the body is attempting to return the pH to its normal range.[13,16]

BOX 14-4 Compensated Arterial Blood Gas Values

Example 1
PaO_2: 90 mm Hg
pH: 7.37
$PaCO_2$: 60 mm Hg
HCO_3^-: 38 mEq/L
Interpretation: Compensated respiratory acidosis with metabolic alkalosis. (The acidosis is considered the main disorder, and the alkalosis the compensatory response, because the pH is on the acid side of 7.40.)

Example 2
PaO_2: 90 mm Hg
pH: 7.42
$PaCO_2$: 48 mm Hg
HCO_3^-: 35 mEq/L
Interpretation: Compensated metabolic alkalosis with respiratory acidosis. (The alkalosis is considered the main disorder, and the acidosis the compensatory response, because the pH is on the alkaline side of 7.40.)

Table 14-3 summarizes the changes in the acid–base components that accompany various acid–base disorders.[13,14,16] In addition to the parameters previously discussed, other factors must be considered when reviewing a patient's ABGs, including oxygen saturation, oxygen content, and base excess and deficit.

Oxygen Saturation

Oxygen saturation is a measure of the amount of oxygen bound to hemoglobin, compared with hemoglobin's maximal capability for binding oxygen. It can be assessed as a component of the ABG (SaO_2) or can be measured noninvasively using a pulse oximeter (SpO_2).[17,18] Oxygen saturation is reported as a percentage or as a decimal; normal values are greater than 95% when the patient is on room air. Normally, the saturation level cannot reach 100% (on room air) because of physiologic shunting.[10] However, when supplemental oxygen is administered, oxygen saturation may approach 100% so closely that it is reported as 100%.

Proper evaluation of the oxygen saturation level is vital. For example, an SaO_2 of 97% means that 97% of the available hemoglobin is bound with oxygen. The word *available* is essential to evaluating the SaO_2 level because the hemoglobin level is not always within normal limits and oxygen can bind only with what is available. A 97% saturation level associated with 10 g/dL of hemoglobin does not deliver as much oxygen to the tissues as does a 97% saturation level associated with 15 g/dL of hemoglobin. Assessing only the SaO_2 level and finding it within normal limits does not ensure that the patient's oxygenation status is normal. The hemoglobin level must also be evaluated before a decision on oxygenation status can be made.[10,17,18]

Oxygen Content

Oxygen content (CaO_2) is a measure of the total amount of oxygen carried in the blood, including the amount dissolved

TABLE 14-3 Arterial Blood Gas Assessment

DISORDER	pH	$PaCO_2$	HCO_3^-
Respiratory Acidosis			
Uncompensated	<7.35	>45 mm Hg	22-26 mEq/L
Partially compensated	<7.35	>45 mm Hg	>26 mEq/L
Compensated	7.35-7.39	>45 mm Hg	>26 mEq/L
Respiratory Alkalosis			
Uncompensated	>7.45	<35 mm Hg	22-26 mEq/L
Partially compensated	>7.45	<35 mm Hg	<22 mEq/L
Compensated	7.41-7.45	<35 mm Hg	<22 mEq/L
Metabolic Acidosis			
Uncompensated	<7.35	35-45 mm Hg	<22 mEq/L
Partially compensated	<7.35	<35 mm Hg	<22 mEq/L
Compensated	7.35-7.39	<35 mm Hg	<22 mEq/L
Combined (or mixed) respiratory and metabolic acidosis	<7.35	>45 mm Hg	<22 mEq/L
Metabolic Alkalosis			
Uncompensated	>7.45	35-45 mm Hg	>26 mEq/L
Partially compensated	>7.45	>45 mm Hg	>26 mEq/L
Compensated	7.41-7.45	>45 mm Hg	>26 mEq/L
Combined (or mixed) respiratory and metabolic alkalosis	>7.45	<35 mm Hg	>26 mEq/L

in plasma (measured by the PaO_2) and the amount bound to the hemoglobin molecule (measured by the SaO_2). CaO_2 is reported in milliliters of oxygen carried per 100 mL of blood. The normal value is 20 mL of oxygen per 100 mL of blood. To calculate the oxygen content, the PaO_2, the SaO_2, and the hemoglobin level are used (see Appendix B). A change in any one of these parameters will affect the CaO_2.[10]

Base Excess and Base Deficit

Base excess and base deficit reflect the nonrespiratory contribution to acid–base balance and are reported in milliequivalents per liter (mEq/L) above or below the normal range of −2 mEq/L to +2 mEq/L. A negative base level is reported as a *base deficit*, which correlates with *metabolic acidosis*, whereas a positive base level is reported as a *base excess*, which correlates with *metabolic alkalosis*.[10,13,16]

Classic Shunt Equation and Oxygen Tension Indices

The efficiency of oxygenation can be assessed by measuring the degree of intrapulmonary shunting that occurs in a patient at any one time, using the classic shunt equation and oxygen tension indices. *Intrapulmonary shunting* (QS/QT [the portion of cardiac output not exchanging with alveolar blood divided by the total cardiac output]) refers to venous blood that flows to the lungs without being oxygenated because of nonfunctioning alveoli.[10] Other names for this condition include shunt effect, low V/Q, wasted blood flow, and venous admixture.[10,11,12] Direct determination of intrapulmonary shunting requires the use of the classic shunt equation, which is invasive and cumbersome. A shunt greater than 10% is considered abnormal and indicative of a shunt-producing disorder. A shunt greater than 30% is a serious and potentially life-threatening condition, which requires pulmonary intervention.[1,19,20]

Often, intrapulmonary shunting is estimated by using the oxygen tension indices. One advantage to these methods is the ease of performance, although they have been found to be unreliable in critically ill patients.[10,19] An estimate of intrapulmonary shunting can be determined by computing the difference between the alveolar and arterial oxygen concentrations. Normally, alveolar (A) and arterial (a) PO_2 values are approximately equal. When they are not, it indicates that venous blood is passing malfunctioning alveoli and returning unoxygenated to the left side of the heart.[10,19] The most common oxygen tension indices used to estimate intrapulmonary shunting are the PaO_2/FiO_2 ratio, the PaO_2/PAO_2 ratio, and the A-a gradient ($P[A - a]O_2$) (See Appendix B for formulas).

PaO_2/FiO_2 Ratio

The PaO_2/FiO_2 ratio is clinically the easiest formula to calculate because it does not call for the computation of the alveolar PO_2. Normally, the PaO_2/FiO_2 ratio is greater than 286; the lower the value, the worse the lung function.[10,17,19]

PaO_2/PAO_2 Ratio

The PaO_2/PAO_2 ratio (arterial/alveolar O_2 ratio) is normally greater than 60%. The disadvantage to using this formula is that it calls for the computation of the alveolar PO_2, but the advantage is that it is unaffected by changes in the FiO_2, as long as the underlying lung condition is stable.[10,19]

Alveolar-Arterial Gradient

The A-a gradient ($P[A - a]O_2$) is normally less than 20 mm Hg on room air for patients younger than 61 years. This estimate of intrapulmonary shunting is the least reliable clinically, but it is used often in clinical decision making. One of the major disadvantages to using this formula is that it is greatly influenced by the amount of oxygen the patient is receiving.[10,19-21] Serial determinations of the estimates of intrapulmonary shunting provide the practitioner with objective data on which to base clinical decisions.[10,19,20]

Dead Space Equation

The efficiency of ventilation can be measured using the clinical dead space (V_D/V_T) equation (see Appendix B). The formula measures the fraction of tidal volume not participating in gas exchange. A dead space value greater than 0.6 indicates a dead space-producing disorder and is considered abnormal. The major limitations to using this formula are that it requires the measurement of exhaled carbon dioxide to complete and that the work of breathing by patients must remain stable during the collection.[20,22]

Sputum Studies

Careful analysis of sputum specimens is crucial for the rapid identification and treatment of pulmonary infections. The most difficult aspect of sputum examination is proper collection of the specimen. Collection of a good sputum sample requires a conscious, cooperative, and sufficiently hydrated patient.[20] When the patient has difficulty producing sputum, heated, nebulized saline may help to loosen secretions for expectoration.[20] Chest physiotherapy combined with nebulization improves the success rate. Collection of a sputum specimen is best done in the morning because a greater volume of secretions is present as a result of nighttime pooling. Brushing the teeth and rinsing the oropharyngeal airway is recommended to reduce contamination before collecting a sample.[20,23]

Many critically ill patients cannot cough effectively, and sputum collection by other means is required. These methods include tracheobronchial aspiration, transtracheal aspiration, and the use of a fiberoptic bronchoscopy with a protected brush catheter. Because each method has its own benefits and risks, the patient's clinical condition determines the appropriate technique.[20] Many critically ill patients have endotracheal or tracheostomy tubes already in place. Collecting sputum specimens from these patients requires special attention to technique (Box 14-5). Deep specimens are obtained to avoid collecting specimens that contain resident upper airway flora that may have migrated down the tube. Colonization of the lower airways with upper airway flora can occur within 48 hours of intubation.[2]

After a sputum specimen is obtained, it is examined for volume, physical properties, mucopurulence, and color. Next, a microscopic examination is done to identify the source of the specimen. If a bacterial infection is suspected, a Gram stain is performed, followed by culture and sensitivity (C&S) assessments.[20,23,24]

DIAGNOSTIC PROCEDURES

Table 14-4 presents an overview of the various diagnostic procedures used to evaluate the patient with pulmonary dysfunction.

BOX 14-5 Procedure for Collection of Tracheal or Endotracheal Sputum Specimen

- Clear the endotracheal or tracheostomy tube of all local secretions, avoiding deep airway penetration.
- Attach a sputum trap to a sterile suction catheter and advance the catheter into the trachea while trying to avoid contact with the endotracheal tube or tracheostomy tube (Figure 14-4).
- After the catheter is fully advanced, apply suction until secretions return to the sputum trap. When enough secretions are collected, discontinue suctioning and remove the catheter.
- Do not apply suction while the catheter is being withdrawn because this can contaminate the sample with sputum from the upper airway.
- Do not flush the catheter with sterile water because this dilutes the sample.
- If the catheter becomes plugged with secretions, place it in a sterile container and send it to the laboratory. The specimen must be transported immediately or refrigerated if a delay is necessary.

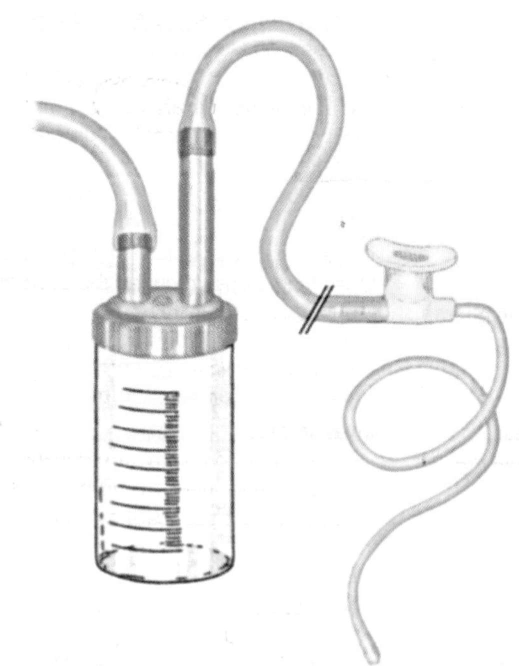

FIG 14-4 Specimen Container. (From Kacmarek RM, et al, eds. *Egan's Fundamentals of Respiratory Care.* 10th ed. St. Louis: Mosby; 2013.)

Nursing Management

Nursing management of a patient undergoing a diagnostic procedure involves a variety of interventions. **Priorities are directed toward 1) preparing the patient psychologically and physically for the procedure, 2) monitoring the patient's responses to the procedure, and 3) assessing the patient after the procedure.** Preparing the patient includes teaching the patient about the procedure, answering any questions, and positioning the patient for the procedure. Monitoring the patient's responses to the procedure includes observing the patient for signs of pain, anxiety, or respiratory decompensation (Box 14-6) and monitoring vital signs, breath sounds, and oxygen saturation. Assessing the patient after the procedure includes observing for complications of the procedure and medicating the patient for any postprocedural discomfort. **Any evidence of respiratory distress should be immediately reported to the physician, and emergency measures to maintain breathing must be initiated.**

BOX 14-6 Clinical Manifestations of Respiratory Decompensation

Inadequate Airway
Stridor
Noisy respirations
Supraclavicular and intercostal retractions
Flaring of nares
Labored breathing with use of accessory muscles

Inadequate Ventilation
Absence of air exchange at nose and mouth (breathlessness)
Minimal/absent chest wall motion
Manifestations of obstructed airway
Central cyanosis
Decreased or absent breath sounds (bilateral, unilateral)
Restlessness, anxiety, confusion
Paradoxical motion involving significant portion of chest wall
Decreased PaO_2, increased $PaCO_2$, decreased pH

Inadequate Gas Exchange
Tachypnea
Decreased PaO_2
Increased dead space
Central cyanosis
Chest infiltrates on radiographic evaluation

BEDSIDE MONITORING

Capnography

Capnography is the measurement of exhaled carbon dioxide (CO_2) gas; it is also known as *end-tidal CO_2* monitoring. Normally, alveolar and arterial CO_2 concentrations are equal in the presence of normal V/Q relationships. In a patient who is hemodynamically stable, the end-tidal CO_2 ($P_{ET}CO_2$) can be used to estimate the $PaCO_2$, with the $P_{ET}CO_2$ levels 1 to 5 mm Hg less than $PaCO_2$ levels. The practitioner must determine first that a normal V/Q relationship exists before correlation of the $P_{ET}CO_2$ and the $PaCO_2$ can be assumed.[20,25] Causes of increased $P_{ET}CO_2$ include situations in which CO_2 production is increased, such as hyperthermia, sepsis, and seizures, or in which alveolar ventilation is decreased, such as respiratory depression. Causes of decreased $P_{ET}CO_2$ include situations in which CO_2 production is decreased, such as hypothermia, cardiac arrest, and pulmonary embolism, or in which alveolar ventilation is increased, such as hyperventilation.[20,25]

In the critical care area, continuous capnography is used for assessment and monitoring of the patient's ventilatory status in a variety of situations, including weaning from mechanical ventilation and undergoing procedural sedation.

TABLE 14-4 Pulmonary Diagnostic Studies

STUDY	EVALUATION	COMMENTS
Bronchography	Detect obstruction or malformation of the tracheobronchial tree.	Patient inspires radiopaque substance and then x-rays are taken. Inquire about possibility of pregnancy.
Chest x-ray	Detect pathological lung condition (e.g., pneumonia, pulmonary edema, atelectasis, tuberculosis, etc.). Determine size and location of lung lesions and tumors. Verify placement of endotracheal tube, central venous catheters, and chest tubes.	Noninvasive test with minimal radiation exposure. Inquire about possibility of pregnancy. Posteroanterior (PA) and lateral films are done most commonly, but in critical care areas, anteroposterior (AP) portable films are frequently necessary because of inability to transport patient. Lateral decubitus films aid in identification of pleural effusion.
Exercise testing	Identify early disability. Differentiates between cardiac and pulmonary disease.	Monitor for changes in SpO_2 during exercise. Monitor closely for exercise-induced hypotension or ventricular dysrhythmias.
Laryngoscopy, bronchoscopy, mediastinoscopy	Obtain cytological specimen or biopsy. Identify tumors, obstructions, secretions, or foreign bodies in tracheobronchial tree. Locate a bleeding site. May be used therapeutically to remove secretions, foreign bodies, and other contaminants.	Patient is sedated before the procedure, usually with a benzodiazepine (e.g., diazepam, midazolam). Monitor the patient for subcutaneous emphysema after study; indicates tracheal or bronchial tear. Monitor for hemoptysis; some blood in sputum is normal after biopsy, but frank hemoptysis requires immediate attention.
Lung biopsy Transthoracic needle lung biopsy Open lung biopsy	Obtain specimen for cytological evaluation.	Transthoracic needle biopsy performed under fluoroscopy. Inquire about possibility of pregnancy. Open lung biopsy requires thoracotomy.
Magnetic resonance imaging (MRI)	Distinguishes tumors from other structures (e.g., tumor, pleural thickening, fibrosis).	Noninvasive test. Contraindicated for patients with pacemakers or implanted metallic devices.
Pulmonary angiography	Detects changes in lung tissue (e.g., masses). Diagnoses abnormalities in pulmonary vasculature including thrombi and emboli. Identifies congenital abnormalities of the circulation.	Invasive test. Inquire about possibility of pregnancy. Contrast media injected into pulmonary artery; ensure adequate hydration after study. Monitor arterial puncture point for hematoma or hemorrhage.
Pulmonary function studies • Spirometry • Ventilator mechanics • Flow-volume loop • Diffusing capacity	Measures lung volumes, capacities, and flow rates. Identifies features of restrictive or obstructive lung disease. Evaluates responsiveness to bronchodilator therapy. Aids in evaluation of surgical risk. Documents a disability or cause of dyspnea.	Noninvasive studies. Frequently repeated after bronchodilator therapy.
Sleep studies	Diagnose and differentiate between obstructive, central, and cardiac sleep apnea.	Restrict caffeine before testing. Usually done during normal sleep hours.
Thoracentesis (may include pleural biopsy)	Obtain pleural fluid and/or tissue specimen. May be used therapeutically to remove pleural fluid.	Monitor patient for indications of pneumothorax. Monitor for leakage from puncture point.
Thoracic computerized tomography (CT)	Defines lesions, masses, cavities, or shadows seen on normal chest x-rays. Evaluates tracheal or bronchial narrowing. Aids in planning radiation therapy.	X-rays are taken at different angles.

Continued

TABLE 14-4 Pulmonary Diagnostic Studies—cont'd

STUDY	EVALUATION	COMMENTS
Ultrasonography	Evaluates pleural disease. Visualizes diaphragm and detects disease around diaphragm (e.g., subphrenic hematoma or abscess).	Noninvasive test.
Ventilation scan Lung perfusion scan Ventilation/perfusion scan	Diagnoses ventilation and/or perfusion abnormalities including emphysema and pulmonary emboli.	Invasive test: radioisotope inspired and injected intravascularly. Inquire about possibility of pregnancy. Nuclear scan study: assure patient that amount of radioactive material is minimal.

Modified from Dennison RD: *Pass CCRN!*, ed 4, St Louis, 2013, Mosby.

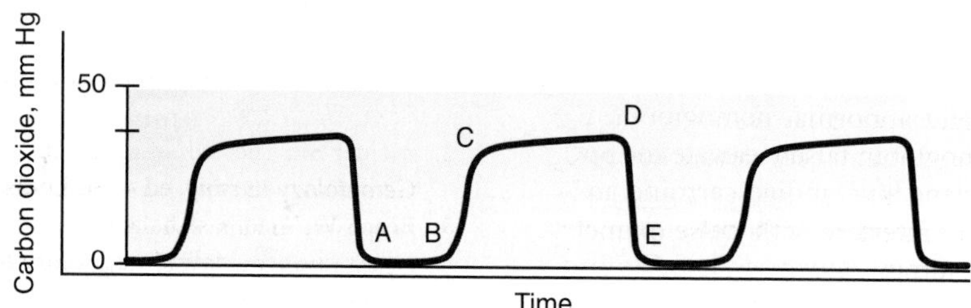

FIG 14-5 Normal Findings on a Capnogram. *A* → *B* indicates the baseline; *B* → *C*, the expiratory upstroke; *C* → *D*, the alveolar plateau; *D*, the partial pressure of end-tidal carbon dioxide; and *D* → *E*, the inspiratory downstroke. (From Frakes M. Measuring end-tidal carbon dioxide: clinical applications and usefulness. *Crit Care Nurse.* 2001;21[5]:23.)

Assessment of changes in physiologic dead space can be carried out with end-tidal CO_2 monitoring, based on the degree of difference between the $PaCO_2$ and the $P_{ET}CO_2$. As the severity of pulmonary impairment increases, so does the disparity between the $PaCO_2$ and the $P_{ET}CO_2$, as indicated by an increased gradient. A gradient of greater than 5 mm Hg can be seen with underperfused alveolar-capillary units (dead space-producing situations) and nonperfused alveolar-capillary units (alveolar dead space). Increased dead space ventilation is a result of decreased pulmonary blood flow or cardiac output and lung disease. This leads to an abnormality in the transfer of CO_2 from the blood to the lung. The result is a $P_{ET}CO_2$ level that is lower than the $PaCO_2$ because of the mixing of carbon dioxide between perfused and nonperfused units. The end result is an increased or widened $PaCO_2$/$P_{ET}CO_2$ gradient.[20,25]

The noninvasive measurement of $P_{ET}CO_2$ enables assessment of the adequacy of cardiopulmonary resuscitation and endotracheal tube placement. Decreased pulmonary blood flow is associated with lower $P_{ET}CO_2$ values, reflected clinically by decreased cardiac output, as in the case of cardiopulmonary resuscitation.[20,25] During endotracheal intubation, a low $P_{ET}CO_2$ reading indicates that the tube is positioned in the stomach because the amount of carbon dioxide in the esophagus is expected to be low.[20,25]

There are three forms of capnography: microstream, side-stream, and proximal diverting. All forms can be used in intubated patients, but side-stream and microstream capnography can also be used in nonintubated patients, broadening the application of end-tidal CO_2 monitoring. Mainstream capnography measures the CO_2 level directly by a sensor in the exhalation port of the ventilator tubing. During exhalation, gas passes over the sensor, and the information is transferred by an electrical cable to the display unit. The display unit produces a waveform, called a *capnogram* (Figure 14-5), and a numeric recording ($P_{ET}CO_2$). Disadvantages to this form of capnography include the weight of the sensor on the ventilator tubing and possible obstruction of the sensor by secretions and condensation. In side-stream capnography, the CO_2 gas is continuously aspirated through a side port in the ventilator tubing or nasal cannula and is measured and analyzed by a side unit. Disadvantages to this form of capnography include obstruction of the sampling tube with secretions and slow response time. Proximal diverting capnography is a newer and improved version of side-stream capnography that transports gas a short distance from the airway to a site where the sensor is located thereby reducing the bulkiness at the airway.[25]

Capnography and partial pressure of end-tidal carbon dioxide ($P_{ET}CO_2$) analysis have many diverse applications in the critical care area, but the practitioner must never assume the $P_{ET}CO_2$ values reflect arterial values of the partial pressure of carbon dioxide ($PaCO_2$) without waveform analysis. Any change in the waveform can indicate a change in the patient's pulmonary status and warrants further evaluation. Loss of the waveform may signal loss of effective respirations.[20,25]

Pulse Oximetry

Pulse oximetry is a noninvasive method for monitoring oxygen saturation (SpO_2). It is indicated in any situation in which the patient's oxygenation status requires continuous observation. It consists of a microprocessor and a probe that attaches to the patient's forehead, finger, ear, toe, or nose. The probe consists of two light-emitting diodes and a photodetector. The diodes transmit red and infrared light wavelengths through the pulsating arterial vascular bed to the photodetector on the other side. The percentage of oxygen saturation is determined by the difference in absorbance of the red and infrared light caused by the difference in color between oxygen-bound (bright red) and oxygen-unbound (dark red) hemoglobin. The photodetector converts the light signals into an electric signal that is sent to the microprocessor, which converts it to a digital reading. The pulse oximeter is considered very accurate; readings vary less than 4% to 5% at a saturation level greater than 70%. However, several physiologic and technical factors limit the monitoring system.[17,20]

Physiologic limitations of pulse oximetry include elevated levels of abnormal hemoglobins, presence of vascular dyes, and poor tissue perfusion. The pulse oximeter cannot differentiate between normal and abnormal hemoglobin. Elevated levels of abnormal hemoglobin falsely elevate the SpO_2. Vascular dyes such as methylene blue, indigo carmine, indocyanine green, and fluorescein interfere with pulse oximetry and can lead to falsely low readings. Poor tissue perfusion to the area with the probe leads to loss of pulsatile flow and signal failure.[17,20] In the critically ill patient, pulse oximetry is reliable only for monitoring the patient's oxygenation status. It is not a reliable method for monitoring the patient's ventilatory status. The ability of a pulse oximeter to detect hypoventilation is accurate only when the patient is breathing room air.[17] Because most critically ill patients require some form of oxygen therapy, pulse oximetry is not a reliable method of detecting hypercapnia and should *not* be used for this purpose.

Technical limitations of pulse oximetry include bright lights, excessive motion, and incorrect placement of the probe. Bright lights may interfere with the photodetector and cause inaccurate results. The probe must be covered to limit optical interference. Excessive motion can mimic arterial pulsations and can lead to false readings. Incorrect placement of the probe can lead to inaccurate results because part of the light can reach the photodetector without having passed through blood (optical shunting).[17,20] Interventions to limit these problems include using the proper probe in the appropriate spot (e.g., not using a finger probe on the ear), applying the probe according to the directions, and ensuring that the area being monitored has adequate perfusion.[17,20]

REFERENCES

1. Baid H: The process of conducting a physical assessment: a nursing perspective, *Br J Nurs* 15:710, 2006.
2. Simpson H: Respiratory assessment, *Br J Nurs* 15:484, 2006.
3. Reinke LF: Respiratory assessment. In Geiger-Bronksy M, Wilson DJ, editors: *Respiratory nursing: A core curriculum*, New York, 2008, Springer.
4. Finesilver C: Pulmonary assessment: what you need to know, *Prog Cardiovasc Nurs* 18:83, 2003.
5. Kallet RH: Bedside assessment of the patient. In Kacmarek RM, et al, editors: *Egan's fundamentals of respiratory care*, ed 10, St. Louis, 2013, Mosby.
6. Higginson R, Jones B: Respiratory assessment in critically ill patients: airway and breathing, *Br J Nurs* 18:456, 2009.
7. Schraufnagel DE, Murray JF: History and physical examination. In Mason RJ, et al, editors: *Murray and nadel's textbook of respiratory medicine*, ed 5, Philadelphia, 2010, Elsevier.
8. Ball JW, et al: *Seidel's guide to physical examination*, ed 8, St. Louis, 2015, Elsevier.
9. Wilkins RL, et al: *Fundamentals of lung and heart sounds*, ed 3, St. Louis, 2004, Mosby.
10. Hirsch CA: Gas exchange and transport. In Kacmarek RM, et al, editors: *Egan's fundamentals of respiratory care*, ed 10, St. Louis, 2013, Mosby.
11. Goldsmith J, Karotkin E: Appendix. In Goldsmith J, Karotkin E, editors: *Assisted ventilation of the neonate*, ed 5, St. Louis, 2011, Saunders.
12. Meiner SE: Theories of aging. In Meiner SE, editor: *Gerontology nursing*, ed 4, St. Louis, 2011, Mosby.
13. Beach W: Acid base balance. In Kacmarek RM, et al, editors: *Egan's fundamentals of respiratory care*, ed 10, St. Louis, 2013, Mosby.
14. Noble K: The ABC's of arterial blood gases, *J Perianesth Nurs* 24:401, 2009.
15. Ruholl L: Arterial blood gases: analysis and responses, *Medsurg Nurs* 15:343, 2006.
16. Sood P, et al: Interpretation of arterial blood gas, *Indian J Crit Care Med* 14(2):57, 2010.
17. Siobal MS: Analysis and monitoring of gas exchange. In Kacmarek RM, et al, editors: *Egan's fundamentals of respiratory care*, ed 10, St. Louis, 2013, Mosby.
18. Schultz S: Oxygen saturation monitoring with pulse oximetry. In Wiegand DJHM, editor: *AACN's procedure manual for critical care*, ed 6, St. Louis, 2011, Elsevier.
19. Burns S: Shunt calculation. In Wiegand DJHM, editor: *AACN's procedure manual for critical care*, ed 6, St. Louis, 2011, Elsevier.
20. Pierce LNB: *Management of the mechanically ventilated patient*, ed 2, St. Louis, 2007, Saunders.
21. Kacmarek RM, Volsko TA: Physiology of ventilatory support. In Kacmarek RM, et al, editors: *Egan's fundamentals of respiratory care*, ed 10, St. Louis, 2013, Mosby.
22. Vines DL: Respiratory monitoring in the intensive care unit. In Heuer AJ, Scanlan CL, editors: *Wilkins' clinical assessment in respiratory care*, ed 7, Maryland Heights, MO, 2014, Elsevier.
23. Fink J, Arzu A: Humidity and bland aerosol. In Kacmarek RM, et al, editors: *Egan's fundamentals of respiratory care*, ed 10, St. Louis, 2013, Mosby.
24. Hirsch CA: Airway clearance therapy. In Kacmarek RM, et al, editors: *Egan's fundamentals of respiratory care*, ed 10, St. Louis, 2013, Mosby.
25. Adams AB: Monitoring the patient in the intensive care unit. In Kacmarek RM, et al, editors: *Egan's fundamentals of respiratory care*, ed 10, St. Louis, 2013, Mosby.

15 CHAPTER

Pulmonary Disorders

Kathleen M. Stacy

Be sure to check out the bonus mzaterial, including review questions, on the Evolve website at http://evolve.elsevier.com/Urden/priorities/.

ACUTE LUNG FAILURE

Description and Etiology

Acute lung failure (ALF),[1] also known as acute respiratory failure, is a clinical condition in which the pulmonary system fails to maintain adequate gas exchange.[1,2] It is the most common type of organ failure seen in the critical care unit, with approximately 56% of the patients in the critical care unit experiencing it.[1] The mortality rate for patients with ALF is between 30% to 40%, with more than one-third of patients not surviving to discharge.[3]

ALF results from a deficiency in the performance of the pulmonary system (Figure 15-1).[2,4] It usually occurs secondary to another disorder that has altered the normal function of the pulmonary system in such a way as to decrease the ventilatory drive, decrease muscle strength, decrease chest wall elasticity, decrease the lung's capacity for gas exchange, increase airway resistance, or increase metabolic oxygen requirements.[1,5]

ALF can be classified as hypoxemic normocapnic respiratory failure (type I) or hypoxemic hypercapnic respiratory failure (type II), depending on analysis of the patient's arterial blood gases (ABGs). In type I respiratory failure, the patient presents with a low PaO_2 and a normal $PaCO_2$, whereas in type II respiratory failure, PaO_2 is low, and $PaCO_2$ is high.[2,4] The etiologies of ALF may be classified as *extrapulmonary* or *intrapulmonary,* depending on the component of the respiratory system that is affected. Extrapulmonary causes include disorders that affect the brain, the spinal cord, the neuromuscular system, the thorax, the pleura, and the upper airways. Intrapulmonary causes include disorders that affect the lower airways and alveoli, the pulmonary circulation, and the alveolar-capillary membrane.[1,6] Table 15-1 lists the different etiologies of ALF and their associated disorders.

Pathophysiology

Hypoxemia is the result of impaired gas exchange and is the hallmark of ALF. Hypercapnia may be present, depending on the underlying cause of the problem. The main causes of hypoxemia are alveolar hypoventilation, ventilation/perfusion (V/Q) mismatching, and intrapulmonary shunting.[1,2,7] Type I respiratory failure usually results from V/Q mismatching and intrapulmonary shunting, whereas type II respiratory failure usually results from alveolar hypoventilation, which may or may not be accompanied by V/Q mismatching and intrapulmonary shunting.[2]

Alveolar Hypoventilation

Alveolar hypoventilation occurs when the amount of oxygen being brought into the alveoli is insufficient to meet the metabolic needs of the body.[6] This can be the result of increasing metabolic oxygen needs or decreasing ventilation.[5] Hypoxemia caused by alveolar hypoventilation is associated with hypercapnia and commonly results from extrapulmonary disorders.[1,2,7]

Ventilation/Perfusion Mismatching

V/Q mismatching occurs when ventilation and blood flow are mismatched in various regions of the lung in excess of what is normal. Blood passes through alveoli that are underventilated for the given amount of perfusion, leaving these areas with a lower-than-normal amount of oxygen. V/Q mismatching is the most common cause of hypoxemia and is usually the result of alveoli that are partially collapsed or partially filled with fluid.[1,2,7]

Intrapulmonary Shunting

The extreme form of V/Q mismatching, intrapulmonary shunting, occurs when blood reaches the arterial system without participating in gas exchange. The mixing of unoxygenated (shunted) blood and oxygenated blood lowers the average level of oxygen present in the blood. Intrapulmonary shunting occurs when blood passes through a portion of a lung that is not ventilated. This may be the result of 1) alveolar collapse secondary to atelectasis or 2) alveolar flooding with pus, blood, or fluid.[1,2,7]

If allowed to progress, hypoxemia can result in a deficit of oxygen at the cellular level. As the tissue demands for oxygen continue and the supply diminishes, an oxygen supply/demand imbalance occurs, and tissue hypoxia develops. Decreased oxygen to the cells contributes to impaired tissue perfusion and the development of lactic acidosis and multiple organ dysfunction syndrome.[8]

Assessment and Diagnosis

The patient with ALF may experience a variety of clinical manifestations, depending on the underlying cause and the extent of tissue hypoxia. The clinical manifestations

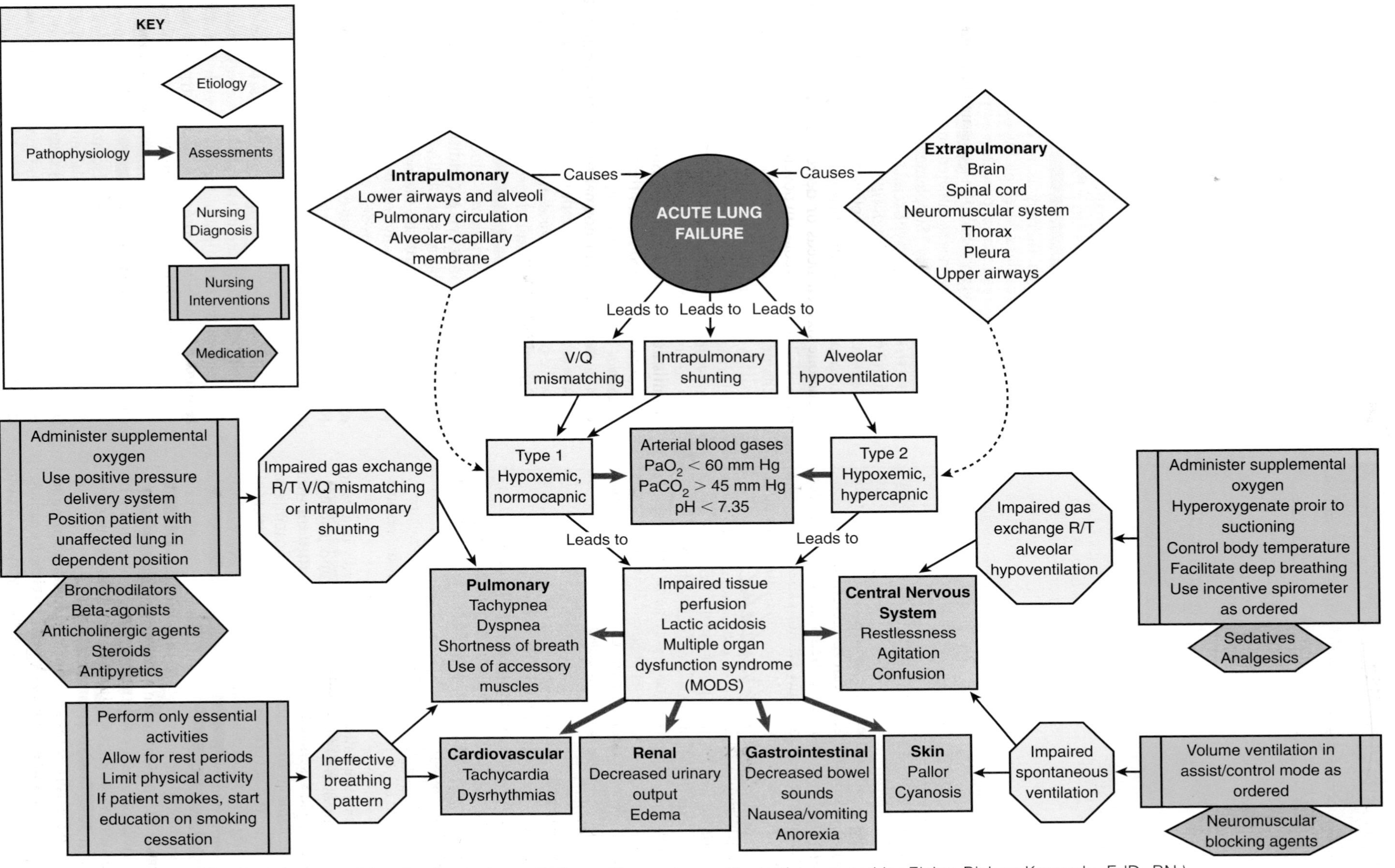

FIG 15-1 Concept Map for Acute Lung Failure. (Concept map illustration created by Elaine Bishop Kennedy, EdD, RN.)

TABLE 15-1 Etiologies of Acute Lung Failure

AFFECTED AREA	DISORDERS*
Extrapulmonary	
Brain	Drug overdose Central alveolar hypoventilation syndrome Brain trauma or lesion Postoperative anesthesia depression
Spinal cord	Guillain-Barré syndrome Poliomyelitis Amyotrophic lateral sclerosis Spinal cord trauma or lesion
Neuromuscular system	Myasthenia gravis Multiple sclerosis Neuromuscular-blocking antibiotics Organophosphate poisoning Muscular dystrophy
Thorax	Massive obesity Chest trauma
Pleura	Pleural effusion Pneumothorax
Upper airways	Sleep apnea Tracheal obstruction Epiglottitis
Intrapulmonary	
Lower airways and alveoli	Chronic obstructive pulmonary disease (COPD) Asthma Bronchiolitis Cystic fibrosis Pneumonia
Pulmonary circulation	Pulmonary emboli
Alveolar-capillary membrane	Acute respiratory distress syndrome (ARDS) Inhalation of toxic gases Near-drowning

*Not an inclusive list.
From Urden LU et al: *Critical care nursing: Diagnosis and management*, ed. 7, St Louis, 2014, Elsevier.

commonly seen in the patient with ALF are usually related to the development of hypoxemia, hypercapnia, and acidosis.[9] Because the clinical symptoms are so varied, they are not considered reliable in predicting the degree of hypoxemia or hypercapnia[2] or the severity of ALF.

Diagnosing and following the course of respiratory failure is best accomplished by ABG analysis. ABG analysis confirms the level of $PaCO_2$, PaO_2, and blood pH. ALF is generally accepted as being present when the PaO_2 is less than 60 mm Hg. If the patient is also experiencing hypercapnia, the $PaCO_2$ will be greater than 50 mm Hg. In patients with chronically elevated $PaCO_2$ levels, these criteria must be broadened to include a pH less than 7.35.[9]

A variety of additional tests are performed depending on the patient's underlying condition. These include bronchoscopy for airway surveillance or specimen retrieval, chest radiography, thoracic ultrasound, thoracic computed tomography (CT), and selected lung function studies.[10]

Medical Management

Medical management of the patient with ALF is aimed at treating the underlying cause, promoting adequate gas exchange, correcting acidosis, initiating nutrition support, and preventing complications. Medical interventions to promote gas exchange are aimed at improving oxygenation and ventilation.[1]

Oxygenation

Actions to improve oxygenation include supplemental oxygen administration, either with a low flow system or a high flow system,[11] and the use of positive airway pressure.[12] The purpose of oxygen therapy is to correct hypoxemia, and although the absolute level of hypoxemia varies in each patient, most treatment approaches aim to keep the arterial hemoglobin oxygen saturation greater than 90%.[9] The goal is to keep the tissues' needs satisfied but not produce hypercapnia or oxygen toxicity.[9] Supplemental oxygen administration is effective in treating hypoxemia related to alveolar hypoventilation and V/Q mismatching. When intrapulmonary shunting exists, supplemental oxygen alone is ineffective.[11] In this situation, positive pressure is necessary to open collapsed alveoli and facilitate their participation in gas exchange. Positive pressure is delivered via invasive and noninvasive mechanical ventilation. To avoid intubation, positive pressure is usually administered initially noninvasively via a mask.[13] For further information on supplemental oxygen therapy and noninvasive ventilation, see Chapter 16.

Ventilation

Interventions to improve ventilation include the use of noninvasive and invasive mechanical ventilation. Depending on the underlying cause and the severity of the ALF, the patient may be treated initially with noninvasive ventilation.[13] However, one study found that those patients with a pH of less than 7.25 at initial presentation had an increased likelihood of the need for invasive mechanical ventilation.[14] The selection of ventilatory mode and settings depends on the patient's underlying condition, severity of respiratory failure, and body size. Initially the patient is started on volume ventilation in the assist/control mode. In the patient with chronic hypercapnia, the settings should be adjusted to keep the ABG values within the parameters expected to be maintained by the patient after extubation.[15] For further information on mechanical ventilation, see Chapter 16.

Pharmacology

Medications to facilitate dilation of the airways may also be of benefit in the treatment of the patient with ALF. Bronchodilators, such as beta₂-agonists and anticholinergic agents, aid in smooth muscle relaxation and are of particular benefit to patients with airflow limitations. Methylxanthines, such as aminophylline, are no longer recommended because of their negative side effects. Steroids also are often administered to decrease airway inflammation and enhance the effects of the beta₂-agonists. Mucolytics and expectorants are also no longer used since they have been found to be of no benefit in this patient population.[16]

Sedation is necessary in many patients to assist with maintaining adequate ventilation. It can be used to comfort the patient and decrease the work of breathing, particularly if the patient is fighting the ventilator. Analgesics should be administered for pain control.[17,18] In some patients, sedation does not decrease spontaneous respiratory efforts enough to allow adequate ventilation. Neuromuscular paralysis may be necessary to facilitate optimal ventilation. Paralysis also may be necessary to decrease oxygen consumption in the severely compromised patient.[18]

Acidosis

Acidosis may occur in the patient for a number of reasons. Hypoxemia causes impaired tissue perfusion, which leads to the production of lactic acid and the development of metabolic acidosis. Impaired ventilation leads to the accumulation of carbon dioxide and the development of respiratory acidosis. Once the patient is adequately oxygenated and ventilated, the acidosis should correct itself. The use of sodium bicarbonate to correct the acidosis has been shown to be of minimal benefit to the patient and thus is no longer recommended as first-line treatment. Bicarbonate therapy shifts the oxygen-hemoglobin dissociation curve to the left and can worsen tissue hypoxia. Sodium bicarbonate may be used if the acidosis is severe (pH less than 7.1), refractory to therapy, and causing dysrhythmias or hemodynamic instability.[19]

Nutrition Support

The initiation of nutrition support is of utmost importance in the management of the patient with ALF. The goals of nutrition support are to meet the overall nutritional needs of the patient while avoiding overfeeding, to prevent nutrition delivery-related complications, and to improve patient outcomes.[20] Failure to provide the patient with adequate nutrition support results in the development of malnutrition. Both malnutrition and overfeeding can interfere with the performance of the pulmonary system, further perpetuating ALF. Malnutrition decreases the patient's ventilatory drive and muscle strength, whereas overfeeding increases carbon dioxide production, which then increases the patient's ventilatory demand, resulting in respiratory muscle fatigue.[21]

The enteral route is the preferred method of nutrition administration. If the patient cannot tolerate enteral feedings or cannot receive enough nutrients enterally, he or she will be started on parenteral nutrition. Because the parenteral route is associated with a higher rate of complications, the goal is to switch to enteral feedings as soon as the patient can tolerate them.[20,21] Nutrition support should be initiated before the third day of mechanical ventilation for the well-nourished patient and within 24 hours for the malnourished patient.[20,21]

Complications

The patient with ALF may experience a number of complications including delirum,[22] cardiac dysrhythmias,[23] venous thromboembolism (VTE),[24] and gastrointestinal bleeding due to stress ulcers.[25] Delirium results from a variety of factors including hypoxemia, hypercapnia, and acidosis.[22] Dysrhythmias are precipitated by hypoxemia, acidosis, electrolyte imbalances, and the administration of beta$_2$-agonists.[23] Maintaining oxygenation, normalizing electrolytes, and monitoring medication levels will facilitate the prevention and treatment of delirium and dysrhythmias.[22,23] VTE is precipitated by venous stasis resulting from immobility and can be prevented through the use of intermittent pneumatic compression devices and low-dose unfractionated heparin (UFH) or low-molecular-weight heparin (LMWH).[24] In addition, stress ulcer prophylaxis is initiated with histamine receptor antagonists, cytoprotective agents, or proton pump inhibitors, though recently this practice has been called into question as there is minimal evidence to support the use of stress ulcer prophylaxis in the critically ill patient.[25] In addition, the patient is at risk for the complications associated with an artificial airway, mechanical ventilation, enteral and parenteral nutrition, and peripheral arterial cannulation.

BOX 15-1 NURSING DIAGNOSIS PRIORITIES

Acute Lung Failure

- Impaired Gas Exchange related to alveolar hypoventilation, p. 593
- Impaired Gas Exchange related to ventilation/perfusion mismatching or intrapulmonary shunting, p. 594
- Risk for Aspiration, p. 602
- Imbalanced Nutrition: Less Than Body Requirements related to lack of exogenous nutrients or increased metabolic demand, p. 593
- Risk for Infection, p. 607
- Anxiety related to threat to biologic, psychologic or social integrity, p. 576
- Deficient Knowledge: Discharge Regimen related to lack of previous exposure to information, p. 585 (See Box 15-2, Patient Education for Acute Lung Failure)

Nursing Management

Nursing management of the patient with ALF incorporates a variety of nursing diagnoses (Box 15-1). Nursing care is directed by the specific cause of the respiratory failure, although some common interventions are used. **Nursing priorities are directed toward 1) optimizing oxygenation and ventilation, 2) providing comfort and emotional support, 3) maintaining surveillance for complications, and 4) educating the patient and family.**

Optimizing Oxygenation and Ventilation

Nursing interventions to optimize oxygenation and ventilation include positioning, preventing desaturation, and promoting secretion clearance.

Positioning. Positioning of the patient with ALF depends on the type of lung injury and the underlying cause of hypoxemia. For those patients with V/Q mismatching, positioning is used to facilitate better matching of ventilation with perfusion to optimize gas exchange.[26] Because gravity normally facilitates preferential ventilation and perfusion to the dependent areas of the lungs, the best gas exchange would take place in the dependent areas of the lungs. Thus, the goal of positioning is to place the least affected area of the patient's lung in the most dependent position. Patients with unilateral lung disease should be positioned with the healthy lung in a dependent position.[26,27] Patients with diffuse lung disease may benefit from being positioned with the right lung down because it is larger and more vascular than the left lung.[27,28]

"Good lung down"

For those patients with alveolar hypoventilation, the goal of positioning is to facilitate ventilation. These patients benefit from nonrecumbent positions such as sitting or a semierect position.[29] In addition, semirecumbency (head of the bed elevated 30 to 45 degrees) is believed to decrease the risk of aspiration and inhibit the development of hospital-associated pneumonia.[30] Frequent repositioning (at least every 2 hours) is beneficial in optimizing the patient's ventilatory pattern and V/Q matching.[31]

Preventing desaturation. A number of activities can prevent desaturation from occurring. These include performing procedures only as needed, hyperoxygenating the patient before suctioning, providing adequate rest and recovery time between various procedures, and minimizing oxygen consumption. Interventions to minimize oxygen consumption include limiting the patient's physical activity, administering sedation to control anxiety, and providing measures to control fever.[29] The patient should be continuously monitored with a pulse oximeter to warn of signs of desaturation.

Promoting secretion clearance. Interventions to promote secretion clearance include providing adequate systemic hydration, humidifying supplemental oxygen, coughing, and suctioning. Postural drainage and chest percussion and vibration have been found to be of little benefit in the critically ill patient[32,33] and thus are not discussed here. To facilitate deep breathing, the patient's thorax should be maintained in alignment and the head of the bed elevated 30 to 45 degrees. This position best accommodates diaphragmatic descent and intercostal muscle action.

Once the patient is extubated, deep breathing and incentive spirometry should be started as soon as possible. Deep breathing involves having the patient take a deep breath and holding it for approximately 3 seconds or longer. Incentive spirometry involves having the patient take at least 10 deep, effective breaths per hour using an incentive spirometer. These actions help prevent atelectasis and re-expand any collapsed lung tissue. The chest should be auscultated during inflation to ensure that all dependent parts of the lung are well-ventilated and to help the patient understand the depth of breath necessary for optimal effect. Coughing should be avoided unless secretions are present because it promotes collapse of the smaller airways.

Educating the Patient and Family

Early in the patient's hospital stay, the patient and family should be taught about ALF, its etiologies, and its treatment. As the patient moves toward discharge, teaching should focus on the interventions necessary for preventing the reoccurrence of the precipitating disorder (Box 15-2). If the patient smokes, he or she should be encouraged to stop smoking and be referred to a smoking cessation program (Box 15-3). In addition, the importance of participating in a pulmonary rehabilitation program should be stressed.

Collaborative management of the patient with ALF is outlined in Box 15-4.

BOX 15-2 PATIENT EDUCATION PRIORITIES

Acute Lung Failure

- Pathophysiology of disease
- Specific etiology
- Precipitating factor modification
- Importance of taking medications
- Breathing techniques (e.g., pursed-lip breathing, diaphragmatic breathing)
- Energy conservation techniques
- Measures to prevent pulmonary infections (e.g., proper nutrition, hand washing, immunization against *Streptococcus pneumoniae* and influenza viruses)
- Signs and symptoms of pulmonary infections (e.g., sputum color change, shortness of breath, fever)
- Cough enhancement techniques (e.g., cascade cough, huff cough, end-expiratory cough, augmented cough)

Additional information for the patient can be found at the following websites:

American Lung Association: http://www.lung.org
Smokefree.gov: http://smokefree.gov
Healthfinder—U.S. Department of Health and Human Services: http://healthfinder.gov
WebMD: http://www.webmd.com
NHLBI ARDS Network: http://www.ardsnet.org
The ARDS Foundation: http://www.ardsusa.org/facts.htm

ACUTE RESPIRATORY DISTRESS SYNDROME

Description and Etiology

Acute respiratory distress syndrome (ARDS) is a systemic process that is considered to be the pulmonary manifestation of multiple organ dysfunction syndrome.[34] It is characterized by noncardiac pulmonary edema and disruption of the alveolar-capillary membrane as a result of injury to either the pulmonary vasculature or the airways.[35]

Many different diagnostic criteria have been used to identify ARDS, which has led to confusion, particularly among researchers. In 2012, in an attempt to address the limitations of the existing definition of ARDS, the ARDS Definition Task Force drafted a new definition (known as the Berlin Definition) of ARDS. This definition eliminated the term "acute lung injury" and proposed three distinct categories (mild, moderate, and severe) of ARDS based on the severity of hypoxemia. The Berlin Definition of ARDS is as follows:

- Timing—within 1 week of known clinical insult or new or worsening respiratory symptoms
- Chest imaging—bilateral opacities not fully explained by effusions, lobar/lung collapse, or nodules
- Origin of edema—respiratory failure not fully explained by heart failure or fluid overload; need objective assessment to exclude hydrostatic edema if no risk factor present
- Oxygenation—mild (200 mg Hg less than PaO_2/FiO_2 less than or equal to 300 mm Hg with positive end-respiratory airway pressure [PEEP] or constant positive airway pressure [CPAP] greater than or equal to 5 cm H_2O), moderate (100 mg Hg less than PaO_2/FiO_2 less than or equal to 200 mm Hg with PEEP greater than or equal to 5 cm H_2O), or severe (PaO_2/FiO_2 less than or equal to 100 mm Hg with PEEP greater than or equal to 5 cm H_2O).[36]

The mortality rate for ARDS is estimated to be 34% to 58%.[37]

A wide variety of clinical conditions is associated with the development of ARDS. These are categorized as *direct* or *indirect,* depending on the primary site of injury (Box 15-5).[35,38]

BOX 15-3 EVIDENCE-BASED PRACTICE SMOKING CESSATION GUIDELINES (QSEN)

The following are the key recommendations of the updated guideline *Treating Tobacco Use and Dependence,* based on the literature review and expert panel opinion:

1. Tobacco dependence is a chronic disease that often requires repeated intervention and multiple attempts to quit. Effective treatments exist, however, that can significantly increase rates of long-term abstinence.
2. It is essential that clinicians and health care delivery systems consistently identify and document tobacco use status and treat every tobacco user seen in a health care setting.
3. Tobacco dependence treatments are effective across a broad range of populations. Clinicians should encourage every patient willing to make a quit attempt to use the counseling treatments and medications recommended in this Guideline.
4. Brief tobacco dependence treatment is effective. Clinicians should offer every patient who uses tobacco at least the brief treatments shown to be effective in this Guideline.
5. Individual, group, and telephone counseling are effective, and their effectiveness increases with treatment intensity. Two components of counseling are especially effective, and clinicians should use these when counseling patients making a quit attempt:
   - Practical counseling (problem solving/skills training)
   - Social support delivered as part of treatment
6. Numerous effective medications are available for tobacco dependence, and clinicians should encourage their use by all patients attempting to quit smoking—except when medically contraindicated or with specific populations for which there is insufficient evidence of effectiveness (i.e., pregnant women, smokeless tobacco users, light smokers, and adolescents).
   - Seven first-line medications (5 nicotine and 2 non-nicotine) reliably increase long-term smoking abstinence rates:
     - Bupropion SR
     - Nicotine gum
     - Nicotine inhaler
     - Nicotine lozenge
     - Nicotine nasal spray
     - Nicotine patch
     - Varenicline
   - Clinicians also should consider the use of certain combinations of medications identified as effective in this Guideline.
7. Counseling and medication are effective when used by themselves for treating tobacco dependence. The combination of counseling and medication, however, is more effective than either alone. Thus, clinicians should encourage all individuals making a quit attempt to use both counseling and medication.
8. Telephone quitline counseling is effective with diverse populations and has broad reach. Therefore, clinicians and health care delivery systems should both ensure patient access to quitlines and promote quitline use.
9. If a tobacco user currently is unwilling to make a quit attempt, clinicians should use the motivational treatments shown in this Guideline to be effective in increasing future quit attempts.
10. Tobacco dependence treatments are both clinically effective and highly cost-effective relative to interventions for other clinical disorders. Providing coverage for these treatments increases quit rates. Insurers and purchasers should ensure that all insurance plans include the counseling and medication identified as effective in this Guideline as covered benefits.

From Fiore MC, et al. *Treating Tobacco Use and Dependence: 2008 Update* (Clinical Practice Guideline). Rockville, MD: U.S. Department of Health and Human Services, Public Health Service; 2008. Available from http://www.ncbi.nlm.nih.gov/books/NBK63952/.

Direct injuries are those in which the lung epithelium sustains a direct insult. Indirect injuries are those in which the insult occurs elsewhere in the body and mediators are transmitted via the bloodstream to the lungs. Sepsis, aspiration of gastric contents, diffuse pneumonia, and trauma were found to be major risk factors for the development of ARDS.[37]

Pathophysiology

The progression of ARDS can be described in three phases: exudative, fibroproliferative, and resolution. ARDS is initiated with stimulation of the inflammatory-immune system as a result of a direct or indirect injury (Figure 15-2). Inflammatory mediators are released from the site of injury, resulting in the activation and accumulation of the neutrophils, macrophages, and platelets in the pulmonary capillaries. These cellular mediators initiate the release of humoral mediators that cause damage to the alveolar-capillary membrane.[38]

Exudative Phase

Within the first 72 hours after the initial insult, the exudative phase or acute phase ensues. Once released, the mediators cause injury to the pulmonary capillaries, resulting in increased capillary membrane permeability leading to the leakage of fluid filled with protein, blood cells, fibrin, and activated cellular and humoral mediators into the pulmonary interstitium. Damage to the pulmonary capillaries also causes the development of microthrombi and elevation of pulmonary artery pressures. As fluid enters the pulmonary interstitium, the lymphatics are overwhelmed and unable to drain all the accumulating fluid, resulting in the development of interstitial edema. Fluid is then forced from the interstitial space into the alveoli, resulting in alveolar edema. Pulmonary interstitial edema also causes compression of the alveoli and small airways. Alveolar edema causes swelling of the type I alveolar epithelial cells and flooding of the alveoli.

BOX 15-4 COLLABORATIVE MANAGEMENT

Acute Lung Failure

- Identify and treat underlying cause.
- Administer oxygen therapy.
- Intubate patient.
- Initiate mechanical ventilation.
- Administer medications:
  - Bronchodilators
  - Steroids
  - Sedatives
  - Analgesics
- Position patient to optimize ventilation/perfusion matching.
- Suction as needed.
- Provide adequate rest and recovery time between various procedures.
- Correct acidosis.
- Initiate nutritional support.
- Maintain surveillance for complications:
  - Encephalopathy
  - Cardiac dysrhythmias
  - Venous thromboembolism
  - Gastrointestinal bleeding
- Provide comfort and emotional support.

BOX 15-5 Risk Factors for Acute Respiratory Distress Syndrome

Direct Injury
Aspiration
Near-drowning
Toxic inhalation
Pulmonary contusion
Pneumonia
Oxygen toxicity
Transthoracic radiation

Indirect Injury
Sepsis
Nonthoracic trauma
Hypertransfusion
Cardiopulmonary bypass
Severe pancreatitis
Embolism—air, fat, amniotic fluid
Disseminated intravascular coagulation (DIC)
Shock states

Protein and fibrin in the edema fluid precipitate the formation of hyaline membranes over the alveoli. Eventually, the type II alveolar epithelial cells are also damaged, leading to impaired surfactant production. Injury to the alveolar epithelial cells and the loss of surfactant lead to further alveolar collapse.[38,39]

Hypoxemia occurs as a result of intrapulmonary shunting and V/Q mismatching secondary to compression, collapse, and flooding of the alveoli and small airways. Increased work of breathing occurs as a result of increased airway resistance, decreased functional residual capacity (FRC), and decreased lung compliance secondary to atelectasis and compression of the small airways. Hypoxemia and the increased work of breathing lead to patient fatigue and the development of alveolar hypoventilation. Pulmonary hypertension occurs as a result of damage to the pulmonary capillaries, microthrombi, and hypoxic vasoconstriction leading to the development of increased alveolar dead space and right ventricular afterload. Hypoxemia worsens as a result of alveolar hypoventilation and increased alveolar dead space. Right ventricular afterload increases and leads to right ventricular dysfunction and a decrease in cardiac output (CO).[38]

Fibroproliferative Phase

This phase begins as disordered healing and starts in the lungs. Cellular granulation and collagen deposition occur within the alveolar-capillary membrane. The alveoli become enlarged and irregularly shaped (fibrotic), and the pulmonary capillaries become scarred and obliterated. This leads to further stiffening of the lungs, increasing pulmonary hypertension, and continued hypoxemia.[38,39]

Resolution Phase

Recovery occurs over several weeks as structural and vascular remodeling take place to re-establish the alveolar-capillary membrane. The hyaline membranes are cleared, and intra-alveolar fluid is transported out of the alveolus into the interstitium. The type II alveolar epithelial cells multiply, some of which differentiate to type I alveolar epithelial cells, facilitating the restoration of the alveolus. Alveolar macrophages remove cellular debris.[38,39]

Assessment and Diagnosis

Initially the patient with ARDS may be seen with a variety of clinical manifestations, depending on the precipitating event. As the disorder progresses, the patient's signs and symptoms can be associated with the phase of ARDS that he or she is experiencing (Table 15-2). During the exudative phase, the patient presents with tachypnea, restlessness, apprehension, and moderate increase in accessory muscle use. During the fibroproliferative phase, the patient's signs and symptoms progress to agitation, dyspnea, fatigue, excessive accessory muscle use, and fine crackles as respiratory failure develops.[40,41]

Arterial blood-gas analysis reveals a low PaO_2, despite increases in supplemental oxygen administration (refractory hypoxemia).[40] Initially the $PaCO_2$ is low as a result of hyperventilation, but eventually the $PaCO_2$ increases as the patient fatigues. The pH is high initially but decreases as respiratory acidosis develops.[40,41] Initially the chest x-ray film may be normal because changes in the lungs do not become evident for up to 24 hours. As the pulmonary edema becomes apparent, diffuse, patchy interstitial and alveolar infiltrates appear. This progresses to multifocal consolidation of the lungs, which appears as a "whiteout" on the chest x-ray film.[40]

Medical Management

Medical management of the patient with ARDS involves a multifaceted approach. This strategy includes treating the underlying cause, promoting gas exchange, supporting tissue oxygenation, and preventing complications. Given the severity of hypoxemia, the patient is intubated and mechanically ventilated to facilitate adequate gas exchange.[42]

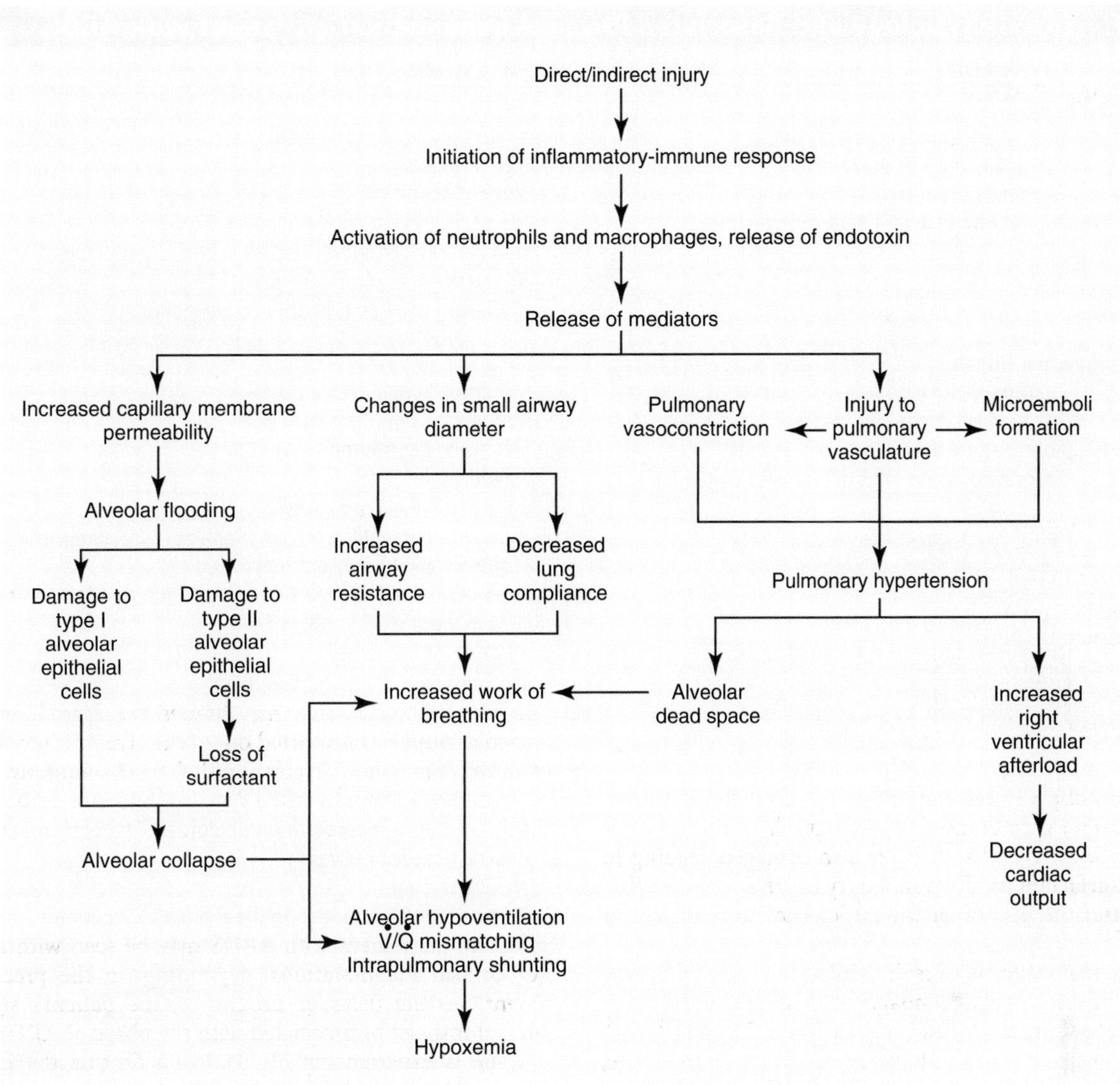

FIG 15-2 Pathophysiology of Acute Respiratory Distress Syndrome.

Ventilation

Traditionally the patient with ARDS was ventilated with a mode of volume ventilation, such as assist/control ventilation (A/CV) or synchronized intermittent mandatory ventilation (SIMV), with tidal volumes adjusted to deliver 10 to 15 mL/kg. Current research now indicates that this approach may have actually led to further lung injury. It is now known that repeated opening and closing of the alveoli cause injury to the lung units (atelectrauma), resulting in inhibited surfactant production, and increased inflammation (biotrauma), resulting in the release of mediators and an increase in pulmonary capillary membrane permeability. In addition, excessive pressure in the alveoli (barotrauma) or excessive volume in the alveoli (volutrauma) leads to excessive alveolar wall stress and damage to the alveolar-capillary membrane, resulting in air escaping into the surrounding spaces.[42] Thus, several different approaches have been developed to facilitate the mechanical ventilation of the patient with ARDS.

Low tidal volume. Low tidal volume ventilation uses smaller tidal volumes (6 mL/kg) to ventilate the patient in an attempt to limit the effects of barotrauma and volutrauma. The goal is to provide the maximum tidal volume possible while maintaining end-inspiratory plateau pressure less than 30 cm H_2O. To allow for adequate carbon dioxide elimination, the respiratory rate is increased to 20 to 30 breaths/min.[42,43]

Permissive hypercapnia. Permissive hypercapnia uses low tidal volume ventilation in conjunction with normal respiratory rates in an attempt to limit the effects of atelectrauma and biotrauma. Normally, to maintain normocapnia, the patient's respiratory rate would have to be increased to compensate for the small tidal volume. In ARDS though, increasing the respiratory rate can lead to worsening alveolar damage. Thus, the patient's carbon dioxide level is allowed to rise, and the patient becomes hypercapnic. As a general rule, the patient's $PaCO_2$ should not rise faster than 10 mm Hg per hour and overall should not exceed 80 to 100 mg Hg. Because of the negative cardiopulmonary effects of severe acidosis, the arterial pH is generally maintained at 7.20 or greater. To maintain the pH, the patient is given intravenous sodium bicarbonate, or the respiratory rate and/or tidal volume are increased. Permissive hypercapnia is contraindicated in

TABLE 15-2 Physiology and Associated Physical Examination of Patient with ARDS

PHASE	PHYSIOLOGY	PHYSICAL EXAMINATION
Exudative Phase		
	Parenchymal surface hemorrhage	Restless, apprehensive, tachypneic
	Interstitial or alveolar edema	Respiratory alkalosis
	Compression of terminal bronchioles	PaO_2 normal
	Destruction of type I alveolar cells	CXR: normal
		Chest examination: moderate use of accessory muscles, lungs clear
		Pulmonary artery pressures: elevated
		Pulmonary artery occlusion pressure: normal or low
Fibroproliferative Phase		
	Destruction of type II alveolar cells	Pulmonary artery pressures: elevated
	Gas exchange compromised	Increased workload on right ventricle
	Increased peak inspiratory pressure	Increased use of accessory muscles
	Decreased compliance (static and dynamic)	Fine crackles
		Increasing agitation related to hypoxia
	Refractory hypoxemia:	CXR: interstitial or alveolar infiltrates; elevated diaphragm
	• Intra-alveolar atelectasis	Hyperventilation; hypercarbia
	• Increased shunt fraction	Decreased SvO_2
	• Decreased diffusion	Widening alveolar-arterial gradient
	Decreased functional residual capacity	Increased work of breathing
	Interstitial fibrosis	Worsening hypercarbia and hypoxemia
	Increased dead space ventilation	Lactic acidosis (related to aerobic metabolism)
		Alteration in perfusion:
		• Increased heart rate
		• Decreased blood pressure
		• Change in skin temperature and color
		• Decreased capillary filling
		End-organ dysfunction:
		• Brain: change in mentation, agitation, hallucinations
		• Heart: decreased cardiac output→angina, HF, papillary muscle dysfunction, dysrhythmias, MI
		• Renal: decreased urinary or GFR
		• Skin: mottled, ischemic
		• Liver: elevated SGOT, bilirubin, alkaline phosphatase, PT/PTT; decreased albumin

Modified from Phillips JK. Management of patients with acute respiratory distress syndrome. *Crit Care Nurs Clin North Am.*1999; 11:233.
ARDS, acute respiratory distress syndrome; *PaO_2,* arterial oxygen pressure; *CXR,* chest radiograph; *SvO_2,* venous oxygen saturation; *HF,* heart failure; *MI,* myocardial infarction; *GFR,* glomerular filtration rate; *SGOT,* serum glutamate oxaloacetate transaminase; *PT,* prothrombin time; *PTT,* partial thromboplastin time.

patients with increased intracranial pressure, pulmonary hypertension, seizures, and heart failure.[44]

Pressure control ventilation. In pressure control ventilation (PCV) mode, each breath is delivered or augmented with a preset amount of inspiratory pressure as opposed to tidal volume, which is used in volume ventilation. Thus, the actual tidal volume the patient receives varies from breath to breath. PCV is used to limit and control the amount of pressure in the lungs and decrease the incidence of volutrauma. The goal is to keep the patient's plateau pressure (end-inspiratory static pressure) lower than 30 cm H_2O. A known problem with this mode of ventilation is that as the patient's lungs get stiffer, it becomes harder and harder to maintain an adequate tidal volume, and severe hypercapnia can occur.[42,43]

Inverse ratio ventilation. Another alternative ventilatory mode that is used in managing the patient with ARDS is inverse ratio ventilation (IRV), either pressure-controlled or volume-controlled. IRV prolongs the inspiratory (I) time and shortens the expiratory (E) time, thus reversing the normal I:E ratio. The goal of IRV is to maintain a more constant mean airway pressure throughout the ventilatory cycle, which helps keep alveoli open and participating in gas exchange. It also increases FRC and decreases the work of breathing. In addition, as the breath is delivered over a longer period of time, the peak inspiratory pressure in the lungs is decreased. A major disadvantage to IRV is the development of auto-PEEP. As the expiratory phase of ventilation is shortened, air can become trapped in the lower airways, creating unintentional PEEP (or auto-PEEP), which can cause hemodynamic compromise and worsening gas exchange. Patients on IRV usually require heavy sedation with neuromuscular blockade to prevent them from fighting the ventilator.[42,43]

High-frequency oscillatory ventilation. Another alternative ventilatory mode that is used in patients who remain severely hypoxemic despite the treatments previously described is high-frequency oscillatory ventilation (HFOV). The goal of this method of ventilation is similar to that of IRV in that it uses a constant airway pressure to promote alveolar recruitment while avoiding overdistention of the alveoli. HFOV uses a piston pump to deliver very low tidal volumes at very high rates or oscillations (300 to 3000 breaths/min).[45]

Oxygen Therapy

Oxygen is administered at the lowest level possible to support tissue oxygenation. Continued exposure to high levels of oxygen can lead to oxygen toxicity, which perpetuates the entire process. The goal of oxygen therapy is to maintain an arterial hemoglobin oxygen saturation of 90% or greater using the lowest level of oxygen—preferably less than 0.50.[35]

Positive end-expiratory pressure. Because the hypoxemia that develops with ARDS is often refractory or unresponsive to oxygen therapy, it is necessary to facilitate oxygenation with PEEP. The purpose of using PEEP in the patient with ARDS is to improve oxygenation while reducing FiO_2 to less toxic levels. PEEP has several positive effects on the lungs, including opening collapsed alveoli, stabilizing flooded alveoli, and increasing FRC. Thus, PEEP decreases intrapulmonary shunting and increases compliance. PEEP also has several negative effects including 1) decreasing CO as a result of decreasing venous return secondary to increased intrathoracic pressure and 2) barotrauma as a result of gas escaping into the surrounding spaces secondary to alveolar rupture. The amount of PEEP a patient requires is determined by evaluating both arterial hemoglobin oxygen saturation and CO. In most cases, a PEEP of 10 to 15 cm H_2O is adequate. If PEEP is too high, it can result in overdistention of the alveoli, which can impede pulmonary capillary blood flow, decrease surfactant production, and worsen intrapulmonary shunting. If PEEP is too low, it allows the alveoli to collapse during expiration, which can result in more damage to alveoli.[42]

Extracorporeal gas exchange. Extracorporeal gas exchanges are last-resort techniques used in the treatment of severe ARDS when conventional therapy has failed.[46] These methods allow the lungs to rest by facilitating the removal of carbon dioxide and providing oxygen external to the lungs by means of an "artificial lung" or membrane/fiber oxygenator. Extracorporeal membrane oxygenation (ECMO) and extracorporeal carbon dioxide removal ($ECCO_2R$) are two techniques that employ this type of technology. ECMO is similar to cardiopulmonary bypass in that blood is removed from the body and pumped through a membrane oxygenator, where CO_2 is removed and O_2 is added, and then returned to the body. $ECCO_2R$ is a variation of ECMO in which the primary focus is removal of CO_2. Both of these techniques pose serious bleeding problems to the patient, and none has been shown to improve patient outcome.[47]

Tissue Perfusion

Adequate tissue perfusion depends on an adequate supply of oxygen being transported to the tissues. An adequate CO and hemoglobin level is critical to oxygen transport. CO depends on heart rate, preload, afterload, and contractility. A variety of fluids and medications are used to manipulate this parameter. Newer approaches to fluid management include maintaining a very low intravascular volume (pulmonary artery occlusion pressure of 5 to 8 mm Hg) with fluid restriction and diuretics, while supporting the CO with vasoactive and inotropic medications. The goal is to decrease the amount of fluid leakage into the lungs.[48]

BOX 15-6 NURSING DIAGNOSIS PRIORITIES

Acute Respiratory Distress Syndrome

- Impaired Gas Exchange related to ventilation/perfusion mismatching or intrapulmonary shunting, p. 594
- Decreased Cardiac Output related to alterations in preload, p. 579
- Imbalanced Nutrition: Less Than Body Requirements related to lack of exogenous nutrients or increased metabolic demand, p. 593
- Risk for Infection, p. 607
- Compromised Family Coping related to critically ill family member, p. 578

Nursing Management

Nursing management of the patient with ARDS incorporates a variety of nursing diagnoses (Box 15-6). **Nursing priorities are directed toward 1) optimizing oxygenation and ventilation, 2) providing comfort and emotional support, and 3) maintaining surveillance for complications.**

Optimizing Oxygenation and Ventilation

Nursing interventions to optimize oxygenation and ventilation include positioning, preventing desaturation, and promoting secretion clearance. For further discussion on these interventions, see Nursing Management of Acute Lung Failure earlier in this chapter. One additional nursing intervention that can be used to improve the oxygenation and ventilation of the patient with ARDS is prone positioning.

Prone positioning. A number of studies have shown that prone positioning the patient with ARDS results in an improvement in oxygenation. Although a number of theories propose how prone positioning improves oxygenation, the discovery that with ARDS there is greater damage to the dependent areas of the lungs probably provides the best explanation. It was originally thought that ARDS was a diffuse homogenous disease that affected all areas of the lungs equally. It is now known that the dependent lung areas are more heavily damaged than the nondependent lung areas. Turning the patient prone improves perfusion to less damaged parts of lungs and improves V/Q matching and decreases intrapulmonary shunting. Prone positioning appears to be more effective when initiated during the early phases of ARDS.[49] For more information on prone positioning, see Chapter 16.

Collaborative management of the patient with ARDS is outlined in Box 15-7.

PNEUMONIA

Description and Etiology

Pneumonia is an acute inflammation of the lung parenchyma that is caused by an infectious agent that can lead to alveolar consolidation. Pneumonia can be classified as community-acquired pneumonia (CAP), hospital-associated pneumonia (HAP), or health care-associated pneumonia (HCAP).[50]

BOX 15-7 COLLABORATIVE MANAGEMENT

Acute Respiratory Distress Syndrome

- Administer oxygen therapy.
- Intubate patient.
- Initiate mechanical ventilation:
  - Permissive hypercapnia
  - Pressure control ventilation
  - Inverse ratio ventilation
- Use PEEP.
- Administer medications:
  - Bronchodilators
  - Sedatives
  - Analgesics
  - Neuromuscular blocking agents
- Maximize cardiac output:
  - Preload
  - Afterload
  - Contractility
- Prone patient.
- Suction as needed.
- Provide adequate rest and recovery time between various procedures.
- Initiate nutritional support.
- Maintain surveillance for complications:
  - Encephalopathy
  - Cardiac dysrhythmias
  - Venous thromboembolism
  - Gastrointestinal bleeding
  - Atelectrauma
  - Biotrauma
  - Volutrauma
  - Barotrauma
  - Oxygen toxicity
- Provide comfort and emotional support.

Pneumonia is referred to as community-acquired when it occurs outside of the hospital or within 48 hours of admission to the hospital.[51] Severe CAP requires admission to the critical care unit and accounts for about 22% of all patients with pneumonia. The mortality for this patient group is approximately 18% to 56%, with increasing age as a major risk factor.[52] Pneumonia is referred to as hospital-associated when it occurs while in the hospital for at least 48 hours.[50] Ventilator-associated pneumonia (VAP) is a subgrouping of HAP that refers to development of pneumonia after the insertion of an artificial airway.[50] VAP is the most common critical care unit-acquired infection.[53] Pneumonia is referred to as health care-associated when it is acquired in health care environments outside of the traditional hospital setting.[54] The spectra of etiologic pathogens of pneumonia vary with the type of pneumonia, as do the risk factors for the disease.

Severe Community-Acquired Pneumonia

Pathogens that can cause severe CAP include *Streptococcus pneumoniae, Legionella species, Haemophilus influenzae, Moraxella catarrhalis, Staphylococcus aureus, Mycoplasma pneumoniae,* respiratory viruses, fungi, *Chlamydia pneumoniae, Pseudomonas aeruginosa,* and Enterobacteriaceae.[51]

BOX 15-8 Risk Factors for Hospital-Acquired Pneumonia

Host-Related
Advanced age
Altered level of consciousness
Chronic obstructive pulmonary disease
Altered immune system
Severity of illness
Poor nutrition
Hemodynamic compromise
Trauma
Smoking
Dental plaque

Treatment-Related
Mechanical ventilation
Endotracheal intubation
Unintentional extubation
Bronchoscopy
Nasogastric tube
Previous antibiotic therapy
Elevated gastric pH secondary to histamine receptor antagonists, proton pump inhibitors, and enteral feedings
Upper abdominal surgery
Thoracic surgery
Supine position

Infection Control-Related
Poor hand-washing practices

A number of factors increase the risk for developing CAP, including alcoholism, chronic obstructive pulmonary disease (COPD), and comorbid conditions such as diabetes, malignancy, and coronary artery disease. Impaired swallowing and altered mental status also contribute to the development of CAP because they result in an increased exposure to the various pathogens due to chronic aspiration of oropharyngeal secretions.[51]

Hospital-Associated Pneumonia

Pathogens that can cause HAP include *Escherichia coli, H. influenzae,* methicillin-sensitive *S. aureus, S. pneumoniae, P. aeruginosa, Acinetobacter baumannii,* methicillin-resistant *S. aureus* (MRSA), *Klebsiella* spp., and *Enterobacter* spp. Two of the pathogens most frequently associated with VAP are *S. aureus* and *P. aeruginosa.* Risk factors for HAP can be categorized as host-related, treatment-related, and infection control-related (Box 15-8).[55]

Health Care-Associated Pneumonia

Pathogens that can cause HCAP are similar to those causing both CAP and HAP, with *P. aeruginosa* and MRSA being the most common in the United States.[54] Risk factors for HCAP include prior hospitalization (hospitalized for 2 or more days within the last 90 days), receiving hemodialysis, receiving intravenous antibiotic therapy, chemotherapy or wound care within 30 days, residing in a long-term care facility or with family member with multidrug-resistant infection, and an immunocompromised state. These patients are at a higher risk of developing multidrug-resistant organisms.[56]

Pathophysiology

Development of acute pneumonia implies a defect in host defenses, a particularly virulent organism, or an overwhelming inoculation event. Bacterial invasion of the lower respiratory tract can occur by inhalation of aerosolized infectious particles, aspiration of organisms colonizing the oropharynx, migration of organisms from adjacent sites of colonization, direct inoculation of organisms into the lower airway, spread of infection to the lungs from adjacent structures, spread of infection to the lung through the blood, and reactivation of latent infection (usually in the setting of immunosuppression). The most common mechanism appears to be aspiration of oropharyngeal organisms.[57] Table 15-3 lists the precipitating conditions that can facilitate the development of pneumonia.

Figure 15-3 depicts the pathophysiology of HAP. Colonization of the patient's oropharynx with infectious organisms is a major contributor to the development of HAP. Normally, the oropharynx has a stable population of resident flora that may be anaerobic or aerobic. When stress occurs, such as with illness, surgery, or infection, pathogenic organisms replace normal resident flora. Previous antibiotic therapy also affects the resident flora population, making replacement by pathologic organisms more likely. The pathogens are then able to invade the sterile lower respiratory tract.[55]

Disruption of the gag and cough reflexes, altered consciousness, abnormal swallowing, and artificial airways all predispose the patient to aspiration and colonization of the lungs and subsequent infection. Histamine$_2$ agonists, antacids, and enteral feedings also contribute to this problem because they raise the pH of the stomach and promote bacterial overgrowth. The nasogastric tube then acts as a wick, facilitating the movement of bacteria from the stomach to the pharynx, where the bacteria can be aspirated.[55]

Infection results in pulmonary inflammation with or without significant exudates. Increased capillary permeability occurs, leading to increased interstitial and alveolar fluid. V/Q mismatching and intrapulmonary shunting occurs, resulting in hypoxemia as lung consolidation progresses. Untreated pneumonia can result in ALF and initiation of the inflammatory-immune response. In addition, the patient may develop a pleural effusion. This is the result of the vascular response to inflammation, whereby capillary permeability is increased and fluid from the pulmonary capillaries diffuses into the pleural space.[58]

TABLE 15-3 Precipitating Conditions of Pneumonia

CONDITION	ETIOLOGIES
Depressed epiglottal and cough reflexes	Unconsciousness, neurologic disease, endotracheal or tracheal tubes, anesthesia, aging
Decreased cilia activity	Smoke inhalation, smoking history, oxygen toxicity, hypoventilation, intubation, viral infections, aging, COPD
Increased secretion	COPD, viral infections, bronchiectasis, general anesthesia, endotracheal intubation, smoking
Atelectasis	Trauma, foreign body obstruction, tumor, splinting, shallow ventilations, general anesthesia
Decreased lymphatic flow	Heart failure, tumor
Fluid in alveoli	Heart failure, aspiration, trauma
Abnormal phagocytosis and humoral activity	Neutropenia, immunocompetent disorders, patients receiving chemotherapy
Impaired alveolar macrophages	Hypoxemia, metabolic acidosis, cigarette smoking history, hypoxia, alcohol use, viral infections, aging

COPD, Chronic obstructive pulmonary disease.

Assessment and Diagnosis

The clinical manifestations of pneumonia will vary with the offending pathogen. The patient may first be seen with a variety of signs and symptoms including dyspnea, fever, and cough (productive or nonproductive). Coarse crackles on auscultation and dullness to percussion may also be present.[53] Patients with severe CAP may manifest confusion and disorientation, tachypnea, hypoxemia, uremia, leukopenia, thrombocytopenia, hypothermia, and hypotension.[57]

Chest radiography is used to evaluate the patient with suspected pneumonia. The diagnosis is established by the presence of a new pulmonary infiltrate. The radiographic pattern of the infiltrates will vary with the organism.[51] A sputum Gram stain and culture are done to facilitate the identification of the infectious pathogen. In 50% of cases, though, a causative agent is not identified.[51] A diagnostic bronchoscopy may be needed, particularly if the diagnosis is unclear or current therapy is not working.[55] In addition, a complete blood count with differential, chemistry panel, blood cultures, and ABGs is obtained.[51]

Medical Management

Medical management of the patient with pneumonia should include antibiotic therapy, oxygen therapy for hypoxemia, mechanical ventilation if ALF develops, fluid management for hydration, nutritional support, and treatment of associated medical problems and complications. For patients having difficulty mobilizing secretions, a therapeutic bronchoscopy may be necessary.[58]

Antibiotic Therapy

Although bacteria-specific antibiotic therapy is the goal, this may not always be possible because of difficulties in identifying the organism and the seriousness of the patient's condition. The time involved obtaining cultures should be balanced against the need to begin some treatment based on the patient's condition. Empiric therapy has become a generally acceptable approach. In this approach, choice of antibiotic treatment is based on the most likely etiologic organism while avoiding toxicity, superinfection, and unnecessary cost. If available, Gram stain results should be used to guide choices of antibiotics. Antibiotics should be chosen that offer broad coverage of the usual pathogens in the hospital or community. Failure to respond to such therapy may indicate that the chosen antibiotic regimen does not appropriately cover all of the etiologic pathogens or that a new source of infection has developed.[51,55]

Currently the Centers for Medicare and Medicaid Services (CMS) and The Joint Commission (TJC) standards for

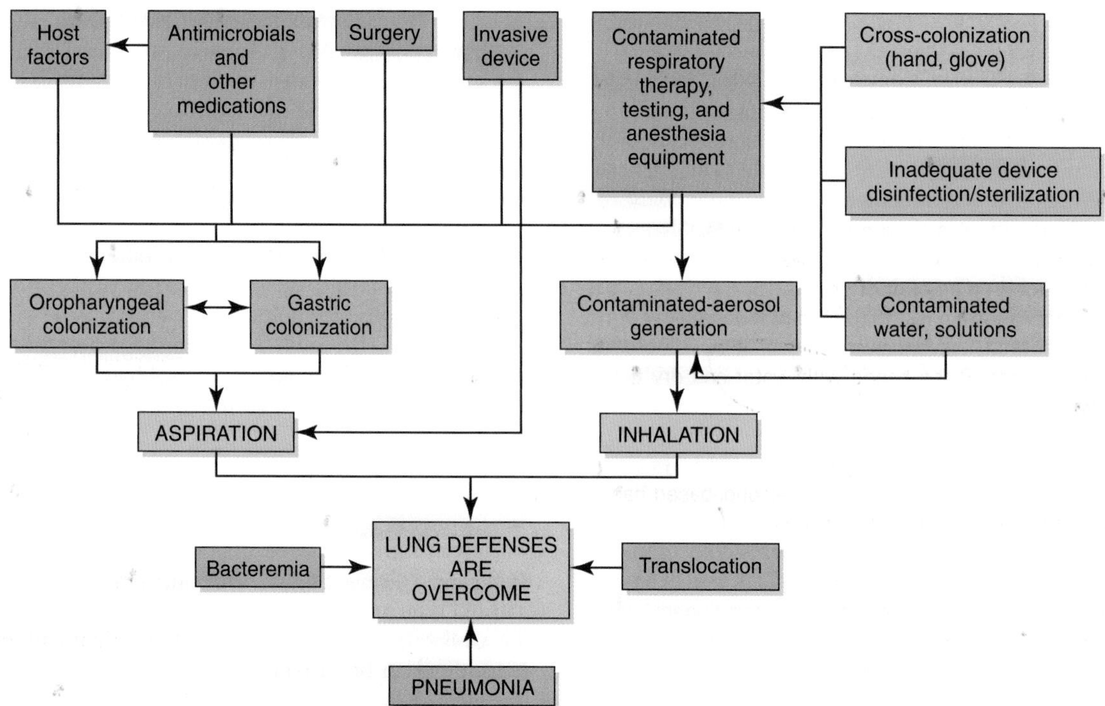

FIG 15-3 Pathophysiology of Pneumonia. (From Tablan OC, et al. Guideline for prevention of nosocomial pneumonia. The Hospital Infection Control Practices Advisory Committee, Centers for Disease Control and Prevention. *Am J Infect Control.* 1994;22:247.)

managing patients with CAP require that the first dose of antibiotics be administered within 6 hours of arrival to the hospital. This timeframe is very controversial and has been the subject of much debate. Those in favor of the standard believe that early antibiotic administration leads to improved outcomes, while those not in favor of the standard believe it leads to the overuse of antibiotics. More research is needed to clarify the issue.[59]

Independent Lung Ventilation

In patients with unilateral pneumonia or severely asymmetric pneumonia, this alternative mode of mechanical ventilation may be necessary to facilitate oxygenation. As the alveoli in the affected lung become flooded with pus, the lung becomes less compliant and difficult to ventilate. This results in a shifting of ventilation to the good lung without a concomitant shift in perfusion and thus an increase in V/Q mismatching. Independent lung ventilation (ILV) allows each lung to be ventilated separately, thus controlling the amount of flow, volume, and pressure each lung receives. A double-lumen endotracheal tube is inserted, and each lumen is usually attached to a separate mechanical ventilator. The ventilator settings are then customized to the needs of each lung to facilitate optimal oxygenation and ventilation.[60]

Nursing Management

Nursing management of the patient with pneumonia incorporates a variety of nursing diagnoses (Box 15-9). **Nursing priorities are directed toward 1) optimizing oxygenation and ventilation, 2) preventing the spread of infection, 3) providing comfort and emotional support, and 4) maintaining surveillance for complications.** The patient's response to the antibiotic therapy should be monitored for adverse effects.

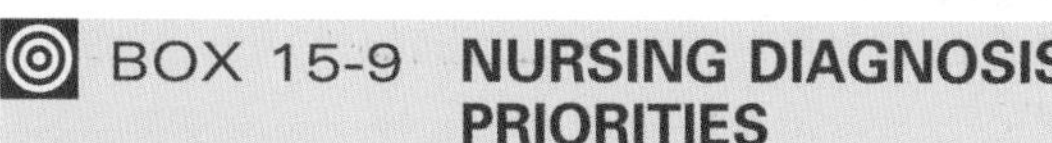

BOX 15-9 NURSING DIAGNOSIS PRIORITIES

Pneumonia

- Ineffective Airway Clearance related to excessive secretions or abnormal viscosity of mucus, p. 597
- Impaired Gas Exchange related to ventilation/perfusion mismatching or intrapulmonary shunting, p. 594
- Imbalanced Nutrition: Less Than Body Requirements related to lack of exogenous nutrients or increased metabolic demand, p. 593
- Risk for Aspiration, p. 602
- Risk for Infection, p. 607
- Anxiety related to threat to biologic, psychologic, or social integrity, p. 576
- Powerlessness related to lack of control over current situation or disease progression, p. 600
- Compromised Family Coping related to critically ill family member, p. 578

Optimizing Oxygenation and Ventilation

Nursing interventions to optimize oxygenation and ventilation include positioning, preventing desaturation, and promoting secretion clearance. For further discussion on these interventions, see Nursing Management of Acute Lung Failure earlier in this chapter.

Preventing the Spread of Infection

Prevention should be directed at eradicating pathogens from the environment and interrupting the spread of organisms

BOX 15-10 Quality Improvement (QSEN) Hand Hygiene Guidelines

The following are the key recommendations of the Hand Hygiene Task Force, based on the literature review and expert panel opinion:

- Wash hands with soap and water when visibly dirty or contaminated with blood and other body fluids.
- When washing hands with soap and water, wet hands first with water, apply an amount of product recommended by the manufacturer to hands, and rub hands together vigorously for at least 15 seconds, covering all surfaces of the hands and fingers. Rinse hands with water and dry thoroughly with a disposable towel. Use towel to turn off the faucet. Avoid using hot water because repeated exposure to hot water may increase the risk of dermatitis.
- If hands are not visibly soiled, use an alcohol-based hand rub for routinely decontaminating hands.
- When decontaminating hands with an alcohol-based hand rub, apply product to palm of one hand and rub hands together, covering all surfaces of hands and fingers, until hands are dry (Follow the manufacturer's recommendations regarding the volume of product to use.).
- Decontaminate hands before and after having direct contact with patients.
- Decontaminate hands before and after donning gloves.
- Wear gloves when contact with blood or other potentially infectious materials, mucous membranes, or non-intact skin could occur.
- Change gloves during patient care if moving from a contaminated body site to a clean body site.
- Remove gloves after caring for a patient. Do not wear the same pair of gloves for the care of more than one patient and do not wash gloves between uses with different patients.
- Decontaminate hands after contact with inanimate objects (including medical equipment).
- Do not wear artificial fingernails or extenders when having direct contact with patients at high risk (e.g., those in critical care units or operating rooms).
- Keep natural nails tips less than 1/4-inch long.

From Boyce JM, et al, Advisory Committee, and the HICPAC/SHEA/APIC/IDSA Hand Hygiene Task Force. Recommendations of the Healthcare Infection Control Practices Advisory Committee. *MMWR Recomm Rep.* 2002; 51(RR16):1.

from person to person. Significant progress has been made in removing contaminants from the patient environment through proper disinfection of respiratory equipment and increased use of disposable supplies. Other possible environmental sources of pathogens include suctioning equipment and indwelling lines. These invasive tools must be given proper aseptic care.[55]

Proper hand hygiene is the single most important measure available to prevent the spread of bacteria from person to person (Box 15-10). Hand hygiene should occur before and after touching a patient or their surroundings, before performing a procedure, and after exposure to any body fluids.[61] In addition, meticulous oral care, including suctioning of the secretions pooling above the cuff of the artificial airway, is critical to decreasing the bacterial colonization of the oropharynx.[55] Prevention of VAP and oral care is further discussed in Chapter 16.

BOX 15-11 COLLABORATIVE MANAGEMENT

Pneumonia

- Administer oxygen therapy.
- Initiate mechanical ventilation as required.
- Administer medications:
  - Antibiotics
  - Bronchodilators
- Position patient to optimize ventilation/perfusion matching.
- Suction as needed.
- Provide adequate rest and recovery time between various procedures.
- Maintain surveillance for complications:
  - Acute lung failure
- Provide comfort and emotional support.

Collaborative management of the patient with pneumonia is outlined in Box 15-11.

ASPIRATION PNEUMONITIS

Description and Etiology

The presence of abnormal substances in the airways and alveoli as a result of aspiration is misleadingly called *aspiration pneumonia.* This term is misleading because the aspiration of toxic substances into the lung may or may not involve an infection. *Aspiration pneumonitis* is a more accurate title because injury to the lung can result from the chemical, mechanical, and/or bacterial characteristics of the aspirate.[62]

A number of factors have been identified that place the patient at risk for aspiration (Table 15-4). Gastric contents and oropharyngeal bacteria (see Pneumonia earlier in this chapter) are the most common aspirates of the critically ill patient.[62-64] The effects of gastric contents on the lungs will vary based on the pH of the liquid. If the pH is less than 2.5, the patient will develop a severe chemical pneumonitis resulting in hypoxemia. If the pH is greater than 2.5, the immediate damage to the lungs will be lessened, but the elevated pH may have promoted bacterial overgrowth of the stomach.[62,63] Once the bacteria-laden gastric contents are aspirated into the lungs, overwhelming bacterial pneumonia can develop.[63]

Pathophysiology

The type of lung injury that develops after aspiration is determined by a number of factors, including the quality of the aspirate and the status of the patient's respiratory defense mechanisms.

Acid Liquid

The aspiration of acid (pH less than 2.5) liquid gastric contents results in the development of bronchospasm and atelectasis almost immediately. Over the next 4 hours, tracheal damage, bronchitis, bronchiolitis, alveolar-capillary breakdown, interstitial edema, and alveolar congestion and hemorrhage occur.[64] Severe hypoxemia develops as a result of intrapulmonary shunting and V/Q mismatching. As the disorder progresses, necrotic debris and fibrin fill the alveoli,

TABLE 15-4 Risk Factors for Aspiration/Aspiration-Related Pneumonia

RISK FACTOR	RATIONALE
Decreased LOC, either because of CNS problems or use of sedatives	Decreased ability to protect airway from oropharyngeal secretions and regurgitated gastric contents Cough and gag reflexes diminish as LOC diminishes, whether from CNS disorder or sedation. Slowed gastric emptying Decreased tone of lower esophageal sphincter
Supine position	Increases probability of gastroesophageal reflux
Presence of a nasogastric tube	Interferes with closure of lower esophageal sphincter Biofilm on tube predisposes to aspiration of pathogenic organisms.
Vomiting	Sudden and forceful entry of gastric contents into oropharynx predisposes to aspiration. Predisposes to displacement of feeding tube ports into esophagus
Feeding tube ports positioned in esophagus	Infused feedings reflux into oropharynx
Tracheal intubation	Reduction in upper airway defense related to ineffective cough, desensitization of the oropharynx and larynx, disuse atrophy of laryngeal muscles, and esophageal compression by an inflated cuff
Mechanical ventilation	Positive abdominal pressure predisposes to aspiration of gastric contents, probably by increasing gastroesophageal reflux.
Accumulation of subglottic secretions above endotracheal cuff	Subglottic secretions can leak around cuff into the lower respiratory tract, especially when cuff is deflated.
Inadequate cuff inflation of tracheal devices	Persistent low cuff pressure (e.g., 20 cm H_2O) predisposes to aspiration of oropharyngeal secretions and refluxed gastric contents.
Gastric feeding site when gastric emptying significantly impaired	Accumulation of formula and gastrointestinal secretions predisposes to gastroesophageal reflux and aspiration.
High GRVs	High GRVs predispose to gastroesophageal reflux and aspiration.
Bolus feedings	Volume of infused formula may exceed the tolerance of patients who have poor cough and gag reflexes.
Poor oral health	Colonized oropharyngeal secretions may be aspirated into respiratory tract.
Advanced age	Older patients tend to have a reduced swallowing ability and are more likely to have neurologic disorders that increase aspiration risks. Strong association between advanced age and probability of developing pneumonia once aspiration has occurred
Hyperglycemia	Even mild hyperglycemia can cause delayed gastric emptying by disrupting postprandial antral contractions.

CNS, central nervous system; *GRVs,* gastric residual volumes; *LOC,* level of consciousness.
From Metheny NA. Strategies to prevent aspiration-related pneumonia in tube-fed patients. *Respir Care Clin N Am.* 2006; 12:603.

hyaline membranes form, and hypoxic vasoconstriction occurs, resulting in elevated pulmonary artery pressures.[63,64] The clinical course will follow one of three patterns: 1) rapid improvement in 1 week, 2) initial improvement followed by deterioration and development of ARDS or pneumonia, or 3) rapid death from progressive ALF.[64]

Acid Food Particles

The aspiration of acid (pH less than 2.5) nonobstructing food particles can produce the most severe pulmonary reaction because of extensive pulmonary damage. Severe hypoxemia, hypercapnia, and acidosis occur.[63,64]

Nonacid Liquid

The aspiration of nonacid (pH greater than 2.5) liquid gastric contents is similar to acid liquid aspiration initially, but minimal structural damage occurs. Intrapulmonary shunting and V/Q mismatching usually start to reverse within 4 hours, and hypoxemia clears within 24 hours.[63,64]

Nonacid Food Particles

The aspiration of nonacid (pH greater than 2.5) nonobstructing food particles is similar to acid aspiration initially, with significant edema and hemorrhage occurring within 6 hours. After the initial reaction, the response changes to a foreign-body-type reaction, with granuloma formation occurring around the food particles within 1 to 5 days.[64] In addition to hypoxemia, hypercapnia and acidosis occur as a result of hypoventilation.[62,63]

Assessment and Diagnosis

Clinically, the patient presents with signs of acute respiratory distress, and gastric contents may be present in the oropharynx. The patient will have shortness of breath, coughing, wheezing, cyanosis, and signs of hypoxemia. Tachypnea, tachycardia, hypotension, fever, and crackles also are present. Copious amounts of sputum are produced as alveolar edema develops.[62,63]

ABGs reflect severe hypoxemia. Chest x-ray film changes appear 12 to 24 hours after the initial aspiration, with no one pattern being diagnostic of the event. Infiltrates will appear in a variety of distribution patterns, depending on the position of the patient during aspiration and the volume of the aspirate. If bacterial infection becomes established, leukocytosis and positive sputum cultures occur.[63]

Medical Management

Management of the patient with aspiration lung disorder includes both emergency and follow-up treatment. When aspiration is witnessed, emergency treatment should be instituted to secure the airway and minimize pulmonary damage. The patient's head should be turned to the side, and the oral cavity and upper airway should be suctioned immediately to remove the gastric contents.[63,64] Direct visualization by bronchoscopy is indicated to remove large particulate aspirate or to confirm an unwitnessed aspiration event. Bronchoalveolar lavage is not recommended because this practice disseminates the aspirate in lungs and increases damage.[64]

After airway clearance, attention should be given to supporting oxygenation and hemodynamics. Hypoxemia should be corrected with supplemental oxygen or mechanical ventilation with PEEP, if necessary.[63,64] Hemodynamic changes result from fluid shifts into the lungs that can occur after massive aspirations. Monitoring intravascular volume is essential, and judicious amounts of replacement fluids should be instituted to maintain adequate urinary output and vital signs.[63,64]

Empiric antibiotic therapy is usually not indicated following aspiration of gastric contents. However, if VAP is suspected or the aspiration event occurred in the presence of a small bowel obstruction or colonized gastric contents, then antibiotic therapy should be considered.[64] Corticosteroids have not demonstrated to be of any benefit in the treatment of aspiration pneumonitis and thus are not recommended.[63,64]

Nursing Management

Nursing management of the patient with aspiration lung disorder incorporates a variety of nursing diagnoses (Box 15-12). **Nursing priorities are directed toward 1) optimizing oxygenation and ventilation, 2) preventing further aspiration events, 3) providing comfort and emotional support, and 4) maintaining surveillance for complications.**

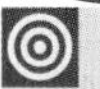 BOX 15-12 NURSING DIAGNOSES PRIORITIES

Aspiration Pneumonitis

- Impaired Gas Exchange related to ventilation/perfusion mismatching or intrapulmonary shunting, p. 594
- Ineffective Airway Clearance related to excessive secretions or abnormal viscosity of mucus, p. 597
- Risk for Aspiration, p. 602
- Risk for Infection, p. 607
- Anxiety related to threat to biologic, psychologic, or social integrity, p. 576
- Ineffective Coping related to situational crisis and personal vulnerability, p. 599
- Compromised Family Coping related to critically ill family member, p. 578

Optimizing Oxygenation and Ventilation

Nursing interventions to optimize oxygenation and ventilation include positioning, preventing desaturation, and promoting secretion clearance. For further discussion on these interventions, see Nursing Management of Acute Lung Failure earlier in this chapter.

Preventing Further Aspiration Events

One of the most important interventions for preventing aspiration is identifying the patient at risk for aspiration (Box 15-13). Actions to prevent aspiration include confirming feeding tube placement, checking for signs and symptoms of feeding intolerance, elevating the head of the bed at least 30 to 45 degrees, feeding the patient via a small-bore feeding tube or gastrostomy tube, avoiding the use of a large-bore

BOX 15-13 EVIDENCE-BASED (QSEN) PRACTICE ASPIRATION PREVENTION GUIDELINES

The following are the expected practice guidelines from the updated AACN Practice Alert: *Preventing Aspiration:*

1. Maintain head-of-bed elevation at an angle of 30 to 45 degrees, unless contraindicated. [Level B]
2. Use sedatives as sparingly as feasible. [Level C]
3. For tube-fed patients, assess placement of the feeding tube at 4-hour intervals. [Level C]
4. For patients receiving gastric tube feedings, assess for gastrointestinal intolerance to the feedings at 4-hour intervals. [Level C]
5. For tube-fed patients, avoid bolus feedings in those at high risk for aspiration. [Level E]
6. Consult with physician about obtaining a swallowing assessment before oral feedings are started for recently extubated patients who have experienced prolonged intubation. [Level C]
7. Maintain endotracheal cuff pressures at an appropriate level and ensure that secretions are cleared from above the cuff before it is deflated. [Level B]

Levels of Evidence:

Level A—Meta-analysis of quantitative studies or metasynthesis of qualitative studies with results that consistently support a specific action, intervention, or treatment

Level B—Well-designed, controlled studies with results that consistently support a specific action, intervention, or treatment

Level C—Qualitative studies, descriptive or correlational studies, integrative reviews, systematic reviews, or randomized controlled trials with inconsistent results

Level D—Peer-reviewed professional and organizational standards with the support of clinical study recommendations

Level E—Multiple case reports, theory-based evidence from expert opinions, or peer-reviewed professional organizational standards without clinical studies to support recommendations

Level M—Manufacturer's recommendations only

Modified from American Association of Critical-Care Nurses. *AACN Practice Alert: Preventing Aspiration.* http://www.aacn.org/wd/practice/content/practicealerts/aspiration-practice-alert.pcms?menu=practice; 2011. Accessed May 14, 2014.

BOX 15-14 COLLABORATIVE MANAGEMENT

Aspiration Pneumonitis

- Administer oxygen therapy.
- Secure the patient's airway.
- Place patient in slight Trendelenburg position.
- Turn patient to right lateral decubitus position.
- Suction patient's oropharyngeal area.
- Initiate mechanical ventilation as required.
- Maintain surveillance for complications:
  - Pneumonia
  - Acute lung failure
  - Acute respiratory distress syndrome
- Provide comfort and emotional support.

nasogastric tube, ensuring proper inflation of artificial airway cuffs, and frequent suctioning of the oropharynx of an intubated patient to prevent secretions from pooling above the cuff of the tube. For patients at risk for aspiration or intolerant of gastric feedings, the feeding tube should be placed in the distal duodenum or jejunum.[65]

Collaborative management of the patient with aspiration pneumonitis is outlined in Box 15-14.

ACUTE PULMONARY EMBOLISM

Description and Etiology

A pulmonary embolism (PE) occurs when a clot (thrombotic embolus) or other matter (nonthrombotic embolus) lodges in the pulmonary arterial system, disrupting the blood flow to a region of the lungs (Figure 15-4). The majority of thrombotic emboli arise from the deep leg veins, particularly the iliac and femoral veins.[66] Other sources include the right ventricle, the upper extremities, and the pelvic veins. Nonthrombotic emboli arise from fat, tumors, amniotic fluid, air, and foreign bodies. This section of the chapter focuses on thrombotic emboli.

A number of predisposing factors and precipitating conditions put a patient at risk for developing a PE (Box 15-15). Of the three predisposing factors (i.e., hypercoagulability, injury to vascular endothelium, and venous stasis [Virchow's triad]), endothelial injury appears to be the most significant.[66]

The American Heart Association (AHA) has developed a classification for an acute PE, which stratifies the patients into one of three categories: massive, submassive, or low-risk. A massive PE is defined as an acute PE with sustained hypotension (systolic blood pressure <90 mm Hg) for greater than 15 minutes, the need for inotropes not based on other causes, or signs of shock. A submassive PE is defined as an acute PE with evidence of right ventricular (RV) dysfunction or myocardial necrosis. A patient with none of these conditions is defined as low-risk.[67]

Pathophysiology

A massive PE occurs with the blockage of a lobar or larger artery, resulting in occlusion of the pulmonary vascular bed. Blockage of the pulmonary arterial system has both pulmonary and hemodynamic consequences.[66] The effects on the pulmonary system are increased alveolar dead space, bronchoconstriction, and compensatory shunting.[68] The hemodynamic effects include an increase in pulmonary vascular resistance and right ventricular workload.[69,70]

BOX 15-15 Risk Factors for Pulmonary Thromboembolism

Predisposing Factors

Venous stasis
- Atrial fibrillation
- Decreased cardiac output (CO)
- Immobility

Injury to vascular endothelium
- Local vessel injury
- Infection
- Incision
- Atherosclerosis

Hypercoagulability
- Polycythemia

Precipitating Conditions

Previous pulmonary embolus

Cardiovascular disease
- Heart failure
- Right ventricular infarction
- Cardiomyopathy
- Cor pulmonale

Surgery
- Orthopedic
- Vascular
- Abdominal

Cancer
- Ovarian
- Pancreatic
- Stomach
- Extrahepatic bile duct system

Trauma (injury or burns)
- Lower extremities
- Pelvis
- Hips

Gynecologic status
- Pregnancy
- Postpartum
- Birth control pills
- Estrogen replacement therapy

Increased Dead Space

An increase in alveolar dead space occurs because an area of the lung is receiving ventilation without being perfused. The ventilation to this area is known as *wasted ventilation* because it does not participate in gas exchange. This effect leads to alveolar dead space ventilation and an increase in the work of breathing. To limit the amount of dead space ventilation, localized bronchoconstriction occurs.[70]

Bronchoconstriction

Bronchoconstriction develops as a result of alveolar hypocarbia, hypoxia, and the release of mediators. Alveolar hypocarbia occurs as a consequence of decreased carbon dioxide in the affected area and leads to constriction of the local airways, increased airway resistance, and redistribution of ventilation to perfused areas of the lungs. A variety of mediators are released

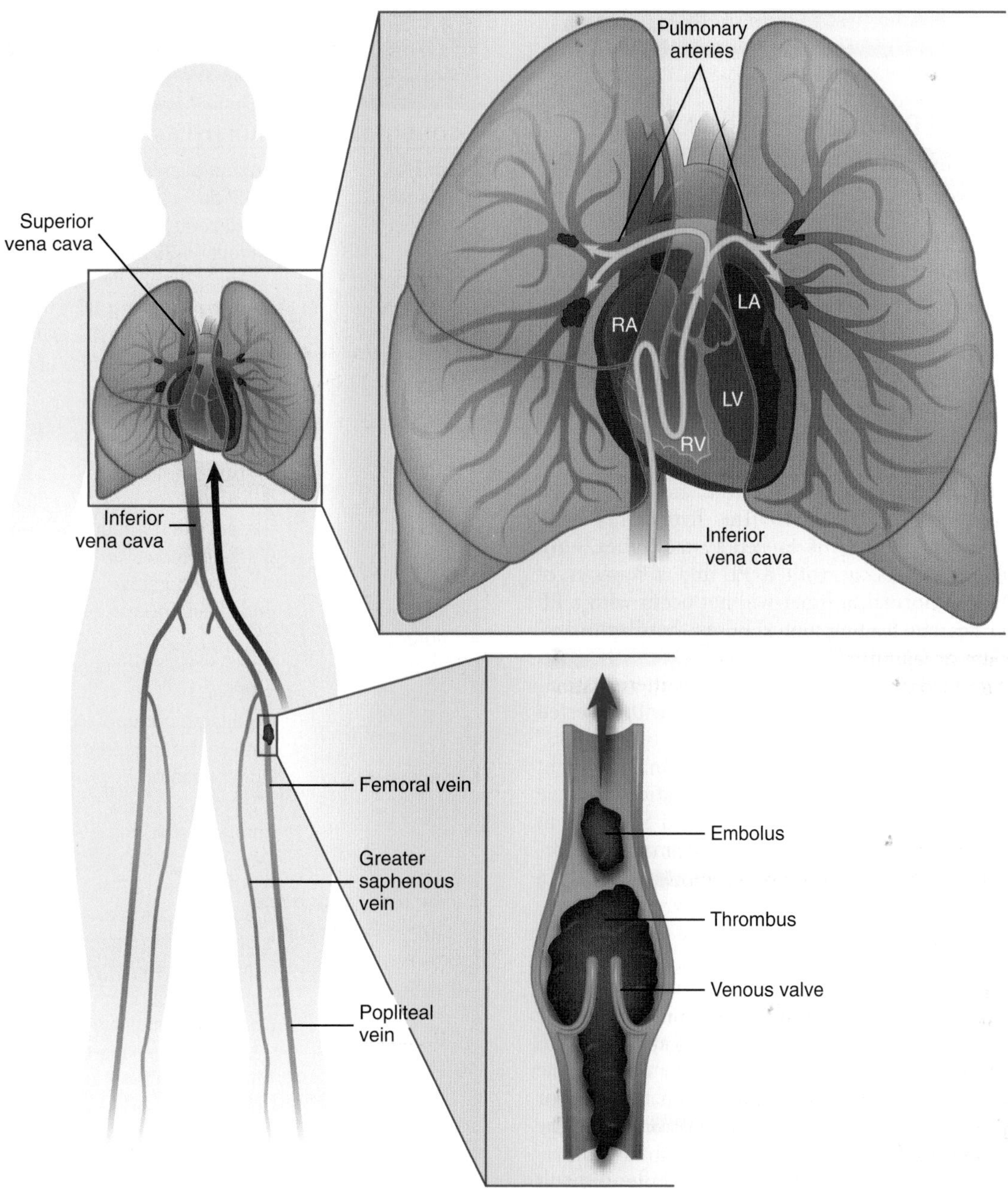

FIG 15-4 Pathophysiology of Pulmonary Embolism. Pulmonary embolism usually originates from the deep veins of the legs, most commonly the calf veins. These venous thrombi originate predominantly in venous valve pockets and at other sites of presumed venous stasis (inset, bottom). If a clot propagates to the knee vein or above, or if it originates above the knee, the risk of embolism increases. Thromboemboli travel through the right side of the heart to reach the lungs. *LA,* left atrium; *LV,* left ventricle; *RA,* right atrium; *RV,* right ventricle. (Modified from Tapson VF. Acute pulmonary embolism. *N Engl J Med.* 2008;358:1037.)

from the site of the injury, either from the clot or the surrounding lung tissue, which further causes constriction of the airways. Bronchoconstriction promotes the development of atelectasis.[70]

Compensatory Shunting

Compensatory shunting occurs as a result of the unaffected areas of the lungs having to accommodate the entire CO. This creates a situation in which perfusion exceeds ventilation and blood is returned to the left side of the heart without participating in gas exchange. This leads to the development of hypoxemia.[70]

Hemodynamic Consequences

The major hemodynamic consequence of a PE is the development of pulmonary hypertension, which is part of the effect of a mechanical obstruction when more than 50% of the vascular bed is occluded. In addition, the mediators released at the injury site and the development of hypoxia cause pulmonary vasoconstriction, which further exacerbates pulmonary hypertension. As the pulmonary vascular resistance increases, so does the workload of the right ventricle as reflected by a rise in pulmonary artery (PA) pressures.

Consequently, right ventricular failure occurs, which can lead to decreases in left ventricular preload, CO, and blood pressure, and to shock.[66,68-70]

Assessment and Diagnosis

The patient with a PE may have any number of presenting signs and symptoms, with the most common being tachycardia and tachypnea. Additional signs and symptoms that may be present include dyspnea, apprehension, increased pulmonic component of the second heart sound (P_1), fever, crackles, pleuritic chest pain, cough, evidence of deep vein thrombosis (DVT), and hemoptysis.[66] Syncope and hemodynamic instability can occur as a result of right ventricular failure.[69]

Initial laboratory studies and diagnostic procedures that may be done are ABG analysis, D-dimer, electrocardiogram (ECG), chest radiography, and echocardiography (ECHO). ABGs may show a low PaO_2, indicating hypoxemia; a low $PaCO_2$, indicating hypocarbia, and a high pH, indicating a respiratory alkalosis. The hypocarbia with resulting respiratory alkalosis is caused by tachypnea.[68] An elevated D-dimer will occur with a PE and a number of other disorders. A normal D-dimer will not occur with a PE and thus can be used to rule out a PE as the diagnosis.[66] The most frequent ECG finding seen in the patient with a PE is sinus tachycardia.[66] The classic ECG pattern associated with a PE—S wave in lead I and Q wave with inverted T wave in lead III—is seen in fewer than 20% of patients.[69] Other ECG findings associated with a PE include right bundle branch block, new-onset atrial fibrillation, T-wave inversion in the anterior or inferior leads, and ST segment changes.[70] Chest x-ray findings vary from normal to abnormal and are of little value in confirming the presence of a PE. Abnormal findings include cardiomegaly, pleural effusion, elevated hemidiaphragm, enlargement of the right descending pulmonary artery (Palla's sign), a wedge-shaped density above the diaphragm (Hampton's hump), and the presence of atelectasis.[68] An ECHO, either transthoracic or transesophageal, is also useful in the identification of a PE because it can provide visualization of any emboli in the central pulmonary arteries. In addition, it can be used for assessing the hemodynamic consequences of the PE on the right side of the heart.[70]

Differentiating a PE from other illnesses can be difficult because many of its clinical manifestations are found in a variety of other disorders.[67] Thus, a variety of other tests may be necessary, including a V/Q scintigraphy, pulmonary angiogram, and DVT studies.[66,78,70] Given the advent of more sophisticated CT scanners, the spiral CT is also being used to diagnose a PE.[68-70] A definitive diagnosis of a PE requires confirmation by a high-probability V/Q scan, an abnormal pulmonary angiogram or CT, or strong clinical suspicion coupled with abnormal findings on lower extremity DVT studies.[68]

Medical Management

Medical management of the patient with a PE involves both prevention and treatment strategies. Prevention strategies include the use of prophylactic anticoagulation with low-dose or adjusted-dose heparin, LMWH, or oral anticoagulants (Table 15-5). The use of pneumatic compression has also been demonstrated as an effective method of prophylaxis in low-risk patients.[24]

TABLE 15-5 Regimens for Venous Thromboembolism Prophylaxis

CONDITION	PROPHYLAXIS
General surgery	Unfractionated heparin 5000 units SC TID or Enoxaparin 40 mg SC QD or Dalteparin 2500 or 5000 units SC QD
Orthopedic surgery	Warfarin (target INR 2.0 to 3.0) or Enoxaparin 30 mg SC BID or Enoxaparin 40 mg SC QD or Dalteparin 2500 or 5000 units SC QD or Fondaparinux 2.5 mg SC QD
Neurosurgery	Unfractionated heparin 5000 units SC BID or Enoxaparin 40 mg SC QD and Graduated compression stockings/ intermittent pneumatic compression Consider surveillance lower extremity ultrasonography
Oncological surgery	Enoxaparin 40 mg SC QD
Thoracic surgery	Unfractionated heparin 5000 units SC TID and Graduated compression stockings/ intermittent pneumatic compression
Medical patients	Unfractionated heparin 5000 units SC TID or Enoxaparin 40 mg SC QD or Dalteparin 5000 units SC QD or Fondaparinux 2.5 mg SC QD or Graduated compression stockings/ intermittent pneumatic compression for patients with contraindications to anticoagulation Consider combination pharmacological and mechanical prophylaxis for very high-risk patients Consider surveillance lower extremity ultrasonography for intensive care unit patients

INR, International normalized ratio; *SC*, subcutaneous; *TID*, 3 times daily; *QD*, daily; *BID*, twice daily.
From Piazza G, Goldhaber SZ. Acute pulmonary embolism: part II treatment and prophylaxis. *Circulation.* 2006; 114(3):e42.

Treatment strategies include preventing the recurrence of a PE, facilitating clot dissolution, reversing the effects of pulmonary hypertension, promoting gas exchange, and preventing complications. Medical interventions to promote gas exchange include supplemental oxygen administration, intubation, and mechanical ventilation.[67]

Prevention of Recurrence

Interventions to prevent the recurrence of a PE include the administration of UFH, fondaparinux, LMWH, and warfarin (Coumadin).[69] Heparin is administered to prevent further clots from forming and has no effect on the existing clot. The heparin should be adjusted to maintain the activated partial thromboplastin time (aPTT) in the range of 2 to 3 times of upper normal.[69] Warfarin should be started at the same time, and when the international normalized ratio (INR) reaches 3.0, the heparin should be discontinued. The INR should be maintained between 2.0 and 3.0. The patient should remain on warfarin for 3 to 12 months, depending on his or her risk for thromboembolic disease.[69]

Interruption of the inferior vena cava is reserved for patients in whom anticoagulation is contraindicated. The procedure involves placement of a percutaneous venous filter (e.g., Greenfield filter) into the vena cava, usually below the renal arteries. The filter prevents further thrombotic emboli from migrating into the lungs.[71]

Clot Dissolution

The administration of fibrinolytic agents in the treatment of PE has had limited success. Currently, fibrinolytic therapy is reserved for the patient with a massive acute PE. Either recombinant tissue-type plasminogen activator (rt-PA) or streptokinase may be used. The therapeutic window for using fibrinolytic therapy is up to 14 days, though the most benefit is usually obtained when given within 48 hours.[72]

If the fibrinolytic therapy is contraindicated, a pulmonary embolectomy may be performed to remove the clot. Generally, it is performed as an open procedure while the patient is on cardiopulmonary bypass. An emerging alternative to surgical embolectomy is catheter embolectomy. It appears to be particularly useful if surgical embolectomy is not available or is contraindicated. It appears to be most successful when performed within 5 days of the occurrence of the PE.[73]

Reversal of Pulmonary Hypertension

To reverse the hemodynamic effects of pulmonary hypertension, additional measures may be taken. These include the administration of inotropic agents and fluid. Fluids should be administered to increase right ventricular preload, which would stretch the right ventricle and increase contractility, thus overcoming the elevated pulmonary arterial pressures. Inotropic agents also can be used to increase contractility to facilitate an increase in CO.[69,70]

Nursing Management

Prevention of PE should be a major nursing focus because the majority of critically ill patients are at risk for this disorder. Nursing actions are aimed at preventing the development of DVT (Box 15-16), which is a major complication of immobility and a leading cause of PE. These measures include the use of pneumatic compression devices, active/passive range-of-motion exercises involving foot extension, adequate hydration, and progressive ambulation.[24]

Nursing management of the patient with a PE incorporates a variety of nursing diagnoses (Box 15-17). **Nursing priorities are directed toward 1) optimizing oxygenation and ventilation, 2) monitoring for bleeding, 3) providing comfort and emotional support, 4) maintaining surveillance for complications, and 5) educating the patient and family.**

Optimizing Oxygenation and Ventilation

Nursing interventions to optimize oxygenation and ventilation include positioning, preventing desaturation, and promoting secretion clearance. For further discussion on these

BOX 15-16 EVIDENCE-BASED (QSEN) PRACTICE VENOUS THROMBOEMBOLISM PREVENTION GUIDELINES

The following are the expected practice guidelines from the updated AACN Practice Alert: *Venous Thromboembolism Prevention:*

1. Assess all patients upon admission to the critical care unit for risk factors of venous thromboembolism (VTE) and anticipate orders for VTE prophylaxis based on risk assessment. [Level D]
2. Clinical eligibility and regimens for VTE prophylaxis include
   - Moderate-risk patients (medically ill and postoperative patients): low-dose unfractionated heparin, LMWH, or fondaparinux [Level B]
   - High-risk patients (major trauma, spinal cord injury, or orthopedic surgery): LMWH, fondaparinux, or oral vitamin K antagonist [Level B]
   - Patients with high risk for bleeding: mechanical prophylaxis including graduated compression stockings and/or intermittent pneumatic compression devices [Level B]
   - Mechanical prophylaxis may also be anticipated in conjunction with anticoagulant-based prophylaxis regimens.
3. Review daily—with the physician and during multidisciplinary rounds—each patient's current VTE risk factors including clinical status, necessity for central venous catheter (CVC), current status of VTE prophylaxis, risk for bleeding, and response to treatment. [Level E]
4. Maximize patient mobility whenever possible and take measures to reduce the amount of time the patient is immobile because of the effects of treatment (e.g., pain, sedation, neuromuscular blockade, mechanical ventilation). [Level E]
5. Ensure that mechanical prophylaxis devices are fitted properly and in use at all times except when being removed for cleaning and/or inspection of skin. [Level E]

Levels of Evidence:

Level A—Meta-analysis of quantitative studies or metasynthesis of qualitative studies with results that consistently support a specific action, intervention, or treatment

Level B—Well-designed, controlled studies with results that consistently support a specific action, intervention, or treatment

Level C—Qualitative studies, descriptive or correlational studies, integrative reviews, systematic reviews, or randomized controlled trials with inconsistent results

Level D—Peer-reviewed professional and organizational standards with the support of clinical study recommendations

Level E—Multiple case reports, theory-based evidence from expert opinions, or peer-reviewed professional organizational standards without clinical studies to support recommendations

Level M—Manufacturer's recommendations only

Modified from American Association of Critical-Care Nurses. *AACN Practice Alert: Venous Thromboembolism Prevention.* http://www.aacn.org/WD/Practice/Docs/PracticeAlerts/VTE%20Prevention%2004-2010%20final.pdf; 2010. Accessed May 14, 2014.

BOX 15-17 NURSING DIAGNOSIS PRIORITIES

Pulmonary Embolus

- Impaired Gas Exchange related to ventilation/perfusion mismatching or intrapulmonary shunting, p. 594
- Decreased cardiac output related to afterload, p. 580
- Acute Pain related to transmission and perception of cutaneous, visceral, muscular, or ischemic impulses, p. 574
- Anxiety related to threat to biologic, psychologic, or social integrity, p. 576
- Deficient Knowledge: Discharge Regimen related to lack of previous exposure to information, p. 585 (see Box 15-18, Patient Education for Pulmonary Embolus).

BOX 15-18 PATIENT EDUCATION PRIORITIES

Pulmonary Embolus

- Pathophysiology of disease
- Specific etiology
- Precipitating factor modification
- Measures to prevent deep vein thrombosis (DVT) (e.g., avoid tight-fitting clothes, crossing legs, and prolonged sitting or standing; elevate legs when sitting; exercise)
- Signs and symptoms of DVT (e.g., redness, swelling, sharp or deep leg pain)
- Importance of taking medications
- Signs and symptoms of anticoagulant complications (e.g., excessive bruising, discoloration of the skin, changes in color of urine or stools)
- Measures to prevent bleeding (e.g., use soft-bristle toothbrush, caution when shaving)

Additional information for the patient can be found at the following websites:

Vascular Web: http://www.vascularweb.org/vascularhealth/Pages/pulmonary-embolism.aspx

Healthfinder—U.S. Department of Health and Human Services: http://healthfinder.gov

WebMD: http://www.webmd.com

interventions, see Nursing Management of Acute Lung Failure earlier in this chapter.

Monitoring for Bleeding

The patient receiving anticoagulant or fibrinolytic therapy should be observed for signs of bleeding. The patient's gums, skin, urine, stool, and emesis should be screened for signs of overt or covert bleeding. In addition, monitoring the patient's INR or aPTT is critical to managing the anticoagulation therapy.

Educating the Patient and Family

Early in the patient's hospital stay, the patient and family should be taught about pulmonary embolus, its etiologies, and its treatment (Box 15-18). As the patient moves toward discharge, teaching should focus on the interventions necessary for preventing the reoccurrence of DVT and subsequent emboli, signs and symptoms of DVT and anticoagulant

BOX 15-19 COLLABORATIVE MANAGEMENT

Pulmonary Embolus

- Administer oxygen therapy.
- Intubate patient.
- Initiate mechanical ventilation.
- Administer medications:
  - Fibrinolytic therapy
  - Anticoagulants
  - Bronchodilators
  - Inotropic agents
  - Sedatives
  - Analgesics
- Administer fluids.
- Position patient to optimize ventilation/perfusion matching.
- Maintain surveillance for complications:
  - Bleeding
  - Acute respiratory distress syndrome
- Provide comfort and emotional support.

complications, and measures to prevent bleeding. If the patient smokes, he or she should be encouraged to stop smoking and be referred to a smoking cessation program.

Collaborative management of the patient with a pulmonary embolus is outlined Box 15-19.

STATUS ASTHMATICUS

Description and Etiology

Asthma is a COPD that is characterized by partially reversible airflow obstruction, airway inflammation, and hyperresponsiveness to a variety of stimuli.[74] Status asthmaticus is a severe asthma attack that fails to respond to conventional therapy with bronchodilators, which may result in ALF.[75,76] The precipitating cause of the attack is usually an upper respiratory infection, allergen exposure, or a decrease in anti-inflammatory medications. Other factors that have been implicated include overreliance on bronchodilators, environmental pollutants, lack of access to health care, failure to identify worsening airflow obstruction, and noncompliance with the health care regimen.[75]

Pathophysiology

An asthma attack is initiated when exposure to an irritant or trigger occurs, resulting in the initiation of the inflammatory-immune response in the airways. Bronchospasm occurs along with increased vascular permeability and increased mucus production. Mucosal edema and thick, tenacious mucus further increase airway responsiveness. The combination of bronchospasm, airway inflammation, and hyperresponsiveness results in narrowing of the airways and airflow obstruction. These changes have significant effects on the pulmonary and cardiovascular systems.[75]

Pulmonary Effects

As the diameter of the airways decreases, airway resistance increases, resulting in increased residual volume, hyperinflation of the lungs, increased work of breathing, and abnormal distribution of ventilation. V/Q mismatching occurs, which results in hypoxemia. Alveolar dead space also increases as hypoxic vasoconstriction occurs, resulting in hypercapnia.[75]

Cardiovascular Effects

Inspiratory muscle force also increases in an attempt to ventilate the hyperinflated lungs. This results in a significant increase in negative intrapleural pressure, leading to an increase in venous return and pooling of blood in the right ventricle. The stretched right ventricle causes the intraventricular septum to shift, thereby impinging on the left ventricle. In addition, the left ventricle has to work harder to pump blood from the markedly negative pressure in the thorax to elevated pressure in systemic circulation. This leads to a decrease in CO and a fall in systolic blood pressure on inspiration (pulsus paradoxus).[75]

Assessment and Diagnosis

Initially, the patient may present with a cough, wheezing, and dyspnea. As the attack continues, the patient develops tachypnea, tachycardia, diaphoresis, increased accessory muscle use, and pulsus paradoxus greater than 25 mm Hg. Decreased level of consciousness, inability to speak, significantly diminished or absent breath sounds, and inability to lie supine herald the onset of ALF.[74-76]

Initial ABGs indicate hypocapnia and respiratory alkalosis caused by hyperventilation. As the attack continues and the patient starts to fatigue, hypoxemia and hypercapnia develop.[76] Lactic acidosis also may occur as a result of lactate overproduction by the respiratory muscles. The end result is the development of respiratory and metabolic acidosis.[77]

Deterioration of pulmonary function tests despite aggressive bronchodilator therapy is diagnostic of status asthmaticus and indicates the potential need for intubation. A peak expiratory flow rate (PEFR) less than 40% of predicted or forced expiratory volume in 1 second (FEV_1; maximum volume of gas that the patient can exhale in 1 second) less than 20% of predicted indicates severe airflow obstruction, and the need for intubation with mechanical ventilation may be imminent.[78]

Medical Management

Medical management of the patient with status asthmaticus is directed toward supporting oxygenation and ventilation. Bronchodilators, corticosteroids, oxygen therapy, and intubation and mechanical ventilation are the mainstays of therapy.[76]

Bronchodilators

Inhaled $beta_2$-agonists and anticholinergics are the bronchodilators of choice for status asthmaticus. $Beta_2$-agonists promote bronchodilation and can be administered by nebulizer or metered-dose inhaler (MDI). Usually larger and more frequent doses are given, and the medication is titrated to the patient's response. Anticholinergics that inhibit bronchoconstriction are not very effective by themselves, but in conjunction with $beta_2$-agonists, they have a synergistic effect and produce a greater improvement in airflow. The routine use of xanthines is not recommended in the treatment of status asthmaticus because they have been shown to have no therapeutic benefit.[75-78]

A number of studies have focused on the bronchodilator abilities of magnesium. Although it has been demonstrated that magnesium is inferior to $beta_2$-agonists as a bronchodilator, in patients who are refractory to conventional treatment, magnesium may be beneficial. A bolus of 1 to 4 g of intravenous magnesium given over 10 to 40 minutes has been reported to produce desirable effects.[75,76,78]

A number of other studies are evaluating the effects of leukotriene inhibitors, such as zafirlukast, montelukast, and zileuton, in the treatment of status asthmaticus. Leukotrienes are inflammatory mediators known to cause bronchoconstriction and airway inflammation. Research suggests that these agents may be beneficial as bronchodilators in those patients who are refractory to $beta_2$-agonists.[78]

Systemic Corticosteroids

Intravenous or oral corticosteroids also are used in the treatment of status asthmaticus. Their anti-inflammatory effects limit mucosal edema, decrease mucus production, and potentiate $beta_2$-agonists. It usually takes 6 to 8 hours for the effects of the corticosteroids to become evident.[76] The use of inhaled corticosteroids for the treatment of status asthmaticus remains undecided at this time.[75,76] Initial studies indicate they may be beneficial in certain patient populations.[76]

Oxygen Therapy

Initial treatment of hypoxemia is with supplemental oxygen. High-flow oxygen therapy is administered to keep the patient's SpO_2 greater than 92%.[75] Another therapy currently under investigation is the use of heliox. A mixture of helium and oxygen, heliox has a lower density and higher viscosity than an oxygen and air mixture. Heliox is believed to reduce the work of breathing and improve gas exchange because it flows more easily through constricted areas. Studies have shown that it reduces air trapping and carbon dioxide and helps relieve respiratory acidosis.[75]

Intubation and Mechanical Ventilation

Indications for mechanical ventilation include cardiac or respiratory arrest, disorientation, failure to respond to bronchodilator therapy, and exhaustion.[75,77,78] A large endotracheal tube (8 mm) should be used to decrease airway resistance and to facilitate suctioning of secretions. Ventilating the patient with status asthmaticus can be very difficult. High inflation pressures should be avoided because they can result in barotrauma. The use of PEEP should be monitored closely because the patient is prone to developing air trapping. Patient–ventilator asynchrony also can be a major problem. Sedation and neuromuscular paralysis may be necessary to allow for adequate ventilation of the patient.[75,77]

Nursing Management

Nursing management of the patient with status asthmaticus incorporates a variety of nursing diagnoses (Box 15-20). **Nursing priorities are directed toward 1) optimizing oxygenation and ventilation, 2) providing comfort and emotional support, 3) maintaining surveillance for complications, and 4) educating the patient and family.**

Optimizing Oxygenation and Ventilation

Nursing interventions to optimize oxygenation and ventilation include positioning, preventing desaturation, and promoting secretion clearance. For further discussion on these interventions, see Nursing Management of Acute Lung Failure earlier in this chapter.

BOX 15-20 NURSING DIAGNOSIS PRIORITIES

Status Asthmaticus

- Impaired Gas Exchange related to alveolar hypoventilation, p. 593
- Impaired Gas Exchange related to ventilation/perfusion mismatching or intrapulmonary shunting, p. 594
- Ineffective Airway Clearance related to excessive secretions or abnormal viscosity of mucus, p. 597
- Anxiety related to threat to biologic, psychologic, or social integrity, p. 576
- Deficient Knowledge: Discharge Regimen related to lack of previous exposure to information, p. 585 (see Box 15-21, Patient Education for Status Asthmaticus)

BOX 15-21 PATIENT EDUCATION PRIORITIES

Status Asthmaticus

- Pathophysiology of disease
- Specific etiology
- Early warning signs of worsening airflow obstruction (20% drop in peak expiratory flow rate [PEFR] below predicted or personal best, increase in cough, shortness of breath, chest tightness, wheezing)
- Treatment of attacks
- Importance of taking prescribed medications and avoidance of over-the-counter asthma medications
- Correct use of an inhaler (with and without spacer device)
- Correct use of a peak flow meter
- Removal or avoidance of environmental triggers (e.g., pollen; dust; mold spores; cat and dog dander; cold, dry air; strong odors; household aerosols; tobacco smoke; air pollution)
- Measures to prevent pulmonary infections (e.g., proper nutrition and hand washing, immunization against *Streptococcus pneumoniae* and influenza viruses)
- Signs and symptoms of pulmonary infection (e.g., sputum color change, shortness of breath, fever)
- Importance of participating in pulmonary rehabilitation program

Additional information for the patient can be found at the following websites:

Asthma and Allergy Foundation of America: http://www.aafa.org

American Lung Association: http://www.lung.org

Healthfinder—US Department of Health and Human Services: http://healthfinder.gov

WebMD: http://www.webmd.com

Educating the Patient and Family

Early in the patient's hospital stay, the patient and family should be taught about asthma, its triggers, and its treatment (Box 15-21). As the patient moves toward discharge, teaching should focus on the interventions necessary for preventing the recurrence of status asthmaticus, early warning signs of worsening airflow obstruction, correct use of an inhaler and a peak flowmeter, measures to prevent pulmonary infections,

BOX 15-22 COLLABORATIVE MANAGEMENT

Status Asthmaticus

- Administer oxygen therapy. Intubate patient.
- Initiate mechanical ventilation.
- Administer medications:
  - Bronchodilators
  - Corticosteroids
  - Sedatives
- Maintain surveillance for complications:
  - Acute lung failure
- Provide comfort and emotional support.

and signs and symptoms of a pulmonary infection. If the patient smokes, he or she should be encouraged to stop smoking and be referred to a smoking cessation program. In addition, the importance of participating in a pulmonary rehabilitation program should be stressed.

Collaborative management of the patient with status asthmaticus is outlined in Box 15-22.

LONG-TERM MECHANICAL VENTILATOR DEPENDENCE

Description and Etiology

Long-term mechanical ventilator dependence (LTMVD) is a secondary disorder that occurs when a patient requires assisted ventilation longer than expected, given the patient's underlying condition.[79] It is the result of complex medical problems that do not allow the weaning process to take place in a normal and timely manner. A review of the literature reveals a great deal of confusion regarding an exact definition of LTMVD, particularly in regard to an actual time frame. In 2005, the National Association for Medical Direction of Respiratory Care (NAMDRC) Consensus Panel recommended that LTMVD (which they referred to as prolonged mechanical ventilation) be defined as "the need for ≥21 consecutive days of mechanical ventilation for ≥6 hours per day."[80]

Pathophysiology

A wide variety of physiologic and psychologic factors contribute to the development of LTMVD. Physiologic factors include those conditions that result in decreased gas exchange, increased ventilatory workload, increased ventilatory demand, decreased ventilatory drive, and increased respiratory muscle fatigue (Box 15-23).[79,81] Psychologic factors include those conditions that result in loss of breathing pattern control, lack of motivation and confidence, and delirium (Box 15-24).[82] The development of LTMVD also is affected by the severity and duration of the patient's current illness and any underlying chronic health problems.[83]

Medical and Nursing Management

The goal of medical and nursing management of the patient with LTMVD is successful weaning. The Third National Study Group on Weaning from Mechanical Ventilation, sponsored by the American Association of Critical-Care Nurses,

BOX 15-23 Physiologic Factors Contributing to Long-Term Mechanical Ventilation Dependence

- Decreased gas exchange
  - Ventilation/perfusion mismatching
  - Intrapulmonary shunting
  - Alveolar hypoventilation
  - Anemia
  - Acute heart failure
- Increased ventilatory workload
  - Decreased lung compliance
  - Increased airway resistance
  - Small endotracheal tube
  - Decreased ventilatory sensitivity
  - Improper positioning
  - Abdominal distention
  - Dyspnea
- Increased ventilatory demand
  - Increased pulmonary dead space
  - Increased metabolic demands
  - Improper ventilator mode/settings
  - Metabolic acidosis
  - Overfeeding
- Decreased ventilatory drive
  - Respiratory alkalosis
  - Metabolic alkalosis
  - Hypothyroidism
  - Sedatives
- Malnutrition
- Increased respiratory muscle fatigue
  - Increased ventilatory workload
  - Increased ventilatory demand
  - Malnutrition
  - Hypokalemia
  - Hypomagnesemia
  - Hypophosphatemia
  - Hypothyroidism
  - Critical illness polyneuropathy
  - Inadequate muscle rest

BOX 15-24 Psychologic Factors Contributing to Long-Term Mechanical Ventilation Dependence

- Loss of breathing pattern control
  - Anxiety
  - Fear
  - Dyspnea
  - Pain
  - Ventilator asynchrony
  - Lack of confidence in ability to breathe
- Lack of motivation and confidence
  - Inadequate trust in staff
  - Depersonalization
  - Hopelessness
  - Powerlessness
  - Depression
  - Inadequate communication
- Delirium
  - Sensory overload
  - Sensory deprivation
  - Sleep deprivation
  - Pain
  - Medications

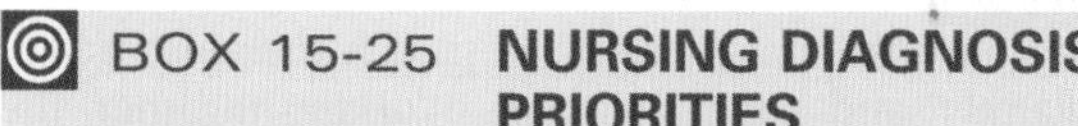

BOX 15-25 NURSING DIAGNOSIS PRIORITIES

Long-Term Mechanical Ventilation Dependence

- Impaired Spontaneous Ventilation related to respiratory muscle fatigue or neuromuscular impairment, p. 594
- Dysfunctional Ventilatory Weaning Response related to physical, psychosocial, or situational factors, p. 588
- Imbalanced Nutrition: Less Than Body Requirements related to lack of exogenous nutrients or increased metabolic demand, p. 593
- Risk for Infection, p. 607
- Relocation Stress Syndrome related to transfer out of the intensive care unit, p. 601

proposed the Weaning Continuum Model, which divides weaning into three stages: preweaning, weaning process, and weaning outcome.[84] It is within this framework that the management of the long-term ventilator-dependent patient is described. In addition, priority nursing diagnoses for this patient population are listed in Box 15-25.

Preweaning Stage

For the long-term ventilator-dependent patient, the preweaning phase consists of resolving the precipitating event that necessitated ventilatory assistance and preventing the physiologic and psychologic factors that can interfere with weaning. Before any attempts at weaning, the patient should be assessed for weaning readiness, an approach should be determined, and a method should be selected.[82,83]

The patient should be physiologically and psychologically prepared to initiate the weaning process by addressing those factors that can interfere with weaning. Aggressive medical management to prevent and treat V/Q mismatching, intrapulmonary shunting, anemia, heart failure, decreased lung compliance, increased airway resistance, acid–base disturbances, hypothyroidism, abdominal distention, and electrolyte imbalances should be initiated. In addition, interventions to decrease the work of breathing should be implemented, such as replacing a small endotracheal tube with a larger tube or a tracheostomy, suctioning airway secretions, administering bronchodilators, optimizing the ventilator settings and trigger sensitivity, and positioning the patient in straight alignment with the head of the bed elevated at least 30 degrees. Enteral or parenteral nutrition should be started and the patient's nutritional state optimized. Physical therapy should be initiated for the patient with critical illness polyneuropathy because increased mobility facilitates weaning. A means of communication should be established with the patient. Sedatives can be administered to provide anxiety control, but the avoidance of respiratory depression is critical.[85]

Although a variety of different methods for assessing weaning readiness have been developed, none has proved to be very accurate in predicting weaning success in the patient with LTMVD. One study did indicate that the presence of left ventricular dysfunction, fluid imbalance, and nutritional deficiency increased the duration of mechanical ventilation. Another study suggested that the upward trending of the albumin level may be predictive of weaning success. Because so many variables can affect the patient's ability to wean, any assessment of weaning readiness should incorporate these variables. Cardiac function, gas exchange, pulmonary mechanics, nutritional status, electrolyte and fluid balance, and motivation should all be considered when making the decision to wean. This assessment should be ongoing to reflect the dynamic nature of the process.[86]

Although weaning the patient requiring short-term mechanical ventilation is a relatively simple process that can usually be accomplished with a nurse and respiratory therapist, weaning the patient with LTMVD is a much more complex process that usually requires a multidisciplinary team approach. Multidisciplinary weaning teams that use a coordinated and collaborative approach to weaning have demonstrated improved patient outcomes and decreased weaning times. The team should consist of a physician, a nurse, a respiratory therapist, a dietitian, a physical therapist, and a case manager, a clinical outcomes manager, or a clinical nurse specialist. Additional members, if possible, should include an occupational therapist, a speech therapist, a discharge planner, and a social worker. Working together, the team members should develop a comprehensive plan of care for the patient that is efficient, consistent, progressive, and cost-effective.[87] Several studies have demonstrated successful weaning through the use of nurse and respiratory therapist-managed protocols.[88]

A variety of weaning methods are available, but no one method has consistently proved to be superior to the others. These methods include T-tube (T-piece), CPAP, pressure support ventilation (PSV), and SIMV. One recent multicenter study lends evidence to support the use of PSV for weaning over T-tube or SIMV weaning. Often these weaning methods are used in combination with each other, such as SIMV with PSV, CPAP with PSV, or SIMV with CPAP.[81,83]

Weaning Process Stage

For the long-term ventilator patient, the weaning process phase consists of initiating the weaning method selected and minimizing the physiologic and psychologic factors that can interfere with weaning.[81,82] It is imperative that the patient not become exhausted during this phase because this can result in a setback in the weaning process.[85] During this phase, the patient is assessed for weaning progress and signs of weaning intolerance.[83]

Weaning should be initiated in the morning while the patient is rested. Before starting the weaning process, the patient is provided with an explanation of how the process works, a description of the sensations to expect, and reassurances that he or she will be closely monitored and returned to the original ventilator mode and settings if any difficulty occurs.[83] This information should be reinforced with each weaning attempt. One study showed that family presence during the weaning trial was beneficial and that the trials were longer when the family was present.[89]

T-tube and CPAP weaning are accomplished by removing the patient from the ventilator and then placing the patient on a T-tube or by placing the patient on CPAP mode for a specified duration of time, known as a weaning trial, for a specified number of times per day. When the weaning trial is over, the patient is placed on the assist-control mode or similar mode and allowed to rest to prevent respiratory muscle fatigue. Gradually, the duration of time spent weaning is increased, as is the frequency, until the patient is able to breathe spontaneously for 24 hours. If PSV is used in conjunction with CPAP, the PSV is initially set to provide the patient with an assisted tidal volume of 10 to 12 mL/kg, and this is gradually weaned until a level of 6 to 8 cm H_2O of pressure support is achieved. SIMV and PSV weaning are accomplished by gradually decreasing the number of breaths or the amount of pressure support the patient receives by a specified amount until the patient is able to breathe spontaneously for 24 hours.[83]

Weaning progress can be evaluated using various methods. Evaluation of weaning progress when using a weaning method that gradually withdraws ventilatory support, such as SIMV or PSV, can be accomplished by measuring the percentage of the minute ventilation requirement that is provided by the ventilator. If the percentage steadily decreases, weaning is progressing. Evaluation of weaning progress when using a weaning method that removes ventilatory support, such as T-tube or CPAP, can be accomplished by measuring the amount of time the patient remains free from support. If the time steadily increases, weaning is progressing.[83]

Once the weaning process has begun, the patient should be continuously assessed for signs of intolerance. When present, these signs indicate when to place the patient back on the ventilator or to return the patient to the previous ventilator settings. Commonly used indicators include dyspnea; accessory muscle use; restlessness; anxiety; change in facial expression; changes in heart rate and blood pressure; rapid, shallow breathing; and discomfort.[86] Table 15-6 lists the different weaning intolerance indicators and actions that can be taken to control or prevent them.

Additional therapies may be needed to facilitate weaning in the patient who is having difficulty making weaning progress. These therapies include ventilatory muscle training and biofeedback. Inspiratory muscle training is used to enhance the strength and endurance of the respiratory muscles. Biofeedback can be used to promote relaxation and assist in the management of dyspnea and anxiety.[83]

Weaning Outcome Stage

Two outcomes are possible for a patient with LTMVD: weaning completed and incomplete weaning.[83] Weaning is deemed successful when a patient is able to breathe spontaneously for 24 hours without ventilatory support. Once this occurs, the patient may be extubated or decannulated at any time, though this is not necessary for weaning to be considered successful.[84] Weaning is deemed incomplete when a patient has reached a plateau (5 days at the same ventilatory support level without any changes) in the weaning process despite managing the physiologic and psychologic factors that impede weaning. Thus, the patient is unable to breathe spontaneously for 24 hours without full or partial ventilatory support. Once this occurs, the patient should be placed in a subacute ventilator facility or discharged home on a ventilator with home care nursing follow-up.[84] See Box 15-26 for Internet Resources.

TABLE 15-6 Weaning Intolerance Indications and Interventions

INDICATOR	ETIOLOGY	INTERVENTION
Pulmonary Signs (Emotional)		
Altered breathing pattern	Inadequate understanding of weaning process	Build trust in staff; consistent care providers
Dyspnea intensity		Encouragement; concrete goals for extubation
Change in facial expression	Inability to control breathing pattern	Involve patient in process and planning daily activities.
		Efficient communication established
	Environmental factors	Organize care; avoid interruptions during weaning.
		Adequate sleep
		Calm, caring presence of nurse; nonsedating anxiolytics
		Measure dyspnea.
		Fan; music
		Biofeedback; relaxation; breathing control
		Family involvement; normalizing daily activities
Pulmonary Signs (Physiologic)		
Accessory muscle use	Airway obstruction	Suction/air-mask bag unit ventilation; manually ventilate patient
Prolonged expiration	Secretions/atelectasis	
Asynchronous movements of chest and abdomen	Bronchospasm	Bronchodilators
	Patient position/kinked	Sitting upright in bed or chair or per patient preference
Retractions	ET tube	
Facial expression changes	Increased workload of muscle	
Dyspnea	Fatigue	
Shortened inspiratory time	Caloric intake	Dietary assessment
Increased breathing frequency, decreased V_T	Electrolyte imbalances	Assess electrolytes; give replacements as necessary.
	Inadequate rest	Rest between weaning trials (i.e., SIMV frequency rate >5).
	Patient/ventilator interactions	Assess ventilator settings (i.e., flow rate, trigger sensitivity).
	Increased V_E requirement	Muscle training if appropriate
	Infection	Check for infection (treat if indicated).
	Overfeeding	Appropriate caloric intake
	Respiratory alkalosis	Baseline ABGs achieved (ventilate according to pH)
	Anxiety	Coaching to regularize breathing pattern; give nonsedating anxiolytics
	Pain	Judicious use of analgesics
CNS Changes		
Restless/irritable	Hypoxemia/hypercarbia	Increase FiO_2.
Decreased responsiveness		Return to mechanical ventilation.
		Discern etiology and treat.
CV Deterioration		
Excessive change in BP or HR	Heart failure	Diuretics as ordered
	Increase venous return	Beta-blockers
Dysrhythmias	Ischemia	Increase FiO_2.
Angina		Return to mechanical ventilation.
Dyspnea		Discern etiology and treat.

ET, endotracheal; *SIMV,* synchronized intermittent mandatory ventilation; V_E, respiratory minute volume; V_T, tidal volume; *ABGs,* arterial blood gases; FiO_2, fraction of inspired oxygen; *CNS,* central nervous system; *CV,* cardiovascular; *BP,* blood pressure; *HR,* heart rate.
Modified from Knebel AR. When weaning from mechanical ventilation fails. *Am J Crit Care.* 1992; 1:19.

FiO2 is % of inspired oxygen
(fraction of inspired oxygen) – higher than atmospheric O2

BOX 15-26 INTERNET RESOURCES

American Association of Critical-Care Nurses: http://www.aacn.org
Society for Critical Care Medicine: http://www.sccm.org
Respiratory Nursing Society: http://respiratorynursingsociety.org
American Association of Respiratory Care: http://www.aarc.org
American College of Chest Physicians: http://www.chestnet.org/accp
NHLBI ARDS Network: http://www.ardsnet.org
American College of Physicians: http://www.acponline.org
American Lung Association: http://www.lung.org
American Medical Association: http://www.ama-assn.org
American Thoracic Society: http://www.thoracic.org
Centers for Disease Control and Prevention: http://www.cdc.gov
National Institutes for Health: http://www.nih.gov
PubMed Health: http://www.ncbi.nlm.nih.gov/pubmedhealth
American Society for Parenteral and Enteral Nutrition: http://www.nutritioncare.org

REFERENCES

1. Mac Sweeney R, et al: Acute lung failure, *Semin Respir Crit Care Med* 32:607, 2011.
2. Aboussouan LS: Respiratory failure and the need for ventilatory support. In Kacmarek RM, et al, editors: *Egan's fundamentals of respiratory care*, ed 10, St. Louis, 2013, Mosby.
3. Linderman DJ, Janssen WJ: Critical care medicine for the hospitalist, *Med Clin North Am* 92:467, 2008.
4. Balk R, Bone RC: Classification of acute respiratory failure, *Med Clin North Am* 67:551, 1983.
5. Curtis JR, Hudson LD: Emergent assessment and management of acute respiratory failure in COPD, *Clin Chest Med* 15:481, 1994.
6. Raju P, Manthous CA: The pathogenesis of respiratory failure: an overview, *Respir Care Clin N Am* 6:195, 2000.
7. Del Sorbo L, et al: Hypoxemic respiratory failure. In Mason RJ, et al, editors: *Murray and nadel's textbook of respiratory medicine*, ed 5, Philadelphia, 2010, Saunders.
8. Loiacono LA, Shapiro DS: Detection of hypoxia at the cellular level, *Crit Care Clin* 26:409, 2010.
9. Sigillito RJ, DeBlieux PM: Evaluation and initial management of the patient in respiratory distress, *Emerg Med Clin North Am* 21:239, 2003.
10. Dakin J, Griffiths M: The pulmonary physician in critical care 1: pulmonary investigations for acute respiratory failure, *Thorax* 57:79, 2002.
11. Martin DS, Grocott MPW: Oxygen therapy in critical illness: precise control of arterial oxygenation and permissive hypoxemia, *Crit Care Med* 41:423, 2013.
12. Kernick J, Magarey J: What is the evidence for the use of high flow nasal cannula oxygen in adult patients admitted to critical care units? A systematic review, *Aust Crit Care* 23:53, 2010.
13. Hess D: Noninvasive ventilation for acute respiratory failure, *Resp Care* 58:950, 2013.
14. Soo Hoo GW, Hakimian N, Santiago SM: Hypercapnic respiratory failure in COPD patients: response to therapy, *Chest* 117:169, 2000.
15. Ward NS, Dushay KM: Clinical concise review: mechanical ventilation of patients with chronic obstructive pulmonary disease, *Crit Care Med* 36:1614, 2008.
16. Make B, Belfer MH: Primary care perspective on chronic obstructive pulmonary disease management, *Postgrad Med* 123:145, 2011.
17. Barr J, et al: Clinical practice guidelines for the management of pain, agitation, and delirium in adult patients in the intensive care unit, *Crit Care Med* 41:263, 2013.
18. Greenberg SB, Vender J: The use of neuromuscular blocking agents in the ICU: where are we now?, *Crit Care Med* 41:1332, 2013.
19. Kraut JA, Madias NE: Metabolic acidosis: pathophysiology, diagnosis and management, *Nat Rev Nephrol* 6:274, 2010.
20. Martindale RG, et al: Guidelines for the provision and assessment of nutrition support therapy in the adult critically ill patient: Society of Critical Care Medicine and American Society for Parenteral and enteral Nutrition: Executive Summary, *Crit Care Med* 37:1757, 2009.
21. Casaer MP, Van den Berghe G: Nurtrition in the acute phase of critical illness, *N Engl J Med* 370:1227, 2014.
22. Olson T: Delirium in the intensive care unit: role of the critical care nurse in early detection and treatment, *Dynamics* 23:32, 2012.
23. van der Jagt M, Miranda DR: Beta-blockers in intensive care medicine: potential benefit in acute brain injury and acute respiratory distress syndrome, *Recent Pat Cardiovascu Drug Discov* 7:141, 2012.
24. McLeod AG, Geerts W: Venous thromboembolism prophylaxis in critically ill patients, *Crit Care Clin* 27:765, 2011.
25. Krag M, et al: Stress ulcer prophylaxis versus placebo or no prophylaxis in critically ill patients. A systematic review of randomized clinical trials with meta-analysis and trial sequential analysis, *Intensive Care Med* 40:11, 2014.
26. Wong WP: Use of body positioning in the mechanically ventilated patient with acute respiratory failure: application of Sackett's rules of evidence, *Physiother Theory Pract* 15:25, 1999.
27. Johnson KL, Meyenburg T: Physiological rationale and current evidence for therapeutic positioning of critically ill patients, *AACN Adv Crit Care* 20:228, 2009.
28. Lasater-Erhard M: The effect of patient position on arterial oxygen saturation, *Crit Care Nurse* 15:31, 1995.
29. Cosenza JJ, Norton LC: Secretion clearance: state-of-the-art from a nursing perspective, *Crit Care Nurse* 6(4):23, 1986.
30. Metheny NA, Frantz RA: Head-of-bed elevation in critically ill patients: a review, *Crit Care Nurse* 33:53, 2013.
31. Krishnagopalan S, et al: Body positioning of intensive care patients: clinical practice versus standards, *Crit Care Med* 30:2588, 2002.
32. Stiller K: Physiotherapy in intensive care: towards an evidence-based practice, *Chest* 118:1801, 2000.
33. McCool FD, Rosen M: Nonpharmacologic airway clearance therapies: ACCP evidence-based clinical practice guidelines, *Chest* 129(Suppl 1):250S, 2006.
34. Krau SD: Making sense of multiple organ dysfunction syndrome, *Crit Care Nurs Clin North Am* 19:87, 2007.

35. Crouser ED, et al: Acute lung injury, pulmonary edema, and multiple system organ failure. In Kacmarek RM, et al, editors: *Egan's fundamentals of respiratory care*, ed 10, St. Louis, 2013, Mosby.
36. The ARDS Definition Task Force: Acute respiratory distress syndrome: the Berlin Definition, *JAMA* 307:2526, 2012.
37. Blank R, Napolitano LM: Epidemiology of ARDS and ALI, *Crit Care Clin* 27:439, 2011.
38. Dechert RE, et al: Current knowledge of acute lung injury and acute respiratory distress syndrome, *Crit Care Nurs Clin N Am* 24:377, 2012.
39. Matthay MA, Zemans RL: The acute respiratory distress syndrome: pathogenesis and treatment, *Annu Rev Path* 6:147, 2011.
40. Ragaller M, Richter T: Acute lung injury and acute respiratory distress syndrome, *J Emerg Trauma Shock* 3:43, 2010.
41. Matthay MA, et al: The acute respiratory distress syndrome, *J Clin Invest* 122:2731, 2012.
42. Bieh M, et al: Ventilator-induced lung injury: minimizing its impact in patients with or at risk for ARDS, *Resp Care* 58:927, 2013.
43. Haas CF: Mechanical ventilation with lung protective strategies: what works?, *Crit Care Clin* 27:469, 2011.
44. Yilmaz M, Gajic O: Optimal ventilator settings in acute lung injury and acute respiratory distress syndrome, *Eur J Anaesthesiol* 25:89, 2008.
45. Ali A, Ferguson ND: High-frequency oscillatory ventilation in ALI/ARDS, *Crit Care Clin* 27:487, 2011.
46. Turner DA, Cheifetz IM: Extracorporeal membrane oxygenation for adult respiratory failure, *Resp Care* 58:1038, 2013.
47. Park PK, et al: Extracorporeal membrane oxygenation in adult acute respiratory distress syndrome, *Crit Care Clin* 27:627, 2011.
48. York NL, Kane C: Trends in caring for adult respiratory distress syndrome patients, *Dimens Crit Care Nurs* 31:153, 2012.
49. Dirkes S, et al: Prone positioning: is it safe and effective?, *Crit Care Nurs Q* 25:64, 2012.
50. American Thoracic Society, Infectious Diseases Society of America: Guidelines for the management of adults with hospital-acquired, ventilator-associated, and healthcare-associated pneumonia, *Am J Respir Crit Care Med* 171:388, 2005.
51. Sligi WI, Marrie TJ: Severe community-acquired pneumonia, *Crit Care Clin* 29:2013. 2013; 95:563.
52. Sligl WI, et al: Age still matters: prognosticating short- and long-term mortality for critically ill patients with pneumonia, *Crit Care Med* 38:2126, 2010.
53. Shorr AF, et al: Diagnostics and epidemiology in ventilator-associated pneumonia, *Ther Adv Resp Dis* 5:121, 2011.
54. Labelle A, Kollef MH: Healthcare-associated pneumonia: approach to management, *Clin Chest Med* 32:507, 2011.
55. Nair GB, Niederman MS: Nosocomial pneumonia: lessons learned, *Crit Care Clin* 29:521, 2013.
56. Lopez A, et al: Does health care associated pneumonia really exist?, *Eur J Intern Med* 23:47, 2012.
57. Mandell LA, et al: Infectious Diseases Society of America/American Thoracic Society consensus guidelines on the management of community-acquired pneumonia in adults, *Clin Infect Dis* 44(Suppl 2):S27, 2007.
58. Miskovich-Riddle L, Keresztes PA: CAP management guidelines, *Nurse Pract* 31(1):43, 2006.
59. Pines JM: Timing of antibiotics for acute, severe infections, *Emerg Med Clin North Am* 26:245, 2008.
60. Anantham D, Jagadesan R, Tiew PE: Clinical review: independent lung ventilation in critical care, *Crit Care* 9:594, 2005.
61. Kendall A, et al: Point-of-care hand hygiene: preventing infection behind the curtain, *Am J Infect Control* 40(4 Suppl 1):S3, 2012.
62. Paintal HS, Kuschner WG: Aspiration syndromes: 10 clinical pearls every physician should know, *Int J Clin Prac* 61:846, 2007.
63. Marik PE: Pulmonary aspiration syndrome, *Curr Opin Pulm Med* 17:148, 2011.
64. Raghavendran K, et al: Aspiration-induced lung injury, *Crit Care Med* 39:818, 2011.
65. Schallom M, et al: Gastroesophageal reflux in critically ill patients, *Dimens Crit Care Nurs* 32:69, 2013.
66. Smithburger PL, et al: Alteplase treatment of acute pulmonary embolism in the intensive care unit, *Crit Care Nurse* 33(2):17, 2013.
67. Jaff MR, et al: Management of massive and submassive pulmonary embolism, iliofemoral deep vein thrombosis, and chronic thromboembolic pulmonary hypertension: a scientific statement from the American Heart Association, *Circulation* 123:1788, 2011.
68. Dweik RA, Arroliga AC: Pulmonary vascular disease. In Kacmarek RM, et al, editors: *Egan's fundamentals of respiratory care*, ed 10, St. Louis, 2013, Mosby.
69. Tapson VF: Acute pulmonary embolism, *N Eng J Med* 358:1037, 2008.
70. Wood KE: Major pulmonary embolism, *Crit Care Clin* 27:885, 2011.
71. Fairfax LM, Sing RF: Vena cava interruption, *Crit Care Clin* 27:781, 2011.
72. Kearon C, et al: Antithrombotic therapy for venous thromboembolic disease: American College of Chest Physicians Evidence-Based Clinical Practice Guidelines (9th Edition), *Chest* 141(Suppl 2):419S, 2012.
73. Samoukovic G, et al: The role of pulmonary embolectomy in the treatment of acute pulmonary embolism: a literature review from 1968 to 2008, *Interact Cardiovasc Thorac Surg* 11:265, 2010.
74. Fanta CH: Asthma, *N Engl J Med* 360:1002, 2009.
75. Mannam P, Siegel MD: Analytic review: management of life-threatening asthma in adults, *J Intensive Care Med* 25:3, 2010.
76. Murata A, Ling PM: Asthma diagnosis and management, *Emerg Med Clin N Am* 30:203, 2012.
77. Cairns CB: Acute asthma exacerbations: phenotypes and management, *Clin Chest Med* 27:99, 2006.
78. Restrepo RD, Peters J: Near-fatal asthma: recognition and management, *Curr Opin Pulm Med* 14:13, 2008.
79. White AC: Long-term mechanical ventilation: management strategies, *Respir Care* 57:889, 2012.
80. MacIntyre NR, et al: Management of patients requiring prolonged mechanical ventilation: report of a NAMDRC Consensus Conference, *Chest* 128:3937, 2005.
81. Caroleo S, et al: Weaning from mechanical ventilation: an open issue, *Minerva Anestesiol* 73:417, 2007.

82. MacIntyre NR: Psychological factors in weaning from mechanical ventilatory support, *Respir Care* 40:277, 1995.
83. Burns SM: Weaning from mechanical ventilation. In Burns SM, editor: *Care of mechanically ventilated patients*, ed 2, Sudbury, MD, 2007, Jones and Bartlett.
84. Knebel AR, et al: Weaning from mechanical ventilatory support: refinement of a model, *Am J Crit Care* 7:149, 1998.
85. El-Khatib MF, Bou-Khalil P: Clinical review: Liberation from mechanical ventilation, *Crit Care* 12:221, 2008.
86. Cox CE, Carson SS: Prolonged mechanical ventilation. In MacIntyre NR, Branson RD, editors: *Mechanical ventilation*, ed 2, St. Louis, 2009, Saunders.
87. White V, et al: Multidisciplinary team developed and implemented protocols to assist mechanical ventilation weaning: a systematic review of literature, *Worldviews Evid Based Nurs* 8:51, 2011.
88. Hass CF, Loik PS: Ventilator discontinuation protocols, *Respir Care* 57:1649, 2012.
89. Happ MB, et al: Family presence and surveillance during weaning from prolonged mechanical ventilation, *Heart Lung* 36:47, 2007.

CHAPTER 16

Pulmonary Therapeutic Management

Kathleen M. Stacy

Be sure to check out the bonus material, including review questions, on the Evolve website at http://evolve.elsevier.com/Urden/priorities/.

OXYGEN THERAPY

Normal cellular function depends on the delivery of an adequate supply of oxygen to the cells to meet their metabolic needs. The goal of oxygen therapy is to provide a sufficient concentration of inspired oxygen to permit full use of the oxygen-carrying capacity of the arterial blood; this ensures adequate cellular oxygenation, provided the cardiac output and hemoglobin concentration are adequate.[1,2]

Principles of Therapy

Oxygen is an atmospheric gas that must also be considered a medication because, like most other medications, it has detrimental as well as beneficial effects. Oxygen is one of the most commonly used and misused medications. As a medication, it must be administered for good reason and in a proper, safe manner. Oxygen is usually ordered in liters per minute (L/min), as a concentration of oxygen expressed as a percentage (e.g., 40%), or as a fraction of inspired oxygen (FiO_2) such as 0.4.

The primary indication for oxygen therapy is hypoxemia.[3] The amount of oxygen administered depends on the pathophysiologic mechanisms affecting the patient's oxygenation status. In most cases, the amount required should provide an arterial partial pressure of oxygen (PaO_2) of greater than 60 mm Hg or an arterial hemoglobin saturation (SaO_2) of greater than 90% during rest and exercise.[2] The concentration of oxygen given to an individual patient is a clinical judgment based on the many factors that influence oxygen transport, such as hemoglobin concentration, cardiac output, and arterial oxygen tension.[1,2]

After oxygen therapy has begun, the patient is continuously assessed for level of oxygenation and the factors affecting it. The patient's oxygenation status is evaluated several times daily until the desired oxygen level has been reached and has stabilized. If the desired response to the amount of oxygen delivered is not achieved, the oxygen supplementation is adjusted, and the patient's condition is re-evaluated. It is important to use this dose-response method so that the lowest possible level of oxygen is administered that will still achieve a satisfactory PaO_2 or SaO_2.[2,3]

Methods of Delivery

Oxygen therapy can be delivered by many different devices (Table 16-1). Common problems with these devices include system leaks and obstructions, device displacement, and skin irritation. These devices are classified as low-flow, reservoir, or high-flow systems.[3]

Low-Flow Systems

A low-flow oxygen delivery system provides supplemental oxygen directly into the patient's airway at a flow of 8 L/min or less. Because this flow is insufficient to meet the patient's inspiratory volume requirements, it results in a variable FiO_2 as the supplemental oxygen is mixed with room air. The patient's ventilatory pattern affects the FiO_2 of a low-flow system: as this pattern changes, differing amounts of room air gas are mixed with the constant flow of oxygen. A nasal cannula is an example of a low-flow device.[3]

Reservoir Systems

A reservoir system incorporates some type of device to collect and store oxygen between breaths. When the patient's inspiratory flow exceeds the oxygen flow of the oxygen delivery system, the patient is able to draw from the reservoir of oxygen to meet his or her inspiratory volume needs. Less mixing of the inspired oxygen occurs with room air than in a low-flow system. A reservoir oxygen delivery system can deliver a higher FiO_2 than a low-flow system. Examples of reservoir systems are simple face masks, partial rebreathing masks, and nonrebreathing masks.[3]

High-Flow Systems

With a high-flow system, the oxygen flows out of the device and into the patient's airways in an amount sufficient to meet all inspiratory volume requirements. This type of system is not affected by the patient's ventilatory pattern. A high-flow system uses either an air-entrainment system or blending system to mix air and oxygen to achieve the desired FiO_2. An air-entrainment mask is an example of a high-flow system that delivers precisely controlled oxygen at the lower FiO_2 range.[3]

One of the newest high-flow systems is the high-flow nasal cannula. With this system, warmed and humidified oxygen is delivered to the patient via a nasal cannula using a blending system. This system has been shown to improve oxygenation and ventilation and decrease the work of breathing in the patient with acute lung failure. It also is more comfortable and better tolerated than similar therapies.[4]

Complications of Oxygen Therapy

Oxygen, like most medications, has adverse effects and complications resulting from its use. The adage, "If a little is good,

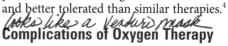

TABLE 16-1 Oxygen Therapy Systems

CATEGORY	DEVICE	FLOW	FiO_2 RANGE (%)	FiO_2 STABILITY	ADVANTAGES	DISADVANTAGES	BEST USE
Low-flow	Nasal cannula	0.25-8 L/min (adults) ≤2 L/min (infants)	22-45	Variable	Use on adults, children, infants; easy to apply; disposable, low-cost; well- tolerated	Unstable, easily dislodged; high flows uncomfortable; can cause dryness or bleeding; polyps, deviated septum may block flow	Stable patient needing low FiO_2; home care patient requiring long-term therapy
	Nasal catheter	0.25-8 L/min	22-45	Variable	Use on adults, children, infants; good stability; disposable, low-cost	Difficult to insert; high flows increase back pressure; needs regular changing; polyps, deviated septum may block insertion; may provoke gagging, air swallowing, aspiration	Procedures in which cannula is difficult to use (bronchoscopy); long-term care for infants
	Transtracheal catheter	0.25-4 L/min	22-35	Variable	Lower oxygen usage or cost; eliminates nasal/skin irritation; improved compliance; increased exercise tolerance; increased mobility; enhanced image	High cost; surgical complications; infection; mucus plugging; lost tract	Home care or ambulatory patients who need increased mobility or who do not accept nasal oxygen
Reservoir	Reservoir cannula	0.25-4 L/min	22-35	Variable	Lower oxygen usage/cost; increased mobility; less discomfort because of lower flows	Unattractive, cumbersome; poor compliance; must be regularly replaced; breathing pattern affects performance	Home care or ambulatory patients who need increased mobility
	Simple mask	5-12 L/min	35-50	Variable	Use on adults, children, infants; quick, easy to apply; disposable, inexpensive	Uncomfortable; must be removed for eating; prevents radiant heat loss; blocks vomitus in unconscious patients	Emergencies, short-term therapy requiring moderate FiO_2
	Partial rebreathing mask	6-10 L/min (prevent bag collapse on inspiration)	35-60	Variable	Same as simple mask; moderate-to-high FiO_2	Same as simple mask; potential suffocation hazard	Emergencies, short-term therapy requiring moderate- to-high FiO_2
	Nonrebreathing mask	6-10 L/min (prevent bag collapse on inspiration)	55-70	Variable	Same as simple mask; high FiO_2	Same as simple mask; potential suffocation hazard	Emergencies, short-term therapy requiring high FiO_2
	Nonrebreathing circuit (closed)	$3 \times V_E$ (prevent bag collapse on inspiration)	21-100	Fixed	Full range of FiO_2	Potential suffocation hazard; requires 50 psi air or oxygen; blender failure common	Patients requiring precise FiO_2 at any level (21%-100%)
High-flow	Air-entrainment mask (AEM)	Varies; should provide output flow >60 L/min	24-50	Fixed	Easy to apply; disposable, inexpensive; stable, precise FiO_2	Limited to adult use; uncomfortable, noisy; must be removed for eating; FiO_2 >0.40 not ensured; FiO_2 varies with back-pressure	Unstable patients requiring precise low FiO_2
	Air-entrainment nebulizer	10-15 L/min input; should provide output flow of at least 60 L/min	28-100	Fixed	Provides temperature control and extra humidification	FiO_2 <28% or >0.40 not ensured; FiO_2 varies with back-pressure; high infection risk	Patients with artificial airways requiring low-to- moderate FiO_2
	Blending system (open)	Should provide output flow of at least 60 L/min	21-100	Fixed	Full range of FiO_2	Requires 50 psi air + oxygen; blender failure or inaccuracy common	Patient with high V_E who needs high FiO_2
	High-flow cannula system	Up to 40 L/min (depending on system)	35-90	Variable or fixed depending on system and input flow	Wide range of FiO_2 and relative or absolute humidity; use on adults, children, infants	FiO_2 not ensured depending on input flow and patient breathing pattern; infection risk	Patients of all ages with high or variable V_E who need supplemental oxygen, positive pressure, or humidity

FiO_2, Fraction of inspired oxygen; V_E, minute volume.

a lot is better" does not apply to oxygen. The lung is designed to handle a concentration of 21% oxygen, with some adaptability to higher concentrations, but adverse effects and oxygen toxicity can result if a high concentration is administered for too long.[5]

Oxygen Toxicity

The most detrimental effect of breathing a high concentration of oxygen is the development of oxygen toxicity. It can occur in any patient who breathes oxygen concentrations of greater than 50% for longer than 24 hours. Patients most likely to develop oxygen toxicity are those who require intubation, mechanical ventilation, and high oxygen concentrations for extended periods.[3]

Hyperoxia, or the administration of higher-than-normal oxygen concentrations, produces an overabundance of oxygen free radicals. These radicals are responsible for the initial damage to the alveolar-capillary membrane. Oxygen free radicals are toxic metabolites of oxygen metabolism. Normally, enzymes neutralize the radicals, preventing any damage from occurring. During the administration of high levels of oxygen, the large number of oxygen free radicals produced exhausts the supply of neutralizing enzymes. Damage to the lung parenchyma and vasculature occurs, resulting in the initiation of acute respiratory distress syndrome (ARDS).[2,5]

A number of clinical manifestations are associated with oxygen toxicity. The first symptom is substernal chest pain that is exacerbated by deep breathing. A dry cough and tracheal irritation follow. Eventually, definite pleuritic pain occurs on inhalation, followed by dyspnea. Upper airway changes may include a sensation of nasal stuffiness, sore throat, and eye and ear discomforts. Chest radiographs and pulmonary function tests show no abnormalities until symptoms are severe. Complete, rapid reversal of these symptoms occurs as soon as normal oxygen concentrations are restored.[5]

Carbon Dioxide Retention

In patients with severe chronic obstructive pulmonary disease (COPD), carbon dioxide (CO_2) retention may occur as a result of administration of oxygen in high concentrations. A number of theories have been proposed for this phenomenon. One states that the normal stimulus to breathe (i.e., increasing CO_2 levels) is muted in patients with COPD and that decreasing oxygen levels become the stimulus to breathe. If hypoxemia is corrected by the administration of oxygen, the stimulus to breathe is abolished; hypoventilation develops, resulting in a further increase in the arterial partial pressure of carbon dioxide ($PaCO_2$).[2,3] Another theory is that the administration of oxygen abolishes the compensatory response of hypoxic pulmonary vasoconstriction. This results in an increase in perfusion of underventilated alveoli and the development of dead space, producing ventilation–perfusion mismatch. As alveolar dead space increases, so does the retention of CO_2.[2,3] One further theory states that the rise in CO_2 is related to the ratio of deoxygenated to oxygenated hemoglobin (Haldane effect). Deoxygenated hemoglobin carries more CO_2 compared with oxygenated hemoglobin. Administration of oxygen increases the proportion of oxygenated hemoglobin, which causes increased release of CO_2 at the lung level.[5] Because of the risk of CO_2 accumulation, all patients who are chronically hypercapnic require careful low-flow oxygen administration.[3]

Absorption Atelectasis

Another adverse effect of high concentrations of oxygen is absorption atelectasis. Breathing high concentrations of oxygen washes out the nitrogen that normally fills the alveoli and helps hold them open (residual volume). As oxygen replaces the nitrogen in the alveoli, the alveoli start to shrink and collapse. This occurs because oxygen is absorbed into the bloodstream faster than it can be replaced in the alveoli, particularly in areas of the lungs that are minimally ventilated.[2,3]

Nursing Management

Nursing priorities for the patient receiving oxygen focus on 1) ensuring the oxygen is being administered as ordered and 2) observing for complications of the therapy. Confirming that the oxygen therapy device is properly positioned and replacing it after removal is important. During meals, an oxygen mask should be changed to a nasal cannula if the patient can tolerate one. The patient receiving oxygen therapy should also be transported with the oxygen. In addition, oxygen saturation should be periodically monitored using a pulse oximeter.

ARTIFICIAL AIRWAYS

Pharyngeal Airways

Pharyngeal airways are used to maintain airway patency by keeping the tongue from obstructing the upper airway. The two types of pharyngeal airways are *oropharyngeal* and *nasopharyngeal airways*. Complications of these airways include trauma to the oral or nasal cavity, obstruction of the airway, laryngospasm, gagging, and vomiting.[6,7]

Oropharyngeal Airway

An oropharyngeal airway is made of plastic and is available in various sizes. The proper size is selected by holding the airway against the side of the patient's face and ensuring that it extends from the corner of the mouth to the angle of the jaw. If the airway is improperly sized, it will occlude the airway.[6,7] An oral airway is placed by inserting a tongue depressor into the patient's mouth to displace the tongue downward and then passing the airway into the patient's mouth, slipping it over the patient's tongue.[7] When properly placed, the tip of the airway lies above the epiglottis at the base of the tongue. It should be used only in an unconscious patient who has an absent or diminished gag reflex.[6,7]

Nasopharyngeal Airway

A nasopharyngeal airway is usually made of plastic or rubber and is available in various sizes. The proper size is selected by holding the airway against the side of the patient's face and ensuring that it extends from the tip of the nose to the ear lobe.[6,7] A nasal airway is placed by lubricating the tube and inserting it midline along the floor of the naris into the posterior pharynx.[7] When properly placed, the tip of the airway lies above the epiglottis at the base of the tongue.[6,7]

Endotracheal Tubes

An endotracheal tube (ETT) is the most commonly used artificial airway for providing short-term airway management. Indications for endotracheal intubation include

TABLE 16-2 Advantages of Orotracheal, Nasotracheal, and Tracheostomy Tubes

OROTRACHEAL TUBES	NASOTRACHEAL TUBES	TRACHEOSTOMY TUBES
Easier access Avoids nasal and sinus complications Allows for larger-diameter tube, which facilitates • Work of breathing • Suctioning • Fiberoptic bronchoscopy	Easily secured and stabilized Reduces risk of unintentional extubation Well-tolerated by patient Enables swallowing and oral hygiene Facilitates communication Avoids need for bite block	Easily secured and stabilized Reduces risk of unintentional decannulation Well-tolerated by patient Enables swallowing, speech, and oral hygiene Avoids upper airway complications Allows for larger-diameter tube, which facilitates • Work of breathing • Suctioning • Fiberoptic bronchoscopy

maintenance of airway patency, protection of the airway from aspiration, application of positive-pressure ventilation, facilitation of pulmonary toilet, and use of high oxygen concentrations.[8] An ETT may be placed through the orotracheal or the nasotracheal route.[9,10] In most situations involving emergency placement, the orotracheal route is used because it is simpler and allows the use of a larger-diameter ETT.[10,11] Nasotracheal intubation provides greater patient comfort over time and is preferred in patients with a jaw fracture.[9,11,12] The advantages of orotracheal and nasotracheal intubation are presented in Table 16-2.

ETTs are available in various sizes, which are based on the inner diameters of the tubes, and have a radiopaque marker that runs the length of the tube. On one end of the tube is a cuff that is inflated with the use of the pilot balloon. Because of the high incidence of cuff-related problems, low-pressure, high-volume cuffs are preferred. On the other end of the tube is a 15-mm adaptor that facilitates connection of the tube to a manual resuscitation bag (MRB), T-tube, or ventilator (Figure 16-1).[13]

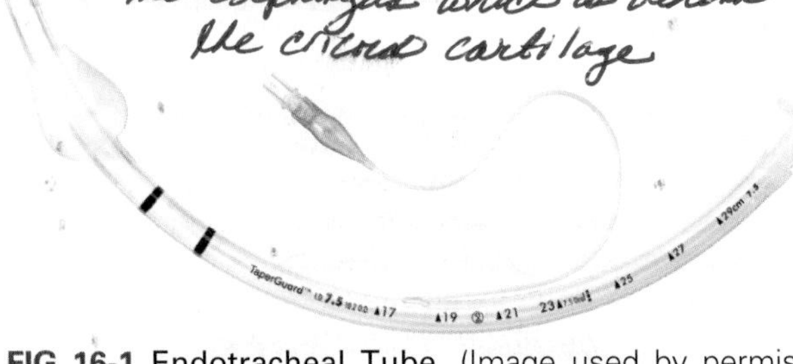

FIG 16-1 Endotracheal Tube. (Image used by permission from Nellcor Puritan Bennett LLC, Boulder, CO.)

Rapid Sequence Intubation

Rapid sequence intubation (RSI) is a seven-step process that is often used to intubate the critically ill patient. It is considered safer for the patient as it decreases the risk of aspiration.[14]

Step 1. Preparation. Before intubation, the necessary equipment is gathered and organized to facilitate the procedure. Readily available equipment should include a suction system with catheters and tonsil suction, an MRB with a mask connected to 100% oxygen, a laryngoscope handle with assorted blades, a variety of sizes of ETTs, and a stylet. Before the procedure is initiated, all equipment is inspected to ensure that it is in working order. The patient should be prepared for the procedure, if possible, with an intravenous catheter in place and should be monitored with a pulse oximeter.[14]

Step 2. Preoxygenation. Once everything is ready, the patient is preoxygenated with 100% oxygen for 3 to 5 minutes via a tight-fitting face mask. If the patient is unable to maintain adequate spontaneous ventilations, then assisted ventilations are initiated with an MRB. The goal is to avoid positive-pressure ventilation, if possible, as this intervention increases the chances of gastric distention and the risk of aspiration. If an MRB is used, cricoid pressure should be initiated.[14]

Step 3. Pretreatment. While the patient is being preoxygenated, the patient is pretreated with adjunct medications to decrease the physiologic response to intubation. These medications include lidocaine, fentanyl, and atropine. A very low dose of a paralytic agent may be administered to prevent fasciculations. The use of these medications is dependent on the patient's underlying condition. If possible, pretreatment should occur 3 minutes prior to the next step.[14]

Step 4. Paralysis with induction. Next, a sedative agent and a paralytic agent are administered in "rapid sequence" to achieve induction and paralysis. A variety of sedative agents, including etomidate, midazolam, ketamine, and propofol, are used to facilitate rapid loss of consciousness. Induction dosages for these medications are usually slightly higher than the typical dosages used for sedation. The two most administered neuromuscular blocking agents used to facilitate skeletal muscle relaxation are succinylcholine and rocuronium.[14]

Step 5. Protection and positioning. The procedure is initiated by positioning the patient with the neck flexed and head slightly extended in the "sniff" position. The oral cavity and pharynx are suctioned, and any dental devices are removed. Next cricoid pressure is applied to protect the airway by preventing vomiting and subsequent aspiration of gastric contents.[14]

Step 6. Placement of the endotracheal tube. Next, the ETT is inserted into the trachea (Figure 16-2), and placement is confirmed.[14] Each intubation attempt is limited to 30 seconds to prevent hypoxemia. After the ETT is inserted, the patient is assessed for bilateral breath sounds and chest movement. Absence of breath sounds is indicative of an esophageal intubation, whereas breath sounds heard over only one side is indicative of a main stem intubation. A disposable end-tidal CO_2 detector is used to verify correct airway placement initially, after which the cuff of the tube is inflated and the tube is secured. Finally, a chest radiograph is obtained to confirm placement.[9-11] The tip of the ETT should be approximately 3

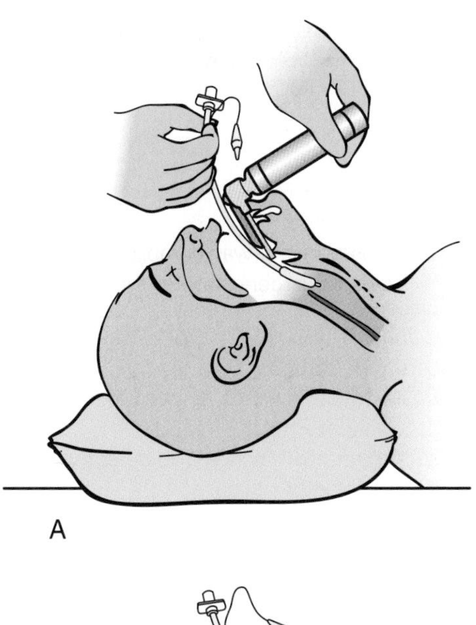

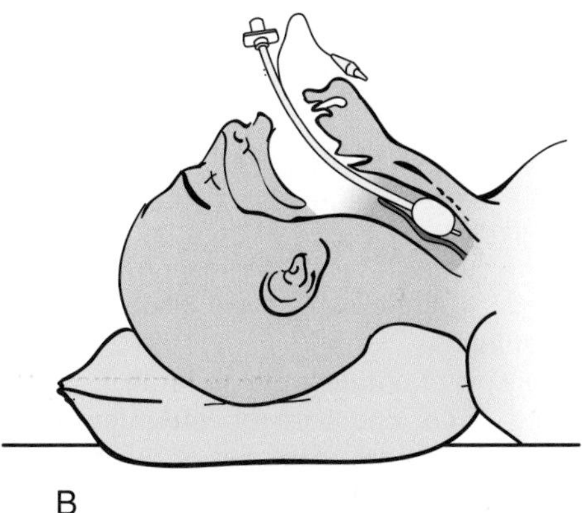

FIG 16-2 Insertion of Tube with Laryngoscope in Place. *A,* Insert the tube with the tip initially against the right buccal mucosa so that a clear view of the vocal cords can be maintained at all times. As it advances, watch the tube pass through the cord. *B,* The tube is correctly placed when the tip is 2 to 3 cm beyond the vocal cords. (From Savage S. Tracheal intubation. In: Pfenninger JL, Fowler GC, eds. *Pfenninger and Fowler's Procedures for Primary Care.* 3rd ed. Philadelphia: Elsevier; 2011.)

to 4 cm above the carina when the patient's head is in the neutral position.[10]

Step 7. Post-intubation management. After final adjustment of the position is complete, the level of insertion (marked in centimeters on the side of the tube) at the teeth is noted. The ETT is then secured to patient's face using tape or a commercial tube holder (Figure 16-3). Securing the tube stabilizes it to prevent movement and potential dislodgement.[9,10,15]

Complications

A number of complications can occur during the intubation procedure, including nasal and oral trauma, pharyngeal and hypopharyngeal trauma, vomiting with aspiration, and cardiac arrest.[15] Tracheal rupture is a rare and often fatal complication that is associated with emergent intubation.[16] Hypoxemia and hypercapnia can also occur, resulting in bradycardia, tachycardia, dysrhythmias, hypertension, and hypotension.[8,12,15]

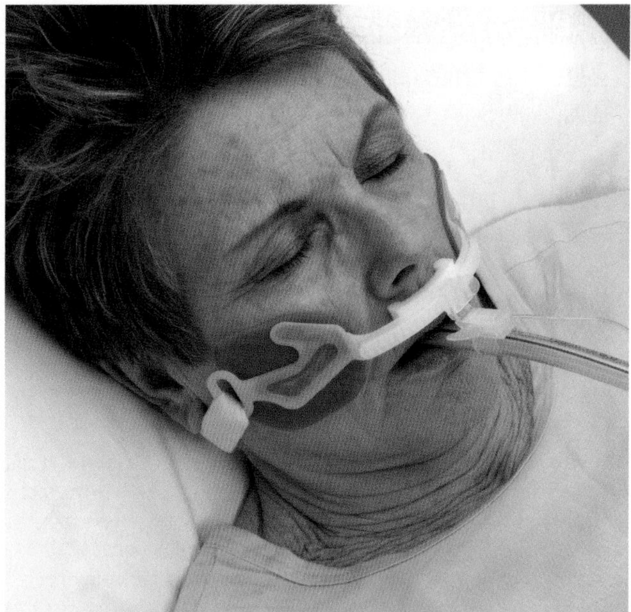

FIG 16-3 Commercial Tube Holder—Anchor Fast oral endotracheal tube fastener. (Courtesy Hollister Incorporated, Libertyville, IL.)

Several complications can occur while the ETT is in place, including nasal and oral inflammation and ulceration, sinusitis and otitis, laryngeal and tracheal injuries, and tube obstruction and displacement. Other complications can occur days to weeks after the ETT is removed, including laryngeal and tracheal stenosis and a cricoid abscess (Table 16-3). Delayed complications usually require some form of surgical intervention.[17,18]

Tracheostomy Tubes

A tracheostomy tube is the preferred method of airway maintenance in the patient who requires long-term intubation. Although no ideal time to perform the procedure has been identified, it is commonly accepted that if a patient has been intubated or is anticipated to be intubated for longer than 7 to 10 days, a tracheostomy should be performed.[19] A tracheostomy is also indicated in several other situations such as the presence of an upper airway obstruction due to trauma, tumors, or swelling and the need to facilitate airway clearance due to spinal cord injury, neuromuscular disease, or severe debilitation.[20,21]

A tracheostomy tube provides the best route for long-term airway maintenance because it avoids the oral, nasal, pharyngeal, and laryngeal complications associated with an ETT. The tube is shorter, of wider diameter, and less curved than an ETT; the resistance to air flow is less, and breathing is easier. Additional advantages of a tracheostomy tube include easier secretion removal, increased patient acceptance and comfort, capability of the patient to eat and talk if possible, and easier ventilator weaning.[11,20] See Table 16-2 for a list of the advantages of a tracheostomy tube.

Tracheostomy tubes are made of plastic or metal and may have one or two lumens. Single-lumen tubes consist of the tube; a built-in cuff, which is connected to a pilot balloon for inflation purposes; and an obturator, which is used during tube insertion. The double-lumen tubes consist of the tube

TABLE 16-3 Complications of Endotracheal Tubes

COMPLICATIONS	CAUSES	PREVENTION AND TREATMENT
Tube obstruction	Patient biting tube Tube kinking during repositioning Cuff herniation Dried secretions, blood, or lubricant Tissue from tumor Trauma Foreign body	*Prevention:* Place bite block. Sedate patient PRN. Suction PRN. Humidify inspired gases. *Treatment:* Replace tube.
Tube displacement	Movement of patient's head Movement of tube by patient's tongue Traction on tube from ventilator tubing Self-extubation	*Prevention:* Secure tube to upper lip. Restrain patient's hands as needed. Sedate patient PRN. Ensure that only 2 inches of tube extend beyond lip. Support ventilator tubing. *Treatment:* Replace tube.
Sinusitis and nasal injury	Obstruction of the paranasal sinus drainage Pressure necrosis of nares	*Prevention:* Avoid nasal intubations. Cushion nares from tube and tape or ties. *Treatment:* Remove all tubes from nasal passages. Administer antibiotics.
Tracheoesophageal fistula	Pressure necrosis of posterior tracheal wall, resulting from overinflated cuff and rigid nasogastric tube	*Prevention:* Inflate cuff with minimal amount of air necessary. Monitor cuff pressures every 8 hours. *Treatment:* Position cuff of tube distal to fistula. Place gastrostomy tube for enteral feedings. Place esophageal tube for secretion clearance proximal to fistula.
Mucosal lesions	Pressure at tube and mucosal interface	*Prevention:* Inflate cuff with minimal amount of air necessary. Monitor cuff pressures every 8 hours. Use appropriate size tube. *Treatment:* May resolve spontaneously. Perform surgical intervention.
Laryngeal or tracheal stenosis	Injury to area from end of tube or cuff, resulting in scar tissue formation and narrowing of airway	*Prevention:* Inflate cuff with minimal amount of air necessary. Monitor cuff pressures every 8 hours. Suction area above cuff frequently. *Treatment:* Perform tracheostomy. Place laryngeal stent. Perform surgical repair.
Cricoid abscess	Mucosal injury with bacterial invasion	*Prevention:* Inflate cuff with minimal amount of air necessary. Monitor cuff pressures every 8 hours. Suction area above cuff frequently. *Treatment:* Perform incision and drainage of area. Administer antibiotics.

PRN, As needed.

with the attached cuff, the obturator, and an inner cannula that can be removed for cleaning and then reinserted or, if disposable, replaced by a new sterile inner cannula. The inner cannula can quickly be removed if it becomes obstructed, making the system safer for patients with significant secretion problems. Single-lumen tubes provide a larger internal diameter for airflow, so airflow resistance is reduced, and the patient can ventilate through the tube with greater ease. Plastic tracheostomy tubes also have a 15-mm adapter on the end (Figure 16-4).[20,21]

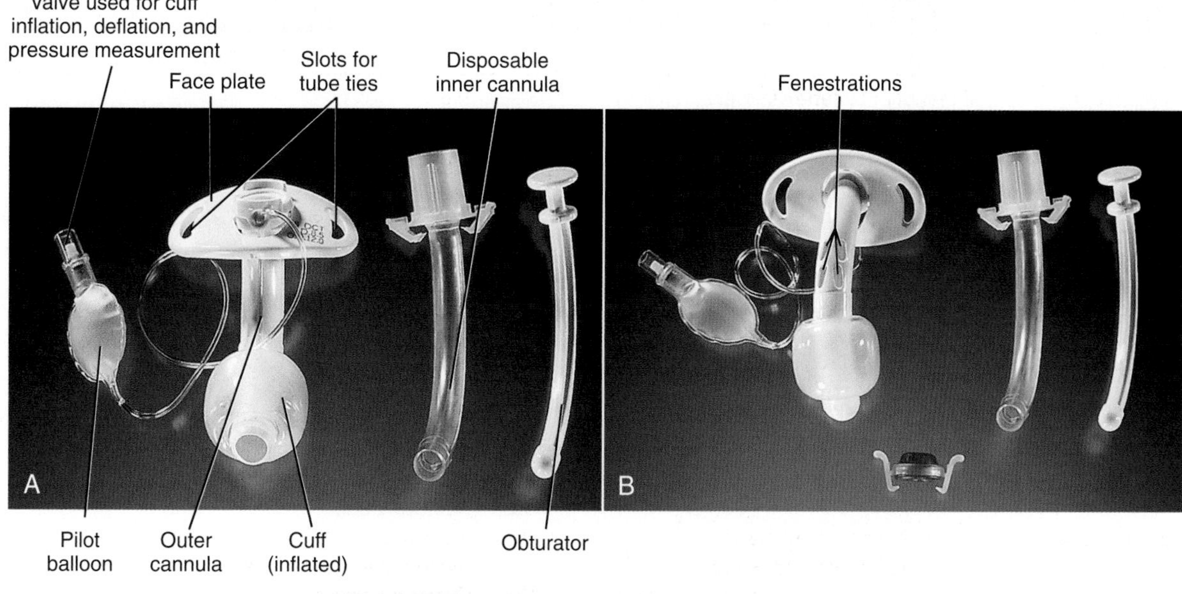

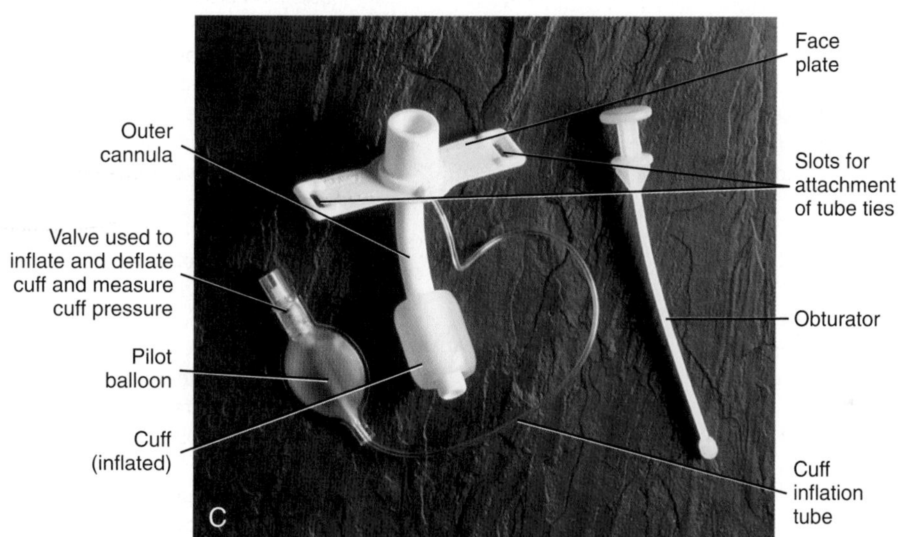

FIG 16-4 Tracheostomy Tubes. *A,* Dual-lumen cuffed tracheostomy tube with disposable inner cannula. *B,* Dual-lumen cuffed fenestrated tracheostomy tube. *C,* Single-lumen cannula cuffed tracheostomy tube. (From Rees HC. Care of patients requiring oxygen therapy or tracheostomy. In: Ignatavicius DD, Workman ML, eds. *Medical-Surgical Nursing.* 7th ed. St. Louis: Elsevier; 2013.)

Tracheostomy Procedure

A tracheostomy tube is inserted by an open procedure or a percutaneous procedure. An open procedure is usually performed in the operating room, whereas a percutaneous procedure can be done at the patient's bedside.[21-23]

Complications

A number of complications can occur during the tracheostomy procedure, including misplacement of the tracheal tube, hemorrhage, laryngeal nerve injury, pneumothorax, pneumomediastinum, and cardiac arrest.[17,21,22] Several complications can occur while the tracheostomy tube is in place, including stomal infection, hemorrhage, tracheomalacia, tracheoesophageal fistula, tracheoinnominate artery fistula, and tube obstruction and displacement.[21,22] A number of complications can occur days to weeks after the tracheostomy tube is removed, including tracheal stenosis and tracheocutaneous fistula (Table 16-4). Delayed complications usually require some form of surgical intervention.[21]

Nursing Management

Nursing management of the patient with an endotracheal or tracheostomy tube requires some additional measures to address the effects associated with tube placement on the respiratory and other body systems. **Nursing priorities for the patient with an artificial airway focus on 1) providing humidification, 2) maintaining cuff management, 3) suctioning, 4) establishing a method of communication, and 5) providing oral hygiene.** Because the tube bypasses the upper airway system, warming and humidifying of air must be performed by external means. Because the cuff of the tube can cause damage to the walls of the trachea, proper cuff inflation and management are imperative. In addition, the

TABLE 16-4 Complications of Tracheostomy Tubes

COMPLICATIONS	CAUSES	PREVENTION AND TREATMENT
Hemorrhage	Vessel opening after surgery Vessel erosion caused by tube	*Prevention:* Use appropriate size tube. Treat local infection. Suction gently. Humidify inspired gases. Position tracheal window not lower than third tracheal ring. *Treatment:* Pack lightly. Perform surgical intervention.
Wound infection	Colonization of stoma with hospital flora	*Prevention:* Perform routine stoma care. *Treatment:* Remove tube, if necessary. Perform aggressive wound care and débridement. Administer antibiotics.
Subcutaneous emphysema	Positive-pressure ventilation Coughing against a tight, occlusive dressing or sutured or packed wound	*Prevention:* Avoid suturing or packing wound closed around tube. *Treatment:* Remove any sutures or packing, if present.
Tube obstruction	Dried blood or secretions False passage into soft tissues Opening of cannula positioned against tracheal wall Foreign body Tissue from tumor	*Prevention:* Suction PRN. Humidify inspired gases. Use a tube with a removable inner cannula. Position tube so that opening does not press against tracheal wall. *Treatment:* Remove or replace inner cannula. Replace tube.
Tube displacement	Patient movement Coughing Traction on ventilatory tubing	*Prevention:* Use commercial tube holder. Use tubes with adjustable neck plates for patients with short necks. Support ventilatory tubing. Sedate patient PRN. Restrain patient, as needed. *Treatment:* Cover stoma and manually ventilate patient by mouth. Replace tube.
Tracheal stenosis	Injury to area from end of tube or cuff, resulting in scar tissue formation and narrowing of airway	*Prevention:* Inflate cuff with minimal amount of air necessary. Monitor cuff pressures every 8 hours. *Treatment:* Perform surgical repair.
Tracheoesophageal fistula	Pressure necrosis of posterior tracheal wall, resulting from overinflated cuff and rigid nasogastric tube	*Prevention:* Inflate cuff with minimal amount of air necessary. Monitor cuff pressures every 8 hours. *Treatment:* Perform surgical repair.
Tracheoinnominate artery fistula	Direct pressure from the elbow of the cannula against the innominate artery Placement of tracheal stoma below fourth tracheal ring Downward migration of the tracheal stoma, resulting from traction on tube High-lying innominate artery	*Prevention:* Position tracheal window not lower than third tracheal ring. *Treatment:* Hyperinflate cuff to control bleeding. Remove tube, replace with endotracheal tube, and apply digital pressure through stoma against the sternum. Perform surgical repair.
Tracheocutaneous fistula	Failure of stoma to close after removal of tube	*Treatment:* Perform surgical repair.

PRN, As needed.

normal defense mechanisms are impaired, and secretions may accumulate; thus, suctioning may be needed to promote secretion clearance. Because the tube does not allow air flow over the vocal cords, developing a method of communication is also very important. Last, observing the patient to ensure proper placement of the tube and patency of the airway is essential.

Patient safety is critically important when caring for a patient with an artificial airway, as loss of the tube can result in loss of the patient's airway. In the event of unintentional extubation or decannulation, the patient's airway should be opened with the head tilt–chin lift maneuver and maintained with an oropharyngeal or nasopharyngeal airway. If the patient is not breathing, he or she should be manually ventilated with a manual resuscitation bag and face mask with 100% oxygen. In the case of a tracheostomy, the stoma should be covered to prevent air from escaping through it. If the tracheostomy remains open, then consideration should be given to ventilating the patient through the stoma instead of the mouth.

One recent study examined patients' perception of endotracheal tube–related discomforts. Forty-six percent of the patients reported remembering having the endotracheal tube while in the critical care unit. The majority of these patients found the discomfort associated with the ETT and the inability to speak very stressful. In addition, some of the patients continued to have problems with hoarseness, sore throat, and voice changes days to months later.[24]

Humidification

Humidification of air normally is performed by the mucosal layer of the upper respiratory tract. When this area is bypassed, as occurs with ETT and tracheostomy tubes or when supplemental oxygen is used, humidification by external means is necessary. Various humidification devices add water to inhaled gas to prevent drying and irritation of the respiratory tract, to prevent undue loss of body water, and to facilitate secretion removal.[25,26] The humidification device should provide inspired gas conditioned (heated) to body temperature and saturated with water vapor.[27]

Cuff Management

Because the cuff of the ETT or tracheostomy tube is a major source of the complications associated with artificial airways, proper cuff management is essential. To prevent the complications associated with cuff design, only low-pressure, high-volume cuffed tubes are used in clinical practice.[13,28] Even with these tubes, cuff pressures can be generated that are high enough to lead to tracheal ischemia and injury. Proper cuff inflation techniques and cuff pressure monitoring are critical components of the care of the patient with an artificial airway.[10,28]

Cuff inflation techniques. Two cuff inflation techniques are used: 1) the minimal leak (ML) technique and 2) the minimal occlusion volume (MOV) technique. The ML technique consists of injecting air into the cuff until no leak is heard and then withdrawing the air until a small leak is heard on inspiration. Problems with this technique include difficulty maintaining positive end-expiratory pressure (PEEP) and aspiration around the cuff. The MOV technique consists of injecting air into the cuff until no leak is heard at peak inspiration. This technique generates higher cuff pressures than does the ML technique. The selection of one technique over the other is determined by individual patient needs. If the patient needs a seal to provide adequate ventilation or is at high risk for aspiration, the MOV technique is used. If these are not concerns, usually the ML technique is used.[10,11,28]

Cuff pressure monitoring. Cuff pressures are monitored at least every shift with a cuff pressure manometer. Cuff pressures should be maintained at 20 to 25 mm Hg (24 to 30 cm H_2O) because greater pressures decrease blood flow to the capillaries in the tracheal wall and lesser pressures increase the risk of aspiration. Pressures in excess of 25 mm Hg (30 cm H_2O) should be reported to the physician. Cuffs are not routinely deflated because this increases the risk of aspiration.[10,28]

Subglottic secretion removal. The cuff has also been implicated in the development of ventilator-associated pneumonia. Fluids can leak around the cuff into the airway, resulting in microaspiration. Bacteria-laden oral secretions trickle down the larynx and pool above the cuff of the artificial airway. These secretions are referred to as subglottic secretions. Subglottic secretions can then leak into the lower airways around the cuff via the longitudinal folds that form in the cuff as it accommodates for the shape of the airway, an underinflated cuff that fails to form a proper seal in the airway, or inadvertent movement of the endotracheal tube within airway. Thus, the use of established cuff inflation techniques, monitoring of cuff pressures, using an appropriate method of tube stabilization, and oral hygiene are important interventions for preventing this problem.[29] Deep oropharyngeal suctioning to remove subglottic secretions should be performed at least every 12 hours and prior to deflating the cuff or moving the tube.[30]

Specialized tubes are available to allow for the continuous removal of subglottic secretions. These tubes have an additional lumen, with an opening above the cuff, which is connected to continuous (−20 to −30 cm H_2O) suction.[11] These tubes are recommended for patients who are expected to be intubated for longer than 72 hours.[31] One issue with these tubes is that the aspiration lumen can become clogged and, thus, requires a small amount of air to be injected into the aspiration port every 4 hours.

Suctioning

Suctioning is often required to maintain a patent airway in the patient with an ETT or tracheostomy tube. Suctioning is a sterile procedure that is performed only when the patient needs it and not on a routine schedule.[10,32,33] Indications for suctioning include coughing, secretions in the airway, respiratory distress, presence of rhonchi on auscultation, increased peak airway pressures on the ventilator, and decreasing oxygenation saturation.[11] Complications associated with suctioning include hypoxemia, atelectasis, bronchospasms, dysrhythmias, increased intracranial pressure, and airway trauma.[11,32]

Complications. Hypoxemia can result because the oxygen source is disconnected from the patient or the oxygen is removed from the patient's airways when the suction is applied. Atelectasis is thought to occur when the suction catheter is larger than one-half of the diameter of the ETT. Excessive negative pressure occurs when suction is applied, promoting collapse of the distal airways. Bronchospasms are the result of stimulation of the airways with the suction catheter. Cardiac dysrhythmias, particularly bradycardias, are attributed to vagal stimulation. Airway trauma occurs with impaction of the catheter in the airways and excessive negative pressure applied to the catheter.[10,11,32]

Suctioning protocol. A number of protocols regarding suctioning have been developed. Several practices have been found helpful in limiting the complications of suctioning. Hypoxemia can be minimized by giving the patient three hyperoxygenation breaths (breaths at 100% FiO_2) with the ventilator before the procedure begins and again after each pass of the suction catheter.[10,33,34] If the patient exhibits signs of desaturation, hyperinflation (breaths at 150% tidal volume) should be added to the procedure.[10] Atelectasis can be avoided by using a suction catheter with an external diameter of less than one-half of the internal diameter of the ETT.[32,33] Using no greater than 120 mm Hg of suction decreases the chances of hypoxemia, atelectasis, and airway trauma.[10,33] Limiting the duration of each suction pass to 10 to 15 seconds[10,32,33] and the number of passes to a maximum of three also helps minimize hypoxemia, airway trauma, and cardiac dysrhythmias.[35] The process of applying intermittent (instead of continuous) suction has been shown to be of no benefit.[33,36] The instillation of normal saline to help remove secretions has not proved to be of any benefit,[32,33,37] and it may actually contribute to the development of hypoxemia, as well as lower airway colonization, resulting in ventilator-associated pneumonia (VAP).[10,38,39]

Closed tracheal suction system. One device to facilitate the suctioning of a patient on a ventilator is the closed tracheal suction system (CTSS) (Figure 16-5). This device consists of a suction catheter in a plastic sleeve that attaches directly to the ventilator tubing. It allows the patient to be suctioned while remaining on the ventilator. Advantages of the CTSS include maintenance of oxygenation and PEEP during suctioning, reduction of hypoxemia-related complications, and protection of staff members from the patient's secretions. The CTSS is convenient to use, requiring only one person to perform the procedure.[11]

Concerns related to the CTSS include autocontamination, inadequate removal of secretions, and increased risk of unintentional extubation resulting from the extra weight of the system on the ventilator tubing. Autocontamination has been shown not to be an issue if the catheter is cleaned properly after every use. Inadequate removal of secretions may or may not be a problem, and further investigation is required to settle this issue.[11] Although recommendations for changing the catheter vary, one study indicated that the catheter could be changed on an as-needed basis without increasing the incidence of VAP.[40] One recent study found that suctioning with the CTSS caused massive aspiration of fluid around the tracheal tube cuff as a result of a significant drop in airway pressure.[41]

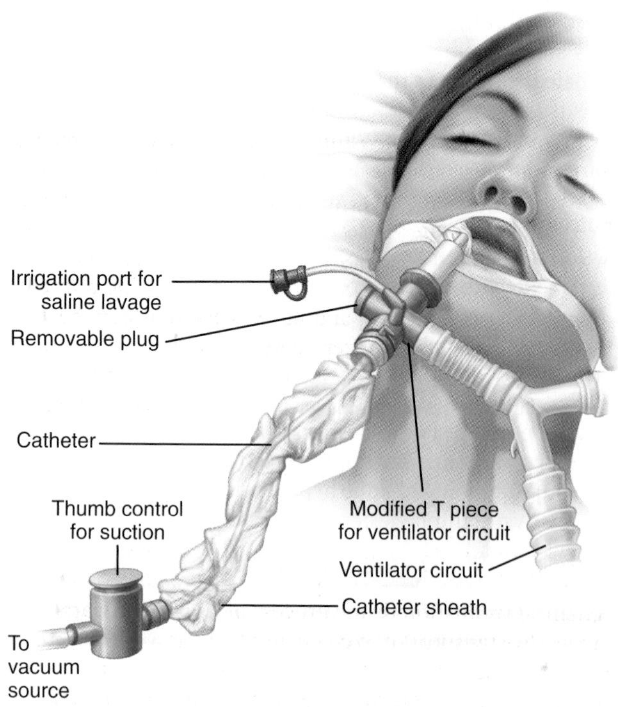

FIG 16-5 Closed Tracheal Suction System. (Modified from Sills JR. *Entry-Level Respiratory Therapist Exam Guide.* St. Louis: Mosby; 2000.)

Communication

One of the major stressors for the patient with an artificial airway is impaired communication. This is related to the inability to speak, insufficient explanations from staff members, inadequate understanding, fear of being unable to communicate, and difficulty with communication methods.[42] A number of interventions can facilitate communication in the patient with an ETT or tracheostomy tube. These include establishing an environment that fosters communication, performing a complete assessment of the patient's ability to communicate, anticipating the patient's needs, teaching the patient and family how to communicate, using a variety of methods to communicate, and facilitating the patient's ability to communicate by providing the patient with his or her eyeglasses or hearing aid.[43]

Methods to facilitate communication in this patient population include the use of verbal and nonverbal language and a variety of devices to assist the patient on short-term and long-term ventilator assistance. Nonverbal communication may include the use of sign language, gestures, lip reading, pointing, facial expressions, or eye blinking. Simple devices available include pencil and paper; Magic Slates; magnetic boards with plastic letters; picture, alphabet, or symbol boards; and flash cards. More sophisticated devices include typewriters, computers, talking ETT and tracheostomy tubes, and external handheld vibrators. Regardless of the method selected, the patient must be taught how to use the device.[10,43]

Passy-muir valve. One device used to assist the mechanically ventilated patient with a tracheostomy to speak is the Passy-Muir valve. This one-way valve opens on inhalation, allowing air to enter the lungs through the tracheostomy tube, and closes on exhalation, forcing air over the vocal cords and out the mouth, permitting the patient to speak (Figure 16-6). Before the valve can be placed on a tracheostomy tube, the cuff must be deflated to allow air to pass around the tube, and the tidal volume of the ventilator must be increased to compensate for the air leak. In addition to aiding communication, the Passy-Muir valve can assist the ventilator-dependent patient with relearning normal breathing patterns. The valve is contraindicated in patients with laryngeal or pharyngeal dysfunction, excessive secretions, or poor lung compliance.[43]

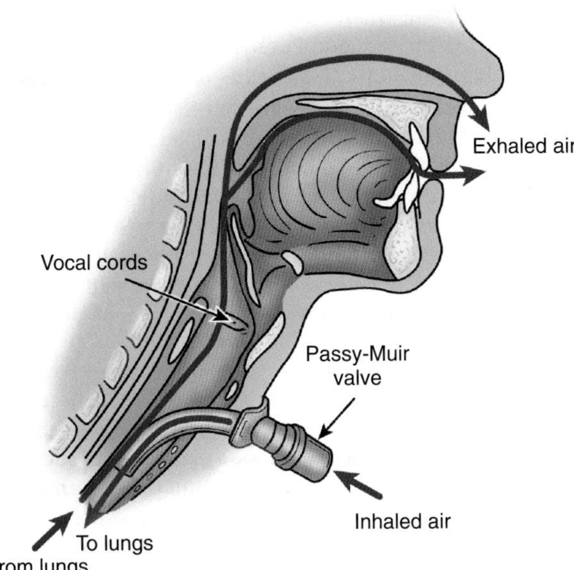

FIG 16-6 Passy-Muir Valve Mechanism of Action. (From Hodder RV. A 55-year-old patient with advanced COPD, tracheostomy tube, and sudden respiratory distress. *Chest.* 2002;121[1]:279.)

Oral Hygiene

Patients with artificial airways are extremely susceptible to developing VAP because of microaspiration of subglottic secretions. These secretions are full of microorganisms from the patient's mouth. Because the cuff of the artificial airway does not form a tight seal in the patient's airway, these secretions seep around the cuff into the patient's lungs, promoting the development of VAP.[44] Although bacteria are normally present in a patient's mouth, in the critically ill patient, increased amounts of bacteria and more resistant bacteria are present. Decreased salivary flow, poor mucosal status, and dental plaque all contribute to this problem.[45]

Proper oral hygiene has the potential to decrease the incidence of VAP.[30,45] However, recent studies have shown that routine oral care is not a priority intervention for many nurses.[46] Currently, no evidence-based protocol exists for oral care. Research studies are lacking, particularly with regard to frequency and effectiveness of different procedures.[47] Most experts agree, however, that oral care should consist of brushing the patient's teeth with a soft toothbrush to reduce plaque, brushing the patient's tongue and gums with a foam swab to stimulate the tissue, and performing deep oropharyngeal suctioning to remove any secretions that have pooled above the patient's cuff.[30,48] A sample oral care protocol is outlined in Box 16-1. One intervention that has evidence supporting its use is rinsing or swabbing the patient's mouth with 15 mL of 0.12% chlorhexidine every 12 hours.[49] This procedure has been shown to reduce oral colonization of bacteria and to decrease the incidence of ventilator-associated pneumonia, particularly in patients who have undergone cardiac surgery or trauma.[39,50]

Extubation and Decannulation

After the airway is no longer needed, it is removed. Extubation is the process of removing an ETT. It is a simple procedure that can be accomplished at the bedside.[10,11] Before the cuff of an ETT or tracheostomy tube is deflated in preparation for removal, it is very important to ensure that secretions are cleared from above the tube cuff. Complications of extubation include sore throat, stridor, hoarseness, odynophagia, vocal cord immobility, pulmonary aspiration, and cough.[17] Decannulation is the process of removing a tracheostomy tube. It is also a simple process that can be performed at the bedside. After removal of the tracheostomy tube, the stoma is usually covered with a dry dressing, with the expectation that it will close within several days.[10,11] Difficulty removing the tracheostomy tube because of a tight stoma is usually the only complication associated with decannulation.[17]

BOX 16-1 Sample Oral Care Protocol

Standard of Care

1. The oral cavity is assessed initially and daily by a registered nurse.
2. Unconscious patients and those with artificial airways (endotracheal or tracheostomy tubes) are provided oral care every 4 hours and as needed.
3. Patients with cuffed artificial airways have oropharyngeal and subglottic secretions suctioned at least every 12 hours and before repositioning of the tube or deflation of the cuff.

Procedure

1. Set up suction equipment.
2. Position patient's head to the side or place in semi-Fowler's position.
3. Provide suction, as needed, to patients with an artificial airway to remove any oropharyngeal and subglottic secretions (those secretions that migrate down the tube and settle on top of the cuff).
4. Brush teeth using suction toothbrush and small amounts of water and alcohol-free antiseptic oral rinse.
   - Brush for approximately 1 to 2 minutes.
   - Exert gentle pressure while moving in short horizontal or circular strokes.
5. Gently brush surface of tongue.
6. Use suction swab to clean the teeth and tongue if brushing causes discomfort or bleeding.
   - Place swab perpendicular to gum line, applying gentle mechanical action for 1 to 2 minutes.
   - Turn swab in clockwise rotation to remove mucus and debris.
7. Swab mouth with 15 mL of 0.12% chlorhexidine every 12 hours.
8. Apply mouth moisturizer inside mouth.
9. Apply lip balm, if needed.

INVASIVE MECHANICAL VENTILATION

Mechanical ventilation is the process of using an apparatus to facilitate the transport of oxygen and CO_2 between the atmosphere and the alveoli for the purpose of enhancing pulmonary gas exchange. It is indicated for physiologic and clinical reasons. Physiologic objectives include supporting cardiopulmonary gas exchange (alveolar ventilation and arterial oxygenation), increasing lung volume (end-expiratory lung inflation and functional residual capacity), and reducing the work of breathing. Clinical objectives include reversing hypoxemia and acute respiratory acidosis, relieving respiratory distress, preventing or reversing atelectasis and respiratory muscle fatigue, permitting sedation and neuromuscular blockade, decreasing oxygen consumption, reducing intracranial pressure, and stabilizing the chest wall.[51,52]

Types of Ventilators

The two main types of ventilators currently available are 1) positive-pressure ventilators and 2) negative-pressure ventilators. Negative-pressure ventilators are applied externally to the patient and decrease the atmospheric pressure surrounding the thorax to initiate inspiration. They generally are not used in the critical care environment. Positive-pressure ventilators use a mechanical drive mechanism to force air into the patient's lungs through an ETT or tracheostomy tube.[53]

Ventilator Mechanics

The ventilator must complete four phases of ventilation to ventilate the patient properly: 1) change from exhalation to inspiration, 2) inspiration, 3) change from inspiration to exhalation, and 4) exhalation. The ventilator uses four different variables to begin, sustain, and terminate each of these phases. These variables are described in terms of *volume, pressure, flow,* and *time*.[7,51,54,55]

Trigger

The phase variable that initiates the change from exhalation to inspiration is called the *trigger*. Breaths may be pressure-triggered or flow-triggered, depending on the sensitivity setting of the ventilator and the patient's inspiratory effort; or they may be time-triggered, depending on the rate setting of the ventilator. A breath that is initiated by the patient is known as a *patient-triggered* or *patient-assisted* breath, whereas a breath that is initiated by the ventilator is known as a *machine-triggered* or *machine-controlled* breath.[54]

A *time-triggered breath* is a machine-controlled breath that is initiated by the ventilator after a preset length of time has elapsed. It is controlled by the rate setting on the ventilator (e.g., a rate of 10 breaths per minute yields 1 breath every 6 seconds). *Flow-triggered* and *pressure-triggered* breaths are patient-assisted breaths that are initiated by decreased flow or pressure, respectively, within the breathing circuit. Flow-triggering (also known as *flow-by)* is controlled by adjusting the flow-sensitivity setting of the ventilator, whereas pressure-triggering is controlled by adjusting the pressure-sensitivity setting. Many ventilators offer the various types of triggers in combination. For example, a breath may be time-triggered and flow-triggered, depending on the patient's ability to interact with the ventilator and initiate a breath.[7,53,54]

Limit

The variable that maintains inspiration is called the *limit* or *target*. Inspiration can be pressure- limited, flow-limited, or volume-limited. A *pressure-limited breath* is one in which a preset pressure is attained and maintained during inspiration. *A flow-limited breath* is one in which a preset flow is reached before the end of inspiration. A *volume-limited breath* is one in which a preset volume is delivered during the inspiration. However, the limit variable does not end inspiration; it only sustains it.[7,53,54]

Cycle

The variable that ends inspiration is called the *cycle*. The classification of positive-pressure ventilators is based on this variable: volume-cycled, pressure-cycled, flow-cycled, and time-cycled ventilators. *Volume-cycled ventilators* are designed to deliver a breath until a preset volume is delivered. *Pressure-cycled ventilators* deliver a breath until a preset pressure is reached within the patient's airways. *Flow-cycled ventilators* deliver a breath until a preset inspiratory flow rate is achieved. *Time-cycled ventilators* deliver a breath over a preset time interval.[7,53,54]

Baseline

The variable that is controlled during exhalation is called the *baseline*. Pressure is almost always used to adjust this variable. The patient exhales to a certain baseline pressure that is set on the ventilator. It may be set at zero (i.e., atmospheric pressure) or above atmospheric pressure (i.e., PEEP).[7,53,54]

Modes of Ventilation

The term *ventilator mode* refers to how the machine ventilates the patient. Selection of a particular mode of ventilation determines how much the patient will participate in his or her own ventilatory pattern. The choice depends on the patient's situation and the goals of treatment. The mode is determined by the combination of phase variables selected. Many modes are available (Table 16-5), and some may be used in conjunction with others.[7,51-55] Because brands of ventilators vary in their ability to perform certain functions, not all modes are available on all ventilators.[54]

Ventilator Settings

Settings on the ventilator allow the ventilator parameters to be individualized to the patient and also allow selection of the desired ventilation mode (Table 16-6). Each ventilator has a patient-monitoring system that allows all aspects of the patient's ventilatory pattern to be assessed, monitored, and displayed.[51,53,56]

Complications

Mechanical ventilation is often life-saving, but, like other interventions, it is not without complications. Some complications are preventable, whereas others can be minimized but not eradicated. Physiologic complications associated with mechanical ventilation include ventilator-induced lung injury, cardiovascular compromise, gastrointestinal disturbances, patient-ventilator dyssynchrony, and HAP.

Ventilator-Induced Lung Injury

Mechanical ventilation can cause two different types of injury to the lungs: 1) air leaks and 2) biotrauma.[55,57] Air leaks related to mechanical ventilation are the result of excessive pressure in the alveoli (barotrauma), excessive volume in the alveoli (volutrauma), or shearing due to repeated opening and closing of the alveoli (atelectrauma).[55,58] Barotrauma, volutrauma, and atelectrauma can lead to excessive alveolar wall stress and damage to the alveolar–capillary membrane, resulting in air leakage into the surrounding spaces. The air then travels out through the hilum and into the mediastinum (pneumomediastinum), pleural space (pneumothorax), subcutaneous tissues (subcutaneous emphysema), pericardium

TABLE 16-5 **Modes of Mechanical Ventilation**

MODE OF VENTILATION	CLINICAL APPLICATION	NURSING IMPLICATIONS
Continuous mandatory (volume or pressure) ventilation (CMV), also known as assist-control (AC) ventilation: delivers gas at preset tidal volume or pressure (depending on selected cycling variable) in response to patient's inspirator or efforts and initiates breath if patient fails to do so within preset time.	Volume-controlled (VC) CMV is used as the primary mode of ventilation in spontaneously breathing patients with weak respiratory muscles. Pressure-controlled (PC) CMV is used in patients with decreased lung compliance or increased airway resistance, particularly when the patient is at risk for volutrauma.	Hyperventilation can occur in patients with increased respiratory rates. Sedation may be necessary to limit the number of spontaneous breaths. Patient on VC-CMV should be monitored for volutrauma. Patient on PC-CMV should be monitored for hypercapnia.
Pressure-regulated volume- control ventilation (PRVCV): a variation of CMV that combines volume and pressure features; delivers a preset tidal volume using the lowest possible airway pressure; airway pressure will not exceed preset maximum pressure limit.	PRVCV is used in patients with rapidly changing pulmonary mechanics (airway resistance and lung compliance), limiting potential complications.	
Pressure-controlled inverse-ratio ventilation (PC-IRV): PC-CMV mode in which the inspiratory-to-expiratory (I:E) time ratio is greater than 1:1.	PC-IRV is used in patients with hypoxemia refractory to positive end-expiratory pressure (PEEP); the longer inspiratory time increases functional residual capacity and improves oxygenation by opening collapsed alveoli, and the shorter expiratory time induces auto-PEEP that prevents alveoli from recollapsing.	Requires sedation or pharmacologic paralysis, or both because of discomfort. Increased intrathoracic pressure can result in excessive air trapping and decreased cardiac output.
Intermittent mandatory (volume or pressure) ventilation (IMV), also known as synchronous intermittent mandatory ventilation (SIMV): delivers gas at preset tidal volume or pressure (depending on selected cycling variable) and rate while allowing patient to breathe spontaneously; ventilator breaths are synchronized to patient's respiratory effort.	VC-IMV is used as a primary mode of ventilation in many clinical situations and as a weaning mode. PC-IMV is used in patients with decreased lung compliance or increased airway resistance when the need to preserve the patient's spontaneous effects is important.	May increase the work of breathing and promote respiratory muscle fatigue. Patient should be monitored for hypercapnia, particularly with PC-IMV.
Adaptive support ventilation (ASV): ventilator automatically adjusts settings to maintain 100 mL/min/kg of minute ventilation; pressure support.	ASV is a computerized mode of ventilation that increases or decreases ventilatory support based on patient needs; can be used with any patient requiring volume-controlled ventilation.	Not intended as a weaning mode. Adapts to changes in patient position.
Constant positive airway pressure (CPAP): positive pressure applied during spontaneous breaths; patient controls rate, inspiratory flow, and tidal volume.	CPAP is a spontaneous breathing mode used in patients to increase functional residual capacity and improve oxygenation by opening collapsed alveoli at end expiration; it is also used for weaning.	Side effects include decreased cardiac output, volutrauma, and increased intracranial pressure. No ventilator breaths are delivered in PEEP or CPAP mode unless used with CMV or IMV.
Airway pressure release ventilation (APRV): two different levels of CPAP (inspiratory and expiratory) are applied for set periods of time, allowing spontaneous breathing to occur at both levels.	APRV is a spontaneous breathing mode used to maintain alveolar recruitment without imposing additional peak inspiratory pressures that could lead to barotrauma.	Patient needs to be monitored for hypercapnia.
Pressure support ventilation (PSV): preset positive pressure used to augment patient's inspiratory efforts; patient controls rate, inspiratory flow, and tidal volume.	PSV is a spontaneous breathing mode used as the primary mode of ventilation in patients with stable respiratory drive to overcome any imposed mechanical resistance (e.g., artificial airway).	Patient should be monitored for hypercapnia. Advantages include reduced patient work of breathing and improved patient-ventilator synchrony.

Continued

TABLE 16-5 Modes of Mechanical Ventilation—cont'd

MODE OF VENTILATION	CLINICAL APPLICATION	NURSING IMPLICATIONS
	PSV can also be used with IMV to support spontaneous breaths.	
Volume-assured pressure support ventilation (VAPSV), also known as pressure augmentation (PA): a variation of PSV with a set tidal volume to ensure that patient receives minimum tidal volume with each pressure support breath	VAPSV is a spontaneous breathing mode used to treat acute respiratory illness and to facilitate weaning.	Advantages include increased patient comfort, decreased work of breathing, decreased respiratory muscle fatigue, and promotion of respiratory muscle conditioning.
Neurally adjusted ventilatory assist (NAVA): a partial ventilatory support mode that uses the electrical activity of the diaphragm (Edi) to control patient-ventilator interaction	NAVA delivers an assisted breath in proportion to and in synchrony with the patient's respiratory effort.	Requires an esophageal catheter (similar to a nasogastric tube) that measures the electrical signal to the diaphragm (Edi)
Independent lung ventilation (ILV): each lung is ventilated separately.	ILV is used in patients with unilateral lung disease, bronchopleural fistulas, or bilateral asymmetric lung disease.	Requires a double-lumen endotracheal tube, two ventilators, sedation, pharmacologic paralysis, or all
High-frequency ventilation (HFV): delivers a small volume of gas at a rapid rate. *High-frequency positive-pressure ventilation (HFPPV)* delivers 60-100 breaths/mm. *High-frequency jet ventilation (HFJV)* delivers 100-600 cycles/min. *High-frequency oscillation (HFO)* delivers 900-3000 cycles/min.	HFV is used in situations in which conventional mechanical ventilation compromises hemodynamic stability, in patients with bronchopleural fistulas, during short-term procedures, and with diseases that create a risk of volutrauma.	Patients require sedation, pharmacologic paralysis, or both. Inadequate humidification can compromise airway patency. Assessment of breath sounds is difficult.

TABLE 16-6 Ventilator Settings

PARAMETER	DESCRIPTION	TYPICAL SETTINGS
Respiratory rate or Frequency (f)	Number of breaths the ventilator delivers per minute	6-20 breaths/min
Tidal volume (Vt)	Volume of gas delivered to patient during each ventilator breath	6-10 mL/kg 4-8 mL/kg in acute respiratory distress syndrome (ARDS)
Oxygen concentration (FiO_2)	Fraction of inspired oxygen delivered to patient	May be set between 21% and 100%; adjusted to maintain PaO_2 (arterial partial pressure of oxygen) level greater than 60 mm Hg or SpO_2 (oxygen saturation based on pulse oximeter) level greater than 92%
Positive end-expiratory pressure (PEEP)	Positive pressure applied at the end of expiration of ventilator breaths	3-5 cm H_2O
Pressure support (PS)	Positive pressure used to augment patient's inspiratory efforts	5-10 cm H_2O
Inspiratory flow rate and time	Speed with which the tidal volume is delivered	40-80 L/min Time: 0.8-1.2 sec
I:E ratio	Ratio of duration of inspiration to duration of expiration	1:2 to 1:1.5 unless inverse ratio ventilation is desired
Sensitivity	Determines the amount of effort the patient must generate to initiate a ventilator breath; it may be set for pressure-triggering or flow-triggering.	Pressure trigger: 0.5-1.5 cm H_2O below baseline pressure Flow trigger: 1-3 L/min below baseline flow
High-pressure limit	Regulates the maximal pressure the ventilator can generate to deliver the tidal volume; when the pressure limit is reached, the ventilator terminates the breath and spills the undelivered volume into the atmosphere.	10-20 cm H_2O above peak inspiratory pressure

(pneumopericardium), peritoneum (pneumoperitoneum), and retroperitoneum (pneumoretroperitoneum). The resultant disorders vary from the fairly benign to the potentially lethal—the most lethal of which is a pneumothorax or pneumopericardium resulting in cardiac tamponade.[55,59]

Barotrauma, volutrauma, and atelectrauma can also cause the release of cellular mediators and initiation of the inflammatory-immune response. This type of ventilator-induced injury is known as *biotrauma*.[55,60] Biotrauma can result in the development of ARDS.[61] To limit ventilator-induced lung injury, the plateau pressure (pressure needed to inflate the alveoli) should be kept at less than 32 cm H_2O, PEEP should be used to avoid end-expiratory collapse and reopening, and the tidal volume should be set at 6 to 10 mL/kg.[57,60]

Cardiovascular Compromise

Positive-pressure ventilation increases intrathoracic pressure, which decreases venous return to the right side of the heart. Impaired venous return decreases preload, which results in a decrease in cardiac output. As a secondary consequence, hepatic and renal dysfunction may occur. Positive-pressure ventilation impairs cerebral venous return. In patients with impaired autoregulation, positive-pressure ventilation can result in increased intracranial pressure.[55,62]

Gastrointestinal Disturbances

Gastrointestinal disturbances can occur as a result of positive-pressure ventilation. Gastric distention occurs when air leaks around the ETT or tracheostomy tube cuff and overcomes the resistance of the lower esophageal sphincter.[7] Vomiting can occur as a result of pharyngeal stimulation from the artificial airway.[17] These problems can be prevented by inserting a nasogastric tube and ensuring appropriate cuff inflation. Hypomotility and constipation may occur as a result of immobility and the administration of paralytic agents, analgesics, and sedatives.[7]

Patient–Ventilator Dyssynchrony

Because the ventilatory pattern is normally initiated by the establishment of negative pressure within the chest, the application of positive pressure can lead to patient difficulties in breathing while on the ventilator. To achieve optimal ventilatory assistance, the patient should breathe in synchrony with the machine. The selected mode of ventilation, the settings, and the type of ventilatory circuitry used can increase the work of breathing and lead to breathing out of synchrony with the ventilator. Patient–ventilator dyssynchrony can result in decreased effectiveness of mechanical ventilation, the development of auto-PEEP, and psychologic distress. Patients who are not breathing in synchrony with the ventilator appear to be fighting or "bucking" the ventilator. To minimize this problem, the ventilator is adjusted to accommodate the patient's spontaneous breathing pattern and to work with the patient. If this is not possible, the patient may need to be sedated or pharmacologically paralyzed.[63-65]

Ventilator-Associated Pneumonia

Ventilator-associated pneumonia (VAP) is a subgroup of hospital-acquired pneumonia that refers to the development of pneumonia 48 to 72 hours after endotracheal intubation.[66] A great potential for the development of pneumonia exists after placement of an artificial airway because the tube bypasses or impairs many of the lung's normal defense mechanisms. After an artificial airway has been placed, contamination of the lower airways follows within 24 hours. This results from a number of factors that directly and indirectly promote airway colonization. The use of respiratory therapy devices (e.g., ventilators, nebulizers, intermittent positive-pressure breathing machines) also can increase the risk of pneumonia. The severity of the patient's illness and the presence of ARDS or malnutrition significantly increase the likelihood that an infection will ensue. Therapeutic measures such as nasogastric intubation and gastric alkalization with enteral feedings or medications facilitate the development of pneumonia. Nasogastric tubes promote aspiration by acting as a wick for stomach contents, whereas enteral feedings, antacids, histamine inhibitors, and proton-pump inhibitors increase the pH level of the stomach, promoting the growth of bacteria that can then be aspirated (Figure 16-7).[66,67] Additional information on managing the patient with pneumonia is provided in Chapter 15.

Prevention of VAP is critical. The Institute for Healthcare Improvement (IHI) identified five interventions that, when consistently implemented together, have been shown to improve patient outcomes. Known as the "IHI Ventilator Bundle" these interventions are 1) elevation of the head of the bed, 2) daily "sedation vacations" and assessment of readiness to extubate, 3) peptic ulcer disease prophylaxis, 4) deep venous thrombosis prophylaxis, and 5) daily oral care with chlorhexidine.[68]

Semirecumbency. Positioning of the patient who requires mechanical ventilation is very important. Semirecumbent positioning (elevation of the head of the bed 30 to 45 degrees) reduces the incidence of gastroesophageal reflux and subsequent aspiration and decreases the incidence of VAP. The head of the patient's bed should be elevated to 30 to 45 degrees at all times unless contraindicated (e.g., hemodynamic instability, presence of intra-aortic balloon pump, physician's order to the contrary). However, this intervention does increase the risk of skin shear on the coccyx, and extra surveillance is mandatory for prevention of pressure ulcers.[69,70]

Sedation vacation. Many patients receiving mechanical ventilation require sedation to ameliorate symptoms of anxiety and stress associated with critical illness. However, the prolonged use of sedation has been shown to contribute to the development of complications, including oversedation, prolonged mechanical ventilation, and delirium. To decrease the incidence of these complications the concept of a "sedation vacation" has been developed. A "sedation vacation" is simply the daily interruption of sedation to evaluate the patient and their need for continued sedation and mechanical ventilation. Not every patient is a candidate for this procedure. Contraindications include hemodynamic instability, increased intracranial pressure, ongoing agitation, seizures, or alcohol withdrawal, and patient's receiving neuromuscular blocking agents. If the patient is able to tolerate being off the sedation for more than 4 hours (this number varies depending on the protocol being used), then the sedation is discontinued. Signs of intolerance include ongoing agitation, increased respiratory rate, decreasing oxygen saturation, cardiac dysrhythmias, and signs of respiratory distress.[71]

Other measures to reduce the incidence of ventilator-associated pneumonia. Recent studies have shown that use

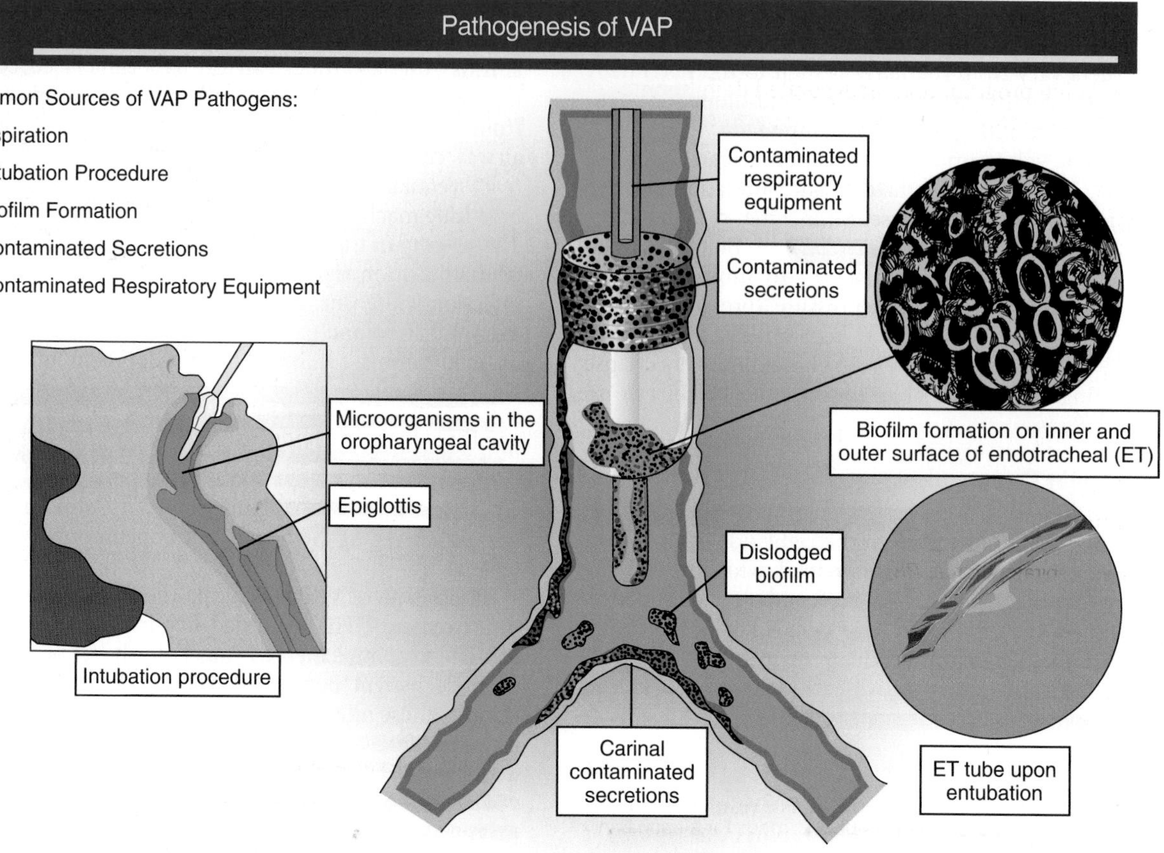

FIG 16-7 Pathogenesis of Ventilator-Associated Pneumonia. (Redrawn from Sachdev G, Napolitano LM. Postoperative pulmonary complications: pneumonia and acute respiratory failure. *Surg Clin N Am.* 2012;92:321.)

of an ETT with a polyurethane cuff may decrease the incidence of VAP. A traditional ETT has a polyvinyl low-pressure high-volume cuff. When the cuff is inflated, folds form in the cuff, allowing fluids and air to leak around the cuff and into the lungs. This is why subglottic secretion removal is so important. Polyurethane cuffs are much thinner than the traditional polyvinyl cuffs and do not form folds when they are inflated. No leakage of fluids into the lungs occurs.[72,73] In addition, some evidence suggests that the shape of the cuff may also impact this issue. A taper-shaped cuff appears to prevent fluid leakage better when compared with a cylindrical cuff commonly found on most tubes.[74]

Another recent study found that the use of silver-coated ETTs significantly reduced the incidence and delayed the onset of VAP, compared with a regular ETT. The tube decreased the incidence of VAP by preventing bacterial colonization and biofilm formation.[75] Biofilm is formed when bacteria cling to the inner lumen of the ETT and then secrete an exopolysaccharide substance. This substance forms a gelatinous matrix that allows bacteria to thrive on a nonbiologic surface.[72]

Weaning

Weaning is the gradual withdrawal of the mechanical ventilator and the re-establishment of spontaneous breathing. Weaning should begin only after the original process for which ventilator support was required has been corrected and patient stability has been achieved. Other factors to consider when weaning are length of time on ventilator, sleep deprivation, and nutritional status. Major factors that affect the patient's ability to wean include the ability of the lungs to participate in ventilation and respiration, cardiovascular performance, and psychologic readiness.[76] This discussion focuses on weaning of the patient from short-term (≤3 days) mechanical ventilation. Management of weaning in the patient on long-term mechanical ventilation is discussed in Chapter 15.

Readiness to Wean

Patients should be screened every day for their readiness to be weaned. The screen should include an evaluation of the patient's level of consciousness, physiologic and hemodynamic stability, adequacy of oxygenation and ventilation, spontaneous breathing capability, and respiratory rate and pattern.[76] Routine parameters that are usually assessed are presented in Table 16-7.

The rapid, shallow breathing index (RSBI) can predict weaning success. To calculate an RSBI, the patient's respiratory rate and minute ventilation are measured for 1 minute during spontaneous breathing. The measured respiratory rate is then divided by the tidal volume (expressed in liters). An RSBI of less than 105 is considered predictive of weaning success. If the patient is receiving sedation, the medication should be discontinued at least 1 hour before the RSBI is measured. If the patient meets criteria for weaning readiness and has an RSBI of less than 105, a spontaneous breathing trial can be performed.[77] One study showed that implementation of a weaning program that incorporated daily spontaneous breathing trials (SBT) had a positive impact on extubation rates and no effect on reintubation rates.[78] Figure 16-8 outlines one approach for an SBT.

TABLE 16-7 Conventional Weaning Parameters

PARAMETERS	WEANABLE VALUES	NORMAL RANGES
NIF (cm of water)	<–20	<–50
VC (mL/kg)	>10	>65-75
V_T (mL/kg)	<5	>5-7
RR (breaths/min)	<32	12-20
V_E (L/min)	>10	>10
Rapid shallow breathing index (RSBI) (RR/V_T)	<105	<40

NIF, Negative inspiratory force; *RR*, respiratory rate; *VC*, vital capacity; V_E, minute ventilation; V_T, tidal volume.
From Casserly B, Rounds S. Essentials in critical care medicine. In: Andreoli TE, ed. *Andreoli and Carpenter's Cecil Essentials of Medicine*. 8th ed. Philadelphia: Saunders; 2010.

After the patient's readiness to be weaned has been established, the patient is prepared for the weaning trial. The patient is positioned upright to facilitate breathing and suctioned to ensure airway patency. The process is explained to the patient, and the patient is offered reassurance and diversional activities. The patient is assessed immediately before the start of the trial and frequently during the weaning period for signs of weaning intolerance (Box 16-2).[76,77,79,80]

Weaning Methods

A number of methods can be used to wean a patient from the ventilator. The method selected depends on the patient, his or her pulmonary status, and length of time on the ventilator. The three main methods for weaning are 1) T-tube (T-piece) trials, 2) synchronized intermittent mandatory ventilation (SIMV), and 3) pressure-support ventilation (PSV).[76,79,81] Regardless of the method selected, evidence shows that using a standardized approach decreases weaning time and length of stay in the critical care unit.[82]

T-piece trials. T-piece weaning trials consist of alternating periods of ventilatory support (usually assist-control ventilation [ACV] or continuous mandatory ventilation

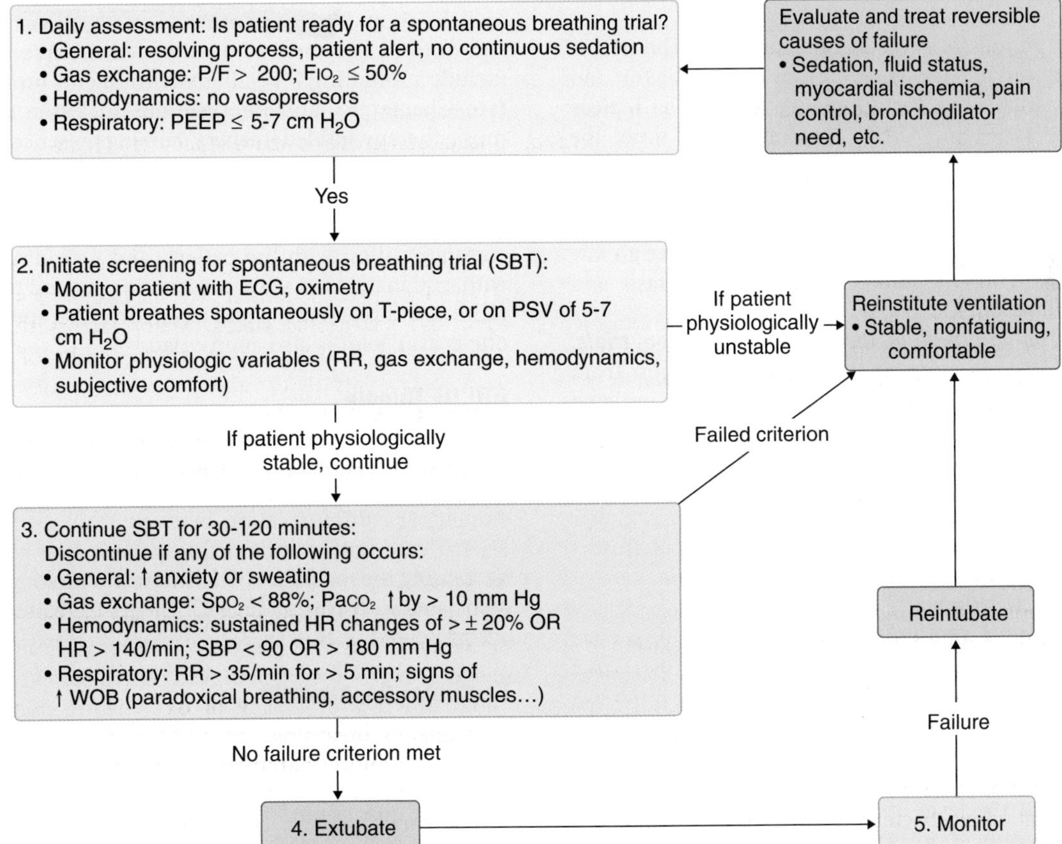

FIG 16-8 Algorithm for Assessing Whether a Patient is Ready to be Liberated from Mechanical Ventilation and Extubated. *ECG*, Electrocardiogram; *HR*, heart rate; *P/F*, PaO_2/FIO_2 ratio; *PSV*, pressure support ventilation; *RR*, respiratory rate; *SBP*, systolic blood pressure; SpO_2, oxygen saturation based on pulse oximeter; *WOB*, work of breathing. (From Slutsky AS, Hudson LD. Mechanical ventilation. In: Goldman L, Scharfer AI, eds. *Goldman's Cecil Medicine*. 24th ed. Philadelphia: Elsevier; 2012.)

BOX 16-2 Weaning Intolerance Indicators

- Decrease in level of consciousness
- Systolic blood pressure increased or decreased by 20 mm Hg
- Diastolic blood pressure greater than 100 mm Hg
- Heart rate increased by 20 beats per minute
- Premature ventricular contractions greater than 6 per minute, couplets, or runs of ventricular tachycardia
- Changes in ST segment (usually elevation)
- Respiratory rate greater than 30 breaths per minute or less than 10 breaths per minute
- Respiratory rate increased by 10 breaths per minute
- Spontaneous tidal volume less than 250 mL
- Arterial partial pressure of carbon dioxide ($PaCO_2$) increased by 5 to 8 mm Hg, pH less than 7.30, or both
- Oxygen saturation based on pulse oximeter (SpO_2) less than 90%
- Use of accessory muscles of ventilation
- Complaints of dyspnea, fatigue, or pain
- Paradoxical chest wall motion or chest abdominal asynchrony
- Diaphoresis
- Severe agitation or anxiety unrelieved by reassurance

[CMV]) with periods of spontaneous breathing. The trial is initiated by removing the patient from the ventilator and having the patient breathe spontaneously on a T-piece oxygen delivery system. After a set amount of time, the patient is placed back on the ventilator. The goal is to increase the duration of time spent off the ventilator progressively. During the weaning process, the patient is observed closely for respiratory muscle fatigue.[76-79,81] Constant positive airway pressure (CPAP) may be added to prevent atelectasis and improve oxygenation.[79,81]

Synchronized intermittent mandatory ventilation trials. The goal of SIMV weaning is the gradual transition from ventilatory support to spontaneous breathing. It is initiated by placing the ventilator in the SIMV mode and slowly decreasing the rate, usually one to three breaths at a time, until a rate of zero or near-zero is reached. An arterial blood gas (ABG) sample is usually obtained 30 minutes after the trial. This method of weaning can increase the work of breathing, and the patient must be closely monitored for signs of respiratory muscle fatigue.[76,79,81]

Pressure-support ventilation trials. PSV weaning consists of placing the patient on the pressure-support mode and setting the pressure support at a level that facilitates the patient's achieving a spontaneous tidal volume of 10 to 12 mL/kg. PSV augments the patient's spontaneous breaths with a positive-pressure boost during inspiration. During the weaning process, the level of pressure support is gradually decreased in increments of 3 to 6 cm H_2O, while the tidal volume is maintained at 10 to 15 mL/kg, until a level of 5 cm H_2O is achieved. If the patient is able to maintain adequate spontaneous respirations at this level, extubation is considered. PSV also can be used with SIMV weaning to help overcome the resistance in the ventilator system.[76,79,81]

Nursing Management

Nursing priorities for the patient with invasive mechanical ventilation focus on 1) evaluating the patient for patient-related complications and 2) monitoring the patient for ventilator-related complications.

Patient Assessment

It includes a total patient assessment, with particular emphasis on the pulmonary system, placement of the ETT or tracheostomy tube, and observation for subcutaneous emphysema and dyssynchrony with the ventilator. Bedside evaluation of vital capacity, minute ventilation, ABG values, and other pulmonary function tests may be warranted, according to the patient's condition. The use of pulse oximetry can facilitate continuous, noninvasive assessment of oxygenation. The use of capnography may facilitate continuous noninvasive assessment of ventilation. Static and dynamic compliance should also be monitored to assess for changes in lung compliance (see Appendix B).[83]

Symptom Management

Patients requiring mechanical ventilation may present with a variety of disturbing symptoms, including anxiety, pain, shortness of breath, confusion and agitation, and sleep disturbances. These symptoms are often managed with sedation and analgesic medications. As discussed earlier, these medications could contribute to prolonged mechanical ventilation and delirium. Nonpharmacologic interventions have been shown to be of benefit to these patients. These interventions include promoting a healing environment, promoting sleep (see Chapter 5), and interventions to lessen anxiety (e.g., music therapy, guided imagery, nursing presence, and animal-assisted therapy). Nursing activities to promote a healing environment include minimizing noise levels, ensuring the patient has access to natural light, establishing a method of communication with the patient, and providing the patient with explanations of what is occurring around them.[84] Referral to a complementary and alternative therapy specialist (if one is available) is also appropriate.

ABCDE Bundle

Another bundle that has recently been proposed is the Awakening and Breathing Coordination, Delirium Monitoring, and Early Mobility (ABCDE) bundle. This bundle focuses on enhancing communication between team members in the critical care unit, standardizing patient care processes, and decreasing the incidence of delirium and prolonged weakness associated with critical illness.[85] The ABCDE bundle activities are presented in Box 16-3.

Ventilator Assessment

Assessment of the ventilator includes a review of all the ventilator settings and alarms. A clear understanding of the alarms and their related problems is important (Table 16-8). The peak inspiratory pressure, exhaled tidal volume, and ABGs are also monitored.

Patient Safety

Several measures are required to maintain a trouble-free ventilator system. These include maintaining a functional manual resuscitation bag connected to oxygen at the bedside,

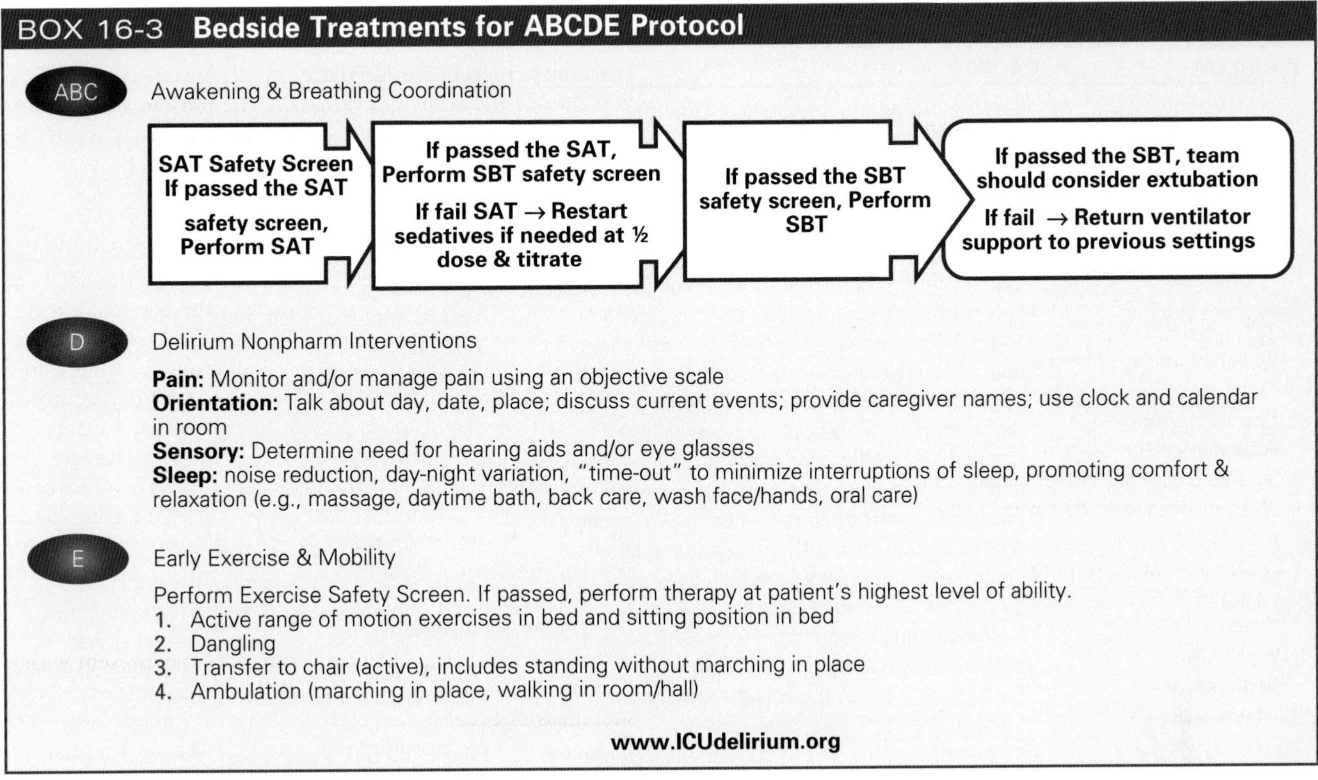

BOX 16-3 Bedside Treatments for ABCDE Protocol

ABC
Awakening & Breathing Coordination
SAT Safety Screen
If passed the SAT
safety screen,
Perform SAT
If passed the SAT,
Perform SBT safety screen
If fail SAT → Restart
sedatives if needed at ½
dose & titrate
If passed the SBT
safety screen, Perform
SBT
If passed the SBT, team
should consider extubation
If fail → Return ventilator
support to previous settings

D Delirium Nonpharm Interventions

Pain: Monitor and/or manage pain using an objective scale
Orientation: Talk about day, date, place; discuss current events; provide caregiver names; use clock and calendar in room
Sensory: Determine need for hearing aids and/or eye glasses
Sleep: noise reduction, day-night variation, "time-out" to minimize interruptions of sleep, promoting comfort & relaxation (e.g., massage, daytime bath, back care, wash face/hands, oral care)

E Early Exercise & Mobility

Perform Exercise Safety Screen. If passed, perform therapy at patient's highest level of ability.

1. Active range of motion exercises in bed and sitting position in bed
2. Dangling
3. Transfer to chair (active), includes standing without marching in place
4. Ambulation (marching in place, walking in room/hall)

www.ICUdelirium.org

ensuring that the ventilator tubing is free of water, positioning the ventilator tubing to avoid kinking, maintaining the patency of ventilator tubing and connections, changing ventilator tubing per hospital policy, and monitoring the temperature of the inspired air. If the ventilator malfunctions, the patient is removed from the ventilator and ventilated manually with a manual resuscitation bag. Alarms should be sufficiently audible with respect to distance and competing noise within the unit. Issues regarding patient transport are addressed in Box 16-4.

NONINVASIVE VENTILATION

Noninvasive ventilation (NIV) is an alternative method of ventilation that uses a mask instead of an ETT to deliver the therapy. Advantages of this type of ventilation include decreased frequency of hospital-acquired pneumonia, increased comfort, and the noninvasive nature of the procedure, which allows easy application and removal. It is indicated in type I and type II acute respiratory failure, cardiogenic pulmonary edema, and other situations in which intubation is not an option. Contraindications to NIV include hemodynamic instability, dysrhythmias, apnea, uncooperativeness, intolerance of the mask, recent upper airway or esophageal surgery, and inability to maintain a patent airway, clear secretions, or properly fit the mask.[86]

NIV can be applied with a total face, nasal, or facial mask and ventilator or with a BiPAP machine (Respironics Inc., Murrysville, PA) (Figure 16-9). One study found that a full-face mask is better tolerated than a nasal mask.[87] This type of ventilation uses a combination of PSV and PEEP supplied by a ventilator, or inspiratory and expiratory positive airway pressure (IPAP and EPAP, respectively) supplied by a BiPAP machine, to assist the spontaneously breathing patient with ventilation. On inspiration, the patient receives PSV or IPAP to increase tidal volume and minute ventilation, resulting in increased alveolar ventilation, a decreased $PaCO_2$ level, relief of dyspnea, and reduced accessory muscle use. On expiration, the patient receives PEEP or EPAP to increase functional residual capacity, resulting in an increased PaO_2 level. Humidified supplemental oxygen is administered to maintain a clinically acceptable PaO_2 level, and timed breaths may be added, if necessary.[52]

Nursing Management

Nursing priorities for the patient with noninvasive mechanical ventilation focus on 1) evaluating the patient for patient-related complications and 2) monitoring the patient for ventilator-related complications. Routine assessment of these patients includes monitoring for patient-related and ventilator-related complications. As with invasive mechanical ventilation, the patient must be closely monitored. Respiratory rate, accessory muscle use, and oxygenation status are continually assessed to ensure that the patient is tolerating this method of ventilation. Continuous pulse oximetry is also used.[88,89]

The key to ensuring adequate ventilatory support is a properly fitted mask. A nasal mask, face mask, or a full-face mask may be used, depending on the patient. A properly fitted mask minimizes air leakage and discomfort for the patient. Transparent dressings placed over the pressure points of the face help minimize air leakage and prevent facial skin necrosis caused by the mask. The BiPAP machine is able to compensate for air leaks.[89]

The patient is positioned with the head of the bed elevated at 30 to 45 degrees to minimize the risk of aspiration and to facilitate breathing. Insufflation of the stomach is a complication of this mode of therapy and places the patient at risk for

TABLE 16-8 Troubleshooting Ventilator Alarms

PROBLEM	CAUSES	INTERVENTIONS
Low exhaled VT	Altered settings; any condition that triggers high- or low-pressure alarm; patient stops spontaneous respirations; leak in system preventing VT from being delivered; cuff insufficiently inflated; leak through chest tube; airway secretions; decreased lung compliance; spirometer disconnected or malfunctioning	Check settings; evaluate patient, check respiratory rate; check all connections for leaks; suction patient's airway; check cuff pressure; calibrate spirometer.
Low inspiratory pressure	Altered settings; unattached tubing or leak around ETT; ETT displaced into pharynx or esophagus; poor cuff inflation or leak; tracheoesophageal fistula; peak flows that are too low; low VT; decreased airway resistance resulting from decreased secretions or relief of bronchospasm; increased lung compliance resulting from decreased atelectasis; reduction in pulmonary edema; resolution of ARDS; change in position	Reset alarm; reconnect tubing; modify cuff pressures; tighten humidifier; check chest tube; adjust peak flow to meet or exceed patient demand and correct for the patient's VT; reposition or change ETT.
Low exhaled minute volume	Altered settings; leak in system; airway secretions; decreased lung compliance; malfunctioning spirometer; decreased patient-triggered respiratory rate resulting from medications, sleep, hypocapnia, alkalosis, fatigue, change in neurologic status	Check settings; assess patient's respiratory rate, mental status, and work of breathing; evaluate system for leaks; suction airway; assess patient for changes in disease state; calibrate spirometer.
Low PEEP/CPAP pressure	Altered settings; increased patient inspirator/flows; leak; decreased expiratory flows from ventilator	Check settings and correct; observe for leaks in system; if unable to correct problem, increase PEEP settings.
High respiratory rate	Increased metabolic demand; medication administration; hypoxia; hypercapnia; acidosis; shock; pain; fear; anxiety	Evaluate ABGs; assess patient; calm and reassure patient.
High-pressure limit	Improper alarm setting; airway obstruction resulting from patient fighting ventilator (holding breath as ventilator delivers VT); patient circuit collapse; tubing kinked; ETT in right main stem bronchus or against carina; cuff herniation; increased airway resistance resulting from bronchospasm, airway secretions, plugs, and coughing; water from humidifier in ventilator tubing; decreased lung compliance resulting from tension pneumothorax, change in patient position, ARDS, pulmonary edema, atelectasis, pneumonia, or abdominal distention	Reset alarms; clear obstruction from tubing; unkink and reposition patient off of tubing; empty water from tubing; check breath sounds; reassure patient and sedate if necessary; check ABGs for hypoxemia; observe for abdominal distention that would put pressure on the diaphragm; check cuff pressures; obtain chest radiograph and evaluate for ETT position, pneumothorax, and pneumonia; reposition ETT; give bronchodilator therapy.
Low-pressure oxygen inlet	Improper oxygen alarm setting; oxygen not connected to ventilator; dirty oxygen intake filter	Correct alarm setting; reconnect or connect oxygen line to a 50-psi source; clean or replace oxygen filter.
I:E ratio	Inspiratory time longer than expiratory time; use of an inspiratory phase that is too long with a fast rate; peak flow setting too low while rate too high; machine too sensitive	Change inspiratory time or adjust peak flow; check inspiratory phase or hold; check machine sensitivity.
Temperature	Sensor malfunction; overheating resulting from too low or no gas flow; sensor picking up outside airflow (from heater, open door or window, air conditioner); improper water levels	Test or replace sensor; check gas flow; protect sensor from outside source that would interfere with readings; check water levels.

ABGs, Arterial blood gases; *ARDS, acute respiratory distress syndrome*; *CPAP,* constant positive airway pressure; *ETT,* endotracheal tube; *PEEP,* positive end-expiratory pressure; *Vt,* tidal volume.
Modified from Flynn JBM, Bruce NP. *Introduction to Critical Care Nursing Skills.* St. Louis: Mosby; 1993.

BOX 16-4 PATIENT SAFETY (QSEN) ALERT INTRAHOSPITAL TRANSPORT OF CRITICALLY ILL PATIENTS

The following is an excerpt from the *Guidelines for the Inter- and Intrahospital Transport of Critically Ill Patients*:

1. Pretransport Coordination and Communication
   - Confirm receiving unit readiness to receive patient.
   - Nurse-to-nurse handoff (if patient care responsibility is being transferred to a nurse in the receiving area)
   - Notify respiratory therapist and/or other members of the health care team of timing of transport and request equipment support, as needed.
   - Mechanical ventilator in receiving unit (for mechanically ventilated patients)
2. Accompanying Personnel
   - A minimum of two people should accompany a critically ill patient (one of which should be a critical care nurse).
   - Unstable patients should be accompanied by a physician.
3. Accompanying Equipment
   - Blood pressure monitor or cuff
   - Pulse oximeter
   - Cardiac monitor with defibrillator
   - Basic resuscitation medications (Emergency cart should be readily available in receiving unit.)
   - Additional sedatives and narcotic analgesics
   - Additional intravenous fluids and medications
   - Oxygen delivery device attached to oxygen source with at least a 30-minute reserve or manual resuscitation bag and/or transport ventilator (for mechanically ventilated patients)
   - Transport ventilator must have alarms and back-up battery.
4. Monitoring During Transport
   - Continuous electrocardiographic monitoring
   - Continuous pulse oximetry
   - Periodic measurement of blood pressure, pulse rate, and respiratory rate

From Warren J, et al. Guidelines for the inter- and intrahospital transport of critically ill patients. *Crit Care Med.* 2004: 32:256.

aspiration. The patient is closely monitored for gastric distention, and a nasogastric tube is placed for decompression, as necessary. Often, patients are very anxious and have high levels of dyspnea before the initiation of noninvasive mechanical ventilation. After adequate ventilation has been established, anxiety and dyspnea are usually sufficiently relieved. Heavy sedation should be avoided, but if it is needed, it would constitute the need for intubation and invasive mechanical ventilation. It is important to spend 30 minutes with the patient after initiation of noninvasive ventilation because the patient needs reassurance and must learn how to breathe on the machine.[87,89] The patient who requires noninvasive ventilation with a face mask should never be restrained. The patient must be able to remove the mask if it becomes displaced or the patient vomits. A displaced mask can force the patient's bottom jaw inward and occlude the patient's airway.

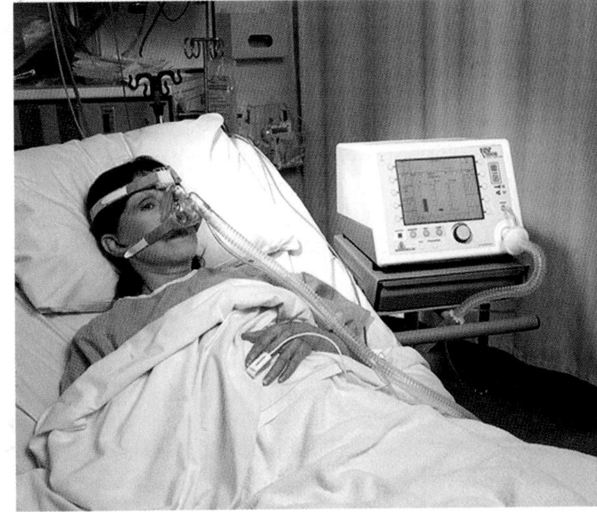

FIG 16-9 Bipap via Face Mask. (Courtesy Respironics Inc., Murrysville, PA.)

POSITIONING THERAPY

Positioning therapy can help match ventilation and perfusion through the redistribution of oxygen and blood flow in the lungs, which improves gas exchange. On the basis of the concept that preferential blood flow occurs to the gravity-dependent areas of the lungs, positioning therapy is used to place the least-damaged portion of the lungs into a dependent position. The least damaged portions of the lungs receive preferential blood flow, resulting in less ventilation–perfusion mismatch.[69] The current two approaches to position therapy are 1) prone positioning and 2) rotation therapy.

Prone Positioning

Prone positioning is a therapeutic modality that is used to improve oxygenation in patients with ARDS.[90-92] It involves turning the patient completely over onto his or her stomach in the face-down position. Although a number of theories have been proposed to explain how prone positioning improves oxygenation, the discovery that ARDS causes greater damage to the dependent areas of the lungs probably provides the best explanation. It was originally thought that ARDS was a diffuse, homogeneous disease that affected all areas of the lungs equally. It is now known that the dependent lung areas are more heavily damaged than the nondependent lung areas. Turning the patient to the prone position improves perfusion to the less-damaged areas of the lungs, improves ventilation–perfusion match, and decreases intrapulmonary shunting. Prone positioning can be used to facilitate the mobilization of secretions and provide pressure relief. Prone positioning is contraindicated in patients with increased intracranial pressure, hemodynamic instability, spinal cord injuries, or abdominal surgery. Patients who are unable to tolerate the face-down position are also not appropriate candidates for this type of therapy.[90-92]

No standard has been established for the length of time a patient should remain in the prone position. A review of the research on this subject revealed a wide variation, anywhere from 30 minutes to 40 hours.[92] The therapy is considered successful if the patient has an improvement in PaO_2 of greater than 10 mm Hg within 30 minutes of being placed in the prone position.[93] The positioning schedule (length of time in the prone position and frequency of turning) is usually based on the patient's tolerance of the procedure, the success of the procedure in improving the patient's PaO_2, and whether the patient is able to sustain improvements in PaO_2 when turned back to the supine position. Prone positioning is discontinued when the patient no longer demonstrates a response to the position change.[93]

The biggest limitation to prone positioning is the actual mechanics of turning the patient. A number of methods have been discussed in the literature, including manually turning the patient and positioning with pillows to support the patient and use of the RotoProne™ Therapy System.[90,92] Regardless of the method used, the abdomen must be allowed to hang free to facilitate diaphragmatic descent.

Before the patient is turned to the prone position, his or her eyes are lubricated and taped closed, tubes and drains are secured, and the procedure is explained to the patient and family. A team is organized to implement the turning procedure, and one member is positioned at the head of the bed to maintain the patient's airway. Complications of the procedure include dislodgment or obstruction of tubes and drains, hemodynamic instability, massive facial edema, pressure ulcers, aspiration, and corneal ulcerations.[90,92]

Rotation Therapy

Automated turning beds to provide rotation therapy are often used in the critical care setting. *Kinetic therapy* and *continuous lateral rotation therapy* (CLRT) are two forms of rotation therapy. The patient is continuously turned from side to side with a rotation of 40 degrees or greater (kinetic therapy) or with a rotation of less than 40 degrees (CLRT).[94] Two types of beds can perform this type of therapy: 1) an oscillation bed, in which the mattress inflates and deflates to provide rotation; and 2) a kinetic bed, in which the entire platform of the bed rotates.[95]

Rotation therapy is thought to improve oxygenation through better matching of ventilation to perfusion and to prevent pulmonary complications associated with bed rest and mechanical ventilation.[96,97] However, to achieve such benefits, rotation must be aggressive, and the patient must be turned at least 40 degrees per side, with a total arc of at least 80 degrees, for at least 18 hours a day.[97,98] CLRT has been shown to be of minimal pulmonary benefit to the critically ill patient.[94] Kinetic therapy decreases the incidence of VAP, particularly in patients with neurologic problems and in those who have undergone surgery.[98] In one study, kinetic therapy decreased the incidence of VAP and lobar atelectasis in medical, surgical, and trauma patients.[97]

Complications of the procedure include dislodgment or obstruction of tubes, drains, and lines; hemodynamic instability; and pressure ulcers. Lateral rotation does not replace manual repositioning to prevent pressure ulcers.[99] Repositioning changes the relationship of the patient's posterior surface to the mattress. This gives the skin a chance to reperfuse and to ventilate. Repositioning shifts weight-bearing points. To prevent pressure ulcers, the patient should be positioned 30 degrees from the surface of the mattress regardless of the degree of rotational turn. One study found that patients receiving rotational therapy still developed pressure ulcers of the sacrum, occiput, and heels.[100]

THORACIC SURGERY

The term *thoracic surgery* refers to a number of surgical procedures that involve opening the thoracic cavity (thoracotomy), the organs of respiration, or both. Indications for thoracic surgery range from tumors and abscesses to repair of the esophagus and thoracic vessels.[101] Table 16-9 describes a variety of thoracic surgical procedures and their indications. This discussion focuses only on the surgical procedures that involve the removal of lung tissue.

Preoperative Care

Before surgery, a complete evaluation of the patient is needed to determine the appropriateness of surgery as a treatment and to determine whether lung tissue can be removed without jeopardizing respiratory function. This is especially important when a lobectomy or pneumonectomy is being considered. When resection is being undertaken for tumor treatment, preoperative care includes evaluation of the type and extent of the tumor and the physical condition of the patient.[102]

The evaluation of the patient's physical status should focus on the adequacy of cardiopulmonary function. The preoperative evaluation should include pulmonary function tests to determine the patient's ability to manage with less lung tissue. Cardiac function also should be evaluated. Uncontrolled dysrhythmias, acute myocardial infarction, severe chronic heart failure, and unstable angina are all contraindications to surgery.[103,104]

Surgical Considerations

The type and location of surgery will dictate the type of surgical approach that is used. The most common approach is the posterolateral thoracotomy, which allows for exposure of both the lung and mediastinum (Figure 16-10). Other approaches that are used include anterolateral thoracotomy and median sternotomy.[101]

Special care is taken to avoid drainage of blood or secretions into the unaffected lung during surgery because such an occurrence could cause hypoxemia and cardiac dysfunction. A double-lumen endotracheal tube is used during the surgery to protect the unaffected lung from secretions and necrotic tumor fragments. To decrease the incidence of hypoxemia during the procedure, 5 to 10 cm H_2O of PEEP is maintained to the deflated lung. In addition, the deflated lung is intermittently ventilated during the procedure.[105]

Complications and Medical Management

A number of complications are associated with a lung resection. These include acute respiratory failure, bronchopleural fistula, hemorrhage, and cardiovascular disturbances.

Acute Lung Failure

In the postoperative period, acute respiratory failure may result from atelectasis or pneumonia. Atelectasis can occur as a result of anesthesia, the surgical procedure, immobilization, and pain. Treatment should be aimed at correcting the underlying problems and supporting gas exchange. Supplemental oxygen and mechanical ventilation with PEEP may be necessary.[106]

Bronchopleural Fistula

Development of a postoperative bronchopleural fistula is a major cause of mortality after a lung resection. A

TABLE 16-9 **Thoracic Surgeries**

PROCEDURE	DEFINITION	INDICATIONS
Pneumonectomy	Removal of entire lung with or without resection of the mediastinal lymph nodes	Malignant lesions Unilateral tuberculosis Extensive unilateral bronchiectasis Multiple lung abscesses Massive hemoptysis Bronchopleural fistula
Lobectomy	Resection of one or more lobes of lung	Lesions confined to a single lobe Pulmonary tuberculosis Bronchiectasis Lung abscesses or cysts Trauma
Segmental resection	Resection of bronchovascular section of lung lobe	Small peripheral lesions Bronchiectasis Congenital cysts or blebs
Wedge resection	Removal of small wedge-shaped section of lung tissue	Small, peripheral lesions (without lymph node involvement) Peripheral granulomas Pulmonary blebs
Bronchoplastic reconstruction (also called *sleeve resection*)	Resection of lung tissue and bronchus with end-to-end reanastomosis of bronchus	Small lesions involving the carina or major bronchus without evidence of metastasis May be combined with lobectomy
Lung volume reduction surgery	Resection of the most damaged portions of lung tissue, allowing more normal chest wall configuration	Severe emphysema
Bullectomy	Resection of a large bulla (an airspace that is greater than 1 cm in diameter that formed as a result of pulmonary tissue destruction)	Severe emphysema with large bullae compressing surrounding tissue
Open lung biopsy	Resection of a small portion of the lung for biopsy	Failure of closed lung biopsy Removal of small lesions
Decortication	Removal of fibrous membrane from pleural surface of lung	Fibrothorax resulting from hemothorax or empyema
Drainage of empyema	Drainage of pus in the pleural space	Acute and chronic infections
Partial rib resection	Removal of one or more ribs to allow healing of underlying lung tissue	Chronic empyemic infections
Video-assisted thoracoscopy (VATS)	Endoscopie procedure performed through small incisions in the chest	Evaluation of pulmonary, pleural, mediastinal, or pericardial conditions Biopsy of lung, pleural, or mediastinal lesions Recurrent spontaneous pneumothorax Evacuation of emphysema, hemothorax, pleural effusion, or pericardial effusion Blebectomy or bullectomy Pleurodesis Sympathectomy Closure of bronchopleural fistula Lysis of adhesions

bronchopleural fistula develops when the suture line fails to secure occlusion of the bronchial stump, and an opening develops into the pleural space.[107] This can result from an imperfect stump closure, perforation of the stump (e.g., with a suction catheter), high pressure within the airways (e.g., caused by mechanical ventilation), or infection.[108,109] During surgery, careful attention is given to isolating and closing the bronchus in an attempt to secure a lasting seal with subsequent stump healing.[101] In addition, early extubation is encouraged to eliminate the possibility of perforation of the stump and high airway pressures.[108] Clinical manifestations of a bronchopleural fistula include shortness of breath and coughing up serosanguineous sputum. Immediate surgery is usually necessary to close the stump and prevent flooding of the remaining lung with fluid from the residual space.[109] If this occurs, the patient should be placed with the operative side down (remaining lung up), and a chest tube should be inserted to drain the residual space.[101]

Hemorrhage

Hemorrhage is an early, life-threatening complication that can occur after a lung resection. It can result from bronchial or intercostal artery bleeding or disruption of a suture or clip around a pulmonary vessel.[108] Excessive chest tube drainage

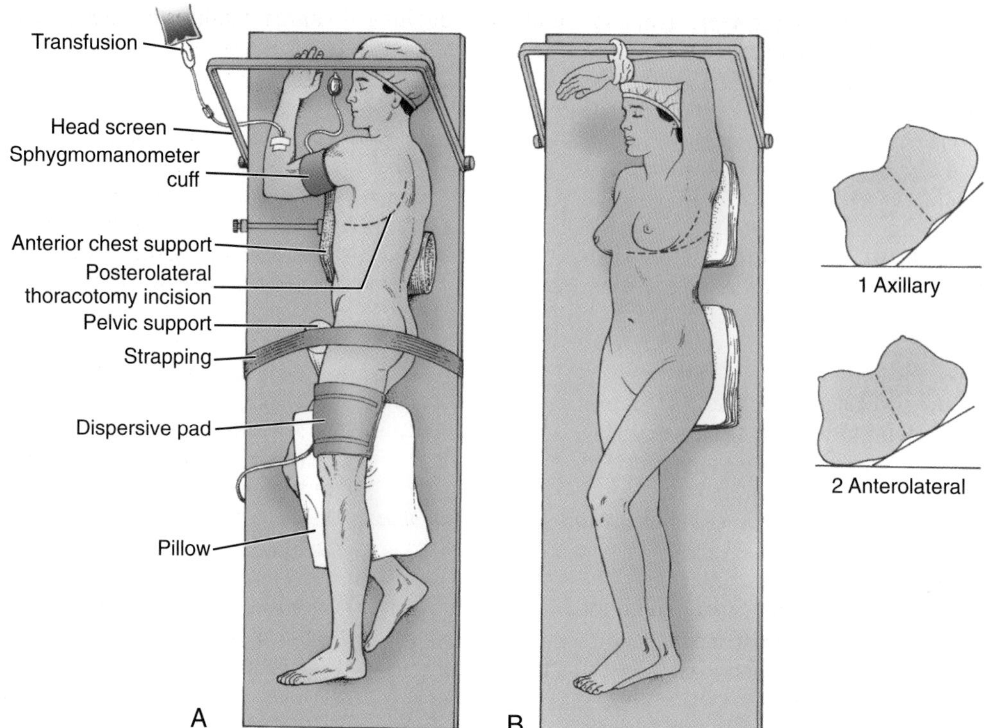

FIG 16-10 Positions for Thoracotomy Incisions. *A,* Lateral position for posterolateral incision. *B,* Semilateral position for axillary or anterolateral position. (From Blanchard B. Thoracic surgery. In: Rothrock JC, McEwen DR, eds. *Alexander's Care of the Patient in Surgery.* 14th ed. St. Louis: Elsevier; 2011.)

can signal excessive bleeding. During the immediate postoperative period, chest tube drainage should be measured every 15 minutes; this frequency should be decreased as the patient stabilizes. If chest tube loss is greater than 100 mL/hr, fresh blood is noted, or a sudden increase in drainage occurs, hemorrhage should be suspected.

Cardiovascular Disturbances

Cardiovascular complications after thoracic surgery include dysrhythmias and pulmonary edema. Resections of a large lung area or a pneumonectomy may be followed by a rise in central venous pressure. With the loss of one lung, the right ventricle must empty its stroke volume into a vascular bed that has been reduced by 50%. This means a higher pressure system is created, which increases right ventricular workload and precipitates right ventricular failure. Depending on previous heart function, acute decompensation of both ventricles can result. Measures are aimed at supporting cardiac function and avoiding intravascular volume excess. These measures include optimizing preload, afterload, and contractility with vasoactive agents.[108]

Postoperative Nursing Management

Nursing care of the patient who has had thoracic surgery incorporates a number of nursing diagnoses (Box 16-5). **Nursing priorities focus on 1) optimizing oxygenation and ventilation, 2) preventing atelectasis, 3) monitoring chest tubes, 4) assisting the patient to return to an adequate activity level, 5) providing comfort and emotional support, and 6) maintaining surveillance for complications.**

BOX 16-5 NURSING DIAGNOSIS PRIORITIES

Thoracic Surgery

- Ineffective Breathing Pattern, related to decreased lung expansion, p. 598
- Impaired Gas Exchange, related to ventilation/perfusion mismatching or intrapulmonary shunting, p. 594
- Impaired Gas Exchange, related to alveolar hypoventilation, p. 593
- Acute Pain, related to transmission and perception of cutaneous, visceral, muscular, or ischemic impulses, p. 574
- Disturbed Body Image, related to actual change in body structures, function, or appearance, p. 586

Optimizing Oxygenation and Ventilation

Nursing interventions to optimize oxygenation and ventilation include positioning, preventing desaturation during procedures, and promoting secretion clearance.

Preventing Atelectasis

Nursing interventions to prevent atelectasis include proper patient positioning and early ambulation, deep-breathing exercises, incentive spirometry (IS), and pain management. The goal is to promote maximal lung ventilation and prevent hypoventilation.

Patient positioning and early ambulation. The nurse should consider the surgical incision site and the type of surgery when positioning the patient. After a lobectomy, the patient should be turned onto the nonoperative side to promote

V/Q matching. When the good lung is dependent and blood flow is greater to the area with better ventilation, V/Q matching is better. V/Q mismatching results when the affected lung is positioned down because of the increase in blood flow to an area with less ventilation. The patient should be turned frequently to promote secretion removal but should have the affected lung dependent as little as possible. The patient who has had a pneumonectomy should be positioned supine or on the operative side during the initial period. Turning onto the operative side promotes splinting of the incision and facilitates deep-breathing exercises. Tilting the patient slightly toward the unaffected side is possible, but the surgeon should indicate when free side-to-side positioning is safe.[109]

When sitting at the bedside or ambulating, patients must be encouraged to keep the thorax in straight alignment while they breathe deeply. This position best accommodates diaphragmatic descent and intercostal muscle action. The sitting or standing position provides enhanced ventilation to areas of the lung that are dependent in the supine position, thus accommodating maximal inflation and promoting gas exchange. Ambulation is essential in restoring lung function and should be initiated as soon as possible.

Deep breathing and incentive spirometry. Deep breathing and incentive spirometry should be performed regularly by patients who have undergone a thoracotomy. Deep breathing involves having the patient take a deep breath and hold it for approximately 3 seconds or longer. Incentive spirometry involves having the patient take at least 10 deep, effective breaths per hour using an incentive spirometer. These activities help re-expand collapsed lung tissue, thus promoting early resolution of the pneumothorax in patients with partial lung resections. The chest should be auscultated during inflation to ensure that all dependent parts of the lung are well-ventilated and to help the patient understand the depth of breath necessary for optimal effect. Coughing, which should be encouraged only when secretions are present, assists in mobilizing secretions for removal.[110]

Pain management. Pain can be a major problem after thoracic surgery. Pain can increase the workload of the heart, precipitate hypoventilation, and inhibit mobilization of secretions. Clinical manifestations of pain include tachypnea, tachycardia, elevated blood pressure, facial grimacing, splinting of the incision, hypoventilation, moaning, and restlessness. Several alternatives for pain management after thoracic surgery can be used. The two most common methods are systemic narcotic administration and epidural narcotic administration. Opioids can be administered intravenously or via the patient-controlled analgesia (PCA) method. In addition, the patient should be assisted with splinting the incision with a pillow or blanket when deep breathing and coughing. Splinting stabilizes the area and reduces pain when moving, deep breathing, or coughing.[106]

Maintaining the Chest Tube System

Chest tubes are placed after most thoracic surgery procedures to remove air and fluid. The drainage will initially appear bloody, becoming serosanguineous and then serous over the first 2 to 3 days postoperatively. Approximately 100 to 300 mL of drainage will occur during the first 2 hours postoperatively, which will decrease to less than 50 mL/hr over the next several hours. Routine stripping of chest tubes is not recommended because excessive negative pressure can be generated in the chest. If blood clots are present in the drainage tubing or an obstruction is present, the chest tubes may be carefully milked. The chest tube may be placed to suction or water seal.[111]

During auscultation of the lungs, air leaks should be evaluated. In the early phase, an air leak is commonly heard over the affected area because the pleura have not yet tightly sealed. As healing occurs, this leak should disappear. An increase in an air leak or the appearance of a new air leak should prompt investigation of the chest drainage system to discover whether air is leaking into the system from outside or whether the leak is originating from the incision. Increased air leaks not related to the thoracic drainage system may indicate disruption of sutures.[108]

Assisting Patient to Return to Adequate Activity Level

Within a few days after surgery, range-of-motion exercises for the shoulder on the operative side should be performed. The patient frequently splints the operative side and avoids shoulder movement because of pain. If immobility is allowed, stiffening of the shoulder joint can result. This is referred to as *frozen shoulder* and may require physical therapy and rehabilitation to regain satisfactory range of motion of the shoulder joint.[109]

Usually on the day after surgery, the patient is able to sit in a chair. Activity should be systematically increased, with attention to the patient's activity tolerance. With adequate pulmonary function before surgery and a surgical approach designed to preserve respiratory function, full return to previous activity levels is possible. This may take as long as 6 months to 1 year, depending on the tissue resected and the patient's general condition.[101]

PHARMACOLOGY

A number of pharmacologic agents are used in the care of the patient with pulmonary dysfunction who is critically ill. Table 16-10 reviews these agents and the special considerations necessary for administering them.

TABLE 16-10 Pharmacologic Management: Pulmonary Disorders

MEDICATION	DOSAGE	ACTIONS	SPECIAL CONSIDERATIONS
Neuromuscular Blocking Agents (NMBAs)			
Vecuronium (Norcuron)	Loading dose: 0.08-0.1 mg/kg IV IV infusion: 0.8-1.2 mcg/kg/min	Used to paralyze patient to decrease oxygen demand and avoid ventilator dyssynchrony	Boxed Warning from FDA: Risk of anaphylactic and anaphylactoid type adverse reactions, including fatalities, reported in association with use of neuromuscular blockers.

Continued

TABLE 16-10 Pharmacologic Management: Pulmonary Disorders—cont'd

MEDICATION	DOSAGE	ACTIONS	SPECIAL CONSIDERATIONS
Pancuronium (Pavulon)	Loading dose: 0.06-0.1 mg/kg IV infusion: 0.02-0.04 mg/kg/hr		Administer sedative and analgesic agents concurrently, because NMBAs have no sedative or analgesic properties.
Rocuronium (Zemuron)	Loading dose: 0.6 mg/kg IV IV infusion: 10-12 mcg/kg/min		Evaluate level of paralysis q4h using a peripheral nerve stimulator.
Atracurium (Tracrium)	Loading dose: 0.30-0.50 mg/kg IV IV infusion: 4-12 mcg/kg/min		Protect patients from the environment because they are unable to respond.
Cisatracurium (Nimbex)	Loading dose: 0.15-0.2 mg/kg IV IV Infusion: 0.5-10.2 mcg/kg/min)		Prolonged muscle paralysis may occur after discontinuation of the paralytic agent.
Mucolytics			
Acetylcysteine (Mucomyst)	Nebulizer, 20% solution: 3-5 mL tid–qid Nebulizer, 10% solution: 6-10 mL tid–qid	Used to decrease viscosity and elasticity of mucus by breaking down disulfide bonds within mucus	May be administered with a bronchodilator because medication can cause bronchospasms and inhibit ciliary function. Treatment is considered effective when bronchorrhea develops and coughing occurs. Antidote for acetaminophen overdose
B_2-Agonists			
Epinephrine (Adrenalin)	Nebulizer, 1% solution: 2.5-5 mg (0.25-0.5 mL) qid	Used to relax bronchial smooth muscle and dilate airways to prevent bronchospasms	May cause skeletal muscle tremors. Higher doses may cause tachycardia, palpitations, increased blood pressure, dysrhythmias, and angina.
Racemic epinephrine	Nebulizer, 2.25% solution: 5.625-11.25 mg (0.25-0.5 mL) qid		
Isoetharine 1% (Bronkosol)	Nebulizer, 1% solution: 2.5-5 mg (0.25-0.5 mL) qid		May increase serum glucose and decrease serum potassium levels.
Terbutaline	MDI, 340 mcg/puff: 1-2 puffs qid MDI, 200 mcg/puff: 2 puffs q4-6h		Treatment is considered effective when breath sounds improve and dyspnea is lessened.
Metaproterenol (Alupent, Metaprel)	Nebulizer, 5% solution: 15 mg (0.3 mL) tid–qid MDI, 650 mcg/puff: 2-3 puffs tid–qid		Only approximately 10% of the administered dose reaches the site of action within the lungs.
Albuterol (Proventil, Ventolin)	Nebulizer, 5% solution: 2.5 mg (0.5 mL) tid–qid MDI, 90 mcg/puff: 2 puffs tid–qid		
Levalbuterol (Xopenex)	Nebulizer: 0.63 mg q6-8h		
Anticholinergic Agents			
Ipratropium (Atrovent)	Nebulizer, 0.02% solution: 0.5 mg (2.5 mL) q6-8h	Used to block the constriction of bronchial smooth muscle and reduce mucus production	There are relatively few adverse effects because systemic absorption is poor.
Xanthines			
Theophylline	Loading dose: 4.6 mg/kg IV IV infusion: 0.4-0.8 mg/kg/hr	Used to dilate bronchial smooth muscle and reverse diaphragmatic muscle fatigue	Administer loading dose over 30 minutes. Monitor serum blood levels; therapeutic level is 10-20 mg/dL.
Aminophylline	Loading dose: 5.7 mg/kg IV IV infusion: 0.5-1 mg/kg/hr		Administer with caution to patients with cardiac, renal, or hepatic disease. Signs of toxicity include central nervous system excitation, seizures, confusion, irritability, hyperglycemia, headache, nausea, hypotension, and dysrhythmias.

TABLE 16-10 Pharmacologic Management: Pulmonary Disorders—cont'd

MEDICATION	DOSAGE	ACTIONS	SPECIAL CONSIDERATIONS
Inhaled Corticosteroids			
Beclomethasone (Vanceril, Beclovent)	MDI, 42 meg/puff: 2 puffs tid-qid	Used to decrease airway inflammation and enhance effectiveness of beta-agonists	Suppresses inflammatory response and interferes with ability to fight infection
Flunisolide (AeroBid)	MDI, 250 meg/puff: 2 puffs bid		Oral candidiasis is a side effect that can be minimized by having patients rinse their mouths after treatment.
Triamcinolone (Azmacort)	MDI, 100 meg/puff: 2 puffs tid-qid		

FDA, U.S. Food and Drug Administration; *MDI*, metered-dose inhaler, *NMBAs*, neuromuscular blocking agents.
Data from *Elsevier/Gold Standard.* http://www.mdconsult.com/das/pharm/lookup/340530070-12?type=alldrugs. Accessed May 17, 2014.

BOX 16-6 INTERNET RESOURCES

- American Association of Critical-Care Nurses: http://www.aacn.org
- Society for Critical Care Medicine: http://www.sccm.org
- Respiratory Nursing Society: http://respiratorynursingsociety.org
- American Holistic Nurses Association: http://www.ahna.org
- American Association of Respiratory Care: http://www.aarc.org
- American College of Chest Physicians: http://www.chestnet.org/accp
- NHLBI ARDS Network: http://www.ardsnet.org
- American College of Physicians: http://www.acponline.org
- American College of Surgeons: http://www.facs.org
- American Lung Association: http://www.lung.org
- American Medical Association: http://www.ama-assn.org
- American Thoracic Society: http://www.thoracic.org
- American Holistic Medical Association: http://www.holisticmedicine.org
- ICU Delirium and Cognitive Impairment Study Group: http://www.icudelirium.org/resources.html
- Centers for Disease Control and Prevention: http://www.cdc.gov
- National Institutes for Health: http://www.nih.gov
- PubMed Health: http://www.ncbi.nlm.nih.gov/pubmedhealth

CASE STUDY Patient with Acute Respiratory Failure

Brief Patient History

Mr. B is a 63-year-old man who is clinically obese. He has a long history of chronic obstructive pulmonary disease (COPD) associated with smoking two packs of cigarettes a day for 40 years. During the past week, Mr. B has experienced a flulike illness with fever, chills, malaise, anorexia, diarrhea, nausea, vomiting, and a productive cough with thick, brownish, purulent sputum.

Clinical Assessment

Mr. B is admitted to the intermediate care unit from the emergency department with acute respiratory insufficiency. He is sitting up in bed, leaning forward, with his elbows resting on the over-the-bed table. Mr. B is breathing through his mouth, taking rapid shallow breaths, using his accessory muscles to ventilate. On inhalation, his nostrils flare, and his accessory muscles retract. During exhalation, Mr. B uses pursed-lip breathing, and his intercostal muscles bulge. He appears anxious and irritable and is able to speak only one or two barely audible words between each breath. Auscultation reveals crackles posteriorly over the right and left lower lung fields.

Diagnostic Procedures

His admission chest radiograph reveals infiltrates in the right lower lobe and left lower lobe. Gram stain of Mr. B's sputum shows numerous gram-positive diplococci. His baseline vital signs are as follows: blood pressure of 110/60 mm Hg, heart rate of 108 beats/min (sinus tachycardia), respiratory rate of 30 breaths/min, and temperature of 101.3°F. His baseline arterial blood gas (ABG) values on a 28% Venturi face mask are as follows: PaO_2 of 58 mm Hg, $PaCO_2$ of 33 mm Hg, pH of 7.52, HCO_3^- level of 28, and O_2 saturation of 88%.

Medical Diagnosis

Mr. B is diagnosed with community-associated pneumococcal pneumonia.

Questions

1. What major outcomes do you expect to achieve for this patient?
2. What problems or risks must be managed to achieve these outcomes?
3. What interventions must be initiated to monitor, prevent, manage, or eliminate the problems and risks identified?
4. What interventions should be initiated to promote optimal functioning, safety, and well-being of the patient?
5. What possible learning needs do you anticipate for this patient?
6. What cultural and age-related factors may have a bearing on the patient's plan of care?

REFERENCES

1. Henderson Y: Delivering oxygen therapy to acutely breathless adults, *Nurs Stand* 22(35):46, 2008.
2. O'Driscoll BR, et al: BTS guideline for emergency oxygen use in adult patients, *Thorax* 63(Suppl 6):vi1, 2008.
3. Heuer AJ: Medical gas therapy. In Kacmarek RM, et al, editors: *Egan's fundamentals of respiratory care*, ed 10, St. Louis, 2013, Mosby.
4. Kernick J, Magarey J: What is the evidence for the use of high flow nasal cannula oxygen in adult patients admitted to critical care units? A systematic review, *Aust Crit Care* 23:53, 2010.
5. White AC: The evaluation and management of hypoxemia in the chronic critically ill patient, *Clin Chest Med* 22:123, 2001.
6. Barnes TA: Emergency cardiovascular life support. In Kacmarek RM, et al, editors: *Egan's fundamentals of respiratory care*, ed 10, St. Louis, 2013, Mosby.
7. Pierce LNB: *Management of the mechanically ventilated patient*, ed 2, St. Louis, 2007, Saunders.
8. McCorstin P, et al: Management of the mechanically ventilated patient in the emergency department, *J Emerg Nurs* 34:121, 2008.
9. Walz JM, Zayaruzny M, Heard SO: Airway management in critical illness, *Chest* 131:608, 2007.
10. St John RE, Seckel MA: Airway management. In Burns SM, editor: *AACN protocols for practice: Care of the mechanically ventilated patient*, ed 2, Sudbury, MA, 2007, Jones and Bartlett.
11. Altobelli N: Airway management. In Kacmarek RM, et al, editors: *Egan's fundamentals of respiratory care*, ed 10, St. Louis, 2013, Mosby.
12. Chethan DB, Hughes RC: Tracheal intubation, tracheal tubes and laryngeal mask airways, *J Perioper Pract* 18:88, 2008.
13. Colice GL: Technical standards for tracheal tubes, *Clin Chest Med* 12:433, 1991.
14. Mace SE: Challenges and advances in intubation: rapid sequence intubation, *Emerg Med Clin N Am* 26:1043, 2008.
15. Kabrhel C, et al: Orotracheal intubation, *N Eng J Med* 356:e15, 2007.
16. Miñambres E, et al: Tracheal rupture after endotracheal intubation: a literature systematic review, *Eur J Cardiothorac Surg* 35:1056, 2009.
17. Feller-Kopman D: Acute complications of artificial airways, *Clin Chest Med* 24:445, 2003.
18. Gaissert HA, Burns J: The compromised airway: tumors, strictures, and tracheomalacia, *Surg Clin N Am* 90:1065, 2010.
19. Durbin CG: Tracheostomy: why, when, and how?, *Respir Care* 55:1056, 2010.
20. St John RE, Malen JF: Contemporary issues in adult tracheostomy management, *Crit Care Nurs Clin North Am* 16:413, 2004.
21. Morris LL, Afifi MS: *Tracheostomies: The complete guide*, New York, 2010, Springer.
22. Vallamkondu V, Visvanathan V: Clinical review of adult tracheostomy, *J Perioper Pract* 21:172, 2011.
23. Cabrini L, et al: Percutaneous tracheostomy, a systematic review, *Acta Anaesthesiol Scand* 56:270, 2012.
24. Samuelson KAM: Adult intensive care patients' perception of endotracheal tube-related discomforts: a prospective evaluation, *Heart Lung* 40:49, 2011.
25. Züchner K: Humidification: measurement and requirements, *Respir Care Clin N Am* 12:149, 2006.
26. Fink J, Ari A: Humidity and bland aerosol therapy. In Kacmarek RM, et al, editors: *Egan's fundamentals of respiratory care*, ed 10, St. Louis, 2013, Mosby.
27. Schulze A: Respiratory gas conditioning and humidification, *Clin Perinatol* 34(1):19, 2007.
28. Wright SE, VanDahm K: Long-term care of the tracheostomy patient, *Clin Chest Med* 24:473, 2003.
29. Hamilton VA, Grap MJ: The role of the endotracheal tube cuff in microaspiration, *Heart Lung* 41:167, 2012.
30. Browne JA, et al: Pursuing excellence: development of an oral hygiene protocol for mechanically ventilated patients, *Crit Care Nurs Q* 34:25, 2011.
31. Muscedere J, et al: Comprehensive evidence-based clinical practice guidelines for ventilatory-associated pneumonia: prevention, *J Crit Care* 23:126, 2008.
32. American Association for Respiratory Care: AARC Clinical Practice Guidelines. Endotracheal suctioning of mechanically ventilated patients with artificial airways 2010, *Respir Care* 55:758, 2010.
33. Pedersen CM, et al: Endotracheal suctioning of the adult intubated patient–what is the evidence, *Intensive Crit Care Nurs* 25:21, 2009.
34. Grap MJ, et al: Endotracheal suctioning: ventilator vs. manual delivery of hyperoxygenation breaths, *Am J Crit Care* 5:192, 1996.
35. Stone KS: Ventilator versus manual resuscitation bag as the method of delivering hyperoxygenation before endotracheal suctioning, *AACN Clin Issues Crit Care Nurs* 1:289, 1990.
36. Czarnik RE, et al: Differential effects of continuous versus intermittent suction on tracheal tissue, *Heart Lung* 20:144, 1991.
37. Raymond SJ: Normal saline instillation before suctioning: helpful or harmful? A review of the literature, *Am J Crit Care* 4:267, 1995.
38. Kinloch D: Instillation of normal saline during endotracheal suctioning: effects on mixed venous oxygen saturation, *Am J Crit Care* 8:231, 1999.
39. Hagler DA, Traver GA: Endotracheal saline and suction catheters: sources of lower airway contamination, *Am J Crit Care* 3:444, 1994.
40. Jelic S, Cunningham JA, Factor P: Clinical review: airway hygiene in the intensive care unit, *Crit Care* 12:209, 2008.
41. Dave MH, et al: Massive aspiration past the tracheal tube cuff caused by closed trachael suction system, *J Intensive Care Med* 26:326, 2011.
42. Jenabzadeh NE, Chlan L: A nurse's experience being intubated and receiving mechanical ventilation, *Crit Care Nurse* 31(6):51, 2011.
43. Grossbach I, et al: Promoting effective communication for patients receiving mechanical ventilation, *Crit Care Nurse* 31:46, 2011.
44. Scherzer R: Subglottic secretion aspiration in the prevention of ventilator-associated pneumonia, *Dimens Crit Care Nurs* 29:276, 2010.
45. Stonecypher K: Ventilator-associated pneumonia: the importance of oral care in intubated adults, *Crit Care Nurs Q* 33:339, 2010.
46. Binkley C, et al: Survey of oral care practices in U.S. intensive care units, *Am J Infect Control* 32:161, 2004.

47. Garcia R: A review of the possible role of oral and dental colonization on the occurrence of health-care associated pneumonia: underappreciated risk and a call for interventions, *Am J Infect Control* 33:527, 2005.
48. Roberts N, Moule P: Chlorhexidine and tooth-brushing as prevention strategies in reducing ventilator-associated pneumonia, *Nurs Crit Care* 16:295, 2011.
49. Chlebicki MP, Safdar N: Topical chlorhexidine for prevention of ventilator-associated pneumonia: a meta-analysis, *Crit Care Med* 35(2):595, 2007.
50. Grap JM, et al: Early, single chlorhexidine application reduces ventilator-associated pneumonia in trauma patients, *Heart Lung* 40:e115, 2011.
51. Kracz M, et al: State-of-the-art mechanical ventilation, *J Cardiothorac Vasc Anesth* 26:486, 2012.
52. Archambault PM, St-Onge M: Invasive and noninvasive ventilation in the emergency department, *Emeg Med Clin N Am* 30:421, 2012.
53. Chatburn RL, Volsko TA: Mechanical ventilators. In Kacmarek RM, et al, editors: *Egan's fundamentals of respiratory care*, ed 10, St. Louis, 2013, Mosby.
54. Cairo JM: *Pilbeam's mechanical ventilation: Physiological and clinical applications*, ed 5, St. Louis, 2012, Elsevier.
55. Maclntyre NR, Branson RD: *Mechanical ventilation*, ed 2, St. Louis, 2009, Saunders.
56. Kacmarek RM: Initiating and adjusting invasive ventilatory support. In Kacmarek RM, et al, editors: *Egan's fundamentals of respiratory care*, ed 10, St. Louis, 2013, Mosby.
57. Gattinoni L, et al: Ventilator-induced lung injury: the anatomical and physiological framework, *Crit Care Med* 38:S539, 2010.
58. Sarge T, Talmor D: Targeting transpulmonary pressure to prevent ventilator induced lung injury, *Minerva Anestesiol* 75:293, 2009.
59. Wahla AS, Khan FZ: Development of massive pneumopericardium after intubation and positive pressure ventilation, *J Coll Physicians Surg Pak* 22:401, 2012.
60. Sarge T, Talmor D: Transpulmonary pressure: its role in preventing ventilator-induced lung injury, *Minerva Anestesiol* 74:335, 2008.
61. Oeckler RA, Hubmayr RD: Cell wounding and repair in ventilator injured lungs, *Respir Physiol Neurobiol* 163:44, 2008.
62. Frazier SK: Cardiovascular effects of mechanical ventilation and weaning, *Nurs Clin North Am* 43:1, 2008.
63. Unroe M, Maclntyre N: Evolving approaches to assessing and monitoring patient-ventilator interactions, *Curr Opin Crit Care* 16:261, 2010.
64. Haas CF, Bauser KA: Advanced ventilator modes and techniques, *Crit Care Nurs Q* 35:27, 2012.
65. Grossbach I, et al: Overview of mechanical ventilator support and management of patient- and ventilator-related responses, *Crit Care Nurse* 31(3):30, 2011.
66. Rebmann T, Green LR: Preventing ventilator-associated pneumonia: An executive summary of the Association for Professionals in Infection Control and Epidemiology, Inc, Elimination Guide, *Am J Infect Control* 38:647, 2010.
67. Kieninger AN, Lipsett PA: Hospital-acquired pneumonia: pathophysiology, diagnosis, and treatment, *Surg Clin N Am* 89:439, 2009.
68. Institute for Healthcare Improvement. Implement the IHI ventilator bundle. http://www.ihi.org/knowledge/pages/changes/implementtheventilatorbundle.aspx. 2012. Accessed July 29, 2012.
69. Johnson KL, Meyenburg T: Physiological rationale and current evidence for therapeutic positioning of critically ill patients, *AACN Adv Crit Care* 20:228, 2009.
70. Niël-Weise B, et al: An evidenc-based recommendation on bed head elevation for mechanically ventilated patients, *Crit Care* 15:R111, 2011.
71. Berry E, Zecca H: Daily interruptions of sedation: a clinical approach to improve outcomes in critically ill patients, *Crit Care Nurse* 32(1):43, 2012.
72. Ramirez P, et al: Measures to prevent nosocomial infections during mechanical ventilation, *Curr Opin Crit Care* 18:86, 2012.
73. Lorente L, et al: Influence of an endotracheal tube with polyurethane cuff and subglottic secretion drainage on pneumonia, *Am J Respir Crit Care Med* 176:1079, 2007.
74. Blot S, et al: What is new in the prevention of ventilator-associated pneumonia?, *Curr Opin Pulm Med* 17:155, 2011.
75. Kollef MH, et al: Silver-coated endotracheal tubes and incidence of ventilator-associated pneumonia: the NASCENT randomized trial, *JAMA* 300:805, 2008.
76. Kacmarek RM: Discontinuing ventilatory support. In Kacmarek RM, et al, editors: *Egan's fundamentals of respiratory care*, ed 10, St. Louis, 2013, Mosby.
77. MacIntyre N: Discontinuing mechanical ventilatory support, *Chest* 132:1049, 2007.
78. Robertson TE, et al: Improved extubation rates and earlier liberation from mechanical ventilation with implementation of a daily spontaneous-breathing trial protocol, *J Am Coll Surg* 206:489, 2008.
79. Burns SM: Weaning from mechanical ventilation. In Burns SM, editor: *AACN protocols for practice: Care of the mechanically ventilated patient*, ed 2, Sudbury, MA, 2007, Jones and Bartlett.
80. Siner JM, Manthous CA: Liberation from mechanical ventilation: what monitoring matters?, *Crit Care Clin* 23:613, 2007.
81. Caroleo S, et al: Weaning from mechanical ventilation: an open issue, *Minerva Anestesiol* 73:417, 2007.
82. Blackwood B, et al: Use of weaning protocols for reducing duration of mechanical ventilation in critically ill adult patients: Cochrane systematic review and meta-analysis, *BMJ* 342:c7237, 2011.
83. Bekos V, Marini JJ: Monitoring the mechanically ventilated patient, *Crit Care Clin* 23:575, 2007.
84. Tracy MF, Chlan L: Nonpharmacological interventions to management common symptoms in patient receiving mechanical ventilation, *Crit Care Nurse* 31(3):19, 2011.
85. Balas MC, et al: Critical care nurse's role in implementing the "ABCDE Bundle" into practice, *Crit Care Nurse* 32(2):35, 2012.
86. McNeill GBS, Glossop AJ: Clinical applications of non-invasive ventilation in critical care, *Cont Edu Anaesth Crit Care & Pain* 12:33, 2012.
87. Holanda MA, et al: Influence of total face, facial and nasal masks on short-term adverse effects during noninvasive ventilation, *J Bras Pneumol* 35:164, 2009.
88. Williams PF: Noninvasive ventilation. In Kacmarek RM, et al, editors: *Egan's fundamentals of respiratory care*, ed 10, St. Louis, 2013, Mosby.

89. Pierce LNB: Invasive and noninvasive modes and methods of mechanical ventilation. In Burns SM, editor: *AACN protocols for practice: Care of the mechanically ventilated patient*, ed 2, Sudbury, MA, 2007, Jones and Bartlett.
90. Dirkes S, et al: Prone positioning: is it safe and effective?, *Crit Care Nurs Q* 35:64, 2012.
91. Alsaghir AH, Martin CM: Effect of prone positioning in patients with acute respiratory distress syndrome: a meta-analysis, *Crit Care Med* 36:603, 2008.
92. Dickinson S, et al: Prone positioning therapy in ARDS, *Crit Care Clin* 27:511, 2011.
93. Wright AD, Flynn M: Using the prone position for ventilated patients with respiratory failure: a review, *Nurs Crit Care* 16:19, 2011.
94. Goldhill DR, et al: Rotational bed therapy to prevent and treat respiratory complications: a review and meta-analysis, *Am J Crit Care* 16:50, 2007.
95. Stiller K: Physiotherapy in intensive care: towards an evidence-based practice, *Chest* 118:1801, 2000.
96. Ranee M: Kinetic therapy positively influences oxygenation in patients with ALI/ARDS, *Nurs Crit Care* 10:35, 2005.
97. Ahrens T, et al: Effect of kinetic therapy on pulmonary complications, *Am J Crit Care* 13:376, 2004.
98. Collard HR: Prevention of ventilator-associated pneumonia: an evidence-based systematic review, *Ann Intern Med* 138:494, 2003.
99. Powers J, Daniels D: Turning points: implementing kinetic therapy in the ICU, *Nurs Manage* 35:1, 2004.
100. Russell T, Logsdon A: Pressure ulcers and lateral rotation beds: a case study, *J Wound Ostomy Continence Nurs* 30:143, 2003.
101. Blanchard B: Thoracic surgery. In Rothrock JC, McEwen DR, editors: *Alexander's care of the patient in surgery*, ed 14, St. Louis, 2011, Elsevier.
102. Banki F: Pulmonary assessment for general thoracic surgery, *Surg Clin N Am* 90:969, 2010.
103. Sweitzer BJ, Smetana GW: Identification and evaluation of the patient with lung disease, *Med Clin N Am* 93:1017, 2009.
104. von Groote-Bidlingmaier F, et al: Functional evaluation before lung resection, *Clin Chest Med* 32:773, 2011.
105. Della Rocca G, Coccia C: Ventilatory management of one-lung ventilation, *Minerva Anestesiol* 77:534, 2011.
106. Sachdev G, Napolitano LM: Postoperative pulmonary complications: pneumonia and acute respiratory failure, *Surg Clin N Am* 92:321, 2012.
107. Shekar K, et al: Bronchopleural fistula: an update for intensivists, *J Crit Care* 25:47, 2010.
108. Kopec SE, et al: The postpneumonectomy state, *Chest* 114:1158, 1998.
109. Brenner Z, Addona C: Caring for the pneumonectomy patient: challenges and changes, *Crit Care Nurse* 15(5):65, 1995.
110. Hirsch CA: Airway clearance therapy. In Kacmarek RM, et al, editors: *Egan's fundamentals of respiratory care*, ed 10, St. Louis, 2013, Mosby.
111. Cerfolio RJ: Advances in thoracostomy tube management, *Surg Clin North Am* 82:833, 2002.

CHAPTER 17

Neurologic Clinical Assessment and Diagnostic Procedures

Darlene M. Burke

Be sure to check out the bonus material, including review questions, on the Evolve website at http://evolve.elsevier.com/Urden/priorities/.

HISTORY

Common to all neurologic assessments is the need to obtain a comprehensive history of events preceding hospitalization. An adequate neurologic history includes information about clinical manifestations, associated complaints, precipitating factors, progression, and familial occurrences (Box 17-1).[1] The ideal historian for recounting this information is someone who is able to provide a detailed description and chronology of events. If the patient is incapable of serving as the historian, family members or significant others who have contact with the patient on a daily basis should be contacted as soon as possible. Through history taking, the caregiver gains valuable information that directs him or her to focus on certain aspects of the patient's clinical assessment.[2]

FOCUSED CLINICAL ASSESSMENT

A thorough clinical assessment of the critically ill patient with neurologic dysfunction is imperative for the early identification and treatment of a neurologic disorder and serves as source of comparison for ongoing assessments of the patient. The most important finding in any neurologic assessment is change, which should be reported promptly. Early identification of neurologic deterioration is vital to preventing secondary brain injury.[3] Other medical conditions, as well as the administration of medications, can affect the clinical assessment and should be taken into consideration when the results of the neurologic examination are abnormal.

Five major components make up the neurologic evaluation of the critically ill patient. Nursing assessment of the patient focuses on five priorities: 1) level of consciousness, 2) motor function, 3) pupillary function, 4) respiratory function, and 5) vital signs. A complete neurologic examination requires assessment of all five components.[2,4]

Level of Consciousness

Assessment of the level of consciousness is the most important aspect of the neurologic examination. In most situations, a patient's level of consciousness deteriorates before any other neurologic changes are noticed. These deteriorations often are subtle and must be monitored carefully. **Nursing priorities in assessment of level of consciousness focus on two areas: 1) evaluation of arousal or alertness and 2) appraisal of content of consciousness or awareness.**[2,5] Although universally accepted definitions for various levels of consciousness do not exist, the categories outlined in Box 17-2 are often used to describe the patient's level of consciousness.[2,4,6]

Evaluation of Arousal

Assessment of the arousal component of consciousness is an evaluation of the reticular activating system and its connection to the thalamus and the cerebral cortex. Arousal is the lowest level of consciousness, and observation centers on the patient's ability to respond to verbal or noxious stimuli in an appropriate manner.[5] To stimulate the patient, the nurse should begin with verbal stimuli in a normal tone. If the patient does not respond, the nurse should increase the stimuli by talking very loudly to the patient. If the patient still does not respond, the nurse should further increase the stimuli by shaking the patient. Noxious stimuli, in the form of peripheral and central stimulation, should follow if previous attempts to arouse the patient are unsuccessful (Box 17-3).[2]

Appraisal of Awareness

Content of consciousness is a higher-level function, and appraisal of awareness is concerned with assessment of the patient's orientation to person, place, time, and situation.[5] Assessment of content of consciousness requires the patient to give appropriate answers to a variety of questions. Changes in the patient's answers that indicate increasing degrees of confusion and disorientation may be the first sign of neurologic deterioration.[1,2]

Glasgow Coma Scale

The most widely recognized tool for assessing level of consciousness is the Glasgow Coma Scale (GCS).[7] This scored scale is based on evaluation of three categories: 1) eye opening, 2) verbal response, and 3) best motor response (Table 17-1).

BOX 17-1 Data Collection

Neurologic History

Common Neurologic Symptoms
- Fainting
- Dizziness
- Blackouts
- Seizures
- Headache
- Memory loss
- Weakness
- Paralysis
- Tremors or other involuntary movements
- Pain
- Numbness
- Tingling
- Speech disturbances
- Vision disturbances

Events Preceding Onset of Symptoms
- Travel
- Animal contact
- Falls
- Infection
- Dental problems or procedures
- Sinus or middle ear infections
- Prodromal symptoms
- Food or drugs ingested

Progression of Symptoms
- Initial onset
- Evolution
- Frequency
- Severity
- Duration
- Associated activities or aggravating factors

Family History
- Stroke (arteriovenous malformation, aneurysm)
- Diabetes mellitus
- Hypertension
- Seizures
- Tumors
- Headaches
- Emotional problems or depression

Medical History

Child
- Birth injuries, congenital defects, encephalitis, meningitis, bedwetting, fainting, seizures, trauma

Adult
- Diabetes; hypertension; cardiovascular, pulmonary, kidney, liver, or endocrine disease; tuberculosis; tropical infection; sinusitis; visual problems; tumors; psychiatric disorders

Surgical History
- Neurologic, ear-nose-throat, dental, eye surgery

Traumatic History
- Motor vehicle accidents, falls, blows to the head, neck or back, being knocked out

Allergies
- Drug, food, environment

Patient Profile
- Personal habits
  - Use of alcohol, recreational drugs, over-the-counter medications, smoking, dietary habits, sleeping patterns, elimination patterns, exercise habits
- Recent life changes
- Living conditions
- Working conditions
- Exposure to toxins, chemicals, fumes; occupational duties
- General temperament

Current Medication Use
- Sedatives, tranquilizers
- Anticonvulsants
- Psychotropics
- Anticoagulants
- Antibiotics
- Calcium channel blockers
- Beta-blockers
- Nitrates
- Oral contraceptives

The highest possible score on the GCS is 15, and the lowest score is 3. A score of 7 or less on the GCS usually indicates coma. The scoring system was developed to assist in general communication concerning the severity of neurologic injury. Recently, however, the usefulness of the GCS has been called into question because of its lack of sensitivity and poor interrater reliability.[8] Several points should therefore be kept in mind when the GCS is used for serial assessment. First, the GCS provides data about level of consciousness only and should never be considered a complete neurologic examination. Second, it is not a sensitive tool for evaluation of an altered sensorium. Third, it does not account for possible aphasia or mechanical intubation. Finally, the GCS is a poor indicator of lateralization of neurologic deterioration.[9] *Lateralization* involves decreasing motor response on one side or unilateral changes in pupillary reaction.

Motor Function

Nursing priorities in assessment of motor function focus on two areas: 1) evaluation of muscle size and tone and 2) estimation of muscle strength. Each side should be assessed individually and then compared with the other.[2,10]

Evaluation of Muscle Size and Tone

Initially, muscles should be inspected for size and shape. The presence of atrophy is noted. Muscle tone is assessed by evaluating opposition to passive movement. The patient is instructed to relax the extremity while the nurse performs passive range-of-motion movements and evaluates the degree of resistance. Muscle tone is appraised for signs of flaccidity (no resistance), hypotonia (little resistance), hypertonia (increased resistance), spasticity, or rigidity.[6]

Estimation of Muscle Strength

Muscle strength in the upper and lower extremities is assessed by having the patient perform a number of movements and movements against resistance. The strength of the movement is then graded on a six-point scale (Box 17-4). The pronator-drift test is a sensitive indicator of upper extremity weakness. In this test, the patient is asked to extend both arms with the palms turned upward and to hold that position with the eyes closed. If the patient has a weaker side, that arm will drift downward and pronate.[6]

Abnormal Motor Responses

If the patient is incapable of comprehending and following a simple command, noxious stimuli are necessary to determine motor responses. The stimulus is applied to each extremity separately to allow evaluation of individual extremity function. Peripheral stimulation is used to assess motor function (Box 17-3).[2,4] Motor responses elicited by noxious stimuli are interpreted differently from those elicited by voluntary demonstration.[3] These responses may be classified as shown in Box 17-5.

Abnormal flexion also is known as *decorticate posturing* (Figure 17-1A). In response to painful stimuli, the upper

BOX 17-2 Categories of Consciousness

Alert	Patient responds immediately to minimal external stimuli.
Confused	Patient is disoriented to time or place but usually oriented to person, with impaired judgment and decision making and decreased attention span.
Delirious	Patient is disoriented to time, place, and person, with loss of contact with reality, and often has auditory or visual hallucinations.
Lethargic	Patient displays a state of drowsiness or inaction, in which the patient needs an increased stimulus to be awakened.
Obtunded	Patient displays dull indifference to external stimuli, and response is minimally maintained. Questions are answered with a minimal response.
Stuporous	Patient can be aroused only by vigorous and continuous external stimuli. Motor response is often withdrawal or localizing to stimulus.
Comatose	Vigorous stimulation fails to produce any voluntary neural response.

From Barker E. *Neuroscience Nursing: A Spectrum of Care*. 3rd ed. St. Louis: Mosby; 2008.

BOX 17-3 Stimulation Techniques in Patient Arousal

Central Stimulation

- *Trapezius pinch:* Squeeze trapezius muscle between thumb and first two fingers.
- *Sternal rub:* Apply firm pressure to sternum with knuckles, using a rubbing motion.

Peripheral Stimulation

- *Nail bed pressure:* Apply firm pressure, using object such as a pen, to nail bed.
- *Pinching of inner aspect of arm or leg:* Firmly pinch small portion of patient's tissue on sensitive inner aspect of arm or leg.

BOX 17-4 Muscle Strength Grading Scale

- 0/5 –No movement or muscle contraction
- 1/5 –Trace contraction
- 2/5 –Active movement with gravity eliminated
- 3/5 –Active movement against gravity
- 4/5 –Active movement with some resistance
- 5/5 –Active movement with full resistance

TABLE 17-1 Glasgow Coma Scale

CATEGORY	SCORE	RESPONSE
Eye Opening	4	Spontaneous: Eyes open spontaneously without stimulation.
	3	To speech: Eyes open with verbal stimulation but not necessarily to command.
	2	To pain: Eyes open with noxious stimuli.
	1	None: No eye opening regardless of stimulation
Verbal Response	5	Oriented: Accurate information about person, place, time, reason for hospitalization, and personal data
	4	Confused: Answers not appropriate to question, but use of language is correct
	3	Inappropriate words: Disorganized, random speech, no sustained conversation
	2	Incomprehensible sounds: Moans, groans, and incomprehensible mumbles
	1	None: No verbalization despite stimulation
Best Motor Response	6	Obeys commands: Performs simple tasks on command; able to repeat performance
	5	Localizes to pain: Organized attempt to localize and remove painful stimuli
	4	Withdraws from pain: Withdraws extremity from source of painful stimuli
	3	Abnormal flexion: Decorticate posturing spontaneously or in response to noxious stimuli
	2	Extension: Decerebrate posturing spontaneously or in response to noxious stimuli
	1	None: No response to noxious stimuli; flaccid

Modified from Teasdale G, Jennett B. Assessment of coma and impaired consciousness—a practical scale, *Lancet* 2:81,1974.

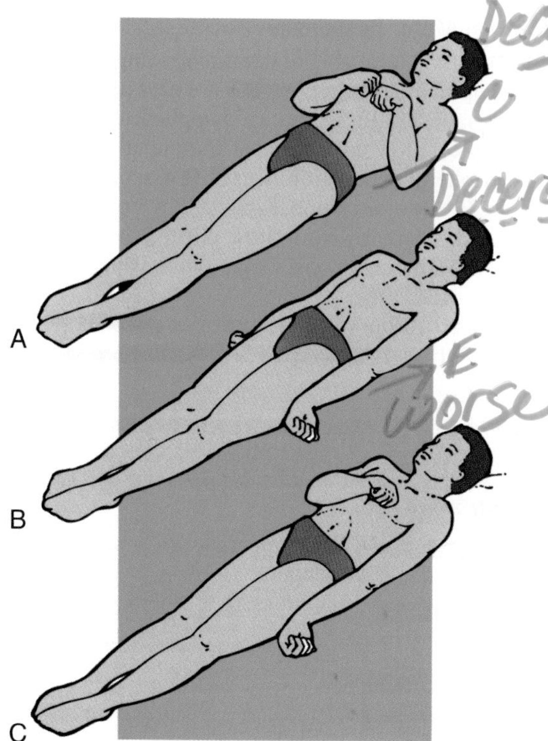

FIG 17-1 Abnormal Motor Responses. *A,* Decorticate posturing. *B,* Decerebrate posturing. *C,* Decorticate posturing on right side and decerebrate posturing on left side of body.

BOX 17-5 Classification of Abnormal Motor Function

Spontaneous	Occurs without regard to external stimuli and may not occur by request
Localization	Occurs when the extremity opposite the extremity receiving pain crosses midline of the body in an attempt to remove the noxious stimulus from the affected limb
Withdrawal	Occurs when the extremity receiving the painful stimulus flexes normally in an attempt to avoid the noxious stimulus
Decortication	Abnormal flexion response that may occur spontaneously or in response to noxious stimuli (see Fig. 17-1A and C)
Decerebration	Abnormal extension response that may occur spontaneously or in response to noxious stimuli (see Fig. 17-1B and C)
Flaccid	No response to painful stimuli

extremities exhibit flexion of the arm, wrist, and fingers, with adduction of the limb. The lower extremity exhibits extension, internal rotation, and plantar flexion. Abnormal flexion occurs with lesions above the midbrain, located in the region of the thalamus or cerebral hemispheres. Abnormal extension is known as *decerebrate rigidity* or *posturing* (see Figure 17-1B). Upon stimulation, the teeth clench; arms are stiffly extended, adducted, and hyperpronated; and legs are stiffly extended with plantar flexion of the feet. Abnormal extension occurs with lesions in the area of the brainstem.[10] Because abnormal flexion and extension appear similar in the lower extremities, the upper extremities are used to determine the presence of these abnormal movements. It is possible for the patient to exhibit abnormal flexion on one side of the body and extension on the other (see Figure 17-1C).[2,4] Outcome studies indicate abnormal flexion, which has a less serious prognosis than does extension, or decerebrate posturing.[10] Onset of posturing or a change from abnormal flexion to abnormal extension requires immediate physician notification.

Pupillary Function

Nursing priorities in assessment of pupillary function focuses on three areas: 1) estimation of pupil size and shape, 2) evaluation of pupillary reaction to light, and 3) assessment of eye movements. Pupillary function is an extension of the autonomic nervous system. Parasympathetic control of the pupil occurs through innervation of the oculomotor nerve (CN III), which exits from the brainstem in the midbrain area. When the parasympathetic fibers are stimulated, the pupil constricts. Sympathetic control originates in the hypothalamus and travels down the entire length of the brainstem. When the sympathetic fibers are stimulated, the pupil dilates. Pupillary changes provide a valuable assessment tool because of pathway locations.[11] The oculomotor nerve lies at the junction of the midbrain and the tentorial notch. Any increase of pressure that exerts force down through the tentorial notch compresses the oculomotor nerve. Oculomotor nerve compression results in a dilated, nonreactive pupil. Sympathetic pathway disruption occurs with involvement in the brainstem. Loss of sympathetic control leads to pinpoint, nonreactive pupils. Control of eye movements occurs with interaction of three cranial nerves: 1) oculomotor (CN III), 2) trochlear (CN IV), and 3) abducens (CN VI). The pathways for these cranial nerves provide integrated function through the internuclear pathway of the medial longitudinal fasciculus (MLF) located in the brainstem. The MLF provides coordination of eye movements with the vestibular nerve (CN VIII) and the reticular formation.[12]

Estimation of Pupil Size and Shape

Pupil diameter should be documented in millimeters (mm) with the use of a pupil gauge to reduce the subjectivity of description. Most people have pupils of equal size, between 2 and 5 mm. A discrepancy up to 1 mm between the two pupils is normal; it is called *anisocoria* and occurs in 16% to 17% of the human population.[13] Change or inequality in pupil size, especially in patients who previously have not shown this discrepancy, is a significant neurologic sign. It may indicate impending danger of herniation and should be reported immediately. With the location of CN III at the notch of the tentorium, pupil size and reactivity play a key role in the physical assessment of intracranial pressure (ICP) changes and herniation syndromes. In addition to CN III compression, changes in pupil size occur for other reasons. Large pupils can result from the instillation of cycloplegic agents such as atropine or scopolamine or can indicate extreme stress. Extremely small pupils can indicate opioid overdose, lower brainstem compression, or bilateral damage to the pons.[13,14]

Pupil shape is included in the assessment of pupils. Although the pupil is normally round, an irregularly shaped

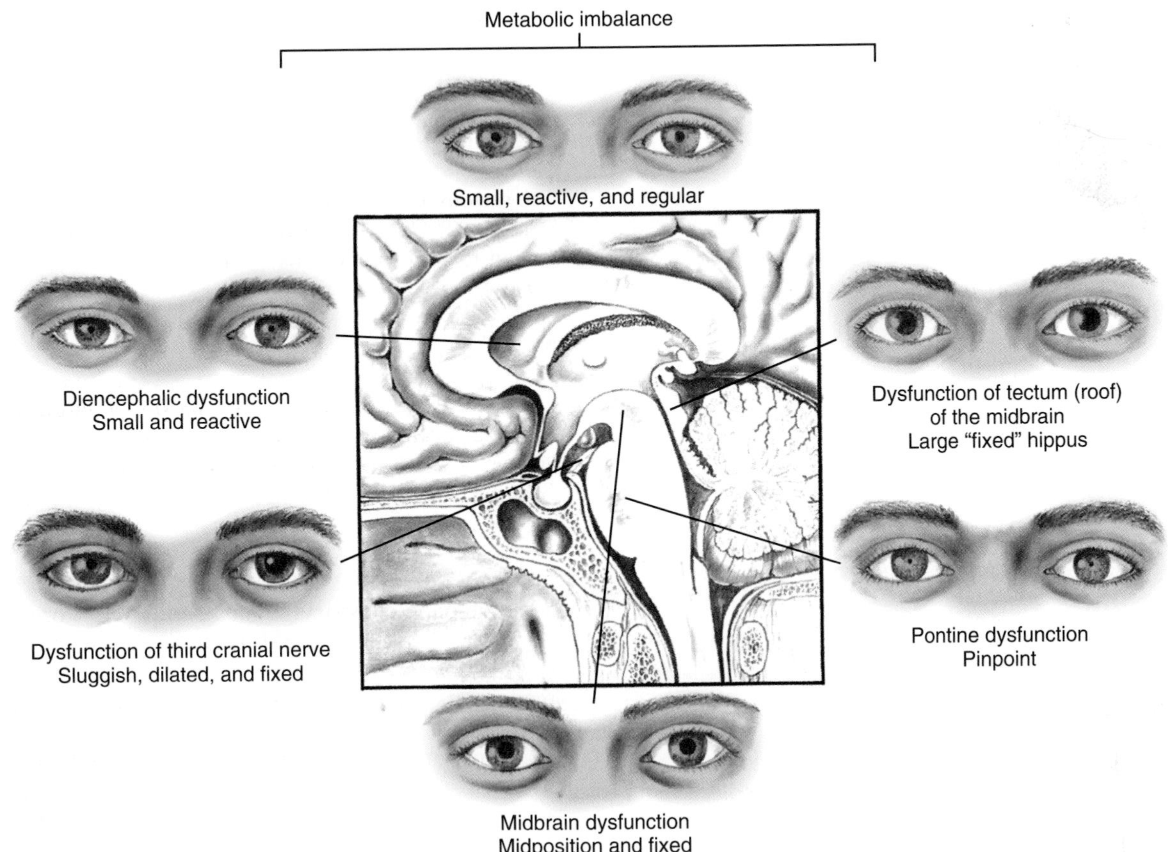

FIG 17-2 Abnormal Pupillary Responses.

or oval pupil may be observed in patients who have undergone eye surgery. Initial stages of CN III compression from elevated ICP also can cause the pupil to have an oval shape.[2,13]

Evaluation of Pupillary Reaction to Light

The pupillary light reflex depends on optic nerve (CN II) and oculomotor nerve (CN III) function (Figure 17-2).[6,13] The technique for evaluation of the pupillary light response involves use of a narrow-beamed bright light shined into the pupil from the outer canthus of the eye. If the light is shined directly onto the pupil, glare or reflection of the light may prevent the assessor's proper visualization. Pupillary reaction to light is identified as brisk, sluggish, or nonreactive or fixed.[2] Each pupil should be evaluated for direct light response and for consensual response. The consensual pupillary response is constriction in response to a light shined into the opposite eye. This reflex occurs as a result of the crossing of nerve fibers at the optic chiasm.[2] Evaluation of consensual response is necessary to rule out optic nerve dysfunction as a cause for lack of a direct light reflex. Because the optic nerve is the afferent pathway for the light reflex, shining a light into a blind eye produces neither a direct light response in that eye nor a consensual response in the opposite eye. A consensual response in the blind eye produced by shining a light into the opposite eye demonstrates an intact oculomotor nerve. Oculomotor compression associated with transtentorial herniation affects the direct light response and the consensual response in the affected pupil.[2,4,12,13]

no reaction – probably wont make it

Assessment of Eye Movement

In the conscious patient, the function of the three cranial nerves of the eye and their MLF innervation can be assessed by asking the patient to follow a finger through the full range of eye motion. If the eyes move together into all six fields, extraocular movements are intact (Figure 17-3).[3,12]

In the unconscious patient, assessment of ocular function and innervation of the MLF is performed by eliciting the oculocephalic reflex (doll's eyes reflex). If the patient is unconscious as a result of trauma, the nurse must ascertain the absence of cervical injury before performing this examination. To assess the oculocephalic reflex, the nurse holds the patient's eyelids open and briskly turns the head to one side while observing the eye movement and then briskly turns the head to the other side and observes the eye movement again. If the eye movement deviates to the opposite direction in which the head is turned, the doll's eyes reflex is present, and the oculocephalic reflex arc is intact (Figure 17-4A). If the oculocephalic reflex arc is not intact, the reflex is absent. This lack of response, in which the eyes remain midline and move with the head, indicates significant brainstem injury (see Figure 17-4C). The reflex may also be absent in severe metabolic coma. An abnormal oculocephalic reflex is present when the eyes rove or move in opposite directions from each other (see Figure 17-4B). Abnormal oculocephalic reflex indicates some degree of brainstem injury.[2,4,12]

Often as one of the final clinical assessments of brainstem function, a physician will perform caloric testing to assess

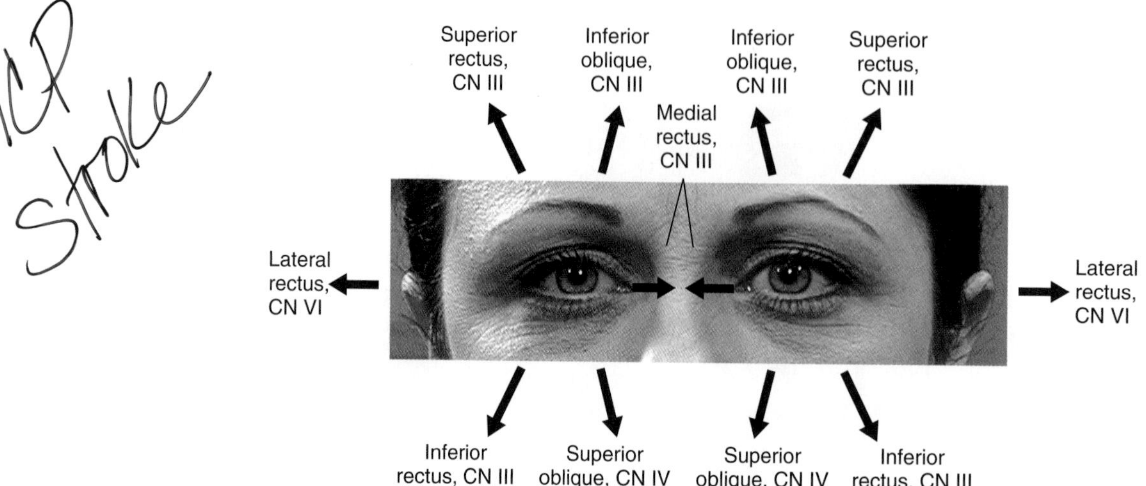

FIG 17-3 Extraocular Eye Movements. (From Ball JW., et al. *Seidel's Guide to Physical Examination.* 8th ed. St. Louis: Mosby; 2015.)

TABLE 17-2 Respiratory Patterns

PATTERN OF RESPIRATION	DESCRIPTION OF PATTERN	SIGNIFICANCE
Cheyne-Stokes breathing	Rhythmic crescendo and decrescendo of rate and depth of respiration; includes brief periods of apnea	Usually seen with bilateral deep cerebral lesions or some cerebellar lesions
Central neurogenic hyperventilation	Very deep, very rapid respirations with no apneic periods	Usually seen with lesions of the midbrain and upper pons
Apneustic breathing	Prolonged inspiratory and/or expiratory pause of 2-3 seconds	Usually seen in lesions of the middle to lower pons
Cluster breathing	Clusters of irregular, gasping respirations separated by long periods of apnea	Usually seen in lesions of the lower pons or upper medulla
Ataxic respirations	Irregular, random pattern of deep and shallow respirations with irregular apneic periods	Usually seen in lesions of the medulla

oculovestibular reflex. After confirmation that the tympanic membrane is intact, the patient's head is raised to a 30-degree angle, and 20 to 100 milliliters (mL) of ice water are injected into the external auditory canal. The normal eye movement response is a conjugate, slow, tonic nystagmus, deviating toward the irrigated ear and lasting 30 to 120 seconds. This response indicates brainstem integrity. Rapid nystagmus returns the eye position to the midline only in a conscious patient with cortical functioning (Figure 17-5).[2,10] An abnormal response is disconjugate eye movement, which indicates a brainstem lesion, or no response, which indicates little or no brainstem function. The oculovestibular reflex may be temporarily absent in reversible metabolic encephalopathy.[8] This test is an extremely noxious stimulation and may produce a decorticate or decerebrate posturing response in a comatose patient. In the conscious patient, this procedure may produce nausea, vomiting, or dizziness.[2,12,14]

Respiratory Function

Nursing priorities in assessment of respiratory function focus on two areas: 1) observation of respiratory pattern and 2) evaluation of airway status. The activity of respiration is a highly integrated function that receives input from the cerebrum, brainstem, and metabolic mechanisms. In clinical assessment, correlations exist among altered levels of consciousness, the level of brain or brainstem injury, and the patient's respiratory pattern. Under the influence of the cerebral cortex and the diencephalon, three brainstem centers control respirations. The lowest center, the *medullary respiratory center*, sends impulses through the vagus nerve to innervate muscles of inspiration and expiration. The *apneustic* and *pneumotaxic centers of the pons* are responsible for the length of inspiration and expiration and the underlying respiratory rate.[2,4,10]

Observation of Respiratory Pattern

Changes in respiratory patterns assist in identifying the level of brainstem dysfunction or injury (Table 17-2). Evaluation of the respiratory pattern must include assessment of the effectiveness of gas exchange in maintaining adequate oxygen and carbon dioxide levels. Hypoventilation is not uncommon in the patient with an altered level of consciousness. Alterations in oxygenation or carbon dioxide levels can result in further neurologic dysfunction. ICP increases with hypoxemia or hypercapnia.[2,4,10]

Evaluation of Airway Status

Evaluation of the respiratory function in a patient with a neurologic deficit must include assessment of airway maintenance and secretion control. Cough, gag, and swallow reflexes responsible for protection of the airway may be absent or diminished.[15]

Vital Signs

Nursing priorities in assessment of vital signs focus on two areas: 1) evaluation of blood pressure and 2) observation

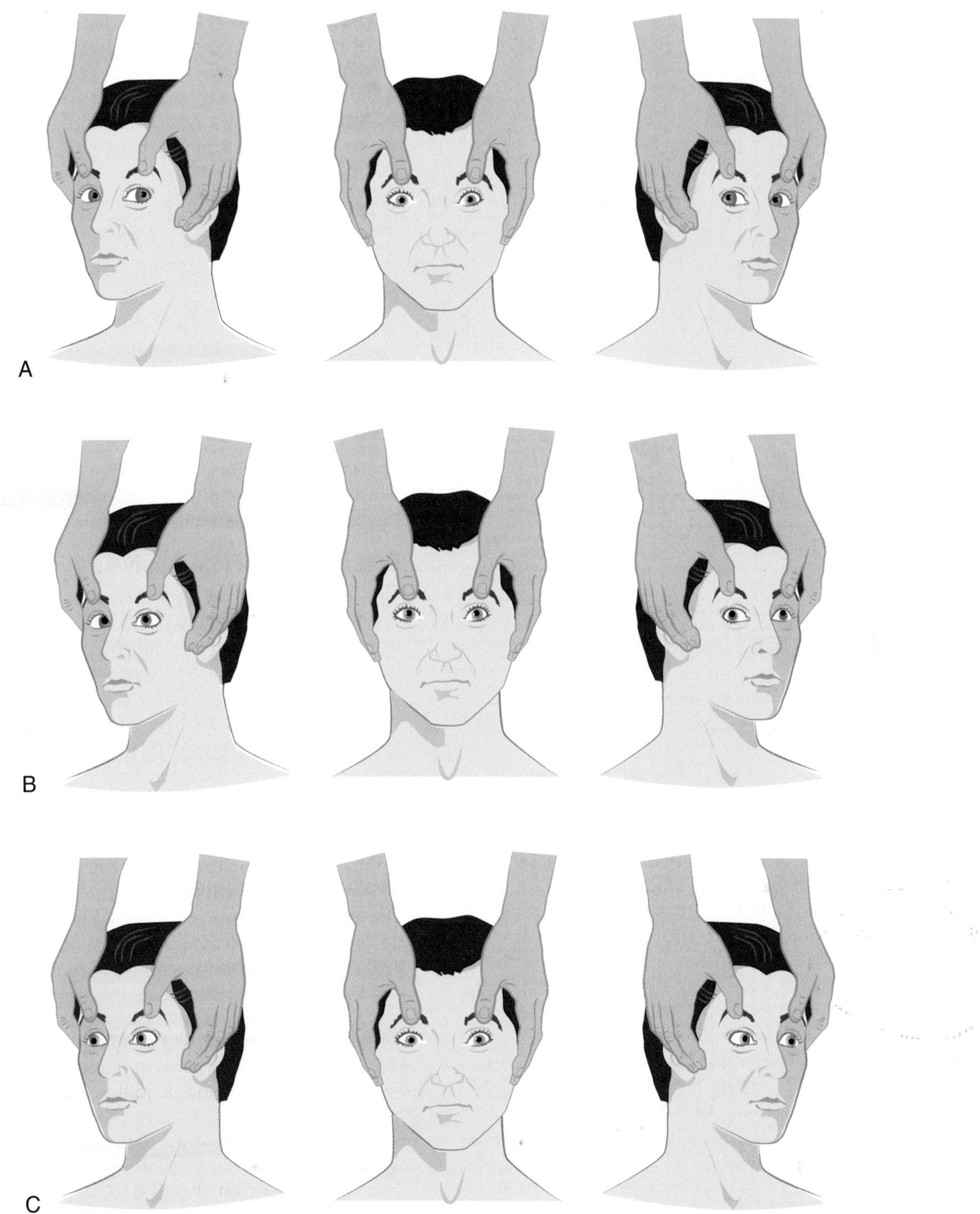

FIG 17-4 Oculocephalic Reflex (Doll's Eyes). *A*, Normal. *B*, Abnormal. *C*, Absent.

of heart rate and rhythm. As a result of the brain and brainstem influences on cardiac, respiratory, and body temperature functions, changes in vital signs could be signs of deterioration in neurologic status.[2,4]

Evaluation of Blood Pressure

A common manifestation of intracranial injury is systemic hypertension. Cerebral autoregulation, responsible for the control of cerebral blood flow (CBF), frequently is lost with any type of intracranial injury. After cerebral injury, the body often is in a hyperdynamic state (increased heart rate, blood pressure, and cardiac output) as part of a compensatory response. With the loss of autoregulation as blood pressure increases, CBF and cerebral blood volume increase, and ICP therefore increases. Control of systemic hypertension is necessary to stop this cycle, but caution must be exercised. The mean arterial pressure must be maintained at a level sufficient to produce adequate CBF in the presence of elevated ICP.

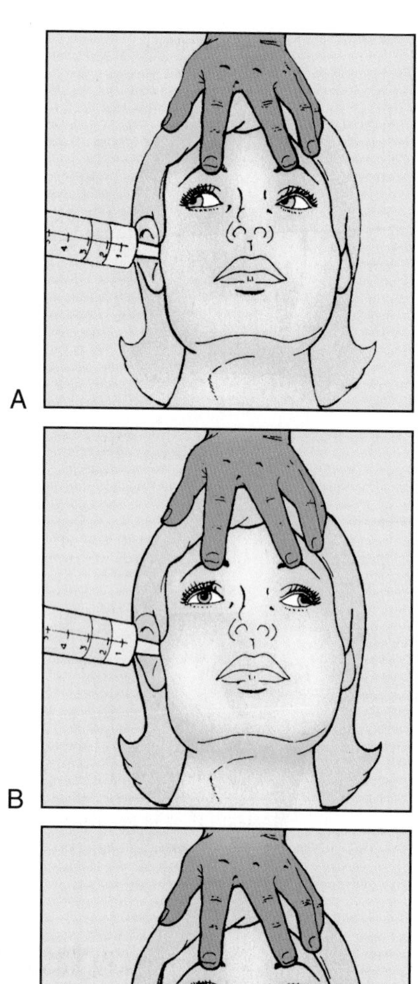

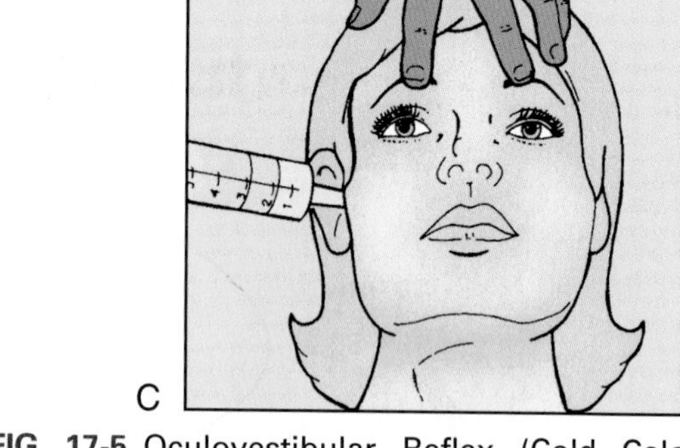

FIG 17-5 Oculovestibular Reflex (Cold Caloric Test). *A*, Normal. *B*, Abnormal. *C*, Absent.

Attention must also be paid to the pulse pressure because widening of this value may occur in the late stages of intracranial hypertension.[15,16]

Observation of Heart Rate and Rhythm

The medulla and the vagus nerve provide parasympathetic control to the heart. When stimulated, this lower brainstem system produces bradycardia. Sympathetic stimulation increases the rate and contractility. Various intracranial pathologies and abrupt ICP changes can produce bradycardia, premature ventricular contractions (PVCs), QT changes, and myocardial damage.[17]

Cushing Reflex

Cushing reflex, also known as *Cushing triad* or *Cushing phenomena*, is a set of three clinical manifestations (systolic hypertension, bradycardia, and abnormal respirations) related to pressure on the medullary area of the brainstem. These signs may occur in response to intracranial hypertension or a herniation syndrome. The appearance of Cushing reflex is a late finding that may be absent in patients with severe neurologic deterioration. Attention should be paid to alteration in each component of the triad and intervention initiated accordingly.[18]

Neurologic Changes Associated with Intracranial Hypertension

Assessment of the patient for signs of increasing ICP is an important responsibility of the critical care nurse. Increasing ICP can be identified by changes in level of consciousness, pupillary reaction, motor response, vital signs, and respiratory patterns (Figure 17-6).[10,19]

LABORATORY STUDIES

The major laboratory study performed in the patient with neurologic dysfunction is analysis of CSF obtained by a lumbar puncture or a ventriculostomy.[2,4]

Cerebrospinal Fluid Analysis

The main purpose of a lumbar puncture is to obtain CSF for analysis. CSF opening pressure may also be obtained. CSF samples are evaluated for the presence of subarachnoid blood or infection, or they are sent for laboratory analysis (Table 17-3).[20]

DIAGNOSTIC PROCEDURES

Table 17-4 presents an overview of the various diagnostic procedures used to evaluate the patient with neurological dysfunction.

Nursing Management

The nursing management of a patient undergoing a diagnostic procedure involves a variety of interventions. **Nursing priorities are directed toward 1) preparing the patient psychologically and physically for the procedure, 2) monitoring the patient's responses to the procedure, and 3) assessing the patient after the procedure.** Preparation includes teaching the patient about the procedure, answering questions, and transporting and positioning the patient for the procedure. During the procedure, the nurse observes the patient for signs of pain, anxiety, or hemorrhage and monitors vital signs. After the procedure, the nurse observes for complications of the procedure and medicates the patient for any postprocedure discomfort. **Any evidence of increasing ICP should be immediately reported to the physician, and emergency measures to decrease intracranial** pressure **must be initiated.**

BEDSIDE MONITORING

Monitoring for secondary injury is a fundamental aspect of caring for the critically ill patient with a neurologic dysfunction. By utilizing more than one monitoring technique, the observer is more likely to determine whether a genuine change in cerebral physiology has occurred and what the most appropriate intervention should be.[15,21]

Text continued on p. 344

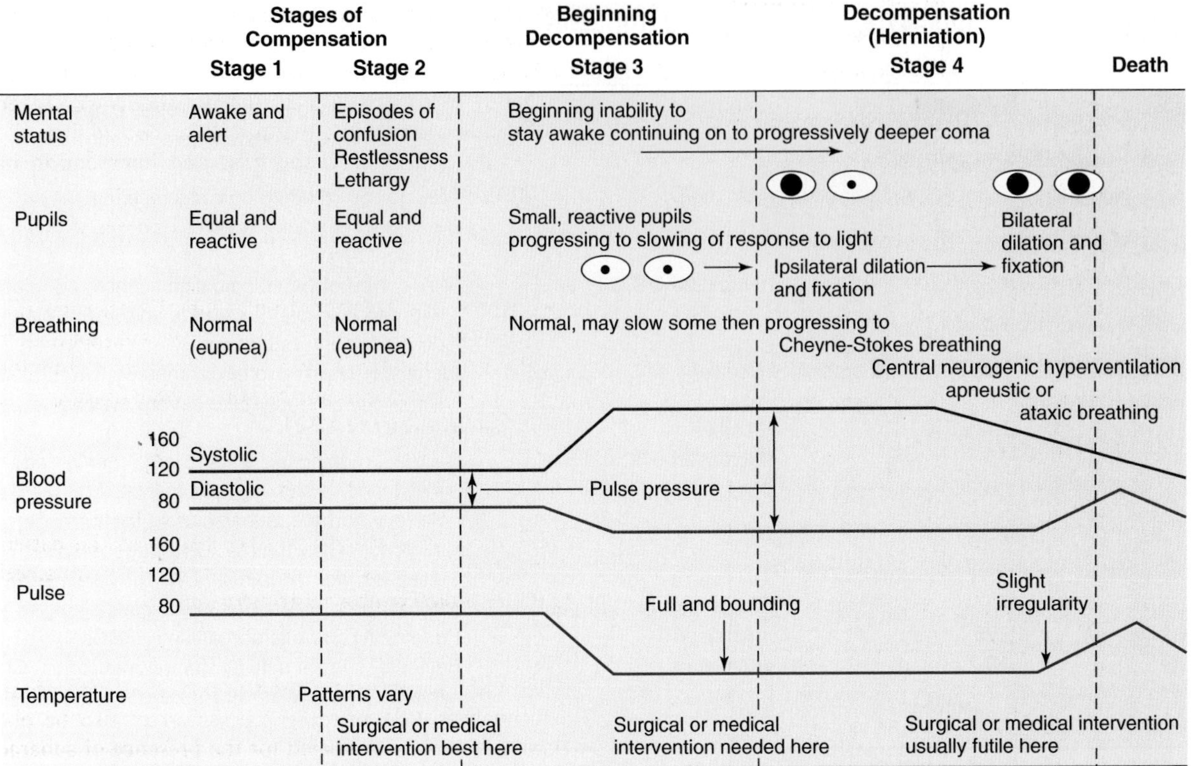

FIG 17-6 Clinical Correlates of Compensated and Decompensated Phases of Intracranial Hypertension. (From Beare PG, Myers JL. *Principles and Practice of Adult Health Nursing.* 3rd ed. St. Louis: Mosby; 1998.)

TABLE 17-3 **Analysis of Cerebrospinal Fluid**

CHARACTERISTIC	NORMAL FINDINGS	ABNORMAL FINDINGS	POSSIBLE CAUSES AND COMMENTS
Pressure	<200 mm H_2O	<60 mm H_2O	Faulty needle placement Dehydration Spinal block along subarachnoid space Block of foramen magnum Hydrocephalus
		>200 mm H_2O	Muscle tension Abdominal compression Brain tumor Subdural hematoma Brain abscess Brain cyst Cerebral edema (any cause)
Color	Clear, colorless	Cloudy or turbid	Cloudy as a result of microorganisms (e.g., WBCs) Turbid as a result of increased cell count
		Yellow (xanthochromic)	Breakdown of RBCs with RBC pigments, high-protein count
		Smoky	RBCs
Blood	None	Red blood cells: blood-tinged	Traumatic tap: Bloody in first sample
		Grossly bloody	Traumatic tap: Bloody in all samples
Volume	150 mL	Increase	Hydrocephalus
Specific gravity	1.007	Increase	Infection, presence of cells or protein
WBCs	0-5 cells/mm^3	<500 cells/mm^3	Bacterial or viral infections of meninges, neurosyphilis, subarachnoid hemorrhage, infarction, abscess, tuberculous meningitis, metastatic lesions
		>500 cells/mm^3	Purulent infection

Continued

TABLE 17-3 Analysis of Cerebrospinal Fluid—cont'd

CHARACTERISTIC	NORMAL FINDINGS	ABNORMAL FINDINGS	POSSIBLE CAUSES AND COMMENTS
Glucose	50-75 mg/dL or 60%-70% of blood glucose	<40 mg/dL	Bacterial meningitis, tuberculosis, parasitic, fungal carcinomatous, subarachnoid hemorrhage
		>80 mg/Dl	May not be of neurologic significance
Chloride	700-750 mg/dL	Decreased (<625 mg/dL)	Meningeal infection, tuberculosis meningitis, hypochloremia
		Increased (>800 mg/dL)	May not be of neurologic significance; correlated with blood levels of chloride and not routine; done only on request
Culture and sensitivity	No organisms present	*Neisseria* or *Streptococcus*	Identify organisms to begin therapy; Gram stain for some cultures may take several weeks.
Serology for syphilis	Negative	Positive	Syphilis
Protein*	15-50 mg/dL	Increased (>60 mg/dL)	Bacterial meningitis, brain tumors (benign and malignant), complete spinal block, ALS, Guillain-Barré syndrome, subarachnoid hemorrhage, infarction, CNS trauma, CNS degenerative diseases, herniated disk, DM with polyneuropathy
		Decreased (<10 mg/dL)	May not be of neurologic significance
Osmolality	295 Osm/L	Increased	Protein, WBCs, microorganisms, RBCs
Lactate	10-20 mg/dL	Increased	Bacterial, seizure activity, fungal meningitis, CNS trauma, coma related to toxic or metabolic causes

ALS, Amyotrophic lateral sclerosis; *CNS*, central nervous system; *CSF*, cerebrospinal fluid; *DM*, diabetes mellitus; *RBC*, red blood cell; *WBC*, white blood cell.
*Blood in the CSF will raise the protein level.
From Barker E. *Neuroscience Nursing: A Spectrum of Care*. 3rd ed. St. Louis: Mosby; 2008.

TABLE 17-4 Neurological Diagnostic Studies

STUDY	PURPOSES	COMMENTS
Angiography	Visualizes extracranial and intracranial vasculature. Identifies aneurysm, AVM, vasospasm, and vascular tumors. Detects arterial occlusion and allows delivery of intraarterial therapy to restore blood flow.	May cause local hematoma, vasospasm, vessel occlusion, allergic reaction to contrast media, and transient or permanent neurological dysfunction Prior to test: Keep patient NPO for 4 hours and provide sedation before the study. Check for allergy to iodine. Evaluate renal function. After the test Ensure hydration postprocedure (contrast medium used). • Maintain bed rest for 8-12 hours. • Monitor arterial puncture point for hemorrhage or hematoma. • Monitor neurovascular status of affected limb. • Monitor for indications of systemic emboli. • Reevaluate renal function.
Cisternogram	Views CSF flow. Identifies hydrocephalus. Evaluates CSF leakage through a dural tear. Evaluates abnormality of structures at the base of the brain and upper cervical cord region.	Contraindicated in intracranial hypertension

TABLE 17-4 Neurological Diagnostic Studies—cont'd

STUDY	PURPOSES	COMMENTS
CT computerized axial tomography (CAT)	Views intracranial structures: size, shape, location, shifts. Differentiates between tumors, hemorrhage, and infarction. Identifies hydrocephalus, brain edema, infectious processes, trauma, aneurysm, hematoma, AVM, brain atrophy, and subacute and old brain infarction. Evaluates arterial system if CT angiography studies performed.	Patient must be cooperative. Contrast media may be used; contrast media may be used after a noncontrast CT. • Check for allergy to iodine or seafood before study. • Patient will be NPO for 4-8 hours before the study. • Sedation may be given. • Monitor for signs of allergic reaction. • Encourage fluid intake. • Evaluate renal function when contrast media used.
Digital subtraction angiography: brain; spine	Visualizes the vasculature, especially carotid and larger cerebral arteries. Evaluates occlusive vascular disease. Identifies tumors, aneurysms, AVM, vascular abnormalities.	May be done IV or intraarterially. • If IV, is less invasive with fewer complications than cerebral angiography • If intraarterially, care as for angiogram • Contrast media are used. • Check for allergy to iodine, seafood before study. • Patient will be NPO for 4-8 hours before the study. • Monitor for signs of allergic reaction. • Encourage fluid intake.
Electroencephalography	Differentiates epilepsy from mass lesion. Detects focus of seizure activity. Evaluates drug intoxication. Evaluates electrical function of the brain, which may be abnormal in the presence of cerebrovascular alterations. Localizes tumor, abscess, and other mass lesions. May be used in designation of brain death.	Stimulants, anticonvulsants, tranquilizer, and antidepressants may be withheld for 24-48 hours before the study. Hair shampooed before and after study
Electromyography; nerve conduction velocity studies	Detects muscle disease. Identifies peripheral neuropathies, nerve compression. Identifies nerve regeneration and muscle recovery.	Patient must be cooperative. Contraindicated in patients taking anticoagulants, with bleeding disorders or skin infection. May be uncomfortable for patient.
Electronystagmography	Detects nystagmus, which may aid in identification of cerebellar or vestibular problem.	
Evoked potential studies	Evaluates electrical potentials (responses) of brain to external stimuli; evaluates sensory and somatosensory neurological pathways. Identifies neuromuscular disease, cerebrovascular disease, spinal cord injury, traumatic brain injury, peripheral nerve disease, and tumors. Determines prognosis in traumatic brain injury. Contributes to diagnosis of multiple sclerosis and brainstem injury.	Hair shampooed before and after study
Isotope ventriculography	Visualizes CSF circulation system.	No CSF withdrawn May cause meningeal irritation and aseptic meningitis.

Continued

TABLE 17-4 Neurological Diagnostic Studies—cont'd

STUDY	PURPOSES	COMMENTS
Lumbar puncture or cisternal puncture	Obtains CSF for analysis. Measures CSF opening pressure (roughly equivalent to intracranial pressure for most patients if done recumbent and no blockage is present).	Cisternal puncture is higher risk but may be used if scar tissue prevents LP. Patient must be cooperative. Contraindicated in patients with intracranial hypertension because herniation may occur. Contraindicated in bleeding disorders and in patients receiving anticoagulants. Patient kept flat for 4-8 hours to prevent headache. May cause headache, low back pain, meningitis, abscess, CSF leak, or puncture of spinal cord.
Magnetic resonance angiography/magnetic resonance imaging	As for CT Visualizes tissue state (diffusion and perfusion) so that early ischemic changes are apparent (CT cannot visualize most early changes). Identifies vascular lesions, tissue abnormalities, hemorrhage, infarction, epileptic foci, and multiple sclerosis. Identifies patency of large veins and venous sinuses. Identifies brainstem abnormalities. Identifies type, location, and extent of brain injury.	Patient must be cooperative. Contraindicated in patients with any implanted metallic device, including pacemakers. Tends to overestimate degree of stenosis.
Magnetic resonance spectroscopy (also known as nuclear magnetic resonance [NMR] spectroscopy	Measures biochemical changes in the brain tissue. Detects abnormal changes as in brain tumors, epilepsy, stroke, and traumatic brain injury.	Patient must be cooperative. Contraindicated in patients with any implanted metallic device, including pacemakers.
Myelography	Visualizes spinal subarachnoid space. Detects spinal cord lesions and cord or nerve root compression. Detects pressure on spinal nerve roots.	If done with oil-based iophendylate (Pantopaque), patient must lie flat for 4-8 hours after study. May cause headache, nerve root irritation, allergic reaction, or adhesive arachnoiditis. If done with water-soluble metrizamide (Amipaque), patient should have head of bed elevated. May cause headache, nausea, vomiting, backache and neck ache, chest pain, seizures, hallucinations, speech disorders, dysrhythmias, or allergic reaction. Encourage fluid intake with either type of dye.
Nerve conduction velocity studies	Identifies peripheral neuropathies and nerve compression.	Needle electrodes are used.
Oculoplethysmography (OPG)	Indirectly measures ocular artery pressure. Reflects adequacy of cerebrovascular blood flow in the carotid artery.	Contraindicated in patients who have undergone eye surgery within the last 6 months, who have had lens implants or cataracts, or who have had retinal detachment. May cause conjunctival hemorrhage, corneal abrasions, or transient photophobia.
Pneumoencephalography	Visualizes ventricular system and subarachnoid space. Identifies intracranial tumors. Identifies brain atrophy.	Care as for LP Contraindicated in patients with intracranial hypertension. May cause headache, nausea, vomiting, autonomic dysfunction, herniation, subdural hematoma, air embolus, or seizures. Keep patient flat for 12-24 hours after the study.

TABLE 17-4 **Neurological Diagnostic Studies—cont'd**

STUDY	PURPOSES	COMMENTS
Positron emission tomography or single-photon emission computed tomography	Evaluates oxygen and glucose metabolism. Measures cerebral blood flow, which may be altered by traumatic brain injury, seizure, ischemia, stroke, or neoplasm. Also used to evaluate dementia, depression, schizophrenia, and Alzheimer's disease.	Patient must be cooperative. Contraindicated in pregnant and breastfeeding patients.
Radioisotope brain scan	Identifies tumors, cerebrovascular disease, infarction, trauma, infectious processes, and seizures.	Generally replaced by CT scan Reassure patient that amount of radioactive material is minimal. Patient must be cooperative. Contraindicated in pregnant and breastfeeding patients.
Regional cerebral blood flow (xenon [133Xe] inhalation)	Evaluates blood flow to the cerebral cortex material. Identifies cerebrovascular disease. Detects regions of increased or decreased perfusion. Determines presence of collateral blood flow Evaluates the effect of vasospasm on tissue perfusion.	Assure patient that amount of radioactive material is minimal. Contraindicated in pregnant and breastfeeding patients.
Skull x-rays	Detects skull fracture, facial fracture, tumor, bone erosion, cranial anomalies, air-fluid level in sinuses, abnormal intracranial calcification, and radiopaque foreign bodies.	Linear and basal fractures frequently missed by routine x-rays Contraindicated in pregnant patients.
Somatosensory evoked potentials (SSEP)	Evaluates neural pathways involving spinal cord, brainstem, thalamus, and cerebral cortex. Useful in diagnosis of multiple sclerosis, brain tumor, and spinal cord injury Useful in determination of brain death	
Somnography	Records electroencephalogram (EEG) during sleep. Evaluates sleep and sleep disorders.	
Spinal cord arteriography	Differentiates between spinal AVM, angioma, tumor, and ischemia.	As for angiogram May cause thrombosis of spinal vessels and allergy to contrast agent.
Spine x-rays	Detects vertebral dislocation or fracture, degenerative disease, tumor, bone erosion, or calcification. Identifies structural spinal deficits and rules out associated cervical spine injuries.	Care must be taken to prevent fracture displacement and spinal cord injury. C1-C2 view best obtained via open mouth; C6-C7 best obtained with arms pulled down.
Suboccipital puncture	Obtains CSF for analysis. Measures CSF pressure. Rarely performed but may be useful when LP is contraindicated.	May cause trauma to the medulla.
Transcranial Doppler	Measures blood flow velocity through the cerebral arteries. Identifies vasospasm, emboli, vascular stenosis, and brain death.	Quality of findings and interpretation vary with user Transtemporal window required (lacking in 14% of general population)
Ventriculography	Obtains CSF for analysis. Measures CSF pressure. Is used especially when intracranial hypertension contraindicates LP.	May cause meningeal irritation, seizures, herniation, intracerebral or intraventricular hemorrhage.

From Dennison RD: *Pass CCRN!* Ed. 4, St Louis, 2013, Mosby.

AVM, Arteriovenous malformation; *CSF*, cerebrospinal fluid; *CT*, computed tomography; *IV*, intravenous; *LP*, lumbar puncture; *NPO*, nothing by mouth.

Intracranial Pressure Monitoring

In the patient with suspected intracranial hypertension, a device may be placed within the cranium to quantify and monitor ICP and possibly drain excess CSF. Under normal physiologic conditions, mean ICP is maintained below 15 mm Hg.[22] An increase in ICP can decrease blood flow to the brain, causing brain damage. Persistent ICP elevation above 20 mm Hg remains the most significant factor associated with a fatal outcome.[22,23]

Types of Catheters

A variety of catheters are available to monitor ICP. They can be separated into two categories: 1) those that facilitate drainage and 2) those that do not allow for drainage. Catheters that allow for drainage are attached to a fluid-filled pressure monitoring system and an external transducer. Catheters that do not allow for drainage are of two types: 1) fiberoptic (using a light sensor to facilitate measurement of ICP) and 2) microsensor (using a microchip on the end of the catheter to facilitate measurement of ICP).[24] Also available is a device with a combination intraventricular/fiberoptic catheter that combines the capability of external ventricular drainage of CSF with ICP monitoring.[25]

Monitoring Sites

The five sites for monitoring ICP are 1) the intraventricular space, 2) the subarachnoid space, 3) the epidural space, 4) the subdural space, and 5) the parenchyma (Figure 17-7). The type of monitor and site chosen depends on the suspected pathologic condition and the physician's preference.[15,26,27] Nursing considerations for each type of device are discussed in Table 17-5.

Intraventricular space. ICP monitoring is accomplished by placing a small catheter into the ventricular system; this procedure is known as a ventriculostomy. With the patient under local anesthesia, the catheter is inserted through a burr hole and usually placed in the anterior horn of the lateral ventricle. If possible, the side chosen for placement of the ventriculostomy is the nondominant hemisphere.[26] Any of

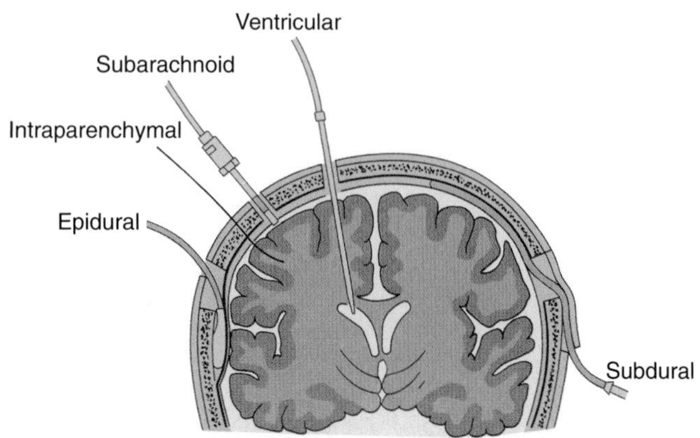

FIG 17-7 Intracranial Pressure Monitoring Sites. (From Lewis SL, et al. *Medical-Surgical Nursing: Assessment and Management of Clinical Problems.* 9th ed. St. Louis: Elsevier; 2014.)

TABLE 17-5 Advantages, Disadvantages, and Nursing Considerations of ICP Monitoring Techniques

MONITORING DEVICE	ADVANTAGES	DISADVANTAGES	NURSING CONSIDERATIONS
Intraventricular catheter (ventriculostomy)	Allows accurate ICP measurement.	Provides an additional site for infection.	Provide appropriate sedatives or analgesics during catheter insertion.
	Provides access to CSF for drainage or sampling.	Is most invasive ICP monitoring technique.	Do baseline and serial neurologic assessments. Measure patient's temperature at least every 4 hours.
	Provides access for instillation of contrast media.	Requires frequent transducer balancing or recalibration.	Note character, amount, and turbidity of CSF drainage.
	Allows reliable evaluation of intracranial compliances (volume–pressure relationships).	Catheter may be occluded by blood clot or tissue debris.	Document ICP and CPP measurements, response to stimulation, and nursing care activities per hospital or unit protocol.
		Insertion difficult if ventricles are small, compressed, or displaced	Monitor quality of ICP waveform. Monitor system and tubing for air bubbles and flush or purge system, as appropriate.
		Is associated with risk for CSF leakage around insertion site.	Drain CSF, as indicated for treatment of ICP elevation. Notify physician if CSF drainage is not within prescribed parameters.
		Is associated with increased risk for infection.	Monitor insertion site for bleeding, drainage, swelling, and CSF leakage.

TABLE 17-5 Advantages, Disadvantages, and Nursing Considerations of ICP Monitoring Techniques—cont'd

MONITORING DEVICE	ADVANTAGES	DISADVANTAGES	NURSING CONSIDERATIONS
			Set to zero or calibrate device per hospital or unit protocol. Level transducer at the foramen of Monro. External landmarks include the tragus of the patient's ear and the external auditory canal, among others. All ICP measurements should be made with the transducer at a consistent level relative to external landmarks. Administer sedatives or analgesics as appropriate to decrease risk of catheter being dislodged by patient's movements. Educate patient's family, as indicated. Notify physician if ICP or CPP is not within specified parameters.
Subarachnoid bolt or screw	Is associated with lower infection rates than is ventriculostomy.	Has potential for dampened waveform (cerebral edema, blood or tissue debris).	Administer appropriate sedatives or analgesics during insertion. Do baseline and serial neurologic assessments.
		Is quickly and easily placed.	Measure patient's temperature at least every 4 hours.
	Can be used with small or collapsed ventricles.	Is less accurate at high ICP elevations.	Monitor insertion site for bleeding, drainage, swelling, and CSF leakage.
	Requires no penetration of brain tissue.	Requires frequent balancing or recalibration (e.g., with position changes).	Monitor quality of ICP waveform. Document ICP and CPP measurements and response to stimulation per hospital or unit protocol.
		Provides no access for CSF sampling.	Administer sedatives or analgesics as appropriate to decrease risk of catheter being dislodged by patient's movements. Set to zero or calibrate device per hospital or unit protocol. Level transducer at the foramen of Monro. External landmarks include the tragus of the patient's ear and the external auditory canal, among others. All ICP measurements should be made with the transducer at a consistent level relative to external landmarks. Educate patient's family as indicated. Notify physician if ICP or CPP is not within specified parameters.
Subdural or epidural catheter or sensor	Is least invasive. Is associated with decreased risk of infection.	Increase in baseline drift over time means possible loss of reliability or accuracy.	Administer appropriate sedatives or analgesics during insertion. Do baseline and serial neurologic assessments.

Continued

TABLE 17-5 Advantages, Disadvantages, and Nursing Considerations of ICP Monitoring Techniques—cont'd

MONITORING DEVICE	ADVANTAGES	DISADVANTAGES	NURSING CONSIDERATIONS
	Is easily and quickly placed.	Provides no access for CSF drainage or sampling.	Measure patient's temperature at least every 4 hours. Monitor insertion site for bleeding, drainage, and swelling. Monitor quality of ICP waveform and drift over time. Document ICP and CPP measurements and response to stimulation per hospital or unit protocol. Administer sedatives or analgesics, as appropriate, to decrease risk of catheter being dislodged or damaged by patient's movements. Educate patient's family as indicated. Notify physician if ICP or CPP is not within specified parameters.
Fiberoptic transducer–tipped catheter	Can be placed in subdural or subarachnoid space, in a ventricle, or directly within brain tissue. Is easily transported.	Provides no access for CSF sampling or drainage.	Administer appropriate sedatives or analgesics during insertion. Do baseline and serial neurologic assessments.
		Cannot be recalibrated after placement.	Measure patient's temperature at least every 4 hours.
	Requires setting to zero only once (during insertion).	Requires periodic replacement of probe.	Monitor insertion site for bleeding, drainage, swelling, and CSF leakage.
	Has baseline drift of up to 1 mm Hg per day. Is associated with decreased risk for infection when brain tissue is not penetrated. Provides good-quality ICP waveforms (less artifact than with other devices).	Is easily damaged.	Monitor quality of ICP waveform and drift over time. Document ICP and CPP measurements and response to stimulation per hospital or unit protocol. Administer sedatives or analgesics as appropriate to decrease risk of catheter being dislodged or damaged by patient's movements.
	Requires no adjustment in level of transducer with patient's change of position.		Educate patient's family, as indicated. Notify physician if ICP or CPP is not within specified parameters.

CPP, Cerebral perfusion pressure; *CSF*, cerebrospinal fluid; *ICP*, intracranial pressure.
From Arbour R. Intracranial hypertension: monitoring and nursing assessment. *Crit Care Nurse*. 2004: 24(5):19.

the catheters mentioned above can be used in the intraventricular space.[28]

Subarachnoid space. ICP monitoring is accomplished by placing a small hollow bolt or screw with a sensor at the tip into the subarachnoid space. With the patient under local anesthesia, it is inserted through a burr hole and usually placed in the front of the skull behind the hairline. Inserting this device is easier than inserting the ventriculostomy catheter.[27,28]

Epidural space. ICP monitoring is accomplished by placing a small fiberoptic sensor into the epidural space. It is inserted through a burr hole while the patient is under local anesthesia. The physician strips the dura away from the inner table of the skull before inserting the epidural monitor.[27,28]

Subdural space. ICP monitoring is accomplished by placing a fiberoptic or microsensor catheter into the subdural space. It is inserted through a burr hole while the patient is under local anesthesia.[27,28]

Intraparenchymal site. ICP monitoring is accomplished by placing a fiberoptic catheter or microsensor catheter into the parenchymal tissue. After placing a subarachnoid bolt (as previously described), a hole is punched in the dura, and the catheter is inserted approximately 1 cm into the brain's white matter.[27,28] The intraventricular space is considered the

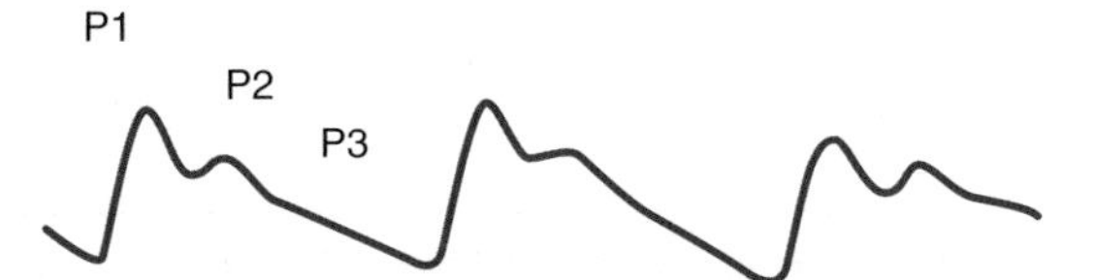

FIG 17-8 Normal Intracranial Pressure Waveform. (From Bader MK, *Littlejohns LR. AANN Core Curriculum for Neuroscience Nursing.* 4th ed. St. Louis: Elsevier; 2004.)

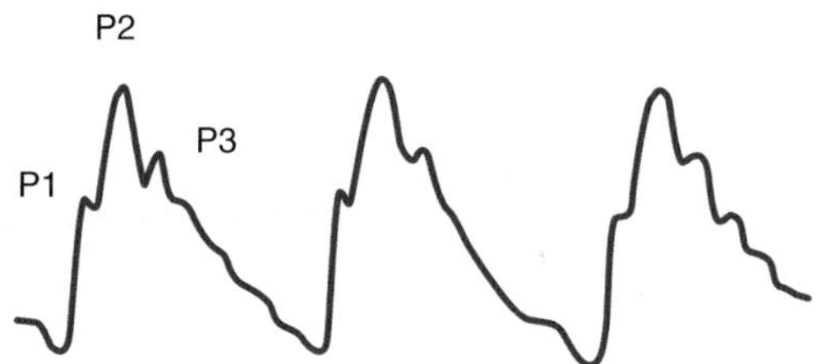

FIG 17-9 Abnormal Intracranial Pressure Waveform. (From Bader MK, Littlejohns LR. *AANN Core Curriculum for Neuroscience Nursing.* 4th ed. St. Louis: Elsevier; 2004.)

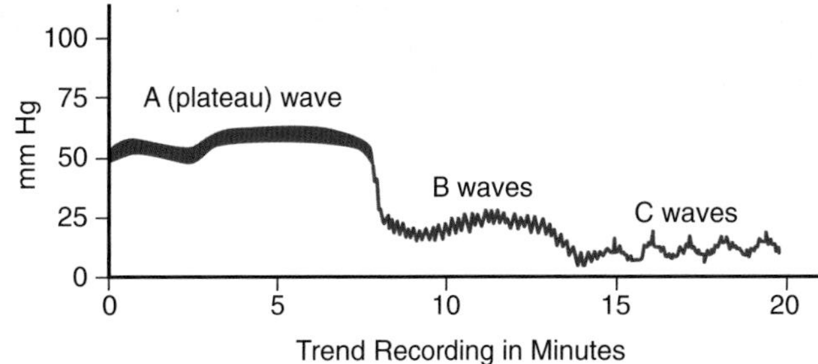

FIG 17-10 Intracranial Pressure Waves. Composite diagram of A-waves (plateau waves), B-waves (sawtooth waves), and C-waves (small rhythmic waves). (From Barker E. *Neuroscience Nursing: A Spectrum of Care.* 3rd ed. St. Louis: Mosby; 2008.)

gold standard for monitoring of ICP, since it is the most accurate of all methods.[26] However, a recent study found that an intraparenchymal catheter was better than an intraventricular catheter unless CSF drainage was required. The intraparenchymal catheter was associated with decreased monitoring time, decreased length of stay, and decreased device-related complications.[29]

Intracranial Pressure Waves

The ICP pulse waveform is observed on a continuous, real-time pressure display, and it corresponds to each heartbeat. The waveform arises primarily from pulsations of the major intracranial arteries but also receives retrograde venous pulsations.[26]

Normal intracranial pressure waveform. The normal ICP wave has three or more defined peaks (Figure 17-8). The first peak (P1) is called the percussion wave. Originating from the pulsations of the choroid plexus, it has a sharp peak and is fairly consistent in its amplitude. The second peak (P2) is called the tidal wave. The tidal wave varies more in shape and amplitude, ending on the dicrotic notch. The P2 portion of the pulse waveform has been most directly linked to the state of decreased compliance. When the P2 component is equal to or higher than P1, decreased compliance occurs (Figure 17-9). Immediately after the dicrotic notch is the third wave (P3), which is called the dicrotic wave. After the dicrotic wave, the pressure usually tapers down to the diastolic position unless retrograde venous pulsations add a few more peaks.[26,30,31]

Abnormal intracranial pressure waveforms. A, B, and C pressure waves are not true waveforms (Figure 17-10). Rather, they are the graphically displayed trend data of ICP over time. These waves reflect spontaneous alterations in ICP associated with respiration, systemic blood pressure, and deteriorating neurologic status. A-waves, also called *plateau waves* because of their distinctive shape, are the most clinically significant of the three types. They usually occur in an already elevated baseline ICP (>20 mm Hg) and are characterized by sharp increases in ICP of 30 to 69 mm Hg, which plateau for 2 to 20 minutes and then return to baseline. The cause of A-waves is unknown, but they may result from vasodilation and increased CBF, decreased venous outflow (and, therefore, increased cerebral blood volume), fluctuations in $PaCO_2$ (and, therefore, changes in cerebral blood volume), or decreased CSF absorption. B-waves often precede A-waves. Plateau waves are considered significant because of the reduced cerebral perfusion pressure associated with ICP, in the range of 50 to 100 mm Hg. Transient signs of intracranial hypertension such as a decreased level of consciousness, bradycardia, pupillary changes, or respiratory changes may accompany these waves. Some research suggests that prolonged increases in ICP associated with plateau waves may result in transient and permanent cell damage from ischemia.[4,26] B-waves are sharp, rhythmic oscillations with a sawtooth appearance that occur every 30 seconds to 2 minutes and that can raise the ICP from 5 to 70 mm Hg. They are a normal physiologic phenomenon that can occur in any patient, but they are amplified in states of low intracranial compliance. B-waves appear to reflect fluctuations in cerebral blood volume.[4,26] C-waves are small, rhythmic waves that occur every 4 to 8 minutes at normal levels of ICP. They are related to normal fluctuations in respiration and systemic arterial pressure.[4,26]

Pupillometry

Quantitative measurement and classification of pupillary reactivity using a handheld pupillometer and the Neurological Pupil index (NPi) are emerging techniques to trend increased ICP in patients with severe traumatic brain injury (TBI), aneurysmal subarachnoid hemorrhage, or intracerebral hemorrhage (ICH). The pupillometer is a handheld infrared system that automatically tracks and analyzes pupil dynamics over a 3-second period.[32] A detachable headrest facilitates the correct and consistent placement of the pupillometer in front of the eye. The device has been specifically designed to minimize possible interobserver variability in the pupillary evaluation.[33] NPi classifies pupil reactivity through the use of an algorithm. An inverse relationship between decreasing pupil reactivity and increasing ICP has been identified with the use of pupillometry and NPi.[33]

Cerebral Perfusion Pressure Monitoring

Measurement of ICP allows for an estimation of cerebral perfusion pressure (CPP). CPP is the blood pressure gradient across the brain, and it is calculated as the difference between the incoming mean arterial pressure (MAP) and the opposing ICP on the arteries: (CPP = MAP − ICP). Over the last two decades, treatment approaches have emphasized maintaining the CPP near 80 mm Hg to provide an adequate of supply to the brain and, thus, avoid secondary cerebral ischemia.[34] However, recent studies have emphasized that individual patients may have different CPP thresholds, depending on the degree of autoregulation and intracranial compliance.[35] The 2007 Brain Trauma Foundation guidelines now recommend a CPP in the range of 50 to 70 mm Hg and consideration of cerebral autoregulation status when selecting a CPP target in a specific patient.[36]

Cerebral Oxygenation and Metabolic Monitoring

Jugular Venous Oxygen Saturation

Jugular venous oxygen saturation ($SjvO_2$) is an indicator of global oxygen extraction of the brain. Jugular venous desaturation suggests an increase in cerebral oxygen extraction, which indirectly implies that a decrease has occurred in cerebral oxygen delivery and, hence, perfusion.[21] Any disorder that increases the cerebral metabolic rate of oxygen ($CMRO_2$) or decreases oxygen delivery may decrease $SjvO_2$. Conversely, any disorder that decreases $CMRO_2$ or increases oxygen delivery may increase $SjvO_2$.[37,38]

To measure $SjvO_2$, a fiberoptic catheter is placed retrograde through the internal jugular vein into the jugular bulb and attached to a bedside monitor. The normal value is 55% to 75%. Patients with values less than 54% are hypoxemic or oligemic (low CBF compared with metabolic rate). Oligemia occurs as a result of decreased blood flow due to hypotension, vasospasm, or intracranial hypertension or as a result of increased brain metabolic requirements due to fever or seizures. $SjvO_2$ values below 45% are indicative of severe cerebral hypoxia. Patients with values above 75% are considered hyperemic (high CBF compared with metabolic need).[21] $SjvO_2$ also increases if the brain is so severely injured that the neurons are unable to extract oxygen. As a global measure, $SjvO_2$ monitoring is complementary to focal monitoring of brain tissue oxygen pressure ($PbtO_2$).[34]

$SjvO_2$ monitoring has several limitations. The most significant limitation is that $SjvO_2$ does not reflect metabolic inadequacies in the focal areas of brain injury and, therefore, may miss regional areas of ischemia.[21] Another limitation is that $SjvO_2$ readings are affected by the position and movement of the patient's head.[38] Inaccuracies with $SjvO_2$ monitoring can occur with catheter misplacement, contamination with extra cerebral blood, when the catheter abuts the blood vessel wall, or if thrombosis occurs around the catheter tip.[21]

Brain Tissue Oxygen Pressure

Monitoring $PbtO_2$ has been shown to be a reliable and sensitive diagnostic method to monitor cerebral oxygenation. $PbtO_2$ uses a device similar to pulse oximetry that allows continuous monitoring of regional tissue oxygenation and, in particular, areas of high ischemic risk.[21,39] The device consists of a monitoring probe on the end of a catheter, which is inserted into the brain parenchyma and attached to a bedside monitor. The probe may be inserted into the damaged portion of the brain to measure regional oxygenation or inserted into the undamaged portion of the brain to measure global oxygenation. One risk associated with insertion of the catheter is bleeding and hematoma formation.[40] Although no consensus on normal values exists because values vary from device to device, it has been concluded that the probability of death increases with prolonged periods of $PbtO_2$ less than 15 mm Hg and any episode of $PbtO_2$ less than 6 mm Hg.[39]

In the patient with head injury, the goal of treatment is to maintain the $PbtO_2$ greater than 20 mm Hg. Factors that decrease $PbtO_2$ include tissue hypoxia, hypocapnia, hypovolemia, decreased blood pressure, low hemoglobin levels, intracranial hypertension, and hyperthermia.[40] Treatment is directed at the underlying cause.

Continuous Electroencephalography Monitoring

Continuous electroencephalography (cEEG) in the critical care unit is increasingly recognized as an important diagnostic and prognostic tool.[41] Continuous EEG monitoring provides dynamic information about brain function, permitting early detection of changes in neurologic status. This is especially useful when the clinical examination is limited. The principal applications for cEEG are monitoring for seizures and ischemia, guiding therapy for seizures and ischemia (especially vasospasm), adjusting levels of sedation for paralyzed or delirious patients, and charting trends in brain function and prognosis.[42] The drawbacks to the use of cEEG are that it is an expensive, labor-intensive program that requires expertise for interpretation and is subject to artifact from the ICU environment.[42]

REFERENCES

1. Daroff RB, et al: Diagnosis of neurological disease. In Daroff RB, et al, editors: *Bradley's neurology in clinical practice*, ed 6, Philadelphia, 2012, Elsevier.
2. Barker E: *Neuroscience nursing: a spectrum of care*, ed 3, St. Louis, 2008, Mosby.
3. McGlinsey A, Kirk A: Neurological assessment: early identification of neurological deterioration is vital to preventing secondary brain injury. Available at:: http://nursing.advanceweb.com/Continuing-Education/CE-Articles/Neurological-Assessment.aspx. Accessed May 3 2014.
4. Bader MK, Littlejohns LR, editors: *AANN core curriculum for neuroscience nursing*, ed 5, Glenview, 2010, American Association of Neuroscience Nurses.
5. Koita J, et al: The mental status examination in emergency practice, *Emerg Med Clin North Am* 28:439, 2010.
6. Seidel HM, et al: *Mosby's guide to physical examination*, ed 7, St. Louis, 2011, Mosby.
7. Teasdale G, Jennett W: Assessment of coma and impaired consciousness—a practical scale, *Lancet* 2:81, 1974.
8. Green SM: Cheerio, laddie! Bidding farewell to the Glasgow Coma Scale, *Ann Emer Med* 58:427, 2011.
9. Kornbluth J, Bhardwaj A: Evaluation of coma: a critical appraisal of popular scoring systems, *Neurocrit Care* 14:134, 2011.
10. Berger JR: Stupor and coma. In Daroff RB, et al, editors: *Bradley's neurology in clinical practice*, ed 6, Philadelphia, 2012, Elsevier.
11. McGee S: *Evidence-based physical diagnosis*, ed 3, Philadelphia, 2012, Elsevier.
12. Rucker JC: Pupillary and eyelid abnormalities. In Daroff RB, et al, editors: *Bradley's neurology in clinical practice*, ed 6, Philadelphia, 2012, Elsevier.

13. Adoni A, McNett M: The pupillary response in traumatic brain injury: a guide for trauma nurses, *Trauma Nurs* 14:191, 2007.
14. Bishop BS: Pathologic papillary signs: self-learning module. Part II, *Crit Care Nurs* 11(7):58, 1991.
15. Haddad SH, Arabi YM: Critical care management of severe traumatic brain injury in adults, *Scand J Trauma Resusc Emerg Med* 20:12, 2012.
16. Saiki RL: Current and evolving management of traumatic brain injury, *Crit Care Nurs Clin North Am* 21:549, 2009.
17. Samuels MA: The brain-heart connection, *Circulation* 116:77, 2007.
18. Fodstad H: History of the Cushing reflex, *Neurosurgery* 59:1132, 2006.
19. Yuh EL, Dillon WP: Intracranial hypotension and intracranial hypertension, *Neuroimaging Clin N Am* 20:597, 2010.
20. Welch H, Hasbun R: Lumbar puncture and cerebrospinal fluid analysis, *Handb Clin Neurol* 96:31, 2010.
21. Kitchener N, et al: *The flying publisher guide to critical care in neurology*, 2012. Available at: http://www.operationflyingpublisher.com/pdf/FPG_007_CriticalCareinNeurology_2012.pdf. Accessed May 3, 2014.
22. Balasteri M, et al: Impact of intracranial pressure and cerebral perfusion pressure on severe disability and mortality after head injury, *Neurocrit Care* 4:8, 2006.
23. Narotam PK, et al: Brain tissue monitoring in traumatic brain injury and major trauma: Outcome analysis of a brain tissue oxygen-directed therapy, *J Neurosurg* 111:672, 2009.
24. Chin LS: ICP monitors. Available at: http://emedicine.medscape.com/article/1983045-overview#a3. Accessed May 3 2014.
25. Slazinski T: Combination intraventricular/fiberoptic catheter insertion (assist), monitoring, nursing care, troubleshooting, and removal. In Lynn-McHale Wiegand DJ, editor: *AACN procedure manual for critical care*, ed 6, St. Louis, 2011, Saunders.
26. American Association of Neuroscience Nurses: *Guide to the care of the patient undergoing intracranial pressure monitoring/external ventricular drainage or lumbar drainage: aann clinical practice guideline series*, Glenview, 2011, The Association.
27. Arbour R: Intracranial hypertension: monitoring and nursing assessment, *Crit Care Nurse* 24(5):19, 2004.
28. Brain Trauma Foundation, et al: Guidelines for the management of severe traumatic brain injury. VII. Intracranial pressure monitoring, *J Neurotrauma* 24(Suppl 1):S45, 2007.
29. Kasotakis G, et al: Intraperechymal vs extracranial ventricular drain intracranial pressure monitors in traumatic brain injury: less is more?, *J Am Coll Surg* 214:950, 2012.
30. Rangel-Castillo L, Robertson CS: Management of intracranial hypertension, *Crit Care Clin* 22:713, 2006.
31. Bhatia A, Gupta AK: Neuromonitoring in the intensive care unit. I. Intracranial pressure and cerebral blood flow monitoring, *Intensive Care Med* 33:1263, 2007.
32. Cecil S, et al: Traumatic brain injury: advanced multimodal neuromonitoring from theory to practice, *Crit Care Nurse* 31(2):25, 2011.
33. Chen JW, et al: Pupillary reactivity as an early indicator of increased intracranial pressure: The introduction of the Neurological Pupil Index, *Surg Neurol Int* 2:82, 2011.
34. Hemphill JC, et al: Mulitmodal monitoring and neurocritical care bioinformatics, *Nat Rev Neurol* 7:451, 2011.
35. Naval NS, et al: Controversies in the management of aneurysmal subarachnoid hemorrhage, *Crit Care Med* 34:511, 2006.
36. Brain Trauma Foundation, et al: Guidelines for the management of severe traumatic brain injury. IX. Cerebral perfusion thresholds, *J Neurotrauma* 24(Suppl 1):S59, 2007.
37. Smith M: Perioperative uses of transcranial perfusion monitoring, *Anesthesiol Clin* 25:557, 2007.
38. Slazinski T: Jugular venous oxygen saturation monitoring: insertion (assist), patient care, troubleshooting, and removal. In Lynn-McHale Wiegand DJ, editor: *AACN procedure manual for critical care*, ed 6, St. Louis, 2011, Saunders.
39. Bader MK: Recognizing and treating ischemic insults to the brain: the role of brain tissue oxygen monitoring, *Crit Care Nurs Clin North Am* 18:243, 2006.
40. Wartenberg KE, et al: Multimodality monitoring in neurocritical care, *Crit Care Clin* 23:507, 2007.
41. Vulliemoz S, et al: Imaging compatible electrodes for continuous electroencephalogram monitoring in the intensive care unit, *J Clin Neurophysiol* 26:236, 2009.
42. Young GB: Continuous EEG monitoring in the ICU: challenges and opportunities, *Can J Neurol Sci* 2:89, 2009.

18 CHAPTER

Neurologic Disorders and Therapeutic Management

Lourdes Januszewicz, Barbara Buesch

Be sure to check out the bonus material, including review questions, on the Evolve website at http://evolve.elsevier.com/Urden/priorities/.

COMA

Description and Etiology

Normal consciousness requires awareness and arousal. Awareness is the combination of cognition (mental and intellectual) and affect (mood) that can be construed based on the patient's interaction with the environment.[1] Alterations of consciousness may be the result of deficits in awareness, arousal, or both.[2] The four discrete disorders of consciousness are 1) coma, 2) vegetative state, 3) minimally conscious state, and 4) locked-in syndrome. *Coma* is characterized by the absence of both wakefulness and awareness, whereas a *vegetative state* is characterized by the presence of wakefulness with the absence of awareness. In the *minimally conscious state*, wakefulness is present, and awareness is severely diminished but not absent. *Locked-in syndrome* is characterized by the presence of wakefulness and awareness, but with quadriplegia and the inability to communicate verbally; thus, the patient appears to be unconscious.[3] Box 18-1 lists the disorders of consciousness in descending order of wakefulness.

Coma is the deepest state of unconsciousness; arousal and awareness are lacking.[1-3] The patient cannot be aroused and does not demonstrate any purposeful response to the surrounding environment.[4] Coma is a symptom rather than a disease, and it occurs as a result of some underlying process.[1,2] The incidence of coma is difficult to ascertain because a wide variety of conditions can induce coma.[1,2] This state of unconsciousness is, unfortunately, very commonly encountered in the critical care unit, and it is the focus of the following discussion.

The causes of coma can be divided into two general categories: 1) structural or surgical and 2) metabolic or medical. Structural causes of coma include ischemic stroke, intracerebral hemorrhage (ICH), trauma, and brain tumors.[5] Metabolic causes of coma include drug overdose, infectious diseases, endocrine disorders, and poisonings.[5] Coma demands immediate attention, resulting in a high percentage of admissions to all hospital services.[6] Box 18-2 and Table 18-1 provides a list of the possible causes of coma.

Pathophysiology

Consciousness involves arousal, or wakefulness, and awareness. Neither of these functions is present in the patient in coma. Ascending fibers of the reticular activating system (ARAS) in the pons, hypothalamus, and thalamus maintain arousal as an autonomic function. Neurons in the cerebral cortex are responsible for awareness. Diffuse dysfunction of both cerebral hemispheres and diffuse or focal dysfunction of the reticular activating system can produce coma.[1,6,7] Structural causes usually produce compression or dysfunction in the area of the ARAS, whereas most medical causes lead to general dysfunction of both cerebral hemispheres.[8] Trauma, hemorrhage, and tumor can damage the ARAS, leading to coma. Destruction of large regions of bilateral cerebral hemispheres can be the result of seizures or viral agents. Toxic drugs, toxins, or metabolic abnormalities can suppress cerebral function.[5-7]

Assessment and Diagnosis

The clinical diagnosis of the comatose state is readily established by assessment of the level of consciousness. However, determining the full nature and cause of coma requires a thorough history and physical examination. A medical history is essential because events immediately preceding the change in the level of consciousness can often provide valuable clues to the origin of the coma. When limited information is available and the coma is profound, the response of the patient to emergent treatment may provide clues to the underlying diagnosis; for example, the patient who becomes responsive with the administration of naloxone can be presumed to have ingested some type of opiate.[6]

Detailed serial neurologic examinations are essential for all patients in coma. Assessment of pupillary size and reaction to light (normal, sluggish, or fixed), extraocular eye movements (normal, asymmetric, or absent), motor response to pain (normal, decorticate, decerebrate, or flaccid), and breathing pattern yields important clues for determining whether the cause of coma is structural or metabolic.[1,6]

The areas of the brainstem that control consciousness and pupillary responses are anatomically adjacent. The sympathetic and parasympathetic nervous systems control pupillary dilation and constriction, respectively. The anatomic directions of these pathways are known, and changes in pupillary responses can help identify where a lesion may be located (see Fig. 17-2 in Chapter 17). For example, if damage occurs in the midbrain region, pupils will be slightly enlarged and unresponsive to light. Lesions that compress the third nerve result in a fixed and dilated pupil on the same side as the neurologic insult. Pupillary responses are usually preserved when the cause of coma is metabolic in origin. Pupillary light

BOX 18-1 Continuum of Descending States of Consciousness

Consciousness
↓
Wakefulness
↓
Arousal
↓
Drowsiness
↓
Confusion
↓
Inattentiveness
↓
Delirium
↓
Stupor
↓
Vegetative state
↓
Coma

BOX 18-2 Causes of Coma

STRUCTURAL OR SURGICAL COMA	METABOLIC OR MEDICAL COMA
Trauma	Infection
Epidural hematoma	Meningitis
Subdural hematoma	Encephalitis
Diffuse axonal injury	Metabolic encephalopathy
Brain contusion	Metabolic conditions
Intracerebral hemorrhage	Hypoglycemia
Subarachnoid hemorrhage	Hyperglycemia
Posterior fossa hemorrhage	Hyperosmolar states
Supratentorial hemorrhage	Uremia
Hydrocephalus	Hepatic encephalopathy
Ischemic stroke	Hypertensive encephalopathy
Tumor	Hypoxic encephalopathy
Other causes	Hyponatremia
	Hypercalcemia
	Myxedema
	Intoxication
	Opioid overdose
	Alcohol
	Poisonings
	Psychogenic causes

TABLE 18-1 Blood Pressure Management for Stroke According to the American Stroke Association Guidelines

BLOOD PRESSURE*	TREATMENT
Nonthrombolytic Candidates	
DBP >140 mm Hg	Sodium nitroprusside (0.5 mcg/kg/min); aim for 10%-20% reduction in DBP
SBP >220 mm Hg, DBP 121-140 mm Hg, or MAP† >130 mm Hg	10-20 mg of labetalol‡ given by IVP over 1-2 min; may repeat or double labetalol every 20 min to a maximum dose of 300 mg
SBP <220 mm Hg, DBP = 120 mm Hg, or MAP† <130 mm Hg	Emergency antihypertensive therapy is deferred in the absence of aortic dissection, acute myocardial infarction, severe congestive heart failure, or hypertensive encephalopathy.
Thrombolytic Candidates	
Pretreatment	
SBP >185 mm Hg or DBP >110 mm Hg	1-2 inches of nitroglycerine paste (Nitropaste) or 1-2 doses of 10-20 mg of labetalol‡ given by IVP; if BP is not reduced and maintained to <185/110 mm Hg, the patient should not be treated with tPA.
During and After Treatment	
Monitor BP	BP is monitored every 15 min for 2 hr, then every 30 min for 6 hr, and then hourly for 16 hr.
DBP >140 mm Hg	Sodium nitroprusside (0.5 mcg/kg/min)
SBP >230 mm Hg or DBP 121-140 mm Hg	10 mg of labetalol‡ given by IVP over 1-2 min; may repeat or double labetalol every 10 min to a maximum dose of 300 mg or give initial labetalol bolus and then start a labetalol drip at 2-8 mg/min. If BP not controlled by labetalol, consider sodium nitroprusside.
SBP 180-230 mm Hg or DBP 105-120 mm Hg	10 mg of labetalol‡ given by IVP; may repeat or double labetalol every 10-20 min to a maximum dose of 300 mg or give initial labetalol bolus and then start a labetalol drip at 2-8 mg/min.

*All initial blood pressures should be verified before treatment by repeating reading in 5 minutes.
†As estimated by one-third of the sum of systolic and double diastolic pressure.
‡Labetalol should be avoided in patients with asthma, cardiac failure, or severe abnormalities in cardiac conduction. For refractory hypertension, alternative therapy may be considered with sodium nitroprusside or enalapril.
BP, Blood pressure; *DBP*, diastolic blood pressure; *IVP*, intravenous push; *MAP*, mean arterial pressure; *SBP*, systolic blood pressure; *tPA*, tissue-type plasminogen activator.
From Bader MK, Littlejohns LR. *AANN Core Curriculum for Neuroscience Nursing.* 4th ed. St. Louis: Elsevier; 2004.

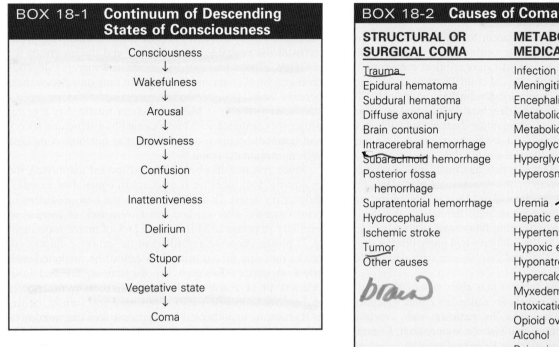

responses are often the key to differentiating between structural and metabolic causes of coma.[1,6,7,9]

Areas of the brainstem adjacent to those responsible for consciousness also control the oculomotor eye movement. The ability to maintain conjugate gaze requires preservation of the internuclear connections of cranial nerves III, VI, and VIII by means of the medial longitudinal fasciculus (MLF).[8] As with pupillary responses, structural lesions that impinge on these pathways cause oculomotor dysfunction such as a disconjugate gaze. Deficits in extraocular eye movements usually accompany a structural cause.[1,5,9]

Focal or asymmetric motor deficits usually indicate structural lesions.[1,5] Abnormal motor movements may also help pinpoint the location of a lesion. Decorticate posturing (abnormal flexion) can be seen with damage to the diencephalon. Decerebrate posturing (abnormal extension) can be seen with damage to the midbrain and pons. Flaccid posturing is an ominous sign and can be seen with damage to the medulla.[9]

Abnormal breathing patterns may also assist in differentiating structural from metabolic causes of coma. Cheyne-Stokes respirations are seen in patients with cerebral hemispheric dysfunction or metabolic suppression. Central neurogenic hyperventilation, or Kussmaul breathing, occurs with metabolic acidosis or damage to the midbrain and upper pons. Apneustic breathing may occur with damage to the pons, hypoglycemia, and anoxia. Ataxic breathing occurs with damage to the medulla. Agonal breathing occurs with failure of the respiratory centers in the medulla.[6,9]

In addition to physical assessment, laboratory studies and diagnostic procedures are done. Structural causes of coma are usually readily apparent with computed tomography (CT) or magnetic resonance imaging (MRI).[4,8] Laboratory studies are also used to identify metabolic or endocrine abnormalities.[7] Evoked potentials are also useful in facilitating a differential diagnosis between the disorders of consciousness and in evaluating a patient's prognosis. Generally, a patient in coma, with absence of brainstem auditory evoked responses (BAERs), is considered to have a poor prognosis of recovery.[3] Occasionally, the cause of coma is never clearly determined.

Medical Management

The goal of medical management of the patient in coma is identification and treatment of the underlying cause of the condition. Initial medical management includes emergency measures to support vital functions and prevent further neurologic deterioration. Protection of the airway and ventilatory assistance are often needed. Administration of thiamine (at least 100 milligrams [mg]), glucose, and a opioid antagonist is suggested when the cause of coma is not immediately known.[1,6] Thiamine is administered before glucose because the coma produced by thiamine deficiency, Wernicke encephalopathy, can be precipitated by a glucose load.[1]

The patient who remains in coma after emergent treatment requires supportive measures to maintain physiologic body functions and prevent complications. Intubation for continued airway protection and nutritional support are essential. Fluid and electrolyte management is often complex because of alterations in the neurohormonal system. Anticonvulsant therapy may be necessary to prevent further ischemic damage to the brain.[1,5,6]

The health care team and the patient's family make decisions jointly regarding the level of medical management to be provided. Family members require informational support in terms of the probable cause of coma and the prognosis for recovery of consciousness and function. Prognosis depends on the cause of coma and the length of time unconsciousness persists. Only 15% of patients in nontraumatic coma make a satisfactory recovery.[7] Metabolic coma usually has a better prognosis compared with coma caused by a structural lesion, and traumatic coma usually has a better outcome compared with nontraumatic coma.[5,7]

Much research has been directed toward identifying the prognostic indicators for the patient in coma after a cardiopulmonary arrest. In a meta-analysis, the best predictors of poor outcome after cardiac arrest were lack of corneal or papillary response at 24 hours and lack of motor movement at 72 hours. However, regardless of the cause or duration of coma, outcome for an individual cannot be predicted with 100% accuracy.[10] Research has focused on induced (also referred to as *therapeutic)* hypothermia in patients after in-hospital or out-of -hospital cardiac arrest. While the use of therapeutic hypothermia has demonstrated improved neurologic outcomes and survival rates in some studies,[11] the data supporting its use are rather weak, and more randomized control trials are needed.[12]

Nursing Management

Nursing management of the patient in coma incorporates a variety of nursing diagnoses (Box 18-3) and is directed by the specific cause of the coma, although some common interventions are used. The patient in coma totally depends on the health care team. **Nursing priorities are directed toward 1) monitoring for changes in neurological status and clues to the origin of the coma, 2) supporting all body functions, 3) maintaining surveillance for complications, 4) providing comfort and emotional support, and 5) initiating rehabilitation measures.**[1] Measures to support body functions include promoting pulmonary hygiene, maintaining skin integrity, initiating range-of-motion exercises, managing bowel and bladder functions, and ensuring adequate nutritional support.[1]

Eye Care

The blink reflex is often diminished or absent in the patient in coma. The eyelids may be flaccid and may depend on body

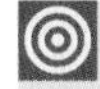 BOX 18-3 **NURSING DIAGNOSIS PRIORITIES**

Coma

- Ineffective Airway Clearance, related to excessive secretions or abnormal viscosity of mucus, p. 597
- Ineffective Breathing Pattern, related to decreased lung expansion, p. 598
- Imbalanced Nutrition: Less Than Body Requirements, related to lack of exogenous nutrients or increased metabolic demand, p. 593
- Risk for Aspiration, p. 602
- Compromised Family Coping, related to critically ill family member, p. 578

BOX 18-4 Collaborative Management

Coma

- Identify and treat the underlying cause.
- Protect the airway.
- Provide ventilatory assistance, as required.
- Support circulation, as required.
- Initiate nutritional support.
- Provide eye care.
- Protect skin integrity.
- Initiate range-of-motion exercises.
- Maintain surveillance for complications:
  - Infections
  - Metabolic alterations
  - Cardiac dysrhythmias
  - Temperature alterations
- Provide comfort and emotional support.
- Plan for the rehabilitation program.

positioning to remain in a closed position, and edema may prevent complete closure. Loss of these protective mechanisms results in drying and ulceration of the cornea, which can lead to permanent scarring and blindness.[1]

Two interventions that are commonly used to protect the eyes are instilling saline or methylcellulose lubricating drops and taping the eyelids in the shut position. Evidence suggests that an alternative technique may be more effective in preventing corneal epithelial breakdown. In addition to instilling saline drops every 2 hours, a polyethylene film is taped over the eyes, extending beyond the orbits and eyebrows. The film creates a moisture chamber around the cornea and assists in keeping the eyes moist and in the closed position. This technique also prevents damage to the eyes that results from tape or gauze being placed directly on the delicate skin of the eyelids.[13]

Collaborative management of the patient in coma is outlined in Box 18-4.

STROKE

Stroke is a descriptive term for the sudden onset of acute neurologic deficit persisting for more than 24 hours and caused by the interruption of blood flow to the brain. Stroke is the fourth leading cause of death in the United States, preceded by heart disease, cancer, and chronic respiratory disease. Each year, approximately 795,000 people have a stroke; 610,000 of these are first attacks, and 185,000 are recurrent attacks.[14]

Strokes are classified as ischemic and hemorrhagic (Figure 18-1). Hemorrhagic strokes can be further categorized as subarachnoid hemorrhages (SAHs) and intracerebral hemorrhages (ICHs). Approximately 87% of all strokes are ischemic, 10% are ICHs, and 3% are SAHs. Although less common, hemorrhagic strokes (ICHs and SAHs) have a higher mortality rate compared with ischemic strokes. Approximately 8% to 12% of ischemic strokes and 37% to 38% of hemorrhagic strokes result in death within 30 days.[14] The annual cost for care and loss of productivity was estimated to be $76.6 billion in 2012.[14]

The national concern for the incidence and effects of stroke is illustrated by the inclusion of emergent stroke care in the American Heart Association (AHA) guidelines for basic and advanced life support. Major public education programs, stroke appraisal screening programs, development of stroke centers, and algorithms for stroke management are based on the success that these same approaches have had with coronary artery disease.

Ischemic Stroke

Description and Etiology

Ischemic stroke results from interruption of blood flow to the brain and accounts for 80% to 85% of all strokes. The interruption can be the result of a thrombotic or embolic event. Thrombosis can form in large vessels (large-vessel thrombotic strokes) or small vessels (small-vessel thrombotic strokes). Embolic sources include the heart (cardioembolic strokes) and atherosclerotic plaques in larger vessels (atheroembolic strokes). In 30% of the cases, the underlying cause of the stroke is unknown (cryptogenic strokes).[15]

Strokes are preventable. Most thrombotic strokes are the result of the accumulation of atherosclerotic plaque in the vessel lumen, especially at the bifurcations or curves of the vessel. The pathogenesis of cerebrovascular disease is identical to that of coronary vasculature. The greatest risk factor for ischemic stroke is hypertension.[15,16] Other risk factors are dyslipidemia, diabetes, smoking, and carotid atherosclerotic disease.[14,17] Common sites of atherosclerotic plaque are the bifurcation of the common carotid artery, the origins of the middle and anterior cerebral arteries, and the origins of the vertebral arteries.[16] Ischemic strokes resulting from vertebral artery dissection have been reported after chiropractic manipulation of the cervical spine.[18]

An embolic stroke occurs when an embolus from the heart or lower circulation travels distally and lodges in a small vessel, obstructing the blood supply. At least 20% of ischemic strokes are attributed to a cardioembolic phenomenon.[19] The most common cause of cardiac emboli is atrial fibrillation. It is responsible for about 50% of all cardiac emboli.[19] Other sources of cardiac emboli are from mitral stenosis, mechanical valves, atrial myxoma, endocarditis, and recent myocardial infarction.[16] Researchers hypothesize that a patent foramen ovale or atrial septal aneurysms may be the cause of cryptogenic stroke.[20]

Pathophysiology

Ischemic stroke is a cerebral hemodynamic insult. When cerebral blood flow is reduced to a level insufficient to maintain neuronal viability, ischemic injury occurs. In focal stroke, an area of hypoperfused tissue, the ischemic penumbra, surrounds a core of ischemic cells. The ischemic penumbra can be salvaged with return of blood flow. However, sustained anoxic insult initiates a chain of biochemical events leading to apoptosis, or cellular death.[21]

The phenomenon of a focal ischemic stroke is identical to that associated with myocardial infarction, which is why the term *brain attack* is used in public education strategies. Often, a history of transient ischemic attacks (TIAs), brief episodes of neurologic symptoms that last less than 24 hours, offers a warning that stroke is likely to occur. Sudden onset indicates embolism as the final insult to flow.[15,16] The size of the stroke depends on the size and location of the occluded vessel and the availability of collateral blood flow. Global ischemia results when severe hypotension or cardiopulmonary arrest

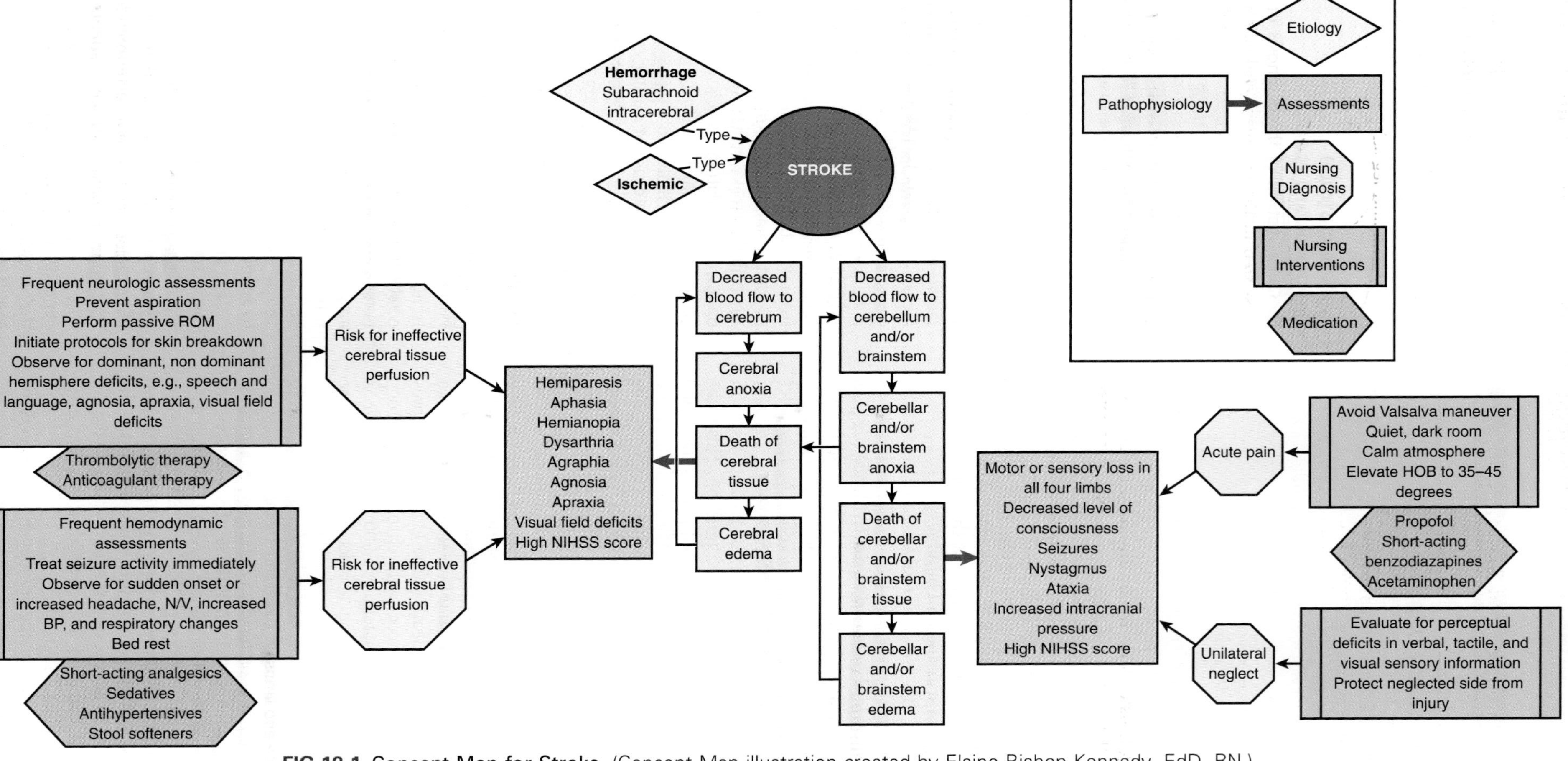

FIG 18-1 Concept Map for Stroke. (Concept Map illustration created by Elaine Bishop Kennedy, EdD, RN.)

provokes a transient drop in blood flow to all areas of the brain.[21]

Cerebral edema sufficient to produce clinical deterioration develops in 10% to 20% of patients with ischemic stroke and can result in intracranial hypertension. The edema results from a loss of normal metabolic function of the cells and peaks at 4 days.[15] This process is commonly the cause of death during the first week after a stroke.[22] Secondary hemorrhage at the site of the stroke lesion, known as *hemorrhagic conversion*, and seizures are the two other major acute neurologic complications of ischemic stroke.[22,23]

Assessment and Diagnosis

The characteristic sign of an ischemic stroke is the sudden onset of focal neurologic signs persisting for more than 24 hours.[15] These signs usually occur in combination. Box 18-5 lists common patterns of neurologic symptoms associated with an ischemic stroke. Hemiparesis, aphasia, and hemianopia are common. Changes in the level of consciousness usually occur only with brainstem or cerebellar involvement, seizure, hypoxia, hemorrhage, or elevated intracranial pressure (ICP). These changes may be exhibited as stupor, coma, confusion, and agitation.[1] The reported frequency of seizures in patients with ischemic stroke ranges from 3% to 8%. If seizures occur, they are usually seen within 24 hours of an insult.[23]

The National Institutes of Health Stroke Scale (NIHSS) is often used as the basis of the focused neurologic examination.

BOX 18-5 Neurologic Abnormalities in Acute Ischemic Strokes

Left (Dominant) Hemisphere
Aphasia, right hemiparesis, right-sided sensory loss, right visual field defect, poor right conjugate gaze, dysarthria, difficulty in reading, writing, or calculating

Right (Nondominant) Hemisphere
Neglect of the left visual space, left visual field defect, left hemiparesis, left-sided sensory loss, poor left conjugate gaze, extinction of left-sided stimuli, dysarthria, spatial disorientation

Brainstem, Cerebellum, and Posterior Hemisphere
Motor or sensory loss in all four limbs, crossed signs, limb or gait ataxia, dysarthria, disconjugate gaze, nystagmus, amnesia, bilateral visual field defects

Small Subcortical Hemisphere or Brainstem (Pure Motor Stroke)
Weakness of face and limbs on one side of the body without abnormalities of higher brain function, sensation, or vision

Small Subcortical Hemisphere or Brainstem (Pure Sensory Stroke)
Decreased sensation of face and limbs on one side of the body without abnormalities of higher brain function, motor function, or vision

From Adams HP, et al. Guidelines for the management of patients with acute ischemic stroke: a statement for healthcare professionals from a special writing group of the Stroke Council, American Heart Association. *Circulation.* 1994: 90(3):1588.

The score ranges from 0 to 42 points; the higher the score, the more neurologically impaired the patient is. A change of 4 points on the scale indicates significant neurologic change. The components of the NIHSS include level of consciousness (LOC); LOC questions; LOC commands; gaze; visual fields; face, arm, and leg strength; sensation; limb ataxia, and language function.[15] A copy of the NIHSS with complete instructions is available at http://www.ninds.nih.gov/disorders/stroke/strokescales.htm.

Confirmation of the diagnosis of ischemic stroke is the first step in the emergent evaluation of these patients. Differentiation from intracranial hemorrhage is vital. Noncontrast computed tomography (CT) scanning is the method of choice for this purpose, and it is considered the most important initial diagnostic study. In addition to excluding intracranial hemorrhage, CT can assist in identifying early neurologic complications and the cause of the insult.[15] Magnetic resonance imaging (MRI) can demonstrate infarction of cerebral tissue earlier than can CT but is less useful in the emergent differential diagnosis.[24] Because of the strong correlation between acute ischemic stroke and heart disease, 12-lead electrocardiography (ECG), chest radiography, and continuous cardiac monitoring are suggested to detect a cardiac cause or coexisting condition. Echocardiography is valuable in identifying a cardioembolic phenomenon when a sufficient index of suspicion warrants its use.[1] Laboratory evaluation of hematologic function, electrolyte and glucose levels, and renal and hepatic function is also recommended. Arterial blood gas analysis is performed if hypoxia is suspected, and electroencephalography (EEG) is performed if seizures are suspected. Lumbar puncture is performed only if SAH is suspected, and the CT scan is normal.[1]

Medical Management

Major changes have taken place in the medical management of ischemic stroke since 1996. Based on results of the National Institute of Neurologic Disorders and Stroke (NINDS) recombinant tissue plasminogen activator (rtPA) Stroke Study, fibrinolytic therapy with intravenous rtPA is recommended within 3 hours of onset of ischemic stroke.[20] This time frame has now been expanded from 3 hours to 4.5 hours.[25] Patients who should be considered for fibrinolysis are listed in Box 18-6. Confirmation of diagnosis with CT must be accomplished before rtPA administration. The recommended dose of rtPA is 0.9 milligram per kilogram (mg/kg) up to a maximum dose of 90 mg. Ten percent of the total dose is administered as an initial intravenous bolus, and the remaining 90% is administered by intravenous infusion over 60 minutes.[20,24]

The desired result of fibrinolytic therapy is to dissolve the clot and reperfuse the ischemic brain. The goal is to reverse or minimize the effects of stroke. The major risk and complication of rtPA therapy is bleeding, especially intracranial hemorrhage. Unlike fibrinolytic protocols for acute myocardial infarction, subsequent therapy with anticoagulant or antiplatelet agents is not recommended after rtPA administration in ischemic stroke. Patients receiving fibrinolytic therapy for stroke should not receive aspirin, heparin, warfarin, ticlopidine, dabigatran, rivaroxaban, or any other antithrombotic or antiplatelet medications for at least 24 hours after treatment.[15,20]

BOX 18-6 Characteristics of Patients with Ischemic Stroke Who Could be Treated with rtPA

Diagnosis of Ischemic Stroke Causing Measurable Neurologic Deficit

- The neurologic signs should not be clearing spontaneously.
- The neurologic signs should not be minor and isolated.
- Caution should be exercised in treating a patient with major deficits.
- The symptoms of stroke should not be suggestive of subarachnoid hemorrhage.
- Onset of symptoms less than 3 hours before beginning treatment
- No head trauma or prior stroke in previous 3 months
- No myocardial infarction in the previous 3 months
- No gastrointestinal or urinary tract hemorrhage in previous 21 days
- No major surgery in the previous 14 days
- No arterial puncture at a noncompressible site in the previous 7 days
- No history of previous intracranial hemorrhage
- Blood pressure not elevated (systolic <185 mm Hg and diastolic <110 mm Hg)
- No evidence of active bleeding or acute trauma (fracture) on examination
- Not taking an oral anticoagulant or, if anticoagulant being taken, international normalized ratio (INR) 1.7 or less
- If receiving heparin in previous 48 hours, aPTT must be in normal range.
- Platelet count 100 000 mm^3 or greater
- Blood glucose concentration less than 40 mg/dL or greater than 400
- No seizure with postictal residual neurologic impairments
- Computed tomography does not show a multilobar infarction (hypodensity >1/3 cerebral hemisphere).
- The patient or family members understand the potential risks and benefits from treatment.

aPTT, Activated partial thromboplastin time; *INR*, international normalized ratio.

From Adams HP, Jr. et al. Guidelines for the early management of adults with ischemic stroke: a guideline from the American Heart Association/American Stroke Association Stroke Council, Clinical Cardiology Council, Cardiovascular Radiology and Intervention Council, and the Atherosclerotic Peripheral Vascular Disease and Quality of Care Outcomes in Research Interdisciplinary Working Groups: the American Academy of Neurology affirms the value of this guideline as an educational tool for neurologists. *Stroke.* 2007: 38:1655.

The major barriers to effective application of fibrinolytic therapy for ischemic stroke are prehospital and in-hospital delays.[26] To help decrease delays, the public needs to be educated about stroke symptoms and activation of emergency medical system (EMS). EMS responders need adequate education and training on managing a patient with an acute ischemic stroke, focusing on stabilization and transport of the patient quickly to the emergency department. The receiving hospital should ideally have certification for primary stroke treatment and have expert staff and the infrastructure to care for the patient with complex stroke.[20,24]

Other emergent care of the patient with ischemic stroke must include airway protection and ventilatory assistance to maintain adequate tissue oxygenation.[22] Hypertension is often present in the early period as a compensatory response, and in most cases, blood pressure (BP) must not be lowered (Table 18-1). For the patient who has not received fibrinolytic therapy, antihypertensive therapy is considered only if the diastolic blood pressure is greater than 120 mm Hg or the systolic blood pressure is greater than 220 mm Hg.[15,20] Criteria are different for patients who have received rtPA. Their blood pressure is kept below 180/105 mm Hg to prevent intracranial hemorrhage. Intravenous labetalol or nicardipine is used to achieve blood pressure control. If these agents are not effective, nitroprusside, hydralazine, or enalaprilat should be considered.[15] Body temperature and glucose levels also must be normalized.[15,22]

Medical management also includes the identification and treatment of acute complications such as cerebral edema or seizure activity. Prophylaxis for these complications is not recommended. Deep vein thrombosis (DVT) prophylaxis, however, should be initiated to decrease the risk of pulmonary embolism.[15] One study demonstrated that improved outcomes for patients with ischemic stroke can be achieved by managing swallowing issues, initiating DVT prophylaxis, and treating hypoxemia.[27] Surgical decompression is recommended if a large cerebellar infarction compresses the brainstem.[22]

Subarachnoid Hemorrhage

Description and Etiology

Subarachnoid hemorrhage (SAH) is bleeding into the subarachnoid space, which usually is caused by rupture of a cerebral aneurysm or arteriovenous malformation (AVM).[22] At the time of autopsy, approximately 4% of the population has been found to have one or more aneurysms.[28] With improvements in imaging techniques, an increased number of incidental intracranial aneurysms has been found. Computed tomographic angiography (CTA) and magnetic resonance angiography (MRA) can detect up to 95% of all aneurysms. Among people younger than 40 years, more men than women are likely to have SAHs, whereas among those older than 40 years, more women have SAHs. Aneurysmal SAH is associated with a mortality rate of 25% to 50%, with most patients dying on the first day after the insult.[28] Hemorrhage from AVM rupture has a better chance of survival and is associated with an overall mortality rate of 10% to 15%.[29] Known risk factors for SAH include hypertension, smoking, and alcohol or stimulant use.[30]

Cerebral aneurysm rupture accounts for approximately 85% of all cases of spontaneous SAH.[28] An aneurysm is an outpouching of the wall of a blood vessel that results from weakening of the wall of the vessel (Table 18-2).[28] Ninety percent of aneurysms are congenital—the cause of which is unknown. The other 10% can be the result of traumatic injury (that stretches and tears the muscular middle layer of the arterial vessel) or infectious material (most often from infectious vegetation on valves of the left side of the heart after bacterial endocarditis) that lodges against a vessel wall and erodes the muscular layer, or they are of undetermined cause.[30] Multiple aneurysms occur in approximately 30% of the cases and often are bilateral, occurring in the same location on both sides of the cerebral vascular system.[31]

TABLE 18-2 Aneurysm Classification According to Type, Shape, Location, and Common Characteristics

TYPES OF ANEURYSMS	CHARACTERISTICS
Berry or saccular	Most common type, usually congenital; appears at a bifurcation in the anterior circulation, primarily at the base of the brain or the circle of Willis and its branches; grows from the base of the arterial wall with a neck or stem; contains blood; thinned dome is usually the site of rupture.
Giant or fusiform	Can have an irregular shape and be larger than 2.5 cm and atherosclerotic; involves mainly the internal carotid or vertebrobasilar artery; rarely ruptures; has no stem; may act like a space-occupying lesion in the brain; difficult to manage
Mycotic	Rare form; usually occurs from septic emboli, usually results from bacterial infection, which weakens the vessel wall, causing dilation involving the distal branches of the middle cerebral arteries
Dissecting	May occur during angiography; caused by trauma, syphilis, arteriosclerosis, or when blood is forced between layers of the arterial wall; intima is pulled away from the medial layer, allowing blood to enter.
Traumatic	Sometimes called a *pseudoaneurysm*, which may resolve after trauma
Charcot-Bouchard	Small aneurysm that can be seen in the area of the basal ganglia or the brainstem in individuals with a history of hypertension; chronic hypertension causes fibrinoid necrosis in the penetrating and subcortical arteries, weakening the arterial walls and causing formation of small aneurysmal outpouching.

AVM rupture is responsible for roughly 6% of all SAHs.[31] An AVM is a tangled mass of arterial and venous blood vessels that shunt blood directly from the arterial side into the venous side, bypassing the capillary system. AVMs may be small, focal lesions or large, diffuse lesions that occupy almost an entire hemisphere.[30] They are always congenital, although the exact embryonic cause for these malformations is unknown. They also occur in the spinal cord and the renal, gastrointestinal, and integumentary systems.[31] Small, superficial AVMs are seen as port-wine stains of the skin. In contrast to the SAH from an aneurysm in the middle-aged population, SAH from an AVM usually occurs in the second to fourth decades of life.[30,31]

Pathophysiology

The pathophysiologies of the two most common causes of SAH, cerebral aneurysm and AVM, are distinctly different.

Cerebral aneurysm. As the individual with a congenital cerebral aneurysm gets older, blood pressure rises, and more stress is placed on the poorly developed and thin vessel wall. Ballooning of the vessel occurs, giving the aneurysm a berry-like appearance. Most cerebral aneurysms are saccular or berrylike, with a stem or neck. Aneurysms are usually small, are 2 to 7 millimeters (mm) in diameter, and often occur at the base of the brain on the circle of Willis.[29] Figure 18-2 illustrates the usual distribution between the vessels. Most cerebral aneurysms occur at the bifurcation of blood vessels.[28,29,32]

The aneurysm becomes clinically significant when the vessel wall becomes so thin that it ruptures, sending arterial blood at a high pressure into the subarachnoid space. For a brief moment after the aneurysm ruptures, ICP is thought to approach mean arterial pressure, and cerebral perfusion decreases.[32] In other situations, the unruptured aneurysm expands and places pressure on surrounding structures. This is particularly true with posterior communicating artery aneurysms because they put pressure on the oculomotor nerve (cranial nerve III), causing ipsilateral pupil dilation and ptosis.[31]

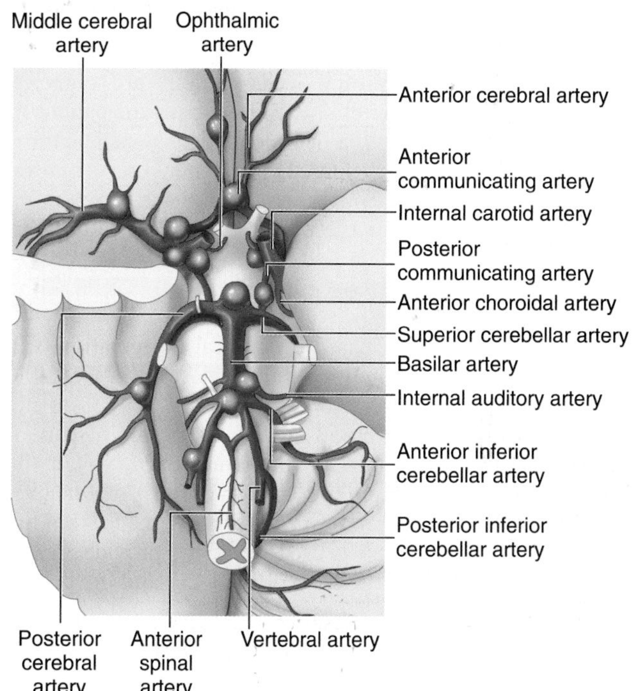

FIG 18-2 Common Sites of Berry Aneurysms. The size of the aneurysm in the drawing is proportional to the frequency of occurrence at the various sites. (From Zivin JA. Hemorrhagic cerebrovascular disease. In: Goldman L, Schafer AI, eds. *Goldman's Cecil Medicine.* 24th ed. St. Louis: Elsevier; 2012.)

Arteriovenous malformation. The pathophysiologic features of an AVM are related to the size and location of the malformation. One or more cerebral arteries, also known as feeders, supply an AVM. These feeder arteries tend to enlarge over time and increase the volume of blood shunted through the malformation and increase the overall mass effect. Large, dilated, tortuous draining veins develop as a result of increasing arterial blood flow being delivered at a higher-than-normal pressure. Normal vascular flow has a mean arterial pressure of 70 to 80 mm Hg, a mean arteriole pressure of 35 to 45 mm Hg, and a mean capillary pressure that drops from 35 to 10 mm Hg as it connects with the venous side. Lack of this capillary bridge allows blood with a mean pressure of 35 to 45 mm Hg to flow into the venous system. Unlike arteries, veins have no muscular layer and become extremely engorged and rupture easily. Some patients with AVMs also have cerebral atrophy. It is the result of chronic ischemia because of the shunting of blood through the AVM and away from normal cerebral circulation.[33]

Assessment and Diagnosis

The patient with an SAH characteristically has an abrupt onset of pain, described as the "worst headache of my life." A brief loss of consciousness, nausea, vomiting, focal neurologic deficits, and a stiff neck may accompany the headache.[28-32] The SAH may result in coma or death.

The patient's history may reveal one or more incidences of sudden onset of headache with vomiting in the weeks preceding a major SAH. These are small "warning leaks" of an aneurysm in which small amounts of blood ooze from the aneurysm into the subarachnoid space. The presence of blood is an irritant to the meninges, particularly the arachnoid membrane, and the irritation causes headache, stiff neck, and photophobia. These warning leaks seldom are detected because the condition is not severe enough for the patient to seek medical attention.[32] If a neurologic deficit such as third cranial nerve palsy develops before aneurysm rupture, medical intervention is sought, and the aneurysm may be surgically secured before the devastation of a rupture can occur. Symptoms of unruptured AVM—headaches with dizziness or syncope or fleeting neurologic deficits—also may be found in the history.[31]

Diagnosis of SAH is based on clinical presentation, CT findings, and lumbar puncture results. Noncontrast CT is the cornerstone of definitive SAH diagnosis.[30-34] In 95% of the cases, CT demonstrates blood in the subarachnoid space if performed within 48 hours of the hemorrhage.[28,32] On the basis of the appearance and the location of the SAH, diagnosis of the cause—aneurysm or AVM—may be made from the CT scan. MRI is not routinely used, but it may provide greater sensitivity for detecting the areas of SAH clot and the potential location of the bleed.[32]

If the initial CT finding is negative, a lumbar puncture is performed to obtain cerebrospinal fluid (CSF) for analysis. CSF after SAH appears bloody and has a red blood cell count greater than 1000 cells/mm^3. If the lumbar puncture is performed more than 5 days after the SAH, the CSF fluid is xanthochromic (dark amber) because the blood products have broken down.[33] Cloudy CSF usually indicates some type of infectious process, such as bacterial meningitis, not SAH.[31]

After the SAH has been documented, cerebral angiography is necessary to identify the exact cause of the hemorrhage. If a cerebral aneurysm rupture is the cause, angiography is essential for identifying the exact location of the aneurysm in preparation for surgery.[31,33,34] After the aneurysm has been located, it is graded using the Hunt and Hess classification scale. This scale categorizes the patient on the basis of the severity of the neurologic deficits associated with the

BOX 18-7 Hunt and Hess Classification of Subarachnoid Hemorrhage

- *Grade I:* Asymptomatic or minimal headache and slight nuchal rigidity
- *Grade II:* Moderate to severe headache, nuchal rigidity, but no neurologic deficit other than cranial nerve palsy
- *Grade III:* Drowsiness, confusion, or mild focal deficit
- *Grade IV:* Stupor, moderate to severe hemiparesis, possible early decerebrate rigidity, and vegetative disturbances
- *Grade V:* Deep coma, decerebrate rigidity, moribund appearance

From Hunt WE, Hess RM. Surgical risks as related to time of intervention in the repair of intracranial aneurysms. *J Neurosurg.* 1968: 28:14.

hemorrhage (Box 18-7).[35] If AVM rupture is the cause, angiography is necessary to identify the feeding arteries and draining veins of the malformation.[30]

Medical Management

SAH is a medical emergency, and time is of the essence. Preservation of neurologic function is the goal, and early diagnosis is crucial. Initial treatment must always support vital functions. Airway management and ventilatory assistance may be necessary.[22] A ventriculostomy is performed to control ICP if the patient's level of consciousness is depressed.[32,34]

Evidence suggests that only 19% of the deaths attributable to aneurysmal SAH are related to the direct effects of the initial hemorrhage.[36] Rebleeding accounts for 22% of deaths from aneurysmal SAH, cerebral vasospasm for 23%, and non-neurologic medical complications for 23%.[36] Principal non-neurologic causes of death are systemic inflammatory response syndrome (SIRS) and secondary organ dysfunction.[37] After initial intervention has provided the necessary support for vital physiologic functions, medical management of acute SAH is aimed primarily toward the prevention and treatment of the complications of SAH, which may produce further neurologic damage and death.[32]

Rebleeding. Rebleeding is the occurrence of a second SAH in an unsecured aneurysm or, less commonly, an AVM.[28] The incidence of rebleeding during the first 24 hours after the first bleed is 4%, with a 1% to 2% chance per day in the following month. The mortality rate associated with aneurysmal rebleeding is approximately 70%.[30,31]

Historically, conservative measures to prevent rebleeding have included blood pressure control and SAH precautions (see "Nursing Management"). An elevation in blood pressure is a normal compensatory response to maintain adequate cerebral perfusion after a neurologic insult. In the belief that hypertension contributes to rebleeding, nitroprusside, metoprolol, or hydralazine has been commonly used to maintain a systolic blood pressure no greater than 140 mm Hg.[32] Individualized guidelines must be determined on the basis of the clinical condition and preexisting values of the patient. Evidence suggests that rebleeding has more to do with variations in blood pressure than it does with absolute values and that blood pressure control does not lower the incidence of rebleeding.[34]

Surgical clipping of aneurysms. Definitive treatment for the prevention of rebleeding is surgical clipping or endovascular coiling with complete obliteration of the aneurysm.[31,32] Timing of the operation is a key medical management issue. Since the introduction of microsurgery and improved surgical techniques, patients commonly are taken to the operating room within the first 48 hours after rupture.[32] This early surgical intervention to secure the aneurysm eliminates the risk of rebleeding and allows more aggressive therapy to be used in the postoperative period for the treatment of vasospasm.[31,32] Early surgery also allows the neurosurgeon to flush out the excess blood and clots from the basal cisterns (reservoir of CSF around the base of the brain and circle of Willis) to reduce the risk of vasospasm.[37] Careful consideration of the patient's clinical situation is necessary in determining the optimal time for surgery.

The surgical procedure involves a craniotomy to expose and isolate the area of aneurysm. A clip is placed over the neck of the aneurysm to eliminate the area of weakness (Figure 18-3). This is a technically difficult procedure that requires the skill of an experienced neurosurgeon. It is not uncommon, particularly in early surgery, for the clot to break away from the aneurysm as it is surgically exposed. Extensive hemorrhage into the craniotomy site results, and cessation of the hemorrhage often causes increased neurologic deficits. Deficits also may occur as a result of surgical manipulation to gain access to the site of the aneurysm.[32]

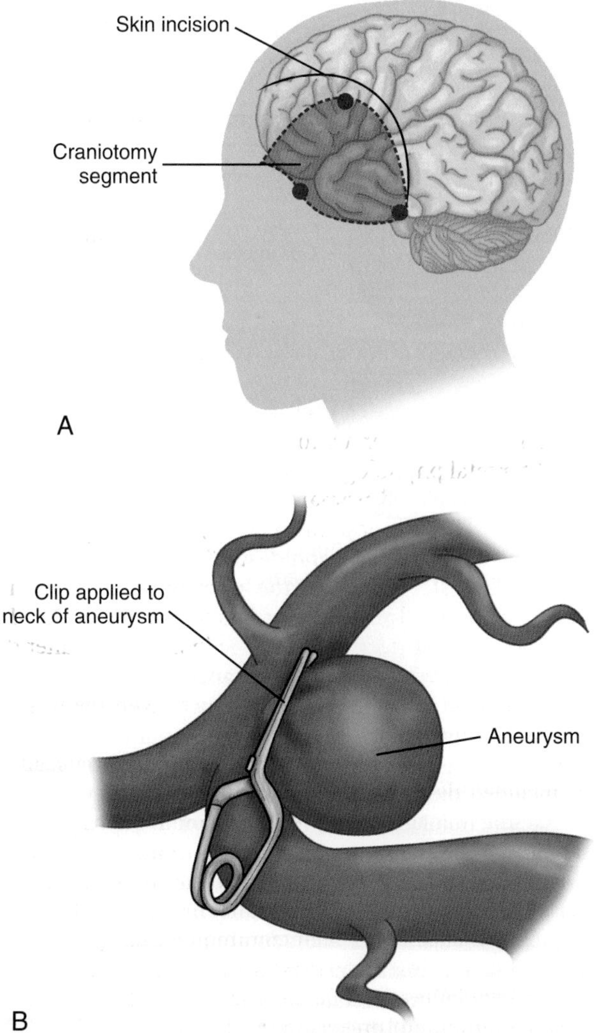

FIG 18-3 Clipping of a Posterior Communicating Artery Aneurysm. *A,* The *solid curved line* shows the typical skin incision, and the *dashed lines* show the craniotomy location. *B,* Application of the clip to the aneurysm.

Surgical excision of arteriovenous malformations. Management of AVM has traditionally involved surgical excision or conservative management of such symptoms as seizures and headache. The decision for surgical excision depends on the location and size of the AVM. Some malformations are located so deep in the cerebral structures (thalamus or midbrain) that attempts to remove the AVM would cause severe neurologic deficits. History of a previous hemorrhage and the patient's age and overall condition are also taken into account when making the decision regarding surgical intervention.[32]

Surgical excision of large AVMs includes the risk of reperfusion bleeding. As feeding arteries of the AVM are clamped off, the arterial blood that usually flowed into the AVM is diverted into the surrounding circulation. In many cases, the surrounding tissue has been in a state of chronic ischemia, and the arterial vessels feeding these areas are maximally dilated. As arterial blood begins to flow at a higher volume and pressure into these dilated arteries, blood may seep from the vessels. Evidence of reperfusion bleeding in the operating room is an indication that no more arterial blood can be diverted from the AVM without risk of serious ICH. In the postoperative phase, a low blood pressure is maintained to prevent further reperfusion bleeding. For large AVMs, two to four stages of surgery may be required over 6 to 12 months.[32]

Embolization. Embolization is used to secure a cerebral aneurysm or AVM that is surgically inaccessible because of size, location, or medical instability of the patient. Embolization involves several new interventional neuroradiology techniques. All of the techniques use a percutaneous transfemoral approach in a manner similar to an angiography. Under fluoroscopy, the catheter is threaded up to the internal carotid artery. Specially developed microcatheters are then manipulated into the area of the vascular anomaly, and embolic materials are placed endovascularly. Three embolization techniques are used, depending on the underlying pathologic derangement.[30]

The first type of embolization is used to embolize an AVM. Small polymeric silicone (Silastic) beads or glue is slowly introduced into the vessels feeding the AVM. Blood flow carries the material to the site, and embolization is achieved. This procedure may be used in combination with surgery. One to three sessions of embolization of the feeding vessels are performed to reduce the size of the lesion before a craniotomy is performed for total excision. The primary risk of this procedure is lodging of the embolic substance in a vessel that feeds normal tissue, which creates an embolic stroke with the immediate onset of neurologic symptoms.[30]

The second type of embolization involves placement of one or more detachable coils into an aneurysm to produce an endovascular thrombus (Figure 18-4). The advantage of this technique is that an electrical current creates a positive charge on the coil, which induces electrothrombosis. Complications include embolic stroke, coil migration, overproduction of the clot, subtotal occlusion and intraprocedural rupture of the vasculature, and death.[30]

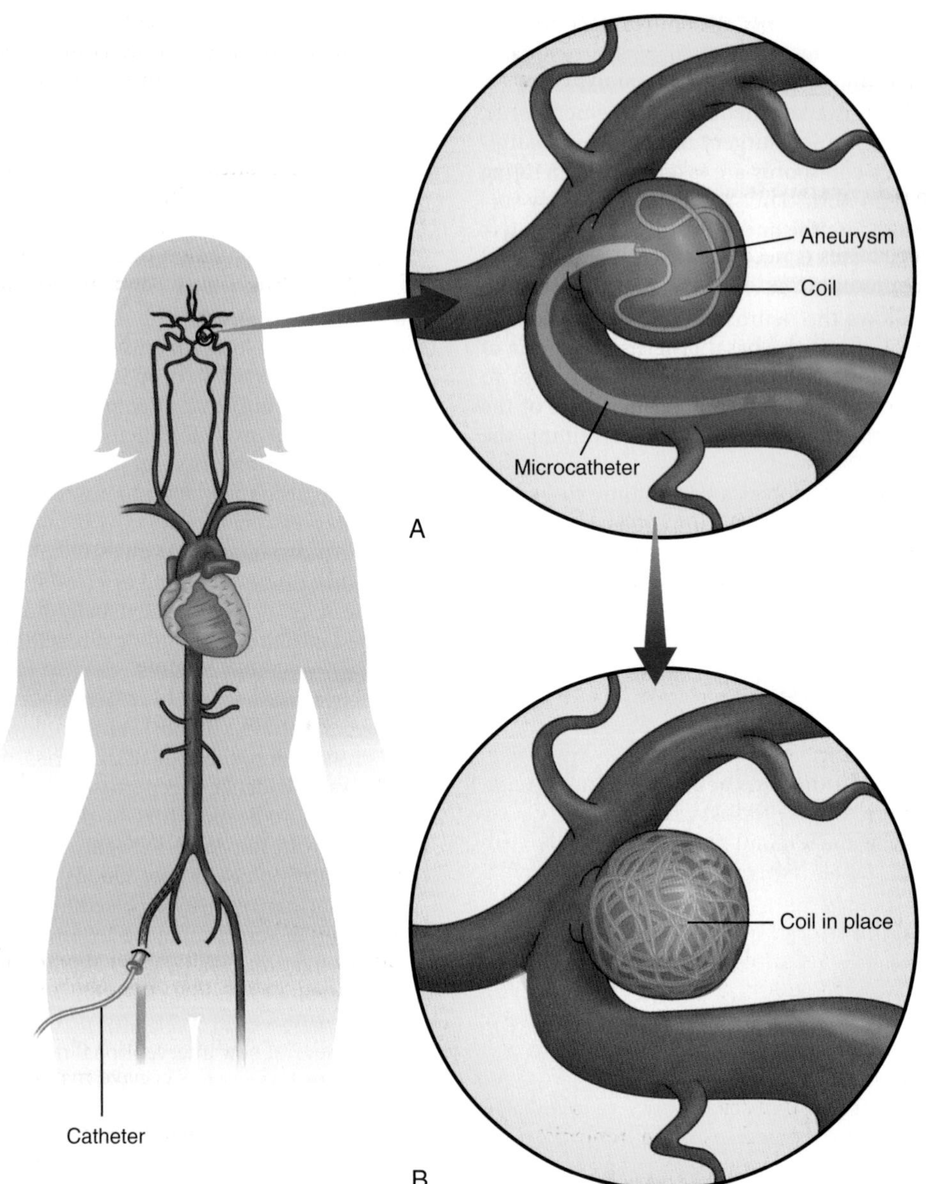

FIG 18-4 Endovascular Occlusion of a Posterior Communicating Artery Aneurysm. *A*, Insertion of the microcatheter into the aneurysm through the right femoral artery, aorta, and left carotid artery. *B*, Occlusion of the aneurysm with coils.

Cerebral vasospasm. The presence or absence of cerebral vasospasm significantly affects the outcome of aneurysmal SAH. This complication does not occur with SAH resulting from AVM rupture. Cerebral vasospasm is a narrowing of the lumen of the cerebral arteries, possibly in response to subarachnoid blood clots coating the outer surface of the blood vessels. Because aneurysms usually occur at the circle of Willis, the major vessels responsible for feeding the cerebral circulation are affected by vasospasm. Depending on the arterial vessels involved in the vasospasm reaction, decreased arterial flow occurs in large areas of the cerebral hemispheres.[30]

It is estimated that 70% of all SAH patients develop vasospasm, which is demonstrable by angiography.[38] Thirty-two percent of these patients develop symptomatic vasospasm, resulting in ischemic stroke or death for up to 23% of them despite the use of maximal therapy.[38] The onset of vasospasm is usually 3 to 12 days after the initial hemorrhage.[22] Three treatments are commonly used: 1) induced hypertensive, hypervolemic, hemodilution (HHH) therapy; 2) oral nimodipine, and 3) transluminal cerebral angioplasty.[34,38]

Hypertensive, hypervolemic, hemodilution therapy. HHH therapy involves increasing the patient's blood pressure and cardiac output with vasoactive medications and diluting the patient's blood with fluid and volume expanders. Systolic blood pressure is maintained between 150 and 160 mm Hg. The increase in volume and pressure forces blood through the vasospastic area at higher pressures. Hemodilution facilitates flow through the area by reducing blood viscosity. Many anecdotal reports exist of patients' neurologic deficits improving as systolic pressure increases from 130 mm Hg to between 150 and 160 mm Hg.[39] The Stroke Council of the AHA has recommended this therapy for prevention and treatment of vasospasm.[34]

The obvious deterrent to the use of induced hypertension is the risk of rebleeding in an unsecured aneurysm. Surgical clipping of the aneurysm before HHH therapy is preferred. Cerebral edema, elevated ICP, heart failure, and electrolyte imbalance are also risks of HHH therapy. Careful monitoring of the patient's neurologic status, hemodynamic parameters, ICP, and serum electrolytes is necessary.[32]

Nimodipine. Nimodipine is strongly recommended to reduce the poor outcomes associated with vasospasm. The exact nature of the effect of nimodipine is not clear, but the use of the medication has demonstrated consistently positive effects on outcome without any demonstrable effect on the incidence or severity of vasospasm.[34,38] A dose of 60 mg of nimodipine is given orally every 4 hours for 21 days. Nimodipine may produce hypotension, especially when administered concurrently with other antihypertensive agents.[38]

Cerebral Angioplasty. Cerebral angioplasty is used when pharmacologic management of cerebral vasospasm has failed. It is performed only when CT or MRI provides evidence that infarction has not occurred. An interventional neuroradiologist performs the procedure, and the patient is placed under local, general, or neuroleptic analgesia. The technique of cerebral angioplasty is very similar to that used in the coronary vasculature. Risks include intimal perforation or rupture, cerebral artery thrombosis or embolism, recurrence of stenosis, and severe, diffuse vasospasm unresponsive to therapy. Hemorrhage at the femoral site also may occur. This procedure is recommended when conventional therapy is unsuccessful.[34,38]

Hyponatremia. Hyponatremia develops in 10% to 43% of patients with SAH as the result of central salt-wasting syndrome. It usually occurs during the same period as vasospasm, several days after the initial hemorrhage.[29] The use of fluid restriction to treat hyponatremia in the SAH patient is associated with a poor outcome. The AHA Stroke Council strongly recommends that fluid restriction not be used in this instance and instead recommends sodium replenishment with isotonic fluids.[34]

Hydrocephalus. Hydrocephalus is a late complication that occurs in approximately 25% of patients after SAH.[30] Blood that has circulated in the subarachnoid space and has been absorbed by the arachnoid villi may obstruct the villi and reduce the rate of CSF absorption. Over time, increasing volumes of CSF in the intracranial space produce communicating hydrocephalus. Treatment consists of placing a drain to remove CSF. This can be accomplished temporarily, by inserting a ventriculostomy, or permanently, by placing a ventriculoperitoneal shunt.[26,31,34]

Intracerebral Hemorrhage

Description and Etiology

Intracerebral hemorrhage (ICH) is bleeding directly into cerebral tissue.[40] ICH destroys cerebral tissue, causes cerebral edema, and increases ICP. The source of intracerebral bleeding is usually a small artery, but it can result also from rupture of an AVM or aneurysm. The most important cause of spontaneous ICH is hypertension, and this section concentrates on spontaneous hypertensive ICH.[41]

Spontaneous ICH accounts for at least 10% of all stroke admissions.[40] The likelihood of death or disability is higher with ICH than with ischemic stroke or SAH. The mortality rate for hemorrhagic stroke is up to 50% within 1 month. Only 20% of patients with ICH return to a functional life at 6 months.[42] The key risk factors for ICH are age-associated cerebral amyloid angiopathy and hypertension.[40]

ICH is most often caused by hypertensive rupture of a cerebral vessel, resulting from a longstanding history of hypertension.[40] Other possible causes of spontaneous ICH are anticoagulation or fibrinolytic therapy, coagulation disorders, drug abuse, and hemorrhage into a cerebral infarct or brain tumors.[31,43] Often, on questioning, the patient with a hypertensive hemorrhage admits to having discontinued antihypertensive medication 2 to 3 weeks before the hemorrhage.

Pathophysiology

The pathophysiology of ICH is caused by continued elevated blood pressure exerting force against smaller arterial vessels that have become damaged from arteriosclerotic changes. Eventually, these arteries break, and blood bursts from the vessels into the surrounding cerebral tissue, creating a hematoma. ICP rises precipitously in response to the increase in overall intracranial volume.[43]

Assessment and Diagnosis

Initial assessment usually reveals a critically ill patient who often is unconscious and requires ventilatory support. History from a relative or significant other describes a sudden onset of focal deficit often accompanied by severe headache, nausea, vomiting, and rapid neurologic deterioration. Signs and symptoms vary, depending on the location of the ICH.[43] Approximately 50% of patients sustain early loss of consciousness, a key feature that differentiates ICH from ischemic stroke. More than one-half of the patients with ICH present with a smooth progression of neurologic symptoms, an uncommon finding in cases of ischemic stroke or SAH.[44] One-third of the patients have maximal symptoms at onset. Assessment of vital signs usually reveals a severely elevated blood pressure (200/100 to 250/150 mm Hg). Signs of increased ICP are often present by the time the patient arrives in the emergency department. Diagnosis is established easily with CT. Angiography is recommended only in patients considered surgical candidates and if a clear cause of hemorrhage is not evident.[40-44]

Medical Management

ICH is a medical emergency. Initial management requires attention to airway, breathing, and circulation. Intubation is usually necessary. Blood pressure management must be based on individual factors. Reduction in blood pressure is usually necessary to decrease ongoing bleeding, but lowering blood pressure too much or too rapidly may compromise cerebral perfusion pressure (CPP), especially in the patient with elevated ICP. National guidelines recommend keeping the *mean* arterial blood pressure below 130 mm Hg in patients with a history of hypertension by moderate blood pressure reduction to a mean arterial pressure below 110 mm Hg.[44] Vasopressor therapy after fluid replenishment is recommended if systolic blood pressure falls below 90 mm Hg.[41]

Increased ICP is common with ICH and is a major contributor to mortality. Recommended management includes mannitol, when indicated; hyperventilation, and

BOX 18-8 EVIDENCE-BASED PRACTICE SPONTANEOUS INTRACEREBRAL HEMORRHAGE MANAGEMENT GUIDELINES (QSEN)

The following are class 1 recommendations from the American Heart Association and American Stroke Association. Class 1 recommendations are conditions for which evidence and general agreement exist that the procedure or treatment is useful and effective.

- Rapid neuroimaging with CT or MRI is recommended to distinguish ischemic stroke from ICH.
- Patients with a severe coagulation factor deficiency or severe thrombocytopenia should receive appropriate factor replacement therapy or platelets, respectively.
- In patients with ICH whose INR is elevated owing to OAC-therapy, warfarin should be withheld, and they should be given therapy to replace vitamin K–dependent factors and correct the INR and should receive intravenous vitamin K.
- Patients with ICH should receive intermittent pneumatic compression for prevention of venous thromboembolism in addition to elastic stockings.
- Initial monitoring and management of patients with ICH should take place in an intensive care unit, preferably one with physician and nursing neuroscience intensive care expertise.
- Blood glucose levels should be monitored, and normoglycemia is recommended.
- Patients with clinical seizures should be treated with antiepileptic medications. Patients with a change in mental status who are found on EEG to have electrographic seizures should be treated with antiepileptic medications.
- Patients with cerebellar hemorrhage who are deteriorating neurologically or who have brainstem compression, hydrocephalus, or both from ventricular obstruction should undergo surgical removal of the hemorrhage as soon as possible.
- After the acute ICH, absent medical contraindications, blood pressure should be well- controlled, particularly for patients with ICH location typical of hypertensive vasculopathy.

CT, Computed tomography; *EEG,* electroencephalography; *ICH,* intracerebral hemorrhage; *INR,* international normalized ratio; *MRI,* magnetic resonance imaging; *OAC,* oral anticoagulant.

Modified from Morgenstern LB, et al. American Heart Association and American Stroke Council on cardiovascular nursing: guidelines for the management of spontaneous intracerebral hemorrhage: a guideline for healthcare professionals from the American Heart Association/American Stroke Association. *Stroke.* 2010: 41:2108.

neuromuscular blockade with sedation. Steroids are avoided. CPP must be kept higher than 70 mm Hg.[41,42]

The goal for fluid management is euvolemia, with a recommended pulmonary artery occlusion pressure (PAOP) of 10 to 14 mm Hg. Body temperature is maintained at less than 38.5° C by using acetaminophen or cooling blankets. Euglycemia, a blood glucose level less than 140 milligram per deciliter (mg/dL), is maintained by using insulin therapy, but hypoglycemia should be avoided. Use of short-acting benzodiazepines or propofol is recommended to treat agitation or hyperactivity. Pneumatic compression devices are used to decrease risk of pulmonary embolism. Prophylactic anticonvulsant therapy is sometimes used.[41,44]

The benefit of surgical treatment for spontaneous ICH is unclear. Recommendations for surgical removal of the clot depend on the size and location of the hematoma, the patient's ICP, and other neurologic symptoms.[44] Medical treatment is recommended if the hemorrhage is small (<10 cm) or neurologic deficit is minimal.[41,44] Likewise, surgery offers no improvement in outcome for patients with a Glasgow Coma Scale (GCS) score of 4 or less. Surgical evacuation of the clot is recommended for patients with cerebellar hemorrhage greater than 3 cm with neurologic deterioration or hydrocephalus with brainstem compression, as well as for young patients with moderate or large lobar hemorrhage with clinical deterioration.[41,44] Numerous techniques are being investigated to lessen the risk of brain damage associated with craniotomy for ICH.

Evidence-based guidelines for the management of the patient with ICH are listed in Box 18-8.

Nursing Management

Nursing management of the patient with stroke incorporates a variety of nursing diagnoses (Box 18-9). **Nursing priorities are directed toward 1) monitoring for changes in neurological and hemodynamic status, 2) maintaining surveillance for complications, 3) providing comfort and emotional support, and 4) educating the patient and family.**

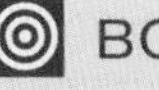

BOX 18-9 NURSING DIAGNOSIS PRIORITIES

Stroke

- Risk for Ineffective Cerebral Tissue Perfusion, p. 604
- Unilateral Neglect, related to perceptual disruption, p. 609
- Impaired Verbal Communication, related to cerebral speech center injury, p. 596
- Impaired Swallowing, related to neuromuscular impairment, fatigue, and limited awareness, p. 595
- Anxiety, related to threat of biologic, psychologic, or social integrity, p. 576
- Deficient Knowledge: Discharge Regimen, related to lack of previous exposure to information, p. 585 (see Box 18-10, Patient Education for Stroke)

Monitoring for Changes in Neurologic and Hemodynamic Status

The goal of frequent assessments is early recognition of neurologic or hemodynamic deterioration. Close monitoring of the patient's neurologic signs and vital signs is essential and requires almost continuous observation. Automatic noninvasive devices such as a blood pressure cuff and a pulse oximeter are helpful. Seizure activity must be identified and treated immediately. It is essential that all personnel working with the patient be aware of the desired hemodynamic and neurologic parameters set by the physician and that the physician be notified at the first sign of any changes.

Maintaining Surveillance for Complications

The patient with stroke should be monitored closely for signs of bleeding, vasospasm, and increased ICP. Other complications of stroke include aspiration, malnutrition, pneumonia, DVT, pulmonary embolism, pressure ulcers, contractures, and joint abnormalities.[29] Nursing measures to prevent these complications are well-known.

Additional complications that may be seen in the patient with stroke are related to the area of the brain that has been damaged. Damage to the temporoparietal area can create a variety of disturbances that affect the patient's ability to interpret sensory information. Damage to the dominant hemisphere (usually left) produces problems with speech and language and abstract and analytic skills. Damage to the nondominant hemisphere (usually right) produces problems with spatial relationships. The resulting deficits include agnosia, apraxia, and visual field defects. Perceptual deficits are not as readily noticeable as are motor deficits, but they may be more debilitating and may lead to inability to perform skilled or purposeful tasks. The patient also may experience impaired swallowing.[30,33]

Bleeding and vasospasm. In the patient with a cerebral aneurysm, sudden onset of, or an increase in, headache and nausea and vomiting, increased blood pressure, and changes in respiration herald the onset of rebleeding. The first indication of vasospasm is usually the appearance of new focal or global neurologic deficits.

SAH precautions must be implemented to prevent any stress or straining that could potentially precipitate rebleeding. Precautions include blood pressure control; bedrest; a dark, quiet environment, and stool softeners. Short-acting analgesics and sedatives are used to relieve pain and anxiety. The patient must be kept calm. Limb restraints cause straining and must therefore be avoided. The head of the bed should be elevated to 35 to 45 degrees at all times. The patient is taught to avoid any activities that correspond to performance of the Valsalva maneuver, such as pushing with the legs to move up in bed, straining for a bowel movement, or holding his or her breath during procedures or discomfort. DVT precautions are routinely implemented. Collaboration with the patient and family is used to establish a visitation plan to meet patient and family needs. Often, family members at the bedside can assist the patient to remain calm.[30,32,33]

Increased intracranial pressure. Numerous signs and symptoms of increased ICP can be observed. A change in the level of consciousness is the most sensitive indicator. Others include unequal pupil size, decreased pupillary response to light, headache, projectile vomiting, altered breathing patterns, Cushing triad (bradycardia, systolic hypertension, and bradypnea), diminished brainstem reflexes, papilledema, and abnormal extension (decerebrate posturing) or flexion (decorticate posturing).[30,32,33]

Impaired swallowing. Normal swallowing occurs in four phases that are controlled by the cranial nerves. Damage to the brain, brainstem, or cranial nerves may result in a variety of swallowing deficits that could place the patient at risk for aspiration. The stroke patient is observed for signs of dysphagia, including drooling; difficulty handling oral secretions; absence of gag, cough, or swallowing reflexes; moist, gurgling voice quality; decreased mouth and tongue movements, and the presence of dysarthria. A speech therapy consult is initiated if any of these signs are present, and the patient must not be orally fed. In the absence of these warning signs, the patient may be fed, as ordered by the physician, although he or she must be continually monitored for signs of aspiration.[30,32,33]

BOX 18-10 PATIENT EDUCATION PRIORITIES

Stroke

- Pathophysiology of disease
- Specific cause
- Risk factor modification
- Importance of taking medications
- Activities of daily living
- Measures to prevent injuries of impaired limbs
- Measures to compensate for residual deficits
- Basic rehabilitation techniques
- Importance of participating in neurologic rehabilitation program or support group

Additional information for the patient and family can be found at the National Stroke Association website (http://www.stroke.org) and the American Stroke Association website (http://www.strokeassociation.org/STROKEORG).

Educating the Patient and Family

Rehabilitation starts in the critical care area, with a multidisciplinary team designing and implementing an individualized plan for maximizing the patient's potential for neurologic rehabilitation. Early in the patient's hospital stay, the patient and family must be taught about stroke, its causes, and its treatment (Box 18-10). As the patient moves toward discharge, teaching focuses on the interventions necessary for preventing the recurrence of the event and on maximizing the patient's rehabilitation potential. The patient's family must be encouraged to participate in the patient's care; learn how to feed, dress, and bathe the patient, and learn some basic rehabilitation techniques. The importance of participating in a neurologic rehabilitation program or a support group, or both, must be stressed.

Collaborative management of the patient with a stroke is outlined in Box 18-11.

GUILLAIN-BARRÉ SYNDROME

Description and Etiology

Guillain-Barré syndrome (GBS), once thought to be a single entity characterized by inflammatory peripheral neuropathy, is a combination of clinical features with various forms of presentation and multiple pathologic processes. A full discussion of this complex condition is beyond the scope of this chapter. Most cases of GBS do not require admission to the critical care unit. However, the prototype of GBS, known as *acute inflammatory demyelinating polyradiculoneuropathy* (AIDP), involves a rapidly progressive, ascending peripheral nerve dysfunction, which leads to paralysis that may produce respiratory failure. Because of the need for ventilatory support, AIDP is one of the few peripheral neurologic diseases that necessitates care in a critical care environment.[45] In this discussion, all references to GBS pertain to the AIDP prototype.

BOX 18-11 COLLABORATIVE MANAGEMENT

Stroke

- Distinguish the cause of the stroke:
  - Ischemic
  - Subarachnoid hemorrhage
  - Cerebral aneurysm
  - Arteriovenous malformation (AVM)
  - Intracerebral bleed
- Implement treatment according to cause of bleed:
  - Ischemic
  - Fibrinolytic therapy
  - Blood pressure control
  - Subarachnoid hemorrhage
  - Surgical aneurysm clipping or AVM excision
  - Embolization
  - Intracerebral bleed
  - Blood pressure control
- Protect patient's airway.
- Provide ventilatory assistance, as required.
- Perform frequent neurologic assessments.
- Maintain surveillance for complications.
- Cerebral edema
  - Cerebral ischemia or vasospasm
  - Rebleeding
  - Impaired swallowing
  - Neurologic deficits
- Provide comfort and emotional support.
- Design and implement appropriate rehabilitation program.
- Educate patient and family.

The annual incidence of GBS is 1.8 cases per 100,000 persons.[45] It occurs more often in males and is the most commonly acquired demyelinating neuropathy. Occasionally, clusters of cases are reported, as occurred following the 1977 swine flu vaccinations.[45] The precise cause of GBS remains unknown, but the syndrome involves an immune-mediated response involving cell-mediated immunity and development of immunoglobulin G (IgG) antibodies. Most patients report a viral infection 1 to 3 weeks before the onset of clinical manifestations, usually involving the upper respiratory tract.[45,46] Numerous antecedent causes, or triggering events, have been associated with GBS. They include viral infections (e.g., influenza virus; cytomegalovirus; hepatitis A, B, or C virus; Epstein-Barr virus; human immunodeficiency virus), bacterial infections (e.g., gastrointestinal *Campylobacter jejuni, Mycoplasma pneumoniae*), vaccines (e.g., rabies, tetanus, influenza), lymphoma, surgery, and trauma.[45,46]

Pathophysiology

GBS affects the motor and sensory pathways of the peripheral nervous system as well as the autonomic nervous system functions of the cranial nerves. The major finding in AIDP-type GBS is a segmental demyelination process of the peripheral nerves. GBS is thought to be an autoimmune response to antibodies formed in response to a recent physiologic event. T cells migrate to the peripheral nerves, resulting in edema and inflammation. Macrophages then invade the area and break down the myelin. Inflammation around this demyelinated area causes further dysfunction. Some axonal damage also occurs.[45,46]

The myelin sheath of the peripheral nerves is generated by Schwann cells and acts as an insulator for the peripheral nerve. Myelin promotes rapid conduction of nerve impulses by allowing the impulses to jump along the nerve by means of the nodes of Ranvier. Disruption of the myelin fiber slows and may eventually stop the conduction of impulses along the peripheral nerves. In GBS, the more thickly myelinated fibers of motor pathways and the cranial nerves are more severely affected than are the thinly myelinated sensory fibers of cutaneous pain, touch, and temperature.[45,46]

After the temporary inflammatory reaction stops, myelin-producing cells begin the process of reinsulating the demyelinated portions of the peripheral nervous system. When remyelination occurs, normal neurologic function should return. In some instances, the axon may be damaged during the inflammatory process. The degree of axonal damage is responsible for the degree of neurologic dysfunction that persists after recovery.[45,46]

Assessment and Diagnosis

Symptoms of GBS include motor weakness, paresthesias and other sensory changes, cranial nerve dysfunction (especially oculomotor, facial, glossopharyngeal, vagal, spinal accessory, and hypoglossal), and some autonomic dysfunction. The usual course of GBS begins with an abrupt onset of lower extremity weakness that progresses to flaccidity and ascends over a period of hours to days. Motor loss usually is symmetric, bilateral, and ascending. In the most severe cases, complete flaccidity of all peripheral nerves, including spinal and cranial nerves, occurs.[46-48]

The patient is admitted to the hospital when lower extremity weakness prevents mobility. Admission to the critical care unit is necessary when progression of the weakness threatens respiratory muscles. As the patient's weakness progresses, close observation is essential. Frequent assessment of the respiratory system, including ventilatory parameters such as inspiratory force and tidal volume, is necessary. The most common cause of death of patients with GBS is respiratory arrest. As the disease progresses and respiratory effort weakens, intubation and mechanical ventilation are necessary. Frequent assessment of neurologic deterioration is continued until the patient reaches the peak of the disease, and a plateau occurs.[46,47]

The diagnosis of GBS is based on clinical findings plus CSF analysis and nerve conduction studies. The diagnostic finding is elevated CSF protein with normal cell count.[46] The increased protein count usually occurs after the first week but does not occur in approximately 10% of all cases. Nerve conduction studies that test the velocity at which nerve impulses are conducted show significant reduction, as the demyelinating process of the disease suggests.[47]

Medical Management

With no curative treatment available, the medical management of GBS is limited. The disease must run its course, which is characterized by ascending paralysis that advances over 1 to 3 weeks and then remains at a plateau for 2 to 4 weeks.[46] The plateau stage is followed by descending paralysis and return to normal or near-normal function. The main focus of medical management is the support of bodily functions and the prevention of complications.[47]

Plasmapheresis and intravenous immune globulin (IVIG) are used to treat GBS.[45,46,49,50] They have been shown to be equally effective.[45] Plasmapheresis involves the removal of venous blood through a catheter, separation of plasma from blood cells, and reinfusion of the cells plus autologous plasma or another replacement solution. Although the number of exchanges may vary, four to six exchanges usually are performed over a 5- to 8-day period.[45] IVIG has emerged as the preferred therapy because of convenience and availability. The usual dose is 0.4 mg/kg for 5 days.[47]

Nursing Management

The nursing management of the patient with GBS incorporates a variety of nursing diagnoses and interventions (Box 18-12). The goal of nursing management is to support all normal body functions until the patient can do so on his or her own. Although the condition is reversible, the patient with GBS requires extensive long-term care because recovery can be a long process. **Nursing priorities are directed toward 1) maintaining surveillance for complications, 2) initiating rehabilitation, 3) facilitating nutritional support, 4) providing comfort and emotional support, and 5) educating the patient and family.**

Maintaining Surveillance for Complications

Continuous assessment of the progressive paralysis associated with GBS is essential to timely intervention and the prevention of respiratory arrest and further neurologic insult. After the patient is intubated and placed on mechanical ventilation, close observation for pulmonary complications such as atelectasis, pneumonia, and pneumothorax is necessary. Autonomic dysfunction (dysautonomia) in the GBS patient can produce variations in heart rate and blood pressure that can reach extreme values.[46,51] Hypertension and tachycardia may require beta-blocker therapy. All patients with GBS must be observed for this phenomenon.[48]

Initiating Rehabilitation

In patients with GBS, immobility may last for months. The usual course of GBS involves an average of 10 days of symptom progression and 10 days of maximal level of dysfunction, followed by 2 to 48 weeks of recovery. Although GBS usually is completely reversible, the patient will require physical and occupational rehabilitation because of the problems of long-term immobility. Rehabilitation starts in the critical care area, with a multidisciplinary team designing and implementing an individualized plan for maximizing the patient's potential for rehabilitation.[51]

Facilitating Nutritional Support

Nutritional support is implemented early in the course of the disease. Because recovery from GBS is a long process, adequate nutritional support will remain a problem for an extended period. Nutritional support usually is accomplished through the use of enteral feeding.

Providing Comfort and Emotional Support

Pain control is another important component in the care of the patient with GBS. Although patients may have minimal to no motor function, most sensory functions remain, causing patients considerable muscle ache and pain. Because of the length of this illness, a safe, effective, long-term solution to pain management must be identified.[51] These patients also require extensive psychologic support. Although the illness is almost 100% reversible, lack of control over the situation, constant pain or discomfort, and the long-term nature of the disorder create coping difficulties for the patient. GBS does not affect the level of consciousness or cerebral function. Patient interaction and communication are essential elements of the nursing management plan.

Educating the Patient and Family

Early in the patient's hospital stay, the patient and family must be taught about GBS and its different treatments (Box 18-13). As the patient moves toward discharge, teaching focuses on the interventions to maximize the patient's rehabilitation potential. The patient's family must be encouraged to participate in the patient's care and to learn some basic rehabilitation techniques. The importance of participating in a neurologic rehabilitation program (if necessary) must be stressed.

Collaborative management of the patient with GBS is outlined in Box 18-14.

CRANIOTOMY

Types of Surgery

A craniotomy is performed to gain access to portions of the central nervous system (CNS) inside the cranium, usually to allow removal of a space-occupying lesion such as a brain tumor (Table 18-3). Common procedures include tumor resection or removal, cerebral decompression, evacuation of hematoma or abscess, and clipping or removal of an aneurysm

BOX 18-12 NURSING DIAGNOSIS PRIORITIES

Guillain-Barré Syndrome

- Ineffective Breathing Pattern, related to musculoskeletal fatigue or neuromuscular impairment, p. 598
- Acute Pain, related to transmission and perception of cutaneous, visceral, muscular, or ischemic impulses, p. 574
- Risk for Aspiration, p. 602
- Powerlessness related to lack of control over current situation or disease progression, p. 600
- Deficient Knowledge: Discharge Regimen, related to lack of previous exposure to information, p. 585 (see Box 18-13, Patient Education for Guillain-Barré Syndrome)

BOX 18-13 PATIENT EDUCATION PRIORITIES

Guillain-Barré Syndrome

- Pathophysiology of disease
- Importance of taking medications
- Measures to compensate for residual deficits
- Basic rehabilitation techniques
- Importance of participating in neurologic rehabilitation program, if necessary

Additional information for the patient and family can be found at the GBS/CIDP Foundation International website (http://www.gbs-cidp.org).

or AVM. Most patients who undergo craniotomy for tumor resection or removal do not require care in a critical care unit. Patients who do usually need intensive monitoring or are at greater risk for complications because of underlying cardiopulmonary dysfunction or the surgical approach used.[52] Box 18-15 provides definitions of common neurosurgical terms.

Preoperative Care

Protection of the integrity of the CNS is a major priority of care for the patient awaiting a craniotomy. Optimal arterial oxygenation, hemodynamic stability, and cerebral perfusion are essential for maintaining adequate cerebral oxygenation. Management of seizure activity is essential for controlling metabolic needs.

Detailed assessment and documentation of the patient's preoperative neurologic status are imperative for accurate postoperative evaluation. Attention is focused on identifying and describing the nature and extent of any preoperative neurologic deficits. When pituitary surgery is planned, a thorough evaluation of endocrine function is necessary to prevent major intraoperative and postoperative complications.[53]

Trends in health care demand judicious use of routine preoperative studies. Depending on the type of surgery to be performed and the general health of the patient, preoperative

BOX 18-14 COLLABORATIVE MANAGEMENT

Guillain-Barré Syndrome

- Support bodily functions.
  - Protect airway.
  - Provide ventilatory assistance, as required.
- Initiate treatments to limit duration of the syndrome.
  - Plasmapheresis
  - Intravenous immunoglobulin
- Initiate nutritional support.
- Maintain surveillance for complications.
  - Infections
  - Cardiac dysrhythmias
  - Blood pressure alterations
  - Temperature alterations
- Provide comfort and emotional support.
- Design and implement appropriate rehabilitation program.
- Educate patient and family.

BOX 18-15 Operative Terms

- *Burr hole:* Hole made into the cranium using a special drill
- *Craniotomy:* Surgical opening of the skull
- *Craniectomy:* Removal of a portion of the skull without replacing it
- *Cranioplasty:* Plastic repair of the skull
- *Supratentorial:* Above the tentorium, separating the cerebrum from the cerebellum
- *Infratentorial:* Below the tentorium; includes the brainstem and the cerebellum; an infratentorial surgical approach may be used for temporal or occipital lesions.
- *Stereotactic:* Minimally invasive surgical intervention that uses a three-dimensional coordinate system to localize a specific area of the brain for ablation, biopsy, dissection, or radiosurgery

TABLE 18-3 Types of Brain Tumors Occurring in Adults

TYPE	PATHOLOGY
Gliomas	
Astrocytomas (grades I to III)	Nonencapsulated, tend to infiltrate brain tissue; arise in any part of brain connective tissue; infiltrate primarily cerebral hemisphere tissue; not well-outlined so difficult to excise completely; grow rapidly—most persons live months to years after diagnosis; tumors assigned grade from I to IV, with IV being most malignant
Glioblastoma multiforme (also called astrocytoma grade IV)	
Oligodendroglioma (grades I to III)	
Ependymoma (grades I to IV)	
Medulloblastoma	
Tumors from Support Structures	
Meningiomas	Arise from meningeal coverings of brain; usually benign but may undergo malignant changes; usually encapsulated, and surgical cure possible; recurrence possible
Neuromas (acoustic neuroma, schwannoma)	Arise from Schwann cells inside auditory meatus on vestibular portion of eighth cranial nerve; usually benign but may undergo cellular change and become malignant; will regrow if not completely excised; surgical resection often difficult because of location
Pituitary adenoma	Arise from various tissues; surgical approach usually successful; recurrence possible
Developmental (Congenital) Tumors	
Dermoid, epidermoid, craniopharyngioma	Arise from embryonic tissue in various sites in brain; success of surgical resection dependent on location and invasiveness
Angiomas	Arise from vascular structures; usually difficult to resect
Metastatic Tumors	Cancer cells spreading to brain via circulatory system; surgical resection difficult; even with treatment, prognosis poor; survival beyond 1-2 yr uncommon

From Monahan FD, et al. *Phipps' Medical-Surgical Nursing: Health and Illness Perspective*. 8th ed. St. Louis: Mosby; 2007.

screening may include a complete blood cell count (CBC); tests for blood urea nitrogen (BUN), creatinine, and fasting blood sugar (FBS); chest radiography, and ECG. A blood type and cross-match may also be ordered.[54]

Preoperative teaching is necessary to prepare the patient and family for what to expect in the postoperative period. A description of the intravascular lines and intracranial catheters used during the postoperative period allows the family to focus on the patient and not be overwhelmed by masses of tubing. Some or all of the patient's hair is shaved off in the operating room, and a large, bulky, turban-like craniotomy dressing is applied. Most patients experience some degree of postoperative eye or facial swelling and periorbital ecchymosis. An explanation of these temporary changes in appearance helps alleviate the shock and fear many patients and families experience in the immediate postoperative period.[54]

All craniotomy patients require instruction to avoid activities known to provoke sudden changes in ICP. These activities include bending, lifting, straining, and the Valsalva maneuver. Patients commonly elicit the Valsalva maneuver during repositioning in bed by holding their breath and straining with a closed epiglottis. This is prevented effectively by teaching the patient to continue to breathe deeply through the mouth during all position changes.[54]

The patient undergoing transsphenoidal surgery requires preparation for the sensations associated with nasal packing. The patient often awakens with alarm because of the inability to breathe through the nose. Preoperative instruction in mouth breathing and avoidance of coughing, sneezing, or blowing of the nose facilitates postoperative cooperation.[53]

The psychosocial issues associated with the prospect of neurosurgery cannot be overemphasized. Few procedures are as threatening as those involving the brain or spinal cord. For some patients, the fear of permanent neurologic impairment may be as ominous as or more ominous than the fear of death. Steps to meet the needs of the patient and the family include collaboration with religious and social services personnel, patient-controlled visitation, and provision of as much privacy as the patient's condition permits. The patient and family must be provided with the opportunity to express their fears and concerns jointly and apart from each other.[52]

Surgical Considerations

Whereas the emphasis in the surgical approach for most other types of surgery is to gain adequate exposure of the surgical site, the neurosurgeon must select a route that also produces the least amount of disruption to the intracranial contents. Neural tissue is unforgiving. A significant portion of neurologic trauma and postoperative deficits is related to the surgical pathway through the brain tissue, rather than to the procedure performed at the site of pathology. Depending on the location of the lesion and the surgical route chosen, a transcranial or a transsphenoidal approach is used to open the skull.

Transcranial Approach

In the transcranial approach, a scalp incision is made, and a series of burr holes is drilled into the skull to form an outline of the area to be opened (Figure 18-5). A special saw is then used to cut between the holes. In most cases, the bone flap is left attached to the muscle to create a hinge effect. In some cases, the bone flap is removed completely and placed in the abdomen for later retrieval and implantation or discarded and replaced with synthetic material. Next, the dura is opened and retracted. After the intracranial procedure, the dura and the bone flap are closed, the muscles and scalp are sutured, and a turbanlike dressing is applied.[52]

Transsphenoidal Approach

The transsphenoidal approach is the technique of choice for removal of a pituitary tumor without extension into the intracranial vault (Figure 18-6).[53,54] This approach involves making a microsurgical entrance into the cranial vault through the nasal cavity. The sphenoid sinus is entered to reach the anterior wall of the sella turcica. The sphenoid bone and the dura are then opened to gain intracranial access. After removal of the tumor, the surgical bed is packed with a small section of adipose tissue grafted from the patient's abdomen or thigh. After closure of the intranasal structures, nasal splints and soft packing or nasal tampons impregnated with antibiotic ointment are placed in the nasal cavities. Occasionally, epistaxis balloons are used instead. A nasal drip pad or mustache-type dressing is placed at the base of the nose to catch surgical drainage.[52]

The patient may be placed in the supine, prone, or sitting position for a craniotomy procedure. A skull clamp connected to skull pins is used to position and secure the patient's head throughout the operation. During a transsphenoidal approach or a transcranial approach into the infratentorial area, the patient's head is elevated during surgery. This position places the patient at risk for an air embolism. Air can enter the vascular system through the edges of the dura or a venous opening. Continuous monitoring of the patient's heart sounds by Doppler signal allows immediate recognition of this complication. If it occurs, an attempt may be made to withdraw the embolus from the right atrium through a central line. Flooding the surgical field with irrigation fluid and placing a moistened sterile surgical sponge over the surgical site creates an immediate barrier to any further air entrance.[52]

Postoperative Medical Management

Definitive management of the postoperative neurosurgical patient varies, depending on the underlying reason for the craniotomy. During the initial postoperative period, management is usually directed toward the prevention of complications. Complications associated with a craniotomy include intracranial hypertension, surgical hemorrhage, fluid imbalance, cerebrospinal fluid leak, and DVT.

Intracranial Hypertension

Postoperative cerebral edema is expected to peak 48 to 72 hours after surgery. If the bone flap is not replaced at the time of surgery, intracranial hypertension will produce bulging at the surgical site. Close monitoring of the surgical site is important so that integrity of the incision can be maintained. Postcraniotomy management of intracranial hypertension is usually accomplished through CSF drainage, patient positioning, and steroid administration.[54]

Surgical Hemorrhage

Surgical hemorrhage after a transcranial procedure can occur in the intracranial vault and manifests as signs and symptoms of increasing ICP. Hemorrhage after a transsphenoidal craniotomy may be evident from external drainage, the patient's complaint of persistent postnasal drip, or excessive

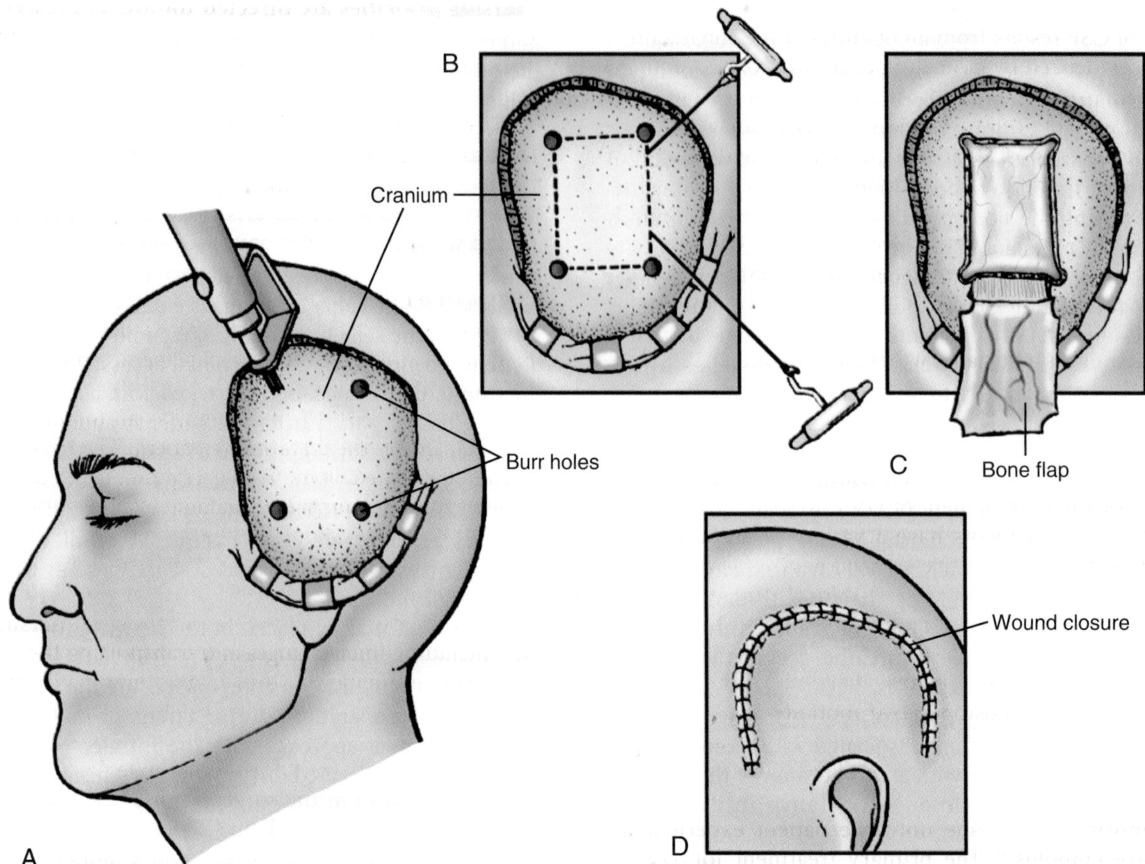

FIG 18-5 Craniotomy Procedure. *A,* Burr holes are drilled into skull. *B,* Skull is cut between burr holes with a surgical saw. *C,* Bone flap is turned back to expose cranial contents. *D,* After surgery, bone flap is replaced, and wound is closed. (From Forsyth LW, Garnett JC. Traumatic and neoplastic problems of the brain. In: Monahan FD, et al, eds. *Phipps' Medical-Surgical Nursing: Health and Illness Perspectives.* 8th ed. St. Louis: Mosby; 2007.)

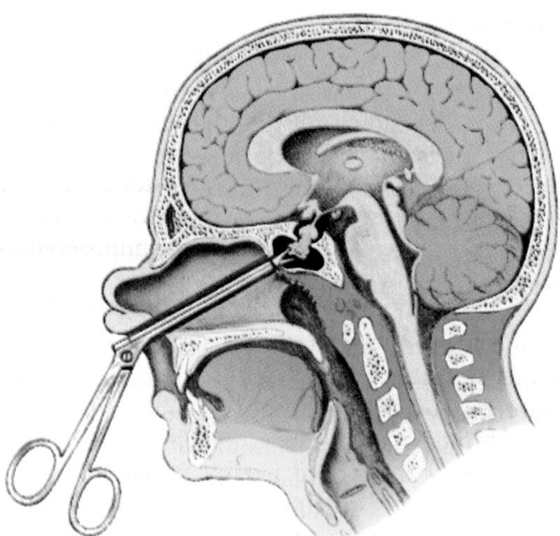

FIG 18-6 Transsphenoidal Hypophysectomy.

swallowing. Loss of vision after pituitary surgery indicates an evolving hemorrhage. Postoperative hemorrhage requires surgical reexploration.[55]

Fluid Imbalance

Fluid imbalance in the postcraniotomy patient usually results from a disturbance in production or secretion of antidiuretic hormone (ADH). ADH is secreted by the posterior pituitary (neurohypophysis) gland. It stimulates the renal tubules and collecting ducts to retain water in response to low circulating blood volume or increased serum osmolality. Inoperative trauma or postoperative edema of the pituitary gland or hypothalamus can result in insufficient ADH secretion. The outcome is unabated renal water loss even when blood volume is low and serum osmolality is high. This condition is known as *diabetes insipidus* (DI). The polyuria associated with DI is often more than 200 milliliters per hour (mL/hr). Urine specific gravity of 1.005 or less and elevated serum osmolality provide evidence of insufficient ADH. The loss of volume may provoke hypotension and inadequate cerebral perfusion. DI is usually self-limiting, and fluid replacement is the only required therapy. In some cases, however, it may be necessary to administer vasopressin intravenously to control the loss of fluid.[56]

The syndrome of inappropriate antidiuretic hormone (SIADH) commonly occurs with neurologic insult and results from excessive ADH secretion. SIADH manifests as inappropriate water retention with hyponatremia in the presence of normal renal function. Urine specific gravity is elevated, and urine osmolality is greater than serum osmolality. The dangers associated with SIADH include circulating volume overload and electrolyte imbalance, both of which may impair neurologic functioning. SIADH is usually self-limiting, with the mainstay of treatment being fluid restriction.[56]

Cerebrospinal Fluid Leak

Leakage of CSF results from an opening in the subarachnoid space, as evidenced by clear fluid draining from the surgical site. When this complication occurs after transsphenoidal surgery, it is evidenced by excessive, clear drainage from the nose or persistent postnasal drip.[57] To differentiate CSF drainage from postoperative serous drainage, a specimen is tested for glucose content. A CSF leak is confirmed by glucose values of 30 mg/dL or greater. Management of the patient with a CSF leak includes bedrest and head elevation. Lumbar puncture or placement of a lumbar subarachnoid catheter may be used to reduce CSF pressure until the dura heals. The risk of meningitis associated with CSF leak often necessitates surgical repair to reseal the opening.[58]

Deep Vein Thrombosis

Patients who have undergone neurosurgery are at particularly high risk for the development of DVT. Research has demonstrated that these patients have a variety of additional risk factors including preoperative leg weakness, longer preoperative and postoperative stay in the critical care unit, longer operative procedure time, prone positioning on frames with flexion of the hips or knees, longer time in the postanesthesia care unit, more days on bedrest, lengthy operative procedures, and delay of postoperative mobility and activity.[59,60] Clinical manifestations of DVT include leg or calf pain and erythema, warmth, and swelling of the affected limb. Unfortunately, the patient with a DVT is often asymptomatic, and the diagnosis is not made until the patient experiences a pulmonary embolus.[61] The primary treatment for DVT is prophylaxis. Following neurosurgery, sequential (intermittent) pneumatic compression boots or stockings are effective in reducing the incidence of DVT. Effectiveness is enhanced when these devices are initiated in the preoperative period. Low-dose unfractionated heparin or low-molecular-weight heparin may also be used prophylactically in high-risk patients once the risk of bleeding has decreased.[62]

Postoperative Nursing Management

The nursing management of the patient following neurosurgery incorporates a variety of nursing diagnoses (Box 18-16). As in preoperative care, the primary goal of postcraniotomy nursing management is protection of the integrity of the CNS.

BOX 18-16 NURSING DIAGNOSIS PRIORITIES

Craniotomy

- Decreased Intracranial Adaptive Capacity, related to failure of normal intracranial compensatory mechanisms, p. 582
- Ineffective Cerebral Tissue Perfusion, related to hemorrhage, p. 604
- Acute Pain, related to transmission and perception of cutaneous, visceral, muscular, or ischemic impulses, p. 574
- Disturbed Body Image, related to actual change in body structure, function, or appearance, p. 586
- Deficient Knowledge: Discharge Regimen, related to lack of previous exposure to information, p. 585 (see Box 18-17, Patient Education for Craniotomy)

Nursing priorities are directed toward 1) preserving adequate CPP, 2) promoting arterial oxygenation, 3) providing comfort and emotional support, 4) maintaining surveillance for complications, 5) initiating early rehabilitation, and 6) educating the patient and family. Frequent neurologic assessment is necessary to evaluate accomplishment of these objectives and to identify problems and quickly intervene if complications do arise. Often, a ventriculostomy is placed to facilitate ICP monitoring and CSF drainage.

Preserving Adequate Cerebral Perfusion

Nursing interventions to preserve cerebral perfusion include patient positioning, fluid management, and avoidance of postoperative vomiting and fever.

Positioning. Patient positioning is an important component of care for the craniotomy patient. The head of the bed should be elevated 30 to 45 degrees at all times to reduce the incidence of hemorrhage, facilitate venous drainage, and control ICP. Other positioning measures to control ICP include maintaining the patient's head in a neutral position at all times and avoiding neck or hip flexion. These rules of positioning must be followed throughout all nursing activities, including linen changes and transporting the patient for diagnostic evaluation. Most craniotomy patients can be turned from side to side within these restrictions, using pillows for support, except in some cases of extensive tumor removal, cranioplasty, and when the bone flap is not replaced. Specific orders from the surgeon must be obtained in these instances. The patient with an infratentorial incision may be restricted to only a very small pillow under the head to prevent strain on the incision. Avoidance of anterior or lateral neck flexion also protects the integrity of this type of incision.

Fluid management. Fluid management is another important component of postcraniotomy care. Hourly monitoring of fluid intake and output facilitates early identification of fluid imbalance. Urine specific gravity must be measured if DI is suspected. Fluid restriction may be ordered as a routine measure to lessen the severity of cerebral edema or as treatment for the fluid and electrolyte imbalances associated with SIADH.[56]

Avoidance of vomiting and fever. Postoperative vomiting must be avoided to prevent sharp spikes in ICP and possibly surgical hemorrhage. Antiemetics are administered as soon as nausea is apparent. Early nutrition in the patient is beneficial. If the patient is unable to eat, enteral hyperalimentation delivered through a feeding tube is the preferred method of nutritional support and can be initiated as early as 24 hours after surgery. Postoperative fever may also adversely affect ICP and increase the metabolic needs of the brain. Acetaminophen is administered orally, rectally, or through a feeding tube. External cooling measures such as a hypothermia blanket may be necessary.

Promoting Arterial Oxygenation

Routine pulmonary care is used to maintain airway clearance and prevent pulmonary complications. To prevent dangerous elevations in ICP, this care measure must be performed using proper technique and at time intervals that are adequately spaced from other patient care activities. If pulmonary complications do arise, consideration must be given to maintaining adequate oxygenation during repositioning. It may be necessary to restrict turning to only the side that places the good lung down.

Providing Comfort and Emotional Support

Pain management in the patient after craniotomy primarily involves control of headache. Small doses of intravenous morphine are used in the critical care setting. Oral analgesics should be started as soon as can be tolerated. Nonopioid medications such as tramadol may be used as an adjunct medication.[63] As opioid analgesics cause constipation, administration of stool softeners and initiation of a bowel program are important components of postcraniotomy care. Constipation is hazardous because straining to have a bowel movement can create significant elevations in blood pressure and ICP.

Maintaining Surveillance for Complications

Following neurosurgery, the patient is at risk for infection, corneal abrasions, and injury from falls or seizures.

Infection. After neurosurgery, patients are at risk for a variety of infections, including meningitis, cerebral abscesses, bone flap infections, and subdural empyema.[64] Care of the incision and surgical dressings is specific to the institution and the physician. The general rule for a craniotomy dressing is to reinforce it, as needed, and change it only on a physician's order. Often, a drain is left in place to facilitate decompression of the surgical site. If a ventriculostomy is present, it is treated as a component of the surgical site. All drainage devices must be secured to the dressing to prevent unintentional displacement with patient movement. Sterile technique is required to prevent infection. Postoperatively, infection should be suspected if the patient exhibits signs of mental status changes, headache, fever, and purulent drainage and swelling around the incision site.[64]

Corneal abrasions. Routine eye care may be necessary to prevent corneal drying and ulceration. Periorbital edema interferes with normal blinking and eyelid closure, which are essential to adequate corneal lubrication. Saline drops are instilled every 2 hours. If the patient remains in a comatose state, covering the eyes with a polyethylene film extending over the orbits and eyebrows may be beneficial.[13,65]

Injury. After craniotomy, the patient may experience periods of altered mentation. Protection from injury may require the use of restraint devices. The side rails of the bed must be padded to protect the patient from injury. Having a family member stay at the bedside or the use of music therapy is often helpful to keep the patient calm during periods of restlessness. In rare circumstances, continuous sedation with or without neuromuscular blockade may be necessary to control patient activity and metabolic needs on a short-term basis.

Initiating Early Rehabilitation

Increased activity, including ambulation, is begun as soon as tolerated by the patient in the postoperative period. Rehabilitation measures and discharge planning may begin in the critical care unit but are beyond the scope of this chapter. Transfer to a general care or rehabilitation unit is usually accomplished as soon as the patient is deemed stable and free of complications.

Educating the Patient and Family

Preoperatively, the patient and family should be taught about the precipitating event necessitating the need for the craniotomy and its expected outcome (Box 18-17). The severity of the disease and the need for critical care management postoperatively must be stressed. As the patient moves toward discharge, teaching focuses on medication instructions; incisional care, including the signs of infection, and the signs and symptoms of increased ICP. If the patient has neurologic deficits, teaching focuses on the interventions to maximize the patient's rehabilitation potential, and the patient's family members must be encouraged to participate in the patient's care and to learn some basic rehabilitation techniques. The importance of participating in a neurologic rehabilitation program must be stressed.

BOX 18-17 PATIENT EDUCATION PRIORITIES

Craniotomy

Before Surgery
- Pathophysiology and expected outcome of underlying disease
- Need for intensive care management after surgery
- Routine preoperative surgical care

After Surgery
- Routine postoperative surgical care
- Discharge medications—purpose, dose, and side effects
- Incisional care
- Signs and symptoms of infection
- Signs and symptoms of increased intracranial pressure
- Measures to compensate for residual deficits
- Basic rehabilitation techniques
- Importance of participating in neurologic rehabilitation program

Additional information for the patient and family can be found at the National Brain Tumor Society website (www.braintumor.org).

INTRACRANIAL HYPERTENSION

Description and Etiology

The intracranial space comprises three components: 1) brain substance (80%), 2) CSF (10%), and 3) blood (10%). Under normal physiologic conditions, the mean ICP is maintained below 15 mm Hg.[33,66] Essential to understanding the pathophysiology of ICP, the Monro-Kellie hypothesis proposes that an increase in volume of one intracranial component must be compensated by a decrease in one or more of the other components so that total volume remains fixed. This compensation, although limited, includes displacing CSF from the intracranial vault to the lumbar cistern, increasing CSF absorption, and compressing the low-pressure venous system.[67,68] Pathophysiologic alterations that can elevate ICP are outlined in Table 18-4.

Pathophysiology

When capable of compliance, the brain can tolerate significant increases in intracranial volume without much increase in ICP. The amount of intracranial compliance, however, does have a limit. After this limit has been reached, a state of decompensation with increased ICP results. As the ICP rises, the relationship between volume and pressure changes, and small increases in volume may cause major elevations in ICP

TABLE 18-4 Mechanisms of Intracranial Pressure Elevation

PATHOPHYSIOLOGY	EXAMPLE	TREATMENT
Disorders of CSF Space		
Overproduction of CSF	Choroid plexus papilloma	Diuretics, surgical removal
Communicating hydrocephalus from obstructed arachnoid	Old subarachnoid hemorrhage	Surgical drainage from lumbar drain
Noncommunicative hydrocephalus	Posterior fossa tumor obstructing aqueduct	Surgical drainage by ventricular drain
Interstitial edema	Any of above	Surgical drainage of CSF
Disorders of Intracranial Blood		
Intracranial hemorrhage causing increased ICP	Epidural hematoma	Surgical drainage
Vasospasm	Subarachnoid hemorrhage	Hypervolemia and hypertensive therapy
Vasodilation	Elevated $PaCO_2$	Hyperventilation
Increasing cerebral blood volume and ICP	Hypoxia	Adequate oxygenation
Disorders of Brain Substance		
Expanding mass lesion with local vasogenic edema causing increased ICP	Brain tumor	Steroids Surgical removal
Ischemic brain injury with cytotoxic edema increasing ICP	Anoxic brain injury from cardiac or respiratory arrest	Resistant to therapy
Increased cerebral metabolic rate increasing cerebral blood flow and ICP	Seizures, hyperthermia	Anticonvulsant medications to control fever

CSF, Cerebrospinal fluid; *ICP*, intracranial pressure.
Modified from Helfaer MA, Kirsch JR. Intracranial vault pathophysiology. *Crit Care Rep.* 1989: 1:12.

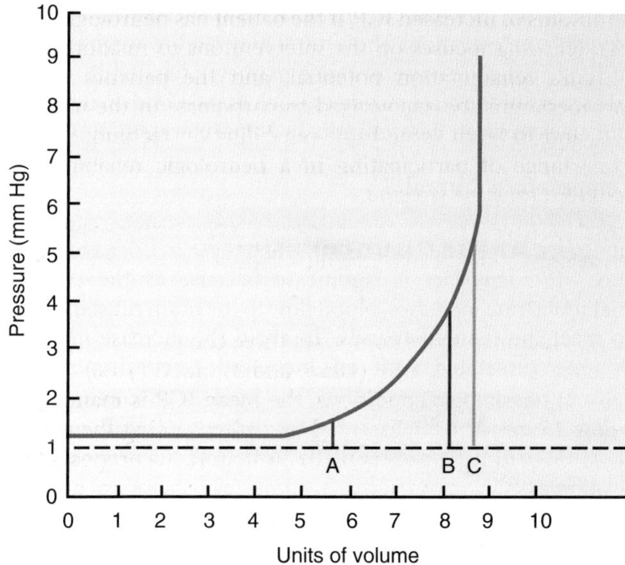

FIG 18-7 Intracranial Volume–Pressure Curve. Pressure is normal *(A)*, and increases in intracranial volume are tolerated without increases in intracranial pressure. Increases in volume *(B)* may cause increases in pressure. Small increases in volume *(C)* may cause larger increases in pressure.

(Figure 18-7).[33,67] The exact configuration of the volume–pressure curve and the point at which the steep rise in pressure occurs vary among patients. The configuration of this curve is also influenced by the cause, and the rate of volume increases within the intracranial vault; for example, neurologic deterioration occurs more rapidly in a patient with an acute epidural hematoma than in a patient with a meningioma of the same size.[66] Regardless of how fast the pressure increases, intracranial hypertension occurs when ICP is greater than 20 mm Hg.[67]

Cerebral blood flow (CBF) corresponds to the metabolic demands of the brain and is normally 50 mL/100 g of brain tissue/min. Although the brain makes up only 2% of body weight, it requires 15% to 20% of the resting cardiac output and 15% of the body's oxygen demands. The normal brain has a complex capacity to maintain constant CBF, despite wide ranges in systemic arterial pressure—an effect known as *autoregulation.* A mean arterial pressure of 50 to 150 mm Hg does not alter CBF when autoregulation is functioning. Outside the limits of this autoregulation, CBF becomes passively dependent on the perfusion pressure.[67]

Factors other than arterial blood pressure that affect CBF are conditions that result in acidosis, alkalosis, and changes in metabolic rate. Conditions that cause acidosis (e.g., hypoxia, hypercapnia, ischemia) result in cerebrovascular dilation. Conditions causing alkalosis (e.g., hypocapnia) result in cerebrovascular constriction. Normally, a reduction in metabolic rate (e.g., from hypothermia or barbiturates) decreases CBF, and increases in metabolic rate (e.g., from hyperthermia) increase CBF.[66,69]

Arterial blood gases exert a profound effect on CBF. Carbon dioxide, which affects the pH of the blood, is a potent vasoactive substance. Carbon dioxide retention (hypercapnia) leads to cerebral vasodilation, with increased cerebral blood volume, whereas hypocapnia leads to cerebral vasoconstriction and a reduction in cerebral blood volume. Prolonged hypocapnia, however, especially at an arterial partial pressure of carbon dioxide ($PaCO_2$) level lower than 20 mm Hg, can lead to cerebral ischemia. Low arterial partial pressure of oxygen (PaO_2) levels, especially below 40 mm Hg, leads to cerebral vasodilation, which increases the intracranial blood volume and can contribute to increased ICP. High PaO_2 levels have not been shown to affect CBF in either direction.[66,69]

Assessment and Diagnosis

The numerous signs and symptoms of increased ICP include decreased level of consciousness, Cushing triad (bradycardia, systolic hypertension, and widening pulse pressure), diminished brainstem reflexes, papilledema, decerebrate posturing (abnormal extension), decorticate posturing (abnormal flexion), unequal pupil size, projectile vomiting, decreased pupillary reaction to light, altered breathing patterns, and headache.[33,70] Patients may exhibit one or all of these symptoms, depending on the underlying cause of the elevation in ICP. One of the earliest and most important signs of increased ICP is a decrease in the level of consciousness. This change must be reported immediately to the physician.[69,70]

In the patient with suspected intracranial hypertension, a monitoring device may be placed within the cranium to quantify ICP. Under normal physiologic conditions, the mean ICP is maintained below 15 mm Hg. The device is used to monitor serial ICPs and assist with the management of intracranial hypertension. An increase in ICP can decrease blood flow to the brain, causing brain damage. The monitoring device can also provide a sterile access for draining excess CSF. The four sites for monitoring ICP are the intraventricular space, the subarachnoid space, the epidural space, and the parenchyma. Each site has advantages and disadvantages for monitoring ICP. The type of monitor chosen depends on the suspected pathologic condition and the physician's preferences.[69-72] Chapter 17 provides a more detailed discussion of ICP monitoring.

Medical and Nursing Management

After intracranial hypertension is documented, therapy must be prompt to prevent secondary insults (Figure 18-8). Although the exact pressure level denoting intracranial hypertension remains uncertain, most current evidence suggests that ICP generally must be treated when it exceeds 20 mm Hg.[33,66,69] All therapies are directed toward reducing the volume of one or more of the components (e.g., blood, brain, CSF) that lie within the intracranial vault. A major goal of therapy is to determine the cause of the elevated pressure and, if possible, to remove the cause.[33,66,69] In the absence of a surgically treatable mass lesion, intracranial hypertension is treated medically. Nursing priorities focus on (1) rapid assessment and (2) implementation of appropriate therapies for reducing ICP.

Positioning and Other Nursing Activities

Positioning of the patient is a significant factor in the prevention and treatment of intracranial hypertension. Head elevation has long been advocated as a conventional nursing intervention to control ICP, presumably by increasing venous return. However, this may decrease CPP. Close monitoring of ICP and CPP should be done with positioning, customizing positioning to maximize CPP and minimize ICP.[68]

Positions that impede venous return from the brain cause elevations in ICP. Obstruction of jugular veins or an increase in intrathoracic or intraabdominal pressure is communicated as increased pressure throughout the open venous system, thereby impeding drainage from the brain and increasing ICP. Positions that decrease venous return from the head (e.g., Trendelenburg, prone, extreme flexion of the hips, angulation of the neck) must be avoided if possible. If changes to positions such as Trendelenburg are necessary to provide adequate pulmonary care, critical care nurses must closely monitor ICP and vital signs.[66]

Some routine nursing activities do affect ICP and may be harmful. Use of positive end-expiratory pressures (PEEP) greater than 20 cm H_2O, coughing, suctioning, tight tracheostomy tube ties, and the Valsalva maneuver have been associated with increases in ICP. Cumulative increases in ICP have been reported when care activities are performed one after another. Conversely, family contact and gentle touch have been associated with decreases in ICP.[66,72]

Hyperventilation

Controlled hyperventilation has been an important adjunct of therapy for the patient with increased ICP. The rationale employed in hyperventilation is that if the $PaCO_2$ can be reduced from its normal level of 35 to 40 mm Hg to a range of 25 to 30 mm Hg in the patient with intracranial hypertension, vasoconstriction of cerebral arteries, reduction of CBF, and increased venous return will result. This practice is being reexamined. Additional research has indicated that severe or prolonged hyperventilation can reduce cerebral perfusion and lead to cerebral ischemia and infarction. The current trend is to maintain $PaCO_2$ levels on the lower side of normal (35 ± 2 mm Hg) by carefully monitoring arterial blood gas measurements and by adjusting ventilator settings.[71-73]

Although hypoxemia must be avoided, excessively high levels of oxygen offer no benefits, and increasing inspired oxygen concentrations above 60% may lead to toxic changes in lung tissue. The use of pulse oximetry has led to greater awareness of the circumstances, such as pain and anxiety, that can cause oxygen desaturation and thus elevate ICP.[33,66]

Temperature Control

Directly proportional to body temperature, cerebral metabolic rate increases 7% per 1° C of increase in body temperature.[68,69,72] This fact is significant because as the cerebral metabolic rate increases, blood flow to the brain must increase to meet the tissue demands. To avoid the increase in blood volume associated with an increased cerebral metabolic rate, nurses must prevent hyperthermia in the patient with a brain injury. Antipyretics and cooling devices must be used when appropriate while the source of the fever is being determined.[68,69]

Blood Pressure Control

Maintenance of arterial blood pressure in the high-normal range is essential in the patient with brain injury. Inadequate perfusion pressure decreases the supply of nutrients and oxygen requirements for cerebral metabolic needs. However, a blood pressure that is too high increases cerebral blood volume and may increase ICP.[69] Figure 18-9 shows the relationship between blood pressure and ICP.

Control of systemic hypertension may require nothing more than the administration of a sedative agent. Small, frequent doses may be sufficient to blunt noxious stimuli and prevent them from triggering increases in blood pressure. When sedation proves inadequate in controlling systemic arterial hypertension, antihypertensive agents are used. Care must be taken in choosing these agents because

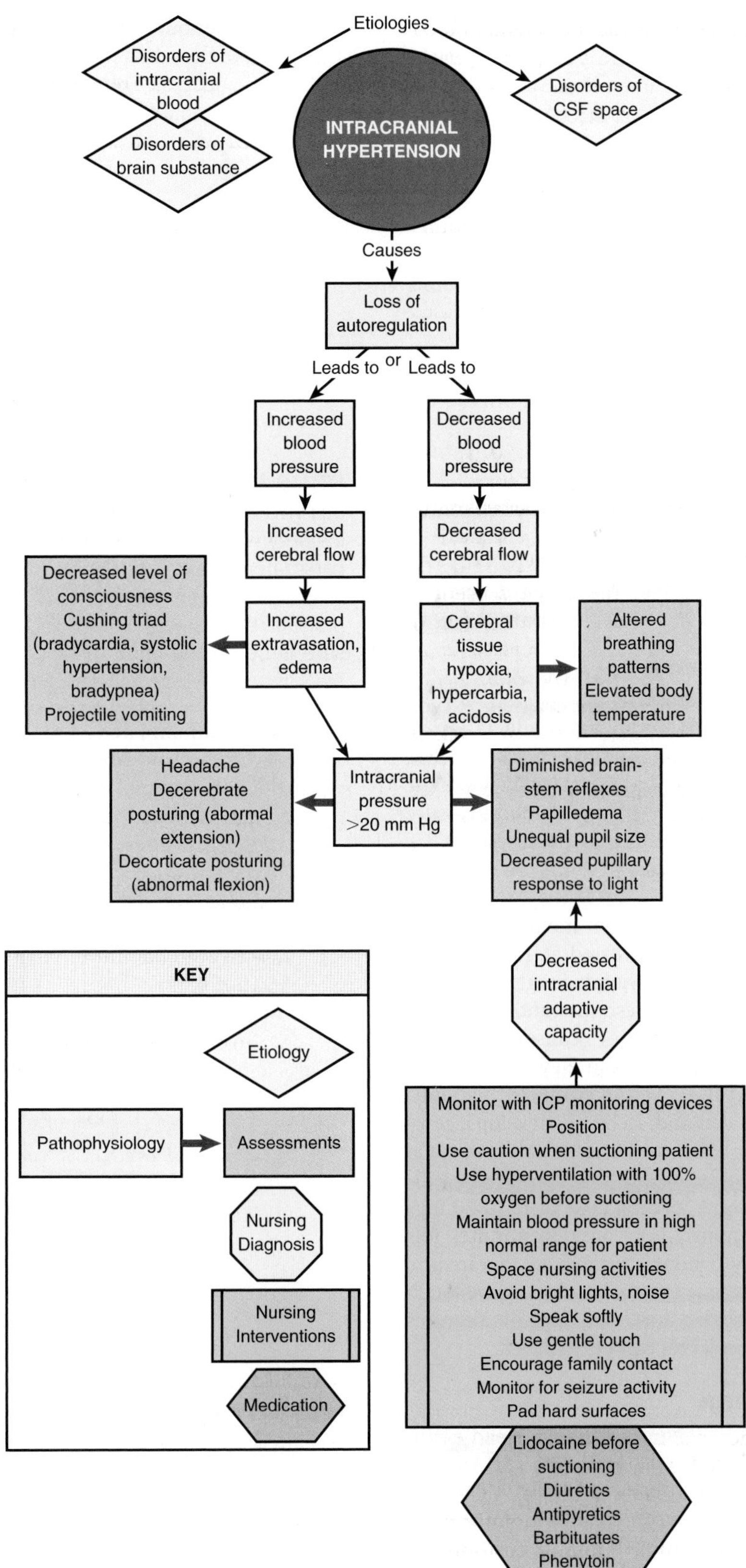

FIG 18-8 Concept Map for Intracranial Hypertension. (Concept map illustration created by Elaine Bishop Kennedy, EdD, RN.)

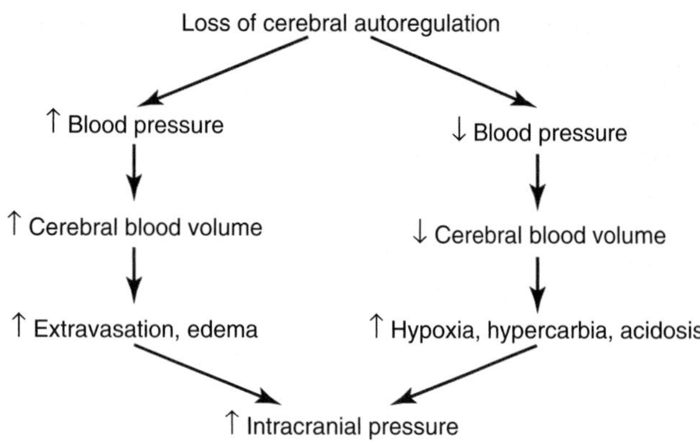

FIG 18-9 Loss of Pressure Autoregulation.

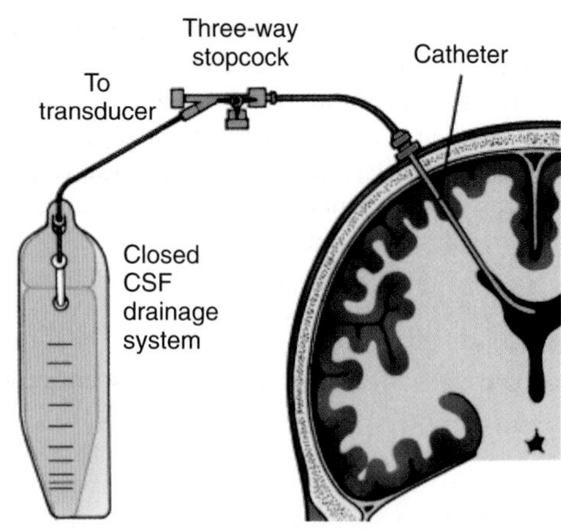

FIG 18-10 Intermittent Drainage System. Intermittent drainage involves draining cerebrospinal fluid (CSF) through a ventriculostomy when intracranial pressure exceeds the upper pressure parameter set by the physician. Intermittent drainage is achieved by opening the three-way stopcock to allow CSF to flow into the drainage bag for brief periods (30 to 120 seconds) until the pressure is below the upper pressure parameter. (From Barker E. *Neuroscience Nursing*. 3rd ed. St. Louis: Mosby; 2008.)

many of the peripheral vasodilators (e.g., nitroprusside, nitroglycerin) also are cerebral vasodilators. All antihypertensives are believed to cause some degree of cerebral vasodilation. To reduce this vasodilating effect, concurrent treatment with beta-blockers (e.g., metoprolol, labetalol) may be beneficial.[66,69]

Systemic hypotension should be treated aggressively with fluids to maintain a systolic blood pressure greater than 90 mm Hg. Crystalloids, colloids, and blood products can be used, depending on the patient's condition. Studies have demonstrated a positive effect on ICP and CPP with hypertonic saline.[73,74] If fluids fail to elevate the patient's blood pressure adequately, the use of inotropic agents may be necessary.[66]

Seizure Control

The incidence of posttraumatic seizures in the patient population with head injury has been estimated at 15% to 20%. Because of the risk of a secondary ischemic insult associated with seizures, many physicians prescribe anticonvulsant medications prophylactically. Seizures cause metabolic requirements to increase, which results in elevation of CBF, cerebral blood volume, and ICP, even in paralyzed patients. If blood flow cannot match demand, ischemia develops, cerebral energy stores are depleted, and irreversible neuronal destruction occurs.[69,75] Phenytoin is the recommended medication for seizure prophylaxis. A loading dose of 15 to 20 mg/kg is administered intravenously (IV) over 30 minutes followed by 100 mg IV every 8 hours, titrated to therapeutic level, for 7 days.[76,77] Fast-acting, short-duration agents such as lorazepam may be indicated for breakthrough seizures until therapeutic medication levels can be achieved.

Cerebrospinal Fluid Drainage

CSF drainage for intracranial hypertension may be used with other treatment modalities (Figures 18-10 and 18-11). CSF drainage is accomplished by the insertion of a pliable catheter into the anterior horn of the lateral ventricle (ventriculostomy), preferably on the nondominant side. This drainage can help support the patient through periods of cerebral edema by controlling spikes in ICP. One of the major advantages of the ventriculostomy is its dual role as a monitoring device and a treatment modality. Care should be taken to avoid infection. However, cleansing ointment such as bacitracin or povidone is not recommended. Ventriculitis occurs in 10% to 17%.[71,78]

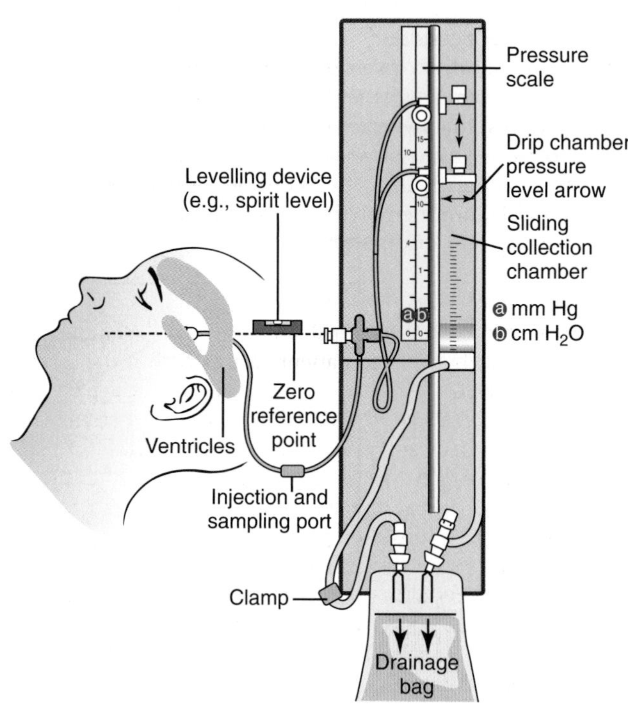

FIG 18-11 Continuous Drainage System. Continuous drainage involves placing the drip chamber of the drainage system at a specified level above the foramen of Monro (usually 15 cm). The system is left open to allow continuous drainage of cerebrospinal fluid into the chamber (which drains into a collection bag) against a pressure gradient that prevents excessive drainage and ventricular collapse.

Hyperosmolar Therapy

Osmotic diuretics and hypertonic saline have also been used to reduce increased ICP. In the presence of an intact blood–brain barrier, hyperosmolar therapy is used to draw water from brain tissue into the intravascular compartment. The direction of flow is from the hypoconcentrated tissue to the hyperconcentrated cerebral vasculature. If the situation becomes reversed and the tissue becomes hyperconcentrated in relation to the cerebral vasculature, a rebound phenomenon may occur. These agents have little direct effect on edematous cerebral tissue situated in an area of a defective blood–brain barrier; instead, they require an intact blood–brain barrier for osmosis to occur.[73,79]

The most widely used osmotic diuretic is mannitol, a large-molecule agent that is retained almost entirely in the extracellular compartment and has little of the rebound effect observed with other osmotic diuretics. Administration of mannitol increases cerebral blood flow and thus induces cerebral vasoconstriction as part of the brain's autoregulatory response to keep blood flow constant.[69,73]

Perhaps the most common difficulty associated with the use of osmotic agents is the provocation of electrolyte disturbances. Careful attention must be paid to body weight and fluid and electrolyte stability. Serum osmolality must be kept between 300 and 320 milliosmoles per liter (mOsm/L). Hypernatremia and hypokalemia often are associated with repeated administration of osmotic agents. Central venous pressure readings must be monitored to prevent hypovolemia. Smaller doses of mannitol simplify fluid and electrolyte management, and their use is encouraged whenever possible.[69,73]

Hypertonic saline, given in concentrations ranging from 3% to 23.4%, can also be used to treat increased ICP. Some studies suggest that hypertonic saline is as equally effective as mannitol for reducing increased ICP.[79] Adverse effects include electrolyte abnormalities, hypotension, pulmonary edema, acute renal failure, hemolysis, central pontine myelinolysis, coagulopathy, and dysrhythmias.[75]

Control of Metabolic Demand

Any treatment modality that increases the incidence of noxious stimulation to the patient carries with it the potential for increasing ICP. Noxious stimuli include pain, the presence of an endotracheal tube, coughing, suctioning, repositioning, bathing, and many other routine nursing interventions. Agents used to reduce metabolic demands include the use of benzodiazepines such as midazolam and lorazepam, intravenous sedative–hypnotics such as propofol, opioid narcotics such as fentanyl and morphine, and neuromuscular blocking agents such as vecuronium and atracurium. These agents may be administered separately or in combination via continuous drip or as an intravenous bolus on an as-needed basis.[66]

The preferred treatment regimen begins with the administration of benzodiazepines for sedation and narcotics for analgesia. If these agents fail to blunt the patient's response to noxious stimuli, propofol or a neuromuscular blocking agent is added. The use of these medications is recommended only in patients who have an ICP monitor in place because sedatives, opioids, and neuromuscular blocking agents affect the reliability of neurologic assessment. The use of neuromuscular blocking agents without sedation is not recommended because these agents can cause skeletal muscle paralysis and because they have no analgesic effect and do not adequately protect the patient from pain and the physiologic responses that can occur from pain-producing procedures.[69,80] If these agents fail to control the patient's ICP, barbiturate therapy is considered.

Barbiturate therapy. Barbiturate therapy is a treatment protocol developed for the management of uncontrolled intracranial hypertension that has not responded to the conventional treatments previously described.[69] The two most commonly used medications in high-dose barbiturate therapy are 1) pentobarbital and 2) thiopental. The goal with either medication is a reduction of ICP to 15 to 20 mm Hg while a mean arterial pressure of 70 to 80 mm Hg is maintained. Patients are maintained on high-dose barbiturate therapy until ICP has been controlled within the normal range for 24 hours. Barbiturates must never be stopped abruptly; they are tapered slowly over approximately 4 days. Despite the theoretical reasons for barbiturate use, clinical trials of its use have not shown improved outcome.[80]

Complications of high-dose barbiturate therapy can be disastrous unless a specific and organized approach is used. The most common complications are hypotension, hypothermia, and myocardial depression. If any complications occur and are allowed to persist unchecked, they may cause secondary insults to an already damaged brain. Hypotension, the most common complication, results from peripheral vasodilation and can be compounded in an already dehydrated patient who has received large doses of an osmotic diuretic in an attempt to control ICP. Careful monitoring of fluid status by central venous pressure or a pulmonary artery catheter can help prevent this complication. Myocardial depression results from cardiac muscle suppression and can be avoided by frequent monitoring of fluid status, cardiac output, and serum drug levels. If an adequate cardiac output cannot be maintained in the presence of normothermia, barbiturates must be reduced, regardless of serum levels.[66,69]

Collaborative management of the patient's intracranial hypertension is outlined in Box 18-18.

Herniation Syndromes

The goal of neurologic evaluation, ICP monitoring, and treatment of increased ICP is to prevent herniation. Herniation of intracerebral contents results in the shifting of tissue from one compartment of the brain to another and places pressure on cerebral vessels and vital function centers of the brain. If

BOX 18-18 COLLABORATIVE MANAGEMENT

Intracranial Hypertension

- Position patient to achieve maximal intracranial pressure (ICP) reduction.
- Reduce environmental stimulation.
- Maintain normothermia.
- Control ventilation to ensure a normal $PaCO_2$ level (35 ± 2 mm Hg).
- Administer diuretic agents, anticonvulsants, sedation, analgesia, paralytic agents, and vasoactive medications to ensure cerebral perfusion pressure (CPP) greater than 70 mm Hg.
- Drain cerebrospinal fluid for ICP greater than 20 mm Hg.

unchecked, herniation rapidly causes death as a result of the cessation of CBF and respirations.[66]

Supratentorial Herniation

The four types of supratentorial herniation syndrome are 1) uncal, 2) central or transtentorial, 3) cingulate, and 4) transcalvarial (Figure 18-12).

Uncal herniation is the most common herniation syndrome. In uncal herniation, a unilateral, expanding mass lesion, usually of the temporal lobe, increases ICP, causing lateral displacement of the tip of the temporal lobe (uncus). Lateral displacement pushes the uncus over the edge of the tentorium, puts pressure on the oculomotor nerve (cranial nerve III) and the posterior cerebral artery ipsilateral to the lesion, and flattens the midbrain against the opposite side. Clinical manifestations of uncal herniation include ipsilateral pupil dilation, decreased level of consciousness, respiratory pattern changes leading to respiratory arrest, and contralateral hemiplegia leading to abnormal flexion (decorticate) or abnormal extension (decerebrate) posturing. If no intervention occurs, uncal herniation results in fixed and dilated pupils, flaccidity, and respiratory arrest.[66,81]

In *central* or *transtentorial herniation*, an expanding mass lesion of the midline, frontal, parietal, or occipital lobe results in downward displacement of the hemispheres, basal ganglia, and diencephalon through the tentorial notch. Central herniation often is preceded by uncal and cingulate herniation. Clinical manifestations of central herniation include loss of consciousness; small, reactive pupils progressing to fixed, dilated pupils; respiratory changes leading to respiratory arrest, and abnormal flexion (decorticate) posturing progressing to flaccidity. In the late stages, uncal and central herniation syndromes affect the brainstem similarly.[66,81]

Cingulate herniation occurs when an expanding lesion of one hemisphere shifts laterally and forces the cingulate gyrus under the falx cerebri. Cingulate herniation occurs often. When a lateral shift is observed on the CT scan, cingulate herniation has occurred. Little is known about the effects of cingulate herniation, and no accompanying clinical manifestations exist to assist in its diagnosis. Cingulate herniation is not in itself a life-threatening condition, but if the expanding mass lesion that caused cingulate herniation is not controlled, uncal or central herniation will follow.[66,81]

Transcalvarial herniation is the extrusion of cerebral tissue through the cranium. In the presence of severe cerebral edema, transcalvarial herniation occurs through an opening from a skull fracture or craniotomy site.[66]

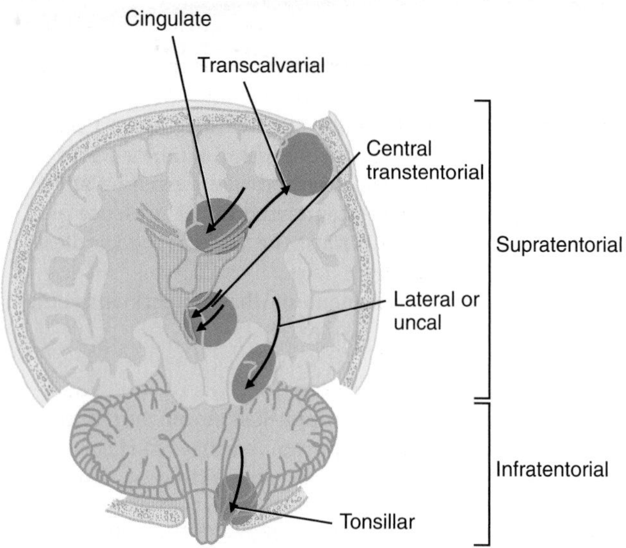

FIG 18-12 Types of Intracranial Herniation. (From Goddard L. Neurological disorders. In: Linton AD. *Introduction to Medical-Surgical Nursing*. St. Louis: Elsevier; 2012.)

Infratentorial Herniation

The two infratentorial herniation syndromes are 1) upward transtentorial herniation and 2) downward cerebellar herniation. *Upward transtentorial herniation* occurs when an expanding mass lesion of the cerebellum causes protrusion of the vermis (central area) of the cerebellum and the midbrain upward through the tentorial notch. Compression of the third cranial nerve and diencephalon occurs. Blockage of the central aqueduct and distortion of the third ventricle obstruct CSF flow. Deterioration progresses rapidly.[66,81] *Downward cerebellar herniation* occurs when an expanding lesion of the cerebellum exerts pressure downward, sending the cerebellar tonsils through the foramen magnum. Compression and displacement of the medulla oblongata occur, rapidly resulting in respiratory and cardiac arrest.[66,81]

PHARMACOLOGIC AGENTS

Many pharmacologic agents are used in the care of patients with neurologic disorders. Table 18-5 reviews the various agents used and any special considerations necessary for administering them. See Box 18-19 for Internet Resources.

BOX 18-19 INTERNET RESOURCES

American Association of Critical-Care Nurses: http://www.aacn.org
American Association of Neuroscience Nurses: http://www.aann.org
Society for Critical Care Medicine: http://www.sccm.org
American Academy of Neurology: http://www.aan.com
American College of Physicians: http://www.acponline.org
American Association of Neurological Surgeons: http://www.aans.org
American College of Surgeons: http://www.facs.org
American Stroke Association: http://www.strokeassociation.org
National Stroke Association: http://www.stroke.org
The Internet Stroke Center: http://www.strokecenter.org
Society for Neuroscience: http://www.sfn.org
American Medical Association: http://www.ama-assn.org
National Institutes for Health: http://www.nih.gov
PubMed Health: http://www.ncbi.nlm.nih.gov/pubmedhealth

CASE STUDY Patient with a Neurologic Problem

Brief Patient History

Mr. P is a 24-year-old man. While he was waterskiing, he was hit by a boat. He was rescued from the water by friends. He was immobilized and transported to the hospital by paramedics called to the scene.

Clinical Assessment

Mr. P is admitted to the emergency department with abrasions and bruising to his head and shoulders. He is having difficulty breathing and is unable to move his extremities. He complains of neck pain, and he has a cervical collar in place. He has urinary and fecal incontinence. He does not have motor, sensory, or deep tendon reflexes from the neck to the feet. He is awake and able to talk.

Diagnostic Procedures

The admission magnetic resonance imaging (MRI) showed an incomplete spinal cord transection. Baseline vital signs include the following: blood pressure of 85/60 mm Hg, heart rate of 48 beats/min (sinus bradycardia), respiratory rate of 8 breaths/min, temperature of 99.3° F, and O_2 saturation of 88%. The Glasgow Coma Scale score was 10.

Medical Diagnosis

Mr. P is diagnosed with an incomplete spinal cord transection and neurogenic shock.

Questions

1. What major outcomes do you expect to achieve for this patient?
2. What problems or risks must be managed to achieve these outcomes?
3. What interventions must be initiated to monitor, prevent, manage, or eliminate the problems and risks identified?
4. What interventions should be initiated to promote optimal functioning, safety, and well-being of the patient?
5. What possible learning needs do you anticipate for this patient?
6. What cultural and age-related factors may have a bearing on the patient's plan of care?

TABLE 18-5 Pharmacologic Management of Neurologic Disorders

MEDICATION	DOSAGE	ACTION	SPECIAL CONSIDERATIONS
Anticonvulsants			
Phenytoin (Dilantin)	Loading dose: 10-20 mg/kg IV Maintenance dose: 100 mg q6-8h IV	Prevents the influx of sodium at the cell membrane	Monitor serum levels closely; therapeutic level is 10-20 mg/L (if hypoalbuminuria, monitor free phenytoin serum levels: therapeutic level of 0.1-0.2 mg/L). Infuse phenytoin no faster than 50 mg/min; administer with normal saline only because it precipitates with other solutions.
Fosphenytoin (Cerebyx)	Loading dose: 15-20 mg/kg IV Maintenance dose: 4-6 mg/kg/24 hr IV	Prevents the influx of sodium at the cell membrane	Monitor serum levels closely; therapeutic level is 10-20 mg/L. Dosage, concentration, and infusion rate of fosphenytoin is expressed as phenytoin sodium equivalents (FE).
Barbiturates			
Phenobarbital	Loading dose: 6-8 mg/kg IV Maintenance dose: 1-3 mg/kg/24 hr IV	Produces central nervous system depression and reduces the spread of an epileptic focus	May depress cardiac and respiratory function. Administer phenobarbital at a rate of 60 mg/min; monitor serum level closely; therapeutic level is 15-40 mcg/mL.
Pentobarbital	Loading dose: 3-10 mg/kg over 30 min Maintenance dose: 0.5-3 mg/kg/hr IV	Induces barbiturate coma	Monitor serum level of pentobarbital closely; therapeutic level for coma is 15-40 mg/L.
Osmotic Diuretics			
Mannitol	1-2 g/kg IV	Treats cerebral edema by pulling fluid from the extravascular space into the intravascular space; requires intact blood–brain barrier	Side effects include hypovolemia and increased serum osmolality. Monitor serum osmolality and notify the physician if >310 mOsm/L. Warm and shake before administering to ensure crystals are dissolved.

Continued

TABLE 18-5 Pharmacologic Management of Neurologic Disorders—cont'd

MEDICATION	DOSAGE	ACTION	SPECIAL CONSIDERATIONS
Calcium Channel Blockers			
Nimodipine (Nimotop)	60 mg q4h NG or PO for 21 days	Decreases cerebral vasospasm	Side effects include hypotension, palpitations, headache, and dizziness. Monitor blood pressure frequently when implementing therapy.
Local Anesthetics			
Lidocaine	50-100 mg IV or 2 mL of 4% solution	Blunts the effects of tracheal stimulation on intracranial pressure	Must be administered not longer than 5 minutes before suctioning.
Thrombolytics			
Tissue-type plasminogen activator (tPA)	0.9 mg/kg total, with 10% of the dose administered as IV bolus over 1 min and 90% of the dose administered as continuous IV infusion over 1 hr	Converts plasminogen to plasmin to dissolve clot	Treatment must start within 4.5 hr of the onset of the symptoms. Do not exceed 90 mg. Do not use anticoagulants during the first 24 hr. Monitor patient for bleeding.

IV, Intravenous; *NG,* nasogastric; *PO,* by mouth.
Data from *Elsevier/Gold Standard.* http://www.mdconsult.com/das/pharm/lookup/340530070-12?type=alldrugs. Accessed May 9, 2014.

REFERENCES

1. Barker E: Altered states of consciousness and sleep. In Barker E, editor: *Neuroscience Nursing: A Spectrum of Care*, ed 3, St. Louis, 2008, Mosby.
2. Hoesch RE, et al: Coma after global ischemic brain injury: pathophysiology and emerging therapies, *Crit Care Clin* 24:25, 2008.
3. Gawryluk JR, et al: Improving the clinical assessment of consciousness with advances in electrophysiological and neuroimaging techniques, *BMC Neurol* 10:11, 2010.
4. Rosenberg RN: Consciousness, coma, and brain death 2009, *JAMA* 301:1172, 2009.
5. Hocker S, Rabinstein AA: Management of the patient with diminished responsiveness, *Neurol Clin* 30:1, 2012.
6. Ropper AH: Coma. In Longo DL, et al, editors: *Harrison's Principles of Internal Medicine*, ed 18, Philadelphia, 2012, McGraw-Hill.
7. Edlow JA, et al: Diagnosis of reversible causes of coma, *Lancet* 2014. [Epub ahead of print].
8. Berger JR: Stupor and coma. In Daroff RB, et al, editors: *Bradley's Neurology in Clinical Practice*, ed 6, Philadelphia, 2012, Elsevier.
9. Boss BJ, Huether SE: Alteration in cognitive systems, cerebral hemodynamics, and motor function. In McCance KL, et al, editors: *Pathophysiology: The Biologic Basis for Disease in Adults and Children*, ed 7, St. Louis, 2014, Mosby.
10. Bruno MA, et al: From unresponsive wakefulness to minimally conscious PLUS and functional locked-in syndromes: recent advances in our understanding of disorders of consciousness, *J Neurol* 258:1373, 2011.
11. Weng Y, Sun S: Therapeutic hypothermia after cardiac arrest in adults: mechanism of neuroprotection, phases of hypothermia, and methods of cooling, *Crit Care Clin* 28:231, 2012.
12. Hessel EA: Therapeutic hypothermia after in-hospital cardiac arrest: A critique, *J Cardiothorac V Anesth* 2014. [Epub ahead of print].
13. Cortese D, et al: Moisture chamber versus lubrication for the prevention of corneal epithelial breakdown, *Am J Crit Care* 4:425, 1995.
14. Go AS, et al: Heart disease and stroke statistics-2014 update: a report from the American Heart Association, *Circulation* 129:E28, 2014.
15. American Association of Neuroscience Nurses: *Guide to the Care of the Hospitalized Patient with Ischemic Stroke: AANN Clinical Practice Guideline Series*, ed 2, Chicago, 2014, The Association.
16. Biller J, et al: Vascular diseases of the nervous system. In Daroff RB, et al, editors: *Bradley's Neurology in Clinical Practice*, ed 6, Philadelphia, 2012, Elsevier.
17. Romano JG, Sacco RL: Progress in secondary stroke prevention, *Ann Neurol* 63:418, 2008.
18. Murphy DR: Current understanding of the relationship between cervical manipulation and stroke: what does it mean for the chiropractic profession?, *Chiropr Osteopat* 18:22, 2010.
19. Amin H, et al: Cardioembolic stroke: Practical considerations for patient risk management, *Postgrad Med* 126:55, 2014.
20. Albers GW, et al: Antithrombotic and thrombolytic therapy for ischemic stroke: American College of Chest Physicians Evidence-Based Clinical Practice Guidelines (9th Edition), *Chest* 141(Suppl 2):e601S, 2012.
21. Boss BJ, Huether SE: Disorders of central and peripheral nervous system and the neuromuscular junction. In McCance KL, Huether SE, editors: *Pathophysiology: The Biologic Basis for Disease in Adults and Children*, ed 7, St. Louis, 2014, Mosby.

22. Seder DB, Mayer SA: Critical care management of subarachnoid hemorrhage and ischemic stroke, *Clin Chest Med* 30:103, 2009.
23. Alvarez V, et al: Acute seizures in acute ischemic stroke: does thrombolysis have a role to play?, *J Neurol* 260:55, 2013.
24. Alexandrov AW: Hyperacute ischemic stroke management: reperfusion and evolving therapies, *Crit Care Nurs Clin N Am* 21:451, 2009.
25. Del Zoppo GJ, et al: Expansion of the time window for treatment of acute ischemic stroke with intravenous tissue plasminogen activator: a science advisory from the American Heart Association/American Stroke Association, *Stroke* 40:2945, 2009.
26. Advisory Working Group on Stroke Center Identification Options of the American Stroke Association: Recommendations for improving the quality of care through stroke centers and systems: an examination of stroke center identification options: multidisciplinary consensus recommendations from the Advisory Working Group on Stroke Center Identification Options of the American Stroke Association, *Stroke* 33:e1, 2002.
27. Bravata DM, et al: Processes of care associated with acute stroke outcomes, *Arch Intern Med* 170:804, 2010.
28. Anderson T: Current and evolving management of subarachnoid hemorrhage, *Crit Care Nurs Clin N Am* 21:529, 2009.
29. Venti M: Subarachnoid and intraventricular hemorrhage, *Front Neurol Neurosci* 30:149, 2012.
30. Pillai P, et al: Management of aneurysms, subarachnoid hemorrhage, and arteriovenous malformations. In Barker E, editor: *Neuroscience Nursing: A Spectrum of Care*, ed 3, St. Louis, 2008, Mosby.
31. Lindsay KW, et al: *Neurology and Neurosurgery Illustrated*, ed 5, London, 2010, Churchill Livingstone.
32. American Association of Neuroscience Nurses: *Care of the Patient with Aneurysmal Subarachnoid Hemorrhage: AANN Clinical Practice Guideline Series*, Chicago, 2009, The Association.
33. Bader MK, Littlejohns LR, editors: *AANN Core Curriculum for Neuroscience Nursing*, ed 5, Glenview, 2010, American Association of Neuroscience Nurses.
34. Benderson JB, et al: Guidelines for the management of aneurysmal sub-arachnoid hemorrhage: a statement for healthcare professionals from a special writing group of the Stroke Council, American Heart Association, *Circulation* 40:994, 2009.
35. Hunt WE, Hess RM: Surgical risks as related to time of intervention in the repair of intracranial aneurysms, *J Neurosurg* 28:14, 1968.
36. Solenski NJ, et al: Medical complications of aneurysmal subarachnoid hemorrhage: a report of the multicenter, cooperative aneurysm study, *Crit Care Med* 23:1007, 1995.
37. Classen J, et al: Effect of acute physiologic derangements on outcome after subarachnoid hemorrhage, *Crit Care Med* 32:832, 2004.
38. Keyrouz SG, Diringer MN: Clinical review: prevention and therapy vasospasm in subarachnoid hemorrhage, *Crit Care* 11:220, 2007.
39. Treggiari MM, et al: Hemodynamic management of subarachnoid hemorrhage, *Neurocrit Care* 15:329, 2011.
40. Rincon F, Mayer SA: Clinical review: critical care management of spontaneous intracerebral hemorrhage, *Crit Care* 12:237, 2008.
41. Hsieh PC, et al: Current updates in perioperative management of intracerebral hemorrhage, *Neurol Clin* 24:745, 2006.
42. Naval NS, Nyquist PA, Carhuapoma JR: Management of spontaneous intracerebral hemorrhage, *Neurol Clin* 26:373, 2008.
43. Zivin JA: Hemorrhagic cerebrovascular disease. In Goldman L, Schafer AI, editors: *Goldman's Cecil Medicine*, ed 24, St. Louis, 2012, Elsevier.
44. Morgenstern LB, et al: American Heart Association Stroke Council and Council on Cardiovascular Nursing: Guidelines for the management of spontaneous intracerebral hemorrhage: A Guideline for Healthcare Professionals from the American Heart Association/American Stroke Association, *Stroke* 41(9):2108, 2010.
45. Yuki N, Hartung HP: Guillain-Barré syndrome, *N Engl J Med* 366:2294, 2012.
46. Van Doorn PA, et al: Clinical features, pathogenesis, and treatment of Guillain-Barré syndrome, *Lancet Neurol* 7:939, 2008.
47. Randall DP: Guillain-Barré syndrome, *Dis Mon* 56:256, 2010.
48. Shah DN: The spectrum of Guillain-Barré syndrome, *Dis Mon* 56:262, 2010.
49. Cortese I, et al: Evidence-based guideline update: plasmapheresis in neurologic disorders: report of the Therapeutics and Technology Assessment Subcommittee of the American Academy of Neurology, *Neurology* 76:294, 2011.
50. Patwa HS, et al: Evidence-based guideline: intravenous immunoglobulin in the treatment of neuromuscular disorders: report of the Therapeutics and Technology Assessment Subcommittee of the American Academy of Neurology, *Neurology* 78:1009, 2012.
51. Mullings KR, et al: Rehabilitation of Guillain-Barré syndrome, *Dis Mon* 56:288, 2010.
52. Ferrara-Hoffman DL, Krizman SJ: Neurosurgery. In Rothrock JC, editor: *Alexander's Care of the Patient in Surgery*, ed 14, St. Louis, 2011, Elsevier.
53. Swearingen B: Update on pituitary surgery, *J Clin Endocrinol Metab* 97:1073, 2012.
54. Yuan W: Managing the patient with transsphenoidal pituitary tumor resection, *J Neurosci Nurs* 45:101, 2013.
55. Seifman MA, et al: Postoperative intracranial haemorrhage: a review, *Neurosurg Rev* 34:393, 2011.
56. Hannon MJ, et al: Clinical review: disorders of water homeostasis in neurosurgical patients, *J Clin Endocrinol Metab* 97:1423, 2012.
57. Ausiello JC, et al: Postoperative assessment of the patient after transsphenoidal pituitary surgery, *Pituitary* 11:391, 2008.
58. Daele JJ, et al: Traumatic, iatrogenic, and spontaneous cerebrospinal fluid (CSF) leak: endoscopic repair, *B-ENT* 7(Suppl 17):47, 2011.
59. Collen JF, et al: Prevention of venous thromboembolism in neurosurgery: a metaanalysis, *Chest* 134:237, 2008.
60. Chibbaro S, Tacconi L: Safety of deep venous thrombosis prophylaxis with low-molecular-weight heparin in brain surgery. Prospective study on 746 patients, *Surg Neurol* 70:117, 2008.
61. Osinbowale O, et al: Venous thromboembolism: a clinical review, *Postgrad Med* 122:54, 2010.
62. Gould MK, et al: Prevention of VTE in nonorthopedic surgical patients: Antithrombotic Therapy and Prevention of Thrombosis, 9th ed. American College of Chest Physicians Evidence-Based Clinical Practice Guidelines, *Chest* 141(Suppl 2):e227S, 2012.

63. Nemergut EC, et al: Pain management after craniotomy, *Best Pract Res Clin Anaesthesiol* 21:557, 2007.
64. Dashti SR, et al: Operative intracranial infection following craniotomy, *Neurosurg Focus* 24(6):E10, 2008.
65. Hang MS, et al: Comparing the effectiveness of polyethylene covers (Gladwrap™) with lanolin (Duratears®) eye ointment to prevent corneal abrasions in critically ill patients: a randomized controlled study, *Internat J Nurs Studies* 45:1565, 2008.
66. Barker E: Intracranial pressure and monitoring. In Barker E, editor: *Neuroscience Nursing: A Spectrum of Care*, ed 3, St. Louis, 2008, Mosby.
67. Eigsti J, Henke K: Anatomy and physiology of neurological compensatory mechanisms, *Dimens Crit Care Nurs* 25:197, 2006.
68. March K, Madden L: Intracranial pressure management. In Littlejohns LR, Bader MK, editors: *AACN-ANNA Protocols for Practice: Monitoring Technologies in Critically Ill Neuroscience Patients*, Sudbury, MA, 2009, Jones & Bartlett.
69. Rangel-Castillo L, Gopinath S, Robertson CS: Management of intracranial hypertension, *Neurol Clin* 26:521, 2008.
70. Latorre JG, Greer DM: Management of acute intracranial hypertension: a review, *Neurologist* 15:193, 2009.
71. Bhatia A, Gupta AK: Neuromonitoring in the intensive care unit. I. Intracranial pressure and cerebral blood flow monitoring, *Intens Care Med* 33:1263, 2007.
72. American Association of Neuroscience Nurses: *Guide to the Care of the Patient with Intracranial Pressure Monitoring: AANN Reference Series for Clinical Practice*, Chicago, 2005, The Association.
73. Rauen CA, et al: Seven evidence-based practice habits: putting some sacred cows out to pasture, *Crit Care Nurse* 28(2):98, 2008.
74. Curley G, Kavanagh BP, Laffey JG: Hypocapnia and the injured brain: more harm than benefit, *Crit Care Med* 38:1348, 2010.
75. Strandvik GF: Hypertonic saline in critical care: a review of the literature and guidelines for use in hypotensive states and raised intracranial pressure, *Anaesthesia* 64:990, 2009.
76. Saiki RL: Current and evolving management of traumatic brain injury, *Crit Care Nurs Clin N Am* 21:549, 2009.
77. Haddad SH, Arabi YM: Critical care management of severe traumatic brain injury in adults, *Scand J Trauma Resusc Emerg Med* 20:12, 75, 2012.
78. Leeper B, Lovasik D: Cerebrospinal drainage systems: external ventricular and lumbar drains. In Littlejohns LR, Bader MK, editors: *AACN-ANNA Protocols for Practice: Monitoring Technologies in Critically Ill Neuroscience Patients*, Sudbury, MA, 2009, Jones & Bartlett.
79. Mortazavi MM, et al: Hypertonic saline for treating raised intracranial pressure: literature review with meta-analysis, *Neurosurg* 116:210, 2012.
80. Cook AM, Weant KA: Pharmacologie strategies for the treatment of elevated intracranial pressure: focus on metabolic suppression, *Adv Emerg Nurs J* 29:309, 2007.
81. Morrison CAM: Brain herniation syndromes, *Crit Care Nurs* 7(5):34, 1987.

CHAPTER 19

Kidney Clinical Assessment and Diagnostic Procedures

Mary E. Lough

Be sure to check out the bonus material, including review questions, on the Evolve website at http://evolve.elsevier.com/Urden/priorities/.

HISTORY

A history begins with a description of the chief complaint, stated in the patient's own words. A description of the chief complaint includes the onset, location, duration, and factors or strategies that lessen or aggravate the problem.[1] A careful history that explores symptoms fully is an essential component of the clinical assessment.

Predisposing factors for acute kidney dysfunction are obtained during the history, including the use of over-the-counter medicines, recent infections requiring antibiotic therapy, antihypertensive medicines, and any diagnostic procedures performed using radiopaque contrast.[2] Nonsteroidal antiinflammatory drugs (e.g., ibuprofen), antibiotics (especially aminoglycosides), antihypertensives (especially medicines that block angiotensin),[3] and iodine-based dyes may cause an acute or chronic decline in kidney function. A history of recent onset of nausea and vomiting or appetite loss caused by taste changes (uremia often causes a metallic taste) may provide clues to the rapid onset of kidney problems.[2] Symptoms such as weight gain of more than 2 pounds per day, sleeping on additional pillows, and sitting in a chair to sleep are signs of fluid accumulation.

PHYSICAL EXAMINATION

Inspection

Nursing priorities for inspection of the patient with kidney dysfunction focus on 1) assessing for bleeding, 2) evaluating volume depletion or overload, and 3) estimating edema.

Assessing for Bleeding

Visual inspection related to the kidneys focuses on the patient's flank and abdomen. Kidney trauma is suspected if a purplish discoloration is present on the flank (Grey-Turner sign) or near the posterior 11th or 12th ribs.[1] Bruising, abdominal distention, and abdominal guarding may also signal kidney trauma or a hematoma around a kidney. Individuals who have experienced a traumatic injury should be carefully assessed for signs of kidney trauma.

Evaluating Volume Depletion or Overload

Fluid volume assessment begins with an inspection of the patient's jugular neck veins (see cardiac assessment section: Box 11-1 and Figures 11-2, 11-3). The supine position facilitates normal jugular venous distention. An absence of distention (flat neck veins) indicates hypovolemia. Assessment continues with the head of the bed elevated 45 to 90 degrees.[1] Fluid overload exists when the neck veins remain distended more than 2 cm above the sternal notch when the bed is at 45 degrees.[4]

Hand vein inspection may be helpful in assessing volume status, and it is performed by observing for venous distention when the hand is held in the dependent position. Venous filling that takes longer than 5 seconds suggests hypovolemia. When the hand is elevated, the distention should disappear within 5 seconds. If distention does not disappear within 5 seconds after the hand is elevated, fluid overload is suspected.

Assessment of skin turgor provides additional data for identifying fluid-related problems. To assess turgor, the skin over the forearm is picked up and released. Normal elasticity and fluid status allow an almost immediate return to shape after the skin is released. In fluid volume deficit, however, the skin remains raised and does not return to its normal position for several seconds. Because of the loss of skin elasticity in older persons, skin turgor assessment is not an accurate fluid assessment for this age group.

Inspection of the oral cavity provides clues to fluid volume status. When a fluid volume deficit exists, the mucous membranes of the mouth become dry. However, mouth breathing and some medicines (e.g., antihistamines) can also dry the mucous membranes temporarily. A more accurate way to assess the oral cavity is to inspect the mouth using a tongue blade. Dryness of the oral cavity is more indicative of fluid volume deficit than are complaints of a dry mouth.[4]

Estimating Edema

Edema is the presence of excess fluid in the interstitial space, and it can be a sign of volume overload. In the presence of volume excess, edema may develop in dependent areas of the

TABLE 19-1 Pitting Edema Scale

RATING	APPROXIMATE EQUIVALENT
+1	2-mm depth
+2	4-mm depth (lasting up to 15 sec)
+3	6-mm depth (lasting up to 60 sec)
+4	8-mm depth (lasting longer than 60 sec)

body, such as the feet and legs of an ambulatory person or the sacrum of an individual confined to bed. However, edema does not always indicate fluid volume overload. A loss of albumin from the vascular space can cause peripheral edema despite hypovolemia or normal fluid states. A critically ill patient may have a low serum albumin level (hypoalbuminemia) because of inadequate nutrition after surgery, a burn, or a head injury and may exhibit edema as a result of the loss of plasma oncotic pressure and not as a result of volume overload. Edema also may signal circulatory difficulties. An individual who is fluid-balanced but who has poor venous return may experience pedal edema after prolonged sitting in a chair with the feet dependent. Similarly, an individual with heart failure may experience edema because the left ventricle is unable to pump blood effectively through the vessels. A key feature that distinguishes edema due to excess volume or hypoalbuminemia from circulatory compromise is that the edema does not reverse with elevation of the extremity.

Edema can be assessed by applying fingertip pressure on the swollen area over a bony prominence, such as the ankles, pretibial areas (shins), and sacrum. If the indentation made by the fingertip does not disappear within 15 seconds, pitting edema exists. Pitting edema indicates increased interstitial volume, and it usually is not evident until significant weight gain has occurred. Edema also may appear in the hands and feet, around the eyes, and in the cheeks. Dependent areas, such as the feet and sacrum, are the areas most likely to demonstrate edema in patients confined to a wheelchair or bed. One way of measuring the extent of edema is by using a subjective scale of 1 to 4, with 1 indicating only minimal pitting and 4 indicating severe pitting (Table 19-1).[1] Other scales for assessing and measuring edema can also be used.

Ausculation

Nursing priorities in auscultation of the patient with kidney dysfunction focus on 1) the heart, 2) blood pressure, and 3) the lungs.

Heart

Auscultation of the heart requires assessing for normal and for extra heart sounds. Fluid overload is often accompanied by a third or fourth heart sound, which is best heard with the bell of the stethoscope.[1] Increased heart rate alone provides little information about fluid volume, but combined with a low blood pressure, it may indicate hypovolemia.

The heart is auscultated for the presence of a pericardial friction rub. A rub can best be heard at the third intercostal space to the left of the sternal border while the individual leans slightly forward.[1] A pericardial friction rub indicates pericarditis, and it may result from uremia in a patient with kidney failure.

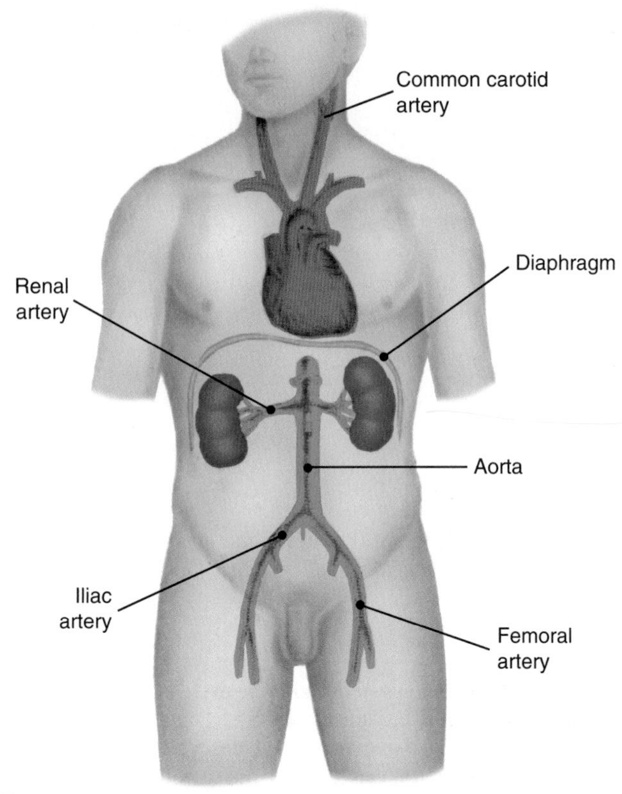

FIG 19-1 Sites for Auscultation of Bruits.

Blood Pressure

In kidney failure the blood pressure is often elevated due to voume overload. Additionally, hypertension is both a cause and a consequence of kidney disease.[5] Hypertension can also occur because of stenosis in a renal artery[6] that decreases flow and activates the renin angiotensin system (see Figure 12-15) with a consequent elevation of blood pressure.

Lungs

Lung assessment is essential in gauging fluid status. Crackles indicate fluid overload. Dyspnea with mild exertion, dyspnea at night that prevents sleeping in a supine position (orthopnea), or dyspnea that awakens the individual from sleep (paroxysmal nocturnal dyspnea) may indicate pooling of fluid in the lungs. Shallow, gasping breaths with periods of apnea reflect severe acid–base imbalances. See Chapter 14 for further information on auscultation of the lungs.

Palpatation

Nursing priorities in percussion of the patient with kidney dysfunction focus on determining the shape and the size of the kidneys.

Although rarely performed in critically ill patients, palpation of the kidneys in stable patients provides information about the kidneys' size and shape. Palpation of the kidneys is achieved through the bimanual capturing approach. Capturing is accomplished by placing one hand posteriorly under the flank of the supine patient with the examiner's fingers pointing to the midline and placing the opposite hand just below the rib cage anteriorly.[1,2] The patient is asked to inhale deeply while pressure is exerted to bring the hands together

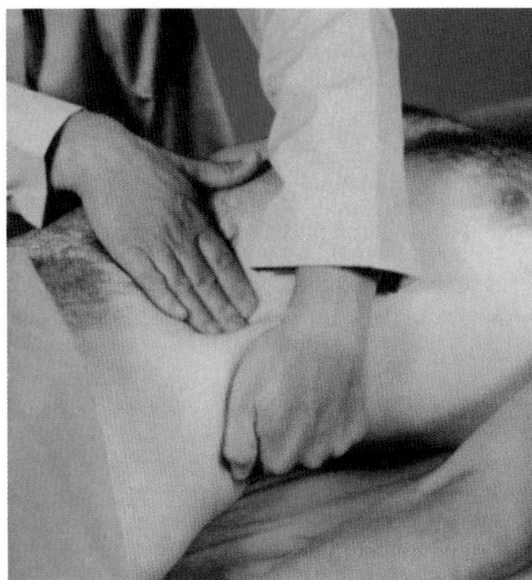

FIG 19-2 Palpation of the Kidney. (From Barkauskas V, et al. *Health & Physical Assessment.* 3rd ed. St. Louis: Mosby; 2002.)

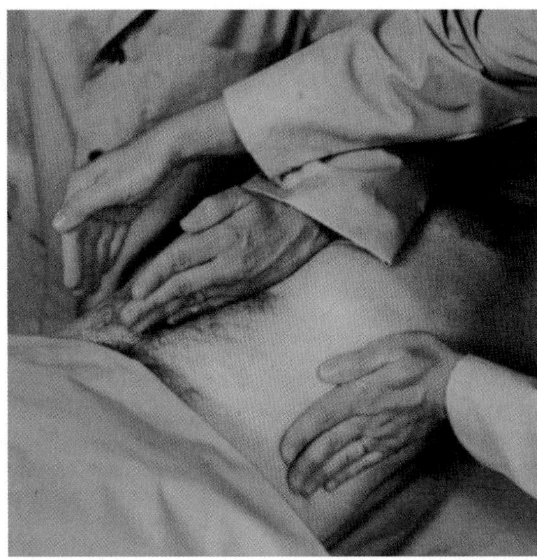

FIG 19-3 Test for the Presence of a Fluid Wave. (From Barkauskas V, et al. *Health & Physical Assessment.* 3rd ed. St. Louis: Mosby; 2002.)

(Figure 19-2). As the patient exhales, the examiner may feel the kidney between the hands. After each kidney is palpated in this manner, the two should be compared for size and shape. Each kidney should be firm and smooth, and the two organs should be of equal size. The examiner is usually unable to palpate a normal left kidney. The right kidney is more easily palpated because of its lower position, caused by downward displacement by the liver. Problems should be suspected if a mass (cancer) or an irregular surface (polycystic kidneys) is palpated, a size difference is detected, or the kidney extends significantly lower than the rib cage on either side.[1]

Percussion

Nursing priorities in percussion of the patient with kidney dysfunction focus on the 1) kidneys and 2) abdomen.

Percussion is performed to detect pain in the area of a kidney or to determine excess accumulation of air, fluid, or solids around the kidneys. Like palpation, percussion of the kidneys is not a routine part of a nursing assessment in critical care.

Kidneys

Percussion of a kidney is performed with the patient in a side-lying or sitting position, with the examiner's hand placed over the costovertebral angle (lower border of the rib cage on the flank).[1] Striking the back of the hand with the opposite fist produces a dull thud, which is normal. Pain may indicate infection (e.g., urinary tract infection that has extended into the kidneys) or injury resulting from trauma.

Abdomen

Observation and percussion of the abdomen may help in assessing fluid status. Percussing the abdomen with the patient in the supine position generally yields a dull sound (solid bowel contents or fluid) or a hollow sound (gaseous bowel).[1]

Ascites, or excess fluid accumulation and distention of the abdominal cavity, is an important observation in determining fluid overload. Differentiating ascites from distortion caused by solid bowel contents is accomplished by producing a fluid wave. A fluid wave is elicited by exerting pressure to the abdominal midline while one hand is placed on the right or left flank.[1] Tapping the opposite flank produces a wave in the accumulated fluid that can be felt under the hands (Figure 19-3). Other signs of ascites include a protuberant, rounded abdomen and abdominal striae.[1]

Individuals with kidney failure may have ascites caused by volume overload, which forces fluid into the abdomen due to increased capillary hydrostatic pressures. However, ascites may or may not represent fluid volume excess. Severe ascites in persons with compromised liver function may result from decreased plasma proteins. The ascites occurs because the increased vascular pressure associated with liver dysfunction forces fluid and plasma proteins from the vascular space into the interstitial space and abdominal cavity. Although the individual may exhibit marked edema, the intravascular space is volume-depleted, and the patient is hypovolemic.

FLUID BALANCE ASSESSMENTS

Nursing priorities for the patient undergoing fluid balance assessment focus on 1) weight monitoring, 2) intake and output management, and **3) hemodynamic monitoring.**

Weight Monitoring

One of the most important assessments of kidney and fluid status is the patient's weight. In the critical care unit, weight is monitored daily. Significant fluctuations in body weight over a 1- to 2-day period indicate fluid gains and losses. Rapid weight gains or losses of more than 2 pounds per day usually indicate fluid rather than nutritional factors. One liter of fluid equals 1 kg or approximately 2.2 pounds.

Whenever possible, the patient is weighed during admission to the critical care unit. It is important to document whether the current weight differs significantly from the weight 1 to 2 weeks before admission to the hospital. The patient is weighed daily for comparison with the previous daily weight. The weight is obtained at the same time each day, with the patient wearing the same amount of clothing and using the same scales. The individual's weight is of critical importance to the dialysis nurse caring for a patient with acute or chronic kidney failure. The differences in weight from day to day are used to calculate the amount of fluid to remove during a dialysis treatment.[7]

Intake and Output Monitoring

Intake and Output Management

Intake and output can be compared with the patient's weight to evaluate fluid gains or losses more accurately. Urinary output plus insensible fluid losses (perspiration, stool, and water vapor from the lungs) can vary by 750 to 2400 mL/day. When intake exceeds output (e.g., excessive intravenous fluid, decreased urine output), a positive fluid balance exists. In impaired kidney function, the positive fluid balance results in fluid volume overload. Conversely, if output exceeds intake (e.g., fever, increased respiration, profuse sweating, vomiting, diarrhea, gastric suction, diuretic therapy), a negative fluid balance exists, and volume deficit results. During a 24-hour period, fever can increase skin and respiratory losses by as much as 75 mL per 1° F increase in temperature.

Adults with *acute kidney injury* (AKI) often exhibit a decrease in urine output or oliguria as urine output declines to less than 0.5 mL/kg/hour. In the early stages of AKI changes may be subtle, with only a slightly decreased urine output that reflects water removal without solute removal. Although urine output is a sensitive indicator, kidney function cannot be accurately determined by urine output alone. Abnormal output of body fluids creates fluid imbalances and causes electrolyte and acid–base disturbances. For example, gastrointestinal suction or loss by diarrhea can result in fluid deficit, sodium and potassium deficits, and metabolic acidosis from excessive loss of bicarbonate. Box 19-1 summarizes important aspects of the fluid status assessment.

In maintaining daily records of intake and output, all gains or losses must be recorded. A standard list of the fluid volume held in various containers (e.g., milk cartons, juice containers) expedites this process. Discussions about the importance of accurate intake and output with the patient and family or friends are necessary and can improve the accuracy of intake and output volume assessment.

Hemodynamic Monitoring

Body fluid status is accurately reflected in measurements of cardiovascular hemodynamics. Measurements such as central venous pressure (CVP), pulmonary artery occlusion pressure (PAOP), cardiac index (CI), and mean arterial pressure (MAP) provide pressure values that have traditionally been used to assess fluid volume status.[8] However, these traditional measures are invasive, and their usefulness in predicting response to a fluid volume challenge has been questioned.[8] The issue of volume responsiveness is of particular importance when the kidneys are not fully fuctional. The use of stroke volume variation (SVV) or pulse pressure variation (PPV) msy be more helpful in assessing fluid requirements in the setting of kidney failure.[8] Other options are to use less invasive devices such as transcutaneous or esophageal Doppler or transcutaneous or esophageal echocardiography and arterial pressure-based systems[8] as described in Table 11-4.

BOX 19-1 Fluid and Electrolyte Assessment

Fluid Status

- Skin turgor
- Mucous membranes
- Intake and output
- Presence of edema or ascites
- Neck and hand vein engorgement
- Lung sounds (crackles)
- Dyspnea
- Central venous pressure (CVP) <2 mm Hg or >12 mm Hg
- Pulmonary artery occlusive pressure (PAOP) <4 mm Hg or >12 mm Hg
- Tachycardia
- Hypertension, hypotension
- Cardiac index (CI) <2.2 L/min/m^2
- S_3, S_4 heart sounds
- Headache
- Blurred vision
- Vertigo on rising
- Papilledema
- Mental changes
- Serum osmolality

Electrolyte and Waste Product Status

- Complete blood cell count (CBC)
- Serum electrolyte levels
- Nitrogen waste products (BUN)
- Electrocardiogram tracings (potassium, calcium, magnesium levels)
- Behavioral and mental changes (sodium, BUN levels)
- Chvostek and Trousseau signs (calcium levels)
- Changes in peripheral sensation (numbness, tremor—sodium, potassium, calcium levels)
- Muscle strength (potassium, BUN)
- Gastrointestinal changes (nausea and vomiting—BUN)
- Itching (calcium, phosphorus, BUN)
- Therapies that can alter electrolyte status (gastrointestinal suction, diuretics, antihypertensives, calcium channel blockers)

LABORATORY ASSESSMENT

Blood Urea Nitrogen

Blood urea nitrogen (BUN), also known as the serum urea, is a byproduct of protein and amino acid metabolism. The normal value for BUN is about 7 to 20 mg/dL, which is increased when kidney function deteriorates. With kidney dysfunction, the BUN is elevated because of a decrease in the glomerular filtration rate (GFR) and resulting decrease in urea excretion. Elevations in the BUN can be correlated with the clinical manifestations of uremia. As the BUN rises, symptoms of uremia become more pronounced.[2] However, a drop in the GFR with an increase in the BUN also may be caused by hypovolemia and dehydration, nephrotoxic drugs, or a sudden hypotensive episode. In these cases, the rise in BUN is caused by a decreased GFR in the presence of normal kidney function. BUN is also increased by changes in protein metabolism that occur with excessive protein intake and catabolism. A catabolic state may occur with chronic poor nutrition, severe infection, surgery, or trauma. The BUN level may be elevated as the result of hematoma resorption, gastrointestinal bleeding, excessive licorice ingestion, or steroid or tetracycline therapy. A decrease in the BUN level may indicate volume overload, liver damage, and inadequate nutrition. Box 19-1 summarizes electrolyte and metabolic waste product assessment.

Serum Creatinine

Creatinine is a by-product of muscle and normal cell metabolism, and it appears in serum in amounts generally proportional to the body muscle mass. Although slightly higher in males than females, the normal serum creatinine level is about 0.5 to 1.3 mg/dL. Creatinine is freely filtered by the glomerulus, easily excreted by the renal tubules, and minimally resorbed or secreted in the tubules.[2] Creatinine levels are fairly constant and are affected by fewer factors than BUN. As a result, the serum creatinine level is a more sensitive and specific indicator of kidney function than BUN. Elevated serum creatinine occurs most often in kidney failure resulting from impaired excretion.

A useful diagnostic parameter in kidney disease is the ratio of serum urea nitrogen to creatinine. The usual ratio of BUN to creatinine is 10 to 1, and a change in the ratio may indicate kidney dysfunction and is often useful in identifying the cause of the acute kidney dysfunction. For example, if BUN and creatinine levels are elevated and maintained at an approximate ratio of 10 to 1, the disorder is intrarenal, or affecting the tubules of the kidneys. If the ratio of BUN to creatinine levels is greater than 10 to 1, the cause is most likely prerenal (e.g., hypovolemia). In prerenal kidney failure, the creatinine is excreted by functioning tubules, but the urea nitrogen is retained because of the poor GFR and hemoconcentration, leading to the increased ratio. In the diagnosis of prerenal failure, the ratio of the two tests is a more useful indicator of kidney function than the separate tests of BUN and creatinine.

Creatinine Clearance (Calculated)

The creatinine clearance measures how well the kidneys remove creatinine in the urine. Because of the relatively constant rate at which creatinine is produced and the nearly complete removal of creatinine by normal kidneys, the ability of the kidneys to remove (clear) creatinine from the blood is an indication of how well the glomeruli and tubules are working. Measuring the creatinine clearance—the amount of creatinine in the excreted urine and the amount of creatinine in the blood over 24 hours—provides a reliable and accurate estimate of glomerular filtration and therefore of kidney function.[2] The normal value for creatinine clearance is 110 to 120 mL/min; values less than 50 mL/min indicate significant kidney dysfunction. The creatinine clearance is most accurate when measured using a 12- or 24-hour urine collection and a concurrent blood sample.

In critical care, creatinine clearance is typically estimated from the serum creatinine level (Box 19-2). As kidney function decreases, creatinine clearance decreases and is useful in monitoring the severity, progression, and recovery of kidney function.[9] The estimated creatinine clearance is widely used to determine changes in medication dosing because so many medications are excreted by the kidneys.

BOX 19-2 Creatinine Clearance Calculations

Measured: 24-Hour Urine*
(Urine creatinine × Volume of urine)/Serum creatinine

Estimated: Adults—Cockcroft-Gault Formula
[(140 − Age) × Body weight (kg)]/[72 × Plasma creatinine (mg/dL)] For women, multiply the result by 0.85.

Estimated: Adults—Modified Modification of Diet in Renal Disease (MDRD) Formula
186 × (Plasma creatinine) − 1.154 × (Age in years) − 0.203
For women, multiply the result by 0.742.
For African Americans, multiply the result by 1.210.†

Estimated: Children

≤10 kg:	0.45 × Height (cm)/Serum creatinine (mg/dL)
>10, <70 kg:	0.55 × Height (cm)/Serum creatinine (mg/dL)
≥70 kg:	[1.55 × Age (yr)] + 0.5 × Height (cm)/Serum creatinine (mg/dL)

*Calculations available from the National Kidney Foundation (www.kidney.org/professionals).
†Both risk factor assessments apply for African American women. The number would be multiplied by both 0.742 (woman) and 1.210 (African American).

Serum Osmolality

The serum osmolality reflects the concentration or dilution of vascular fluid and measures the dissolved particles in the serum. The normal serum osmolality is about 275 to 295 mOsm/L.[4] An elevated osmolality level indicates hemoconcentration or dehydration, and a decreased osmolality level indicates hemodilution or volume overload. When the serum osmolality level increases, antidiuretic hormone (ADH) is released from the posterior pituitary gland and stimulates increased water resorption in the kidney tubules. This expands the vascular space, returns the serum osmolality level to normal, and results in more concentrated urine and an elevated urine osmolality level. The opposite occurs with a decreased serum osmolality level, which inhibits the production of ADH. The decreased ADH results in increased excretion of water in the tubules, producing dilute urine with a low osmolality, and returns the serum osmolality level to normal. Sodium accounts for 85% to 95% of the serum osmolality value; doubling the serum sodium level gives an estimate of the serum osmolality level in healthy individuals. Other particles in the serum can increase the osmolality and need to be considered in individuals with common comorbid conditions. A more precise estimation of serum osmolality can be derived by using the following equation:

$$(\mathrm{Na}^+ \times 2) + (\mathrm{BUN}/3) + (\mathrm{Glucose}/18)$$

The calculated serum osmolality level is a useful tool while awaiting full laboratory results. Measured serum osmolality is a useful parameter in determining fluid balance and fluid replacement therapy for critically ill patients.

Anion Gap (Calculated)

The normal *anion gap* is 8 to 16 mEq/L, a range that has been verified in a healthy population of adults.[10] It is a calculation of the difference between the measurable extracellular plasma cations (sodium and potassium) and the measurable anions (chloride and bicarbonate).[3] The value represents the remaining unmeasurable ions present in the extracellular fluid (phosphates, sulfates, ketones, lactate). In plasma, sodium is the predominant cation, and chloride is the predominant anion. The extracellular potassium concentration in plasma is so small that it is generally ignored, leaving the following equation for calculation of the anion gap:

$$Na^+ - (Cl^- + HCO_3^-)$$

An increased anion gap level reflects overproduction or decreased excretion of acid products and indicates metabolic acidosis; a decreased anion gap indicates metabolic alkalosis.

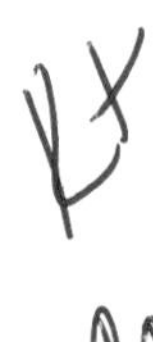

Acute and chronic kidney failure can increase the anion gap because of retention of acids and altered bicarbonate resorption.[11] The anion gap is also increased in diabetic ketoacidosis caused by ketone production. The measurement of the anion gap is a rapid method for identifying acid–base imbalance but cannot be used to pinpoint the source of the acid disturbance specifically.

Hemoglobin and hematocrit. The hemoglobin and hematocrit levels can indicate increases or decreases in intravascular fluid volume.[4]

The hematocrit value is the proportion or concentration of red blood cells (RBCs) in a volume of whole blood and is expressed as a percentage. An increase in the hematocrit value often indicates a fluid volume deficit, which results in hemoconcentration. Conversely, a decreased hematocrit value can indicate fluid volume excess because of the dilutional effect of the extra fluid load. Decreases also can result from anemias, blood loss, liver damage, or hemolytic reactions. In individuals with acute kidney failure, anemia may occur early in the disease.[12]

URINANALYSIS

Analysis of the urine provides excellent information about the patient's kidney function and condition relative to fluids and electrolytes. Specific tests and abnormal indications are presented in Table 19-2. Although often considered routine,

TABLE 19-2 Urinalysis Results

TEST	NORMAL	POSSIBLE CAUSES FOR INCREASED VALUES	POSSIBLE CAUSES FOR DECREASED VALUES
pH	4.5-8.0	Alkalosis	Acidosis Intrarenal AKI
Specific gravity	1.003-1.030*	Volume deficit Glycosuria Proteinuria Prerenal AKI (>1.020)	Volume overload Intrarenal AKI
Osmolality	300-1200 mOsm/kg	Volume deficit Prerenal AKI (urine > serum osmolality)	Volume excess Intrarenal AKI (urine < serum osmolality)
Protein	30-150 mg/24 hr†	Trauma Infection Intrarenal AKI Transient with exercise Glomerulonephritis	
Sodium	40-220 mEq/24 hr	High-sodium diet Intrarenal AKI	Prerenal AKI
Creatinine	1-2 g/24 hr		Intrarenal AKI Chronic kidney failure
Urea	6-17 g/24 hr		Intrarenal AKI Chronic kidney failure
Myoglobin	Absent	Crush injury Rhabdomyolysis	
RBCs	0-5‡	Trauma Intrarenal AKI Infection Strenuous exercise Renal artery thrombus	
WBCs	0-5‡	Infection	
Bacteria	None to few	Infection	
Casts	None to few	RBC: glomerular disease WBC: pyelonephritis Glomerular disease Nephrotic syndrome Epithelial: glomerular disease	

*Adult value; newborn value is slightly lower at 1.001-1.020.
†Higher values usually apply for persons after exercise; lower values apply for persons at rest.
‡Cells per low-power field.
AKI, acute kidney injury; RBCs, red blood cells; WBCs, white blood cells.

TABLE 19-3 Kidney Imaging Tests

TEST	COMMENTS
Kidney-ureter-bladder (KUB) radiograph	Flat-plate x-ray film of the abdomen; determines position, size, and structure of the kidneys, urinary tract, and pelvis; useful for evaluating the presence of calculi and masses; usually followed by additional tests
Intravenous pyelogram (IVP)	Intravenous injection of contrast with radiography; allows visualization of internal kidney tissues
Angiography	Injection of contrast into arterial blood perfusing the kidneys; allows visualization of renal blood flow; may also visualize stenosis, cysts, clots, trauma, and infarctions
Computed tomography (CT)	Radioisotope is administered by intravenous route and absorbed by the kidneys; scintillation photography is then performed in several planes; spiral or helical CT allows rapid imaging; density of the image helps evaluate kidney vessels, perfusion, tumors, cysts, stones/calculi, hemorrhage, necrosis, and trauma.
Ultrasound	High-frequency sound waves are transmitted to the kidneys and urinary tract, and the image is viewed on an oscilloscope; noninvasive; identifies fluid accumulation or obstruction, cysts, stones/calculi, and masses; useful for evaluating kidney before biopsy.
Magnetic resonance imaging (MRI)	A scanner produces three-dimensional images in response to the application of high-energy radiofrequency waves to the tissues; produces clear images; density of the image may indicate trauma, cysts, masses, malformation of the vessels or tubules stones/calculi, and necrosis.

collecting and preserving the urine specimen is important to ensure that results are accurate and not the result of contamination or changes in urine sediment. For most accurate results, the specimen should be collected using sterile technique and examined within 30 minutes of collection.

IMAGING STUDIES

Although laboratory assessment is used most often in diagnosing kidney problems in the critically ill patient, imaging studies can confirm or clarify causes of particular disorders. Imaging assessment includes the use of ultrasound and radiologic techniques. Kidney ultrasound is especially useful in determining the size, shape, and contour of the kidneys, the presence of masses or cysts, and the presence of renal artery stenosis.[6]

Radiologic assessment ranges from basic to more complex (Table 19-3) and provides information about abnormal masses, abnormal fluid collections, obstructions, vascular supply alterations, and other disorders of the kidneys and urinary tract.[2]

Many radiologic studies require the use of contrast, or injection of a radiopaque dye. Because many of the dyes used in radiology are potentially nephrotoxic, they must be used carefully in patients with acute or chronic kidney disease.[13,14] To prevent nephrotoxicity, adequate hydration before and after the test and careful monitoring of both kidney function and fluid volume status are indicated. One recent study used left ventricular end-diastolic pressure (LVEDP) to guide fluid volume administration to preserve kidney function during cardiac catheterization because of the use of contrast dye.[15]

KIDNEY BIOPSY

Kidney biopsy is the definitive tool for diagnosing disease processes of the kidney. Two methods are used: closed biopsy and open biopsy. Percutaneous needle biopsy (closed method) involves inserting a needle through the flank to obtain a specimen of cortical and medullary kidney tissue. An open biopsy is a surgical procedure and is rarely done in critically ill patients. In either case, biopsy is often the last choice for diagnostic assessment in the critically ill patient because of the postprocedural risks of bleeding, hematoma formation, and infection.

REFERENCES

1. Seidel HM, et al: *Mosby's guide to physical examination*, ed 7, St Louis, 2010, Mosby.
2. Schira M, section editor: Assessment of kidney structure and function. In Counts C, editors: *Core ccurriculum for nephrology nursing*, ed 5, Pitman, NJ, 2008, American Nephrology Nurses Association.
3. Wadel HM, Textor SC: The role of the kidney in regulating arterial blood pressure, *Nat Rev Nephrol* 8(10):602, 2012.
4. Parker K: Alterations in fluid, electrolyte, and acid-base balance. In Molzahn A, Butera E, editors: *Contemporary nephrology nursing: principles and practice*, ed 2, Pitman, NJ, 2006, American Nephrology Nurses Association.
5. Tedla FM, Brar A, Browne R, Brown C: Hypertension in chronic kidney disease: navigating the evidence, *Int J Hypertens* 2011:132405, 2011.
6. Weber BR, Dieter RS: Renal artery stenosis: epidemiology and treatment, *Int J Nephrol Renovasc Dis* 7:169–181, 2014.
7. Purcell W, Manias E, Williams A, Walker R: Accurate dry weight assessment: reducing the incidence of hypertension and cardiac disease in patients on hemodialysis, *Nephrol Nurs J* 31(6):631–636, 2004.
8. Davison DL, Patel K, Chawla LS: Hemodynamic monitoring in the critically ill: spanning the range of kidney function, *Am J Kidney Dis* 59(5):715–723, 2012.

9. Israni AK, Kasiske BL: Laboratory assessment of kidney disease: filtration rate, urinalysis, and proteinuria. In Taal MW, et al, editors: *Brenner and Rector's the kidney*, ed 9, Philadelphia, PA, 2011, Elsevier Saunders, pp 868–896.
10. Farwell WR, Taylor EN: Serum anion gap, bicarbonate and biomarkers of inflammation in healthy individuals in a national survey, *CMAJ* 182:137, 2010.
11. Abramowitz MK, Hostetter TH, Melamed ML: The serum anion gap is altered in early kidney disease and associates with mortality, *Kidney Internat* 82:701, 2012.
12. Ramanath V, et al: Anemia and chronic kidney disease: making sense of the recent trials, *Recent Clin Trials* 7:187, 2012.
13. Isaac S: Contrast-induced nephropathy: nursing implications, *Crit Care Nurse* 32:41, 2012.
14. Stacul F, et al: Contrast induced nephropathy: updated ESUR Contrast Media Safety Committee guidelines, *Eur Radiol* 21:2527, 2011.
15. Brar SS, et al: Haemodynamic-guided fluid administration for the prevention of contrast-induced acute kidney injury: the POSEIDON randomised controlled trial, *Lancet* 383(9931):1814, 2014.

Kidney Disorders and Therapeutic Management

Mary E. Lough

Be sure to check out the bonus material, including review questions, on the Evolve website at http://evolve.elsevier.com/Urden/priorities/.

ACUTE KIDNEY INJURY

Acute kidney injury (AKI) is a relatively new term used to describe the spectrum of acute-onset kidney disorders that can range from mild impairment of kidney function through acute kidney failure that requires renal replacement therapy (dialysis).[1,2] Severe AKI is characterized by a sudden decline in glomerular filtration rate (GFR), with subsequent retention of products in the blood that are normally excreted by the kidneys; this disrupts electrolyte balance, acid–base homeostasis, and fluid volume equilibrium. A transition to greater use of the word *kidney* rather than *renal* reflects a trend in the nephrology literature that emphasizes the vulnerability of the kidney during critical illness.[1,2]

Critical Illness and Acute Kidney Injury

Critical care patients with AKI have a longer length of hospital stay, more complications, and higher mortality.[1,2] AKI-associated mortality ranges from 15% to 60%.[2] One of the reasons for poor survival is that critical care patients often have coexisting nonkidney conditions that increase their susceptibility to the development of AKI. High-risk diagnoses include heart failure, shock, respiratory failure, and sepsis. An observational study that examined the incidence and course of severe AKI in 618 patients in six academic medical centers in the United States found that AKI was accompanied by multiorgan failure in most patients, even those who did not require dialysis.[3] In this observational study 64% of patients required dialysis, the in-hospital mortality rate was 37%, and the rate of nonrecovery of kidney function (permanent dialysis) or death was 50%.[3] The mortality rate exceeded 50% when four or more body systems had failed.[3] Other clinical studies report similar findings with equally high mortality.[2] Today the most frequent causes of AKI in the critically ill are associated with sepsis and cardiac surgery.[1]

Typically, a patient is not admitted to the critical care unit with a diagnosis of AKI alone; there is always coexisting hemodynamic, cardiac, pulmonary, or neurologic compromise. Many patients come into the hospital with underlying changes in kidney function, such as an elevated serum creatinine level, although they have no symptoms and are often unaware of their compromised kidney function. The lack of kidney reserve places these patients at increased risk for AKI if complications occur in any other organ systems. As a result, the picture of AKI in the modern critical care unit has changed to encompass patients with kidney injury who also have multisystem dysfunction that complicates their clinical course.

Definitions of Acute Kidney Injury

One of the challenges of estimating the incidence of AKI in the critical care unit has been the wide variation in definitions that have been used. Measurement of kidney function is indirect, and the diagnosis of AKI is predominantly derived from changes in urine output and elevation of serum creatinine level, with the understanding that changes in these values reflect a decline in the GFR.[1,2] Urine output is sometimes a problematic measure to use because diuretics artificially increase the urine output but may not alter the course of kidney failure. The clinical insult may have direct effects on the kidney, such as the inflammation associated with sepsis, which accounts for almost 50% of the AKI seen in critical care units.[1]

RIFLE Criteria

The risk of critically ill patients developing AKI has been classified by a multinational group of nephrologists.[1,2] The classification uses the acronym RIFLE—*r*isk, *i*njury, *f*ailure, *l*oss, and *e*nd-stage kidney disease (ESKD).[2] The *RIFLE* system classifies AKI in three categories of increasing severity (R, I, F) and two outcome criteria (L, E) based on GFR status reflected by the change in urine output or loss of kidney function[2] (Table 20-1). If AKI is superimposed on a kidney that is already compromised, the term *chronic* is added to the RIFLE criteria to denote the cause as acute-on-chronic kidney failure.[2]

Acute Kidney Injury Network Criteria

The *Acute Kidney Injury Network* (AKIN) criteria are listed in Box 20-1. These criteria are similar to those proposed by the RIFLE group, and both groups intend to make the point that in the acutely ill patient, small changes in the serum creatinine level and urine output may signal important declines in the GFR and kidney function. The combined elements of the RIFLE criteria and AKIN criteria are shown in Figure 20-1.[2]

Types of Acute Kidney Injury

Previously, acute renal failure was predominantly classified by the location of the insult relative to the kidney: *prerenal* (before), *intrarenal* (within), and *postrenal* (after) (Box 20-2). This remains a useful way to imagine the relationship between anatomy and functional insults to the kidney, although it is not evident that insults classified in this manner have any impact on outcomes of patients with AKI.

Prerenal Acute Kidney Injury

Any condition that decreases blood flow, blood pressure, or kidney perfusion before arterial blood reaches the renal artery that supplies the kidney may be anatomically described as *prerenal* AKI.[1] When arterial hypoperfusion due to low cardiac output, hemorrhage, vasodilation, thrombosis, or

TABLE 20-1 Rifle Criteria for Acute Kidney Dysfunction

RIFLE	SERUM CREATININE CRITERIA*	URINE OUTPUT CRITERIA
Risk	Serum Cr increased 1.5 times above normal *or* Serum Cr increase ≥0.3 mg/dL	UO <0.5 mL/kg/hr for 6 hr
Injury	Serum Cr increased 2 times above normal	UO <0.5 mL/kg/hr for 12 hr
Failure	Serum Cr increased 3 times above normal *or* Serum Cr ≥4 mg/dL *or* Serum Cr acute rise ≥0.5 mg/dL	UO <0.3 mL/kg/hr for 24 hr *or* anuria for 12 hr (oliguria)
Loss	Persistent AKI = complete loss of kidney function for more than 4 wk	
ESKD	End-stage kidney disease	

AKI, Acute kidney injury; *Cr*, creatinine; *UO*, urine output.
*All serum creatinine references are based on changes from baseline.Data from Kellum JA, et al. Definition and classification of acute kidney injury. *Nephron Clin Pract.* 2008: 109(4):c182.

BOX 20-1 Acute Kidney Injury Network (AKIN) Criteria for the Diagnosis of Acute Kidney Injury

- *Definition:* Acute kidney injury (AKI) is an abrupt (within 48 hours) reduction in kidney function defined as
  - An absolute increase in the serum creatinine level of more than or equal to 0.3 mg/dL (≥26.4 μmol/L)
  - A percentage increase in serum creatinine of more than or equal to 50% (1.5-fold from baseline)
  - A reduction in urine output (documented oliguria of less than 0.5 mL/kg/hr for more than 6 hours)

Explanatory Notes

- *Serum creatinine:* These criteria include an absolute and a percentage change in creatinine to accommodate variations related to age, gender, and body mass index and to reduce the need for a baseline creatinine level, but they do require at least two serum creatinine values within 48 hours.
- *Urine output:* The urine output criterion was included based on the predictive importance of this measure but with the awareness that urine outputs may not be measured routinely in noncritical care unit settings. It is assumed that the diagnosis based on the urine output criterion alone will require exclusion of urinary tract obstructions that reduce urine output or of other easily reversible causes of reduced urine output.
- *Clinical context:* These criteria should be used in the context of the clinical presentation and after adequate fluid resuscitation when applicable. Many acute kidney diseases exist, and some may result in AKI. Because diagnostic criteria are not documented, some cases of AKI may not be diagnosed.
- *Physiologic state:* AKI may be superimposed on or lead to chronic kidney disease.

Data from Mehta RL, et al. for the Acute Kidney Injury Network. Report of an initiative to improve outcomes in acute kidney injury. *Crit Care.* 2007: 11(2):R31.

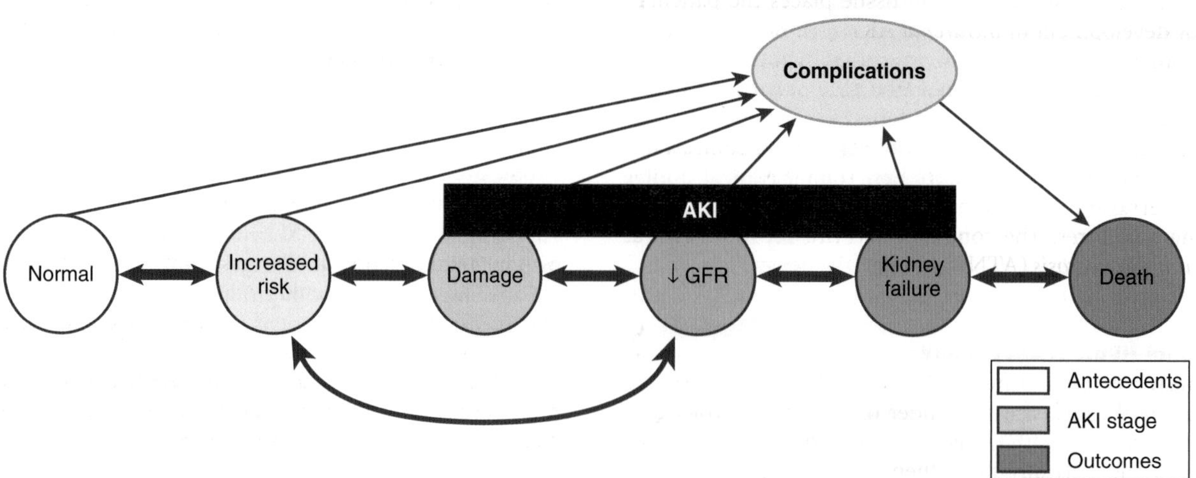

FIG 20-1 Model of the Components of Acute Kidney Injury. (Modified from Acute Kidney Injury Network. AKI Conceptual Model, developed at the Vancouver Summit 2006. http://www.akinet.org.)

BOX 20-2 Acute Kidney Injury

Prerenal Acute Kidney Injury
- Prolonged hypotension (sepsis, vasodilation)
- Prolonged low cardiac output (heart failure, cardiogenic shock)
- Prolonged volume depletion (dehydration, hemorrhage)
- Renovascular thrombosis (thromboemboli)

Intrarenal Acute Kidney Injury
- Kidney ischemia (advanced stage of prerenal acute kidney injury)
- Endogenous toxins (rhabdomyolysis, tumor lysis syndrome)
- Exogenous toxins (radiocontrast dye, nephrotoxic medications)
- Infection (acute glomerulonephritis, interstitial nephritis)

Postrenal Acute Kidney Injury
- Obstruction (urethra, prostate, or bladder)
- Rare as a cause of acute kidney injury in critical care

other cause reduces the blood flow to the kidney, glomerular filtration decreases, and consequently, urine output decreases (see Box 20-2). This is a major reason the critical care nurse monitors the urine output on an hourly basis.[4,5] Initially, in prerenal states, the integrity of the kidney's nephron structure and function may be preserved. If normal perfusion and cardiac output are restored quickly, the kidney will recover and not suffer permanent injury. However, if the prerenal insult is not corrected, the GFR will decline, the blood urea nitrogen (BUN) concentration will rise (prerenal azotemia),[1] and the patient will develop oliguria and be at risk for significant kidney damage. *Oliguria*, defined as urine output less than 400 mL/day, or urine output less than 0.5 mL/kg/hr,[4] with an elevated serum creatinine, is a classic finding in AKI. Prerenal azotemia is associated with a lower mortality than other forms of AKI.[6]

Intrarenal Acute Kidney Injury

Any condition that produces an ischemic or toxic insult directly at parenchymal nephron tissue places the patient at risk for development of *intrarenal* AKI[1] (see Box 20-2). Ischemic damage may be caused by prolonged hypotension or low cardiac output. Toxic injury reaction may occur in response to substances that damage the kidney tubular endothelium, such as some antimicrobial medications and the contrast dye used in radiologic diagnostic studies. The insult may involve the glomeruli and the tubular epithelium and disrupt internal filtering structures. The condition was previously known as *acute tubular necrosis* (ATN), although the newer term of AKI is now more often used.[1]

Postrenal Acute Kidney Injury

Any obstruction that hinders the flow of urine from beyond the kidney through the remainder of the urinary tract may lead to *postrenal* AKI. This is not a common cause of kidney failure in the critically ill.[1] When monitoring of the urine output reveals a sudden decrease in the patient's urine output from the urinary catheter, a blockage may be responsible. Sudden development of *anuria* (urine output less than 100 mL/24 hr) should prompt verification that the urinary catheter is not occluded.

TABLE 20-2 Normal Serum Electrolyte Values

ELECTROLYTE	NORMAL VALUE
Sodium	135-145 mEq/L
Potassium	3.5-4.5 mEq/L
Chloride	98-108 mEq/L
Calcium	8.5-10.5 mg/dL or 4.5-5.8 mEq/L
Phosphorus	2.7-4.5 mg/dL
Magnesium	1.5-2.5 mEq/L
Bicarbonate	24-28 mEq/L

Azotemia

The term *azotemia* is used to describe an acute rise in the BUN level often associated with prerenal AKI.[1,6] *Uremia* is another term used to describe an elevated BUN value.

Assessment and Diagnosis

Laboratory Assessment

After AKI is suspected, the degree of injury is assessed using blood analysis. Most serum levels of electrolytes become increasingly elevated as AKI develops (Table 20-2). Urinalysis values are also altered by AKI although these values are not predictive of outcome in critical illness. Consequently, urinary electrolytes are rarely measured[1] (Table 20-3). Clinical findings associated with AKI are listed in Table 20-4. Normal and abnormal urinalysis findings and reasons for their significance are summarized in Chapter 19.

Acidosis

Acidosis (pH less than 7.35) is one of the trademarks of severe acute kidney injury. Metabolic acidosis occurs as a result of the accumulation of unexcreted waste products. The acid waste products consist of strong negative ions (anions), elevated serum phosphorus levels (hyperphosphatemia), and other normally unmeasured ions (e.g., sulfate, urate, lactate) that decrease the serum pH. A low serum albumin concentration, which often occurs in AKI, has a slight alkalinizing effect, but it is not enough to offset the metabolic acidosis. Even respiratory compensation and mechanical ventilatory support are rarely sufficient to reverse the metabolic acidosis.

Blood Urea Nitrogen

The BUN level is not a reliable indicator of kidney injury as an individual test.[1] The BUN concentration is changed by protein intake, blood in the gastrointestinal tract, and cell catabolism, and it is diluted by fluid administration. A BUN-to-creatinine ratio may be calculated to determine the cause of the AKI (see Table 20-3). The BUN-to-creatinine ratio is most useful in diagnosing prerenal AKI, also described as prerenal azotemia, in which the BUN level is greatly elevated relative to the serum creatinine value.[6]

Serum Creatinine

Creatinine is a byproduct of muscle metabolism that is formed nonenzymatically from creatine in muscles.[7] Creatinine is

TABLE 20-3 Initial Urine Laboratory Analysis Findings in Acute Kidney Injury*

ASSESSMENT	PRERENAL†	INTRARENAL‡	POSTRENAL§
Urine volume	Normal	Oliguria or nonoliguria	Oliguria to anuria
Urine specific gravity	>1.020	1.010	1.000-1.010
Urine osmolality (mOsm/kg)	>350	<300	300-400
Urine sodium (mEq/L)	<20	>30	20-40
FENa (%)	<1%	>2%-3%	1%-3%
BUN/Cr ratio	20:1	Ischemic: 20:1 Toxic: 10:1	10:1
Urine microscopy (sediment)	Normal	Dark granular casts, hyaline casts, kidney epithelial cells	Normal

Anuria, Urine volume less than 100 mL/24 hr; *BUN*, blood urea nitrogen; *Cr*, creatinine; *FENa*, fractional excretion of sodium; *oliguria*, urine volume of 100-400 mL/24 hr; *polyuria*, urine volume excessive over 24 hours.
*Results of urine laboratory tests are valid only in the absence of diuretics.
†Urine in prerenal failure is concentrated, with low sodium.
‡Urine in intrarenal failure shows kidney damage because the nephron cannot concentrate urine or conserve sodium, and evidence of kidney damage (casts) is seen.
§Urine test results in postrenal failure vary because the findings initially depend on the hydration status of the patient rather than the status of the kidney.

TABLE 20-4 Serum Electrolytes in Acute Kidney Failure

ELECTROLYTE DISTURBANCE	SERUM VALUE	CLINICAL FINDINGS
Potassium		
Hypokalemia	<3.5 mEq/L	Muscular weakness Cardiac irregularities on ECG Abdominal distention and flatulence Paresthesia Decreased reflexes Anorexia Dizziness, confusion Increased sensitivity to digitalis
Hyperkalemia	>4.5 mEq/L	Irritability and restlessness Anxiety Nausea and vomiting Abdominal cramps Weakness Numbness and tingling (fingertips and circumoral) Cardiac irregularities on ECG
Sodium		
Hyponatremia	<135 mEq/L	Disorientation Muscle twitching Nausea, vomiting, abdominal cramps Headaches, dizziness Seizures, postural hypotension Cold, clammy skin Decreased skin turgor Tachycardia Oliguria
Hypernatremia	>145 mEq/L	Extreme thirst Dry, sticky mucous membranes Altered mentation Seizures (later stages)

TABLE 20-4 Serum Electrolytes in Acute Kidney Failure—cont'd

ELECTROLYTE DISTURBANCE	SERUM VALUE	CLINICAL FINDINGS
Calcium		
Hypocalcemia	<8.5 mg/dL or <4.5 mEq/L	Irritability Muscular tetany, muscle cramps Decreased cardiac output (decreased contractions) Bleeding (decreased ability to coagulate) Changes on ECG Positive Chvostek or Trousseau signs
Hypercalcemia	>10.5 mg/dL or >5.8 mEq/L	Deep bone pain Excessive thirst Anorexia Lethargy, weakened muscles
Magnesium		
Hypomagnesemia	<1.4 mEq/L	Choroid or athetoid muscle activity Facial tics, spasticity Cardiac dysrhythmias
Hypermagnesemia	>2.5 mEq/L	CNS depression Respiratory depression Lethargy Coma Bradycardia Changes on ECG
Phosphorus		
Hypophosphatemia	<3.0 mg/dL	Hemolytic anemias Depressed white blood cell function Bleeding (decreased platelet aggregation) Nausea, vomiting Anorexia
Hyperphosphatemia	>4.5 mg/dL	Tachycardia Nausea, diarrhea, abdominal cramps Muscle weakness, flaccid paralysis Increased reflexes
Chloride		
Hypochloremia	<98 mEq/L	Hyperirritability Tetany or muscular excitability Slow respirations
Hyperchloremia	>108 mEq/L	Weakness, lethargy Deep, rapid breathing Possible unconsciousness (later stages)
Albumin		
Hypoalbuminemia	<3.8 g/dL	Muscle-wasting Peripheral edema (fluid shift) Decreased resistance to infection Poorly healing wounds

CNS, Central nervous system; *ECG*, electrocardiogram.

completely excreted when kidney function is normal.[7] Consequently, when the kidneys are not functioning normally, the serum creatinine level in the bloodstream rises. Even small increases in serum creatinine represent a significant decrease in GFR.[7] Serum creatinine level is assessed daily to follow the trend of kidney function and to determine whether it is stable, getting better, or getting worse.

Creatinine Clearance

If the patient is making sufficient urine, the urinary creatinine clearance can be measured. A normal urinary creatinine clearance rate is 120 mL/min, but this value decreases with kidney failure. Critical care patients with severe AKI will manifest elevated serum creatinine and may be oliguric. Consequently, the urinary creatinine clearance rate is rarely measured during critical illness.[7] Box 19-2 shows how to calculate the ceatinine clearance using blood sample data (serum creatinine).

Fractional Excretion of Sodium

The fractional excretion of sodium (FENa) in the urine can be measured early in the AKI course to differentiate between prerenal AKI and interrenal AKI (parenchymal). A FENa value below 1% (in the absence of diuretics) suggests prerenal compromise because *resorption* of almost all the filtered sodium is an appropriate response to decreased perfusion to the kidneys. If diuretics are administered, the test is meaningless. A FENa value above 2% implies the kidney cannot concentrate the sodium and that the damage is intrarenal (ATN). FENa values do not have any predictive benefit in critical illness and are rarely measured.[1]

Urinary sodium is measured in milliequivalents per liter (mEq/L). The interpretation of results is similar to the FENa. A urinary sodium concentration less than 10 mEq/L (low) suggests a prerenal condition. A urinary sodium level greater than 40 mEq/L (in the presence of an elevated serum creatinine and the absence of a high sodium load) suggests intrarenal damage has occurred (see Table 20-2). As with other urinalysis tests, the use of diuretics invalidates any results. Because the diuretics alter resorption of water and produce dilute urine, the test result will not reflect actual kidney function.

AT-RISK DISEASE STATES AND ACUTE KIDNEY INJURY

Many patients come into the critical care unit with disease states that predispose them to the development of AKI. Many others already have kidney damage but are unaware of this condition (Figure 20-2).

Underlying Chronic Kidney Disease

The incidence of chronic kidney disease (CKD) in the United States is about 10%, or 1 in 10 people.[8] Clinical practice guidelines for the management of ESKD categorize kidney dysfunction into five stages. Because of the large numbers of adults with kidney dysfunction (diagnosed or not), kidney function must be assessed on all critically ill patients at risk for fluid and electrolyte imbalance. The GFR associated with each stage and the numeric population estimates for each stage of kidney dysfunction are shown in Table 20-5.

Most people in the early stages of kidney disease are unaware of their condition.[9] A national health survey queried individuals about whether they had ever been told by their physician that they had "weak or failing kidneys." The answer to this question was correlated with the individual's GFR and the presence of albuminuria by urine test to stratify them according to the five stages of CKD (see Table 20-5). The results showed that more than one-half of the respondents were unaware that they had kidney dysfunction until they reached stage 5 or ESKD, when they would become dialysis-dependent.[9] In contrast, the prevalence of CKD in individuals between 18 and 39 years of age is only 0.5%.[8] CKD results, categorized by stage of CKD, are listed in Table 20-5.

Older Age and Acute Kidney Injury

Among adults older than 60 years, the prevalence of CKD in the United States is close to 25%.[8] The numbers of older adults with CKD is increasing in tandem with the increase in diabetes and hypertension in the U.S. population.[10]

Heart Failure and Acute Kidney Injury

There is a strong association between kidney failure and heart failure.[11] In studies of critically ill patients with AKI, 54%[3] have acute kidney failure and heart failure. Not all patients with kidney failure and heart failure have the same pathology, and this variation has been recognized. Heart-kidney interactions have been categorized into five subtypes under the term *cardiorenal syndromes*.[12] The purpose of the new classification system is to identify relevant biomarkers, treatments, and future avenues for research.[12]

Several of the risk factors for atherosclerotic cardiovascular disease are also detrimental to the kidney over the long term, notably hypertension and diabetes. Maintenance of a BP below 130/80 mm Hg and a blood glucose within the normal range decrease the risk of both developing CKD and atherosclerotic cardiovascular disease.

Respiratory Failure and Acute Kidney Injury

There is a significant association between respiratory failure and kidney failure. In studies of critically ill patients with kidney failure, over 50% have respiratory failure.[3] Mechanical ventilation can alter kidney function. Positive-pressure ventilation reduces blood flow to the kidney, lowers the GFR, and decreases urine output.[13] These effects are intensified with the addition of positive end-expiratory pressure (PEEP).[13] AKI increases inflammation, causes the lung vasculature to become more permeable, and contributes to the development of acute respiratory distress syndrome (ARDS). Patients with AKI are more likely to require prolonged mechanical ventilatory support.[14,15]

Sepsis and Acute Kidney Injury

Sepsis causes almost 50% of the cases of AKI in the critically ill.[1] Sepsis and septic shock create hemodynamic instability and reduce perfusion to the kidney. Immunologic, toxic, and inflammatory factors may alter the function of the kidney microvasculature and tubular cells. Clinical guidelines for hemodynamic support in sepsis emphasize the need for adequate fluid resuscitation because reversal of hypotension and restoration of hemodynamic stability can often be achieved with fluids alone.[16] Unfortunately, in severely septic patients, inflammation increases vascular permeability, and much of this fluid may move into the third space (interstitial space). If the blood pressure remains low, the use of vasopressors is recommended to raise refractory low blood pressure after volume resuscitation.[16] Vasopressors raise blood pressure and increase systemic vascular resistance (SVR), but they also may raise the vascular resistance within the kidney microvasculature. Other practices aimed at reversing the deleterious effects of sepsis include maintaining the patient's hemoglobin level at 7 to 9 g/dL and blood glucose level below 150 mg/dL, and ensuring optimal hydration.[16]

Trauma and Acute Kidney Injury

Trauma Admissions

Trauma patients have different demographics from those of other critical care populations. They are always emergency admissions, are younger, are more often male, and have fewer coexisting illnesses.[17] A 5-year retrospective study of 9449

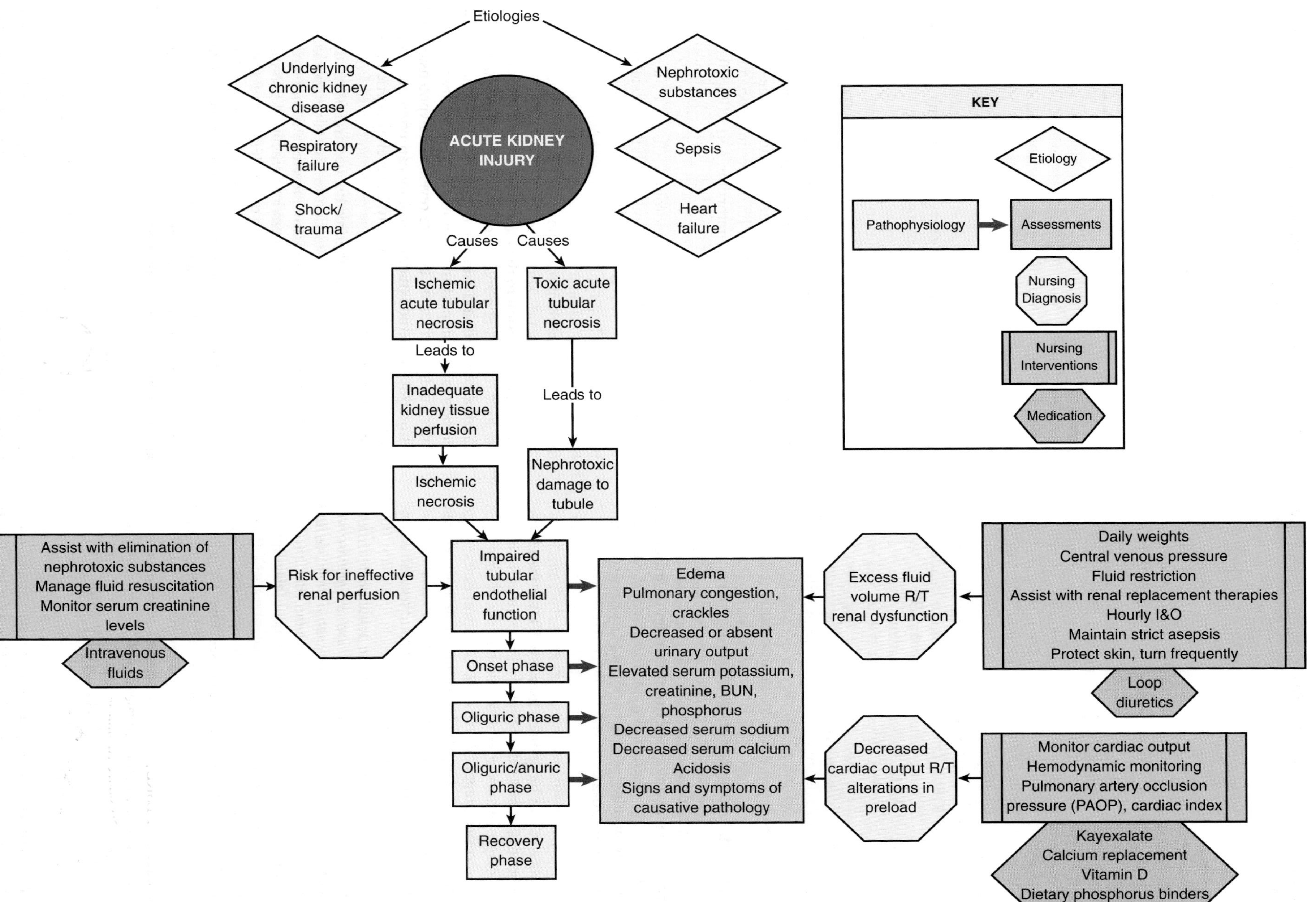

FIG 20-2 Concept Map for Acute Kidney Injury. (Concept map illustration created by Elaine Bishop Kennedy, EdD, RN.)

TABLE 20-5 Decreased Kidney Function by Stage in Adult U.S. Population

STAGE*	POPULATION AFFECTED*	GFR AND DIAGNOSIS*	PERCENTAGE WHO KNOW THEY HAVE KIDNEY DYSFUNCTION (%)†
1	9 million (3.3%)	Normal; persistent albuminuria	40.5
2	5.3 million (3.0%)	60 to 89; persistent albuminuria	29.3
3	7.6 million (4.3%)	30 to 59	22.0
4	400,000 (0.2%)	15 to 29	44.5
5	300,000 (0.2%)	Below 15: ESKD	100

ESKD, End-stage kidney disease; *GFR*, glomerular filtration rate (mL/min/1.73 m^2 of body surface area).
*Data from Coresh J, et al. Prevalence of chronic kidney disease and decreased kidney function in the adult US population: Third National Health and Nutrition Examination Survey. *Am J Kidney Dis.* 2003: 41(1):1.
†Data from Nickolas TL, et al. Awareness of kidney disease in the US population: findings from the National Health and Nutrition Examination Survey (NHANES) 1999 to 2000. *Am J Kidney Dis.* 2004: 44(2):185.

trauma admissions to critical care units in Australia and New Zealand used the RIFLE criteria to determine incidence of AKI in the first 24 hours after admission; 18% of trauma patients developed AKI.[17] However, if patients were older or had preexisting comorbid illnesses, their risk of AKI rose to 35%.[17] Although these AKI numbers are high, they likely underestimate the true incidence because the study did not include patients who developed AKI later than 24 hours after admission to the critical care unit.[17]

Rhabdomyolysis

Trauma patients with major crush injuries have an elevated risk of kidney failure because of the release of creatine and myoglobin from damaged muscle cells, a condition called *rhabdomyolysis*.[18] Myoglobin in large quantities is toxic to the kidney. A major goal of treatment is to prevent rhabdomyolysis-induced AKI. Mortality rate is low, provided adequate crystalloid volume is administered early in the course of treatment.[19] It is important to trend the serum potassium levels. Life-threatening hyperkalemia can occur as cell lysis permits intracellular potassium to be released into the bloodstream.[20]

The level of creatine kinase (CK), a marker of systemic muscle damage, increases in patients with rhabdomyolysis. One trauma service reported that of 2083 critical care trauma admissions, 85% had elevated CK levels, and 10% developed AKI resulting from rhabdomyolysis.[21] A CK level of 5000 units/L was the lowest abnormal value in patients who developed AKI associated with rhabdomyolysis.[21]

Crystalloid volume resuscitation is the primary treatment for preservation of adequate kidney function and prevention of AKI. In many hospitals, the intravenous (IV) fluids are alkalinized by the addition of sodium bicarbonate, and the urine output is increased by IV administration of the diuretic mannitol. A bicarbonate and mannitol regimen is instituted to prevent acidosis and hyperkalemia because both are frequent complications of rhabdomyolysis. Close attention is paid to hourly urine output that can be dark brown or tea-colored,[19] CK levels, serum creatinine levels, serum potassium levels, and any signs of compartment syndrome in all patients admitted with this diagnosis.

Contrast-Induced Nephrotoxic Injury and Acute Kidney Injury

More than 1 million radiologic studies or procedures that involve use of IV radiopaque contrast are performed every year. Approximately 1% of those patients will require dialysis as a result of contrast-induced nephrotoxicity (CIN).[22] Patients at highest risk are those with preexisting CKD, baseline serum creatinine levels more than 1.5 mg/dL, dehydration, diabetes, heart failure, or advanced age (older than 75 years).[23,24] The clinical definition of CIN is an increase in serum creatinine concentration of 0.5 mg/dL or more, or a 25% increase from the patient's baseline within 3 days of contrast medium exposure, without an alternative clinical explanation for development of AKI.[23] The effects of reversible, contrast-induced AKI may not be limited to the immediate hospitalization; it has been linked to increased mortality in the 5-year period after the reversible AKI, compared with similar patients who did not have kidney injury.[25]

Radiopaque Contrast

High–molecular-weight contrast medium is a potential cause of nephrotoxicity. A recommended strategy to prevent CIN involves use of a lower quantity of contrast per study and use of nonionic, low-osmolar or iso-osmolar (iohexol) contrast media that are less nephrotoxic.[23]

Promote Hydration and Avoid Dehydration

The best method of prevention is aggressive hydration with IV normal saline during and after the procedure.[23] After some diagnostic intravascular catheterization procedures, the alert patient is asked to drink several liters of water over a 12-hour period to protect the kidney. Avoiding dehydration is vital.

Medications

The addition of sodium bicarbonate, because of its alkalinizing effect, may confer protection to the vulnerable kidney beyond hydration with normal saline only.[23] Other strategies such as adjunctive use of *N*-acetylcysteine or hemofiltration have shown conflicting results in research studies and are not recommended.[23]

Potentially nephrotoxic medications are also stopped before the procedure. Metformin, a medication that decreases insulin resistance in type 2 diabetes, has been associated with lactic acidosis in rare instances.[23] For patients with elevated serum creatinine, Metformin is stopped the day before any procedure involving contrast and not started again for 48 hours when serum creatinine has returned to baseline.[24]

In summary, the mainstay measures to protect the kidney from contrast-induced AKI are to use the smallest dose of low- or iso-osmolar contrast media possible, provide vigorous fluid volume expansion, stop all nephrotoxic medications, and avoid repeat contrast media injections within 48 hours.

Catheter-Associated Urinary Tract Infection

The majority of critically ill patients have a urinary drainage catheter inserted to record urine output accurately.[26] This is an appropriate use of a urinary catheter. However, because of the risk of catheter-associated urinary tract infection (CAUTI), the catheter should be removed as soon as clinically feasible.[27] Critically ill patients who have a protracted illness have a significant risk of contracting a CAUTI, especially if the catheter is required for several days.[28] Additionally, critically ill patients who have developed a CAUTI have a higher mortality and longer lengths of stay.[29]

The focus on prevention of CAUTI has gained considerable momentum. The Centers for Medicare and Medicaid Services (CMS) will no longer provide reimbursement for hospital-acquired CAUTI because it is considered a preventable infection. The Joint Commission has added prevention of CAUTI as a national patient safety goal.[30] Until recently, only 40% of hospitals routinely collected data on the rates of CAUTI in critical care units.[31,32] Prevention is the best cure, and many critical care units have adopted a "bundle" approach to eliminate CAUTI.[33,34] The key components of CAUTI prevention are listed below:[26]

1. Avoid unnecessary use of urinary catheters.
2. Insert urinary catheters using aseptic technique.
3. Adopt evidence-based standards for maintenance of urinary catheters.
4. Review the need for the urinary catheter daily and remove promptly.

Interventions to prevent CAUTI are listed in Box 20-3.

Hemodynamic Monitoring and Fluid Balance

Hemodynamic monitoring is important for the analysis of fluid volume status in the critically ill patient with AKI.

Hemodynamic Monitoring

Hemodynamic monitoring includes surveillance of fluid volume status, and the monitoring is preferentially minimally invasive or noninvasive.[35]

Daily Weight

A less high-tech method but also important is a daily weight and focused physical assessment. The daily weight, combined with accurate intake and output monitoring, is a powerful indicator of fluid gains or losses over 24 hours. A 1-kg weight gain over 24 hours represents 1000 mL (1 liter) of additional fluid retention.

Physical Assessment

Physical signs and symptoms are used to assess fluid balance. Signs that suggest extracellular fluid (ECF) depletion include thirst, decreased skin turgor, and lethargy. Signs that imply intravascular fluid volume overload include pulmonary congestion, increasing heart failure, and rising blood pressure. The patient with untreated AKI is edematous. Several factors contribute to this state:

1. Fluid retention caused by inadequate urine output
2. Low serum albumin levels create a lower oncotic pressure in the vasculature, and more fluid seeps out into the interstitial spaces to cause peripheral edema.
3. Inflammation associated with AKI or a coexisting nonrenal disease increases vascular permeability, facilitating fluid movement from the vessels into interstitial spaces.

In critical illness, even though there is peripheral edema, and the patient may have gained 8 L of fluid over his or her "dry-weight" baseline, the patient may remain "intravascularly dry" and hemodynamically unstable because the retained fluid is not inside a vascular compartment and cannot contribute to maintenance of hemodynamic stability. The patient with AKI is assessed frequently for pitting edema over bony prominences and in dependent body areas.

Electrolyte Balance

Potassium

Electrolyte levels require frequent observation, especially in the critical phases of AKI when potassium can quickly reach levels of 6.0 mEq/L or higher (see Table 20-4). Specific electrocardiographic changes are associated with hyperkalemia: peaked T waves, a widening of the QRS interval, and, ultimately, ventricular tachycardia or fibrillation.[36] If hyperkalemia is identified, all potassium supplements are stopped. If the patient is producing urine, IV diuretics can be administered. Acute hyperkalemia can be treated temporarily by IV administration of insulin and glucose. An infusion of 50 mL of 50% dextrose accompanied by 10 units of regular insulin forces potassium out of the serum and into the cells.

To treat smaller increases in serum potassium, nonabsorbable potassium-binding resins may be used.[37] The binding resins can be administered orally, through a nasogastric tube, or rectally, to treat hyperkalemia. Cation exchange resins employ either sodium (Kayexalate) or calcium (Sorbisterit, Ca-Resonium, Argamate) and exchange the cation for potassium across the gastrointestinal wall.[38] The potassium is contained in the lower gastrointestinal tract and is eliminated with the stool. Potassium-binding resins and dialysis are the only permanent methods of potassium removal to treat hyperkalemia.

Sodium

Alterations in sodium level are an expected finding in kidney failure (see Table 20-4). Both hypernatremia (elevated serum sodium) and hyponatremia (low serum sodium) are associated with increased mortality with kidney failure;[39] this is unrelated to whether the patient has a diagnosis of heart failure or not.[39]

Calcium and Phosphorus

Serum calcium levels are reduced (hypocalcemia) in kidney failure (see Table 20-4). This reduction results from multiple factors, including hyperphosphatemia. Chronically elevated serum phosphorus levels, above 5.5 mg/dL, are associated with higher mortality rates for patients with kidney failure.[40,41] Calcium and phosphorus levels are regulated by a complex physiologic feedback mechanism involving parathyroid hormone (PTH) and fibroblast growth factor (FGF-23).[42] Normally, PTH helps calcium be resorbed back into the bloodstream at the proximal tubule and distal nephron, and it promotes excretion of phosphorus by the kidney to maintain homeostasis. In kidney failure, this mechanism is nonfunctional; the serum phosphorus level rises, and the serum calcium level falls.[40,41]

BOX 20-3 PATIENT SAFETY ALERT PREVENTION OF CATHETER-ASSOCIATED URINARY TRACT INFECTIONS (CAUTI) QSEN

1. Avoid Unnecessary Use of Indwelling Urinary Catheters

Critical Care Indications

Accurate measurements of urinary output

Prolonged immobilization (e.g., potentially unstable thoracic or lumbar spine, multiple traumatic injuries such as pelvic fractures)

Perioperative Indications

Urologic or genitourinary tract surgery

Prolonged duration of surgery. Catheters inserted for this reason should be removed in the postanesthesia care unit (PACU)

Large-volume infusions or diuretics administered during surgery

Intraoperative monitoring of urinary output

Other Indications

Acute urinary retention or bladder outlet obstruction

Assist in healing of open sacral or perineal wounds in incontinent patients

Improve comfort for end-of-life care if needed

2. Inset Urinary Catheters Using Aseptic Technique

Hand Hygiene

Wash hands thoroughly before or after any patient-care activity.

Use gloves when touching the catheter site or meatus.

Sterile Technique and Sterile Equipment

Use standard supply kits that contain all necessary items:

- Sterile gloves, drape, sponges, antiseptic solution for cleaning the meatus, single-use packet of lubricant jelly for insertion
- Use as small a catheter as possible to minimize urethral trauma.
- Single attempt to insert urinary catheter
- Use new catheter if second attempt at catheterization is required.

3. Adopt Evidence-Based Standards for Maintenance of Urinary Catheters

Maintenance of a Closed Drainage System

Maintain a sterile closed drainage system.

Maintain unobstructed urine flow (avoid dependent loops).

Keep drainage bag below the level of the bladder at all times.

Do not allow drainage bag to touch the floor.

Empty the collection bag regularly, using a separate container for each patient.

Do not allow the drainage spigot to touch the collection container.

Do not break the system to collect a urine sample. Collect from sampling port in the tubing drainage system, disinfecting the port and aspirating using aseptic technique.

Avoid catheter irrigation except in the case of an obstructed catheter; use a bladder ultrasound scan to determine if there is urine in the bladder.

Routine scheduled replacement of catheters is not recommended.

Catheter Securement and Hygiene

Keep urinary catheter secured to prevent catheter movement and urethral friction.

Do not clean periurethral area with antiseptics. Urethral cleansing during a bath is appropriate.

4. Review the Need for the Urinary Catheter Daily and Remove Promptly

Documentation and Monitoring

Document when the catheter was inserted.

Nurses and physicians should review the need for the urinary catheter for every patient every day.

Hospital Strategies to Ensure Early Removal of Urinary Catheters

Ensure clinicians are aware that longer duration of catheter use increases CAUTI risk. This awareness can be reinforced by

- Alerts in computerized ordering systems
- Automatic stops on catheter orders at 24, 48, 72 hours, depending on the clinical situation
- Development of standardized nursing protocols that allow nurses to remove urinary catheters if predetermined criteria are met

Know Your Own CAUTI Data

Each critical care unit should make sure that all nurses and physicians are aware of their unit/patient statistics on CAUTI per 1000 catheter days.

Publicize the strategies used to prevent CAUTI.

Based on data from Gould CV, et al. *Guideline for prevention of catheter associated urinary tract infections 2009.* Centers for Disease Control and Prevention. http://www.cdc.gov/hicpac/pdf/cauti/cautiguideline2009final.pdf. 2009. Accessed October 15, 2014.

Calcium Replacement

Most calcium in the bloodstream is bound to protein. Calcium levels can be measured in two ways: total calcium (tCa) or ionized calcium (iCa). Unfortunately, protein–calcium binding confounds the measurement of accurate calcium levels. In the past, calculations were used to estimate the amounts of protein-bound versus unbound calcium, but these calculations have been shown to produce inaccurate results. The metabolically active, non–protein-bound portion is known as the *ionized calcium* and is the preferred method of measurement.[43] Without adequate levels of serum calcium, a compensatory mechanism "steals" calcium from the bones, making the patient with kidney failure more vulnerable to fractures. Maintaining adequate calcium stores in the body is important and is achieved by administration of calcium supplements and vitamin D.[41]

Dietary–Phosphorus-Binding Medications

A second method used in tandem with calcium supplements to achieve normal calcium levels is to lower the level of phosphorus in the bloodstream.[40] Phosphorus occurs in many foods, especially those with a high protein content or food additives such as dairy products, processed meats, some carbonated drinks, and nuts.[44] After eating these foods, free phosphorus passes from the gastrointestinal tract into the bloodstream and raises the serum level. Medications that bind dietary phosphorus in the gastrointestinal tract are administered orally or by nasogastric tube. The binding agent must be taken at the same time as a meal. After the dietary phosphorus is bound to the binding substance in the bowel, it is eliminated from the intestine with stool.[40] This lowers the serum phosphorus level.

Medical Management

Treatment Goals

Treatment goals for patients with AKI focus on prevention, compensation for the deterioration of kidney function, and regeneration of kidney functional capacity. Key treatment areas include prevention strategies, fluid balance, anemia, medications, and electrolyte imbalance.

Prevention

The only truly effective remedy for AKI is prevention. Effective prevention requires assessment of the patient's risk for AKI. Knowledge of the most frequent causes of AKI in the critically ill is essential if prevention strategies are to be enacted. The critical care team collaborates closely with the clinical pharmacist to avoid medications with nephrotoxic side effects in patients with AKI or CKD.[23] Nonsteroidal anti-inflammatory medications (NSAIDs) for pain relief are avoided in patients with elevated creatinine levels. The use of intravascular contrast dye is preferably delayed until the patient is fully rehydrated.

Fluid Resuscitation

Prerenal failure is caused by decreased perfusion and flow to the kidney. It is often associated with trauma, hemorrhage, hypotension, and major fluid losses. If contrast dye is used, aggressive fluid resuscitation with normal saline (NaCl) is recommended. The objectives of volume replacement are to replace fluid and electrolyte losses and to prevent ongoing loss. Maintenance IV fluid therapy is initiated when oral fluid intake is inadvisable. Maintenance fluids are calculated with consideration for individual body surface area. Adults require approximately 1500 mL/m^2/24 hr; fever, burns, and trauma significantly increase fluid requirements. Other important criteria when calculating fluid volume replacement include baseline metabolism, environmental temperature, and humidity. The rate of replacement depends on cardiopulmonary reserve, adequacy of kidney function, urine output, fluid balance, ongoing loss, and type of fluid replaced.

Crystalloids and Colloids

Crystalloids and colloids refer to two different types of IV fluids used for volume management in critically ill patients. These IV solutions are used on all types of patients, not just those with acute kidney failure. Adequacy of IV fluid replacement depends on strict, ongoing evaluation and frequent adjustment. Frequent monitoring of serum electrolyte levels is required, and strictly regulated intake and output are correlated with daily weight records. In septic shock, hemodynamic readings are frequently undertaken. After a fluid challenge, a merely minimal increase in central venous pressure implies that additional fluid replacement is required. Continued decreases in central venous pressure, pulmonary artery occlusion pressure, and the cardiac index indicate ongoing volume losses.

Which IV fluid to select to resuscitate hemodynamically unstable patients successfully has been a controversial topic in critical care. The debate centers on the differences between crystalloid and colloid solutions.

Crystalloids. Crystalloid solutions, which are balanced salt solutions, are in widespread use for maintenance infusion and replacement therapy. Crystalloid fluids include normal saline solution (0.9 NaCl), half-strength saline solution (0.45 NaCl), and lactated Ringer (LR) solution (Table 20-6). LR solution usually is avoided in patients with kidney failure because it contains potassium. A noncrystalloid solution that may be infused is dextrose (5% or 10%) in water (D_5W, $D_{10}W$).

Colloids. Colloids are solutions containing oncotically active particles that are used to expand intravascular volume to achieve and maintain hemodynamic stability. Albumin (5% and 25%) and hetastarch are colloid solutions (see Table 20-6). Colloids expand intravascular volume, and the effect can last as long as 24 hours, although the use of colloids in critical care volume resuscitation is discouraged because of increased cost without evidence of increased benefit.[45]

The controversy over whether colloids or crystalloid IV fluids are most effective for volume resuscitation appears to have been put to rest by a series of randomized clinical trials and metaanalytic reviews. The SAFE study (saline versus *a*lbumin *f*luid *e*valuation) was a randomized, prospective, double-blind trial that examined whether the selection of resuscitation fluid in the critical care unit affected survival at 28 days.[45] This was a huge study, with almost 7000 critical care patients randomized to two similar groups. One group received 4% albumin, and the other group received 0.9 normal saline (NaCl) for fluid resuscitation.[45] The patients in both groups were similar in terms of organ dysfunction, mechanical ventilator support (64% of patients), and renal replacement therapy (1% of patients). The SAFE results showed that there was no difference in the mortality rate, time in the critical care unit, ventilator days, or renal replacement therapy days.[45] The researchers concluded that albumin and saline should be considered clinically equivalent treatments for intravascular volume expansion in critically ill patients.[45] The exception was for patients with traumatic brain injury (TBI), in which case albumin was associated with a higher mortality rate.[46]

The findings of the SAFE study investigators have been validated by a systematic review of randomized trials of crystalloids versus colloids that reported no difference in mortality rates for the critically ill and injured based on resuscitation fluid.[47] Consequently, colloids are not favored because of their higher cost, and crystalloids are the recommended fluid to use for resuscitation in critical care.

Fluid Restriction

Fluid restriction constitutes a large part of the medical treatment for acute kidney failure. Fluid restriction is used to prevent circulatory overload and the development of interstitial edema when the kidneys cannot remove excess volume. The fluid requirements are calculated on the basis of daily urine volumes and insensible losses. Obtaining daily weight measurements and keeping accurate intake and output records are essential. Patients with kidney failure are

TABLE 20-6 Frequently Used Intravenous Solutions

SOLUTION	ELECTROLYTES	INDICATIONS
Crystalloids*		
Dextrose in water (D_5W), isotonic	None	Maintain volume Replace mild loss Provide minimal calories
Normal saline solution (0.9% NaCl)	Sodium: 154 mEq/L Chloride: 154 mEq/L Osmolality: 308 mEq/L	Maintain volume Replace mild loss Correct mild hyponatremia
Half-strength saline solution (0.45% NaCl)	Sodium: 77 mEq/L Chloride: 77 mEq/L	Free water replacement Correct mild hyponatremia Free water and electrolyte replacement (fluid- and electrolyte-restricted conditions)
Lactated Ringer solution	Sodium: 130 mEq/L Potassium: 4 mEq/L Calcium: 2.7 mEq/L Chloride: 107 mEq/L Lactate: 27 mEq/L pH: 6.5	Fluid and electrolyte replacement (contraindicated for patients with kidney or liver disease or in lactic acidosis)
Colloids		
5% Albumin (Albumisol)	Albumin: 50 g/L Sodium: 130-160 mEq/L Potassium: 1 mEq/L Osmolality: 300 mOsm/L Osmotic pressure: 20 mm Hg pH: 6.4 to 7.4	Volume expansion Moderate protein replacement Achievement of hemodynamic stability in shock states
25% Albumin (salt-poor)	Albumin: 240 g/L Globulins: 10 g/L Sodium: 130-160 mEq/L Osmolality: 1500 mOsm/L pH: 6.4 to 7.4	Concentrated form of albumin sometimes used with diuretics to move fluid from tissues into the vascular space for diuresis
Hetastarch	Sodium: 154 mEq/L Chloride: 154 mEq/L Osmolality: 310 mOsm/L Colloid osmotic pressure: 30-35 mm Hg	Synthetic polymer (6% solution) used for volume expansion Hemodynamic volume replacement after cardiac surgery, burns, sepsis
Low–molecular-weight dextran (LMWD)	Glucose polysaccharide molecules with average molecular weight of 40,000; no electrolytes	Volume expansion and support (contraindicated for patients with bleeding disorders)
High–molecular-weight dextran (HMWD)	Glucose polysaccharide molecules with average molecular weight of 70,000; no electrolytes	Used prophylactically in some cases to prevent platelet aggregation; available in saline and glucose solutions

*For crystalloid solutions that contain electrolytes, specific concentrations of electrolytes and pH vary according to the manufacturer.

usually restricted to 1 L of fluid per 24 hours if the urine output is 500 mL or less. Insensible losses range from 500 to 750 mL/day.

Fluid Removal

Acute kidney failure results in retention of water, solutes, and potential toxins in the circulation, and prompt measures are needed to decrease their levels. Diuretics are used to stimulate the urine output in the early stages of AKI. Renal replacement therapy (hemodialysis or hemofiltration) is another choice, particularly if volume overload exacerbates pulmonary edema or heart failure.

Pharmacologic Management

The first step is to stop all nephrotoxic medications. Second, if medications are eliminated through the kidneys, it is important to decrease the frequency of administration (e.g., from every 6 hours to every 12 or 24 hours) or to decrease the dose and to monitor the concentration by measuring serum medication levels.

Diuretics

Diuretics are used to stimulate urinary output in the fluid-overloaded patient with functioning kidneys. Care must be taken in their use to avoid the creation of secondary electrolyte abnormalities (Table 20-7). Diuretics reduce volume overload and are helpful for symptoms such as pulmonary edema, but they have not been shown to prevent AKI.[48] Diuretics are used in many patient populations other than those with incipient kidney failure.

Loop diuretics. Loop diuretics include furosemide (Lasix), bumetanide (Bumex), and torsemide (Torsemide).[49]

TABLE 20-7 **Pharmacologic Management**

Kidney-Related Medications

MEDICATION	DOSAGE	ACTION	SPECIAL CONSIDERATIONS
Diuretics			
Loop Diuretics			
Furosemide Bumetanide	20-80 mg/day (Lasix) 0.5-2 mg/day (Bumex)	Acts on loop of Henle to inhibit sodium and chloride resorption (natriuresis)	Ototoxicity if administered too rapidly or with other ototoxic medications Monitor intake and output, hydration; monitor for hypotension
Thiazide Diuretics			
Chlorothiazide (Diuril)	500 mg-1 g/day PO/IV	Inhibits sodium, chloride resorption in distal tubule	Enhanced with low-sodium diet Synergistic effect with loop diuretics
Metolazone (Zaroxolyn)	2.5-10 mg/day PO initial dose May increase to 20 mg/day with edema	Inhibits sodium, chloride resorption in distal tubule	Effective to a creatinine clearance of 10 mL/min
Osmotic Diuretics			
Mannitol	0.25-1.0 g/kg IV infusion as a 15%-20% solution over 30-90 min	Increases urine output because of higher plasma osmolality Increases flow of water from tissues, causing increased GFR Increases serum sodium, potassium levels	Often used in head injury to decrease cerebral edema Can be used to promote urinary secretion of toxic substances At low temperatures mannitol may crystallize, use inline 5-micron IV filter with >15% (>15 g/100 mL) solutions
Potassium-Sparing Diuretics			
Spironolactone (Aldactone)	100 mg/day for 5 days PO	Exert effects on collecting duct; retains potassium, increases sodium diuresis	Weak diuretic effect Potassium supplements not required; monitor for hyperkalemia Used as an aldosterone blocker to treat heart failure
Vaptans			
Conivaptan (Vaprisol)	Loading dose: 20 mg IV as 30 min infusion Continuous IV infusion: 20 mg over 24 hours After first day, can be increased to 40 mg/24 hours Maximum infusion is 4 days	Blocks V2 aquaporin channels in collecting tubules	Used only in hyponatremia with hypervolemia Monitor volume status and serum sodium frequently

BP, Blood pressure; *ECG*, electrocardiogram; *GFR*, glomerular filtration rate; *GI*, gastrointestinal; *IV*, intravenous; *PO*, by mouth.

Furosemide is the most frequently used diuretic in critical care patients. It may be administered orally, as an IV bolus, or as a continuous IV infusion. Electrolytic abnormalities are frequently encountered, and close monitoring of serum potassium, magnesium, and sodium is essential. Loop diuretics block the Na-K-2Cl transporter in the nephron on ascending limb of the loop of Henle, where most sodium is reabsorbed (Figure 20-3). This diuresis is also a natriuresis as sodium is excreted in the urine. Diuretic resistance can develop over time in patients with chronic heart failure or kidney failure who were taking loop diuretics at home before they were admitted to the hospital.[50] Their higher diuretic medication dosages are a reflection of diuretic resistance.[50]

Thiazide diuretics. Diuretics from different classes may be prescribed in combination. A thiazide diuretic such as chlorothiazide (Diuril) or metolazone (Zaroxolyn) may be administered and followed by a loop diuretic to take advantage of the fact that these medications work on different parts of the nephron[51] (see Figure 20-3). Creatinine clearance impacts the efficacy of thiazide diuretics. Metolazone is a more effective diuretic in kidney failure when the creatinine clearance is below 30 mL/min. A normal creatinine clearance is 120 mL/min (see Table 20-7). Sometimes a thiazide diuretic is added to a loop diuretic to compensate for the development of loop diuretic resistance.[50]

Osmotic diuretics. Osmotic diuretics, such as mannitol, are prescribed to increase urine output and decrease fluid overload. It is important to use an inline 5-micron filter when administering this IV medication. Mannitol is frequently administered for patients with brain injury and increased

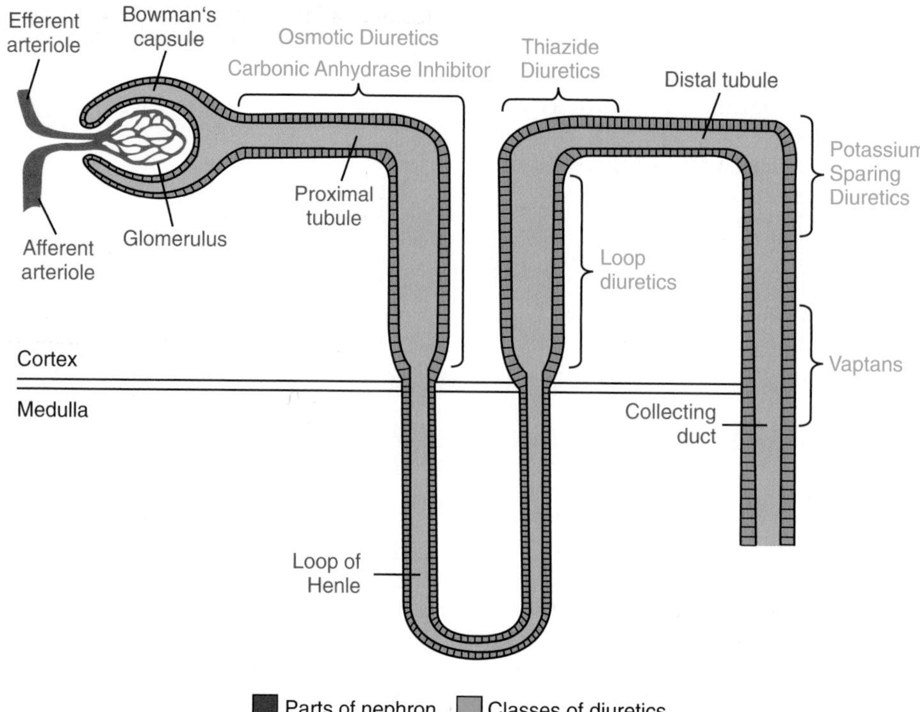

FIG 20-3 Pharmacologic Site of Action of Diuretics in the Nephron.

intracranial pressure (ICP). More information on the use of mannitol in the neuroscience population can be found in Chapter 24. Mannitol is filtered by the glomerulus, not absorbed by the nephron, and works in the proximal tubule and the descending section of the loop of Henle via aquaporin water channels[49] (see Figure 20-3).

Carbonic anhydrase inhibitor diuretics. Only one carbonic anhydrase inhibitor acts as a diuretic, and it is used in very specific clinical circumstances. Acetazolamide (Diamox) acts on the proximal tubule where it inhibits the carbonic anhydrase enzyme allowing more bicarbonate (HCO_3^-) to be released into the filtrate resulting in an alkaline diuresis (see Figure 20-3). Acetazolamide is administered to treat the metabolic alkalosis that sometimes occurs following aggressive diuresis with loop diuretics.[52] Acid–base balance and serum bicarbonate levels are frequently monitored when acetazolamide is used to treat metabolic alkalosis (see Table 20-7).

Potassium sparing diuretics. Spironolactone (Aldactone) is a "potassium sparing" diuretic. Spironolactone inhibits the aldosterone mineralocorticoid receptor in the late distal tubule and collecting duct of the kidneys causing potassium to be retained and sodium to be excreted (see Figure 20-3). At high dosages it has a diuretic action, although that is rarely the rationale behind its use today. Spironolactone is most often administered as an aldosterone antagonist in the management of heart failure.

Vaptans. A new class of medications collectively described as vaptans inhibit the effect of antidiuretic hormone (vasopressin) on the V2 aquaporin channels in the collecting ducts of the kidney (see Figure 20-3). Blockage of the aquaporin channels renders the collecting ducts impermeable, resulting in solute-free water excretion or aquadiuresis.[53] Vaptans are used to correct symptomatic hypervolemic hyponatremic (dilutional) states. The clinical intent is to eliminate water and retain sodium. These medications must not be administered for hypovolemic hyponatremia or anuria. Conditions that can cause dilutional hyponatremia include Syndrome of Inappropriate Antidiuretic Hormone Secretion (SIADH) described in Chapter 23, liver cirrhosis with ascites, and heart failure. Only two vaptans are FDA-approved in the United States. Conivaptan (Vaprisol), which is administered IV, is approved for short-term use in the hospital only (see Table 20-7). Tolvaptan (Samsca) is only available as an oral medication.[53]

Dopamine

Low-dose dopamine (2 to 3 mcg/kg/min), previously known as renal-dose dopamine, is frequently infused to stimulate blood flow to the kidney. Dopamine is effective in increasing urine output in the short term, but tolerance of the dopamine renal receptor to the medication is theorized to develop in the critically ill patients who are most at risk for AKI. Renal-dose dopamine does not prevent onset of AKI, decrease the need for dialysis, or reduce mortality.[1] At this point, the support for routine use of low-dose dopamine for the prevention of AKI remains anecdotal only, although low-dose dopamine infusions may have other therapeutic uses, such as increasing urine output, in combination with furosemide, in heart failure patients.[54]

Acetylcysteine

N-Acetylcysteine (Mucomyst, Mucosil) is an *N*-acetyl derivative of the amino acid l-cysteine. It has been used for many years as a mucolytic agent to assist with expectoration of thick pulmonary secretions. It is also frequently prescribed for patients with mildly elevated serum creatinine levels before a radiologic study using contrast dye.[24] In research trials, the addition of *N*-acetylcysteine to normal saline hydration did not reduce the incidence of contrast-induced AKI.[23]

Dietary-Phosphorus Binders

Many patients with kidney failure are prescribed a dietary-phosphorus-binding medication (see earlier section on Dietary–Phosphorus-Binding Medications).[40,41] Many dietary-phosphorus binders are available, and some important issues concern all of them. The dietary-phosphorus binder must be taken at the time of the meal. If it is taken 2 hours later, it will increase only the level of the binding substance (e.g., calcium) in the bloodstream and will not lower the serum phosphorus level. Related issues such as the quantity of phosphorus in the diet should be discussed with a clinical nutritionist (dietitian).

Nutrition

Diet or nutritional supplementation for the patient with AKI in the critical care unit is designed to account for the diminished excretory capacity of the kidney. The recommended energy intake is between 20 and 30 kilocalories/kg per day, with 1.2 to 1.5 grams/kg of protein per day to control azotemia (increased BUN level).[55] Oral nutrition is preferred, and if the patient cannot eat, enteral nutrition is recommended over parenteral (intravenous) nutrition.[56] Fluids are limited, and monitoring of blood glucose levels is recommended. The electrolytes potassium, sodium, and phosphorus are strictly limited.

Nursing Management

Nursing management with AKI patients involves a variety of nursing diagnoses (Box 20-4). "Prevention is the best cure" is an old saying that captures the role of the critical care nurse, who evaluates all patients for level of kidney function, risk of infection, fluid imbalance, electrolyte disturbances, anemia, readiness to learn, and need for education.

Risk Factors for Acute Kidney Injury

Some individuals are at increased risk for AKI as a complication during hospitalization, and the alert critical care nurse recognizes potential risk factors and acts as a patient advocate. Patients at risk include older persons because their GFR may be decreased, dehydrated patients with kidney hypoperfusion, patients with increased creatinine levels before their hospitalization, and patients undergoing a radiologic procedure involving contrast dye.

Infectious Complications

The critical care patient with infectious complications is at risk for AKI. Signs of infection such as an increased white blood cell (WBC) count, redness at a wound or IV line site, or increased temperature are always a cause for concern. A urinary catheter is inserted to facilitate accurate urine measurement and patient comfort. However, any indwelling catheter is a potential source for infection. When the patient no longer makes large quantities of urine and is hemodynamically stable, the catheter must be removed promptly. If the patient cannot void urine spontaneously, a scheduled intermittent urinary catheterization is performed to minimize the risk of infection from an indwelling catheter and drainage system. This method allows the patient's bladder to be emptied, but the catheter does not remain in place.

Fluid Balance

Intravascular fluid balance is often assessed on an hourly basis for the critically ill patient who has hemodynamic lines inserted. Hemodynamic values (heart rate, blood pressure, central venous pressure, pulmonary artery occlusion pressure, cardiac output, and cardiac index) and daily weight measurements are correlated with the intake and output. Urine output is measured hourly by means of a urinary catheter and drainage bag throughout all phases of AKI, particularly in response to diuretics. Any fluid removed with dialysis is included in the daily fluid balance. Recognition of the clinical signs and symptoms of fluid overload is important. Excess fluid moves from the vascular system into the peripheral tissues (dependent edema), abdomen (ascites), and lungs (crackles, pulmonary edema, and pulmonary effusions),, around the heart (pericardial effusions), and into the brain (increased intracranial swelling).

Electrolyte Imbalance

Hyperkalemia, hypocalcemia, hyponatremia, hyperphosphatemia, and acid–base imbalances occur during AKI (see Table 20-4). Clinical manifestations of these electrolyte imbalances must be prevented and their associated side effects controlled. The more likely imbalances are hyperkalemia and hypocalcemia, which can result in life-threatening cardiac dysrhythmias.[36] Dilutional hyponatremia may develop as fluid overload worsens in the patient with oliguria. Monitoring the serum sodium level is important to prevent this complication. Hyperphosphatemia results in severe pruritus. Nursing care is directed at soothing the itching by performing frequent skin care with emollients, discouraging scratching, and administering phosphate-binding medications. The acid–base imbalances that occur with AKI are monitored by arterial blood gas (ABG) analyses. The goal of treatment is to maintain the pH within the normal range.

Preventing Anemia

Anemia is an expected side effect of kidney failure that occurs because the kidney no longer produces the hormone *erythropoietin*.[57] As a result, the bone marrow is not stimulated to produce erythrocytes, also known as red blood cells (RBCs). Additionally, the normal erythrocyte survival of 80 to 120

BOX 20-4 NURSING DIAGNOSES ACUTE KIDNEY INJURY

- Excess Fluid Volume related to renal dysfunction, p. 590
- Risk for Ineffective Renal Perfusion, p. 606
- Anxiety related to threat to biologic, psychological, or social integrity, p. 576
- Decreased Cardiac Output related to alterations in preload, p. 579
- Risk for Infection, p. 607
- Disturbed Body Image related to functional dependence on life-sustaining technology, p. 587
- Ineffective Coping related to situational crisis and personal vulnerability, p. 599
- Disturbed Sleep Pattern related to fragmented sleep, p. 587
- Deficient Knowledge related to lack of previous exposure to information, p. 585 (see Box 20-5, Patient Education for Acute Kidney Injury)

days is decreased, in CKD patients on dialysis, to 70 to 80 days increasing their risk for anemia.[57] Care is taken to prevent blood loss in patients with AKI, and blood withdrawal is minimized as much as possible. Irritation of the gastrointestinal tract from metabolic waste accumulation is expected, and stress ulcer prophylaxis must be prescribed. Gastrointestinal bleeding remains a possibility. Stool, nasogastric tube drainage, and emesis are routinely tested for occult blood.

Erythropoiesis-stimulating medications. Anemia associated with CKD may be treated pharmacologically by the administration of recombinant human erythropoietin. Three medications are FDA-approved for treatment of CKD-associated anemia in the United States: epoetin alfa (Procrit, Epogen), darbepoetin alfa (Aranesp), and methoxy polyethylene glycol-epoetin beta (Mircera).[57] These agents stimulate erythrocyte production by the bone marrow.[57] Adjunctive treatments include administration of iron supplements, vitamin B_{12}, vitamin B_6, and folate. With symptomatic anemia, RBC transfusion may be required.[57,58]

Patient Education

Accurate and uncomplicated information must be provided to the patient and family about AKI, including its prognosis, treatment, and possible complications.[9] Education of the patient can be challenging because elevations of BUN and creatinine levels can negatively affect the level of consciousness. Sleep-rest disorders and emotional upset often occur as complications of AKI and can disrupt short-term memory. Encouraging the patient and family to voice concerns, frustrations, or fears and allowing the patient to control some aspects of the acute care environment and treatment also are essential (Box 20-5).

BOX 20-5 PATIENT EDUCATION PRIORITIES: ACUTE KIDNEY INJURY

- Explain the pathophysiology.
  - Severe acute kidney injury (AKI) is a sudden decline in kidney function that causes an acute buildup of toxins in the blood.
- Explain the cause.
  - Prerenal (before the kidney)
  - Intrarenal (within the kidney)
  - Postrenal (after the kidney)
- Identify predisposing factors; explain the level of kidney function after the acute phase is over.
- Explain diet and fluid restrictions.
- Demonstrate how to check blood pressure, pulse, respirations, and weight.
- Discuss personal hygiene and how to avoid infections.
- Emphasize need for exercise and rest.
- Describe medications and adverse effects.
- Explain need for ongoing follow-up with health care professional.
- Explain purpose of dialysis and importance of regular treatments.

RENAL REPLACEMENT THERAPY: DIALYSIS

Two types of renal replacement therapy are available for the treatment of AKI. They are intermittent hemodialysis (IHD) therapy and continuous renal replacement therapy (CRRT).

Hemodialysis

Hemodialysis roughly translates as "separating from the blood." Indications and contraindications for hemodialysis are listed in Box 20-6. As a treatment, hemodialysis separates and removes from the blood the excess electrolytes, fluids, and toxins by means of a hemodialyzer (Figure 20-4). Hemodialysis is efficient in removing solutes. Because levels of electrolytes, toxins, and fluids increase between treatments, hemodialysis occurs on a regular basis. Traditional hemodialysis treatments last for 3 to 4 hours. A newer option is the use of *Sustained Low-Efficiency Dialysis* (SLED) that is run daily for 8 hours or 12 hours. Sometimes in critical illness this mode is run continuously (C-SLED). In the acute phase of kidney failure, hemodialysis is performed daily. The dialysis frequency gradually decreases to three times per week should the patient's condition progress to chronic kidney failure.

Hemodialyzer

Hemodialysis works by circulating blood outside the body through synthetic tubing to a dialyzer, which consists of hollow-fiber tubes. The dialyzer is sometimes described as an artificial kidney (Figure 20-5). While the blood flows through the membranes, which are semipermeable, a fluid (dialysate bath) bathes the membranes and, through osmosis and diffusion, performs exchanges of fluid, electrolytes, and toxins from the blood to the bath, where toxins and dialysate then pass out of the artificial kidney. The blood and the dialysate bath are shunted in opposite directions (countercurrent flow) through the dialyzer to match the osmotic and chemical gradients at the most efficient level for effective dialysis.

BOX 20-6 Indications and Contraindications for Hemodialysis

Indications
- Blood urea nitrogen (BUN) level exceeds 90 mg/dL
- Serum creatinine level of 9 mg/dL
- Hyperkalemia
- Medication toxicity
- Intravascular and extravascular fluid overload
- Metabolic acidosis
- Symptoms of uremia
  - Pericarditis
  - Gastrointestinal bleeding
- Changes in mentation
- Contraindications to other forms of dialysis

Contraindications
- Hemodynamic instability
- Inability to anticoagulate
- Lack of access to circulation

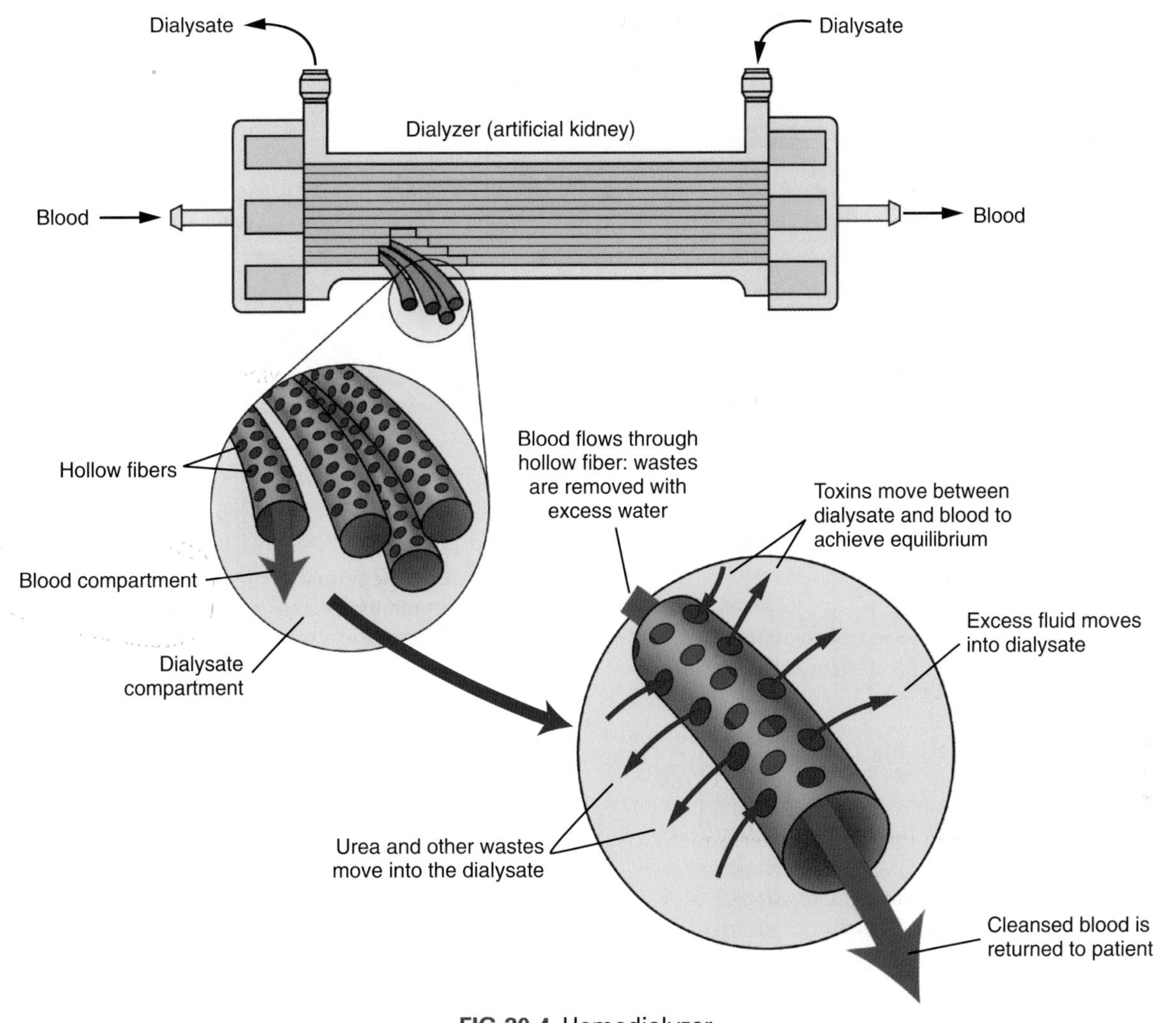
Dialysate
Dialysate
Dialyzer (artificial kidney)
Blood
Blood
Hollow fibers
Blood flows through hollow fiber: wastes are removed with excess water
Toxins move between dialysate and blood to achieve equilibrium
Blood compartment
Excess fluid moves into dialysate
Dialysate compartment
Urea and other wastes move into the dialysate
Cleansed blood is returned to patient

FIG 20-4 Hemodialyzer.

Ultrafiltration

To remove fluid, a positive hydrostatic pressure is applied to the blood, and a negative hydrostatic pressure is applied to the dialysate bath. The two forces together, called *transmembrane pressure*, pull and squeeze the excess fluid from the blood. The difference between the two values, expressed in millimeters of mercury (mm Hg), represents the transmembrane pressure and results in fluid extraction, known as *ultrafiltration*, from the vascular space.

Anticoagulation

Heparin or sodium citrate is added to the system just before the blood enters the dialyzer to anticoagulate the blood within the dialysis tubing.[59] Without an anticoagulant, the blood clots because its passage through the foreign tubular substances of the dialysis machine activates the clotting mechanism. Heparin can be administered by bolus injection or intermittent infusion. It has a short half-life, and its effects subside within 2 to 4 hours. If necessary, the effects of heparin are easily reversed with the antidote protamine sulfate. When there is concern about the development of heparin-induced thrombocytopenia (HIT), alternative anticoagulants can be used. Sodium citrate can be infused as an anticoagulant by intermittent bolus or continuous infusion.

Vascular Access

Hemodialysis requires access to the bloodstream. Various types of temporary and permanent devices are in clinical use. It is important for patient safety to be able to recognize these different vascular access devices and to care for them properly. The following section discusses temporary vascular access catheters used in the acute care hospital environment and permanent methods used for long-term hemodialysis.

Temporary vascular access. Subclavian and femoral veins are catheterized when short-term access is required or when a graft or fistula vascular access is nonfunctional in a patient requiring immediate hemodialysis. Subclavian and femoral catheters are routinely inserted at the bedside. Most temporary catheters are venous lines only. Blood flows out toward the dialyzer and flows back to the patient through the same catheterized vein. A dual-lumen venous catheter is most commonly used. It has a central partition running the length of the catheter. The outflow catheter section pulls the blood flow through openings that are proximal to the inflow openings on the opposite side (Figure 20-6). This design helps prevent dialyzing the same blood just returned to the area (recirculation), which would severely reduce the procedure's efficiency. A silicone rubber, dual-lumen catheter with a

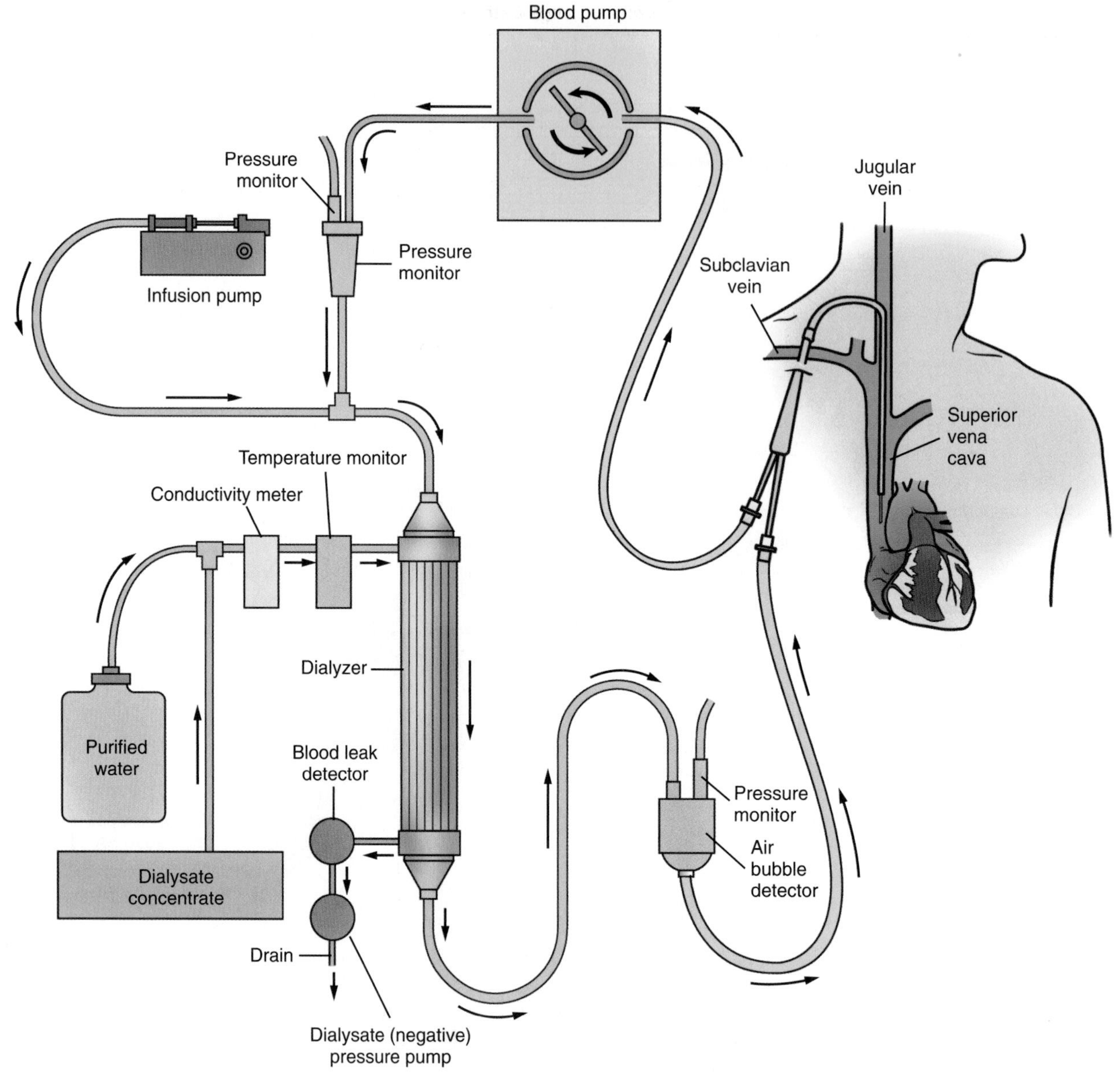

FIG 20-5 Components of a Hemodialysis System.

polyester cuff designed to decrease catheter-related infections is also available.

Permanent vascular access. The common denominator in permanent vascular access devices is a conduit connection between the arterial circulation and the venous circulation.

Arteriovenous fistula. The arteriovenous fistula is created by surgically exposing a peripheral artery and vein, creating a side-by-side opening in the artery and the vein to join the two vessels together. The high arterial flow creates a swelling of the vein, or a pseudoaneurysm, at which point (when healed) a large-bore needle can be inserted to obtain arterial outflow to the dialyzer. Inflow is accomplished through a second large-bore needle inserted into a peripheral vein distal to the fistula (Figure 20-7A). Fistulas are the preferred mode of access because of the durability of blood vessels, relatively few complications, and less need for revision compared with other access methods. An initial disadvantage of a fistula concerns the time required for development of sufficient arterial flow to enlarge the new access. The minimum reported length of time before a fistula can be cannulated for dialysis is 14 days, but the time lag for many patients can be longer. Ideally, the fistula should be established 6 months to ensure it is usable for dialysis when required.[60]

In caring for a patient with a fistula, there are some important nursing priorities to ensure the ongoing viability of the vascular access and safety of the limb (Table 20-8). The critical care nurse frequently assesses the quality of blood flow through the fistula. A patent fistula has a thrill when palpated gently with the fingers and has a bruit if auscultated with a stethoscope. The extremity should be pink and warm to the touch. No blood pressure measurements, IV infusions, or laboratory phlebotomy procedures are performed on the arm with the fistula.

Arteriovenous grafts. Arteriovenous grafts connect a vein and artery to allow vascular access for dialysis in chronic kidney failure.[61] The graft is a tube made of synthetic material,

Double Lumen Catheter

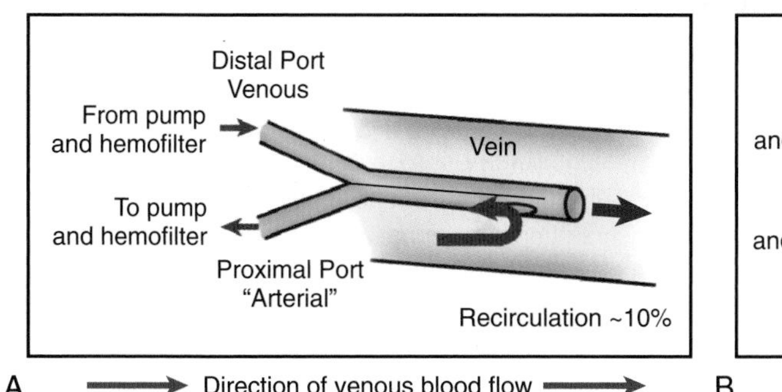

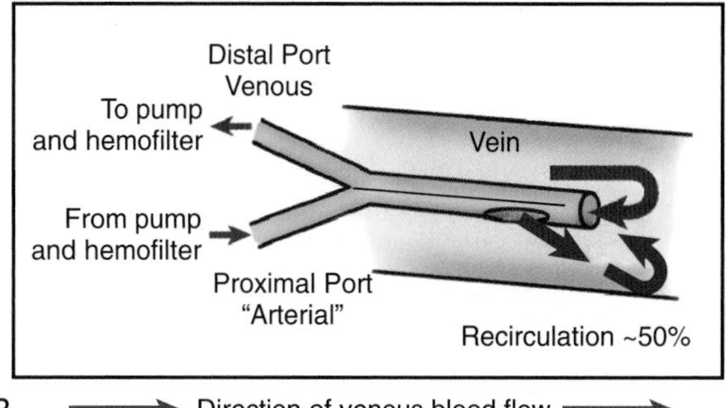

FIG 20-6 Temporary Dialysis Venous Access Catheter.

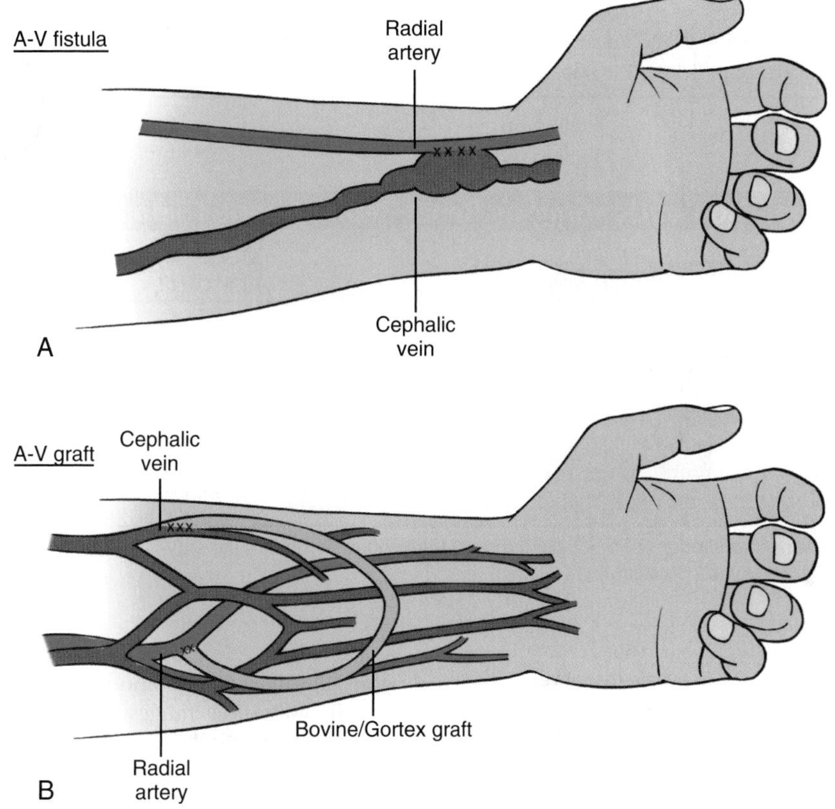

FIG 20-7 Vascular Access for Hemodialysis. *A*, Arteriovenous fistula between the vein and artery. *B*, Internal synthetic graft corrects the artery and vein.

which is surgically implanted inside the limb. The area is surgically opened, and an artery and a vein are located. A tunnel is created in the tissue where the graft is placed. Anastomoses are made with the graft ends connected to the artery and vein. The blood is allowed to flow through the graft, and the surgical area is closed. The graft creates a raised area that looks like a large peripheral vein just under the skin (see Figure 20-7B). Two large-bore needles are used for outflow from and inflow to the graft during dialysis. For grafts and fistulas, after needle removal at the end of the hemodialysis treatment, firm pressure must be applied to stop any bleeding (see Table 20-8).

Tunneled catheters. While waiting for the fistula or graft to mature to be ready for access, some patients with CKD may have a tunneled, cuffed catheter placed in either the internal or external jugular vein.[62,63] The cuff and tunneling are physical barriers to reduce central venous line infections.[64]

Medical Management

Medical management involves the decision to place a vascular access device and then to choose the most appropriate type and location for each patient. Patients in the critical care setting who require vascular access for hemodialysis typically use a temporary hemodialysis catheter. The exact quantity of fluid and solute removal to be achieved by hemodialysis is determined individually for each patient by clinical examination and review of all relevant laboratory results.

TABLE 20-8 Complications and Nursing Management of Arteriovenous Fistula/Graft

TYPE	COMPLICATIONS	NURSING MANAGEMENT
Fistula	Thrombosis Infection Pseudoaneurysm Vascular steal syndrome Venous hypertension Carpal tunnel syndrome Inadequate blood flow	Teach patients to avoid wearing constrictive clothing on limbs containing access. Teach patients to avoid sleeping on or bending accessed limb for prolonged periods. Use aseptic technique when cannulating access. Avoid repetitious cannulation of one segment of access. Offer comfort measures, such as warm compresses and ordered analgesics, to lessen pain of vascular steal. Teach patients to develop blood flow in the fistulas through exercises (squeezing a rubber ball) while applying mild impedance to flow just distal to the access (at least once per day for 10-15 min). Avoid too-early cannulation of new access.
Graft	Bleeding Thrombosis False aneurysm formation Infection Arterial or venous stenosis Vascular steal syndrome	Teach patients to avoid wearing constrictive clothing on accessed limbs. Avoid repeated cannulation of one segment of access. Use aseptic technique when cannulating access. Monitor for changes in arterial or venous pressure while patients are on dialysis. Provide comfort measures to reduce pain of vascular steal (e.g., warm compresses, analgesics as ordered).

TABLE 20-9 Comparison of Continuous Renal Replacement Therapy Modes

TYPE	ULTRAFILTRATION RATE	FLUID REPLACEMENT	MODE OF SOLUTE REMOVAL	INDICATION
SCUF	100-300 mL/hr	None	None	Fluid removal
CVVH	500-800 mL/hr	Predilution or postdilution, calculating hourly net loss	Convection	Fluid removal, moderate solute removal
CVVHD	500-800 mL/hr	Predilution or postdilution, subtracting dialysate, then calculating hourly net loss	Diffusion	Fluid removal, maximum solute removal
CVVHDF		Predilution or postdilution, subtracting dialysate, then calculating hourly net loss	Convection and diffusion	Maximal fluid removal, maximal solute removal

CVVH, Continuous venovenous hemofiltration; *CVVHD*, continuous venovenous hemodialysis; *CVVHDF*, continuous venovenous hemodiafiltration; *SCUF*, slow continuous ultrafiltration.

Nursing Management

A noncritical care nurse who is specially trained in dialysis manages the IHD. The dialysis nurse typically comes to the patient's bedside with the hemodialysis machine. During the acute phase of treatment, hemodialysis occurs daily. The frequency is reduced to 3 days per week as the patient becomes hemodynamically stable. The essential role of the critical care nurse during dialysis is to monitor the patient's hemodynamic status and ensure the patient remains hemodynamically stable. The AKI patient on hemodialysis depends on a viable venous access catheter. When not in use, the catheter is "heparin-locked" to preserve patency. The critical care nurse provides education about the disease process and treatment plan to patient and family.

Continuous Renal Replacement Therapy

CRRT is a continuous therapy that is monitored by the critical care nurse, and it may continue over many days. The venous blood is circulated through a highly porous hemofilter. As with traditional hemodialysis, access and return of blood are achieved through a large venous catheter (venovenous). The CRRT system allows the continuous removal of fluid from the plasma. The patient's blood flow is 100 to 200 mL/min, and the dialysate flow ranges from 20 to 40 mL/min. The fluid removal rate varies depending on the particular CRRT method used and removal of solutes (urea, creatinine, and electrolytes), as listed in Table 20-9. The removed fluid is described as ***ultrafiltrate***. In an ideal situation, the hydrostatic pressure exerted by a mean arterial pressure (MAP) greater than 70 mm Hg would propel a continuous flow of blood through the hemofilter to remove fluid and solute. However, because many critically ill patients are hypotensive and cannot provide adequate flow through the hemofilter, an electric roller pump "milks" the tubing to augment flow. If large amounts of fluid are to be removed, IV replacement solutions are infused. Indications and contraindications for CRRT are described in Box 20-7.

Controversy exists about when CRRT should be started, the optimal dialysis dose, which patients can derive the greatest benefit, and when CRRT should be discontinued. The debate over the optimal "dose" of dialysis is likely to continue because although two recent clinical trials showed no difference in mortality between critically ill patients receiving intensive or nonintensive dialysis regimens,[65,66] the amount of dialysis in the research studies was greater than that normally achieved in clinical practice.[67] Therefore, the debate continues.

Because controlled removal and replacement of fluid is possible over many hours or days with CRRT, hemodynamic stability is maintained. This makes CRRT highly advantageous for use in the hemodynamically unstable patient with multisystem problems. Several modes of CRRT are used in critical care units, a partial list is provided below:[68]

1. Slow continuous ultrafiltration (SCUF)
2. Continuous venovenous hemofiltration (CVVH)
3. Continuous venovenous hemodialysis (CVVHD)
4. Continuous venovenous hemodiafiltration (CVVHDF)

The decision about which type of therapy to initiate is based on clinical assessment, metabolic status, severity of uremia, whether a particular treatment modality is available at that institution, and other factors.

Continuous Renal Replacement Therapy Terminology

In CRRT, solutes are removed from the blood by *diffusion* or *convection.* Both processes remove fluid, and the two methods remove molecules of different sizes.

Diffusion. Diffusion describes the movement of solutes along a concentration gradient from a high concentration to a low concentration across a semipermeable membrane. This is the main mechanism used in hemodialysis. Solutes such as creatinine and urea cross the dialysis membrane from the blood to the dialysis fluid compartment.

Convection. Convection occurs when a pressure gradient is set up so that the water is pushed or pumped across the dialysis filter and carries the solutes from the bloodstream with it. This method of solute removal is known as solvent drag, and it is commonly employed in CRRT.

Absorption. The filter attracts solute, and molecules attach (adsorb) to the dialysis filter. The size of solute molecules is measured in daltons. The different sizes of molecules that can be removed by convection or diffusion methods are shown in Table 20-9. Tiny molecules such as urea and creatinine are removed by diffusion and convection (all methods). As the molecular size increases above 500 daltons, convection is the more efficient method (Table 20-10).

Ultrafiltrate volume. The fluid that is removed each hour is not called urine; it is known as ultrafiltrate.

Replacement fluid. Typically, some of the ultrafiltrate is replaced through the CRRT circuit by a sterile replacement fluid. The replacement fluid can be added before the filter (prefilter dilution) or after the filter (postfilter dilution). The purpose is to increase the volume of fluid passing through the hemofilter and improve convection of solute.

Anticoagulation. Because the blood outside the body is in contact with artificial tubing and filters, the coagulation cascade and complement cascades are activated. To prevent the hemofilter from becoming obstructed by clotting, or clotting off, low-dose anticoagulation must be used. The dose should be low enough to have no effect on patient anticoagulation parameters. Systemic anticoagulation is not the goal. Typical anticoagulant choices include unfractionated heparin (UFH) and sodium citrate. Citrate is an effective prefilter anticoagulant, which has the side effect that it chelates (binds to and removes) calcium from the blood. Consequently, iCa levels are verified, and calcium is replaced per protocol when sodium citrate is the anticoagulant.

Modes of Continuous Renal Replacement

Because of the design of the CRRT machine, it is not possible to look at the outside and follow the flow of blood and, if used, dialysate. Each of the CRRT modes is described, and diagrams are employed to clarify the mode of CRRT that is used.

Slow continuous ultrafiltration. SCUF slowly removes fluid (100 to 300 mL/hr) through a process of ultrafiltration (Figure 20-8A). This consists of a movement of fluid across a semipermeable membrane. SCUF has minimal impact on solute removal. However, SCUF is an infrequent clinical choice because it requires both arterial and venous access for effective functioning and the circuit is more likely to

BOX 20-7 Indications and Contraindications for Continuous Renal Replacement Therapy

Indications

- Need for large fluid volume removal in hemodynamically unstable patient
- Hypervolemic or edematous patients unresponsive to diuretic therapy
- Patients with multiple organ dysfunction syndrome
- Ease of fluid management in patients requiring large daily fluid volume
  - Replacement for oliguria
  - Administration of total parenteral nutrition
- Contraindication to hemodialysis and peritoneal dialysis
- Inability to be anticoagulated

Contraindications

- Hematocrit >45%
- Terminal illness

TABLE 20-10 Size of Molecules Cleared by Continuous Renal Replacement Therapy

TYPE OF MOLECULE	SIZE OF MOLECULE	SOLUTES	SOLUTE REMOVAL METHOD
Small	<500 daltons	Urea, creatinine	Convection, diffusion
Middle	500-5000 daltons	Vancomycin	Convection better than diffusion
Low–molecular-weight (small) proteins	5000-50,000 daltons	Cytokines, complement	Convection or absorption onto hemofilter
Large proteins	>50,000 daltons	Albumin	Minimal removal

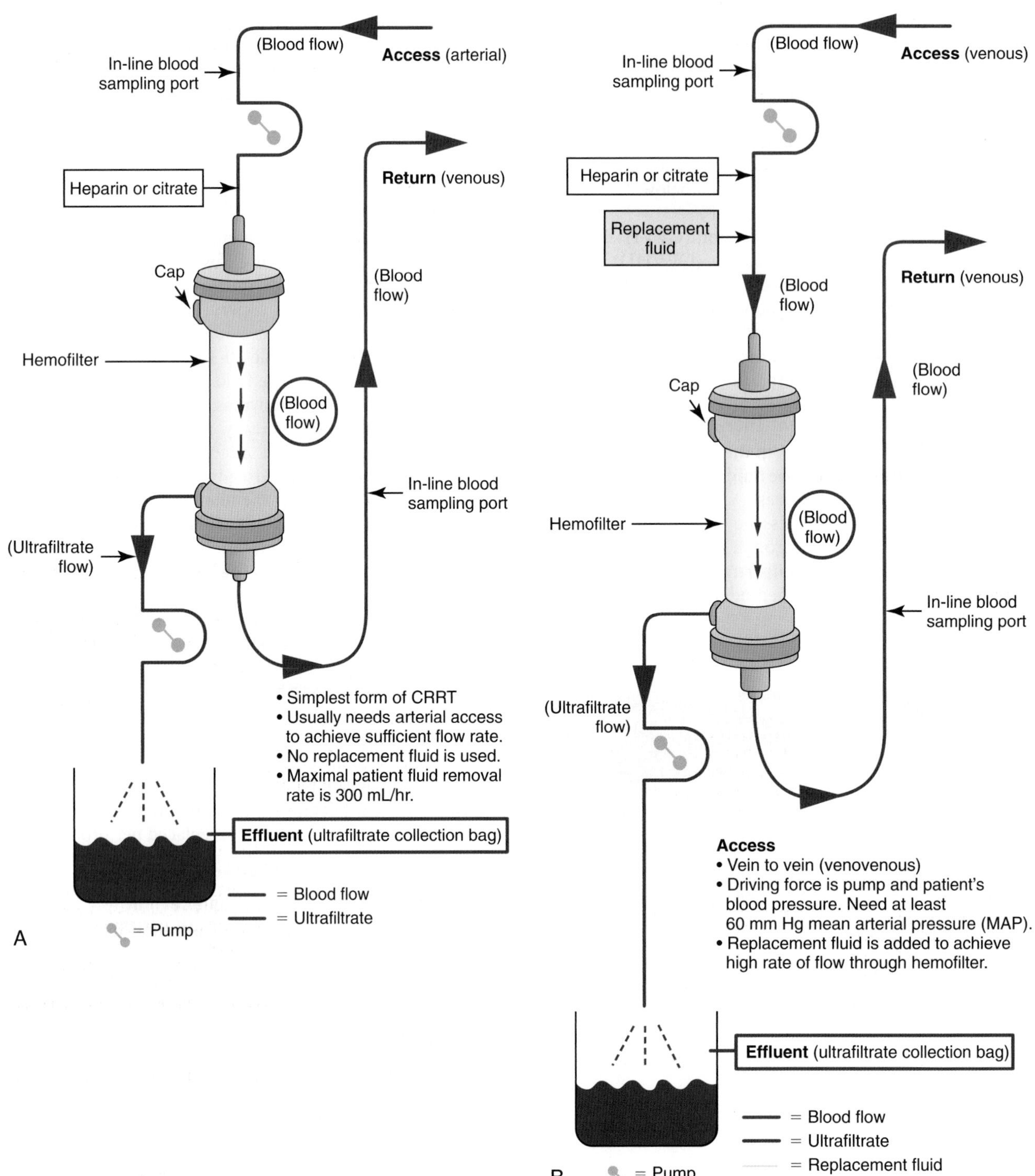

FIG 20-8 Continuous Renal Replacement Therapy (CRRT) Systems. *A*, Slow, continuous ultrafiltration (SCUF). *B*, Continuous venovenous hemofiltration (CVVH).

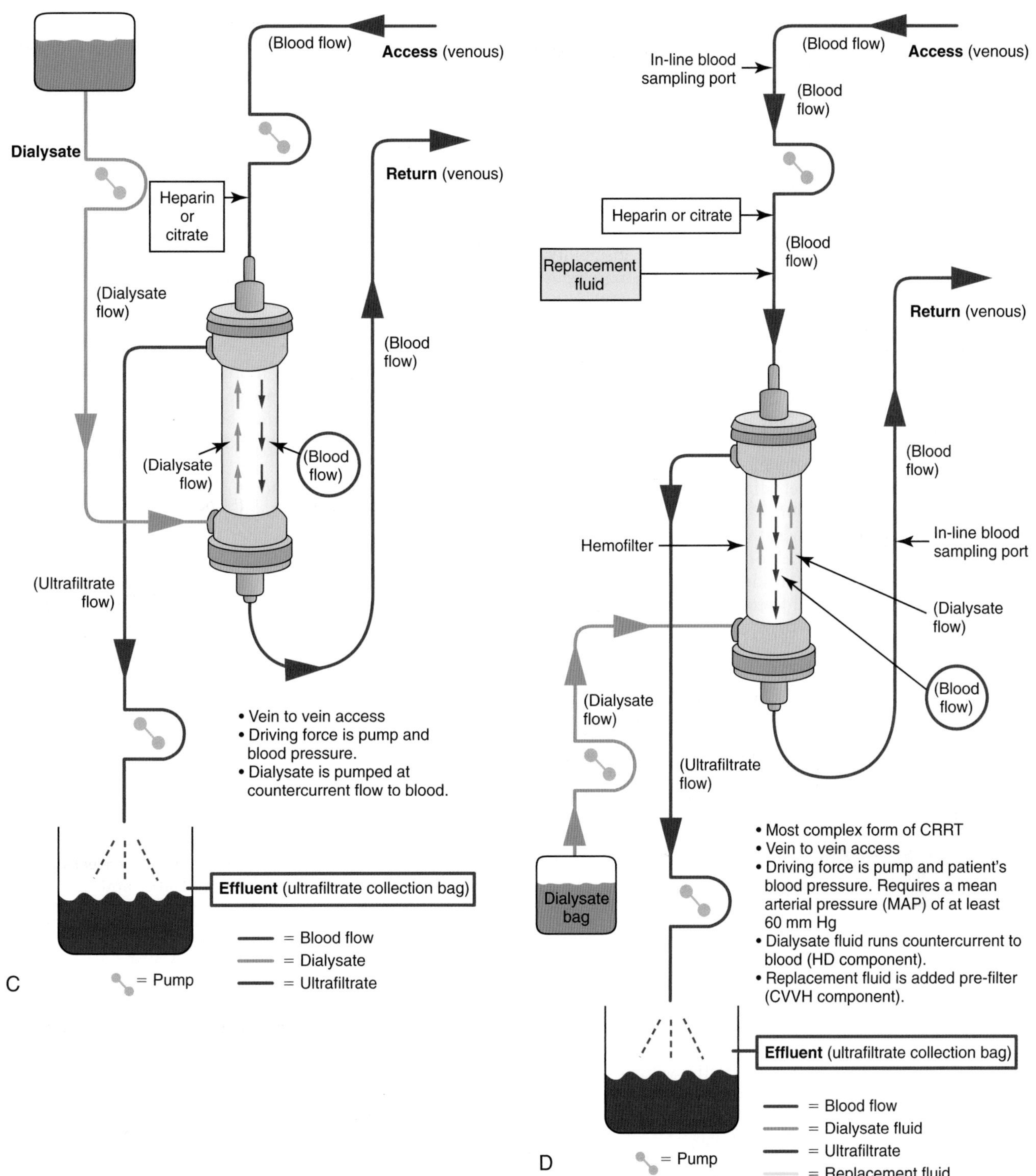

FIG 20-8, cont'd *C*, Continuous venovenous hemofiltration dialysis (CVVHD). *D*, Continuous venovenous hemodiafiltration (CVVHDF).

thrombose (clot off) than other CRRT methods that use higher flows.[69,70]

Continuous venovenous hemofiltration. CVVH is indicated when the patient's clinical condition warrants removal of significant volumes of fluid and solutes. Fluid is removed by ultrafiltration in volumes of 5 to 20 mL/min or up to 7 to 30 L/24 hr. Removal of solutes such as urea, creatinine, and other small non–protein-bound toxins is accomplished by convection. The replacement fluid rate of flow through the CRRT circuit can be altered to achieve desired fluid and solute removal without causing hemodynamic instability. Replacement fluid can be added by the addition of a prehemofilter replacement fluid (see Figure 20-8B) or posthemofilter replacement fluid.

As with other CRRT systems, the blood outside the body is anticoagulated, and the ultrafiltrate is drained off by gravity or by the addition of negative-pressure suction into a large drainage bag. Because large volumes of fluid may be removed in CVVH, some of the removed ultrafiltrate volume must be replaced hourly with a continuous infusion (replacement fluid) to avoid intravascular dehydration. Replacement fluids may consist of standard solutions of bicarbonate, potassium-free LR solution, acetate, or dextrose. Electrolytes such as potassium, sodium, calcium chloride, magnesium sulfate, and sodium bicarbonate may be added. The formula used to calculate the volume removed from the patient follows with an example:

Ultrafiltrate in bag + Other output − (CVVH replacement fluid + IV/oral/NG intake) = Output

1000 mL − 800 mL = 200 mL/hr output

Continuous venovenous hemodialysis. CVVHD is technically like traditional hemodialysis, and it removes solute by diffusion because of a slow (15 to 30 mL/min) countercurrent drainage flow on the membrane side of the hemofilter (see Figure 20-8C). Blood and fluid move by countercurrent flow through the hemofilter. *Countercurrent* means the blood flows in one direction, and the dialysate flows in the opposite direction. As with other types of CRRT and hemodialysis, although arterial access is always possible, venovenous vascular access is the most common choice.

CVVHD is indicated for patients who require large-volume removal for severe uremia or critical acid–base imbalances or for those who are resistant to diuretics. A MAP of at least 70 mm Hg is desirable for effective volume removal and dialysis, and it is most effective when used over days, not hours. The use of replacement fluid is optional and depends on the patient's clinical condition and plan of care.

The critical care nurse is responsible for calculating the hourly intake and output, identifying fluid trends, and replacing excessive losses. This therapy is ideal for hemodynamically unstable patients in the critical care setting because they do not experience the abrupt fluid and solute changes that can accompany standard hemodialysis treatments.

Continuous venovenous hemodiafiltration. Another CRRT option is CVVHDF, which combines two of the previously described methods (CVVH and CVVHD) to achieve maximal fluid and solute removal. A strong transmembrane pressure is applied to the hemofilter to push water across the filter, and a negative pressure is applied at the other side to pull fluid across the membrane and produce large volumes of ultrafiltrate and to create a "solvent drag" (CVVH method). The blood and the dialysate are circulated in a countercurrent flow pattern to remove fluid and solutes by diffusion (hemodialysis method). CVVHDF can remove large volumes of fluid and solute because it employs diffusion gradients and convection.

Complications

Potential problems associated with CRRT and appropriate nursing interventions are listed in Table 20-11. Complications are often related to the rate of flow through the system. If the patient becomes hypotensive or the access lines remain kinked, the ultrafiltration rate will decrease. This can lead to increased clot formation within the hemofilter. As the surface of the hemofilter becomes more clotted, it will not provide effective fluid or solute clearance, and CRRT will be stopped; a new CRRT circuit must then be set up. The most common reasons for interruption in CRRT are clotting and patient clinical issues.[71]

The critical care nurse monitors the pressures displayed on the CRRT machine screen to monitor the positive pressure of fluid going into the hemofilter (inflow) and the pressures coming out of the hemofilter to ensure that resistance to the negative-pressure pull of the fluid across the hemofilter membrane has not developed. Other patient-related complications include fluid and electrolyte alterations, bleeding because of anticoagulation, or problems with the access site, such as dislodgement or infection.[72]

Medical Management

The choice of the method of blood purification to use to treat AKI is a medical decision. There is no clinical or research consensus about whether IHD or CRRT is the most beneficial.[73,74] Age, gender, and preexisting chronic conditions are of little help in determining whether to select IHD or CRRT. Often, the acute clinical diagnosis, physician's preference, availability of the CRRT machine, and knowledgeable nurses and physicians at the hospital are the deciding factors.

The current trend is to start IHD or CRRT earlier rather than later in the course of AKI.[75] Previously, dialysis was not started until the BUN level exceeded 90 mg/dL or the creatinine level exceeded 9 mg/dL. Today, in many critical care units, the threshold to begin treatment is considerably lower.[75] If the patient has severe electrolyte imbalance or fluid overload, even earlier intervention may be required.

Nursing Management

Critical care nurses play a vital role in monitoring the patient receiving CRRT. In many critical care units, the CRRT system is set up by the dialysis staff but is run on a 24-hour basis by critical care nurses with additional training. Complications may be related to the CRRT circuit, the CRRT pump, or to the patient, as shown in Box 20-8. The critical care nurse monitors fluid intake and output, prevents and detects potential complications (e.g., bleeding, hypotension), identifies trends in electrolyte laboratory values, supervises safe operation of the CRRT equipment, and provides patient and family education about the patient's condition and the use of CRRT.

TABLE 20-11 Complications Associated with Continuous Renal Replacement Therapy

PROBLEM	CAUSE	CLINICAL MANIFESTATIONS	NURSING MANAGEMENT
Decreased ultrafiltration rate	Hypotension Dehydration Kinked lines Bending of catheters Clotting of filter	Ultrafiltration rate decreased Minimal flow through blood lines	Observe filter and arteriovenous system. Control blood flow. Control coagulation time. Position patient on back. Lower height of collection container.
Filter clotting	Obstruction Insufficient heparinization	Ultrafiltration rate decreased, despite height of collection container being lower	Control anticoagulation (heparin/citrate). Maintain continuous system anticoagulation. Call physician. Remove system. Prime catheters with anticoagulated solution. Prime new system; connect it. Start predilution with 1000 mL saline 0.9% solution per hour. Do not use three-way stopcocks.
Hypotension	Increased ultrafiltration rate Blood leak Disconnection of one of lines	Bleeding Call physician.	Control amount of ultrafiltration. Control access sites. Clamp lines.
Fluid and electrolyte changes	Too much or too little removal of fluid Inappropriate replacement of electrolytes Inappropriate dialysate	Changes in mentation ↑ or ↓ CVP ↑ or ↓ PAOP ECG changes ↑ or ↓ BP and heart rate Abnormal electrolyte levels	Observe for • Changes in CVP or PAOP. • Changes in vital signs. • ECG change resulting from electrolyte abnormalities. Monitor output values every hour. Control ultrafiltration.
Bleeding	System disconnection ↑ Heparin dose	Oozing from catheter insertion site or connection	Monitor ACT no less than once every hour (heparin). Adjust heparin dose within specifications to maintain ACT. Monitor serum calcium if using citrate as an anticoagulant. Observe dressing on vascular access for blood loss. Observe for blood in filtrate (filter leak).
Access dislodgement or infection	Catheter or connections not secured Break in sterile technique Excessive patient movement	Bleeding from catheter site or connections Inappropriate flow or infusion Fever Drainage at catheter site	Observe access site at least once every 2 hours. Ensure that clamps are available within easy reach at all times. Observe strict sterile technique when dressing vascular access.

ACT, Activated coagulation time; *BP*, blood pressure; *CRRT*, continuous renal replacement therapy; *CVP*, central venous pressure; *ECG*, electrocardiogram; *PAOP*, pulmonary artery occlusion pressure or wedge pressure; ↑, increased; ↓, decreased.

BOX 20-8 Complications of Continuous Renal Replacement Therapy

The Circuit
- Air embolism
- Clotted hemofilter
- Poor ultrafiltration
- Blood leaks
- Broken filter
- Recirculation or disconnection
- Access failure
- Catheter dislodgment

The Pump
- Circuit pressure alarm
  - Decreased inflow pressure
  - Decreased outflow pressure
  - Increased outflow resistance
- Air bubble detector alarm
- Power failure
- Mechanical dysfunction

The Patient
- Code or emergency situation
- Dehydration
- Hypotension
- Electrolyte imbalances
- Acid–base imbalances
- Blood loss or hemorrhage
- Hypothermia
- Infection

CASE STUDY Patient with a Kidney Problem

Brief Patient History
Ms. L is a 32-year-old woman found down in the street near the hospital. She is awake but confused. She is unable to give any medical history and has no idea how long she has been in the street.

Clinical Assessment
Ms. L is admitted to the critical care unit with muscle pain and minimal dark urine output. She continues to be confused, but her neurologic examination results are otherwise normal. She repeatedly tells the nurses that she is tired, has pain everywhere, and just wants to sleep. She is able to move all her extremities and has no signs of injury on skin examination.

Diagnostic Procedures
Laboratory tests show the following results: creatinine phosphokinase (CPK) level of 40,400 U/L, serum myoglobin level of 2.5 mg/L, urinary myoglobin level of 300 mg/L, and serum potassium level of 4.8 mEq/dL. Baseline vital signs were as follows: blood pressure of 85/60 mm Hg, heart rate of 128 beats/min (sinus tachycardia), respiratory rate of 18 breaths/min, temperature of 101.3°F, and O_2 saturation of 98%.

The toxicology screen showed that the patient tested positive for cocaine. The Glasgow Coma Scale score was 14.

Medical Diagnosis
Ms. L is diagnosed with rhabdomyolysis.

Questions
1. What major outcomes do you expect to achieve for this patient?
2. What problems or risks must be managed to achieve these outcomes?
3. What interventions must be initiated to monitor, prevent, manage, or eliminate the problems and risks identified?
4. What interventions should be initiated to promote optimal functioning, safety, and well-being of the patient?
5. What possible learning needs do you anticipate for this patient?
6. What cultural and age-related factors may have a bearing on the patient's plan of care?

REFERENCES

1. Bellomo R: Acute renal failure, *Semin Respir Crit Care Med* 32(5):639, 2011.
2. Singbartl K, Kellum JA: AKI in the ICU: definition, epidemiology, risk stratification, and outcomes, *Kidney Internat* 81(9):819, 2012.
3. Mehta RL, et al: Spectrum of acute renal failure in the intensive care unit: the PICARD experience, *Kidney Internat* 66(4):1613, 2004.
4. Prowle JR, et al: Oliguria as predictive biomarker of acute kidney injury in critically ill patients, *Crit Care* 15(4):R172, 2011.
5. Macedo E, et al: Defining urine output criterion for acute kidney injury in critically ill patients, *Nephrol Dial Transplant* 26(2):509, 2011.
6. Rachoin JS, et al: The fallacy of the BUN:creatinine ratio in critically ill patients, *Nephrol Dial Transplant* 27(6):2248, 2012.
7. Endre ZH, Pickering JW, Walker RJ: Clearance and beyond: the complementary roles of GFR measurement and injury biomarkers in acute kidney injury (AKI), *Am J Physiol Renal Physiol* 301(4):F697, 2011.
8. National Kidney and Urologic Diseases Information Clearinghouse (NKUDIC). http://kidney.niddk.nih.gov/kudiseases/pubs/kustats/. Accessed August 10, 2014.
9. Nickolas TL, et al: Awareness of kidney disease in the US population: findings from the National Health and Nutrition Examination Survey (NHANES) 1999 to 2000, *Am J Kidney Dis* 44(2):185, 2004.
10. Coresh J, et al: Prevalence of chronic kidney disease in the United States, *JAMA* 298(17):2038, 2007.

11. Carubelli V, et al: Renal dysfunction in acute heart failure: epidemiology, mechanisms and assessment, *Heart Failure Rev* 17(2):271, 2012.
12. Ronco C, et al: Cardio-renal syndromes: report from the consensus conference of the acute dialysis quality initiative, *Eur Heart J* 31(6):703, 2010.
13. Koyner JL, Murray PT: Mechanical ventilation and the kidney, *Blood Purif* 29(1):52, 2010.
14. Vieira JM Jr, et al: Effect of acute kidney injury on weaning from mechanical ventilation in critically ill patients, *Crit Care Med* 35(1):184, 2007.
15. Pan SW, et al: Acute kidney injury on ventilator initiation day independently predicts prolonged mechanical ventilation in intensive care unit patients, *J Crit Care* 26(6):586, 2011.
16. Dellinger RP, et al: Surviving Sepsis Campaign: international guidelines for management of severe sepsis and septic shock: 2012, *Crit Care Med* 41(2):580, 2013.
17. Bagshaw SM, George C, Gibney RT, Bellomo R: A multi-center evaluation of early acute kidney injury in critically ill trauma patients, *Ren Fail* 30(6):581, 2008.
18. Delaney KA, Givens ML, Vohra RB: Use of RIFLE criteria to predict the severity and prognosis of acute kidney injury in emergency department patients with rhabdomyolysis, *J Emerg Med* 42(5):521, 2012.
19. Shapiro ML, Baldea A, Luchette FA: Rhabdomyolysis in the intensive care unit, *J Intens Care Med* 2011.
20. Parekh R, Care DA, Tainter CR: Rhabdomyolysis: advances in diagnosis and treatment, *Emerg Med Pract* 14(3):1, 2012.
21. Brown CV, et al: Preventing renal failure in patients with rhabdomyolysis: do bicarbonate and mannitol make a difference?, *J Trauma* 56(6):1191, 2004.
22. Weisbord SD, et al: The incidence of clinically significant contrast-induced nephropathy following non-emergent coronary angiography, *Catheter Cardiovasc Interv* 71(7):879, 2008.
23. Stacul F, et al: Contrast induced nephropathy: updated ESUR Contrast Media Safety Committee guidelines, *Eur Radiol* 21(12):2527, 2011.
24. Isaac S: Contrast-induced nephropathy: nursing implications, *Crit Care Nurse* 32(3):41, 2012.
25. Goldenberg I, Chonchol M, Guetta V: Reversible acute kidney injury following contrast exposure and the risk of long-term mortality, *Am J Nephrol* 29(2):136, 2008.
26. Institute for Healthcare Improvement: Catheter-associated urinary tract infections. http://www.ihi.org/topics/cauti/Pages/default.aspx. Accessed November 3, 2014.
27. Centers for Disease Control and Prevention: Healthcare-associated infections—Catheter associated urinary tract infections. http://www.cdc.gov/HAI/ca_uti/uti.html. Accessed November 3, 2014.
28. Burton DC, et al: Trends in catheter-associated urinary tract infections in adult intensive care units-United States, 1990-2007, *Infect Control Hosp Epidemiol* 32(8):748, 2011.
29. Chant C, Smith OM, Marshall JC, Friedrich JO: Relationship of catheter-associated urinary tract infection to mortality and length of stay in critically ill patients: a systematic review and meta-analysis of observational studies, *Crit Care Med* 39(5):1167, 2011.
30. The Joint Commission: National Patient Safety Goals 2014. http://www.jointcommission.org/assets/1/6/HAP_NPSG_Chapter_2014.pdf. Accessed November 3, 2014.
31. Rosenthal VD, et al: International Nosocomial Infection Control Consortium (INICC) report, data summary of 36 countries, for 2004-2009, *Am J Infect Control* 40(5):396, 2012.
32. Conway LJ, Pogorzelska M, Larson E, Stone PW: Adoption of policies to prevent catheter-associated urinary tract infections in United States intensive care units, *Am J Infect Control* 40(8):705, 2012.
33. Titsworth WL, et al: Reduction of catheter-associated urinary tract infections among patients in a neurological intensive care unit: a single institution's success, *J Neurosurg* 116(4):911, 2012.
34. Marra AR, et al: Preventing catheter-associated urinary tract infection in the zero-tolerance era, *Am J Infect Control* 39(10):817, 2011.
35. Davison DL, Patel K, Chawla LS: Hemodynamic monitoring in the critically ill: spanning the range of kidney function, *Am J Kidney Dis* 59(5):715, 2012.
36. El-Sherif N, Turitto G: Electrolyte disorders and arrhythmogenesis, *Cardiol J* 18(3):233, 2011.
37. Kessler C, Ng J, Valdez K, Geiger B: The use of sodium polystyrene sulfonate in the inpatient management of hyperkalemia, *J Hosp Med* 6(3):136, 2011.
38. Charmot D: Non-systemic drugs: a critical review, *Curr Pharm Des* 18(10):1434, 2012.
39. Kovesdy CP, et al: Hyponatremia, hypernatremia, and mortality in patients with chronic kidney disease with and without congestive heart failure, *Circulation* 125(5):677, 2012.
40. Hutchison AJ, Smith CP, Brenchley PE: Pharmacology, efficacy and safety of oral phosphate binders, *Nature Rev Nephrol* 7(10):578, 2011.
41. Molony DA, Stephens BW: Derangements in phosphate metabolism in chronic kidney diseases/endstage renal disease: therapeutic considerations, *Adv Chronic Kidney Dis* 18(2):120, 2011.
42. Jüppner H: Phosphate and FGF-23, *Kidney Internat (suppl)* (121):S24, 2011.
43. Gauci C, et al: Pitfalls of measuring total blood calcium in patients with CKD, *J Am Soc Nephrol* 19(8):1592, 2008.
44. Kalantar-Zadeh K, et al: Understanding sources of dietary phosphorus in the treatment of patients with chronic kidney disease, *Clin J Am Soc Nephrol* 5(3):519, 2010.
45. The SAFE Study Investigators: A comparison of albumin and saline for fluid resuscitation in the intensive care unit, *N Engl J Med* 350(22):2247, 2004.
46. Investigaors TSS: Saline or albumin for fluid resuscitation in patients with traumatic brain injury, *N Engl J Med* 357(9):874, 2007.
47. Perel P, Roberts I: Colloids versus crystalloids for fluid resuscitation in critically ill patients, *Cochrane Database Syst Rev* (4):Art. No.: CD000567, 2007.
48. Nigwekar SU, Waikar SS: Diuretics in acute kidney injury, *Semin Nephrol* 31(6):523, 2011.
49. Wile D: Diuretics: a review, *Ann Clin Biochem* 49(5):419, 2012.
50. Felker GM: Loop diuretics in heart failure, *Heart Fail Rev* 17(2):305, 2012.
51. Asare K: Management of loop diuretic resistance in the intensive care unit, *Am J Health Syst Pharm* 66(18):1635, 2009.
52. Kassamali R, Sica DA: Acetazolamide: a forgotten diuretic agent, *Cardiol Rev* 19(6):276, 2011.

53. Lehrich RW, Greenberg A: Hyponatremia and the use of vasopressin receptor antagonists in critically ill patients, *J Intens Care Med* 27(4):207, 2012.
54. Giamouzis G, et al: Impact of dopamine infusion on renal function in hospitalized heart failure patients: results of the Dopamine in Acute Decompensated Heart Failure (DAD-HF) Trial, *J Cardiac Failure* 16(12):922, 2010.
55. Casaer MP, Mesotten D, Schetz MR: Bench-to-bedside review: metabolism and nutrition, *Crit Care* 12(4):222, 2008.
56. Gervasio JM, Garmon WP, Holowatyj M: Nutrition support in acute kidney injury, *Nutr Clin Pract* 26(4):374, 2011.
57. Ramanath V, et al: Anemia and chronic kidney disease: making sense of the recent trials, *Rev Recent Clin Trials* 7(3):187, 2012.
58. Besarab A: Anemia and iron management, *Semin Dial* 24(5):498, 2011.
59. Oudemans-van Straaten HM, Kellum JA, Bellomo R: Clinical review: anticoagulation for continuous renal replacement therapy–heparin or citrate?, *Crit Care* 15(1):202, 2011.
60. Kimball TA, et al: Efficiency of the kidney disease outcomes quality initiative guidelines for preemptive vascular access in an academic setting, *J Vasc Surg* 54(3):760, 2011.
61. Schild AF, et al: Arteriovenous fistulae vs. arteriovenous grafts: a retrospective review of 1,700 consecutive vascular access cases, *J Vasc Access* 9(4):231, 2008.
62. Coryell L, et al: The case for primary placement of tunneled hemodialysis catheters in acute kidney injury, *J Vasc Interv Radiol* 20(12):1578, 2009.
63. Vats HS, et al: A comparison between blood flow outcomes of tunneled external jugular and internal jugular hemodialysis catheters, *J Vasc Access* 13(1):51, 2012.
64. Vats HS: Complications of catheters: tunneled and nontunneled, *Adv Chronic Kidney Dis* 19(3):188, 2012.
65. Palevsky PM, et al: Intensity of renal support in critically ill patients with acute kidney injury, *N Engl J Med* 359(1):7, 2008.
66. Bellomo R, et al: Intensity of continuous renal-replacement therapy in critically ill patients, *N Engl J Med* 361(17):1627, 2009.
67. Kellum JA, Ronco C: Dialysis: results of RENAL–what is the optimal CRRT target dose?, *Nat Rev Nephrol* 6(4):191, 2010.
68. Cerdá J, Ronco C: Modalities of continuous renal replacement therapy: technical and clinical considerations, *Semin Dial* 22(2):114, 2009.
69. Felker GM, Mentz RJ: Diuretics and ultrafiltration in acute decompensated heart failure, *JACC* 59(24):2145, 2012.
70. Freda BJ, Slawsky M, Mallidi J, Braden GL: Decongestive treatment of acute decompensated heart failure: cardiorenal implications of ultrafiltration and diuretics, *Am J Kidney Dis* 58(6):1005, 2011.
71. Vesconi S, et al: Delivered dose of renal replacement therapy and mortality in critically ill patients with acute kidney injury, *Crit Care* 13(2):R57, 2009.
72. Finkel KW, Podoll AS: Complications of continuous renal replacement therapy, *Semin Dial* 22(2):155, 2009.
73. Lins RL, et al: Intermittent versus continuous renal replacement therapy for acute kidney injury patients admitted to the intensive care unit: results of a randomized clinical trial, *Nephrol Dial Transplant* 24(2):512, 2009.
74. Karvellas CJ, et al: A comparison of early versus late initiation of renal replacement therapy in critically ill patients with acute kidney injury: a systematic review and meta-analysis, *Crit Care* 15(1):R72, 2011.
75. Macedo E, Mehta RL: When should renal replacement therapy be initiated for acute kidney injury?, *Semin Dial* 24(2):132, 2011.

CHAPTER 21

Gastrointestinal Clinical Assessment and Diagnostic Procedures

Kathleen M. Stacy

Be sure to check out the bonus material, including review questions, on the Evolve website at http://evolve.elsevier.com/Urden/priorities/.

HISTORY

Taking a thorough and accurate history is extremely important to the assessment process. The patient's history provides the foundation and direction for the rest of the assessment. The overall goal of the patient interview is to expose key clinical manifestations that will facilitate the identification of the underlying cause of the illness. This information can then assist in the development of an appropriate management plan.[1,2]

The initial presentation of the patient determines the rapidity and direction of the interview. For a patient in acute distress, the history should be curtailed to a few questions about the patient's chief complaint and the precipitating events. For a patient in no obvious distress, the history should focus on current symptoms, the patient's medical history, and the family's history. Specific items regarding each of these areas are outlined in Box 21-1, Data Collection.[3,4]

FOCUSED CLINICAL ASSESSMENT

The physical examination helps to establish baseline data about the physical dimensions of the patient's situation.[3] The abdomen is divided into four quadrants (left upper, right upper, left lower, and right lower), with the umbilicus as the middle point, to help specify the location of examination findings (Figure 21-1 and Box 21-2). The assessment should proceed when the patient is as comfortable as possible and in the supine position; however, the position may need readjustment if it elicits pain. To prevent stimulation of gastrointestinal activity, the order for the assessment should be changed to inspection, auscultation, percussion, and palpation.[4]

Inspection

Inspection of the patient focuses on three priorities: 1) observation of the oral cavity, 2) assessment of the skin over the abdomen, and 3) evaluation of the shape of the abdomen. The examination should be performed in a warm, well-lighted environment with the patient in a comfortable position and with the abdomen exposed.

Observation of the Oral Cavity

Although assessment of the gastrointestinal system classically begins with inspection of the abdomen, the patient's oral cavity also must be inspected to determine any unusual findings. Abnormal findings of the mouth include joint tenderness, inflammation of the gums, missing teeth, dental caries, ill-fitting dentures, and mouth odor.[5]

Assessment of the Skin over the Abdomen

Observe the skin for pigmentation, lesions, striae, scars, petechiae, signs of dehydration, and venous pattern. Pigmentation may vary considerably and still be within normal limits because of race and ethnic background, although the abdomen usually is a lighter color than other exposed areas of the skin. Abnormal findings include jaundice, skin lesions, and a tense and glistening appearance of the skin. Old striae (stretch marks) usually are silver, whereas pinkish purple striae may indicate Cushing's syndrome.[4] A bluish discoloration of the umbilicus (Cullen's sign) and of the flank (Grey Turner's sign) indicates retroperitoneal bleeding.[1]

Evaluation of the Shape of the Abdomen

Observe the abdomen for contour, noting whether it is flat, slightly concave, or slightly round; observe for symmetry and for movement. Marked distention is an abnormal finding. In particular, ascites may cause generalized distention and bulging flanks. Asymmetric distention may indicate organ enlargement or a mass. Peristaltic waves should not be visible except in very thin patients. In the case of intestinal obstruction, hyperactive peristaltic waves may be observed. Pulsation in the epigastric area is often a normal finding, but increased pulsation may indicate an aortic aneurysm. Symmetric movement of the abdomen with respirations is usually seen in men.[4,5]

Auscultation

Auscultation of the patient focuses on two priorities: 1) evaluation of bowels sounds and 2) assessment of bruits. Auscultation of the abdomen provides clinical data regarding the status of the bowel's motility. Initially, listen with the

BOX 21-1 Data Collection

Gastrointestinal History

Common Gastrointestinal Symptoms
- Oral lesions
- Digestion or indigestion (heartburn)
- Dysphagia
- Nausea
- Vomiting
- Hematemesis
- Change in stool color or contents (e.g., clay-colored, tarry, fresh blood, mucus, undigested food)
- Constipation
- Diarrhea
- Abdominal pain
- Jaundice
- Anal discomfort
- Fecal incontinence

Patient Lifestyle
- Usual height and weight
- Dietary habits
  - Usual number of meals or snacks per day
  - Usual fluid intake per day
- Nutrient intake
  - Types of food usually eaten at each meal or snack
  - Food likes and dislikes
  - Religious or medical food restrictions
  - Food intolerances
  - Patient's perceptions and concerns about adequacy of diet and appropriateness of weight
  - Effects of lifestyle on food intake, weight gain or loss
  - Vitamins or nutritional supplements (e.g., type, amount, frequency)
- Bowel elimination
  - Usual frequency of bowel movements
  - Usual consistency and color of stool
  - Ability to control elimination of gas and stool
  - Any changes in bowel elimination patterns
  - Use of enemas or laxatives (e.g., reason for use, frequency, type, response)
- Alcohol intake (e.g., frequency, usual amounts)
- Exercise patterns

Medical History
- Chronic illnesses
- Previous weight gain or loss
- Tooth extractions or orthodontic work
- Gastrointestinal (GI) disorders (e.g., peptic ulcer, inflammatory bowel disease, polyps, cholelithiasis, diverticular disease, pancreatitis, intestinal obstruction)
- Hepatitis or cirrhosis
- Abdominal surgery
- Abdominal trauma
- Cancer affecting GI system
- Spinal cord injury
- Women: episiotomy or fourth-degree laceration during delivery
- Exposure to infectious agents (e.g., foreign travel, water source)

Family History
- Investigate for history of following disorders and document (+ or −) responses
- Hirschsprung disease
- Obesity
- Metabolic disorders
- Inflammatory disorders
- Malabsorption syndromes
- Familial Mediterranean fever
- Rectal polyps
- Polyposis syndromes
- Cancer of the GI tract

Current Medication Use
- Laxatives
- Stool softeners
- Antiemetics
- Antidiarrheals
- Antacids
- Aspirin
- Acetaminophen
- Nonsteroidal antiinflammatory drugs
- Corticosteroids

diaphragm of the stethoscope below and to the right of the umbilicus. The examination proceeds methodically through all four quadrants, lifting and then replacing the diaphragm of the stethoscope lightly against the abdomen (see Figure 21-1).

Evaluation of Bowel Sounds

Normal bowel sounds include high-pitched, gurgling sounds that occur approximately every 5 to 15 seconds or at a rate of 5 to 34 times per minute. Colonic sounds are low-pitched and have a rumbling quality. A venous hum may be audible sometimes.[6,7] Table 21-1 provides a list of abnormal abdominal sounds.

Abnormal findings include the absence of bowel sounds throughout a 5-minute period, extremely soft and widely separated sounds, and increased sounds with a high-pitched, loud rushing sound (peristaltic rush). Absent bowel sounds may result from inflammation, ileus, electrolyte disturbances, and ischemia. Bowels sounds may be increased with diarrhea and early intestinal obstruction.[6,7]

Assessment of Bruits

The abdomen should be auscultated for the presence of bruits, using the bell of the stethoscope. Bruits are created by turbulent flow over a partially obstructed artery and are always considered an abnormal finding. The aorta, the right and left renal arteries, and the iliac arteries should be auscultated.[5,6]

Percussion

Percussion of the patient focuses on one priority: (1) assessment of the deep organs. Percussion is used to elicit information about deep organs, such as the liver, spleen, and pancreas. Because the abdomen is a sensitive area, muscle tension may interfere with this part of the assessment. Percussion often helps relax tense muscles, and it is performed before palpation. Percussion in the absence of disease helps

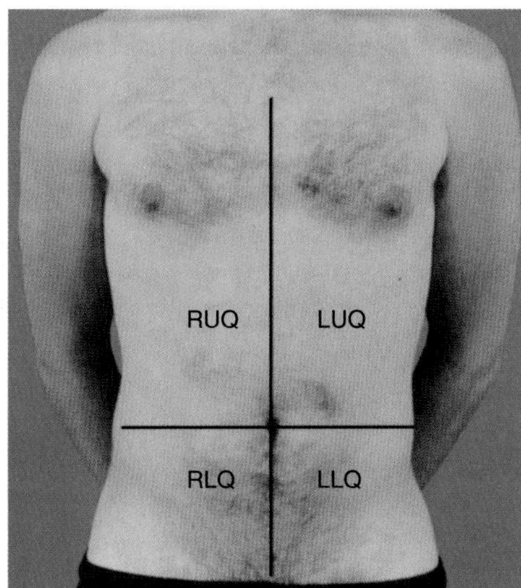

FIG 21-1 Anatomic Mapping of the Four Quadrants of the Abdomen. (From Barkauskas V, et al. *Health & Physical Assessment.* 3rd ed. St. Louis: Mosby; 2002.)

to delineate the position and size of the liver and spleen, and it assists in the detection of fluid, gaseous distention, and masses in the abdomen.[5]

Assessment of Deep Organs

Percussion should proceed systematically and lightly in all four quadrants. Normal findings include tympany over the stomach when empty, tympany or hyperresonance over the intestine, and dullness over the liver and spleen. Abnormal areas of dullness may indicate an underlying mass. Solid masses, enlarged organs, and a distended bladder also produce areas of dullness. Dullness over both flanks may indicate ascites and necessitates further assessment.[6]

Palpation

Palpation of the patient focuses on one priority: (1) detection of abdominal pathological conditions. Both light and deep palpation of each organ and quadrant should be completed. Light palpation, which has a palpation depth of approximately 1 cm, assesses to the depth of the skin and fascia. Deep palpation assesses the *rectus abdominis* muscle and is performed bimanually to a depth of 4 to 5 cm. Deep palpation is most helpful in detecting abdominal masses. Areas in which the patient complains of tenderness should be palpated last.[6]

Detection of Abdominal Pathological Conditions

Normal findings include no areas of tenderness or pain, no masses, and no hardened areas. Persistent involuntary guarding may indicate peritoneal inflammation, particularly if it continues even after relaxation techniques are used. Rebound tenderness, in which pain increases with quick release of a palpated area, indicates an inflamed peritoneum.[4]

LABORATORY STUDIES

The value of various laboratory studies used to diagnose and treat diseases of the gastrointestinal system has been emphasized often. However, no single study provides an overall picture of the various organs' functional state, and no single value is predictive by itself. Laboratory studies used in the assessment of gastrointestinal function, liver function, and pancreatic function are found in Tables 21-2, 21-3, and 21-4, respectively.

BOX 21-2 Anatomic Correlates of the Four Quadrants of the Abdomen

Right Upper Quadrant
- Liver and gallbladder
- Pylorus
- Duodenum
- Head of pancreas
- Right adrenal gland
- Portion of right kidney
- Hepatic flexure of colon
- Portion of ascending and transverse colon

Right Lower Quadrant
- Lower pole of right kidney
- Cecum and appendix
- Portion of ascending colon
- Bladder (if distended)
- Ovary and salpinx
- Uterus (if enlarged)
- Right spermatic cord
- Right ureter

Left Upper Quadrant
- Left lobe of liver
- Spleen
- Stomach
- Body of pancreas
- Left adrenal gland
- Portion of left kidney
- Splenic flexure of colon
- Portions of transverse and descending colon

Left Lower Quadrant
- Lower pole of left kidney
- Sigmoid colon
- Portion of descending colon
- Bladder (if distended)
- Ovary and salpinx
- Uterus (if distended)
- Left spermatic cord
- Left ureter

From Barkauskas V, et al. *Health & Physical Assessment.* 3rd ed. St. Louis: Mosby; 2002.

DIAGNOSTIC PROCEDURES

Table 21-5 presents an overview of the various diagnostic procedures used to evaluate the patient with GI dysfunction.

Nursing Management

The nursing management of a patient undergoing a diagnostic procedure involves a variety of interventions. **Nursing**

Text continued on p. 425

TABLE 21-1 Abnormal Abdominal Sounds

SOUND	CAUSE
Hyperactive bowel sounds (borborygmi), loud and prolonged	Hunger, gastroenteritis, or early intestinal obstruction
High-pitched, tinkling sounds	Intestinal air and fluid under pressure; characteristic of early intestinal obstruction
Decreased (hypoactive) bowel sounds, infrequent and abnormally faint sounds	Possible peritonitis or ileus
Absence of bowel sounds (confirmed only after auscultation of all four quadrants and continuous auscultation for 5 min)	Temporary loss of intestinal motility, as occurs with complete ileus
Friction rubs, high-pitched sounds heard over liver and spleen (RUQ and LUQ), synchronous with respiration	Pathological conditions such as tumors or infection that cause inflammation of organ's peritoneal covering
Bruits, audible swishing sounds that may be heard over aortic, iliac, renal, and femoral arteries	Abnormality of blood flow (requires additional evaluation to determine specific disorder)
Venous hum, low-pitched, continuous sound	Increased collateral circulation between portal and systemic venous systems

LUQ, left upper quadrant; *RUQ*, right upper quadrant.
From Doughty DB, Jackson DB. *Gastrointestinal Disorders.* St. Louis: Mosby; 1993.

TABLE 21-2 Selected Laboratory Studies of Gastrointestinal Function

TEST	NORMAL FINDINGS	CLINICAL SIGNIFICANCE OF ABNORMAL FINDINGS
Stool studies	Resident microorganisms: clostridia, enterococci, *Pseudomonas*, a few yeasts	Detection of *Salmonella typhi* (typhoid fever), *Shigella* (dysentery), *Vibrio cholerae* (cholera), *Yersinia* (enterocolitis), *Escherichia coli* (gastroenteritis), *Staphylococcus aureus* (food poisoning), *Clostridium botulinum* (food poisoning), *Clostridium perfringens* (food poisoning), *Aeromonas* (gastroenteritis)
	Fat: 2-6 g/24 hr	Steatorrhea (increased values) resulting from intestinal malabsorption or pancreatic insufficiency
	Pus: none	Large amounts of pus associated with chronic ulcerative colitis, abscesses, and anorectal fistula
	Occult blood: none (ortho-toluidine or guaiac test)	Positive test results associated with bleeding
	Ova and parasites: none	Detection of *Entamoeba histolytica* (amebiasis), *Giardia lamblia* (giardiasis), and worms
d-Xylose absorption	5-hr urinary excretion: 4.5 g/L Peak blood level: >30 mg/dL	Differentiation of pancreatic steatorrhea (normal d-xylose absorption) from intestinal steatorrhea (impaired d-xylose absorption)
Gastric acid stimulation	11-20 mEq/hr after stimulation	Detection of duodenal ulcers, Zollinger-Ellison syndrome (increased values), gastric atrophy, gastric carcinoma (decreased values)
Manometry*	Values vary at different levels of the intestine.	Inadequate swallowing, motility, sphincter function
Culture and sensitivity of duodenal contents	No pathogens	Detection of *Salmonella typhi* (typhoid fever)
Breath tests		
Glucose or d-xylose breath test	Negative for hydrogen or carbon dioxide	May indicate intestinal bacterial overgrowth
Urea breath test	Negative for isotopically labeled carbon dioxide	Presence of *Helicobacter pylori* infection
Lactose breath test	Negative for exhaled hydrogen	Lactose intolerance

*Use of water-filled catheters connected to pressure transducers passed into the esophagus, stomach, colon, or rectum to evaluate contractility.
From McCance KL, et al, eds. *Pathophysiology: The biologic basis for disease in adults and children.* 7th ed. St Louis: Elsevier; 2014.

TABLE 21-3 Common Laboratory Studies Of Liver Function

TEST	NORMAL VALUE	INTERPRETATION
Serum Enzymes		
Alkaline phosphatase	13-39 units/L	Increases with biliary obstruction and cholestatic hepatitis
Gamma-glutamyltranspeptidase (GGT)	Male 12-38 units/L Female 9-31 units/L	Increases with biliary obstruction and cholestatic hepatitis
Aspartate aminotransferase (AST; previously serum glutamate-oxaloacetate transaminase [SGOT])	5-40 units/L	Increases with hepatocellular injury (and injury in other tissues, i.e., skeletal and cardiac muscle)
Alanine aminotransferase (ALT; previously serum glutamate-pyruvate transaminase [SGPT])	5-35 units/L	Increases with hepatocellular injury and necrosis
Lactate dehydrogenase (LDH)	90-220 units/L	Isoenzyme LD_5 is elevated with hypoxic and primary liver injury.
5′-Nucleotidase	2-11 units/L	Increases with increase in alkaline phosphatase and cholestatic disorders
Bilirubin Metabolism		
Serum bilirubin		
Unconjugated (indirect)	<0.8 mg/dl	Increases with hemolysis (lysis of red blood cells)
Conjugated (direct)	0.2-0.4 mg/dl	Increases with hepatocellular injury or obstruction
Total	<1.0 mg/dl	Increases with biliary obstruction
Urine bilirubin	0	Increases with biliary obstruction
Urine urobilinogen	0-4 mg/24 hr	Increases with hemolysis or shunting of portal blood flow
Serum Proteins		
Albumin	3.5-5.5 g/dl	Reduced with hepatocellular injury
Globulin	2.5-3.5 g/dl	Increases with hepatitis
Total	6-7 g/dl	
Albumin/globulin (A/G) ratio	1.5:1 to 2.5:1	Ratio reverses with chronic hepatitis or other chronic liver disease.
Transferrin	250-300 mcg/dl	Liver damage with decreased values, iron deficiency with increased values
Alpha fetoprotein (AFP)	6-20 ng/ml	Elevated values in primary hepatocellular carcinoma
Blood-Clotting Functions		
Prothrombin time (PT)	11.5-14 sec or 90-100% of control	Increases with chronic liver disease (cirrhosis) or vitamin K deficiency
Partial thromboplastin time (PTT)	25-40 sec	Increases with severe liver disease or heparin therapy
Bromsulphthalein (BSP) excretion	<6% retention in 45 min	Increased retention with hepatocellular injury

From McCance KL, et al., eds. *Pathophysiology: The biologic basis for disease in adults and children.* 7th ed. St Louis: Elsevier; 2014.

TABLE 21-4 Common Laboratory Studies of Pancreatic Function

TEST	NORMAL VALUE	CLINICAL SIGNIFICANCE
Serum amylase	60-180 Somogyi units/mL	Elevated levels with pancreatic inflammation
Serum lipase	1.5 Somogyi units/mL	Elevated levels with pancreatic inflammation (may be elevated with other conditions; differentiates with amylase isoenzyme study)
Urine amylase	35-260 Somogyi units/hr	Elevated levels with pancreatic inflammation
Secretin test	Volume 1.8 mL/kg/hr Bicarbonate concentration: >80 mEq/L Bicarbonate output: >10 mEq/L/30 sec	Decreased volume with pancreatic disease as secretin stimulates pancreatic secretion
Stool fat	2-5 g/24 hr	Measures fatty acids: decreased pancreatic lipase increases stool fat.

From McCance KL, et al., eds. *Pathophysiology: The biologic basis for disease in adults and children.* 7th ed. St Louis: Elsevier; 2014.

TABLE 21-5 **Gastrointestinal Diagnostic Studies**		
STUDY	**EVALUATES**	**COMMENTS**
Angiography: celiac or mesenteric	• Evaluates portal vasculature • Diagnoses source of GI bleeding • Evaluates cirrhosis, portal hypertension, vascular damage resulting from trauma, intestinal ischemia, and tumors • May be used to treat GI bleeding using vasopressin	• Bowel preparation (e.g., cathartics) as prescribed • NPO for 8 hours prior to the study • Sedative usually is prescribed before the procedure. • If contrast media used: • Check for allergy to iodine prior to the study. • Monitor for allergic reaction following procedure. • Ensure hydration following procedure. Postprocedure: • Keep extremity in which catheter was placed immobilized in a straight position for 6-12 hours. • Monitor arterial puncture point for hemorrhage or hematoma. • Monitor neurovascular status of affected limb. • Monitor for indications of systemic emboli.
Barium enema (also called *lower GI series*) NOTE: Meglumine diatrizoate (Gastrografin) may be used especially if bowel perforation is suspected.	• Visualizes the movement, position, and filling of various segments of the colon after instillation of barium by enema • Diagnoses colorectal lesions, diverticulitis, inflammatory bowel disease, strictures, fistulae • Evaluates colon size, length, and patency	• Low-fiber diet for 1 to 3 days prior to the study • Bowel preparation with bowel irrigation (e.g., GoLYTELY) and cathartics • NPO for 8-12 hours prior to study • Cathartics must be given after study. • Contraindicated if bowel perforation or obstruction exists
Barium swallow, upper GI series, and small bowel follow-through NOTE: Tests are ordered according to which area or areas need to be evaluated (e.g., upper GI with small bowel follow-through means stomach, pylorus, duodenum; barium swallow with upper GI evaluates esophagus, stomach, pylorus). NOTE: Meglumine diatrizoate (Gastrografin) may be used especially if bowel perforation is suspected.	• Visualizes the position, shape, and activity of the esophagus, stomach, duodenum, and jejunum • Diagnoses esophageal lesions, varices, or esophageal motility disorders, hiatal hernia, gastric ulcers and tumors, small bowel obstruction, small bowel lesions, Crohn's disease • Evaluates gastric and small bowel motility	• Bowel preparation with bowel irrigation (e.g., GoLYTELY) and cathartics • NPO for 8-12 hours prior to study • Cathartics must be given after study. • Contraindicated if bowel perforation or obstruction exists
Cholecystography (oral, intravenous, percutaneous transhepatic, or common bile duct)	• Assesses gallbladder function, patency of the biliary system, and presence of gallstones • Diagnoses extrahepatic or intrahepatic jaundice, biliary calculi, biliary obstruction, common bile duct injury	• Percutaneous transhepatic cholangiography is contraindicated in patients with bleeding disorders. • Fatty meal the day before the study, but the evening meal is fat-free • Enema may be given the evening prior to the study. • NPO 8-12 hours prior to the study • Contrast medium is administered orally the evening prior to the study, administered intravenous immediately prior to the study, injected percutaneously into the bile duct, or injected directly into the common bile duct during surgery. • Check for allergy to iodine prior to the study. • Monitor for allergic reaction following procedure. • Ensure hydration following procedure. • Monitor for clinical indications of bile leakage, hemorrhage, or peritonitis after percutaneous transhepatic cholangiography.

TABLE 21-5 Gastrointestinal Diagnostic Studies—cont'd

STUDY	EVALUATES	COMMENTS
Computed tomographic (CT) scan of abdomen	• Diagnoses tumors, pancreatic cancer or cysts, pancreatitis, biliary tract disorders, obstructive versus nonobstructive jaundice, cirrhosis, liver metastases, ascites, lymph node metastases, and aneurysm • Evaluates vasculature and focal points found on nuclear scans • Used to direct biopsy of tumors or aspiration of abscess	• No special preparation required • If contrast medium is used: • Check for allergy to iodine prior to the study. • Monitor for allergic reaction postprocedure. • Ensure hydration postprocedure.
Endoscopic retrograde cholangiopancreatography (ERCP)	• Diagnoses biliary stones, ductal stricture, ductal compression, and neoplasms of the pancreas and biliary system • Evaluates patency of biliary and pancreatic ducts, jaundice, pancreatitis, cholecystitis, and hepatitis	• Same as for esophagogastroduodenoscopy • Contraindicated if patient is uncooperative or if bilirubin is greater than 3.5 mg/dL • Monitor for clinical indications of pancreatitis (most common complication) after study. • Monitor for clinical indications of sepsis.
Endoscopy • Esophagogastroduodenoscopy • Colonoscopy • Proctosigmoidoscopy	• Directly visualizes mucosa of areas of the GI tract • Esophagogastroduodenoscopy can be extended to visualize the pancreas and gallbladder. • Esophagogastroduodenoscopy is used to diagnose esophagitis, esophageal ulcers, esophageal strictures, esophageal varices, hiatal hernia, gastritis, gastric ulcers, pyloric obstruction, pernicious anemia, foreign bodies, duodenal inflammation or ulcers and to evaluate esophageal or gastric motility, bleeding, lesions, and status of surgical anastomoses. • Esophagoscopy or gastroscopy also may be used therapeutically for sclerosis of varices. • Proctosigmoidoscopy diagnoses rectosigmoid cancer, strictures, polyps, inflammatory processes, and hemorrhoids and evaluates bleeding from rectosigmoid, surgical anastomoses. • Colonoscopy diagnoses diverticular disease, obstruction, strictures, radiation injury, polyps, neoplasms, bleeding, ischemia. • Colonoscopy or sigmoidoscopy may be used therapeutically for removal of polyps. • Biopsies may be taken during any endoscopy.	• Sedation may be prescribed, especially for colonoscopy. • Bowel preparation with gastric irrigation (e.g., GoLYTELY) and cathartics required before lower GI endoscopy • NPO 4-8 hours prior to study • Keep NPO until gag reflex returns if sedation used. • Monitor closely after procedure for clinical indications of perforation or hemorrhage.
Flat plate of abdomen (may also be referred to as KUB)	• Diagnoses perforated viscus, paralytic ileus, mechanical obstruction, intraabdominal mass • Evaluates the distribution of visceral gas (and identifies free air in the peritoneum indicative of bowel perforation) • Evaluates organ size	• No preparation required

Continued

TABLE 21-5 Gastrointestinal Diagnostic Studies—cont'd

STUDY	EVALUATES	COMMENTS
Liver biopsy	• Obtains tissue specimen for microscopic evaluation • Diagnoses liver disease or malignancy	• May be performed open or closed • Open is done in surgery. • Closed biopsy may be done at bedside. • Clotting profile is evaluated preprocedure. • Closed biopsy is contraindicated if platelet count is less than 100,000 platelets/mm^3. • Patient must be cooperative because he or she must take a deep breath and hold it for closed biopsy. • Type and crossmatch for two units of blood preprocedure • NPO for 4-8 hours before study Postprocedure • Position patient on right side for 2 hours. • Pressure dressing is applied, and the patient is on bedrest for 24 hours. • Observe for the following: • Hemorrhage: hypotension, dyspnea (subphrenic hematoma) • Pneumothorax: dyspnea; chest pain; diminished breath sounds on right; hypoxemia • Sepsis: fever; leukocytosis; rebound tenderness
Liver scan	• Diagnoses cirrhosis, hepatitis, tumors, abscesses, cysts, tuberculosis	• No preparation required
Magnetic resonance imaging (MRI)	• Evaluates liver, biliary tree, pancreas, spleen • Differentiation between cyst and solid mass • Diagnoses hepatic metastasis • Evaluates abscesses, fistulae, source of GI bleeding • Used for staging of colorectal cancer	• Cannot be used in patients with any implanted metallic device, including pacemakers • No special preparation required • Must be able to lie flat and still for 30-60 minutes during the scan; sedation may be necessary.
Paracentesis	• Analysis of fluid removed during peritoneal tap • Diagnoses intraperitoneal bleeding with diagnostic peritoneal lavage	• Monitor for peritoneal leakage after tap. • Monitor for clinical indications of infection or peritonitis after tap.
Percutaneous transhepatic portography	• Diagnoses esophageal varices and visualizes portal venous circulation	• As for angiography
Percutaneous transhepatic cholangiography	• Diagnoses extrahepatic or intrahepatic jaundice, biliary calculi, bile duct obstruction, bile duct injury • Evaluates the patency of the biliary ductal system	• Contraindicated in uncorrected coagulopathy, allergy to iodine, severe ascites, or cholangitis • Monitor closely for clinical indications of bleeding or peritonitis.
Radionuclide imaging (hepatobiliary scintigraphy) • HIDA scan • PIPIDA scan	• Diagnoses hepatocellular disease, hepatic metastasis, biliary disease, lower GI bleeding, gastric reflux	• NPO 2 hours prior to study
Schilling test	• Evaluates ileal absorption of vitamin B_{12} • Diagnoses pernicious anemia caused by intrinsic factor and inadequate ileal absorption of intrinsic factor-vitamin B_{12} complex	• Intramuscular injections of vitamin B_{12} and oral radioactive B_{12} are given, and 24-hour urine specimen is collected.
Ultrasound of abdomen	• Evaluates the pancreas, biliary ducts, gallbladder, and liver • Identifies tumor, abdominal abscesses, hepatocellular disease, splenomegaly, and pancreatic or splenic cysts • Differentiates obstructive from nonobstructive jaundice	• All barium must have been cleared from the GI tract before ultrasonography. • NPO for 8 hours prior to study • If for evaluation of gallbladder: fat-free meal the evening prior to study • Must be able to lie flat and still for 30 minutes during the procedure

GI, Gastrointestinal; *NPO*, nothing by mouth.
Modified from Dennison RD. *Pass CCRN!* 3rd ed. St Louis: Elsevier; 2013.

priorities include 1) preparing the patient psychologically and physically for the procedure, 2) monitoring the patient's responses to the procedure, and 3) assessing the patient after the procedure. Preparing the patient includes teaching the patient about the procedure, answering any questions, and transporting and positioning the patient for the procedure. Monitoring the patient's responses to the procedure includes observing the patient for signs of pain, anxiety, or hemorrhage and monitoring vital signs. Assessing the patient after the procedure includes observing for complications of the procedure and medicating the patient for any postprocedural discomfort. **Any evidence of gastrointestinal bleeding should be immediately reported to the physician, and emergency measures to maintain circulation must be initiated.**[8]

REFERENCES

1. O'Toole MT: Advanced assessment of the abdomen and gastrointestinal problems, *Nurs Clin North Am* 25:771, 1990.
2. Baid H: The process of conducting a physical assessment: a nursing perspective, *Br J Nurs* 15:710, 2006.
3. Ball JW, et al: *Seidel's Guide to Physical Examination*, ed 8, St Louis, 2015, Elsevier.
4. Barkauskas V, et al: *Health and Physical Assessment*, ed 3, St Louis, 2002, Mosby.
5. Thompson JM, et al: *Mosby's Clinical Nursing*, ed 5, St Louis, 2002, Mosby.
6. O'Hanlon-Nicholas T: Basic assessment series: gastrointestinal system, *Am J Nurs* 98:48, 1998.
7. Baid H: A critical review of auscultating bowel sounds, *Br J Nurs* 18(18):1125, 2009.
8. SGNA: *Gastroenterology Nursing: A Core Curriculum*, ed 4, St. Louis, 2008, Society of Gastroenterology Nurses and Associates.

22 CHAPTER

Gastrointestinal Disorders and Therapeutic Management

Sheryl E. Leary

Be sure to check out the bonus material, including review questions, on the Evolve website at http://evolve.elsevier.com/Urden/priorities/.

ACUTE GASTROINTESTINAL HEMORRHAGE

Description and Etiology

GI hemorrhage is a potentially life-threatening emergency that remains a common complication of critical illness and results in over 300,000 hospital admissions yearly.[1] Despite advances in medical knowledge and nursing care, the mortality rate for patients with acute GI bleeding remains at 10% per annum in the United States.[1]

GI hemorrhage occurs from bleeding in the upper or lower GI tract. The ligament of Treitz is the anatomic division used to differentiate between the two areas. Bleeding proximal to the ligament is considered to be from the upper GI tract, and bleeding distal to the ligament is considered to be from the lower GI tract.[1-3] The various causes of acute GI hemorrhage are listed in Box 22-1.[4] Only the three main causes of GI hemorrhage commonly seen in the critical care unit are discussed further.

Peptic Ulcer Disease

Peptic ulcer disease (i.e., gastric and duodenal ulcers), which results from the breakdown of the gastromucosal lining, is the leading cause of upper GI hemorrhage, accounting for approximately 40% of cases.[5,6] Normally, protection of the gastric mucosa from the digestive effects of gastric secretions is accomplished in several ways. First, the gastroduodenal mucosa is coated by a glycoprotein mucous barrier that protects the surface of the epithelium from hydrogen ions and other noxious substances present in the gut lumen.[6-8] Adequate gastric mucosal blood flow is necessary to maintain this mucosal barrier function. Second, gastroduodenal epithelial cells are protected structurally against damage from acid and pepsin because they are connected by tight junctions that help prevent acid penetration. Third, prostaglandins and nitric oxide protect the mucosal barrier by stimulating the secretion of mucus and bicarbonate and inhibiting the secretion of acid.[6-8]

Peptic ulceration occurs when these protective mechanisms cease to function, allowing gastroduodenal mucosal breakdown. After the mucosal lining is penetrated, gastric secretions autodigest the layers of the stomach or duodenum, leading to injury of the mucosal and submucosal layers. This results in damaged blood vessels and subsequent hemorrhage. The two main causes of disruption of gastroduodenal mucosal resistance are the bacterial action of *Helicobacter pylori* and nonsteroidal antiinflammatory drugs (NSAIDs).[9]

Stress-Related Mucosal Disease

Stress-related mucosal disease (SRMD) is an acute erosive gastritis that covers both types of mucosal lesions that are often found in the critically ill patient: stress-related injury and discrete stress ulcers.[10-12] Additional terms used to describe this condition include *stress ulcers, stress erosions, stress gastritis, hemorrhagic gastritis,* and *erosive gastritis.* These abnormalities develop within hours of admission.[11] They range from superficial mucosal erosions to deep focal lesions and usually affect the upper GI tract.[11] SRMD occurs by means of the same pathophysiologic mechanisms as peptic ulcer disease, but the main cause of disruption of gastric mucosal resistance is increased acid production and decreased mucosal blood flow, resulting in ischemia and degeneration of the mucosal lining.[11] Patients at risk include those in situations of high physiologic stress, as occurs with mechanical ventilation, extensive burns, severe trauma, major surgery, shock, sepsis, coagulopathy, or acute neurologic disease.[13] SRMD is decreasing in incidence because of advances in therapeutic techniques and prevention of hypoperfusion of the mucosa.[14]

Esophagogastric Varices

Esophagogastric varices are engorged and distended blood vessels of the esophagus and proximal stomach that develop as a result of portal hypertension caused by hepatic cirrhosis, a chronic disease of the liver, which results in damage to the liver sinusoids (Figure 22-1). Without adequate sinusoid function, resistance to portal blood flow is increased, and pressures within the liver are elevated. This leads to increased portal venous pressure (portal hypertension), causing collateral circulation to divert portal blood from areas of high pressure within the liver to adjacent areas of low pressure outside the liver, such as into the veins of the esophagus, the spleen, the intestines, and the stomach. The tiny, thin-walled vessels of the esophagus and proximal stomach that receive this diverted blood lack sturdy mucosal protection. The vessels become engorged and dilated, forming esophagogastric varices that are vulnerable to damage from gastric secretions and that may result in subsequent rupture and massive hemorrhage.[15] The risk of variceal bleeding increases with

BOX 22-1 Causes of Acute Gastrointestinal Hemorrhage

UPPER GASTROINTESTINAL TRACT	LOWER GASTROINTESTINAL TRACT
• Peptic ulcer disease	• Diverticulosis
• Stress-related erosive syndrome	• Angiodysplasia
• Esophagogastric varices	• Neoplasm
• Mallory-Weiss tear	• Inflammatory bowel disease
• Esophagitis	• Trauma
• Neoplasm	• Infectious colitis
• Aortoenteric fistula	• Radiation colitis
• Angiodysplasia	• Ischemia
	• Aortoenteric fistula
	• Hemorrhoids

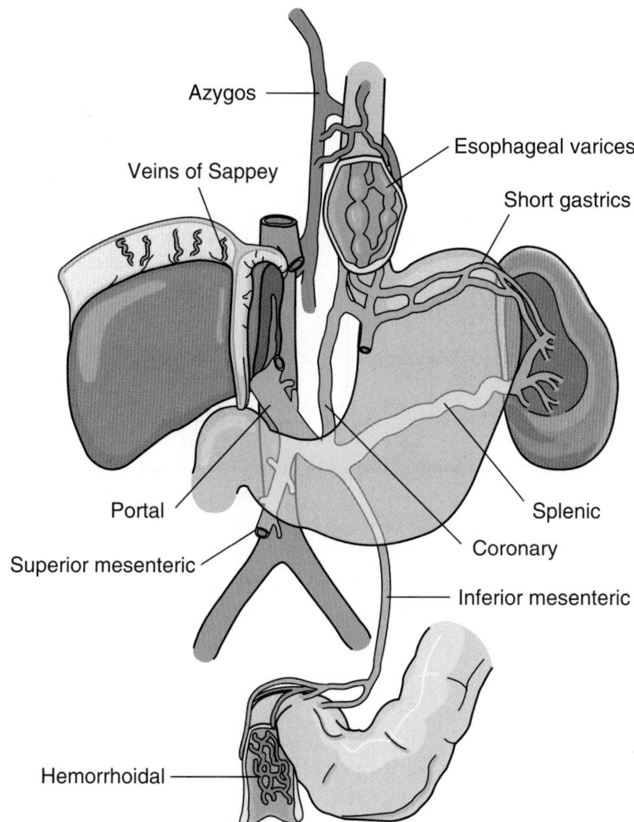

FIG 22-1 Varices Related to Portal Hypertension. Portal vein, its major tributaries, and the most important shunts (collateral veins) between the portal and caval systems. (From Monahan FD, et al. *Phipps' Medical-Surgical Nursing: Concepts and Clinical Practice.* 8th ed. St. Louis: Mosby; 2007.)

disease severity and variceal size, but overall, bleeding occurs in 25% to 30% of patients within 2 years of diagnosis, and 20% to 30% mortality from each bleeding episode.[16,17]

Pathophysiology

GI hemorrhage is a life-threatening disorder that is characterized by acute, massive bleeding. Regardless of the cause, acute GI hemorrhage results in hypovolemic shock, initiation of the shock response, and development of multiple organ dysfunction syndrome if left untreated (Figure 22-2).[7] However, the most common cause of death in cases of GI hemorrhage is exacerbation of the underlying disease, not intractable hypovolemic shock.

TABLE 22-1 Clinical Classification of Hemorrhage

CLASS	BLOOD LOSS (%)	CLINICAL SIGNS AND SYMPTOMS
1	≤15	Pulse rate: normal or <100 beats/min (supine) Capillary refill <3 seconds Urine output: adequate (30-35 mL/hr) Orthostatic hypotension Apprehensive
2	15-30	Pulse rate: increased (>100 beats/min) Capillary refill: sluggish Pulse pressure: decreased Blood pressure: normal (supine) Tachypnea Urine output: low (25-30 mL/hr)
3	30-40	Pulse rate: 120+ beats/min (supine) Hypotension Skin: cool, pale Confused Hyperventilating Urine output: low (5-15 mL/hr)
4	≥40	Profoundly hypotensive Pulse rate: 140+ beats/min Confused, lethargic Urine output minimal

From Klein DG. Physiologic response to traumatic shock. *AACN Clin Issues Crit Care Nurs.* 1990: 1:505.

Assessment and Diagnosis

The initial clinical presentation of the patient with acute GI hemorrhage is that of a patient in hypovolemic shock, and the clinical presentation depends on the amount of blood lost (Table 22-1).[7] Hematemesis (bright red or brown, "coffee grounds" emesis), hematochezia (bright red stools), and melena (black, tarry, or dark red stools) are the hallmarks of GI hemorrhage.[5,18]

Hematemesis

The patient who is vomiting blood is usually bleeding from a source above the duodenojejunal junction; reverse peristalsis is seldom sufficient to cause hematemesis if the bleeding point is below this area. The hematemesis may be bright red or look like coffee grounds, depending on the amount of gastric contents at the time of bleeding and the length of time the blood has been in contact with gastric secretions. Gastric acid converts bright red hemoglobin to brown hematin, accounting for the coffee grounds appearance of the emesis. Bright red emesis results from profuse bleeding with little contact with gastric secretions.[19]

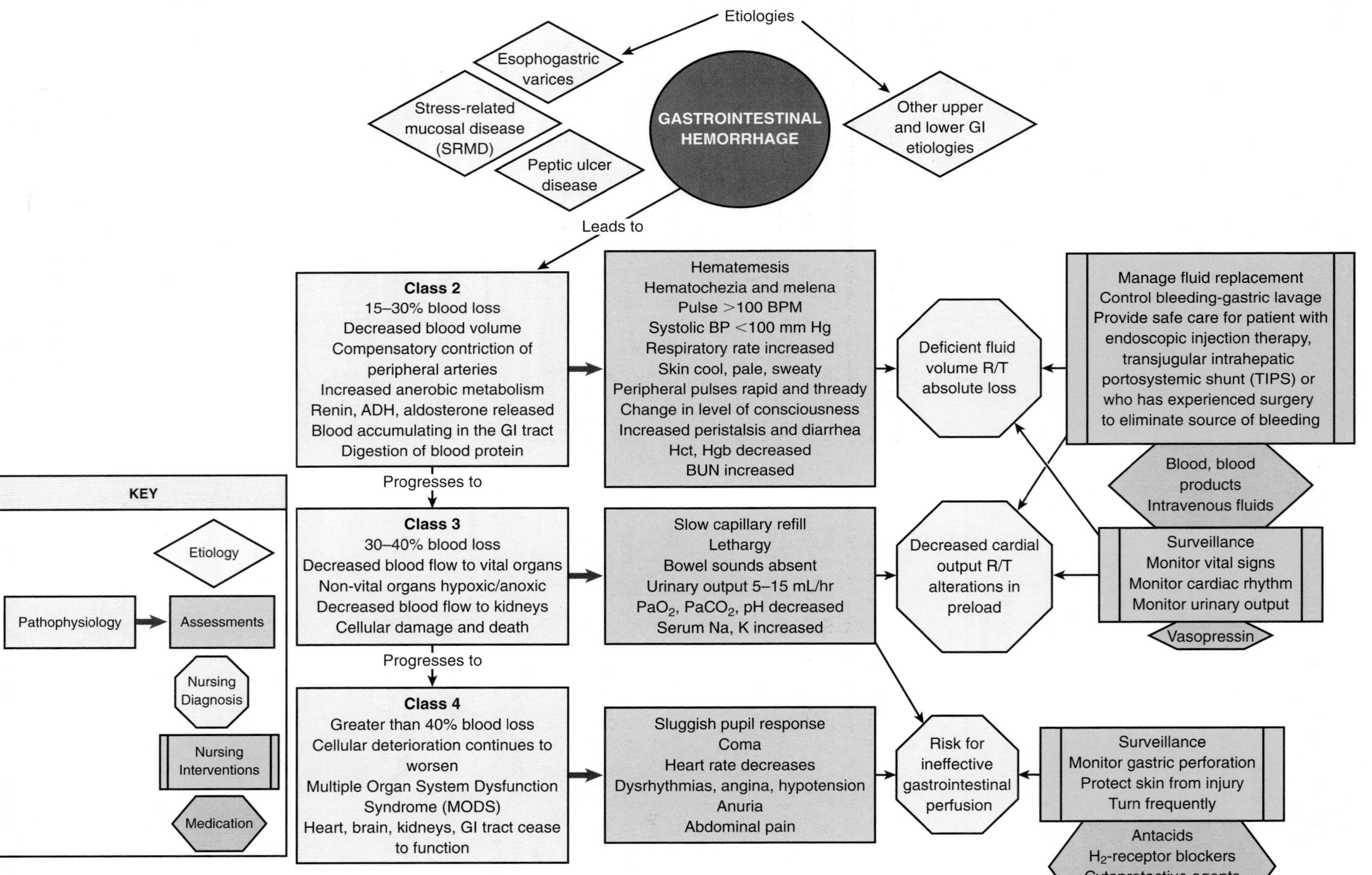

FIG 22-2 Concept Map for Gastrointestinal Hemorrhage. (Illustrated by Elaine B. Kennedy, EdD, RN.)

Hematochezia and Melena

The presence of blood in the GI tract results in increased peristalsis and diarrhea. Hematochezia occurs from massive lower GI hemorrhage and, if rapid enough, upper GI hemorrhage. Melena occurs from digestion of blood from an upper GI hemorrhage and may take several days to clear after the bleeding has stopped.

Laboratory Studies

Laboratory tests can help determine the extent of bleeding, although the patient's hemoglobin level and hematocrit are poor indicators of the severity of blood loss if the bleeding is acute. As whole blood is lost, plasma and red blood cells are lost in the same proportion; if the patient's hematocrit is 45% before a bleeding episode, it will be 45% several hours later.[7] It may take 24 to 72 hours for the redistribution of plasma from the extravascular space to the intravascular space to occur and cause the patient's hemoglobin level and hematocrit value to decrease.[19]

Diagnostic Procedures

To isolate and treat the source of bleeding, an urgent fiberoptic endoscopy is usually undertaken.[20] Before endoscopy, the patient must be hemodynamically stabilized.[21] Tagged red blood cell scanning, angiography, or both may be done to assist with localizing and treating a bleeding lesion in the GI tract when it is impossible to view the GI tract clearly because of continued active bleeding.[19]

Medical Management

To reduce mortality related to GI hemorrhage, patients at risk should be identified early, and interventions should be implemented to reduce gastric acidity and support the gastric mucosal defense mechanisms. Management of the patient at risk for GI hemorrhage should include prophylactic administration of pharmacologic agents for neutralization of gastric acids. These agents include antacids, histamine-2 (H_2) antagonists, cytoprotective agents, and proton pump inhibitors (PPIs).[5,22] Priorities in the medical management of the patient with GI hemorrhage include airway protection, fluid resuscitation to achieve hemodynamic stability, correction of co-morbid conditions (e.g., coagulopathy), therapeutic procedures to control or stop bleeding, and diagnostic procedures to determine the exact cause of the bleeding.[5,21]

Stabilization

The initial treatment priority is the restoration of adequate circulating blood volume to treat or prevent shock. This is accomplished with the administration of intravenous infusions of crystalloids, blood, and blood products.[22] Hemodynamic monitoring can help guide fluid replacement therapy, particularly in patients at risk for heart failure.[7] Supplemental oxygen therapy is initiated to increase oxygen delivery and improve tissue perfusion.[7,22] A large nasogastric tube may be inserted to confirm the diagnosis of active bleeding, to facilitate gastric lavage, decrease the risk for aspiration and to prepare the esophagus, stomach, and proximal duodenum for endoscopic evaluation.[5]

Controlling the Bleeding

Interventions to control bleeding are the second priority for the patient with GI hemorrhage.

Peptic ulcer disease. In the patient with GI hemorrhage related to peptic ulcer disease, bleeding hemostasis may be accomplished by endoscopic injection therapy in conjunction with thermal or hemostatic clips.[20] Endoscopic thermal therapy uses heat to cauterize the bleeding vessel, and endoscopic injection therapy uses a variety of agents such as hypertonic saline, epinephrine, ethanol, and sclerosants to induce localized vasoconstriction of the bleeding vessel.[6] Intraarterial infusion of vasopressin into the gastric artery or intraarterial injection of an embolizing agent (e.g., Gelfoam pledgets, polyvinyl alcohol particles, coils) can be performed during arteriography to control bleeding after the site has been identified.[19]

Stress-related mucosal disease. In the patient with GI hemorrhage caused by SRMD, bleeding hemostasis may be accomplished by intraarterial infusion of vasopressin and intraarterial embolization. Endoscopic therapies provide minimal benefit because of the diffuse nature of the disease.[19]

Esophagogastric varices. In acute variceal hemorrhage, control of bleeding may be initially accomplished through the use of pharmacologic agents and endoscopic therapies. Intravenous vasopressin, somatostatin, and octreotide can reduce portal venous pressure and slow variceal hemorrhaging by constricting the splanchnic arteriolar bed.[16] Two commonly used endoscopic therapies are endoscopic injection sclerotherapy (EIS) and endoscopic variceal ligation (EVL).[23] EIS controls bleeding by the injection of a sclerosing agent in or around the varices. This creates an inflammatory reaction that induces vasoconstriction and results in the formation of a venous thrombosis. During EVL, bands are placed around the varices to create an obstruction to stop the bleeding.[24]

If these initial therapies fail, transjugular intrahepatic portosystemic shunting (TIPS) may be necessary. In a TIPS procedure, a channel between the systemic and portal venous systems is created to redirect portal blood, thereby reducing portal hypertension and decompressing the varices to control bleeding (Figure 22-3).[23,24]

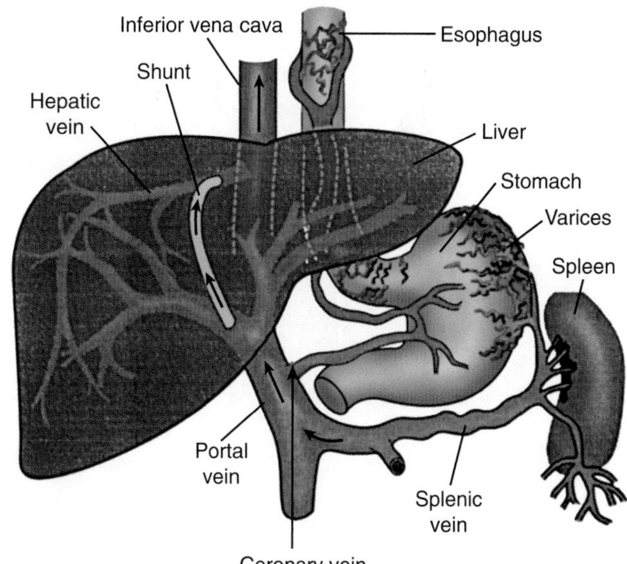

FIG 22-3 Anatomic Location of the Transjugular Intrahepatic Portosystemic Shunt (TIPS). (From Vargas HE, et al. Management of portal hypertension-related bleeding. *Surg Clin North Am.* 1999;79:1.)

Surgical Intervention

The patient who remains hemodynamically unstable despite volume replacement may need urgent surgery.

Peptic ulcer disease. Surgical intervention is required to control bleeding in a minority of patients.[25] The operative procedure of choice to control bleeding from peptic ulcer disease is a vagotomy and pyloroplasty. During this procedure, the vagus nerve to the stomach is severed, eliminating the autonomic stimulus to the gastric cells and reducing hydrochloric acid production. Because the vagus nerve also stimulates motility, a pyloroplasty is performed to provide for gastric emptying.[26]

Stress-related mucosal disease. In the past, several operative procedures were used to control bleeding from SRMD. Because of the advent of stress ulcer prophylaxis, a marked decrease occurs in the incidence of hemorrhage from SRMD.[22]

Esophagogastric varices. If medical treatment is unsuccessful and angiographic interventional TIPS procedure is not available, operative procedures to control bleeding gastroesophageal varices may be undertaken. Though rarely performed, operative interventions focus on some form of shunting (Figure 22-4).[25] These shunt procedures are also referred to as decompression procedures because they result in the diversion of portal blood flow away from the liver and decompression of the portal system. The portacaval shunt procedure has two variations: 1) an end-to-side portacaval shunt procedure, which involves the ligation of the hepatic end of the portal vein with subsequent anastomosis to the vena cava, and 2) a side-to-side portacaval shunt procedure, during which the side of the portal vein is anastomosed to the side of the vena cava. A mesocaval shunt procedure involves the insertion of a graft between the superior mesenteric artery and the vena cava. During a distal splenorenal shunt procedure, the splenic vein is detached from the portal vein and anastomosed to the left renal vein.[27]

Nursing Management

All critically ill patients should be considered at risk for stress ulcers and, therefore, GI hemorrhage. Routine assessment of gastric fluid pH monitoring is controversial.[12,28] Maintaining the pH between 3.5 and 4.5 is a goal of prophylactic therapy. Gastric pH measurements made with litmus paper or direct nasogastric tube probes may be used to assess gastric fluid pH and the effectiveness or need for prophylactic agents.[28] Patients at risk also should be assessed for the presence of bright red or coffee grounds emesis, bloody nasogastric aspirate, and bright red, black, or dark red stools.[4] Any signs of bleeding should be promptly reported to the physician.

Nursing management of a patient experiencing acute GI hemorrhage incorporates a variety of nursing diagnoses (Box 22-2). **Nursing priorities are directed toward 1)**

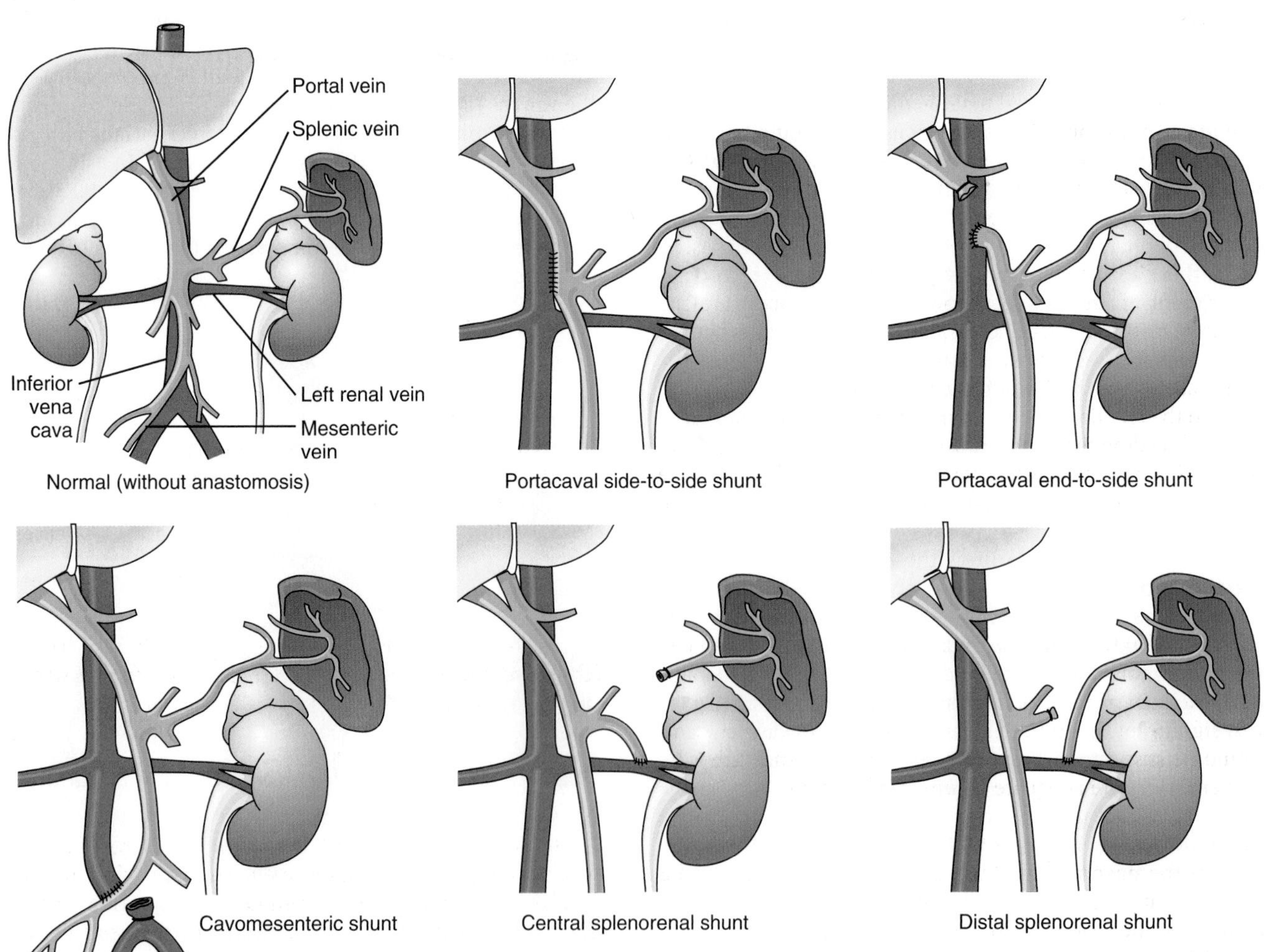

FIG 22-4 **Portosystemic Shunt Operative Procedures.** (From Copstead LC, Banasik JL. *Pathophysiology.* 4th ed. St. Louis: Saunders; 2010.)

 BOX 22-2 **NURSING DIAGNOSIS PRIORITIES**

Acute Gastrointestinal Hemorrhage

- Deficient Fluid Volume, related to absolute loss, p. 583
- Decreased Cardiac Output, related to alterations in preload, p. 579
- Imbalanced Nutrition: Less Than Body Requirements, related to lack of exogenous nutrients and increased metabolic demand, p. 593
- Powerlessness, related to health care environment or illness-related regimen, p. 600
- Deficient Knowledge, related to lack of previous exposure to information, p. 585 (see Patient Education, Box 22-3)

administering volume replacement, 2) controlling the bleeding, 3) providing comfort and emotional support, 4) maintaining surveillance for complications, and 5) educating the patient and family.

Administering Volume Replacement

Measures to facilitate volume replacement include obtaining intravenous access and administering prescribed fluids and blood products. Two large-diameter peripheral intravenous catheters should be inserted to facilitate the rapid administration of prescribed fluids.[1]

Controlling the Bleeding

One measure to control active bleeding is gastric lavage. It is used to decrease gastric mucosal blood flow and evacuate blood from the stomach. Gastric lavage is performed by inserting a large-bore nasogastric tube into the stomach and irrigating it with normal saline or water until the returned solution is clear. It is important to keep accurate records of the amount of fluid instilled and aspirated to ascertain the true amount of bleeding.[1] Historically, iced saline was favored as a lavage irrigant. Research has shown, however, that low-temperature fluids shift the oxyhemoglobin dissociation curve to the left, decrease oxygen delivery to vital organs, and prolong bleeding time and prothrombin time. Iced saline also may further aggravate bleeding; therefore, room-temperature water or saline is the preferred irrigant for use in gastric lavage.[29]

Maintaining Surveillance for Complications

The patient should be continuously observed for signs of gastric perforation. Although a rare complication, gastric perforation constitutes a surgical emergency. Signs and symptoms include sudden, severe, generalized abdominal pain with significant rebound tenderness and rigidity. Perforation should be suspected when fever, leukocytosis, and tachycardia persist despite adequate volume replacement.[30]

Educating the Patient and Family

Early in the hospital stay, the patient and family should be taught about acute GI hemorrhage and its causes and treatments. As the patient moves toward discharge, teaching should focus on the interventions necessary for preventing the recurrence of the precipitating disorder. If an alcohol abuser, the patient should be encouraged to stop drinking and

BOX 22-3 **PATIENT EDUCATION PRIORITIES**

Acute Gastrointestinal Hemorrhage

- Gastrointestinal hemorrhage
- Specific cause
- Precipitating factor modification
- Interventions to reduce further bleeding episodes
- Importance of taking medications
- Lifestyle changes
- Stress management
- Diet modifications
- Alcohol cessation
- Smoking cessation

Additional information for the patient can be found at the following websites:

- Alcoholics Anonymous: http://www.aa.org
- International Foundation for Functional Gastrointestinal Disorders: http://www.iffgd.org
- Healthfinder—U.S. Department of Health and Human Services: http://healthfinder.gov
- Web MD: http://www.webmd.com

BOX 22-4 **COLLABORATIVE MANAGEMENT**

Acute Gastrointestinal Hemorrhage

- Initiate fluid resuscitation to achieve hemodynamic stability.
  - Crystalloids
  - Colloids
  - Blood and blood products
- Determine the cause of the bleeding.
  - Gastric lavage
- Control bleeding.
  - Endoscopic interventions
  - Vasopressin, somatostatin, octreotide
  - Transjugular intrahepatic portosystemic shunting
  - Surgery (last resort)
- Provide comfort and emotional support.
- Maintain surveillance for complications.
  - Hypovolemic shock
  - Gastric perforation

be referred to an alcohol cessation program (Box 22-3). Collaborative management of the patient with acute GI hemorrhage is outlined in Box 22-4.

ACUTE PANCREATITIS

Description and Etiology

Acute pancreatitis is an inflammation of the pancreas that produces exocrine and endocrine dysfunction that may also involve surrounding tissues, remote organ systems, or both. The clinical course can range from a mild, self-limiting disease to a systemic process characterized by organ failure, sepsis, and death. In approximately 80% of patients, it takes the milder form of *edematous interstitial pancreatitis*, whereas

BOX 22-5 Ranson's Criteria for Estimating the Severity of Acute Pancreatitis

At Admission
- Age >55 years
- Hypotension
- Abnormal pulmonary findings
- Abdominal mass
- Hemorrhagic or discolored peritoneal fluid
- Increased serum LDH levels (>350 units/L)
- AST >250 units/L
- Leukocytosis (>16,000/mm^3)
- Hyperglycemia (>200 mg/dL; no diabetes history)
- Neurologic deficit (confusion, localizing signs)

During Initial 48 Hours of Hospitalization
- Fall in hematocrit >10% with hydration or hematocrit <30%
- Necessity for massive fluid and colloid replacement
- Hypocalcemia (<8 mg/dL)
- Arterial PO_2 <60 mm Hg with or without acute respiratory distress syndrome
- Hypoalbuminemia (<3.2 mg/dL)
- Base deficit >4 mEq/L
- Azotemia

AST, Aspartate aminotransferase; *LDH*, lactate dehydrogenase; *PO_2*, partial pressure of oxygen.
From Latifi R, et al. Nutritional management of acute and chronic pancreatitis. *Surg Clin North Am.* 1991: 71:583.

BOX 22-6 Causes of Acute Pancreatitis
- Biliary disease (stones, sludge, common bile duct obstruction)
- Toxins (ethyl alcohol, methyl alcohol, scorpion venom, parathion)
- Smoking
- Medications
- Hypercalcemia (hyperparathyroidism)
- Hyperlipidemia
- Tumors
- Infections (bacterial, viral, parasitic)
- Trauma (abdominal, surgical, endoscopic)
- Hypoperfusion
- Vasculitis
- Pregnancy
- Hypothermia
- Sphincter of Oddi dysfunction
- Autoimmune diseases
- Ampullary stenosis
- Idiopathic cause

the other 20% develop severe *acute necrotizing pancreatitis.*[31] Reported mortality rates for acute pancreatitis range from 2% to 15% overall, with a steadily increasing rate of about 20,000 deaths per year in the United States.[32,33] Several prognostic scoring systems have been developed to predict the severity of acute pancreatitis. One of the most commonly used is Ranson criteria[34] (Box 22-5). If the patient has 0 to 2 factors present, the predicted mortality rate is 2%; with 3 to 4 factors, the rate is 15%; with 5 to 6 factors, the rate is 40%; and with 7 to 8 factors, predicted mortality rate is 100%.[34-36]

The two most common causes of acute pancreatitis are gallstone migration and alcoholism.[36] Together, they account for approximately 80% of cases.[19] Less common causes are quite diverse and include surgical trauma, hypercalcemia, various toxins, ischemia, infections, and the use of certain medications (Box 22-6). In up to 20% of patients with acute pancreatitis, no etiologic factor can be determined.[19,31]

Pathophysiology

In acute pancreatitis, the normally inactive digestive enzymes become prematurely activated within the pancreas itself, leading to autodigestion of pancreatic tissue. The enzymes become activated through various mechanisms, including obstruction of or damage to the pancreatic duct system, alterations in the secretory processes of the acinar cells, infection, ischemia, and other unknown factors.[7,36]

Trypsin is the enzyme that becomes activated first. It initiates the autodigestion process by triggering the secretion of proteolytic enzymes such as kallikrein, chymotrypsin, elastase, phospholipase A, and lipase. Release of kallikrein and chymotrypsin results in increased capillary membrane permeability, leading to leakage of fluid into the interstitium and the development of edema and relative hypovolemia. Elastase is the most harmful enzyme in terms of direct cell damage. It dissolves the elastic fibers of blood vessels and ducts, leading to hemorrhage. Phospholipase A, in the presence of bile, destroys the phospholipids of cell membranes, causing severe pancreatic and adipose tissue necrosis. Lipase flows into the damaged tissue and is absorbed into the systemic circulation, resulting in fat necrosis of the pancreas and surrounding tissues.[7,37]

The extent of injury to the pancreatic cells determines the type of acute pancreatitis that develops. If injury to the pancreatic cells is mild and without necrosis, edematous pancreatitis develops. The acinar cells appear structurally intact, and blood flow is maintained through small capillaries and venules. This form of acute pancreatitis is self-limiting. If injury to the pancreatic cells is severe, acute necrotizing pancreatitis develops.[32,37] Cellular destruction in pancreatic injury results in the release of toxic enzymes and inflammatory mediators into the systemic circulation and causes injury to vessels and other organs distant from the pancreas; this may result in systemic inflammatory response syndrome (SIRS), multiorgan failure, and death.[19,36] Local tissue injury results in infection, abscess and pseudocyst formation, disruption of the pancreatic duct, and severe hemorrhage and shock.[19]

Assessment and Diagnosis

The clinical manifestations of acute pancreatitis range from mild to severe and often mimic those of other disorders (Box 22-7). Acute onset of abdominal pain, nausea, and vomiting are hallmark symptoms.[19,32,37] Epigastric to periumbilical pain may vary from mild and tolerable to severe and incapacitating. Many patients report a twisting or knifelike sensation that radiates to the low dorsal region of the back. The patient may obtain some comfort by leaning forward or assuming a semifetal position. Other clinical findings include fever, diaphoresis, weakness, tachypnea, hypotension, and tachycardia.

BOX 22-7 Presenting Clinical Manifestations of Acute Pancreatitis

- Pain
- Vomiting
- Nausea
- Fever
- Abdominal distention
- Abdominal guarding
- Abdominal tympany
- Hypoactive or absent bowel sounds
- Severe disease
- Peritoneal signs
- Ascites
- Jaundice
- Palpable abdominal mass
- Grey Turner sign
- Cullen sign
- Signs of hypovolemic shock

From Krumberger JM. Acute pancreatitis. *Crit Care Nurs Clin North Am.* 1993: 5:185.

Depending on the extent of fluid loss and hemorrhage, the patient may exhibit signs of hypovolemic shock.[19,37]

The results of physical assessment usually reveal hypoactive bowel sounds and abdominal tenderness, guarding, distention, and tympany. Findings that may indicate pancreatic hemorrhage include Grey Turner sign (gray-blue discoloration of the flanks) and Cullen sign (discoloration of the umbilical region); however, they are rare and usually seen several days into the illness.[19] A palpable abdominal mass indicates the presence of a pseudocyst or abscess.[19]

Laboratory Studies

Assessment of laboratory data usually demonstrates elevated levels of serum amylase and lipase. Serum lipase is more pancreas-specific than amylase and a more accurate marker for acute pancreatitis. Amylase is present in other body tissues, and other disorders (e.g., intraabdominal emergencies, renal insufficiency, salivary gland trauma, liver disease) may contribute to an elevated level. Unlike other serum enzymes, however, amylase is excreted in urine, and this clearance increases with acute pancreatitis. Measurement of urinary versus serum amylase should be considered in light of the patient's creatinine clearance. The serum amylase level may be elevated for only 3 to 5 days; if the patient delays seeking treatment, a normal level (false-negative result) may be detected. A marker of severity may be determined with a serum cross-reactive (C-reactive) protein level.[19,38] Leukocytosis, hypocalcemia, hyperglycemia, hyperbilirubinemia, and hypoalbuminemia may also be present (Table 22-2).[19,36,38]

Diagnostic Procedures

An abdominal ultrasound scan is obtained as part of the diagnostic evaluation to determine the presence of biliary stones. Contrast-enhanced computed tomography (CT) is considered the gold standard for diagnosing pancreatitis and for ascertaining the overall degree of pancreatic inflammation and necrosis.[19,32]

TABLE 22-2 Laboratory Tests and Diagnostic Procedures for Acute Pancreatitis

STUDY	FINDING IN PANCREATITIS
Laboratory Studies	
Serum amylase	Elevated
Serum isoamylase	Elevated
Urine amylase	Elevated
Serum lipase (if available)	Elevated
Serum triglycerides	Elevated
Cross-reactive protein	Elevated
Glucose	Elevated
Calcium	Decreased
Magnesium	Decreased
Potassium	Decreased
Albumin	Decreased or increased
White blood cell count	Elevated
Bilirubin	May be elevated
Liver enzymes	May be elevated
Prothrombin time	Prolonged
Arterial blood gases	Hypoxemia, metabolic acidosis
Diagnostic Procedures	
• Abdominal ultrasonography	
• Computed tomography scan	
• Magnetic resonance imaging	
• Endoscopic retrograde cholangiopancreatography	
• Abdominal radiographs (flat plate and upright or decubitus)	
• Chest radiographs (posteroanterior and lateral)	

Modified from Krumberger JM. Acute pancreatitis. *Crit Care Nurs Clin North Am.* 1993: 5:185.

Medical Management

Initial management of the patient with severe acute pancreatitis includes ensuring adequate fluid and electrolyte replacement, providing nutritional support, and correcting metabolic alterations.[35] Careful monitoring for systemic and local complications is critical.

Fluid Management

Because pancreatitis is often associated with massive fluid shifts, intravenous crystalloids and colloids are administered immediately to prevent hypovolemic shock and maintain hemodynamic stability. Electrolytes are monitored closely, and abnormalities such as hypocalcemia, hypokalemia, and hypomagnesemia are corrected.[37] If hyperglycemia develops, exogenous insulin may be required.

Nutritional Support

Over the past three decades, nutritional support has shifted. Previously, conventional nutritional management was to place the patient on a nothing-by-mouth (NPO) regimen and institute intravenous hydration. The rationale was to rest the inflamed pancreas and prevent enzyme release. Enteral or parenteral support should be initiated if oral intake is withheld more than 5 to 7 days.[39] Randomized clinical trials have demonstrated that enteral feeding (gastric or jejunal) is safe and cost-effective and that it is associated with fewer septic and metabolic complications than other methods.[40-42] Enteral feeding enhances immune modulation and maintenance of the intestinal barrier, and it avoids complications associated with parenteral nutrition. Early initiation of enteral feeding is preferred over TPN.[39] However, TPN still has a role for the critically ill patient with acute pancreatitis who does not tolerate enteral feeding or when nutritional goals are not reached within 2 days.[37,41,42] In the past, nasogastric suction was also recommended, but this intervention has not been shown to be beneficial and should be instituted only if the patient has persistent vomiting, obstruction, or gastric distention.[37]

Systemic Complications

Acute pancreatitis can affect every organ system, and recognition and treatment of systemic complications are crucial to management of the patient (Box 22-8). The most serious complications are hypovolemic shock, acute respiratory distress syndrome (ARDS), acute kidney injury (AKI), and GI hemorrhage. Hypovolemic shock is the result of relative hypovolemia resulting from third spacing of intravascular volume and vasodilation caused by the release of inflammatory immune mediators. These mediators also contribute to the development of ARDS and AKI. Other possible pulmonary complications include pleural effusions, atelectasis, and pneumonia.[37]

Local Complications

Local complications include the development of infected pancreatic necrosis and pancreatic pseudocyst.[19,32,38] The necrotic areas of the pancreas can lead to development of a widespread pancreatic infection (infected pancreatic necrosis), which significantly increases the risk of death.

Prophylactic antibiotics may not reduce mortality in patients suspected of having necrotizing pancreatitis.[43] The use of IV antibiotics should not be used prophylactically but if sepsis, abscess, or biliary calculi are evident.[37] After the patient develops infected necrosis, however, surgical debridement is necessary.[36] The procedure of choice is a minimally invasive necrosectomy, which entails careful debridement of the necrotic tissue in and around the pancreas. A pancreatic pseudocyst is a collection of pancreatic fluid enclosed by a nonepithelialized wall. Cyst formation may result from liquefaction of a pancreatic fluid collection or from direct obstruction in the main pancreatic duct.[37] A pancreatic pseudocyst may 1) resolve spontaneously; 2) rupture, resulting in peritonitis; 3) erode a major blood vessel, resulting in hemorrhage; 4) become infected, resulting in abscess, or 5) invade surrounding structures, resulting in obstruction. Treatment involves drainage of the pseudocyst surgically, endoscopically, or percutaneously.[36,37,44]

Nursing Management

Nursing management of the patient with pancreatitis incorporates a variety of nursing diagnoses (Box 22-9). **Nursing priorities are directed toward 1) providing comfort and emotional support, 2) maintaining surveillance for complications, and 3) educating the patient and family.**

BOX 22-8 Complications of Acute Pancreatitis

Respiratory
- Early hypoxemia
- Pleural effusion
- Atelectasis
- Pulmonary infiltration
- Acute respiratory distress syndrome
- Mediastinal abscess

Cardiovascular
- Hypotension and shock
- Pericardial effusion
- ST-T changes

Renal
- Acute tubular necrosis
- Oliguria
- Renal artery or vein thrombosis

Hematologic
- Disseminated intravascular coagulation
- Thrombocytosis
- Hyperfibrinogenemia

Endocrine
- Hypocalcemia
- Hypertriglyceridemia
- Hyperglycemia

Neurologic
- Fat emboli
- Psychosis
- Encephalopathy and coma

Ophthalmic
- Purtscher's retinopathy (sudden blindness)

Dermatologic
- Subcutaneous fat necrosis

Gastrointestinal or Hepatic
- Hepatic dysfunction
- Obstructive jaundice
- Stress ulceration
- Erosive gastritis
- Paralytic ileus
- Duodenal obstruction
- Pancreatic
  - Pseudocyst
  - Phlegmon
  - Abscess
  - Ascites
- Bowel infarction
- Massive intraperitoneal bleed
- Perforation
  - Stomach
  - Duodenum
  - Small bowel
  - Colon

BOX 22-9 NURSING DIAGNOSIS PRIORITIES

Acute Pancreatitis

- Acute Pain, related to transmission and perception of cutaneous, visceral, muscular, ischemia impulses, p. 574
- Deficient Fluid Volume, related to relative fluid loss, p. 584
- Ineffective Breathing Pattern, related to decreased lung expansion, p. 598
- Anxiety, related to threat to biologic, psychologic, or social integrity, p. 576
- Deficient Knowledge, related to lack of previous exposure to information, p. 585 (see Patient Education, Box 22-10)

Providing Comfort and Emotional Support

Pain management is a major priority in acute pancreatitis. Administration of around-the-clock analgesics to achieve pain relief is essential. Morphine, fentanyl, or hydromorphone are the commonly used narcotics for pain control.[37] Relaxation techniques and the knee-chest position can also assist in pain control.

Maintaining Surveillance for Complications

The patient must be routinely monitored for signs of local or systemic complications (Box 22-8). Intensive monitoring of each of the organ systems is imperative because organ failure is a major indicator of the severity of the disease.[19] The patient must be closely monitored for signs and symptoms of pancreatic infection, which include increased abdominal pain and tenderness, fever, and increased white blood cell count (Box 22-11).[19]

Educating the Patient and Family

Early in the patient's hospital stay, the patient and family should be taught about acute pancreatitis and its causes and treatment. As the patient moves toward discharge, teaching should focus on the interventions necessary for preventing the recurrence of the precipitating disorder. If sustained, permanent damage to the pancreas has occurred, the patient will require teaching specific to diet modification and supplemental pancreatic enzymes. Diabetes education may also be necessary. If an alcohol abuser, the patient should be encouraged to stop drinking and be referred to an alcohol cessation program (Box 22-10). Collaborative management of the patient with pancreatitis is outlined in Box 22-12.

ACUTE LIVER FAILURE

Description and Etiology

Acute liver failure (ALF) is a life-threatening condition characterized by severe and sudden liver cell dysfunction, coagulopathy, and hepatic encephalopathy.[45] Although uncommon, ALF is associated with a mortality rate as high as 40%, and it usually occurs in patients without preexisting liver disease.[45] Because liver transplantation is one of the few definitive treatments, the patient with ALF should be transferred to a critical care unit and strongly considered for referral to a major medical center where transplantation services are available.[45]

BOX 22-10 PATIENT EDUCATION PRIORITIES

Acute Pancreatitis

- Pancreatitis
- Specific cause
- Precipitating factor modification
- Interventions to reduce further episodes
- Importance of taking medications
- Lifestyle changes
- Diet modification
- Stress management
- Alcohol cessation
- Diabetes management, if needed

Additional information for the patient can be found at the following websites:

- The Pancreatitis Association, Inc.: http://pancassociation.org
- Alcoholics Anonymous: http://www.aa.org
- International Foundation for Functional Gastrointestinal Disorders: http://www.iffgd.org
- Healthfinder—U.S. Department of Health and Human Services: http://healthfinder.gov
- Web MD: http://www.webmd.com

BOX 22-11 Signs and Symptoms of Pancreatic Infection

Symptoms
- Persistent abdominal pain
- Abdominal tenderness

Signs
- Prolonged fever
- Abdominal distention
- Palpable abdominal mass
- Vomiting

Diagnostics
- Laboratory findings
  - Increased white blood cell count
  - Persistent elevation of serum amylase
  - Hyperbilirubinemia
  - Elevated alkaline phosphatase level
  - Positive culture and Gram stain
- Radiography or computed tomography findings
  - Pancreatic inflammation or enlargement
  - Necrosis
  - Cystic or mass lesions
  - Fluid accumulations
  - Pseudocyst abscess

Modified from Krumberger JM. Acute pancreatitis. *Crit Care Nurs Clin North Am*. 1993: 5:185.

The causes of ALF include infections, medications, toxins, hypoperfusion, metabolic disorders, and surgery (Box 22-13); however, viral hepatitis and medication-induced liver damage are the predominant causes in North America. Patients are usually healthy before the onset of symptoms because ALF tends to occur in patients with no known liver history. A

BOX 22-12 COLLABORATIVE MANAGEMENT

Acute Pancreatitis

- Ensure adequate circulating volume.
- Provide nutritional support.
- Correct metabolic alterations.
- Minimize pancreatic stimulation.
- Provide comfort and emotional support.
- Maintain surveillance for complications.
  - Multiple organ dysfunction syndrome

thorough medication and health history is imperative to determine a possible cause. The patient should be questioned about exposure to environmental toxins, hepatitis, intravenous drug use, sexual history, viral hepatitis, medication toxicity, and poisoning. Additional vascular causes such as thrombosis, ischemia, and Budd-Chiari syndrome and metabolic disorders such as Reye's syndrome, Wilson disease, galactosemia, and fructose intolerance should be considered.[45]

Pathophysiology

ALF is a syndrome characterized by the development of acute liver failure over 1 to 3 weeks, followed by the development of hepatic encephalopathy within 8 weeks, in a patient with a previously healthy liver. The interval between the failure of the liver and the onset of hepatic encephalopathy usually is less than 2 weeks. The underlying cause is massive necrosis of the hepatocytes.[46]

Acute liver failure results in a number of derangements, including impaired bilirubin conjugation, decreased production of clotting factors, depressed glucose synthesis, and decreased lactate clearance. This results in jaundice, coagulopathies, hypoglycemia, and metabolic acidosis. Other effects of acute liver failure include increased risk of infection and altered carbohydrate, protein, and glucose metabolism. Hypoalbuminemia, fluid and electrolyte imbalances, and acute portal hypertension contribute to the development of ascites.[45] Hepatic encephalopathy is thought to result from failure of the liver to detoxify various substances in the bloodstream, and it may be worsened by metabolic and electrolyte imbalances.[46]

The patient may experience a variety of other complications, including cerebral edema, cardiac dysrhythmias, acute respiratory failure, sepsis, and AKI. Cerebral edema and increased intracranial pressure (ICP) develop as a result of breakdown of the blood–brain barrier and astrocyte swelling. Circulatory failure that mimics sepsis is common in ALF and may exacerbate low cerebral perfusion pressure (CPP).[47] Hypoxemia, acidosis, electrolyte imbalances, and cerebral edema can precipitate the development of cardiac dysrhythmias. Acute respiratory failure, progressing to ARDS, intrapulmonary shunting, ventilation–perfusion mismatch, sepsis, and aspiration may attribute to the universal arterial hypoxemia.[47]

Assessment and Diagnosis

Early recognition of ALF is essential. The diagnosis should include potentially reversible conditions (e.g., autoimmune hepatitis) and should differentiate ALF from decompensating chronic liver disease. Prognostic indicators such as coma grade, serum bilirubin, prothrombin time, coagulation factors, and pH should be assessed and potential causes investigated.[45]

Signs and symptoms of ALF include headache, hyperventilation, jaundice, mental status changes, palmar erythema, spider nevi, bruises, and edema. The patient should be evaluated for the presence of asterixis, or "liver flap," best described as the inability to sustain a fixed position of the extremities voluntarily. Asterixis is best recognized by downward flapping of the hands when the patient extends the arms and dorsiflexes the wrists. Hepatic encephalopathy is assessed by using a grading system that stages the encephalopathy according to the patient's clinical manifestations (Box 22-14).

BOX 22-13 Causes of Acute Liver Failure

Infections
- Hepatitis A, B, C, D, E, non-A, non-B, non-C
- Herpes simplex virus (types 1 and 2)
- Epstein-Barr virus
- Varicella zoster
- Dengue fever virus
- Rift Valley fever virus

Medications or Toxins
- Industrial substances (chlorinated hydrocarbons, phosphorus)
- *Amanita phalloides* (mushrooms)
- Aflatoxin (a toxic metabolite of fungus)
- Medications (isoniazid, rifampin, halothane, methyldopa, tetracycline, valproic acid, monoamine oxidase inhibitors, phenytoin, nicotinic acid, tricyclic antidepressants, isoflurane, ketoconazole, trimethoprim-sulfamethoxazole, sulfasalazine, pyrimethamine, octreotide)
- Acetaminophen toxicity
- Cocaine

Hypoperfusion
- Venous obstructions
- Budd-Chiari syndrome
- Veno-occlusive disease
- Ischemia

Metabolic Disorders
- Wilson disease
- Tyrosinemia
- Heat stroke
- Galactosemia

Surgery
- Jejunoileal bypass
- Partial hepatectomy
- Liver transplantation failure

Other Causes
- Reye's syndrome
- Acute fatty liver of pregnancy
- Massive malignant infiltration
- Autoimmune hepatitis

BOX 22-14 Staging of Hepatic Encephalopathy

I. Euphoria or depression, mild confusion, slurred speech, disordered sleep rhythm; slight asterixis and normal electroencephalogram (EEG)
II. Lethargy, moderate confusion; marked asterixis and abnormal EEG
III. Marked confusion, incoherent speech, sleeping but arousable; asterixis present and abnormal EEG
IV. Coma; initially responsive to noxious stimuli, later unresponsive; asterixis absent and abnormal EEG

Diagnostic findings include prolonged prothrombin times, elevated levels of serum bilirubin, aspartate aminotransferase (AST), alkaline phosphatase, and serum ammonia and decreased levels of serum albumin.[46] Arterial blood gases (ABGs) reveal respiratory alkalosis, metabolic acidosis, or both. Hypoglycemia, hypokalemia, and hyponatremia also may be present.[46,47]

Factors I (fibrinogen), II (prothrombin), V, VII, IX, and X are produced exclusively by the liver. Prothrombin time may be the most useful of tests of these in the evaluation of acute ALF because levels may be 40 to 80 seconds above control values. Test results show decreased levels of plasmin and plasminogen and increased levels of fibrin and fibrin-split products. Platelet counts may be less than 100,000/mm^3.[46]

Medical Management

Medical interventions are directed toward management of the multiple-system impact of ALF.

Ammonia Levels

Antibiotics such as neomycin, metronidazole, rifaximin, or lactulose, which is the gold standard, are administered to remove or decrease production of nitrogenous wastes in the large intestine. Antibiotics reduce bacterial flora of the colon. This aids in decreasing ammonia formation by decreasing bacterial action on the protein in feces. Side effects include renal toxicity and hearing impairment. Lactulose, a synthetic ketoanalogue of lactose split into lactic acid and acetic acid in the intestine, is given orally through a nasogastric tube or as a retention enema. The result is the creation of an acidic environment that results in ammonia being drawn out of the portal circulation. Lactulose has a laxative effect that promotes expulsion.[46,47]

Complications

Bleeding is best controlled through prevention. If an invasive procedure (e.g., central line placement, ICP monitor) will be performed or the patient develops active bleeding, vitamin K, fresh-frozen plasma (to maintain a reasonable prothrombin time), and platelet transfusions are necessary.[25] Metabolic disturbances such as hypoglycemia, metabolic acidosis, hypokalemia, and hyponatremia should be monitored and treated appropriately. Prophylactic antibiotic administration may be initiated because the patient is at high risk for an infection.[25] The development of cerebral edema necessitates ICP monitoring. Treatment with mannitol has been shown to be of benefit in managing ICP in the patient with ALF, but it must be used with caution in patients with renal failure to avoid hyperosmolarity.[47] Other interventions to control ICP include elevating the head of the bed (HOB) to 30 degrees, treating fever and hypertension, minimizing noxious stimulation, and correcting hypercapnia and hypoxemia.[25] Renal failure develops in 70% of patients with ALF, and continuous renal replacement therapy (CRRT) provides renal support.[25] Hemodynamic instability is a common complication necessitating fluid administration and vasoactive medications to prevent prolonged episodes of hypotension. A pulmonary artery catheter may be used to guide clinical management.[46]

If ALF continues and the patient shows no immediate signs of improvement or reversal, the patient should be considered for a liver transplantation. Prompt referral to a transplantation center should be a high priority for patients experiencing ALF.[25,45]

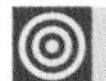
BOX 22-15 NURSING DIAGNOSIS PRIORITIES

Acute Liver Failure

- Impaired Gas Exchange, related to ventilation/perfusion mismatching or intrapulmonary shunting, p. 594
- Decreased Cardiac Output, related to alterations in preload, p. 579
- Risk for Infection, p. 607
- Imbalanced Nutrition: Less Than Body Requirements, related to lack of exogenous nutrients or increased metabolic demand, p. 593
- Disturbed Body Image, related to actual change in body structure, function, or appearance, p. 586
- Deficient Knowledge, related to lack of previous exposure to information, p. 585 (see Patient Education, Box 22-16)

Nursing Management

Nursing management of the patient with ALF incorporates a variety of nursing diagnoses (Box 22-15). **Nursing priorities are directed toward 1) protecting the patient from injury, 2) providing comfort and emotional support, 3) maintaining surveillance for complications, and 4) educating the patient and family.**

Use of benzodiazepines and other sedatives is discouraged in the patient with ALF because pertinent neurologic changes may be masked and hepatic encephalopathy may be exacerbated.[47] These patients are often very difficult to manage because they may be extremely agitated and combative. Physical restraint may be necessary to prevent injury to the patient.

Maintaining Surveillance for Complications

As the neurologic condition worsens, respiratory depression and arrest can occur quickly. Continuous pulse oximetry monitoring and ABG analysis are helpful in assessing adequacy of respiratory efforts. A thorough neurologic assessment should be performed at least every hour.

Educating the Patient and Family

Early in the patient's hospital stay, the patient and family should be taught about ALF and its causes and treatment. As patient discharge is imminent, teaching should focus on the interventions necessary for preventing the recurrence of the

BOX 22-16 PATIENT EDUCATION PRIORITIES

Acute Liver Failure

- Specific cause
- Precipitating factor modification
- Interventions to reduce further episodes
- Importance of taking medications
- Lifestyle changes
- Diet modification
- Alcohol cessation

Additional information for the patient can be found at the following websites:

- American Liver Foundation: http://www.liverfoundation.org
- National Liver Foundation: http://www.nlfindia.com
- Alcoholics Anonymous: http://www.aa.org
- International Foundation for Functional Gastrointestinal Disorders: http://www.iffgd.org
- Healthfinder—U.S. Department of Health and Human Services: http://healthfinder.gov
- Web MD: http://www.webmd.com

BOX 22-17 COLLABORATIVE MANAGEMENT

Acute Liver Failure

- Decrease ammonia levels.
- Control bleeding.
- Correct metabolic alterations.
- Prevent infection.
- Prepare patient for liver transplantation, if necessary.
- Protect patient from injury.
- Provide comfort and emotional support.
- Maintain surveillance for complications:
  - Cerebral edema
  - Renal failure

precipitating cause. If the patient is considered a candidate for liver transplantation, the patient and family will need specific information regarding the procedure and care. Evaluation for liver transplantation may include screening for medical contraindications, human immunodeficiency virus (HIV) serology, anticipated compliance, and assessment of the social support system. Psychiatric and other specialty team consultations are necessary for a thorough evaluation of the patient's suitability for a liver transplantation (Box 22-16). Collaborative management of the patient with ALF is outlined in Box 22-17.

THERAPEUTIC MANAGEMENT

Gastrointestinal Intubation

Because GI intubation is used so often in critical care units, it is important for nurses to know the clinical indications and responsibilities inherent in tube use. The three categories of GI tubes are based on function: 1) nasogastric suction tubes, 2) long intestinal tubes, and 3) feeding tubes (Box 22-18).

Nasogastric Suction Tubes

Nasogastric tubes remove fluid regurgitated into the stomach, prevent accumulation of swallowed air, may partially decompress the bowel, and reduce the patient's risk for aspiration. Nasogastric tubes also can be used for collecting specimens, assessing the presence of blood, and administering tube feedings. The most common nasogastric tubes are the single-lumen Levin tube and the double-lumen Salem sump. The Salem sump has one lumen that is used for suction and drainage and another that allows air to enter the patient's stomach and prevents the tube from adhering to the gastric wall and damaging the mucosa. The tube is passed through the nose into the nasopharynx and then down through the pharynx into the esophagus and stomach. The length of time the nasogastric tube remains in place depends on its use. The tube is then placed to gravity or low continuous suction, and in rare instances, it is clamped.[48]

Nursing management focuses on preventing complications common to this therapy, for example, ulceration and necrosis of the nares, esophageal reflux, esophagitis, esophageal erosion and stricture, gastric erosion, and dry mouth and parotitis from mouth breathing. Interference with ventilation and coughing, aspiration, and loss of fluid and electrolytes can be critical problems. Interventions include irrigating the tube every 4 hours with normal saline, ensuring the blue air vent of the Salem sump is patent and maintained above the level of the patient's stomach, and providing frequent mouth and nares care.[48]

Long Intestinal Tubes

Miller-Abbott, Cantor, and Andersen tubes are examples of long, weighted-tip intestinal tubes that are placed preoperatively or intraoperatively. Their considerable length allows removal of the contents of the intestine to treat an obstruction that cannot be managed by a nasogastric tube. These tubes can decompress the small bowel and can splint the small bowel intraoperatively or postoperatively. Because progression of the tubes depends on bowel peristalsis, their use is contraindicated in patients with paralytic ileus and severe mechanical bowel obstructions.

Interventions used in the care of the patient with a long intestinal tube are similar to those with a nasogastric tube. The patient should be observed for 1) gaseous distention of the balloon section, which makes removal difficult; 2) rupture of the balloon; 3) overinflation of the balloon, which can lead to intestinal rupture, and 4) reverse intussusception if the tube is removed rapidly. Intestinal tubes should be removed slowly; usually 6 inches of the tube is withdrawn every hour.[48]

Feeding Tubes

Small-diameter (8- to 12-Fr [French]) flexible feeding tubes, such as Dobhoff tubes, are commonly placed at the bedside for patients who cannot take nourishment orally. The feeding tube may be inserted orally or nasally so that the tip ends up in the stomach or duodenum. To facilitate passage into the GI tract, these tubes have a weighted tungsten tip, and a guidewire is needed to prevent them from curling up in the back of the patient's throat. A radiograph must be obtained to verify correct placement of the tube before initiating feeding.[49] The tube should also be marked with indelible ink where it exits the mouth or nares so that tube location can be checked at 4-hour intervals.[49]

BOX 22-18 PATIENT SAFETY ALERT QSEN

Tubing Misconnections—A Persistent and Potentially Deadly Occurrence

Tubing and catheter misconnection errors are an important and underreported problem in health care organizations. These errors often are caught and corrected before any injury to the patient occurs. Given the reality of and potential for life-threatening consequences, increased awareness and analysis of these errors—including averted errors—can lead to dramatic improvement in patient safety.

Nine cases involving tubing misconnections have been reported to The Joint Commission's Sentinel Event Database. These errors resulted in 8 deaths and 1 instance of permanent loss of function, and they affected 7 adults and 2 infants. Reports in the media and to such organizations as the ECRI Institute, the U.S. Food and Drug Administration (FDA), the Institute for Safe Medication Practices (ISMP), and the United States Pharmacopeia (USP) indicate that misconnection errors occur with significant frequency and, in a number of instances, lead to deadly consequences.

Types of Misconnections

The types of tubes and catheters involved in the cases reported to The Joint Commission included central intravenous (IV) catheters, peripheral IV catheters, nasogastric feeding tubes, percutaneous enteric feeding tubes, peritoneal dialysis catheters, tracheostomy cuff inflation tubes, and automatic blood pressure cuff insufflation tubes. The specific misconnections involved an enteric tube feeding into an IV catheter; injection of barium sulfate (gastrointestinal contrast medium) into a central venous catheter; an enteric tube feeding into a peritoneal dialysis catheter; a blood pressure insufflator tube connected to an IV catheter; and injection of IV fluid into a tracheostomy cuff inflation tube.

A review by the USP of more than 300 cases reported to its databases found misconnection errors involving the following:

- IV infusions connected to epidural lines and epidural solutions (intended for epidural administration) connected to peripheral or central IV catheters
- Bladder irrigation solutions using primary IV tubing connected as secondary infusions to peripheral or central IV catheters
- Infusions intended for IV administration connected to an indwelling bladder (Foley) catheter
- Infusions intended for IV administration connected to nasogastric tubes
- IV solutions administered with blood administration sets and blood products transfused with primary IV tubing
- Primary IV solutions administered through various other functionally dissimilar catheters such as external dialysis catheters, a ventriculostomy drain, an amnioinfusion catheter, and the distal port of a pulmonary artery catheter

Many of the misconnection cases involved Luer connectors, which are small devices used in the connection of many medical components and accessories. There are two types of Luer connectors: slips and locks. A Luer slip connector consists of a tapered "male" fitting that slips into a wider "female" fitting to create a secure connection. The Luer lock connector has a threaded collar on the male fitting and a flange on the female fitting that screw together to create a more secure connection.

Examples of misconnections involving Luer connectors include the following:

- Capnography sampling tube to an IV cannula
- Enteral feeding set to a central venous catheter
- Enteral feeding set to a hemodialysis line
- Noninvasive blood pressure (NIBP) insufflation tube to a needleless IV port
- Oxygen tubing to a needleless IV port
- Sequential compression device (SCD) hose to a needleless "piggyback" port of an IV administration set

Root Causes Identified

The basic lesson from these cases is that if it *can* happen, it *will* happen. Luer connectors are implicated in or contribute to many of these errors because they enable functionally dissimilar tubes or catheters to be connected. Other causes include the routine use of tubes or catheters for unintended purposes such as using IV extension tubing for epidurals, irrigation, drains, and central lines; using them to extend enteric feeding tubes, and positioning functionally dissimilar tubes used in patient care close to one another. In the cases reported to the Sentinel Event Database, contributing factors included movement of the patient from one setting or service to another and staff fatigue associated with working consecutive shifts.

Risk Reduction Strategies

No standards that specifically restrict the use of Luer connectors to certain medical devices have been published. Consequently, a broad range of medical devices, which have different functions and access the body through different routes, are often outfitted with Luer fittings that can be easily misconnected. Organizations in Europe and the United States are developing standards to restrict the types of devices that use Luer fittings in an attempt to mitigate misconnection hazards. According to Jim Keller, vice-president of Health Technology Evaluation and Safety for the ECRI Institute, and Stephanie Joseph, project engineer for the ECRI Institute, the solution for reducing or eliminating misconnection errors lies in engineering controls respecting how products and devices are designed ("incompatibility by design") and in reengineering work practices.

"A well-designed device should prevent misconnections and should prompt the user to take the correct action," explained Joseph, author of a guidance article published in the March 2006 issue of the ECRI Institute's *Health Devices* journal. As a first step in prevention, Joseph urges hospitals to avoid buying non-IV equipment (e.g., nebulizers, NIBP devices, enteral feeding sets) that can mate with the Luer connectors on patient IV lines. Joseph also emphasizes that the single most important work practice solution for clinicians is to trace all lines back to their origin before connecting or disconnecting any devices or infusions.

Other solutions include specific education and training regarding this problem for all clinicians and having practitioners take simple precautions such as turning on the light in a darkened room before connecting or reconnecting tubes or devices. The risk of waking a sleeping patient is minimal by comparison. Errors have occurred when patients or family members attempted to disconnect and reconnect equipment

Continued

BOX 22-18 PATIENT SAFETY ALERT—cont'd

themselves. Staff should emphasize to all patients the importance of contacting a clinical staff member for assistance when a need to disconnect or reconnect devices is identified.

Some approaches to reducing the risk of misconnections have significant potential for unintended consequences:

- Labeling all tubes and catheters may not always be practical and may therefore lead to inconsistent implementation. However, labeling certain high-risk catheters (e.g., epidural, intrathecal, arterial) should always be done.
- Color-coding tubes and catheters can lead users to rely on the color coding rather than having a clear understanding of which tubes and catheters are connected correctly to which body inlets. Training or educating all staff (including temporary agency and travel staff) about the institution's color-coding system requires ongoing attention. Color-coding schemes often vary across institutions in the same community, creating increased risk when agency and travel staff are used.

Joint Commission Recommendations

The Joint Commission offers the following recommendations and strategies to health care organizations to reduce tubing misconnection errors:

1. Do not purchase non-IV equipment that is equipped with connectors that can physically mate with a female Luer IV line connector.
2. Conduct acceptance testing (for performance, safety, and usability) and, as appropriate, risk assessment (e.g., failure mode and effect analysis) on new tubing and catheter purchases to identify the potential for misconnections and take appropriate preventive measures.
3. Always trace a tube or catheter from the patient to the point of origin before connecting any new device or infusion.
4. Recheck connections and trace all patient tubes and catheters to their sources on the patient's arrival to a new setting or service as part of the handing-off process. Standardize this "line reconciliation" process.
5. Route tubes and catheters having different purposes in different, standardized directions (e.g., IV lines routed toward the head; enteric lines toward the feet). This is especially important in the care of neonates.
6. Inform nonclinical staff, patients, and their families that they must get help from clinical staff in case of a real or perceived need to connect or disconnect devices or infusions.
7. For certain high-risk catheters (e.g., epidural, intrathecal, arterial), label the catheter and do not use catheters that have injection ports.
8. Never use a standard Luer syringe for oral medications or enteric feedings.
9. Emphasize the risk of tubing misconnections in orientation and training curricula.
10. Identify and manage conditions and practices that may contribute to health care worker fatigue and take appropriate action.

The Joint Commission also urges product manufacturers to implement "designed incompatibility," as appropriate, to prevent dangerous misconnections of tubes and catheters.

Resources

- The ECRI Institute. Fatal air embolism caused by the misconnection of a medical device hoses to needleless Luer ports on IV administration sets [hazard report]. *Health Devices.* 2004: 33(6):223.
- The ECRI Institute. Misconnected flowmeter leads to two deaths [special report]. *Health Devices Alerts.* January 25, 2003.
- The ECRI Institute. Preventing misconnections of lines and cables. *Health Devices.* 2006: 35(3):81.
- Safe systems, safe patients: common connectors pose a threat to safe practice. *Texas Board Nurs Bull.* 2006: 37(2):6.
- U.S. Food and Drug Administration. FDA patient safety news, Show #31, September 2004; Show #20, October 2003; Show #46, December 2005. Available at www.accessdata.fda.gov/psn/index.cfm. Accessed May 2009.

Modified from The Joint Commission: Sentinel Event Alert, no. 36, April 3, 2006. Available at http://www.jointcommission.org/assets/1/18/SEA_36.PDF Accessed May 11, 2012.

Nursing priorities for the management of the patient with a feeding tube include prevention of complications and monitoring the tolerance of feeding. Tracheobronchial aspiration of gastric contents is a serious potential complication.[49-51] Before administering medications or feedings, it is important to ensure that the tube is in the patient's stomach or duodenum. Assessing the exit point marked on the tube helps determine whether the tube has maintained the same position. Looking for coiling in the mouth or throat can help detect upward displacement that may have occurred as a result of vomiting. The traditional practice of confirming placement by auscultating air inserted through the tube over the epigastrium is not reliable and is not recommended.[49-52] If any doubt exists about the tube's position, a repeat radiograph should be obtained. During feedings, the head of bed should be elevated at least 30 degrees to minimize the risk of aspiration, and gastric residuals should be checked at least every 4 to 6 hours.[50,51] Large gastric residuals, cramping, and abdominal distention may indicate intolerance of feeding, and the physician should be notified.[51] Other interventions include nares and oral care and flushing the tube with water before and after medication administration to maintain patency.[51]

Endoscopic Injection Therapy

Endoscopic injection therapy is used to control bleeding of ulcers. It may be performed emergently, electively, or prophylactically. An endoscope is introduced through the patient's mouth, and endoscopy of the esophagus and stomach is performed to identify the bleeding varices or ulcers. An injector with a retractable 23- to 25-gauge needle is introduced through the biopsy channel of the endoscope. The needle then is inserted in or around the varices or into the area around the ulcer, and a liquid agent is injected. The most commonly used agent is epinephrine, which results in localized vasoconstriction and enhanced platelet aggregation. Sclerosing agents such as ethanolamine, alcohol, and polidocanol also may be used. These agents cause an inflammatory reaction in the vessel that results in thrombosis and eventually produces a fibrous band. Repeated sclerotherapy results in the development of supportive scar tissue around the varices. Other embolic agents are used, including fibrinogen and thrombin, which when injected together react to form an active fibrin clot, and "glues" (n-butyl cyanoacrylate), which are used as a sealant to stop the bleeding.[20,24,53]

Endoscopic Variceal Ligation

Endoscopic variceal ligation (EVL) involves applying bands or metal clips around the circumference of the bleeding varices to induce venous obstruction and control bleeding. EVL has replaced endoscopic sclerotherapy of variceal hemorrhage. Between 1 and 2 days after the procedure, necrosis and scar formation promote band and tissue sloughing. Fibrinous deposits within the healing ulcer potentiate vessel obliteration. Band ligation is accomplished through endoscopy, with multiple bands placed per session.[16] The procedure may be repeated on an inpatient or outpatient basis every 1 to 2 weeks until all the varices are obliterated.[56] Endoscopic variceal ligation controls bleeding approximately 80% to 90% of the time.[53] The most common complication of endoscopic variceal ligation is the development of superficial mucosal ulcers. Varices may reoccur as local banding does not affect portal pressure.[16,54]

Transjugular Intrahepatic Portosystemic Shunt

TIPS is an angiographic interventional procedure for decreasing portal hypertension. TIPS is advocated for 1) patients with portal hypertension who are also experiencing active bleeding or have poor liver reserve, 2) transplant recipients, and 3) patients with other operative risks.[25,54] The TIPS procedure is usually performed by a gastroenterologist, vascular surgeon, or interventional radiologist.

Portal hypertension is confirmed by direct measurement of the pressure in the portal vein (gradient greater than 10 mm Hg). Cannulation is achieved through the internal jugular vein, and an angiographic catheter is advanced into the middle or right hepatic vein. The midhepatic vein is then catheterized, and a new route is created connecting the portal and hepatic veins using a needle and guidewire with a dilating balloon. A polytetrafluoroethylene (PTFE)–coated stent is then placed in the liver parenchyma to maintain that connection (Figure 22-5). The increased resistance in the liver is bypassed.[25,55] TIPS may be performed on patients with bleeding varices, with refractory bleeding varices, or as a bridge to liver transplantation if the candidate becomes hemodynamically unstable. Postprocedural care should include observation for overt (cannulation site) or covert (intrahepatic site) bleeding, hepatic or portal vein laceration (resulting in rapid loss of blood volume), and inadvertent puncture of surrounding organs. Other complications include hepatic encephalopathy, liver failure, bacteremia, and stent stenosis.[25,55]

Gastrointestinal Surgery

Types of Surgery

GI surgery refers to a wide variety of surgical procedures that involve the esophagus, the stomach, the intestine, the liver, the pancreas, or the biliary tract. Indications for GI surgery are numerous and include bleeding or perforation from peptic ulcer disease, obstruction, trauma, inflammatory bowel disease, and malignancy. Patients may be admitted to the critical care unit for monitoring after GI surgery as a result of their underlying medical condition; however, this portion of the chapter focuses only on several surgical procedures that commonly require postoperative critical care.

Esophagectomy. Esophagectomy is usually performed for cancer of the distal esophagus and gastroesophageal junction. The technically difficult procedure involves the removal of part or the entire esophagus, part of the stomach, and lymph nodes in the surrounding area. The stomach is then pulled up into the chest and connected to the remaining part of the esophagus. If the entire esophagus and stomach must be removed, part of the bowel may be used to form the esophageal replacement (Figures 22-6 and 22-7).[56]

Pancreaticoduodenectomy. The standard operation for pancreatic cancer is a pancreaticoduodenectomy, also called the *Whipple procedure.* In the Whipple procedure, the pancreatic head, the duodenum, part of the jejunum, the common bile duct, the gallbladder, and part of the stomach are removed. The continuity of the GI tract is restored by anastomosing the remaining portion of the pancreas, the bile duct, and the stomach to the jejunum (Figure 22-8).[56]

Bariatric surgery. Bariatric surgery refers to surgical procedures of the GI tract that are performed to induce weight loss. Bariatric procedures are divided into three broad types: 1) restrictive, 2) malabsorptive, and 3) combined restrictive and malabsorptive.[57] Restrictive procedures such as vertical-banded gastroplasty (VBG) (Figure 22-9A) and gastric banding (see Figure 22-9B) reduce the capacity of the stomach and limit the amount of food that can be consumed. Malabsorptive procedures such as the biliopancreatic diversion (BPD) (Figure 22-9C) alter the GI tract to limit the digestion and absorption of food. The Roux-en-Y gastric bypass (RYGBP) (Figure 22-9D) combines both strategies by creating a small gastric pouch and anastomosing the jejunum to the pouch. Food then bypasses the lower stomach and duodenum, resulting in decreased absorption of digestive materials.[57]

Preoperative Care

A thorough preoperative evaluation should be conducted to evaluate the patient's physical status and identify risk factors that may affect the postoperative course. Because obesity is associated with a higher incidence of comorbidities such as cardiovascular disease, hypertension, diabetes, gastroesophageal reflux, obstructive sleep apnea, and heart failure, an extensive workup may be required for the patient who underwent bariatric surgery.[56,58]

Surgical Considerations

Two approaches may be used for esophageal resection: *transhiatal* or *transthoracic* (Figures 22-6 and 22-7). In both approaches, the stomach is mobilized through an abdominal incision and then transposed into the chest. The anastomosis of the stomach to the esophagus is performed in the chest (transthoracic) or in the neck (transhiatal). The approach selected depends on the location of the tumor, the patient's overall health and pulmonary function, and the experience of the surgeon. After surgery, the patient has a nasogastric

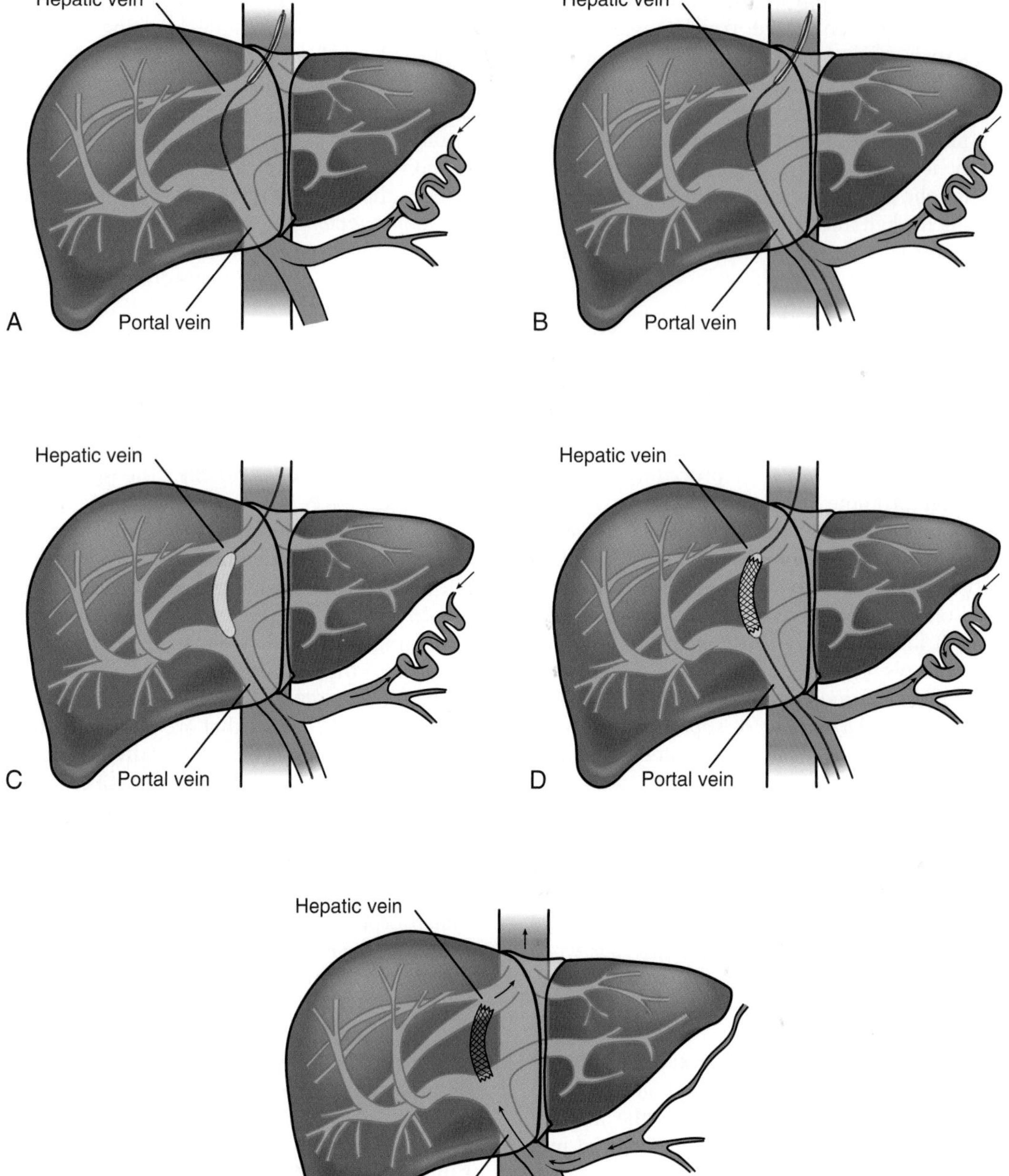

FIG 22-5 Transjugular Intrahepatic Portosystemic Shunt (TIPS). A, Needle directed though liver parenchyma to portal vein. B, Needle and guidewire passed down to midportal vein. C, Balloon dilation. D, Deployment of stent. E, Intrahepatic shunt from portal to hepatic vein. (Modified from Ellis F. Esophagogastrectomy for carcinoma: technical considerations based on anatomic location of lesion. *Surg Clin North Am.* 1980;60:265.)

tube in place, and it should not be manipulated because of the potential to damage the anastomosis. Those who undergo transthoracic esophagectomy have chest tubes.[56]

Most bariatric procedures can be performed using an open or laparoscopic surgical technique. Although laparoscopic approaches are more technically difficult to perform, they have largely replaced open procedures because they are associated with decreased pulmonary complications, less postoperative pain, reduced length of hospital stay, fewer wound complications (e.g., infections, incisional hernia), and an earlier return to full activity.[56,57] Open procedures are performed on patients who have had prior upper abdominal surgery, are morbidly obese, or who may not be able to tolerate the increased abdominal pressure associated with laparoscopic procedures.[56]

Complications and Medical Management

Several complications are associated with GI surgery, including respiratory failure, atelectasis, pneumonia, anastomotic leak, deep vein thrombosis, pulmonary embolus, and

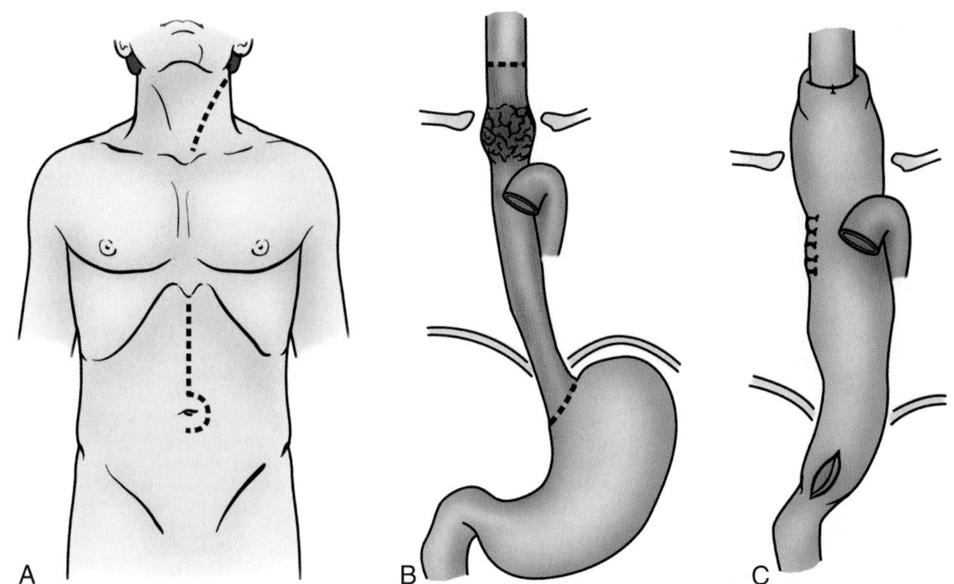

FIG 22-6 Overview of Transhiatal Esophagectomy. *(A)* with gastric mobilization *(B)* and gastric pull-up *(C)* for cervical esophagogastric anastomosis.

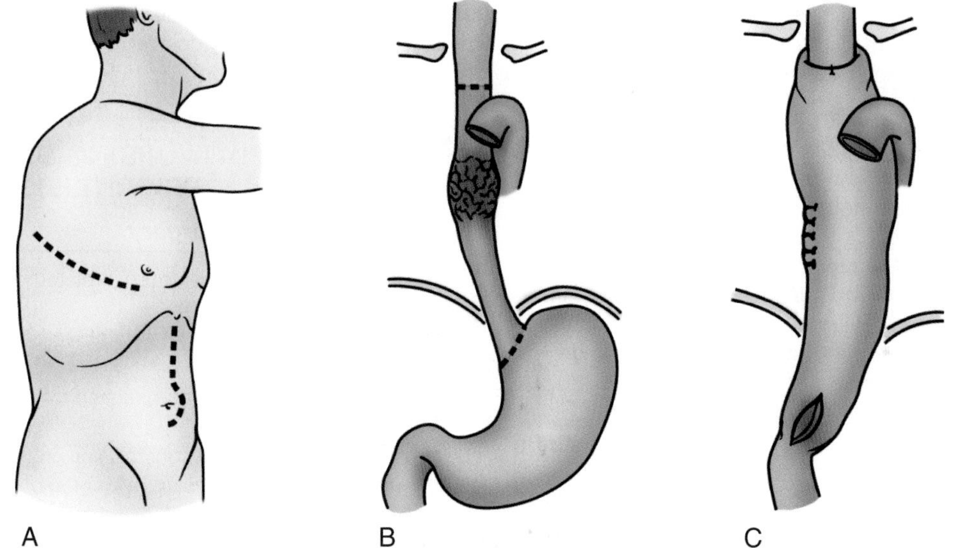

FIG 22-7 Overview of Transthoracic Esophagectomy. *(A)* with esophageal resection, gastric mobilization *(B)*, and intrathoracic anastomosis *(C)* for a midesophageal tumor. (Modified from Ellis FH. Esophagogastrectomy for carcinoma: technical considerations based on anatomic location of lesion. *Surg Clin North Am.* 1980;60:265.)

bleeding. The morbidly obese patient is at even greater risk for many postoperative complications.[57]

Pulmonary complications. The risk for pulmonary complications is substantial after GI surgery, and adverse respiratory events such as atelectasis and pneumonia are twice as likely to occur in the patient who is obese.[58] Aggressive pulmonary exercise should be initiated in the immediate postoperative period. Early ambulation and adequate pain control assist in reducing the risk of atelectasis development. Suctioning, chest physiotherapy, or bronchodilators may be needed to optimize pulmonary function. Patients should be closely monitored for the development of oxygenation problems. Treatment should be aimed at supporting adequate ventilation and gas exchange. Mechanical ventilation may be required in the event of respiratory failure.

Anastomotic leak. An anastomotic leak is a severe complication of GI surgery. It occurs when there is a breakdown of the suture line in a surgical anastomosis and results in leakage of gastric or intestinal contents into the abdomen or mediastinum (transthoracic esophagectomy).[56] The clinical signs and symptoms of a leak can be subtle and often go unrecognized. They include tachycardia, tachypnea, fever, abdominal pain, anxiety, and restlessness.[56] In the patient who had an esophagectomy, a leak of the esophageal anastomosis may manifest as subcutaneous emphysema in the chest and neck.[56] If undetected, a leak can result in sepsis, multiorgan failure, and death. Patients with progressive tachycardia and tachypnea should have a radiologic study (upper GI study with Gastrografin or CT scan with contrast) to rule out an anastomotic leak.[58] The type of treatment depends on the

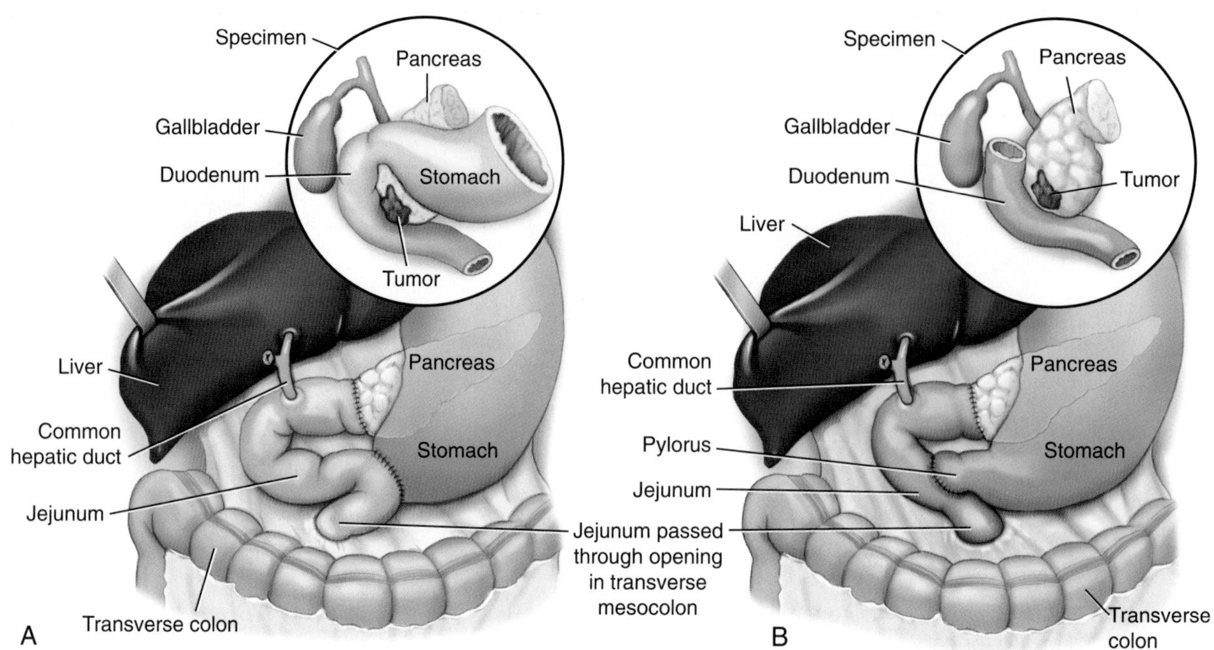

FIG 22-8 Standard and Pylorus-Preserving Whipple Procedures. *A,* The standard Whipple procedure involves resection of the gastric antrum, head of pancreas, distal bile duct, and entire duodenum with reconstruction as shown. *B,* The pylorus-preserving Whipple procedure does not include resection of the distal stomach, pylorus, or proximal duodenum.

severity of the leak. If the leak is small and well-contained, it may be managed conservatively by maintaining the NPO status, administering antibiotics, and draining the fluid percutaneously. If the patient is deteriorating rapidly, an urgent laparotomy is indicated to repair the defect.[56,58]

Deep vein thrombosis and pulmonary embolism. Pulmonary embolism (PE) is a very serious complication of any surgical procedure. Deep vein thrombosis (DVT) prophylaxis should be initiated before surgery and continued until the patient is fully ambulatory to reduce the risk of clot development. Typically, a combination of sequential compression devices and subcutaneous unfractionated heparin or low–molecular-weight heparin is used. Patients determined to be at high risk for PE may benefit from prophylactic inferior vena cava filter placement.[56]

Bleeding. Upper GI bleeding is an uncommon but life-threatening complication of GI surgery. Early bleeding usually occurs at the site of the anastomosis and can usually be treated through endoscopic intervention. Surgical revision may be needed for persistent, uncontrolled bleeding. Late bleeding is usually a result of ulcer development. Medical therapy is aimed at the prevention of this complication through administration of histamine 2 (H_2)–antagonists or PPIs.[5]

Postoperative Nursing Management

Nursing care of the patient who has had GI surgery incorporates a number of nursing diagnoses (Box 22-19). **Nursing priorities are directed toward 1) optimizing oxygenation and ventilation, 2) providing comfort and emotional support, and 3) maintaining surveillance for complications.**

Optimizing oxygenation and ventilation. Nursing interventions in the postoperative period are focused on promoting ventilation and adequate oxygenation and preventing complications such as atelectasis and pneumonia.

BOX 22-19 NURSING DIAGNOSIS PRIORITIES

Gastrointestinal Surgery

- Ineffective Breathing Pattern, related to decreased lung expansion, p. 598
- Impaired Gas Exchange, related to alveolar hypoventilation, p. 593
- Decreased Cardiac Output, related to alterations in preload, p. 579
- Acute Pain, related to transmission and perception of cutaneous, visceral, muscular, or ischemic impulses, p. 574
- Disturbed Body Image, related to actual change in body structure, function, or appearance, p. 586
- Deficient Knowledge, related to lack of previous exposure to information, p. 585

After the patient is extubated, deep-breathing exercises and incentive spirometry should be initiated, and the patient should perform them regularly. Early ambulation is encouraged to promote maximal lung inflation, thereby reducing the risk of pulmonary complications and the potential for pulmonary embolus.

Providing comfort and emotional support. It is imperative to manage the patient's pain after GI surgery appropriately. Adequate analgesia is necessary to promote the mobility of the patient and decrease pulmonary complications. Initial pain management may be accomplished by intravenous opioid (morphine, hydromorphone) administration by means of a patient-controlled analgesia (PCA) pump or through continuous epidural infusion of an opioid and local anesthetic (bupivacaine).[48] Oral pain medications can be started

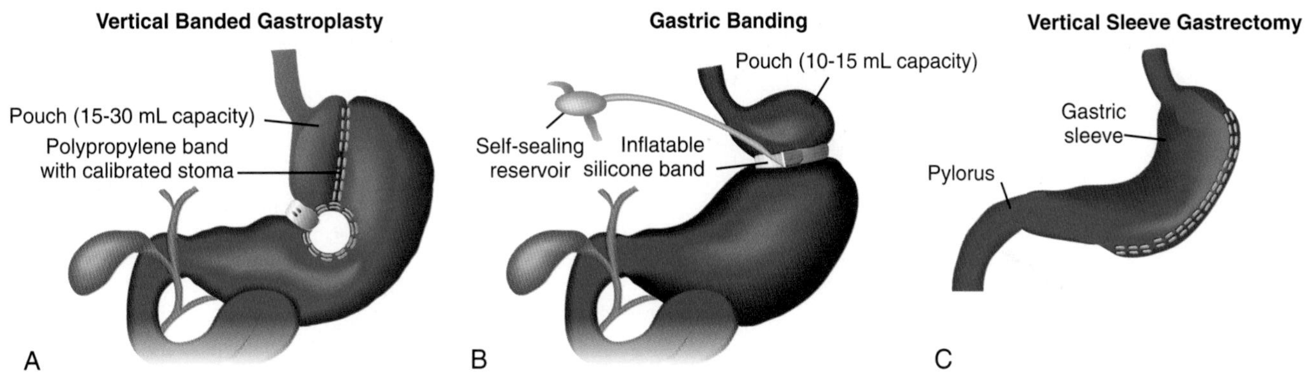

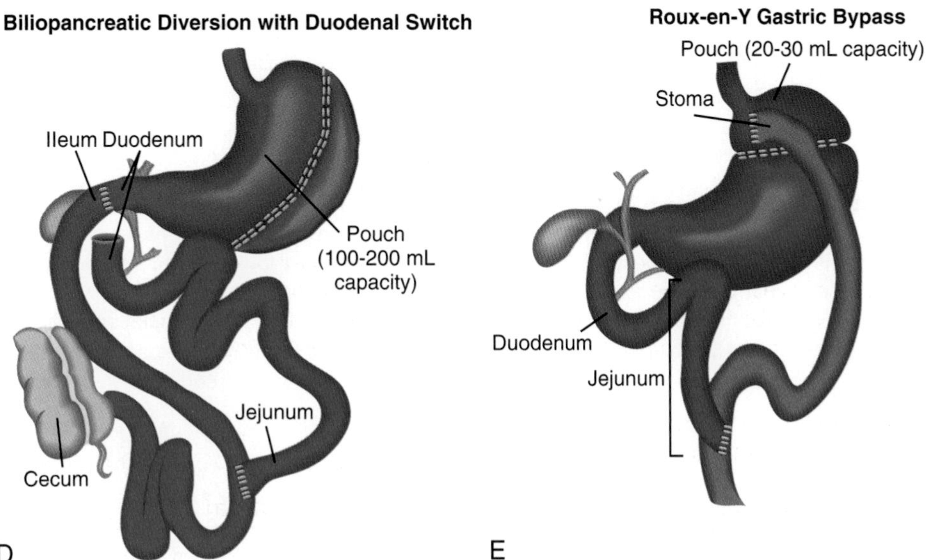

FIG 22-9 Bariatric Surgical Procedures. *A,* Vertical-banded gastroplasty involves creating a small gastric pouch. *B,* Adjustable gastric banding uses a band to create a gastric pouch. *C,* Vertical sleeve gastrectomy involves creating a sleeve-shaped stomach by removing about 80% of the stomach. *D,* Biliopancreatic diversion with duodenal switch procedure creates an anastomosis between the stomach and intestine. *E,* Roux-en-Y gastric bypass procedure involves constructing a gastric pouch whose outlet is a Y-shaped limb of small intestine. (From Lewis SL, et al. *Medical-Surgical Nursing: Assessment and Management of Clinical Problems.* 9th ed. St. Louis: Mosby; 2015.)

BOX 22-20 INTERNET RESOURCES

American Association of Critical-Care Nurses: http://www.aacn.org
Society for Critical Care Medicine: http://www.sccm.org
SGNA—Society of Gastroenterology Nurses and Associates, Inc.: http://www.sgna.org
American Gastroenterological Association: http://www.gastro.org
American College of Gastroenterology: http://gi.org
American Society for Gastrointestinal Endoscopy: http://www.asge.org
American Liver Foundation: http://www.liverfoundation.org
American Association for the Study of Liver Diseases: http://www.aasld.org
American College of Physicians: http://www.acponline.org
American College of Surgeons: http://www.facs.org
American Medical Association: http://www.ama-assn.org
National Digestive Diseases Information Clearinghouse (NDDIC): http://digestive.niddk.nih.gov
National Institutes for Health: http://www.nih.gov
PubMed Health: http://www.ncbi.nlm.nih.gov/pubmedhealth
American Society for Parenteral and Enteral Nutrition: http://www.nutritioncare.org

after an anastomosis leak is ruled out. Nonpharmacologic interventions such as positioning, application of heat or cold, and distraction may also be used. If the patient's pain is not being sufficiently relieved, the pain management service should be consulted.

Pharmacologic Agents

Many pharmacologic agents are used in the care of patients with GI disorders. Table 22-3 reviews the various agents and any special considerations necessary for administering them. See Box 22-20 for Internet Resources.

TABLE 22-3 Pharmacologic Management Gastrointestinal Disorders

MEDICATION	DOSAGE	ACTIONS	SPECIAL CONSIDERATIONS
Antacids	30-90 mL q1-2h PO or NG; possibly titrated to NG pH	Used to buffer stomach acid and raise gastric pH	Can cause diarrhea or constipation and electrolyte disturbances Irrigate NG tube with water after administration because antacids can clog tube.
Histamine$_2$ (H_2) Antagonists			
Cimetidine (Tagamet)	300 mg q6h IV or PO	Used to reduce volume and concentration of gastric secretions	Side effects include CNS toxicity (confusion or delirium) and thrombocytopenia.
Ranitidine (Zantac)	150 mg q12h PO or 50 mg q8h IV		
Famotidine (Pepcid)	40 mg daily PO or 20 mg q12h IV		Separate administration of antacids and PO histamine blocking agents by 1 hour.
Nizatidine (Axid)	150 mg q12h PO or 300 mg q24h		Dosage adjustments recommended for patients with moderate (creatinine clearance <50 mL/min) or severe (creatinine clearance <10 mL/min) renal insufficiency
Gastric Mucosal Agents			
Sucralfate (Carafate)	1 g q6h NG or PO, given 1 hour before meals and at bedtime	Forms an ulcer-adherent complex with proteinaceous exudates Covers the ulcer and protects against acid, pepsin, and bile salts	Requires an acid medium for activation; do not administer within 30 minutes of an antacid. May cause severe constipation May cause decreased absorption of certain medications
Gastric Proton-Pump Inhibitors			
Omeprazole (Prilosec)	20-40 mg q12h PO	Inactivates acid, or hydrogen, acid pump, blocking secretion of hydrochloric acid by gastric parietal cells	Capsules should be swallowed intact. May increase levels of phenytoin, diazepam, warfarin May administer concomitantly with antacids
Lansoprazole (Prevacid)	15-30 mg q24h PO 30 mg over 30 min q24h IV		
Rabeprazole (Aciphex)	20-40 mg q24h PO		
Esomeprazole (Nexium)	40 mg q12-24h PO 20-40 mg q24h IV		
Pantoprazole (Protonix)	20-40 mg q24h PO 80 mg q8-12h IV		
Vasopressin			
(Pitressin Synthetic)	Loading dose of 20 units over 20 min IV, followed by 0.2-0.4 unit/min IV infusion Doses can be increased to 0.9 unit/min, if necessary.	Decreases splanchnic blood flow, reducing portal pressure	Side effects include coronary, mesenteric, and peripheral vasoconstriction. May be administered concurrently with nitroglycerin to minimize side effects
Somatostatin			
Octreotide (Sandostatin)	Bolus dose of 25-50 mcg followed by IV infusion of 25-50 mcg/hr for 48 hours	Decreases splanchnic blood flow, reducing portal pressure	May cause hyperglycemia or hypoglycemia when initiating the drip and changing dosages

CNS, Central nervous system; *IV*, intravenous; *NG*, nasogastric; *PO*, by mouth.
From Gold Standard. Available at: http://www.mdconsult.com/das/pharm/lookup/340530070-12?type=alldrugs. Accessed May 11, 2014.

CASE STUDY Patient with Gastrointestinal Issues

Brief Patient History

Mrs. S is a 70-year-old woman with a long history of chronic back pain. She has been taking nonsteroidal antiinflammatory drugs (NSAIDs) for several years. She was recently started on warfarin for atrial fibrillation.

Clinical Assessment

Mrs. S is admitted to the critical care unit because she is vomiting bright red blood. She is pale and diaphoretic and complains of epigastric pain.

Diagnostic Procedures

Mrs. S's vital signs include the following: blood pressure of 70/40 mm Hg, heart rate of 130 beats/min (sinus tachycardia), respiratory rate of 30 breaths/min, and temperature of 101.3°F. Her urine output is 15 mL/hr, hemoglobin level is 9 g/dL, and international normalized ratio (INR) is 5.3.

Medical Diagnosis

Mrs. S is diagnosed with upper gastrointestinal bleeding.

Questions

1. What major outcomes do you expect to achieve for this patient?
2. What problems or risks must be managed to achieve these outcomes?
3. What interventions must be initiated to monitor, prevent, manage, or eliminate the problems and risks identified?
4. What interventions should be initiated to promote optimal functioning, safety, and well-being of the patient?
5. What possible learning needs do you anticipate for this patient?
6. What cultural and age-related factors may have a bearing on the patient's plan of care?

REFERENCES

1. Cappell MS, Friedel D: Initial management of acute upper gastrointestinal bleeding: from initial evaluation up to gastrointestinal endoscopy, *Med Clin North Am* 92:491, 2008.
2. Tariq SH, Mekjian G: Gastrointestinal bleeding in older adults, *Clin Geriatr Med* 23:769, 2007.
3. Acosta R, Wong R: Differential diagnosis of upper gastrointestinal bleeding proximal to the ligament of Trietz, *Gastrointest Endosc Clin North Am.* 21:555, 2011.
4. Manning-Dimmitt LL, et al: Diagnosis of gastrointestinal bleeding in adults, *Am Fam Physician* 71:1339, 2005.
5. Ghassemi KA, et al: Gastric acid inhibition in the treatment of peptic ulcer hemorrhage, *Curr Gastroenterol Rep* 11:462, 2009.
6. Schubert ML: Gastric secretion, *Curr Opin Gastroenterol* 26:598, 2010.
7. Doig AK, Huether SE: Alterations of digestive function. In McCance KL, et al, editor: *Pathophysiology: The Biologic Basis for Disease in Adults and Children*, ed 7, St. Louis, 2014, Elsevier.
8. Schubert ML, Peura DA: Control of gastric acid secretion in health and disease, *Gastroenterology* 134:1842, 2008.
9. Ferri FF: *Ferri's Clinical Advisor 2014*, Philadelphia, 2014, Elsevier.
10. Marik P, et al: Stress ulcer prophylaxis in the new millennium: a systematic review and meta-analysis, *Crit Care Med* 38:2222, 2010.
11. Porath A: Does stress ulcer prophylaxis explain the association between *Clostridium difficile*-associated disease and mechanical ventilation?, *Chest* 137:1001, 2010.
12. Ali T: Stress-induced ulcer bleeding in critically ill patients, *Gastroenterol Clin North Am* 38:245, 2009.
13. Pilkington KB, et al: Prevention of gastrointestinal bleeding due to stress ulceration: a review of current literature, *Anaesth Intensive Care* 40:253, 2012.
14. Laine L, et al: Gastric mucosal defense and cytoprotection: bench to bedside, *Gastroenterology* 135:60, 2008.
15. Stevens A, et al: *Core Pathology*, ed 3, St. Louis, 2009, Mosby.
16. Cat TB, Liu-DeRyke X: Medical management of variceal hemorrhage, *Crit Care Nurs Clin North Am* 22:381, 2010.
17. Bambha K, et al: Predictors of early re-bleeding and mortality after acute variceal haemorrhage in patients with cirrhosis, *Gut* 57:814, 2008.
18. Jessee MA: Stool studies: tried, true, and new, *Crit Care Nurs Clin Am.* 22:129, 2010.
19. Goldman L, Schafer A: *Goldman's Cecil Medicine*, ed 24, Philadelphia, 2012, Saunders.
20. Huang JH, et al: Guideline: the role of endoscopy in acute non-variceal upper GI bleeding, *Gastrointest Endosc* 75:1132, 2012.
21. Sudheendra D: Radiologic techniques and effectiveness of angiography to diagnose and treat acute upper gastrointestinal bleeding, *Gastrointest Endosc Clin North Am.* 21:697, 2011.
22. Jairath V, Barkun AN: The overall approach to the management of upper gastrointestinal bleeding, *Gastrointest Endosc Clin N Am* 21:657, 2011.
23. Yoshida H, et al: Treatment modalities for bleeding esophagogastric varices, *J Nihon Med Sch.* 79:19, 2012.
24. Opio CK, Garcia-Tsao G: Managing varices: drugs, bands, and shunts, *Gastroenterol Clin North Am* 40:561, 2011.
25. Garcia-Tsao G, Bosch J: Management of varices and variceal hemorrhage in cirrhosis, *N Engl J Med* 362:823, 2010.
26. Lundell L: Acid secretion and gastric surgery, *Dig Dis* 29:487, 2011.
27. Costa G, et al: Surgical shunt versus TIPS for treatment of variceal hemorrhage in the current era of liver and multivisceral transplantation, *Surg Clin North Am* 90:891, 2010.
28. Ghosh T: Review article: methods of measuring gastric acid secretion, *Aliment Pharmacol Ther* 33:768, 2011.
29. Gilbert DA, Saunders DR: Iced saline lavage does not slow bleeding from experimental canine gastric ulcers, *Dig Dis Sci* 26:1065, 1981.
30. Milosavljevic T, et al: Complications of peptic ulcer disease, *Dig Dis* 29:491, 2011.
31. Khan AS, et al: Controversies in the etiologies of acute pancreatitis, *JOP* 11:545, 2010.
32. Tonsi AF, et al: Acute pancreatitis at the beginning of the 21st century: the state of the art, *World J Gastroenterol* 15:2945, 2009.

33. Singla A, et al: National hospital volume in acute pancreatitis: analysis of the Nationwide Inpatient Sample 1998-2006, *HPB (Oxford)* 11:391, 2009.
34. Ranson JH, et al: Prognostic signs and the role of operative management in acute pancreatitis, *Surg Gynecol Obstet* 139:69, 1974.
35. Munsell MA, Buscaglia JM: Acute pancreatitis, *J Hosp Med* 5:241, 2010.
36. Wang G, et al: Acute pancreatitis: etiology and common pathogenesis, *World J Gastroenterol* 15:1427, 2009.
37. Muniraj T, et al: Acute pancreatitis, *Dis Mon* 58:98, 2012.
38. Chernecky CC, Berger BJ: *Laboratory Tests and Diagnostic Procedures*, ed 6, St. Louis, 2013, Elsevier.
39. ASPEN Board of Directors and the Clinical Guidelines Taskforce: Guidelines for the use of parenteral and enteral nutrition in adult and pediatric patients, *JPEN J Parenter Enteral Nutr* 33:259, 2009.
40. Siow E: Enteral versus parenteral nutrition for acute pancreatitis, *Crit Care Nurse* 28(4):19, 2008.
41. Al-Omran M, et al: Enteral versus parenteral nutrition for nutrition for acute pancreatitis, *Cochrane Database Syst Rev* 20(1):CD002837, 2010.
42. Moraes JM, et al: A full solid diet as the initial meal in mild acute pancreatitis is safe and results in a shorter length of hospitalization: results from a prospective, randomized, controlled, double-blind clinical trial, *J Clin Gastroenterol* 44:517, 2010.
43. Dellinger EP, et al: Early antibiotic treatment for severe acute necrotizing pancreatitis. A randomized, double-blind, placebo-controlled study, *Ann Surg* 245:674, 2007.
44. Stevens T, et al: Acute pancreatitis: problems in adherence to guidelines, *Cleve Clin J Med* 76:697, 2009.
45. Foston TP, Carpentar D: Acute liver failure, *Crit Care Nurs Clin North Am* 22:395, 2010.
46. Mahajan A, Lat I: Correction of coagulopathy in the setting of acute liver failure, *Crit Care Nurs Clin North Am* 22:315, 2010.
47. Ginès P, et al: Management of critically-ill cirrhotic patients, *J Hepatol* 56(Suppl 1):S13, 2012.
48. Noble KA: Name that tube, *Nursing* 33:56, 2003.
49. Bourgault AM, Halm MA: Feeding tube placement in adults: safe verification method for blindly inserted tubes, *Am J Crit Care* 18:73, 2009.
50. McClave SA, et al: Guidelines for the provision and assessment of nutrition support therapy in the adult critically ill patient: Society of Critical Care Medicine and American Society for Parenteral and Enteral Nutrition: executive summary, *Crit Care Med* 37:1757, 2009.
51. Guenter P: Safe practices for enteral nutrition in critically ill patients, *Crit Care Nurs Clin North Am* 22:197, 2010.
52. Bankhead R, et al: Enteral nutrition practice recommendations, *JPEN J Parenter Enteral Nutr* 33:122, 2009.
53. Holster IL, Kuipers EJ: Update on the endoscopic management of peptic ulcer bleeding, *Curr Gastroenterol Rep* 13:525, 2011.
54. Cárdenas A: Management of acute variceal bleeding: emphasis on endoscopic therapy, *Clin Liver Dis* 14:251, 2010.
55. Riggio O, et al: Hepatic encephalopathy after transjugular intrahepatic portosystemic shunt, *Clin Liver Dis* 16:133, 2012.
56. Smith CE: Gastrointestinal surgery. In Rothrock JC, editor: *Alexander's Care of the Patient in Surgery*, ed 14, St. Louis, 2011, Mosby.
57. Apau D, Whiteing N: Pre- and post-operative nursing considerations of bariatric surgery, *Gastrointest Nurs.* 9(3):2011.
58. Cannon-Diehl R: Emerging issues for the postbariatric surgical patient, *Crit Care Nurs Q* 33:361, 2010.

CHAPTER 23

Endocrine Clinical Assessment and Diagnostic Procedures

Mary E. Lough

Be sure to check out the bonus material, including review questions, on the Evolve website at http://evolve.elsevier.com/Urden/priorities/.

Assessment of the patient with endocrine dysfunction is a systematic process that incorporates a thorough history and physical examination. Most of the endocrine glands are deeply encased in the human body. Although the placement of the glands provides security for the glandular functions, their resulting inaccessibility means the nurse must understand the metabolic actions of the hormones produced by endocrine glands in order to assess the effects on that gland's target tissue as listed in Figure 23-1. This chapter describes clinical and diagnostic evaluation of the pancreas, the posterior pituitary gland.

HISTORY

The initial presentation of the patient determines the rapidity and direction of the interview. For a patient in acute distress, the history is curtailed to only a few questions about the patient's chief complaint and precipitating events. For the patient without obvious distress, the endocrine history focuses on four areas: 1) current health status, 2) description of the current illness, 3) medical history and general endocrine status, and 4) family history. Data collection in the endocrine history for diabetes complications is outlined in Box 23-1.

PANCREAS

Physical Assessment

Nursing priorities for physical assessment of the patient with pancreatic dysfunction focus on prevention of 1) hyperglycemia and 2) hypoglycemia.

Insulin, which is produced by the pancreas, is responsible for glucose metabolism. The clinical assessment provides information about pancreatic functioning. Clinical manifestations of abnormal glucose metabolism often include hyperglycemia, which is the initial assessment priority for the patient with pancreatic dysfunction.[1,2] Patients with hyperglycemia may ultimately be diagnosed with type 1 or type 2 diabetes or be hyperglycemic in association with a severe critical illness.[1,2] All of these conditions have specific identifying features. More information on the specific pathophysiology and management of each condition is available in Chapter 24.

Hyperglycemia

Because severe hyperglycemia affects a variety of body systems, all systems are assessed. The patient may complain of blurred vision, headache, weakness, fatigue, drowsiness, anorexia, nausea, and abdominal pain. On *inspection*, the patient has flushed skin, polyuria, polydipsia, vomiting, and evidence of dehydration. Progressive deterioration in the level of consciousness, from alert to lethargic or comatose, is observed as the hyperglycemia exacerbates. If ketoacidosis occurs, the patient's breathing becomes deep and rapid (Kussmaul respirations), and the breath may have a fruity odor. *Auscultation* of the abdomen may reveal hypoactive bowel sounds. *Palpation* elicits abdominal tenderness. *Percussion* may reveal diminished deep tendon reflexes. Because hyperglycemia results in osmotic diuresis, the patient's fluid volume status is assessed. Signs of dehydration include tachycardia, orthostatic hypotension, and poor skin turgor. The key laboratory tests that assist in assessment are discussed in the following section.

Laboratory Studies

Pertinent laboratory tests for pancreatic function measure short-term and long-term blood glucose levels, which can identify and diagnose diabetes.

Fasting Plasma Glucose

The fasting plasma glucose (FPG) level provides a "snapshot" of the blood glucose level at a single point in time after a person has not eaten for 8 hours. A normal FPG level is between 70 and 100 milligrams per deciliter (mg/dL).[1] A fasting glucose level between 100 and 125 mg/dL identifies a person who is *prediabetic*.[1] A FPG level of 126 mg/dL (7 millimoles per liter [mmol/L]) or higher is diagnostic of diabetes (Table 23-1). In nonurgent settings, the test is repeated on another day to ensure that the result is accurate. After a meal, the concentration of glucose increases in the

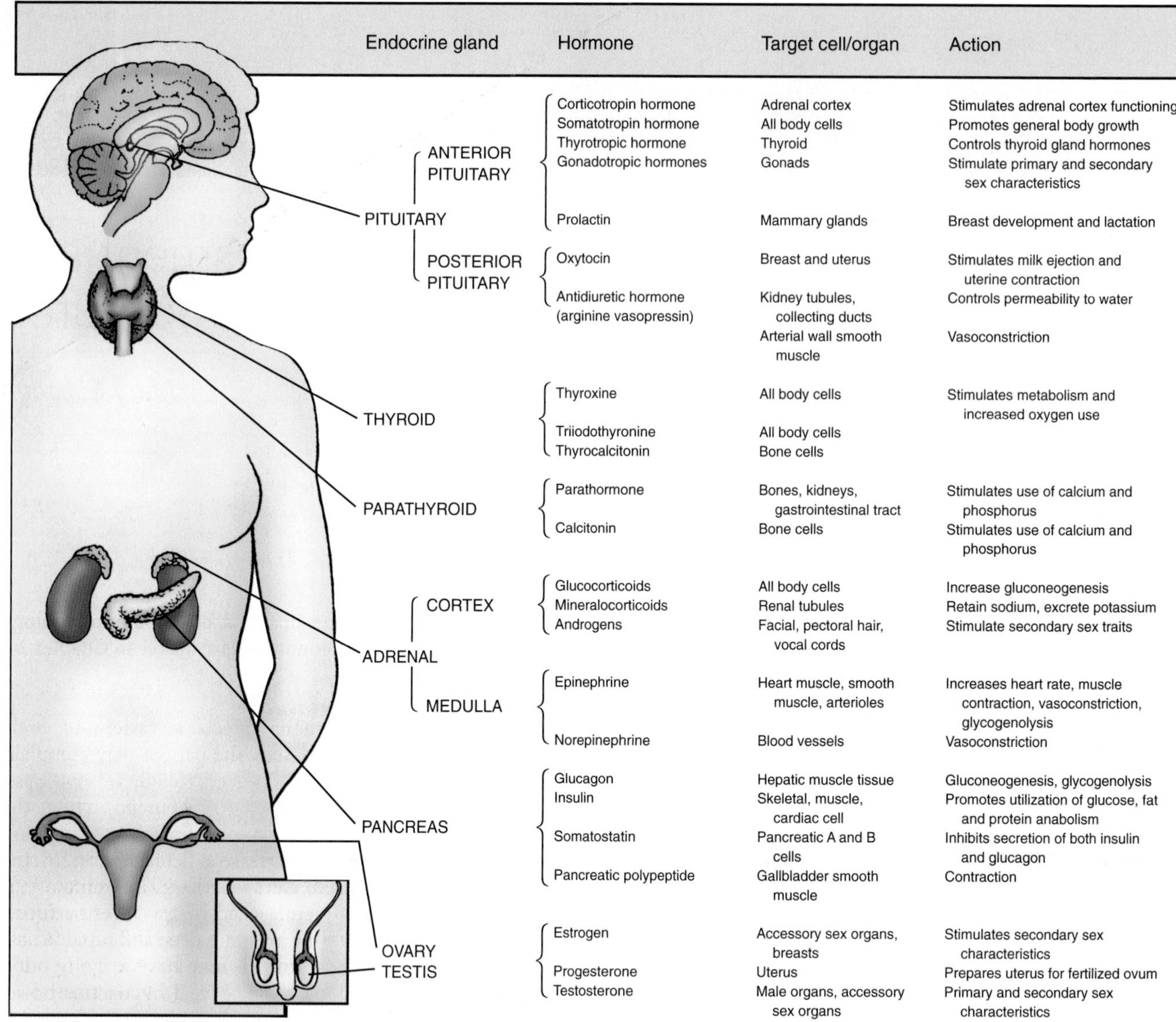

Endocrine gland	Hormone	Target cell/organ	Action
PITUITARY — ANTERIOR PITUITARY	Corticotropin hormone	Adrenal cortex	Stimulates adrenal cortex functioning
	Somatotropin hormone	All body cells	Promotes general body growth
	Thyrotropic hormone	Thyroid	Controls thyroid gland hormones
	Gonadotropic hormones	Gonads	Stimulate primary and secondary sex characteristics
	Prolactin	Mammary glands	Breast development and lactation
PITUITARY — POSTERIOR PITUITARY	Oxytocin	Breast and uterus	Stimulates milk ejection and uterine contraction
	Antidiuretic hormone (arginine vasopressin)	Kidney tubules, collecting ducts	Controls permeability to water
		Arterial wall smooth muscle	Vasoconstriction
THYROID	Thyroxine	All body cells	Stimulates metabolism and increased oxygen use
	Triiodothyronine	All body cells	
	Thyrocalcitonin	Bone cells	
PARATHYROID	Parathormone	Bones, kidneys, gastrointestinal tract	Stimulates use of calcium and phosphorus
	Calcitonin	Bone cells	Stimulates use of calcium and phosphorus
ADRENAL — CORTEX	Glucocorticoids	All body cells	Increase gluconeogenesis
	Mineralocorticoids	Renal tubules	Retain sodium, excrete potassium
	Androgens	Facial, pectoral hair, vocal cords	Stimulate secondary sex traits
ADRENAL — MEDULLA	Epinephrine	Heart muscle, smooth muscle, arterioles	Increases heart rate, muscle contraction, vasoconstriction, glycogenolysis
	Norepinephrine	Blood vessels	Vasoconstriction
PANCREAS	Glucagon	Hepatic muscle tissue	Gluconeogenesis, glycogenolysis
	Insulin	Skeletal, muscle, cardiac cell	Promotes utilization of glucose, fat and protein anabolism
	Somatostatin	Pancreatic A and B cells	Inhibits secretion of both insulin and glucagon
	Pancreatic polypeptide	Gallbladder smooth muscle	Contraction
OVARY / TESTIS	Estrogen	Accessory sex organs, breasts	Stimulates secondary sex characteristics
	Progesterone	Uterus	Prepares uterus for fertilized ovum
	Testosterone	Male organs, accessory sex organs	Primary and secondary sex characteristics

FIG 23-1 Location of endocrine glands with the hormones they produce, target cells or organs, and hormonal actions.

bloodstream; postprandial blood glucose levels should not exceed 180 mg/dL (10 mmol/L).[1]

Point of Care Blood Glucose

At the bedside, a point of care blood glucose value is usually obtained using a drop of whole blood measured by a handheld glucometer. The device provide an immediate result, which allows for rapid assessment and intervention.

All critically ill patients must have their blood glucose levels monitored frequently. Clinical practice guidelines from the American Association of Clinical Endocrinologists (AACE) and the American Diabetes Association (ADA) recommend instituting insulin therapy when the blood glucose is greater than 180 mg/dL in critical illness.[3] A target blood glucose range of 140 to 180 mg/dL is recommended.[3]

When a continuous insulin infusion is administered, point-of-care blood glucose testing is performed hourly or according to hospital protocol to achieve and maintain the blood glucose within the target range.[3]

Hypoglycemia is defined as a blood glucose level below 70 mg/dL (3.9 mmol/L).[1,3] Severe hypoglycemia is a medial emergency where the blood glucose is less than 40 mg/dL. A complication of glucose management with insulin is that hypoglycemic episodes may occur more frequently both in the hospital and with self-management of glucose levels in diabetes.[3]

Before discharge to home, patients with diabetes should be taught to monitor their blood glucose levels.[4] Maintaining blood glucose within the normal range is associated with fewer long-term diabetes-related complications.[4] Laboratory blood tests and point-of-care or self-monitoring of blood glucose represent the standard of care for management of diabetes.

Urine Glucose

Testing the urine for glucose is not recommended for patients with diabetes because too much variation exists in the threshold for glucose when diabetes-related kidney damage has

BOX 23-1 Data Collection Complications of Diabetes

Current Health Status

The body may not be able to adjust to increased insulin needs resulting from sudden physiologic changes such as infection, injury, or surgery. The nurse assesses whether the patient has a severe infection, surgical wound, or traumatic injury.

- Recent or current signs and symptoms:
  - Unexplained changes in weight, thirst, hunger
  - Headache, blurred vision
  - Longstanding, unhealed infection
  - Vaginitis, pruritus
  - Leg pain, numbness
- Unexplained change in urinary patterns (e.g., daytime and nighttime, frequency, volume)
- Energy or stamina changes
- Endurance level
- Weakness
- Unexplained, excessive fatigue
- Behavior or mental changes (also ask family member or significant other for input):
  - Memory loss
  - Orientation

Assessment of Current Illness: Onset, Characteristics, and Course

- Chronic illness: Physiologic or psychologic stress may increase endogenous glucose.
- Recent treatments that could be a source of exogenous glucose:
  - Hyperalimentation
  - Peritoneal dialysis
  - Hemodialysis
- Medications, including prescription and over-the-counter preparations: Pharmacologic agents may alter pancreatic function by increasing or decreasing the release of endocrine hormones. Medications also may interfere with hormonal action at the receptor site on the target cell.

Medical History: Questions

- Have you had prior pancreatic surgery?
- Have you ever been told that any of the following applied to you:
  - Too much sugar in the urine?
  - Too much sugar in the blood?
  - Will probably develop too much sugar in your blood later in life?
- If you answered yes to any of these questions, what treatment, if any, was prescribed?
- Are you currently following such a treatment?

Family History: Questions

- Has a close family member (parent or sibling) been diagnosed with diabetes or "sugar in the blood"?
- If yes, how was this condition treated?

TABLE 23-1 Blood Glucose Levels

PATIENT STATUS	FASTING BG (mg/dL)	FASTING BG (mmol/L)
Hypoglycemia	<70	<3.9
Normal	70-100	>3.9-5.6
Prediabetes	100-125	5.6-6.9
Diabetes	≥126	≥7.0

BG, Blood glucose; *mg/dL*, milligram per deciliter; *mmol/L*, millimole per liter.
Data from American Diabetes Association. Standards of medical care in diabetes—2014, *Diabetes Care*. 2014: 37(suppl 1):S14-S80.

occurred. Urine glucose measurements are affected by variation in fluid intake, reflect an average glucose level, not a specific point in time, and are altered by some medications. Urine glucose testing does not offer any help in the identification of hypoglycemia. For all of these reasons, urine glucose testing is never to be used.

Glycated Hemoglobin

Blood testing of glucose is useful for daily management of diabetes. However, a different blood test is used to achieve an objective measure of blood glucose over an extended period. The *glycated hemoglobin test*, also known as *glycosylated hemoglobin* (*HbA$_{1C}$* or *A$_{1C}$*) provides information about the average amount of glucose that has been present in the patient's bloodstream over the previous 3 to 4 months. During the 120-day life span of red blood cells (RBCs; erythrocytes), the hemoglobin within each cell binds to the available blood glucose through a process known as *glycosylation*. Typically, 4% to 6% of hemoglobin contains the glucose group A$_{1C}$. A normal A$_{1C}$ value is less than 5.4%, with an acceptable target level for diabetic patients below 6.5%.[1,2,5] The A$_{1C}$ value correlates with specific blood glucose levels as shown in Table 23-2.[1,2] The American Diabetes Association recommends use of the A$_{1C}$ value both during initial assessment of diabetes mellitus and for follow-up to monitor treatment effectiveness.[1]

Blood Ketones

Ketone bodies are a byproduct of rapid fat breakdown. Ketone blood levels rise in acute illness, with fasting, and with sustained elevation of blood glucose in type 1 diabetes in the absence of insulin. In diabetic ketoacidosis (DKA), fat breakdown (*lipolysis*) occurs so rapidly that fat metabolism is incomplete, and the ketone bodies (acetone, beta-hydroxybutyric acid, and acetoacetic acid) accumulate in the blood (*ketonemia*) and are excreted in the urine (*ketonuria*). It is recommended that all patients with diabetes perform self-test, or have their blood or urine tested, for the presence of ketones during any alteration in level of consciousness or acute illness with an elevated blood glucose.[6] A blood test that measures *beta-hydroxybutyrate*, the primary metabolite of ketoacidosis, provides the most accurate measurement.[6,7] Self-test point-of-care meters to measure blood ketones from a fingerstick drop of blood are now available.[6]

TABLE 23-2 Correlation Between Hemoglobin A_{1c} Concentration and Plasma Glucose Level

HbA_{1c} (%)	MEAN PLASMA GLUCOSE LEVEL (mg/dL)	MEAN PLASMA GLUCOSE LEVEL (mmol/L)
6	126	7.0
7	154	8.6
8	183	10.2
9	212	11.8
10	240	13.4
11	269	14.9
12	298	16.5

HbA_{1c}, Glycosylated hemoglobin; *mg/dL*, milligram per deciliter; *mmol/L*, millimole per liter.
Data from American Diabetes Association. Standards of medical care in diabetes—2014. *Diabetes Care*. 2014: 37(suppl 1):S14-S80.

Elevated levels of ketones (ketonemia) may be detected by a fruity, sweet-smelling odor on the exhaled breath. This distinctive breath odor derives from the elimination of acetone as part of the compensatory response to maintain a normal pH.

Urine Ketones

Ketones are eliminated in the urine, and urine may be tested for ketones. Ketonuria is retrospective and indicates that blood ketones were or are elevated.[6,7] Ketonuria may also occur in fasting and starvation states.

PITUITARY GLAND

The pituitary gland, recessed in the base of the cranium, is not accessible to physical assessment. The critical care nurse must, therefore, be aware of the systemic effects of a normally functioning pituitary to be able to identify dysfunction. One essential hormone formed in the hypothalamus but secreted through the posterior pituitary gland is *antidiuretic hormone* (ADH), also known as *vasopressin.*

Physical Assessment

Nursing priorities for physical assessment of the patient with pituitary gland dysfunction focus on 1) hydration status, 2) vital signs, and 3) weight change and intake and output.

ADH controls the amount of fluid lost and retained within the body. Acute dysfunction of the posterior pituitary or the hypothalamus may result in insufficient or excessive ADH production. The clinical signs of posterior pituitary dysfunction often manifest as fluid volume deficit (insufficient ADH production) or fluid volume excess (excessive ADH production).

Hydration Status

The nurse determines the effectiveness of ADH production by conducting a hydration assessment. A hydration assessment includes observations of skin integrity, skin turgor, and buccal membrane moisture. Moist, shiny buccal membranes indicate satisfactory fluid balance. Skin turgor that is resilient and returns to its original position in less than 3 seconds after being pinched or lifted indicates adequate skin elasticity. The skin over the forehead, clavicle, and sternum is the most reliable for testing tissue turgor because these areas are less affected by aging and easily assessed for changes related to fluid balance. In older patients, these typical assessment findings may be absent.

Other indicators that the patient's hydration status is adequate for metabolic demands include a balanced intake and output and absence of thirst. Absence of thirst, however, is not a reliable indicator of dehydration in those with decreased thirst mechanisms such as the older or critically ill patients. Absence of abrupt changes in mental status may also indicate normal hydration. Other indicators of normal hydration include absence of edema, stable weight, and urine specific gravity that falls within the normal range (1.005 to 1.030).

Vital Signs

Changes in heart rate, blood pressure, and central venous pressure (when available) are useful to determine fluid volume status. Blood pressure and pulse are monitored frequently. Decreased blood pressure with increased pulse is characteristic of hypovolemia, whereas elevated blood pressure and a rapid, bounding pulse may indicate hypervolemia.

Weight Changes and Intake and Output

Daily weight changes coincide with fluid retention and fluid loss. Sudden changes in weight can result from a change in fluid balance; 1 L of fluid lost or retained is equal to approximately 2.2 pounds (lb), or 1 kilogram (kg), of weight gained or lost. To use weight as a true determinant of the fluid balance, all extraneous variables are eliminated, and the same scale is used at the same time each day. Precise measurement and notation of intake and output are used as criteria for fluid replacement therapy.

Laboratory Assessment

No single diagnostic test identifies dysfunction of the posterior pituitary gland. Diagnosis usually is made through the patient's clinical presentation and history. Although serum measurement of ADH is available, it is rarely obtained in critical illness.

Serum Antidiuretic Hormone

The normal serum ADH range is 1 to 5 picogram per milliliter (pg/mL). Prior to ADH measurement, all medications that may alter the release of ADH are withheld for a minimum of 8 hours. Common medications that affect ADH levels include morphine sulfate, lithium carbonate, chlorothiazide, carbamazepine, oxytocin, and selective serotonin reuptake inhibitors (SSRIs). Nicotine, alcohol, positive-pressure and negative-pressure ventilation, and emotional stress also influence ADH.

Serum ADH levels are then compared with the blood and urine osmolality to differentiate *syndrome of inappropriate antidiuretic hormone* (SIADH) from central *diabetes insipidus* (DI). Increased ADH levels in the bloodstream compared with a low serum osmolality and elevated urine osmolality confirms the diagnosis of SIADH. Reduced levels of serum

ADH in a patient with high serum osmolality, hypernatremia, and reduced urine concentration signal central DI. Chapter 24 provides more information about SIADH and DI.

Serum and Urine Osmolality

Values for serum osmolality in the bloodstream range from 275 to 295 milliosmole per kilogram of water (mOsm/kg H_2O) and the range will vary according to the normal limits established by the clinical laboratory where the test was analyzed. *Osmolality* measurements determine the concentration of dissolved particles in a solution. In a healthy person, a change in the concentration of solutes triggers a chain of events to maintain adequate serum dilution. The most accurate measures of the body's fluid balance are obtained when urine and blood samples are collected simultaneously. Increased serum osmolality stimulates the release of ADH, which reduces the amount of water lost through the kidney. Body fluid is thus retained at the kidney tubules and collecting ducts to dilute the particle concentration in the bloodstream.

Decreased serum osmolality inhibits the release of ADH. The kidney tubules increase their permeability, and fluid is eliminated from the body in an attempt to regain normal concentration of particles in the bloodstream. Urine osmolality in the person with normal kidneys depends on fluid intake. With high fluid intake, particle dilution is low but will increase if fluids are restricted. The expected range for urine osmolality is, therefore, wide, ranging from 50 to 1400 mOsm/kg.

Antidiuretic Hormone Test

The ADH test is used to differentiate *neurogenic* DI (central) from *nephrogenic* (kidney) DI. The patient is challenged with 0.05 to 1.0 mL of intranasally administered ADH in the form of desmopressin (1-deamino-8-D-arginine vasopressin [DDAVP]). A peripheral intravenous catheter is inserted before ADH administration, and urine volume and osmolality are measured every 30 minutes for 2 hours before and after the ADH challenge. Test results in which urine osmolality remains unchanged indicate nephrogenic DI, suggesting kidney dysfunction because the kidneys are no longer responsive to ADH. This test is rarely or never performed in the critical care unit because of the unstable hemodynamic and volume status of most patients.

Serum sodium. Assessment of the serum sodium is essential in any condition that may alter fluid volume status. Sodium is the most abundant electrolyte in the bloodstream with a normal range from 135-145 mEq/L. Any significant alteration in volume status, whether as a consequence of DI, SIADH, neurosurgery or traumatic brain injury, will alter serum sodium levels.[8,9] SIADH, by retaining water, will dilute blood volume, and serum sodium will trend below 135 mEq/L, whereas in DI the extracellular fluid is concentrated, and serum sodium may rise above 145 mEq/L.

Serum osmolality. The serum osmolality is assessed in concordance with the serum sodium. When the serum sodium is low, there are fewer particles (osmoles) in the extracellular fluid, and serum osmolarity will also be low (<285 mOsmo/Kg).[9] In contrast, when the serum sodium is elevated, there are more measurable particles in the extracellular fluid, and serum osmolarity will be high (>295 mOsmo/Kg).[9]

DIAGNOSTIC PROCEDURES

In addition to laboratory tests, radiographic examination, computed tomography (CT), and magnetic resonance imaging (MRI) are used to diagnose structural lesions such as cranial bone fractures, tumors, or blood clots in the region of the pituitary. Although these procedures do not diagnose DI or SIADH, they are useful in uncovering the likely underlying cause.

Radiographic Examination

A basic radiographic examination of the inferior skull views the sella turcica and surrounding bone formation. Bone fractures or tissue swelling at the base of the brain, which are apparent on a radiograph, suggest interference with the vascular supply and nerve impulses to the hypothalamic–pituitary system. Dysfunction may occur if the hypothalamus, infundibular stalk, or pituitary gland is impaired.

Computed Tomography

CT of the base of the skull identifies pituitary tumors, blood clots, cysts, nodules, or other soft tissue masses. This rapid procedure causes no discomfort except that it requires the patient to lie perfectly still. CT studies can be performed with radiopaque contrast or without contrast. The contrast dye is given intravenously to highlight the hypothalamus, infundibular stalk, and pituitary gland. This dye may cause allergic reactions in iodine-sensitive persons, and the patient must be carefully questioned about iodine allergy before the test. The size and shape of the sella turcica and the position of the hypothalamus, infundibular stalk, and pituitary are identified.[10]

Magnetic Resonance Imaging

MRI enables the radiologist to visualize internal organs and cellular characteristics of specific tissues. MRI uses a magnetic field rather than radiation to produce high-resolution, cross-sectional images. The soft brain tissue and surrounding cerebrospinal fluid (CSF) make the brain especially suited to MRI, especially in cases of DI or SIADH.[10]

REFERENCES

1. American Diabetes Association: Standards of medical care in diabetes-2014, *Diabetes Care* 37(Suppl 1):S14, 2014.
2. American Diabetes Association: Diagnosis and classification of diabetes mellitus, *Diabetes Care* 37(Suppl 1):S81, 2014.
3. Moghissi ES, et al: American Association of Clinical Endocrinologists and American Diabetes Association consensus statement on inpatient glycemic control, *Diabetes Care* 32(6):1119, 2009.
4. Cryer PE, et al: Evaluation and management of adult hypoglycemic disorders: an Endocrine Society Clinical Practice Guideline, *J Clin Endocrinol Metab* 94(3):709, 2009.
5. Handelsman Y, et al: American Association of Clinical Endocrinologists Medical Guidelines for Clinical Practice for developing a diabetes mellitus comprehensive care plan, *Endocr Pract* 17(Suppl 2):1, 2011.
6. Kitabchi AE, Umpierrez GE, Miles JM, Fisher JN: Hyperglycemic crises in adult patients with diabetes, *Diabetes Care* 32(7):1335, 2009.

7. Arora S, Henderson SO, Long T, Menchine M: Diagnostic accuracy of point-of-care testing for diabetic ketoacidosis at emergency-department triage: β-hydroxybutyrate versus the urine dipstick, *Diabetes Care* 34(4):852, 2011.
8. John CA, Day MW: Central neurogenic diabetes insipidus, syndrome of inappropriate secretion of antidiuretic hormone, and cerebral salt-wasting syndrome in traumatic brain injury, *Crit Care Nurse* 32(2):e1, 2012.
9. Kirkman MA, Albert AF, Ibrahim A, Doberenz D: Hyponatremia and brain injury: historical and contemporary perspectives, *Neurocrit Care* 18(3):406, 2013.
10. Ouyang T, Rothfus WE, Ng JM, Challinor SM: Imaging of the pituitary, *Radiol Clin North Am* 49(3):549, 2011.

CHAPTER 24

Endocrine Disorders and Therapeutic Management

Mary E. Lough

Be sure to check out the bonus material, including review questions, on the Evolve website at http://evolve.elsevier.com/Urden/priorities/.

The endocrine system is almost invisible when it functions well, but it causes widespread upset when an organ is suppressed, hyperstimulated, or under physiologic stress. This results in a wide spectrum of possible disorders; some are rare, and others are frequently encountered in the critical care unit. This chapter focuses on the neuroendocrine stress associated with critical illness and on disorders of two major endocrine glands: the pancreas and the posterior pituitary gland.

NEUROENDOCRINOLOGY OF STRESS AND CRITICAL ILLNESS

Major neurologic and endocrine changes occur when an individual is confronted with physiologic stress caused by any critical illness, sepsis,[1] trauma, major surgery, or underlying cardiovascular disease.[2] The normal "fight or flight" response that is initiated in times of physiologic or psychologic stress is exacerbated in critical illness through activation of the neuroendocrine system, specifically the hypothalamic-pituitary-adrenal axis (HPA).[3] All endocrine organs are affected by acute critical illness, as shown in Table 24-1.

Acute Neuroendocrine Response to Critical Illness

The fight-or-flight acute response to physiologic threat is a rapid discharge of the catecholamines *norepinephrine* and *epinephrine* into the bloodstream.[3] Norepinephrine is released from the nerve endings of the sympathetic nervous system (SNS).

Hypothalamic-Pituitary-Adrenal Axis in Critical Illness

Epinephrine (adrenalin) is released from the medulla of the adrenal glands. Epinephrine increases cerebral blood flow and cerebral oxygen consumption and may be the trigger for recruitment of the hypothalamic-pituitary axis.[3]

The *posterior pituitary gland* releases antidiuretic hormone (ADH), also known as *vasopressin* (pitressin), as a component of the physiologic stress response. This hormone is an antidiuretic with a powerful vasoconstrictive effect on blood vessels.[3] The combination of epinephrine and vasopressin quickly raises blood pressure; it also decreases gastric motility.[3] Epinephrine increases heart rate, causes ventricular dysrhythmias in susceptible patients, and provides some analgesia or lack of pain awareness during acute physical stress.[3]

The *anterior pituitary gland* produces several hormones including *corticotropin* (also called ACTH), which stimulates release of *cortisol* from the adrenal cortex.[4] Cortisol release is an important protective response to stress. Increased cortisol levels alter carbohydrate, fat, and protein metabolism so that energy is immediately and selectively available to vital organs such as the brain. However, if critical illness is prolonged, the HPA may not be able to respond adequately to prolonged physiologic stress.

The *adrenal gland* produces cortisol from the cortex and epinephrine from the medulla. Diminished adrenal gland function may result from a variety of causes during critical illness:

- *Primary hypoadrenalism* describes an intrinsic failure of the adrenal gland to produce normal endogenous glucocorticosteroid hormones (e.g., cortisol) and mineralocorticosteroid hormones (e.g., aldosterone). Primary adrenal failure is rare.
- *Secondary adrenal dysfunction,* or *Cushing syndrome,* occurs as a result of the administration of therapeutic steroids. In response to exogenous glucocorticosteroids, the adrenal glands stop production of intrinsic hormones. Patients who have taken steroids before their admission to the hospital need their dosage increased during illness.
- *Critical illness–related corticosteroid insufficiency* (CIRCI) describes a situation in which the adrenal gland produces glucocorticosteroids but the quantity is insufficient for the disease process. Peripheral cortisol resistance occurs as inflammatory cytokines induce cellular resistance to cortisol.[5]

Serum Cortisol Level

Clinical assessment of adrenal dysfunction is difficult in the critically ill, and a specialized laboratory assay is necessary for an accurate diagnosis. First, a baseline serum cortisol level is obtained. Adrenal failure is likely if the cortisol level is less than 10 mcg/dL.[5]

Cosyntropin Stimulation Test

Further confirmation of adrenal dysfunction may be obtained by performance of a corticotropin stimulation test *(cosyntropin test).* Cosyntropin is a medication made from the first 24 amino acids of corticotropin. In the test, 250 mcg cosyntropin is administered by the intravenous (IV) route, and serum blood levels are measured 30 minutes later. A serum cortisol rise from baseline of less than 9 mcg/dL after 30 minutes denotes inability of the adrenal gland to respond to a stress stimulus (nonresponder).[5] If the cortisol rise is greater than 9 mcg/dL in response to corticotropin stimulation, the adrenal glands are

TABLE 24-1 Endocrine Responses to Physiologic Stress in Critical Illness

GLAND OR ORGAN	HORMONE	PHYSIOLOGIC RESPONSE and FINDINGS ON CLINICAL AND LABORATORYASSESSMENT
Adrenal cortex	Cortisol	↑ Insulin resistance → ↑ glycogenolysis → ↑ glucose circulation ↑ Hepatic gluconeogenesis → ↑ glucose available ↑ Lipolysis ↑ Protein catabolism ↑ Sodium → ↑ water retention to maintain plasma osmolality by movement of extravascular fluid into the intravascular space ↓ Connective tissue fibroblasts → poor wound healing
	Glucocorticoid	↓ Histamine release → suppression of immune system ↓ Lymphocytes, monocytes, eosinophils, basophils ↑ Polymorphonuclear leukocytes → ↑ infection risk ↑ Glucose ↓ Gastric acid secretion
	Mineralocorticoids	↑ Aldosterone → ↓ sodium excretion → ↓ water excretion → ↑ intravascular volume ↑ Potassium excretion → hypokalemia ↑ Hydrogen ion excretion → metabolic acidosis
Adrenal medulla	Epinephrine	↑ Endorphins → ↓ pain
	Norepinephrine, epinephrine	↑ Metabolic rate to accommodate stress response ↑ Live glycogenolysis → ↑ glucose ↑ Insulin (cells are insulin-resistant) ↑ Cardiac contractility ↑ Cardiac output ↑ Dilation of coronary arteries ↑ Blood pressure ↑ Heart rate ↑ Bronchodilation → ↑ respirations ↑ Perfusion to heart, brain, lungs, liver, and muscle ↓ Perfusion to periphery of body ↓ Peristalsis
	Norepinephrine	↑ Peripheral vasoconstriction ↑ Blood pressure ↑ Sodium retention ↑ Potassium excretion
Pituitary	All hormones	↑ Endogenous opioids → ↓ pain
Anterior pituitary	Corticotropin	↑ Aldosterone → ↓ sodium excretion → ↓ water excretion → ↑ intravascular volume ↑ Cortisol → ↑ blood volume
	Growth hormones	↑ Protein anabolism of amino acids to protein ↑ Lipolysis → ↑ gluconeogenesis
Posterior pituitary	Antidiuretic hormone	↑ Vasoconstriction ↑ Water retention → restoration of circulating blood volume ↓ Urine output ↑ Hypoosmolality
Pancreas	Insulin	↑ Insulin resistance → hyperglycemia
	Glucagon	↑ Glycolysis (directly opposes action of insulin) ↑ Glucose for fuel ↑ Glycogenolysis ↑ Gluconeogenesis ↑ Lipolysis
Thyroid	Thyroxine	↓ Routine metabolic demands during stress

↑, Increased; →, causes; ↓, decreased.

functioning normally (responder).[5] Corticosteroids are given only to nonresponders. The combination of a low baseline cortisol value (less than 10 mcg/dL) with minimal or no rise (less than 9 mcg/dL) after cosyntropin stimulation is evidence of adrenal gland dysfunction with corticosteroid deficiency.[5]

Corticosteroid Replacement

Clinical practice guidelines[5] recommend short-term provision of low-dose hydrocortisone for patients who have a diagnosis of septic shock with refractory vasopressor-dependent hypotension. Hydrocortisone is the recommended replacement because it is the pharmacologic steroid that most resembles endogenous cortisol.

The guidelines recommend use of the cosyntropin stimulation test as described previously. However, the test is not recommended as a stand-alone method to identify patients who might receive low-dose steroids. This apparent contradiction is explained by the fact that several clinical trials of low-dose steroid replacement in sepsis have demonstrated a faster resolution of the shock symptoms but no difference in overall mortality compared with placebo.[5] High-dose steroid replacement is never recommended in the management of sepsis. Corticosteroids are never discontinued abruptly and must be tapered gradually over several days.[5]

Liver and Pancreas in Critical Illness

The liver releases the hormone *glucagon* to stimulate the liver to pour additional glucose into the bloodstream in response to physiologic stress. Glucagon rapidly raises blood glucose levels. Peripheral tissues may become *insulin-resistant*, meaning the tissues are unable to use the available insulin to transport glucose inside the cells. This further raises blood glucose levels, causing persistent stress-induced hyperglycemia.[6] There is a second metabolic system that enables insulin to enter the cell. The insulin-independent *glucose transporters* (GLUT 1, GLUT 2, and GLUT 3) are active during physiologic stress but may be unable to keep up with the massive increase in glucose production by the liver. Continuous infusion of insulin to return and maintain blood glucose levels within a safe, near-normal range reduces morbidity and mortality.[2]

Hyperglycemia in Critical Illness

Normal fasting blood glucose levels range between 70 and 100 mg/dL in a healthy person. Critically ill patients frequently have much higher blood glucose levels, and several retrospective analyses have reported that hyperglycemic patients have a higher mortality rate than patients with normal blood glucose values. In 2001, a landmark prospective, randomized study showed a significant reduction in morbidity and mortality among critically ill surgical patients whose blood glucose concentration was maintained between 80 and 110 mg/dL with a continuous insulin infusion, compared with those whose blood glucose was only treated if it was greater than 180 mg/dL.[7] A study of medical critical care patients by the same group with the same protocol demonstrated a survival benefit after 3 days of tight glucose control with a continuous insulin infusion.[8] These initial studies were greeted with tremendous enthusiasm, and many critical care units adopted stringent glucose control standards to reduce hyperglycemia-associated morbidity and mortality. However, achievement of such tight glucose control outside of a research trial can be challenging as shown by the results of more recent clinical trials.

The NICE-SUGAR trial was a prospective randomized trial of 6014 critically ill patients. It compared continuous insulin infusion to achieve tight glucose control (target 81 to 108 mg/dL) with a conventional glucose control range (target below 180 mg/dL).[9] In the tight glucose control group 6.8% had episodes of severe hypoglycemia (below 40 mg/dL); in the conventional control group only 0.5% experienced severe hypoglycemia.[9] There was a 2.6% higher risk of death in the intensive glucose control group (27.5% died) compared with the conventional control group (24.9% died).[9]

Clinical Practice Guidelines Related to Blood Glucose Management in Critically Ill Patients

As a result of the studies just described, clinical practice guidelines were developed by the American Association of Clinical Endocrinologists (AACE) and the American Diabetes Association (ADA) that recommend the use of continuous insulin infusions to maintain blood glucose in critical care patients between 140 and 180 mg/dL, with frequent monitoring of blood glucose.[2] The 140 to 180 mg/dL level was selected to minimize the risk of hypoglycemia.

Other glucose-control guidelines relevant to critical illness have also been published. The Society of Critical Care Medicine (SCCM) recommends initiating glycemic control when the blood glucose rises above 150 mg/dL.[1,10] Insulin management must be initiated if the blood glucose level is above 180 mg/dL.[2,10] More liberal glucose control represents the current trend of targeted values.

Insulin Management in the Critically Ill

As a result of the research that has highlighted the deleterious effects of hyperglycemia in critical illness, most hospitals have developed an institution-specific glucose–insulin algorithm to lower blood glucose into the targeted range.[11] The vigilance of the critical care nurse is pivotal to the success of any intervention to lower blood glucose using a continuous insulin infusion. As discussed earlier, many glucose control protocols are using less restrictive ranges due to concerns about iatrogenic hypoglycemia.

Frequent Blood Glucose Monitoring

Monitoring the blood glucose with a point-of-care glucometer is the basis of targeted glucose control. As part of the comprehensive initial assessment, the blood sugar is measured by a standard laboratory sample or by a finger-stick capillary blood sample. In many institutions, if the blood sugar is greater than 180 mg/dL, the patient is started on a continuous IV insulin infusion. While the glucose is elevated, blood sample measurements are usually obtained hourly, to allow titration of the insulin drip to lower blood glucose.[11] After the patient is stable, blood glucose measurements can be spaced approximately every 2 hours, based on individual hospital protocols.

Several different blood-sampling methods are available. A capillary finger-stick is perhaps the easiest initial option, although the fingers can become noticeably marked if there are numerous sticks over several days. Trauma to the fingers is also exacerbated if peripheral perfusion is diminished. If a central venous catheter (CVC) or an arterial line with a blood conservation system attached is in place, this can be a highly efficient system for sampling because there is no blood wastage. If a blood conservation setup is not attached, use of the venous or arterial catheter for access is unacceptable because of the quantity of "waste" blood that would be discarded.

Continuous Insulin Infusion

Many hospitals use insulin infusion protocols for management of stress-induced hyperglycemia that are implemented by the critical care nurse.[2,11] Effective glucose protocols gauge the insulin infusion rate based on two parameters: 1) the immediate blood glucose result and 2) the rate of change in the blood glucose level since the last hourly measurement. The following three examples illustrate this concept:

- Patient A receives 3 units of continuous IV regular insulin per hour and has a blood glucose measurement of 110 mg/dL, but 1 hour ago it was 190 mg/dL; this represents a decrease of 80 mg/dL in the blood glucose in one hour. Consequently, the insulin rate must be decreased to avoid sudden hypoglycemia.
- Patient B receives 3 units of continuous IV regular insulin per hour and has a blood glucose measurement of 110 mg/dL, but 1 hour ago it was 112 mg/dL, this represents a decrease of only 2 mg/dL in the blood glucose in one hour; in this situation, no change is made in the insulin infusion rate.
- Patient C receives 3 units of continuous IV regular insulin per hour and has a blood glucose measurement of 190 mg/dL, and 1 hour ago it was 197 mg/dL, this represents a decrease of only 7 mg/dL in the blood glucose in one hour; In this situation, the insulin rate must be increased to more rapidly move the patient's blood sugar toward the targeted glucose range (i.e., 140 to 180 mg/dL, although the target range will vary by individual hospital protocol).

The important point to emphasize is that the *rate of change* of the blood glucose is as important as the *most recent* blood glucose measurement.[11] Each of the patients described in the examples may have the same insulin infusion rate, depending on their catabolic state, but individualization among patients with different diagnoses can be safely achieved as long as the rate of change is also considered.

A person's insulin requirement often fluctuates over the course of an illness. This occurs in response to changes in the clinical condition, such as development of an infection, caloric alterations caused by stopping or starting enteral or parenteral nutrition, administration of therapeutic steroids, or because the person is less catabolic. A method to allow for corrective incremental changes (up or down) to adapt to the reality of clinical developments and maintain the glucose within the target range is essential. Some protocols alter only the infusion rate, whereas others incorporate bolus insulin doses if the glucose concentration is greater than a preestablished threshold (e.g., 180 mg/dL). Typically, after the blood glucose has remained within the target range for a number of hours (varies according to the hospital protocol), the time interval between measurements for blood glucose monitoring may be extended to every 2 hours.

Transition from Continuous to Intermittent Insulin Coverage

The transition from a continuous insulin infusion to intermittent insulin coverage must be handled with care to avoid large fluctuations in blood glucose levels. Before the conversion, the regular insulin infusion should be at a stable and preferably low rate, and the patient's blood glucose level should be maintained consistently within the target range. The transition from IV to subcutaneous administration depends on numerous factors, including whether the patient is able to eat a consistent amount of dietary carbohydrate.[12]

Clinicians use various methods to calculate the quantity of insulin to prescribe during the transition from IV to subcutaneous insulin to maintain stable blood glucose levels. Figure 24-1 depicts hypothetical examples of how a combination of basal and bolus insulin regimens (prandial insulin) can work in clinical practice. The following paragraphs describe the application of one calculation method for a 67-year-old patient, Alice Smith, who is recovering from critical illness and has recently been weaned from the ventilator and extubated.

1. Ms. Smith is in stable condition on a regular insulin drip at 1 unit per hour. She is ready to be transitioned to subcutaneous insulin and will be taking food and liquids by mouth. Her total insulin requirement over the previous 24 hours was 32 units. Ms. Smith will now require basal coverage (provided by subcutaneous intermediate or long-acting insulin) and *prandial* coverage for mealtimes (provided by short-acting subcutaneous insulin).
2. The 30 units of insulin infused during the previous 24 hours is Ms. Smith's required daily insulin dose. To transition to subcutaneous insulin, a proportion of this amount (i.e., 75% to 80%) will be divided between basal and prandial components.[2] In this situation, 75% of the 32 units = 24 units. Half of this amount (12 units) will be administered subcutaneously as intermediate or long-acting insulin; the other half will be administered as short-acting insulin to coincide with meals (i.e., 4 units with each of three meals).
3. The options for insulin administration for Ms. Smith are as follows:
   - *Basal insulin*: 12 units of glargine once daily *or* 6 units twice daily of Neutral Protamine Hagedorn (NPH) administered subcutaneously
   - *Prandial insulin*: 4 units regular insulin given subcutaneously before each meal (short-acting) *or* 4 units Lispro or Aspart given subcutaneously with each meal (ultra–short-acting insulin); verify current blood glucose level.
   - *Supplemental corrective insulin*: A supplemental correction scale can be used to cover any hyperglycemia above the target range, and administration can be combined with scheduled blood glucose measurements; verify current blood glucose level.

After the transition to subcutaneous insulin, the dosage is adjusted based upon the patient's *insulin sensitivity*, or stated another way, according to how much insulin is needed for each 15 grams of carbohydrate intake. Patients who are *insulin-resistant* require more insulin than those who are *insulin-sensitive*.

Table 24-2 describes the various types of insulin available for use. These include ultra–short-acting, short-acting, intermediate-acting, long-acting, and combination insulin replacement options.[13] Even after the transition to subcutaneous insulin is completed, blood glucose is monitored frequently to maintain blood glucose within the target range and detect hyperglycemia or hypoglycemia.[14]

Corrective Insulin Coverage

A patient may be prescribed supplemental or corrective doses of insulin in addition to the basal/prandial insulin combination. The use of the trio of basal, prandial, and corrective insulin is designed to eliminate the use of the traditional sliding scale. Criticisms of the sliding scale method are that the dosages are rarely reevaluated or adjusted once established and that the scales treat hyperglycemia only after it has occurred; they are not proactive in the manner of the basal/bolus/corrective insulin method.[11]

Hypoglycemia Management

It is important to have a protocol for the management of hypoglycemia. The major drawback to use of intensive insulin

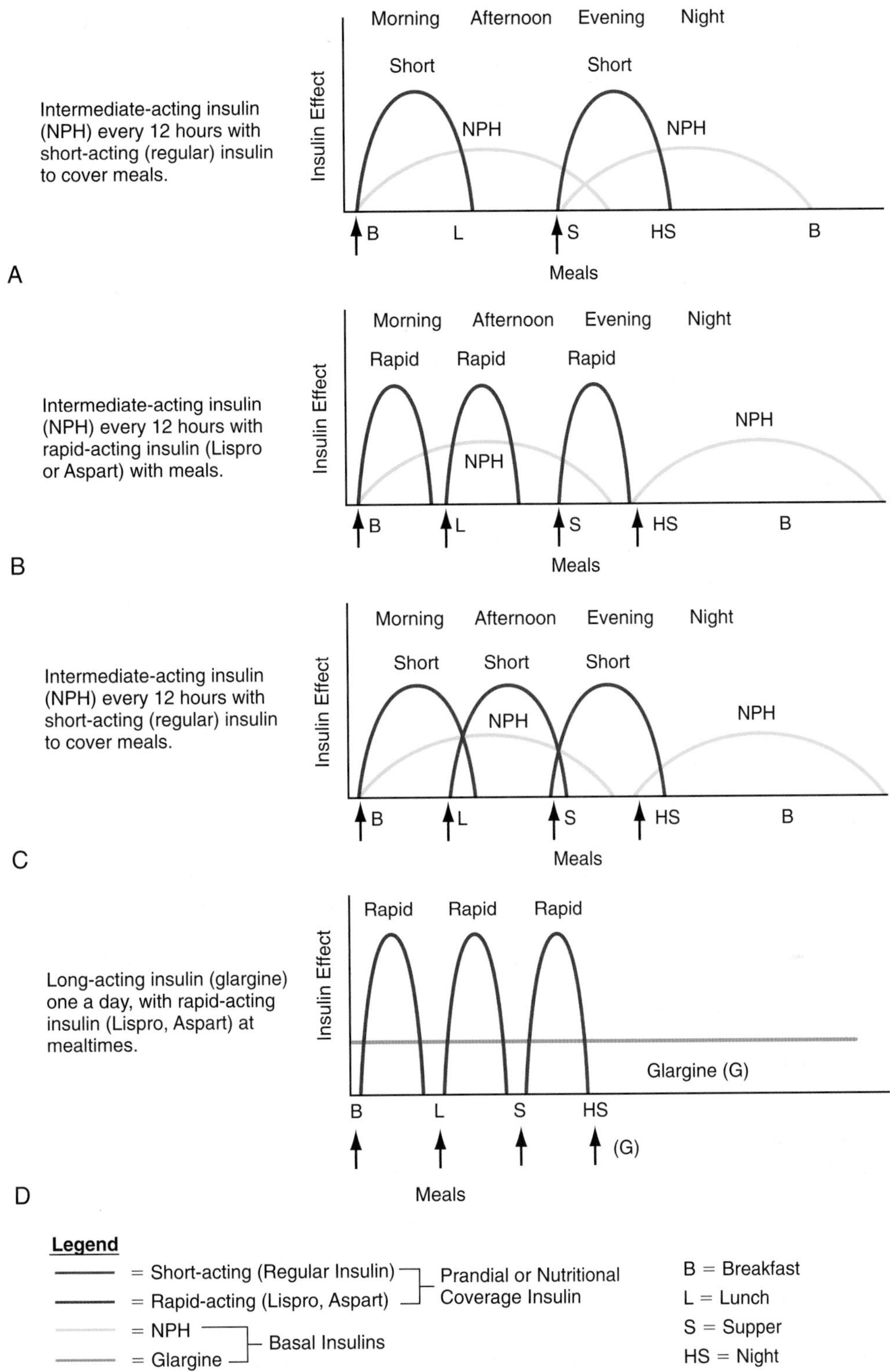

FIG 24-1 Basal and Nutritional Bolus Insulin Combinations.

protocols, as described earlier, is the potential for hypoglycemia.[14] Whenever hypoglycemia is detected, it is important to *stop* any continuous infusion of insulin. An example of one protocol to reverse hypoglycemia follows:

- Blood glucose level lower than 40 mg/dL (severe hypoglycemia): administer 50 mL dextrose (50%) in water ($D_{50}W$) as an IV bolus.
- Blood glucose level between 40 and 70 mg/dL (hypoglycemia): administer 25 mL of $D_{50}W$ as an IV bolus.

In all cases of hypoglycemia, the blood glucose concentration is monitored every 15 minutes until the blood glucose has risen above 70 mg/dL.

Nursing Management

Nursing management of the patient with neuroendocrine stress resulting from critical illness incorporates a variety of nursing diagnoses (Box 24-1). The goals of nursing

TABLE 24-2 Pharmacologic Management

Insulin*

INSULIN	ROUTE[†]	ACTION	ONSET/PEAK/DURATION	SPECIAL CONSIDERATIONS
Ultra–Short-Acting Insulins				
Aspart (NovoLog)	SC	Insulin replacement, rapid onset	5-15 min/30-90 min/<5 hr	Insulin analogue almost *immediately* absorbed; must be taken with food. Insulin appearance should be clear. Must be used in combination with intermediate-acting or long-acting basal insulin regimen. See Figure 24-1.
Lispro (Humalog)	SC	Insulin replacement, rapid onset	5-15 min/30-90 min/<5 hr	Insulin analogue; almost *immediately* absorbed; must be taken with food. Shorter duration of action than regular insulin; should be used with basal longer-acting insulin. See Figure 24-1.
Glulisine (Apidra)	SC	Insulin replacement, rapid onset	5-15 min/30-90 min/<5 hr	Insulin analogue
Short-Acting Insulin				
Regular	IV or SC	Insulin replacement therapy	IV: <15 min SC: 30-60 min/2-3 hr/5-8 hr	Only type of insulin suitable for IV continuous infusion or IV bolus administration
Intermediate-Acting Basal Insulin				
Neutral Protamine Hagedorn (NPH)	SC	Insulin replacement, intermediate action	2-4 hr/4-10 hr/10-16 hr	NPH is not recommended for SC basal insulin because it has a peak with a less predictable time course than the long-acting insulin analogues.
Long-Acting Basal Insulins				
Glargine (Lantus)	SC	Long-acting basal insulin analogue;	2-4 hr until steady state/no peak Concentration relatively constant over 20-24 hours	Synthetic insulin (analogue); differs from human insulin by three amino acids, slow release over 24 hours; no peak. Decrease dose by 20% if switching from NPH to glargine. Must not be diluted or mixed with other insulins. See Figure 24-1.
Detemir (Levemir)	SC	Long-acting basal insulin analogue	3-8 hr until steady state/no peak/5-23 hr	
Combination (Premixed) Insulins				
Various	SC	Rapid plus intermediate or long-acting insulin combination	Varies according to combination used	Many combinations exist; examples (long-acting component/short-acting component) include 70/30 regular (70% NPH with 30% regular), NovoLog mix 70/30 (70% aspart-protamine suspension with 30% aspart), and Humalog mix 75/25 (75% lispro-protamine suspension with 25% lispro).

*Dosages are individualized according to patient's age and size.
[†]Only regular insulin is suitable for intravenous use.
IV, Intravenous; *SC*, subcutaneous.

management are to monitor the hyperglycemic side effects of vasopressor therapy, administer prescribed corticosteroids, monitor blood glucose and insulin effectiveness, avoid hypoglycemia, provide nutrition, and provide education to the patient's family and supportive others (Box 24-2).

Monitor Hyperglycemic Side Effects of Vasopressor Therapy

Two vasopressors frequently used as continuous infusions to counteract hypotension also raise blood glucose. Epinephrine and norepinephrine stimulate gluconeogenesis (creation of new glucose), increase liver glycogenolysis (glucose production),

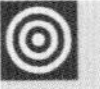

BOX 24-1 NURSING DIAGNOSES: STRESS OF CRITICAL ILLNESS

- Deficient Fluid Volume related to absolute loss, p. 584
- Imbalanced Nutrition: Less Than Body Requirements related to exogenous nutrients and increased metabolic demand, p. 593
- Risk for Infection, p. 607
- Risk for Ineffective Peripheral Tissue Perfusion, p. 605
- Compromised Family Coping related to critically ill family member, p. 578

BOX 24-2 PATIENT EDUCATION PRIORITIES: PHYSIOLOGIC STRESS OF CRITICAL ILLNESS

- Even if the patient is unresponsive because of the underlying critical illness or because of sedation and analgesic medications, brief explanations of procedures are quietly and simply given before interventions.
- During the period of acute illness, questions are answered, and information is provided to the family and significant others.
- After recovery additional information is provided to the patient concerning the trajectory of their illness.

increase lipolysis (fat breakdown), suppress insulin secretion, and increase peripheral insulin resistance. All of these actions increase blood glucose.

Administer Prescribed Corticosteroids

Critically ill patients with below-normal cortisol levels may be prescribed IV hydrocortisone.[1] Therapeutic steroids raise blood glucose levels and can make glycemic control more difficult. Frequent monitoring of the blood glucose concentration is necessary to guide treatment of hyperglycemia in the patient receiving IV corticosteroids. Ongoing monitoring for the presence of new infection is mandatory.

Monitor Blood Glucose—Avoid Hypoglycemia

The critical care nurse is responsible for the hourly monitoring of blood glucose and titration of the insulin infusion according to the hospital's protocol while the patient is hyperglycemic. The use of standardized protocols makes possible a systematic approach to the control of blood glucose. It is essential and recommended that nurses receive effective and ongoing education about the anabolic impact of insulin therapy in critical illness.[2] Hospital protocols to minimize development of hypoglycemia, such as using the 140-180 mg/dL target range,[2] and rapid reversal of any occurrence of severe hypoglycemia (below 40 mg/dL) by provision of IV dextrose ($D_{50}W$) are essential.[10]

Provide Nutrition

Whenever an insulin infusion is started to lower blood glucose, enteral nutritional support should be considered. In the absence of nutrition, a 10% dextrose solution may temporarily be infused. The 10% dextrose offers the advantage of carbohydrate calories for metabolism, limits fluctuations in the blood sugar, and reduces the risk of hypoglycemia. After the patient's metabolic condition is stable, introduction of nonglucose nutrition (protein and fat) is desirable. Referral to a Registered Dietician is recommended to support healthful eating as part of a comprehensive approach to diabetes management.[15]

BOX 24-3 EVIDENCE-BASED PRACTICE: HYPERGLYCEMIA MANAGEMENT IN CRITICAL ILLNESS (QSEN)

Summary of evidence and evidence-based recommendations for controlling hyperglycemic symptoms related to physiologic stress of critical illness

Strong Evidence to Support

- Initiate insulin therapy for persistent hyperglycemia above 180 mg/dL.
- Once a continuous insulin infusion is initiated, maintain the target blood glucose level between 140 and 180 mg/dL.
- Frequent blood glucose monitoring to avoid hypoglycemia, which is defined as a blood glucose below 70 mg/dL; or as severe hypoglycemia <40 mg/dL.
- For patients who are eating, maintain preprandial blood glucose below 130 mg/dL; maintain 2-hour postprandial blood glucose below 180 mg/dL.
- A multidisciplinary team approach to implement institutional guidelines, protocols, and standardized order-sets results in fewer hypoglycemic and hyperglycemic events.

References

American Diabetes Association: Standards of medical care in diabetes—2014, *Diabetes Care* 37(suppl 1):S14–S80, 2014.

Moghissi ES, et al: American Association of Clinical Endocrinologists and American Diabetes Association consensus statement on inpatient glycemic control, *Endocr Pract* 15(4):1, 2009.

Patient Education

While the patient is acutely ill, most of the educational interventions are directed to the family at the bedside. Numerous explications are required to describe the IV medications, the nutritional needs, the purpose of insulin, the role of steroids (if applicable), the ongoing nursing care, prevention of complications, and management of the underlying disease process. Educational issues that may be discussed are listed in Box 24-2.

Collaborative Management

It is well-established that standardized protocols designed to manage the complications of critical illness result in lower morbidity and mortality for patients. Optimally, all disciplines concerned with the endocrine status of the patient will have participated in the hospital's guidelines related to targeted glucose control. Guidelines for blood glucose monitoring in critical illness are described in Box 24-3.[2,16]

DIABETES MELLITUS

Diabetes mellitus is a progressive endocrinopathy associated with carbohydrate intolerance and insulin dysregulation.

Diagnosis of Diabetes

Diabetes mellitus is diagnosed by measurement of the fasting plasma glucose (FPG) or by a glycated hemoglobin above 6.5%.[16] The blood glucose may also be called a fasting blood glucose (FBG). The benchmarks for a normal blood glucose value have been progressively lowered as more knowledge has been gained about the benefits of maintaining the plasma glucose level as close to normal as possible.

Blood glucose values endorsed by the ADA are as follows:[16]

- An FPG level 70 to 100 mg/dL (3.9 to 5.6 mmol/L) signifies normal fasting glucose.
- An FPG level between 100 and 125 mg/dL (5.6 and 6.9 mmol/L) denotes impaired fasting glucose (IFG).
- An FPG level greater than 126 mg/dL (7 mmol/L) provides a diagnosis of diabetes (result is verified by testing more than once).

The benefit and importance of maintaining blood glucose at levels as close to normal as possible has been conclusively demonstrated in patients with type 1 and type 2 diabetes. The Diabetes Control and Complications Trial (DCCT) of 1995 on type 1 diabetes and the United Kingdom Prospective Diabetes Study (UKPDS), published in 1998, on type 2 diabetes demonstrated that lifestyle changes and use of medications that lead to consistently normal glucose levels reduce microvascular diabetes-related complications and decrease mortality.

Types of Diabetes

Two distinct types of diabetes are discussed in this chapter:[17]

- Type 1 diabetes results from beta-cell destruction, usually leading to absolute insulin deficiency.
- Type 2 diabetes results from a progressive insulin secretory defect in addition to insulin resistance.

The two diseases are different in nature, cause, treatment, and prognosis. A further category of *prediabetes* describes patients with impaired fasting glucose (FPG between 100 and 125 mg/dL) who are likely to develop diabetes in the future and who are at increased risk for coronary artery disease and stroke.[16] Other conditions, such as gestational diabetes, are not discussed in this chapter.

Glycated Hemoglobin

For individuals with diabetes, maintenance of blood glucose within a tight normal range is fundamental to avoid the development of microvascular and neuropathic secondary conditions. Although the plasma glucose produces a snapshot of the blood glucose concentration at a single point in time, the *glycated hemoglobin* (HbA_{1C}), also known as a *glycosylated hemoglobin*, measures the percentage of glucose the red cells have absorbed from the plasma over the previous 3-month period. The optimal target for patients with diabetes is an A_{1C} value below 6.5%.[16]

Type 1 Diabetes

Type 1 diabetes mellitus accounts for only about 5% to 10% of the diabetic population.[17] Older names for this condition included insulin-dependent diabetes (IDDM) and juvenile diabetes. Type 1 diabetes is an autoimmune disease that causes progressive destruction of the beta cells of the islets of Langerhans in the pancreas. Autoantibodies that falsely identify self as a foreign invader to be destroyed can now be identified by laboratory analysis. Autoantibodies that contribute to pancreatic destruction include autoantibodies to the islet cell, to insulin, to glutamic acid decarboxylase (GAD_{65}), and to the tyrosine phosphatases IA-2 and IA-2β (beta).[17] One or more of these autoantibodies are present in 85% to 90% of individuals with type 1 diabetes when fasting hyperglycemia is initially detected.[17] Over time, the autoantibodies render the pancreatic beta cells incapable of secreting insulin and regulating intracellular glucose. In type 1 diabetes, the rate of beta-cell destruction is highly variable. It occurs rapidly in some individuals (mainly children) and slowly in others (mainly adults). Some patients, particularly children and adolescents, may have ketoacidosis as the first manifestation of their disease.

Genetic predisposition and unknown environmental factors are also believed to play an important role.[17] Patients with type 1 diabetes are prone to development of other autoimmune disorders such as Graves disease (hyperthyroidism), Hashimoto thyroiditis, Addison's disease, autoimmune hepatitis, myasthenia gravis, and pernicious anemia.[17] Lack of insulin impairs carbohydrate, protein, and fat metabolism.

Management of Type 1 Diabetes

Patients with type 1 diabetes must receive IV or subcutaneous insulin therapy. Treatment with exogenous insulin replacement restores normal entry of glucose into the cells. The range of insulin replacements available is expanding, and it is essential that critical care nurses be knowledgeable about this class of medications (see Table 24-2). Without insulin, the rapid breakdown of noncarbohydrate substrate, particularly fat, leads to ketonemia, ketonuria, and diabetic ketoacidosis (DKA), a life-threatening hyperglycemic emergency that is associated with type 1 diabetes. DKA is discussed later in the chapter.

Type 2 Diabetes

Type 2 diabetes accounts for 90% to 95% of those with diabetes.[17] Previously used names for this condition were non–insulin-dependent diabetes, type II diabetes, or adult-onset diabetes.[17] Type 2 diabetes is identified by *insulin resistance* with a relative, versus absolute, insulin deficiency. Most patients with type 2 diabetes are obese, with excess adipose tissue concentrated in the abdominal area. The onset of hyperglycemia occurs gradually, and many people are unaware that they have diabetes. Initially, type 2 diabetes is managed by oral medications (noninsulin therapies) because the pancreatic beta cells remain functional. Although, as progressive beta cell dysfunction occurs, a basal long-acting insulin is added to the oral noninsulin medications.[18,19]

Insulin resistance describes a complex metabolic situation in which organ and tissue cells deny entry to insulin and glucose. This creates the clinical paradox in which elevated serum insulin levels and hyperglycemia are present at the same time. Insulin resistance has a strong association with obesity.

Lifestyle Management for Type 2 Diabetes

For most patients with type 2 diabetes, a program of weight reduction, increased physical exercise, and a change in diet pattern is the first step.[18] The diet should contain less than 30% of calories from fat, with an increased quantity of whole grains, vegetables, and fruits. Crash diets are discouraged, and a gradual program of weight loss, if needed, is recommended. The exercise program is tailored to the individual but might start with 30 minutes of brisk walking each day if the person was previously sedentary.

Patients who have type 2 diabetes are prone to a wide range of other complications that increase morbidity and mortality. In addition to medications to control blood glucose, patients often require medications to lower their blood pressure, lower their cholesterol and triglyceride levels, treat ischemic heart disease, and manage symptoms of heart failure.[16,19]

Pharmacologic Management of Type 2 Diabetes

If lifestyle changes are unsuccessful in reversing the pattern of type 2 diabetes, oral noninsulin antihyperglycemic medications are prescribed.[16] These medications are not oral forms of insulin because insulin would be destroyed by gastric juices. There are several types of oral agents: sulfonylureas, glinides, biguanides, thiazolidinediones, alpha-glucosidase inhibitors, incretin mimetics, incretin enhancers and sodium-glucose co-transporter 2 (SGLT2) inhibitors. These oral antidiabetic medications work to lower plasma glucose levels by a variety of mechanisms: increasing insulin secretion, increasing sensitivity to insulin, delaying carbohydrate

BOX 24-4 Oral Antihyperglycemic Medication Actions

- Medications that stimulate the pancreas to make more insulin (insulin secretagogues)
  - Sulfonylureas
  - Glinides
- Medications that sensitize the body to insulin (insulin sensitizers)
  - Biguanides
  - Thiazolidinediones
- Medications that delay carbohydrate absorption from small intestine
  - Alpha-glucosidase inhibitors
- Medications that augment gut incretin hormone effects
  - Incretin mimetics
  - Incretin enhancers

TABLE 24-3 Pharmacologic Management

Medications for Type 2 Diabetes

MEDICATION*	DOSAGE	ACTION	ONSET/PEAK/ DURATION	SPECIAL CONSIDERATIONS
Insulin Secretagogues				
Second-Generation Sulfonylureas				
Glipizide (Glucotrol)	*Initial dosage:* Immediate release tablet 5 mg once/day *Maximum dose:* 40 mg bid	Stimulates insulin release	1 hr/1-3 hr/12-24 hr	Administer with breakfast or after first main meal. Also available in an extended extended-release formulation (Glucotrol XL); do not cut, crush, or chew. Extended release: *Initial dosage:* 5 mg, once daily; *maximum dose:* 20 mg/day. Adjust dose if creatinine clearance <50 mL/min.
Glyburide (DiaBeta; Micronase)	*Initial dosage:* 2.5 mg once/day *Maintenance dosage:* 1.5-20 mg/day	Stimulates insulin release	1 hr/4 hr/18-24 hr	Administer with breakfast or first main meal.
Glimepiride (Amaryl)	*Initial dosage:* 1-2 mg once/day *Maximum dosage:* 8 mg once/day	Stimulates insulin release	Duration 24 hours	Administer with breakfast or first main meal of day. Initial dose is lower in patients with kidney dysfunction (1 mg once/day).
Meglitinides				
Nateglinide (Starlix)	*Initial dosage:* 120 mg tid *Maximum dosage:* 120 mg tid	Stimulates insulin release	Peak <1 hour	Administer 15-30 minutes before meals. Cut dose in half (i.e., 60 mg tid) for frail older patients and for those near their HA_{1c} target.
Repaglinide (Prandin)	*Initial dosage:* 1-2 mg tid *Maximum dosage:* 16 mg per day	Stimulates insulin release		Administer 15-30 minutes before meals. Cut dose in half (i.e., 0.5 mg tid) for frail older patients.

Continued

TABLE 24-3 Pharmacologic Management—cont'd

Medications for Type 2 Diabetes

MEDICATION*	DOSAGE	ACTION	ONSET/PEAK/ DURATION	SPECIAL CONSIDERATIONS
Insulin Sensitizers				
Biguanides				
Metformin (Glucophage)	*Initial dosage:* 500 mg bid; or 850 mg in morning *Maximum dosage:* 2550 mg tid	Reduces glucose output from liver. Increases insulin action by decreasing peripheral insulin resistance.	1-3 hr/24 hr/24-48 hr	Temporarily withhold if patient is having contrast radiography. Adverse effects: lactic acidosis (rare) GI upset Use extreme caution in patients with creatinine clearance <50 mL/min.
Thiazolidinediones (TZDs)				
Pioglitazone (Actos)	*Initial dosage:* 15-30 mg bid *Maximum dosage:* 45 mg once/daily	Increases peripheral insulin sensitivity	Peak 2-3 hours	Associated with weight gain, edema and heart failure Bone fractures
Rosiglitazone (Avandia)	*Initial dosage:* 4 mg once/day or 2 mg bid *Maximum dosage:* 8 mg once/day or 4 mg bid	Increases peripheral insulin sensitivity		Associated with weight gain, edema and heart failure LDL cholesterol increase FDA warnings on cardiovascular safety Bone fractures
Carbohydrate Inhibitors				
Alpha-Glucosidase Inhibitors				
Acarbose (Precose)	*Initial dosage:* 25 mg tid *Maximum dosage:* 100 mg tid	Delays carbohydrate digestion by blocking absorption of complete carbohydrates in small intestine	Peak 2-3 hours	Administer with first bite of each meal. GI side effects (flatulence, abdominal pain, diarrhea) Not recommended in severe kidney dysfunction
Miglitol (Glyset)	*Initial dosage:* 25 mg tid *Maximum dosage:* 100 mg tid		Peak 2-3 hours	Administer with first bite of each meal.
Incretin Mimics and Enhancers				
Incretin Mimetics				
Exenatide (Byetta); Exenatide extended-release (Bydureon)	*Initial dosage (immediate release):* 5 mg bid; after 1 month may increase to 10 mg bid *Extended release:* 2 mg once/week	Activates GLP-1 receptors in pancreatic beta cells	Not applicable	SC injection, avoid if creatinine clearance <30 mL/min. GI side effects (nausea, vomiting diarrhea) Pancreatitis has occurred.
Liraglutide (Victoza)	*Initial dosage:* 0.6 mg SC once/day (irrespective of meals) for 7 days, then increase to 1.2 mg once/day	Activates GLP-1 receptors in pancreatic beta cells	Not applicable	Pancreatitis has occurred.
Abiglutide (Tanzeum)	30 mg to 50 mg SC once every 7 days.	Activates GLP-1 receptors in pancreatic beta cells	Not applicable	No dosage adjustment for kidney dysfunction needed.

TABLE 24-3 Pharmacologic Management—cont'd

Medications for Type 2 Diabetes

MEDICATION*	DOSAGE	ACTION	ONSET/PEAK/ DURATION	SPECIAL CONSIDERATIONS
Incretin Enhancers				
Sitagliptin (Januvia) Saxagliptin (Onglyza) Linagliptin (Tradjenta)	100 mg oral once/day 2.5 to 5 mg oral once/ day 5 mg oral once/day	Inhibits DPP-4 hormone activity, prolongs survival of endogenously released incretin hormones	Not applicable	Pancreatitis has occurred. Reduce dosage with kidney dysfunction for Sitagliptin and Saxagliptin. No dosage adjustment for kidney dysfunction needed with Linagliptin
Sodium Glucose Co-Transporter 2 (SGLT2) Inhibitors				
Jardiance (empagliflozin) Invokana (canagliflozin) Farxiga (dapagliflozin)	Start at 10 mg/day. Max dose 25 mg/day. Start at 100 mg per day. Max dose 300 mg/day. Start at 5 mg per day. Max dose 10 mg/day.	Stop glucose, in blood from getting resorbed by the kidneys.	Not applicable	Dosage is adjusted downward to accommodate kidney impairment according to GFR. Increased incidence of urinary tract infections, probably due to increased glucose in urine. Not recommended with liver failure.

bid, Twice daily; *DPP-4*, dipeptidyl peptidase-4; GFR, Glomerular filtration rate; *GI*, gastrointestinal; *GLP-1*, glucagon glucagon-like peptide-1; *LDL*, low-density lipoprotein; mg/day, milligrams per day; *SC* subcutaneous; *tid*, three times daily.

*Combination medications are too numerous to include in this table.

absorption and excreting glucose via the kidneys as described in Table 24-3 and Box 24-4). The pharmacologic management of type 2 diabetes is increasingly complex. Current guidelines recommend a patient-focused, individualized approach that includes pharmacologic management and risk factor modification to reduce early mortality from cardiovascular disease.[19-23]

HYPERGLYCEMIC EMERGENCIES

There are two hyperglycemic emergencies related to diabetes. Diabetic ketoacidosis (DKA) is the hyperglycemic emergency that occurs in patients with type 1 diabetes. Hyperglycemic hyperosmolar state (HHS) is the hyperglycemic emergency that occurs in patients with type 2 diabetes. Both of these conditions are described in detail in the following sections.

DIABETIC KETOACIDOSIS

Epidemiology and Etiology

DKA is a life-threatening complication of diabetes mellitus. Type 1 diabetics who are dependent on insulin are typically affected.

The diagnostic criteria for DKA are as follows:[24]

- Blood glucose greater than 250 mg/dL
- pH less than 7.3
- Serum bicarbonate less than 18 mEq/L
- Moderate or severe ketonemia or ketonuria

DKA is categorized as mild, moderate, or severe depending on the severity of the metabolic acidosis (assessed by blood pH, bicarbonate, ketones) and by the presence of altered mental status (Table 24-4).[24] Hospitalizations for DKA are increasing.[24] DKA accounts for more than 500,000 hospital days per year, with hospital costs that exceed $2.4 billion per year.[24] Infection is the most common precipitating cause of DKA.[24] Symptoms of fatigue and polyuria may precede full-blown DKA, which can develop in less than 24 hours in a person with type 1 diabetes. In a patient with undiagnosed diabetes, it is unknown how long it may take for DKA to develop as the pancreatic beta cells gradually fail. Hospital admission is generally required for DKA related to new-onset type 1 diabetes. With management by experienced clinicians, the mortality rate from DKA in type 1 diabetics is less than 1%.[24]

Changes in the type of insulin, change in dosage, or increased metabolic demand can precipitate DKA in individuals with type 1 diabetes.[24] Life cycle changes, such as growth spurts in the adolescent, require an increase in insulin intake, as do surgery, infection, and trauma. In young persons with diabetes, psychologic problems combined with eating disorders are a contributing factor in up to 20% of cases of recurrent ketoacidosis.[24]

Ketoacidosis also occurs with acute pancreatitis. In addition to elevated glucose and acidosis, the serum amylase and lipase are abnormally high, which helps to establish pancreatitis as a separate diagnosis from type 1 diabetes. Other nondiabetic causes of ketoacidosis are starvation ketosis and alcoholic ketoacidosis. These cases are distinguished from classic DKA by clinical history and usually by a plasma glucose below 200 mg/dL.[24]

Pathophysiology

Insulin Deficiency

Insulin is the metabolic key to the transfer of glucose from the bloodstream into the cell, where it can be used immediately for energy or stored for use at a later time. Without insulin, glucose remains in the bloodstream, and cells are

TABLE 24-4 Diagnostic Criteria for Diabetic Ketoacidosis (DKA) and Hyperglycemic Hyperosmolar Syndrome (HHS)

	DKA			HHS
	MILD (PLASMA GLUCOSE >250 mg/dL)	MODERATE (PLASMA GLUCOSE >250 mg/dL)	SEVERE (PLASMA GLUCOSE >250 mg/dL)	PLASMA GLUCOSE >600 mg/dL
Arterial pH	7.25-7.30	7.00 to <7.24	<7.00	>7.30
Serum bicarbonate (mEq/L)	15-18	10 to <15	<10	>18
Urine ketone*	Positive	Positive	Positive	Small
Serum ketone*	Positive	Positive	Positive	Small
Effective serum osmolality†	Variable	Variable	Variable	>320 mOsm/kg
Anion gap‡	>10	>12	>12	Variable
Mental status	Alert	Alert/drowsy	Stupor/coma	Stupor/coma

*Nitroprusside reaction method.
†Effective serum osmolality: 2[measured Na^+ (mEq/L)] + glucose (mg/dL)18.
‡Anion gap: (Na^+) – (Cl^- + HCO_3^-)mEq/L.
Data from Kitabchi AE, et al. Hyperglycemic crises in adult patients with diabetes: a consensus statement from the American Diabetes Association. *Diabetes Care.* 2009;32(7):1335.

deprived of their energy source. A complex pathophysiologic chain of events follows (Figure 24-2). The release of glucagon from the liver is stimulated when insulin is ineffective in providing the cells with glucose for energy. Glucagon increases the amount of glucose in the bloodstream by breaking down stored glucose (glycogenolysis). Noncarbohydrates (fat and protein) are converted into glucose (gluconeogenesis). Plasma glucose levels for the patient in DKA typically are above 250 mg/dL. Elevated serum glucose levels alone do not define DKA; the other crucial determining factor is the presence of ketoacidosis as listed in Table 24-4.[24] About 10% of patients in DKA present to the hospital with a plasma glucose below 250 mg/dL and with ketoacidosis.[24]

Hyperglycemia

Hyperglycemia increases the plasma osmolality, and the blood becomes hyperosmolar. Cellular dehydration occurs as the hyperosmolar extracellular fluid draws the more dilute intracellular and interstitial fluid into the vascular space in an attempt to return the plasma osmolality to normal. Dehydration stimulates catecholamine production in an effort to provide emergency support. Catecholamine output stimulates further glycogenolysis, lipolysis, and gluconeogenesis, pouring glucose into the bloodstream.

Fluid Volume Deficit

Polyuria (excessive urination) and *glycosuria* (sugar in the urine) occur as a result of the osmotic particle load that occurs with DKA. The excess glucose, filtered at the glomeruli, cannot be resorbed at the renal tubule and spills into the urine. The unresorbed solute exerts its own osmotic pull in the renal tubules, and less water is returned to circulation through the collecting ducts. As a result, large volumes of water, along with sodium, potassium, and phosphorus, are excreted in the urine, causing a fluid volume deficit. The serum sodium concentration may be decreased because of the movement of water from the intracellular to the extracellular (vascular) space.[24]

Ketoacidosis

In the healthy individual, the presence of insulin in the bloodstream suppresses the manufacture of ketones. In insulin deficiency states, fat is rapidly converted into glucose (gluconeogenesis). *Ketoacidosis* occurs when free fatty acids are metabolized into ketones: acetoacetate, β-hydroxybutyrate, and acetone are the three ketone bodies that are produced. During normal metabolism, the ratio of β-hydroxybutyrate to acetoacetate is 1:1, with acetone present in only small amounts. In insulin deficiency, the quantities of all three ketone bodies increase substantially, and the ratio of β-hydroxybutyrate to acetoacetate increases to as much as 10:1. β-Hydroxybutyrate and acetoacetate are the ketones responsible for acidosis in DKA. Acetone does not cause acidosis and is safely excreted in the lungs, causing the characteristic fruity odor.

Ketones are measurable in the bloodstream (ketonemia). Blood tests that measure the quantity of β-hydroxybutyric acid, the predominant ketone body in the blood, are the most useful.[24] Because ketones are excreted by the kidney, they are also measurable in the urine (*ketonuria*). Ketone blood tests are preferred over urine tests for diagnosis and monitoring of DKA in critical care. When the blood and urine become clear of ketones, the DKA is resolved.

Acid–Base Balance

The acid–base balance varies depending on the severity of the DKA. The patient with mild DKA typically has a pH between 7.25 and 7.30. In severe DKA, the pH can drop below 7.00 (see Table 24-4).[24] Acid ketones dissociate and yield hydrogen ions (H^+), which accumulate and precipitate a fall in serum pH. The level of serum bicarbonate also decreases, consistent with a diagnosis of metabolic acidosis. Breathing becomes deep and rapid (Kussmaul respirations) to release carbonic acid in the form of carbon dioxide. Acetone is exhaled, giving the breath its characteristic fruity odor.

Gluconeogenesis

Gluconeogenesis is the process of breaking down fat or protein to make new glucose. Fat is metabolized to ketones, as described earlier. Protein used for gluconeogenesis leaves no reserve protein available for synthesis and repair of vital body tissues. Nitrogen accumulates as protein is metabolized to urea. Urea, added to the bloodstream, increases the osmotic diuresis and accentuates the dehydration.

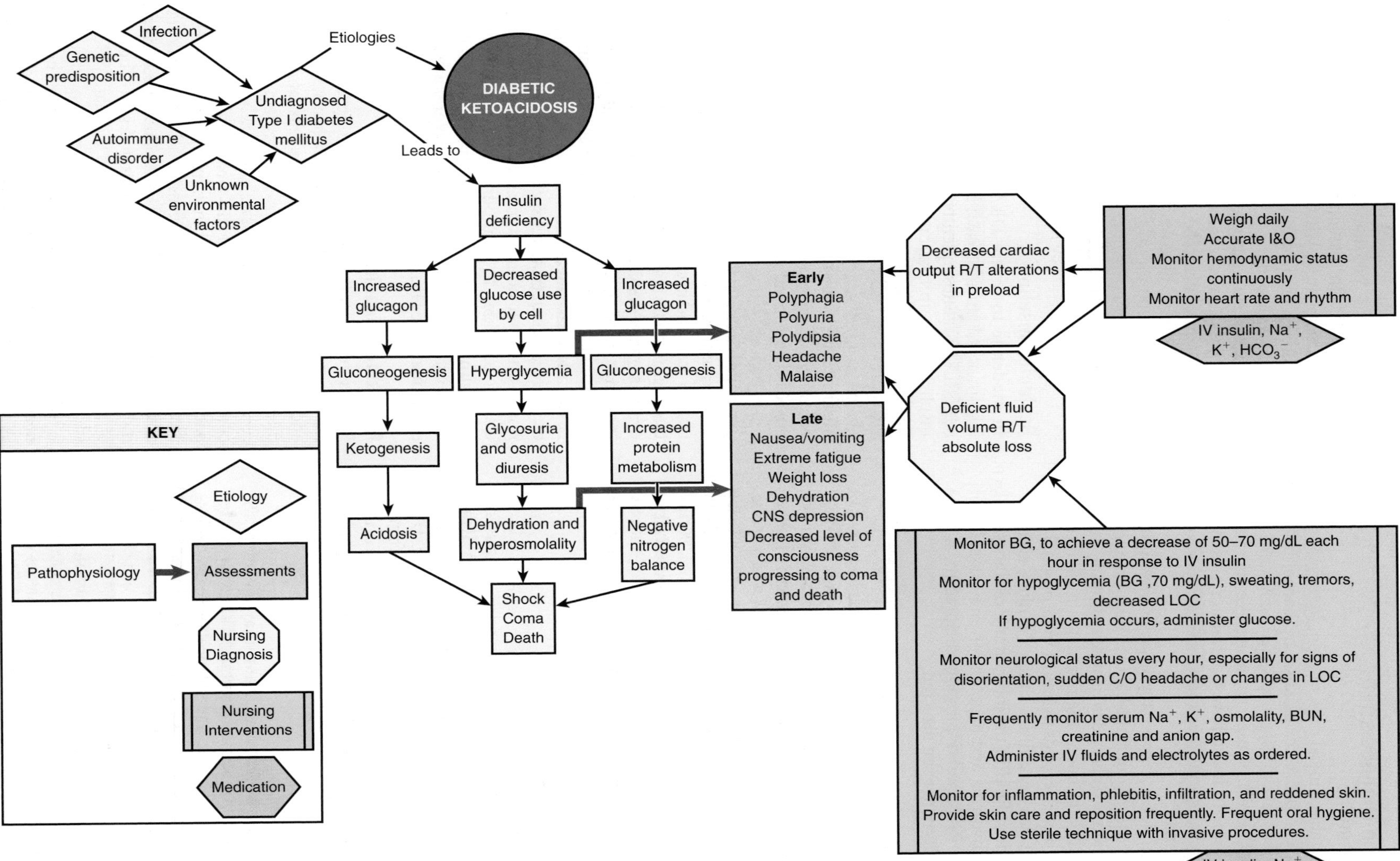

FIG 24-2 Concept Map for Diabetic Ketoacidosis. (Concept map illustration created by Elaine Bishop Kennedy, EdD, RN.)

Assessment and Diagnosis

Clinical Manifestations

DKA has a predictable clinical presentation. It is usually preceded by patient complaints of malaise, headache, polyuria (excessive urination), polydipsia (excessive thirst), and polyphagia (excessive hunger). Nausea, vomiting, extreme fatigue, dehydration, and weight loss follow. Central nervous system depression, with changes in the level of consciousness, can lead quickly to coma.[16,24]

The patient with DKA may be stuporous or unresponsive, depending on the degree of fluid-balance disturbance. The physical examination reveals evidence of dehydration, including flushed dry skin, dry buccal membranes, and skin turgor that takes longer than 3 seconds to return to its original position after the skin has been lifted. Often, "sunken eyeballs," resulting from lack of fluid in the interstitium of the eyeball, are observed. Tachycardia and hypotension may signal profound fluid losses. Kussmaul respirations are present, and the fruity odor of acetone may be detected.

Laboratory Studies

Considering the complexity and potential seriousness of DKA, the laboratory diagnosis is straightforward. With a known type 1 diabetic patient, the presence of hyperglycemia and ketones provides rapid diagnostic confirmation of DKA. A blood gas sample can confirm the acid–base imbalance. Other clues may be gleaned from the venous blood chemistry panel. CO_2, if measured, is low in the presence of uncompensated metabolic acidosis, and the anion gap is elevated. Serum sodium may be low as a result of the movement of water from the intracellular space into the extracellular (vascular) space.[24] The serum potassium level is often normal; a low serum potassium level in DKA suggests a significant potassium deficiency may be present.[24]

Medical Management

Diagnosis of DKA is based on the combination of presenting symptoms, patient history, medical history (type 1 diabetes), precipitating factors (if known), and results of serum glucose and urine ketone testing. After diagnosis, DKA requires aggressive clinical management to prevent progressive decompensation. The goals of treatment are to reverse dehydration, replace insulin, reverse ketoacidosis, and replenish electrolytes.

Reversing Dehydration

The patient with DKA is dehydrated and may have lost 5% to 10% of body weight in fluids. Aggressive IV fluid replacement is provided to rehydrate the intracellular and extracellular compartments and prevent circulatory collapse (Figure 24-3).[24] Assessment of hydration is an important first step in the treatment of DKA.

Intravenous isotonic normal saline (0.9% NaCl) is infused to replenish the vascular deficit and to reverse hypotension. For the severely dehydrated patient, 1 L of normal saline is infused immediately. Laboratory assessment of serum osmolality and the serum sodium concentration can help guide the subsequent interventions. If the serum osmolality is elevated and serum sodium is high (hypernatremia), infusions of hypotonic sodium chloride (0.45) follow the initial saline replacement. The replacement infusion typically includes 20 to 30 mEq of potassium per liter to restore the intracellular potassium debt, provided kidney function is normal (see Figure 24-3).[24] In patients without normally functioning kidneys and in those with cardiopulmonary disease, careful attention must be paid to the volume of fluid replacement to avoid fluid overload.

After the serum glucose level decreases to 200 mg/dL, the infusing solution is changed to a 50/50 mix of hypotonic saline and 5% dextrose. Dextrose is added to replenish depleted cellular glucose as the circulating serum glucose decreases to 200 mg/dL.[24] Dextrose infusion also prevents unexpected hypoglycemia when the insulin infusion is continued but the patient cannot take in sufficient carbohydrate from an oral diet.

Replacing Insulin

In moderate to severe DKA, an initial IV bolus of regular insulin at 0.1 unit for each kilogram of body weight may be administered. Subsequently, a continuous infusion of regular insulin at 0.1 unit/kg/hr is infused simultaneously with IV fluid replacement (see Figure 24-3).[24] In a 70-kg adult, the infusion would be 7 units of insulin per hour. If the plasma glucose concentration does not fall by 50 to 70 mg/dL during the first hour of treatment, the glucose measurement should be rechecked. When the plasma glucose level is decreasing as expected, the insulin infusion will be increased each hour until a steady glucose decline of between 50 and 70 mg/dL per hour is achieved.[24]

Frequent assessment of the patient's blood glucose concentration is mandatory in moderate to severe DKA. Initially, blood glucose tests are performed hourly. The frequency then decreases to every 2 to 4 hours as the patient's blood glucose level stabilizes and approaches normal. After the level has decreased to 200 mg/dL, the acidosis has been corrected, and rehydration has been achieved, the insulin infusion rate may be decreased to 0.05 to 0.1 unit/kg/hr. This usually represents 3 to 6 units per hour in an adult receiving a continuous IV insulin infusion. It is important to verify that the serum potassium concentration is not lower than 3.3 mEq/L and to replace potassium if necessary, before administering the initial insulin bolus.[24]

Reversing Ketoacidosis

Replacement of fluid volume and insulin interrupts the ketotic cycle and reverses the metabolic acidosis. In the presence of insulin, glucose enters the cells, and the body ceases to convert fats into glucose.

Adequate hydration and insulin replacement usually correct the acidosis, and this treatment is sufficient for many patients with DKA. As shown in Figure 24-3, replacement of bicarbonate is no longer routine except for the severely acidotic patient with a serum pH value lower than 7.0.[24] An indwelling arterial line provides access for hourly sampling of arterial blood gases (ABGs) to evaluate pH, bicarbonate, and other laboratory values in the patient with severe DKA.

Hyperglycemia usually resolves before the ketoacidemia does.[24] Type 1 diabetes patients with DKA can require 6 L of IV fluid replacement even for mild DKA.[25] In one clinical report, patients with previously diagnosed type 1 diabetes in DKA took an average of 21 hours after being started on an IV insulin protocol to clear ketones from the urine. The insulin infusion was continued for 36 hours until the patients

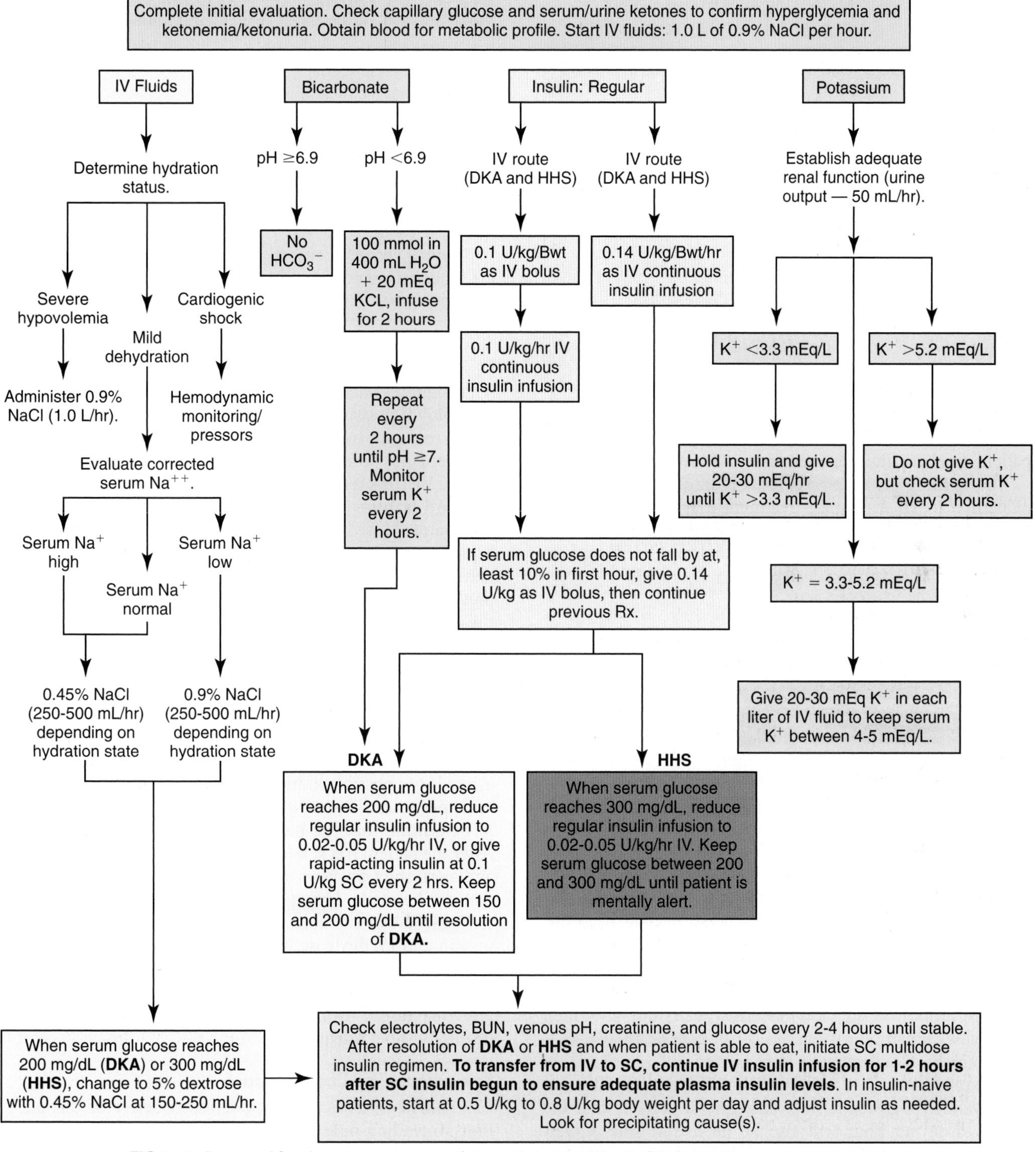

Complete initial evaluation. Check capillary glucose and serum/urine ketones to confirm hyperglycemia and ketonemia/ketonuria. Obtain blood for metabolic profile. Start IV fluids: 1.0 L of 0.9% NaCl per hour.
IV Fluids
Bicarbonate
Insulin: Regular
Potassium
Determine hydration status.
Severe hypovolemia
Mild dehydration
Cardiogenic shock
Administer 0.9% NaCl (1.0 L/hr).
Hemodynamic monitoring/ pressors
Evaluate corrected serum Na++.
Serum Na+ high
Serum Na+ normal
Serum Na+ low
0.45% NaCl (250-500 mL/hr) depending on hydration state
0.9% NaCl (250-500 mL/hr) depending on hydration state
When serum glucose reaches 200 mg/dL (DKA) or 300 mg/dL (HHS), change to 5% dextrose with 0.45% NaCl at 150-250 mL/hr.
pH ≥6.9
pH <6.9
No HCO3−
100 mmol in 400 mL H2O + 20 mEq KCL, infuse for 2 hours
Repeat every 2 hours until pH ≥7. Monitor serum K+ every 2 hours.
IV route (DKA and HHS)
IV route (DKA and HHS)
0.1 U/kg/Bwt as IV bolus
0.14 U/kg/Bwt/hr as IV continuous insulin infusion
0.1 U/kg/hr IV continuous insulin infusion
If serum glucose does not fall by at, least 10% in first hour, give 0.14 U/kg as IV bolus, then continue previous Rx.
DKA
HHS
When serum glucose reaches 200 mg/dL, reduce regular insulin infusion to 0.02-0.05 U/kg/hr IV, or give rapid-acting insulin at 0.1 U/kg SC every 2 hrs. Keep serum glucose between 150 and 200 mg/dL until resolution of DKA.
When serum glucose reaches 300 mg/dL, reduce regular insulin infusion to 0.02-0.05 U/kg/hr IV. Keep serum glucose between 200 and 300 mg/dL until patient is mentally alert.
Establish adequate renal function (urine output — 50 mL/hr).
K+ <3.3 mEq/L
K+ >5.2 mEq/L
Hold insulin and give 20-30 mEq/hr until K+ >3.3 mEq/L.
Do not give K+, but check serum K+ every 2 hours.
K+ = 3.3-5.2 mEq/L
Give 20-30 mEq K+ in each liter of IV fluid to keep serum K+ between 4-5 mEq/L.
Check electrolytes, BUN, venous pH, creatinine, and glucose every 2-4 hours until stable. After resolution of DKA or HHS and when patient is able to eat, initiate SC multidose insulin regimen. To transfer from IV to SC, continue IV insulin infusion for 1-2 hours after SC insulin begun to ensure adequate plasma insulin levels. In insulin-naive patients, start at 0.5 U/kg to 0.8 U/kg body weight per day and adjust insulin as needed. Look for precipitating cause(s).

FIG 24-3 **Protocol for the management of diabetic ketoacidosis (DKA) and hyperglycemic hyperosmolar state (HHS).** (From Kitabchi AE, et al. Hyperglycemic crises in adult patients with diabetes: a consensus statement from the American Diabetes Association. *Diabetes Care.* 2009;32[7]:1335.)

could tolerate an oral diet; during this time, the patients received a total of 9.5 L of normal saline for rehydration.[26] Patients who are newly diagnosed with type 1 diabetes take longer to clear urine ketones and require more insulin to achieve normal glycemic control, compared with long-term diabetics.[26]

Replenishing Electrolytes

Low serum potassium (hypokalemia) occurs as insulin promotes the return of potassium into the cell and metabolic acidosis is reversed. Replacement of potassium by administration of potassium chloride (KCl) begins as soon as the serum potassium falls below normal. Frequent verification of

 BOX 24-5 **NURSING DIAGNOSES: DIABETIC KETOACIDOSIS**

- Decreased Cardiac Output related to alterations in preload, p. 579
- Deficient Fluid Volume related to absolute loss, p. 584
- Anxiety related to threat to biologic, psychologic, and social integrity, p. 576
- Disturbed Body Image related to functional dependence on life-sustaining technology, p. 587
- Ineffective Coping related to situational crisis and personal vulnerability, p. 599
- Powerlessness related to lack of control over current situation or disease progression, p. 600
- Deficient Knowledge related to lack of previous exposure to information, p. 585 (see Box 24-8, Patient Education for Diabetic Ketoacidosis)

the serum potassium concentration is required for the DKA patient receiving fluid resuscitation and insulin therapy.

The serum phosphate level is sometimes low (hypophosphatemia) in DKA. Insulin treatment may make this more obvious as phosphate is returned to the interior of the cell. If the serum phosphate level is less than 1 mg/dL, phosphate replacement is recommended.[24]

Nursing Management

Nursing management of the patient with DKA incorporates a variety of nursing diagnoses (Box 24-5). The goals of nursing management are to administer prescribed fluids, insulin, and electrolytes; monitor response to therapy; maintain surveillance for complications, and provide patient education.

Administering Fluids, Insulin, and Electrolytes

Rapid IV fluid replacement requires the use of a volumetric pump. Insulin is administered intravenously to patients who are severely dehydrated or have poor peripheral perfusion to ensure effective absorption. Patients with DKA are kept on NPO status (nothing by mouth) until the hyperglycemia is under control. The critical care nurse is responsible for monitoring the rate of plasma glucose decline in response to insulin. The goal is to achieve a fall in glucose levels of approximately 50 to 70 mg/dL each hour.[24] The coordination involved in monitoring blood glucose, potassium, and often blood gases on an hourly basis is considerable.

When the blood glucose level falls to 200 mg/dL, a 5% dextrose solution (D_5W) with 0.45% NaCl solution is infused to prevent hypoglycemia.[24] At this time, it is likely that the insulin dose per hour will also be decreased. The regular insulin drip is not discontinued until the ketoacidosis subsides, as identified by absence of ketones and a normal pH by arterial blood gas analysis.[24]

Insulin is given subcutaneously after glucose levels, dehydration, hypotension, and acid–base balance are normalized; the patient is in stable condition and taking an oral diet.

Monitoring Response to Therapy

Accurate intake and output (I&O) measurements must be maintained to monitor reversal of dehydration. Hourly urine output is an indicator of kidney function and provides information to prevent overhydration or insufficient hydration.

BOX 24-6 **Hydration Assessment**

- Hourly intake
- Blood pressure changes
  - Orthostatic hypotension
  - Pulse pressure
  - Pulse rate, character, rhythm
- Neck vein filling
- Skin turgor
- Skin moisture
- Body weight
- Central venous pressure
- Hourly urine output
- Complaints of thirst

Vital signs, especially heart rate (HR), hemodynamic values, and blood pressure (BP), are continuously monitored to assess response to the fluid replacement. Evidence that fluid replacement is effective includes normal central venous pressure (CVP), decreased HR, and normal BP. Box 24-6 lists the standard features to be included in an assessment of hydration status. More invasive hemodynamic monitoring, such as a pulmonary artery catheter, is rarely needed. Further evidence of hydration improvement includes a change from a previously weak, thready pulse to a pulse that is strong and full and a change from hypotension to a gradual elevation of systolic BP. Respirations are assessed frequently for changes in rate, depth, and presence of the fruity acetone odor.

Blood glucose is measured each hour in the initial period. Sometimes potassium is measured just as frequently. The serum osmolality and serum sodium concentration are evaluated, and blood urea nitrogen (BUN) and creatinine levels are assessed for possible kidney impairment related to decreased renal perfusion. The purpose of these frequent assessments is to determine that the patient's clinical status is improving. After the patient has stable laboratory indicators and is awake and alert, the transition to subcutaneous insulin and an oral diet can be made. Hypoglycemia is a risk during the transition period. For example, in anticipation of discontinuing the insulin and IV dextrose infusion, a patient receives a subcutaneous dose of insulin and is expected to eat a meal. However, if the patient is then unable to eat an adequate amount, hypoglycemia results from the administration of subcutaneous insulin without adequate glucose.

Surveillance for Complications

The patient in DKA can experience a variety of complications, including fluid volume overload, hypoglycemia, hypokalemia or hyperkalemia, hyponatremia, cerebral edema, and infection.

Fluid volume overload. Fluid overload from rapid volume infusion is a serious complication that can occur in the patient with a compromised cardiopulmonary system or kidneys. Neck vein engorgement, dyspnea without exertion, and pulmonary crackles on auscultation signal circulatory overload. Reduction in the rate and volume of infusion, elevation of the head of the bed, and provision of oxygen may be required to manage the increased intravascular volume. Hourly urine measurement is mandatory to assess kidney function and adequacy of fluid replacement.

Hypoglycemia. Hypoglycemia is defined as a serum glucose level lower than 70 mg/dL.[24] Most acute care hospitals have specific procedures for management of the hypoglycemic patient. For example, if hypoglycemia is detected by finger-stick point-of-care testing at the bedside, a blood sample is sent to the laboratory for verification, the physician is notified immediately, and replacement glucose is given intravenously or orally, depending on the patient's clinical condition, diagnosis, and level of consciousness.

Unexpected behavior change or decreased level of consciousness, diaphoresis, and tremors are physical warning signs that the patient has become hypoglycemic. These symptoms are especially important to recognize if the frequency of glucose testing has lengthened to 2- to 4-hour intervals. A comparison between the physical symptoms expected with hypoglycemia and those of hyperglycemia is provided in Box 24-7.

Hypokalemia and hyperkalemia. Hypokalemia can occur within the first hours of rehydration and insulin treatment. Continuous cardiac monitoring is required because low serum potassium (hypokalemia) can cause ventricular dysrhythmias.

Hyperkalemia occurs with acidosis or with overaggressive administration of potassium replacement in patients with renal insufficiency. Severe hyperkalemia is demonstrated on the cardiac monitor by a large, peaked T wave; flattened P wave, and widened QRS complex. See Figure 11-46 in Chapter 11. Ventricular fibrillation can follow.

Hyponatremia. Sodium elimination from the body results from the osmotic diuresis and is compounded by the vomiting and diarrhea that can occur during DKA. Clinical manifestations of hyponatremia include abdominal cramping, postural hypotension, and unexpected behavioral changes. Sodium chloride is infused as the initial IV solution. Maintenance of the saline infusion depends on clinical manifestations of sodium imbalance and serum laboratory values.

Risk for cerebral edema. Changes in the patient's neurologic status may be insidious. Alterations in level of consciousness, pupil reaction, and motor function may be the result of fluctuating glucose levels and cerebral fluid shifts. Confusion and sudden complaints of headache are ominous signs that may signal cerebral edema. These observations require immediate action to prevent neurologic damage. Neurologic assessments are performed every hour or as needed during the acute phase of hyperglycemia and rehydration. Assessment of level of consciousness serves as the index of the patient's cerebral response to the rehydration therapy.

Risk for infection. Skin care takes on new dimensions for the patient with DKA. Dehydration, hypovolemia, and hypophosphatemia interfere with oxygen delivery at the cell site and contribute to inadequate perfusion and tissue breakdown. Patients must be repositioned frequently to relieve capillary pressure and promote adequate perfusion to body tissues. The typical patient with type 1 diabetes is of normal weight or underweight. Bony prominences must be assessed for tissue breakdown, and the patient's body weight must be repositioned every 1 to 2 hours. Irritation of skin from adhesive tape, shearing force, and detergents should be avoided. Maintenance of skin integrity prevents unwanted portals of entry for microorganisms.

Oral care, including tooth brushing and use of lip balm, helps keep lips supple and prevents cracking. Prepared sponge sticks or moist gauze pads can be used to moisten oral membranes of the unconscious patient. Swabbing the mouth moistens the tissue and displaces the bacteria that collect when saliva, which has a bacteriostatic action, is curtailed by dehydration. The conscious patient must be provided the means to self-remove oral bacteria by tooth brushing and frequent oral rinsing.

Strict sterile technique is used to maintain all IV systems. All venipuncture sites are checked every 4 hours for signs of inflammation, phlebitis, or infiltration. Strict surgical asepsis is used for all invasive procedures. Sterile technique is used if urinary catheterization is necessary to obtain urine samples for testing. Urinary catheter care is provided every 8 hours.

BOX 24-7 Clinical Manifestations of Hypoglycemia and Hyperglycemia

HYPOGLYCEMIA	HYPERGLYCEMIA
• Restlessness	• Excessive thirst
• Apprehension	• Excessive urination
• Irritability	• Hunger
• Trembling	• Weakness
• Weakness	• Listlessness
• Diaphoresis	• Mental fatigue
• Pallor	• Flushed, dry skin
• Paresthesia	• Itching
• Pallor	• Headache
• Headache	• Nausea
• Hunger	• Vomiting
• Difficulty thinking	• Abdominal cramps
• Loss of coordination	• Dehydration
• Difficulty walking	• Weak, rapid pulse
• Difficulty talking	• Postural hypotension
• Visual disturbances	• Hypotension
• Blurred vision	• Acetone breath odor
• Double vision	• Kussmaul respirations
• Tachycardia	• Rapid breathing
• Shallow respirations	• Changes in level of consciousness
• Hypertension	• Stupor
• Changes in level of consciousness	• Coma
• Seizures	
• Coma	

Patient Education

It is important to be aware of the knowledge level and adherence history of patients with previously diagnosed diabetes to formulate an appropriate teaching plan. Learning objectives include a discussion of target glucose levels, definition of hyperglycemia and its causes, harmful effects, symptoms, and how to manage insulin and diet when one is unwell and unable to eat. Additional objectives include a definition of DKA and its causes, symptoms, and harmful consequences. The patient and family are also expected to learn the principles of diabetes management. Universal precautions must be emphasized for all family caregivers. The patient and family must also learn the warning signs of DKA to report to the attention of a health care practitioner. Education of the patient, family, or other support persons to achieve

*DKA has Ketones

BOX 24-8 PATIENT EDUCATION PRIORITIES: DIABETIC KETOACIDOSIS

Acute Phase
- Explain rationale for critical care unit admission.
- Reduce anxiety associated with critical care unit.

Predischarge
- Assess knowledge level.
- Assess prior adherence to self-monitoring of blood glucose
- Diabetes disease process
- Target glucose levels
- Causes of diabetic ketoacidosis (DKA)
- Pathophysiology of DKA
- Self-care monitoring of blood glucose level
- Insulin regimen
- Sick-day management
- Universal precautions for caregivers
- Signs and symptoms to report to health care practitioner

BOX 24-9 EVIDENCE-BASED (QSEN) PRACTICE: DIABETIC KETOACIDOSIS

Summary of evidence and evidence-based recommendations for controlling symptoms related to diabetic ketoacidosis (DKA)

Strong Evidence to Support
- Regular insulin by continuous infusion is recommended.
- Replace serum potassium if level is lower than 3.3 mEq/L.
- Replace serum phosphate if level is lower than 1.0 mg/dL.

Very Little Evidence to Support
- No support for use of routine bicarbonate to correct low serum pH; use may be considered if pH is below 7.0.

Reference

Kitabchi AE, et al: Hyperglycemic crises in adult patients with diabetes: a consensus statement from the American Diabetes Association, *Diabetes Care* 32(7):1335, 2009.

knowledge-based, independent self-management of blood glucose level and avoidance of diabetes-related complications are the ultimate goals of the teaching process (Box 24-8).

Collaborative Management

In all aspects of patient care management, health care professionals work as a team with the major collaborative goal of providing the best possible outcome for each patient. Current guidelines related to Collaborative Management of patients with hyperglycemia crisis are listed in Box 24-9.

HYPERGLYCEMIC HYPEROSMOLAR STATE

Epidemiology and Etiology

Hyperglycemic hyperosmolar state (HHS) is a potentially lethal complication of type 2 diabetes. The hallmarks of HHS are extremely high levels of plasma glucose with resultant elevation in serum hyperosmolality causing osmotic diuresis. Ketosis is absent or mild. Inability to replace fluids lost through diuresis leads to profound dehydration and changes in level of consciousness. The overall mortality rate from HHS ranges from 5% to 20%.[24] Because patients with HHS have type 2 diabetes as an underlying disorder, they are generally older adults with cardiovascular comorbidities.

The diagnostic criteria for HHS are as follows and as shown in Table 24-4:[24]

- Blood glucose greater than 600 mg/dL
- Arterial pH greater than 7.3
- Serum bicarbonate greater than 18 mEq/L
- Serum osmolality greater than 320 mOsm/kg H_2O (320 mmol/kg)
- Absent or mild ketonuria

Most patients with this level of metabolic disruption experience visual changes, mental status changes, and potentially hypovolemic shock.

HHS occurs when the pancreas produces a relatively insufficient amount of insulin for the high levels of glucose that flood the bloodstream. HHS primarily affects older, obese persons with underlying cardiovascular conditions. Infection is the primary reason that type 2 diabetics develop HHS; the most common infections are pneumonia and urinary tract infections. The patient may have type 2 diabetes treated with diet and oral hypoglycemic agents that is destabilized by an infection. Other precipitating causes of HHS include stroke, myocardial infarction, trauma, major surgery, and the stress of critical illness.

Differences between Hyperglycemic Hyperosmolar State and Diabetic Ketoacidosis

Clinically, HHS is distinguished from DKA by the presence of extremely elevated serum glucose, more profound dehydration, and minimal or absent ketosis (Table 24-5). Another major difference is that protein and fats are not used to create new supplies of glucose in HHS as they are in DKA; as a result, the ketotic cycle is never started or does not occur until the glucose level is extremely elevated.

Pathophysiology

HHS represents a deficit of insulin and an excess of glucagon (Figure 24-4). Reduced insulin levels prevent the movement of glucose into the cells, allowing glucose to accumulate in the plasma. The decreased insulin triggers glucagon release from the liver, and hepatic glucose is poured into the circulation. As the number of glucose particles increases in the blood, serum hyperosmolality increases. In an effort to decrease the serum osmolality, fluid is drawn from the intracellular compartment (inside the cells) into the vascular bed. Profound intracellular volume depletion occurs if the patient's thirst sensation is absent or decreased. HHS may evolve over days or even weeks.[24]

Hemoconcentration persists despite removal of large amounts of glucose in the urine (glycosuria). The glomerular filtration and elimination of glucose by the kidney tubules is ineffective in reducing the serum glucose level sufficiently to maintain normal glucose levels. The hyperosmolality and reduced blood volume stimulate release of ADH to increase the tubular resorption of water. ADH, however, is powerless to overcome the osmotic pull exerted by the glucose load. Excessive fluid volume is lost at the kidney tubule, with

TABLE 24-5 Comparison of Diabetic Ketoacidosis and Hyperglycemic Hyperosmolar State

CHARACTERISTICS AND LABORATORY TESTS	DKA	HHS
Cause	Insufficient exogenous glucose for glucose needs	Insufficient exogenous/endogenous insulin for glucose needs
Onset	Sudden (hours)	Slow, insidious (days, weeks)
Precipitating factors	Noncompliance with type 1 diabetes therapy, illness, surgery, decreased activity	Recent acute illness in an older patient; therapeutic procedures
Mortality (%)	9-14%	10-50%
Population affected	Patients with type 1 diabetes	Patients with type 2 diabetes
Clinical manifestations	Dry mouth, polydipsia, polyuria, polyphagia, dehydration, dry skin, hypotension, weakness	Mental confusion, tachycardia, changes in level of consciousness
	Ketoacidosis; air hunger, acetone breath odor, respirations deep and rapid, nausea, vomiting	No ketosis, no breath odor, respirations rapid and shallow, usually mild nausea/vomiting
Laboratory tests		
Glucose (mg/dL)	300-800	600-2000
Ketones	Strongly positive	Normal or mildly elevated
pH	<7.3	Normal*
Osmolality (mOsm/L)	Variable	>350
Sodium	Normal or low	Normal or elevated
Potassium (K^+)	Normal, low, or elevated (total body K^+ depleted)	Low, normal, or elevated
Bicarbonate	<15 mEq/L	Normal
Phosphorus	Low, normal, or elevated (may decrease after insulin therapy)	Low, normal, or elevated (may decrease after insulin therapy)
Urine acetone	Strong	Absent or mild

DKA, Diabetic ketoacidosis; *HHS*, hyperglycemic hyperosmolar state.
*Exception: In severe HHS, lactic acidosis may develop as a result of dehydration and severe tissue hypoperfusion and ischemia.

simultaneous loss of potassium, sodium, and phosphate in the urine. This chain of events results in progressively worsening hypovolemia.

Hypovolemia reduces perfusion to the kidney, and oliguria develops. Although this process conserves water and preserves the blood volume, it prevents further glucose loss, and hyperosmolality increases. Ketosis is absent or mild in HHS.

The SNS reacts to the body's stress response to try to restore homeostasis. Epinephrine, a potent stimulus for gluconeogenesis, is released, and additional glucose is added to the bloodstream. Unless the glycemic diuresis cycle is broken by aggressive fluid replacement and insulin administration, intracellular dehydration negatively affects fluid and oxygen transport to the brain cells. Central nervous system dysfunction may result and may lead to coma. Hemoconcentration increases the blood viscosity, which may result in clot formation, thromboemboli, and cerebral, cardiac, and pleural infarcts.

Assessment and Diagnosis

Clinical Manifestations

HHS has a slow, subtle onset and develops over several days. Initially, the symptoms may be nonspecific and may be ignored or attributed to the patient's concurrent disease processes. History reveals malaise, blurred vision, polyuria, polydipsia (depending on the patient's thirst sensation), weight loss, and increasing weakness. Medical attention may not be obtained for these nonspecific, nonacute symptoms until the patient is unable to take sufficient fluids to offset the fluid losses. Progressive dehydration follows and leads to mental confusion, convulsions, and eventually coma, especially in older patients.

The physical examination may reveal a profound fluid deficit. Signs of severe dehydration include longitudinal wrinkles in the tongue, decreased salivation, and decreased CVP, with increases in HR and rapid respirations (Kussmaul air hunger does not occur.). In older patients, assessment of clinical signs of dehydration is challenging. Neurologic status is affected as the serum glucose climbs, especially at levels greater than 1500 mg/dL. Without intervention, obtundation and coma occur.

Laboratory Studies

Laboratory findings are used to establish the definitive diagnosis of HHS. Plasma glucose levels are strikingly elevated (greater than 600 mg/dL). Serum osmolality is greater than 320 mOsm/kg. Acidosis is absent (arterial pH greater than 7.3), and the serum bicarbonate concentration is greater than 18 mEq/L. Ketonuria is absent or mild.[24] The patient may have an elevated hematocrit and depleted potassium and phosphorus levels.

Point-of-care finger-stick or arterial-line testing of glucose at the bedside is the usual method for frequent monitoring of the serum blood glucose. Insulin replacement is then prescribed according to the blood glucose result. Some electrolytes also can be tested at the bedside (potassium, sodium, ionized calcium), but usually an arterial line is required for frequent blood access. If point-of-care testing is not available, traditional serial laboratory tests keep the clinician apprised of the fluctuating serum electrolyte levels and provide the

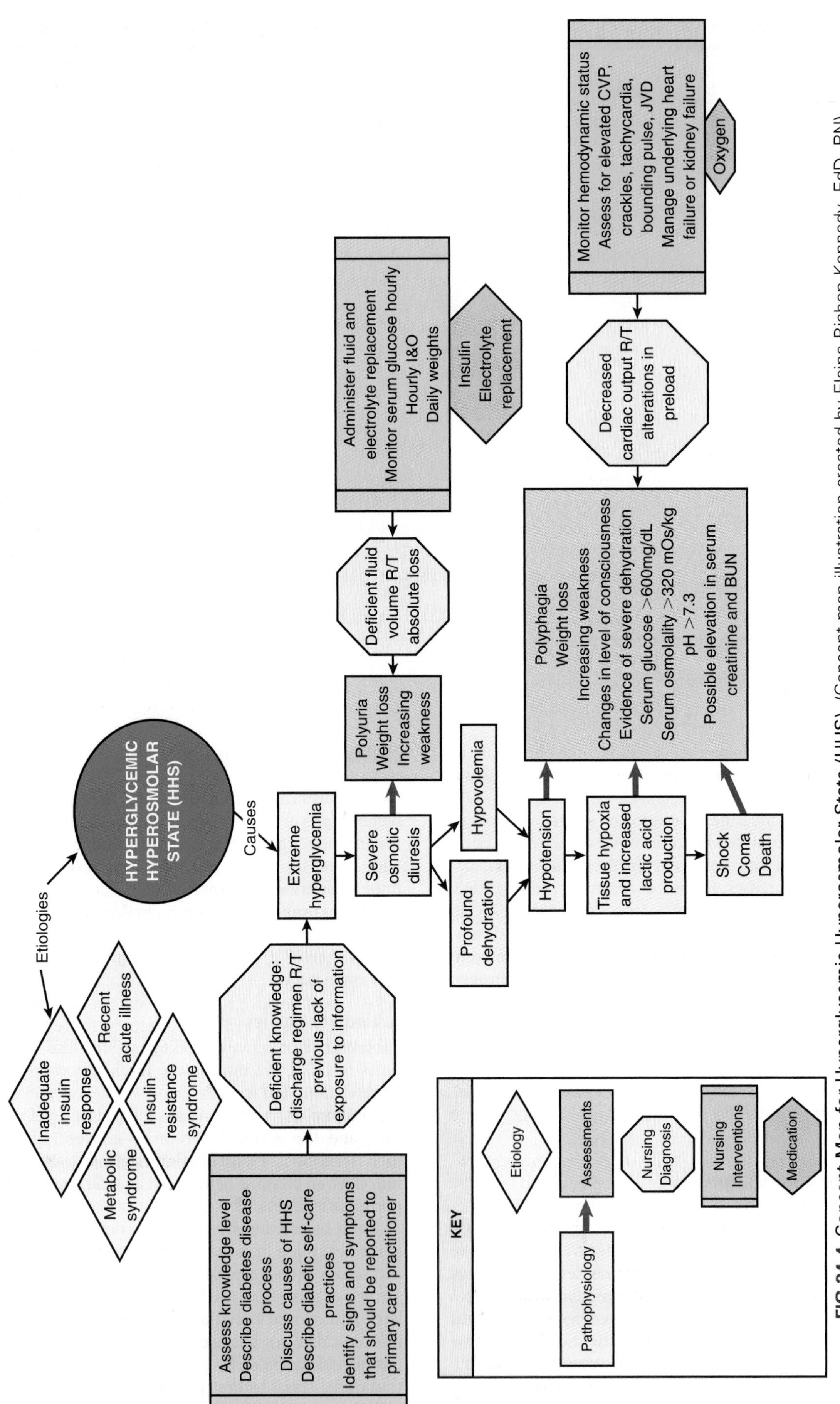

FIG 24-4 Concept Map for Hyperglycemic Hyperosmolar State (HHS). (Concept map illustration created by Elaine Bishop Kennedy, EdD, RN)

basis for electrolyte replacement. Intracellular potassium and phosphate levels usually are depleted as a result of prior osmotic diuresis.[24]

Elevated BUN and creatinine levels suggest kidney impairment as a result of the severe reduction in renal circulation. Metabolic acidosis usually is absent at lower glucose levels. Acidosis may result from starvation ketosis or from an increase in lactic acid production caused by poor tissue perfusion.

Medical Management

The goals of medical management are rapid rehydration, insulin replacement, and correction of electrolyte abnormalities, specifically potassium replacement. The underlying stimulus of HHS must be discovered and treated. The same basic principles used to treat DKA are used for the patient with HHS.

Rapid Rehydration

The primary intervention for HHS is rapid rehydration to restore the intravascular volume. The fluid deficit may be as much as 150 mL/kg of body weight. The average 150-pound adult can lose more than 7 to 10 L of fluid. Physiologic saline solution (0.9%) is infused at 1 L/hr, especially for the patient in hypovolemic shock if there is no cardiovascular contraindication. Several liters of volume replacement may be required to achieve a BP and CVP within normal range. Infusion volumes are adjusted according to the patient's hydration state and sodium level.[24]

The serum sodium concentration is the parameter that is monitored to determine whether to change from isotonic (0.9%) to hypotonic (0.45%) saline. For example, patients with sodium levels equal to or less than 140 mEq/L may be given 0.9% normal saline solution, whereas those with levels greater than 140 mEq/L are given 0.45% saline solution (see Figure 24-3).[24] It is difficult to assess the serum sodium level in the presence of hemoconcentration. Another recommendation is to calculate a *corrected sodium value.* This involves adding 1.6 mEq to the sodium laboratory value for each 100 mg/dL plasma glucose above normal.[24] Sodium input should not exceed the amount required to replace the losses. Careful monitoring of the serum sodium level is recommended to avoid a sodium-water imbalance and hemolysis as the hemoconcentration is reduced.

To prevent hypoglycemia in HHS, when the serum glucose decreases to 300 mg/dL, the hydrating solution is changed to D_5W with 0.45% NaCl at 150 to 250 mL/hr.[24]

Insulin Administration

Volume resuscitation lowers the serum glucose level and improves symptoms even without insulin administration. However, insulin replacement is recommended in the treatment of HHS because acidosis can develop if insulin is withheld, and insulin will facilitate the cellular use of glucose.

Methods to lower the blood glucose level vary. One method is to administer an IV bolus of regular insulin (0.15 unit/kg of body weight) initially, followed by a continuous insulin drip. Regular insulin infusing at an initial rate calculated as 0.1 unit/kg hourly (e.g., 7 units/hr for a person weighing 70 kg) should lower the plasma glucose concentration by 50 to 70 mg/dL during the first hour of treatment. If the measured glucose level does not decrease by this amount, the insulin infusion rate may be doubled until the blood glucose is declining at a rate of 50 to 70 mg/dL per hour.[24]

Insulin resistance. Patients with HHS have underlying type 2 diabetes and may exhibit signs of insulin resistance.[19] In critical illness, the presence of counterregulatory hormones, also known as stress hormones (cortisol, glucagon, epinephrine), increases glucose production and induces insulin resistance. Patients with HHS may require supraphysiologic doses of insulin initially to overcome the hyperglycemia and insulin resistance. Hourly serial monitoring of the blood glucose level permits safe glycemic management and avoids the most common complication, which is hypoglycemia caused by overzealous insulin administration.[24] After the patient has recovered from the hyperglycemic crisis and insulin has been discontinued, oral medications designed to decrease insulin resistance in type 2 diabetics will be part of the treatment plan (see Table 24-3).

Electrolyte Replacement

Increasing the circulating levels of insulin with therapeutic doses of IV insulin promotes the rapid return of potassium and phosphorus into the cell. Serial laboratory tests keep the clinician apprised of the serum electrolyte levels and provide the basis for electrolyte replacement. Potassium typically is added to the IV infusion (see Figure 24-3). If the serum potassium concentration is lower than 3.3 mEq/L, it is essential to replenish the serum potassium before giving insulin.[24] Many hospitals have potassium replacement algorithms that are used to treat hypokalemia. Serum phosphate levels are carefully monitored and phosphate replaced if the level is lower than 1.0 mg/dL.[24]

Nursing Management

Nursing management of the patient with HHS incorporates a variety of nursing diagnoses (Box 24-10). Nursing management goals are similar to those outlined for DKA. The critical care nurse administers prescribed fluids, insulin, and electrolytes; monitors the response to therapy; maintains surveillance for complications, and provides patient education.

Administering Fluids, Insulin, and Electrolytes

Rigorous fluid replacement and continuous IV insulin replacement must be controlled with an electronic volumetric pump. Accurate I&O measurements are maintained to monitor fluid balance. I&O measurements include the total of all fluids administered minus hourly losses, such as urine output and emesis. Hemodynamic monitoring may include use of an arterial line and measurements of CVP if the patient manifests signs of hypovolemic shock. Arterial line access is very helpful in monitoring serial blood glucose and electrolyte values. The use of a blood conservation system on the arterial line is essential to avoid iatrogenic exsanguination of the patient. Most critical care units have developed protocols or guidelines to ensure that patients in hyperglycemic crisis are managed safely (see Figure 24-3). The major responsibility for delivery of insulin, hourly monitoring of blood glucose, and infusion of appropriate crystalloid solutions lies with the critical care nurse. Many hospitals mandate a double-check procedure for medications such as insulin that have the potential to cause harm if wrongly administered.

BOX 24-10 NURSING DIAGNOSES: HYPERGLYCEMIC HYPEROSMOLAR STATE

- Decreased Cardiac Output related to alterations in preload, p. 579
- Deficient Fluid Volume related to absolute loss, p. 584
- Anxiety related to threat to biologic, psychologic, and social integrity, p. 576
- Deficient Knowledge related to previous lack of exposure to information, p. 585 (see Box 24-11, Patient Education for Hyperglycemic Hyperosmolar State)

Monitoring Response to Therapy

The BP, HR, and CVP are monitored to evaluate the degree of dehydration, the effectiveness of hydration therapy, and the patient's fluid tolerance. Because patients with HHS have underlying type 2 diabetes and, if older, are likely have preexisting illnesses such as heart failure and kidney failure, it is important to monitor for symptoms of circulatory overload. Symptoms to anticipate include elevated CVP, tachycardia, bounding pulse, dyspnea, tachypnea, lung crackles, and engorged neck veins. The astute critical care nurse is aware of the clinical manifestations of fluid overload and observes for potential complications when rehydrating the patient with HHS and cardiac, pulmonary, or kidney disease.

The serum glucose level should decrease by 50 to 70 mg/dL per hour with insulin administration.[24] This decrease is monitored by hourly blood glucose determinations. Based on the result, the critical care nurse can alter the infusion of insulin according to hospital protocol (see Figure 24-4).

Surveillance for Complications

The potential complications of HHS are similar to those described for DKA: hypoglycemia, hypokalemia or hyperkalemia, and infection. The patient with HHS is at risk for other complications specific to associated disease entities. A history of cardiovascular, pulmonary, or kidney disease, whether known or latent, places the patient with HHS at high risk for complications.

Patient Education

As the patient's condition improves and the patient demonstrates readiness to learn, education about type 2 diabetes and avoiding a recurrence of HHS becomes a priority (Box 24-11). Most teaching occurs after the patient has left the critical care unit. Teaching topics include a description of type 2 diabetes and how it relates to HHS, dietary restrictions, exercise requirements, medication protocols, home testing of blood glucose, signs and symptoms of hyperglycemia and hypoglycemia, foot care, and lifestyle modifications if cardiovascular disease is present.

Collaborative Management

Because HHS is an acute condition superimposed on the chronic health problem of type 2 diabetes, many health professionals provide care and work collaboratively to restore homeostasis for each patient (Box 24-12).

BOX 24-11 PATIENT EDUCATION PRIORITIES: HYPERGLYCEMIC HYPEROSMOLAR STATE

Acute Phase
- Explain rationale for critical care unit admission.

Predischarge
- Assess knowledge level.
- Assess compliance history.
- Diabetes disease process
- Definition of hyperglycemic hyperosmotic state (HHS)
- Causes of HHS
- Self-care for diabetes
- Signs and symptoms to report to health care practitioner

BOX 24-12 EVIDENCE-BASED QSEN PRACTICE: HYPERGLYCEMIC HYPEROSMOLAR STATE

Summary of evidence and evidence-based recommendations for controlling symptoms related to hyperglycemic hyperosmolar state (HHS)

Strong Evidence to Support
- Regular insulin by continuous infusion is recommended to normalize blood glucose.
- Replace serum potassium if the level is less than 3.3 mEq/L.
- Replace serum phosphate if the level is less than 1 mg/dL.
- A multidisciplinary team approach reduces length of stay and improves clinical outcomes.
- Close follow-up after discharge is recommended to maintain glycosylated hemoglobin (A_{1c}) at less than 6.5% and to prevent diabetes-related complications.

Weak Evidence to Support
- Use of a sliding insulin scale alone is discouraged because it is associated with hyperglycemia and hypoglycemia in hospitalized patients.

Reference

Kitabchi AE, et al: Hyperglycemic crises in adult patients with diabetes: a consensus statement from the American Diabetes Association, *Diabetes Care* 32(7):1335, 2009.

DIABETES INSIPIDUS

Diabetes insipidus (DI) is recognized by the vast quantities of very dilute urine that are produced in susceptible patients. In the critically ill patient, the extreme diuresis is most likely to be caused by a lack of ADH (vasopressin). Any patient who has head trauma,[27] or resection of a pituitary tumor, has an increased risk of developing DI.[28] Normally, ADH is produced in the hypothalamus and stored in the posterior pituitary gland. Physiologically, ADH is released primarily in response to even small elevations in serum osmolality and secondarily in reaction to hypovolemia or hypotension. DI can occur if 1) the hypothalamus produces insufficient ADH,

BOX 24-13 Causes of Diabetes Insipidus

Central Diabetes Insipidus
Primary (Rare in Critical Care)
- ADH deficiency caused by hypothalamic-hypophyseal malformation
  - Congenital defect
  - Idiopathic

Secondary (Most Common in Critical Care)
- ADH deficiency caused by damage to the hypothalamic-hypophyseal system
  - Trauma
  - Infection
  - Surgery
  - Primary neoplasms
  - Metastatic malignancies

Nephrogenic Diabetes Insipidus
- Inability of kidney tubules to respond to circulating ADH
  - Decrease or absence of ADH receptors
  - Cellular damage to nephron, especially loop of Henle
  - Kidney damage (e.g., hydronephrosis, pyelonephritis, polycystic kidney)
  - Untoward response to medication therapy (e.g., lithium carbonate, demeclocycline)

Psychogenic Diabetes Insipidus
- Rare form of water intoxication
- Compulsive water drinking

ADH, Antidiuretic hormone.

2) the posterior pituitary fails to release ADH, or 3) the kidney nephron is resistant (unresponsive) to ADH.

Etiology

DI is divided into three types according to cause: central, nephrogenic, and psychogenic (Box 24-13). Only central DI, also known as neurogenic DI because of its association with the brain, is encountered with any frequency in the critical care unit.

Central Diabetes Insipidus

In central DI, there is an inability to secrete an adequate amount of ADH (arginine vasopressin) in response to an osmotic or nonosmotic stimuli, resulting in inappropriately dilute urine. The synthesis of ADH is incomplete in the hypothalamus, or the release of ADH from the pituitary is interrupted. Central DI can be congenital or acquired.[29] In critical care, the most likely acute cause of central DI is neurosurgery, traumatic head injury, tumors, increased intracranial pressure, brain death, and infections such as encephalitis or meningitis. Among patients undergoing surgery on the pituitary gland, transient DI occurs in approximately 20% to 30%; permanent DI occurs in 2% to 10% of patients.[29] The degree of hormone replacement required after surgery depends the quantity of pituitary tissue that has been surgically or endoscopically removed.

Nephrogenic Diabetes Insipidus

Nephrogenic DI is a rare congenital or an acquired disorder that occurs when the V_2 receptors on the kidney tubule become nonresponsive to the action of ADH. Some medications cause nephrogenic DI by decreasing the responsiveness of the kidney tubules to ADH. Long-term use of lithium carbonate, prescribed for bipolar disorder, was a frequent culprit in the past.[29]

Primary Polydipsia

Primary polydipsia, previously called psychogenic DI, is a rare form of the disease that occurs with compulsive drinking of more than 5 L of water daily. Long-standing psychogenic DI closely mimics nephrogenic DI because the kidney tubules become less responsive to ADH as a result of prolonged conditioning to hypotonic urine.[29]

Pathophysiology

The purpose of ADH is to maintain normal serum osmolality and circulating blood volume. Normally, ADH binds to the V_2 receptors on the kidney collecting tubules, causing insertion of water channels, known as aquaporins, along the luminal surface. Even small increases in plasma osmolality are sufficient to stimulate ADH release. Although there are several types of DI, this discussion focuses on neurogenic (central) DI, the condition encountered in the critical care unit after neurosurgery or head injury (Figure 24-5).

In DI, as free water is eliminated, the urine osmolality and specific gravity decrease (dilute urine). At the same time, in the bloodstream, the serum sodium concentration and serum osmolality rise. Normally, a rise in the serum osmolality to greater than 290 mOsm per kilogram of H_2O (290 mmol/L) triggers synthesis and release of ADH. If the thirst mechanism is intact, thirst sensors are activated in the hypothalamus causing a sensation of thirst that leads the person to drink lots of fluids.[30] In central DI, however, no ADH is released, or the ADH released is insufficient. Without ADH, the kidney collecting tubules are incapable of concentrating urine and retaining water.

As extracellular dehydration ensues, hypotension and hypovolemic shock can occur. If the patient is alert, extreme thirst will lead the person to replace lost fluids by drinking lots of water.[30] This excessive intake of water reduces the serum osmolality to a more normal level and prevents dehydration. In the person with decreased level of consciousness, the polyuria leads to severe hypernatremia, dehydration, decreased cerebral perfusion, seizures, loss of consciousness, and death.

Assessment and Diagnosis
Clinical Manifestations

The clinical diagnosis is based on the clinical increase in dilute urine output occurring in the absence of diuretics, a fluid challenge, or hyperglycemia. Central DI is anticipated in conditions in which the underlying disease process is likely to disrupt pituitary function. Central DI that occurs because of increasing intracranial pressure is life-threatening. It is imperative that the underlying condition be recognized and treated appropriately. In this situation, medications that treat DI are not sufficient.

Laboratory Studies

The core diagnostic tests used to establish the presence of DI and that evaluate the body's ability to balance fluid and electrolytes are not specific to the endocrine system. The most

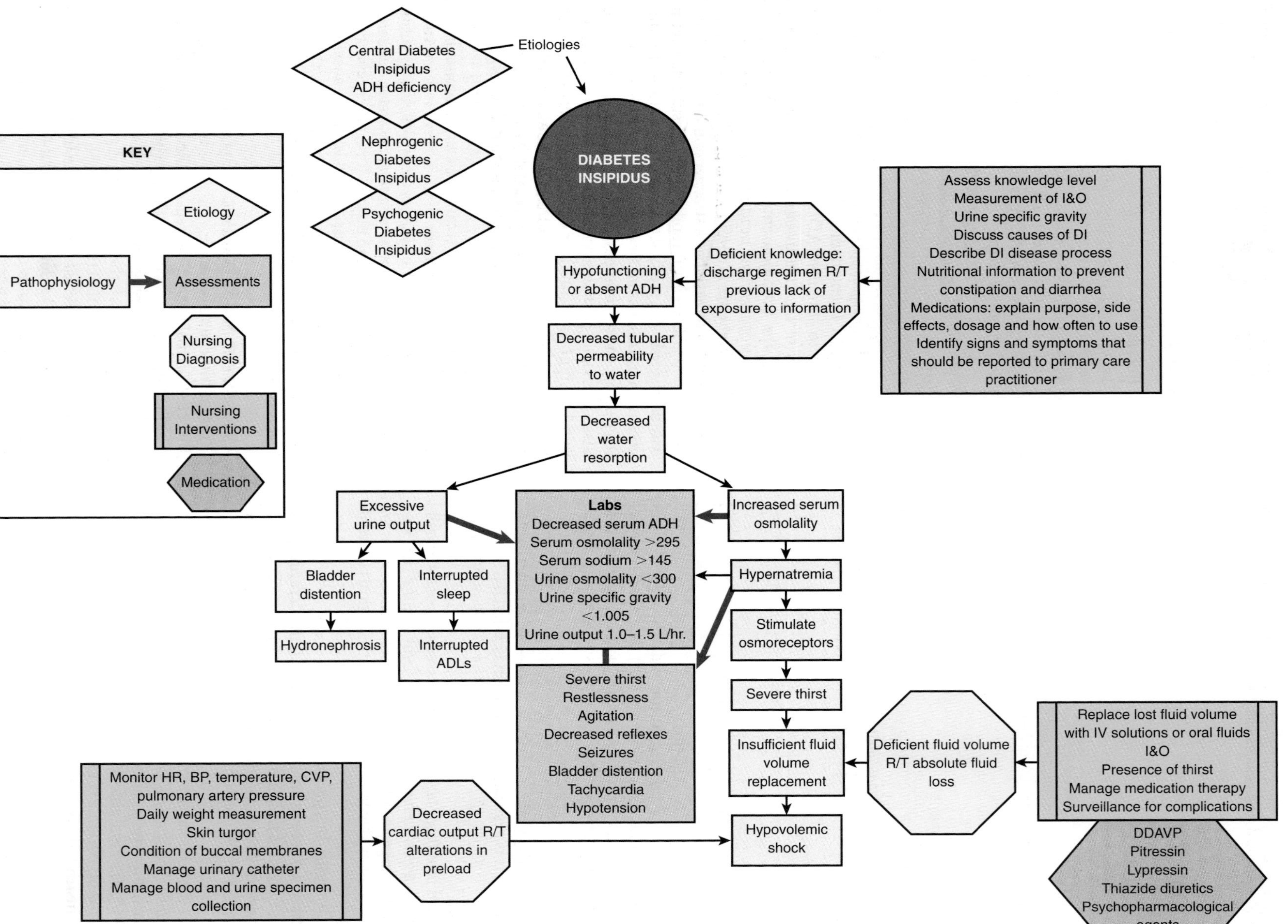

FIG 24-5 Concept Map for Diabetes Insipidus (DI). (Concept map illustration created by Elaine Bishop Kennedy, EdD, RN.)

TABLE 24-6 Laboratory Values for Patients with Diabetes Insipidus and Syndrome of Inappropriate Antidiuretic Hormone

VALUE	NORMAL	DI	SIADH
Serum ADH	1-5 pg/mL	Decreased in central DI	Elevated
Serum osmolality (mOsm/L)	275-295*	>295*	<270
Serum sodium (mEq/L)	135-145	>145	<120
Urine osmolality (mOsm/L)	300-1400	<300	Increased
Urine specific gravity	1.005-1.030	<1.005	>1.030
Urine output	1.0-1.5 L/day	1.0-1.5 L/hr	Below normal

ADH, Antidiuretic hormone; *DI*, diabetes insipidus; *L/day*, liters per day; *pg/mL*, picogram per milliliter; *SIADH*, syndrome of inappropriate antidiuretic hormone.

*Some hospitals use 280-300 mOsm/L as their normal reference value.

common tests are serum sodium concentration, serum osmolality, and urine osmolality (Table 24-6). The combination of an obvious clinical picture with high volumes of hypotonic urine, in the presence of the following laboratory criteria, is sufficient to diagnose central DI:[29,30]

- Serum sodium level greater than 145 mEq/L
- Serum osmolality greater than 295 mOsm/kg H_2O (greater than 295 mmol/L)
- Urine osmolality less than 300 mOsm/kg H_2O (less than 300 mmol/L)
- Urine specific gravity less than 1.005

Serum sodium. The normal serum sodium concentration is 140 mEq/L (range, 135 to 145 mEq/L). In central DI, the serum sodium level can rise precipitously because of the loss of free water. Hypernatremia is usually associated with serum hyperosmolality.

Serum osmolality test. Serum osmolality has a narrow normal range, 275 to 295 mOsm/kg. Severe DI can raise serum osmolality to greater than 320 mOsm/kg.

Urine osmolality. Urine osmolality is low, less than 300 mOsm/kg H_2O (300 mmol/L) in patients with central DI.[29] For greatest accuracy, the urine sample should be collected and tested simultaneously with the blood sample. This test is rarely performed in the critical care unit.

Measurement of antidiuretic hormone. Measurement of the baseline serum ADH level is an additional diagnostic step. This is not typically performed in critical care if the clinical circumstances (e.g., head injury with raised intracranial pressure) make further testing unnecessary. Normal ADH levels range from 1 to 5 picogram/mL (pg/mL). With normal hydration the normal morning fasting serum level is lower than 4 pg/mL.

Medical Management

Immediate management of DI requires an aggressive approach. Treatment goals include restoration of circulating fluid volume, pharmacologic ADH replacement, and treatment of the underlying condition.

Volume Restoration

Fluid replacement is provided in the initial phase of the treatment to prevent circulatory collapse. Patients who are able to drink are given voluminous amounts of fluid orally to balance output. For those who are unable to take sufficient fluids orally, hypotonic IV solutions are infused and carefully monitored to restore the hemodynamic balance.

Medications

Central DI requires immediate pharmacologic management. Table 24-7 presents the medications most frequently prescribed to treat central DI and replace ADH.

Medications used for central diabetes insipidus. Patients with central DI who are unable to synthesize ADH require replacement with ADH (vasopressin) or an ADH analogue. The most commonly prescribed medication is the synthetic analogue of ADH, desmopressin (DDAVP). It is preferred over vasopressin (Pitressin) because it has a stronger antidiuretic action with little effect on BP. DDAVP can be given IV, subcutaneously, or as a nasal spray. A typical DDAVP dose is 1 to 2 mcg administered IV or subcutaneously every 12 hours.[30] Sometimes only 0.5 mcg is given intravenously. The dosage is subsequently titrated according to the patient's antidiuretic response, and close monitoring of urine output is advised.[28] To avoid a medication error, it is important to be aware that DDAVP is also used to control hemorrhage caused by platelet disorders and that the dose ranges for all of these conditions are different.

Vasopressin (Pitressin), 5 units administered subcutaneously every 6 to 8 hours, produces a reduction in urine output.[31] Vasopressin acts on the V_1 receptors in vascular smooth muscle and can elevate systemic BP. Vasopressin can also be prescribed for septic shock states as an IV infusion and for cardiac arrest as an IV push. Dosages for these conditions are very different from that used to treat central DI. Extreme care must be taken to ensure that all medication dosages are accurate for each specific diagnosis.

Medications used for nephrogenic diabetes insipidus. The mainstay of therapy is to stop any medications that are inducing the ADH resistance. Nephrogenic DI is not a diagnosis encountered in critical care unless the patient is admitted with this condition. It is treated with the diuretic hydrochlorothiazide, with the dosage titration based upon the patient's antidiuretic response.

Nursing Management

Nursing management of the patient with DI incorporates a variety of nursing diagnoses (Box 24-14). Nursing management is directed toward administration of prescribed fluids and medications, evaluation of response to therapy, surveillance for complications, and provision of patient education.

Administration of Fluids and Medications

Rapid IV fluid replacement requires the use of a volumetric pump. Initially, a hypotonic IV solution is used to replace

TABLE 24-7 Pharmacologic Management

Central Diabetes Insipidus

MEDICATION	DOSAGE*	ACTIONS	SPECIAL CONSIDERATIONS
Central Diabetes Insipidus			
DDAVP (available IV, as nasal spray, Rhinal tube, Rhinyle drops, Stimate)	Nasal: 10-40 mcg before bed or in divided doses Parenteral: 2-4 mcg twice daily	Central DI Antidiuretic Increases water resorption in nephron. Prevents and controls polydipsia, polyuria.	Few side effects Observe for nasal congestion, upper respiratory infection, allergic rhinitis. Monitor intake and output, urine osmolality, serum sodium level.
Vasopressin (Pitressin)	IV, IM, subcutaneous	Central DI antidiuretic	Monitor fluid volume often, especially in older patients.
	Topical: nasal mucosa	Promotes resorption of water at kidney tubule. Decreases urine output. Increases urine osmolality. Diagnostic aid Increases gastrointestinal peristalsis.	Assess cardiac status. May precipitate angina, hypertension, or myocardial infarction if increased dose is given to patient with cardiac history. Parenteral extravasation can cause skin necrosis.
Lypressin (Diapid)	Intranasal: 1-2 sprays (7-14 mcg) in each nostril four times daily	Central DI Synthetic ADH Increases resorption of sodium and water in nephron.	Proper instillation is important for absorption and action. Patient sits upright while holding bottle upright for administration. Repeat sprays (>2-3) are ineffective and wasteful; if dose is increased to 2-3 sprays, shorten time between dosing. Cough, chest tightness, shortness of breath

ADH, Antidiuretic hormone; *DDAVP*, desmopressin acetate; *DI*, diabetes insipidus; *IM*, intramuscular; *IV*, intravenous; *mcg*, microgram.
*Parenteral indicates intravenous or subcutaneous administration.

BOX 24-14 NURSING DIAGNOSES: DIABETES INSIPIDUS

- Decreased Cardiac Output related to alterations in preload, p. 579
- Deficient Fluid Volume related to absolute fluid loss, p. 584
- Deficient Knowledge related to lack of previous exposure to information, p. 585 (see Box 24-15, Patient Education for Diabetes Insipidus)

fluids lost and lower the serum hyperosmolality. ADH replacement is accomplished with extreme caution in the patient with a history of heart disease because ADH may cause hypertension and overhydration. At the first signs of cardiovascular impairment, the medication is discontinued, and fluid intake is restricted until urine specific gravity is less than 1.015 and polyuria resumes.

Evaluation of Response to Therapy

Critical assessment and management of fluid status are the most important initial concerns for the patient with DI. Monitoring of HR, BP, CVP, and pulmonary artery pressures (if a pulmonary artery catheter is in place) provides early indications of response to fluid volume replacement. I&O measurement, condition of buccal membranes, skin turgor, daily weight measurements, presence of thirst, and temperature provide a basic assessment list that is vital for the patient who is unable to regulate fluid needs and losses. Placement of a urinary catheter is essential to monitor the urinary output accurately. Simultaneous urine and blood specimens for determination of osmolality, serum sodium and serum potassium are obtained, and the results are relayed to the physician as necessary. The patient who is unable to satisfy sensations of thirst or to complete any task or self-care activity without the need to urinate may be confused and frightened. For patients who are able to verbalize their fears, having a caring nurse who is interested and nonjudgmental helps to reduce the emotional turmoil associated with their condition.

Surveillance for Complications

The most dangerous potential complication is hypertension and vasospasm of cardiac, cerebral, or mesenteric arterial vessels in response to vasopressin replacement. In most cases, DDAVP is selected for ADH replacement to avoid this complication. A less serious complication of DI is constipation due to fluid loss; it is treated with dietary fiber, stool softeners, or both. Conversely, diarrhea, abdominal cramping, and intestinal hyperactivity may accompany vasopressin therapy. Untoward effects can be mitigated by modification of the vasopressin dose.

Patient Education

Educating the patient and the family about the disease process and how it affects thirst, urination, and fluid balance encourages patients to participate in their care and reduces the feelings of hopelessness (Box 24-15). For most critical care patients, central DI is a temporary condition that resolves as the underlying medical condition (e.g., brain injury) improves. Patients who are discharged with DI are taught, along with their families, the signs and symptoms of dehydration and

BOX 24-15 PATIENT EDUCATION PRIORITIES: DIABETES INSIPIDUS

Acute Phase
- Explain rationale for critical care unit admission.

Predischarge
- Assess knowledge base.
- Measurement of fluid intake and output
- Urine specific gravity
- Causes of diabetes insipidus
- Disease process of diabetes insipidus
- Nutritional information to prevent constipation and diarrhea
- Medications: explain purpose, side effects, dosage, and how often to use.
- Signs and symptoms to report to health care professional

overhydration and procedures for accurate daily weight and urine specific gravity measurements. Printed information pertaining to medication actions, side effects, dosages, and timetable is provided, as well as an outline of factors that must be reported to the physician.

Collaborative Management

Central DI is a life-threatening condition. The collaborative assessment and clinical skills of all health care professionals and use of a clear plan of care are essential to achieve optimal outcomes for each patient.

SYNDROME OF INAPPROPRIATE SECRETION OF ANTIDIURETIC HORMONE

The opposing syndrome to DI is the *syndrome of inappropriate secretion of antidiuretic hormone* (SIADH), also known as the *syndrome of inappropriate antidiuresis* (SIAD).[32] The patient with SIADH has an excess of ADH secreted into the bloodstream, more than the amount needed to maintain normal blood volume and serum osmolality. Excessive water is resorbed at the kidney tubule, leading to dilutional hyponatremia.

Etiology

Numerous causes of SIADH are observed in patients who are critically ill (Box 24-16). Central nervous system injury, tumors, and diseases that interfere with the normal functioning of the hypothalamic-pituitary system can cause SIADH.[33] A common cause is malignant bronchogenic small cell carcinoma. This type of malignant cell is capable of synthesizing and releasing ADH regardless of the body's needs. With much less frequency, other cancers that involve the brain, head and neck, gastroenteral, gynecologic, and hematologic systems are capable of autonomous production of ADH.

Pathophysiology

ADH is a powerful, complex polypeptide compound. When released into the circulation by the posterior pituitary gland, ADH regulates water and electrolyte balance in the body. In SIADH, profound fluid and electrolyte disturbances result from the unsolicited, continuous release of the hormone into the bloodstream (Figure 24-6). Excessive ADH stimulates the kidney tubules to retain fluid regardless of need. This results in severe overhydration.

Excessive ADH dramatically alters the sodium balance in the extracellular vascular compartment. The overhydration causes a dilutional hyponatremia and reduces the sodium concentration to critically low levels. In the healthy adult, hyponatremia inhibits the release of ADH. In SIADH, however, the increased level of circulating ADH is unrelated to the serum sodium concentration. Aldosterone production from the adrenal glands is also suppressed. Serum hypoosmolality leads to a shift of fluid from the extracellular fluid space into the intracellular fluid compartment (inside the cells) in an attempt to equalize osmotic pressure. Because minimal sodium is present in this fluid, edema usually does not result. Without ADH and aldosterone, water is retained, urine output is diminished, and further sodium is excreted in the urine. The urine has an increased osmolality from the decreased water excretion. Urinary concentration is also elevated by excess sodium in the urine. It is believed that, despite the serum hyponatremia, the increased release of ADH promotes sodium loss through the kidneys into the urine.

Assessment and Diagnosis

Clinical Manifestations

The clinical manifestations of SIADH relate to the excess fluids in the extracellular compartment and the proportionate dilution of the circulating sodium. Edema usually is not present, although slight weight gain may occur from the expanded extracellular fluid volume. Early clinical manifestations of dilutional hyponatremia include lethargy, anorexia, nausea, and vomiting. Severe neurologic symptoms usually do not develop until the serum sodium concentration drops to less than 120 mEq/L. Progressively deteriorating neurologic signs of hyponatremia then predominate, and the patient is admitted to the critical care unit. Symptoms of severe hyponatremia include inability to concentrate, mental confusion, apprehension, seizures, decreased level of consciousness, coma, and death.

Laboratory Values

Patients with SIADH present with very dilute serum and very concentrated urine output. Laboratory values confirm this clinical picture. In SIADH, there is decreased plasma osmolality (less than 275 mOsm/kg H_2O), with increased urine osmolality (greater than 100 mOsm/kg).[32] The low serum sodium (less than 125 mEq/L) is associated with increasing severity of neurologic symptoms. The urine sodium concentration is elevated (greater than 40 mEq/L), congruent with the concentrated urine output of SIADH.[32] Use of diuretics negates the reliability of the urine sodium and urine osmolality levels.[32] See Table 24-6 for comparison of the typical laboratory values associated with SIADH with those of DI.

Medical Management

In the critical care unit, SIADH often occurs as a secondary disease. Ideally, recognition and treatment of the primary disease will reduce the production of ADH. If the patient is receiving any of the medications suspected of causing SIADH,

BOX 24-16 Causes of Syndrome of Inappropriate Secretion of Antidiuretic Hormone

Malignant Disease **Associated with Autonomous Production of ADH**
- Bronchogenic small cell carcinoma
- Pancreatic adenocarcinoma
- Duodenal, bladder, ureter, and prostatic carcinomas
- Lymphosarcoma, Ewing sarcoma
- Acute leukemia, Hodgkin disease
- Cerebral neoplasm, thymoma

Central Nervous System Diseases **That Interfere with the Hypothalamic-Hypophyseal System and Increase the Production or Release of ADH**
- Head injury
- Brain abscess
- Hydrocephalus
- Pituitary adenoma
- Subdural hematoma
- Subarachnoid hemorrhage
- Cerebral atrophy
- Guillain-Barré syndrome

Neurogenic Stimuli **Capable of Increasing ADH**
- Decreased glomerular filtration rate
- Physical or emotional stress
- Pain
- Fear
- Trauma
- Surgery
- Myocardial infarction
- Acute infection
- Hypotension
- Hemorrhage
- Hypovolemia

Pulmonary Diseases **Believed to Stimulate the Baroreceptors and Increase ADH**
- Pulmonary tuberculosis
- Viral and bacterial pneumonia
- Empyema
- Lung abscess
- Chronic obstructive lung disease
- Status asthmaticus
- Cystic fibrosis

Endocrine Disturbances **That Hormonally Influence ADH**
- Myxedema
- Hypothyroidism
- Hypopituitarism
- Adrenal insufficiency—Addison's disease

Medications **That Mimic, Increase the Release of, or Potentiate ADH**
- Hypoglycemics
  - Insulin
  - Tolbutamide
  - Chlorpropamide
- Potassium-depleting thiazide diuretics
- Tricyclic antidepressants
  - Imipramine
  - Amitriptyline
- Phenothiazine
  - Fluphenazine
  - Thioridazine
- Thioxanthenes
  - Thiothixene
  - Chlorprothixene
- Chemotherapeutic agents
  - Vincristine
  - Cyclophosphamide
- Opiates
- Carbamazepine
- Clofibrate
- Acetaminophen
- Nicotine
- Oxytocin
- Vasopressin
- Anesthetics

ADH, Antidiuretic hormone.

discontinuing that medication may return ADH levels to normal.[34] Some of the medications that alter ADH levels are listed in Box 24-16. The goals of medical management are to restore fluid and sodium balance.

Fluid Restriction

Reduction in fluid intake is one component of the treatment plan for SIADH.

Sodium Replacement

Patients with severe hyponatremia (less than 125 mEq/L serum sodium) experience severe neurologic symptoms, even seizures. Too-rapid serum sodium correction must be avoided to reduce the risk of *osmotic demyelination*,[33] which occurs in the white matter of the brain. Severe neurologic damage or death can result.[33] The demyelination complication can be avoided by raising the serum sodium slowly, such as by 8 to 12 mEq/L in 24 hours.[33] Serum sodium levels must be evaluated at least every 4 hours during the acute phase of sodium replacement.

In SIADH an infusion of 3% saline (hypertonic saline) may be used to replenish the serum sodium without adding extra volume. It is imperative to be aware that hypertonic saline solution is dangerous if administered too quickly, as described above. Calculation of the quantity of sodium that will be administered each hour, and over 24 hours, is advised.

Medications

Medications are prescribed when water restriction is ineffective in correcting the SIADH. One pharmacologic action is to increase the action of ADH on the V_2 kidney tubule receptors so that more water is excreted.

Vasopressin receptor antagonists. The vasopressin receptor antagonists are used to treat euvolemic hyponatremia such as SIADH. Medications in this class are also described as "vaptans." Conivaptan (Vaprisol) is approved for

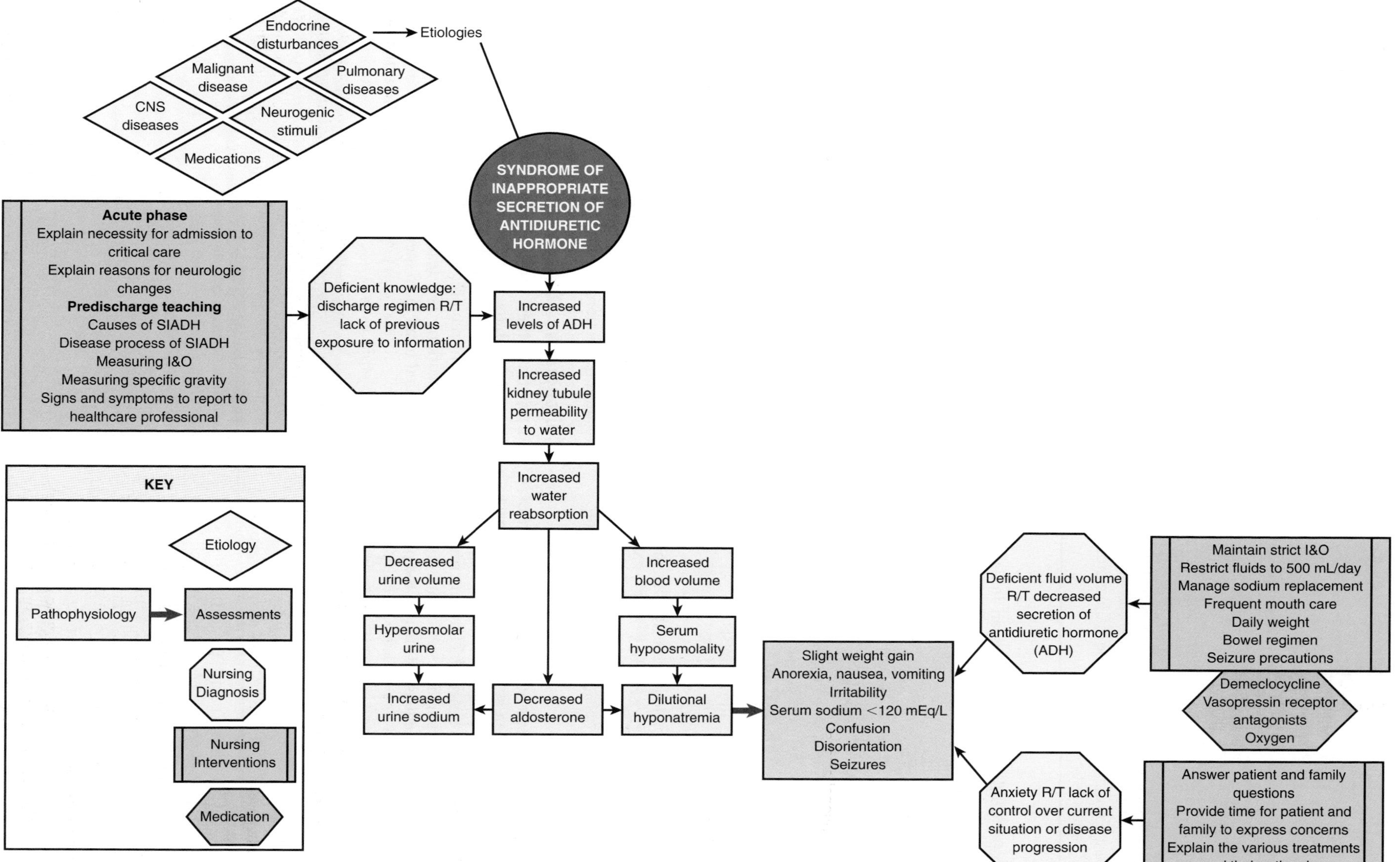

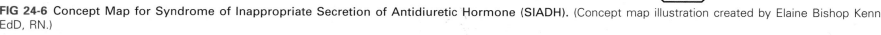

FIG 24-6 Concept Map for Syndrome of Inappropriate Secretion of Antidiuretic Hormone (SIADH). (Concept map illustration created by Elaine Bishop Kennedy, EdD, RN.)

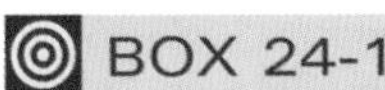

BOX 24-17 NURSING DIAGNOSES: SYNDROME OF INAPPROPRIATE SECRETION OF ANTIDIURETIC HORMONE

- Deficient Fluid Volume related to decreased secretion of antidiuretic hormone (ADH), p. 583
- Anxiety related to threat to biological, psychologic, or social integrity, p. 576
- Deficient Knowledge: Discharge Regimen related to lack of previous exposure to information, p. 585 (see Box 24-18, Patient Education for Syndrome of Inappropriate Secretion of Antidiuretic Hormone)

use only in hospitalized patients. There is an initial 20 mg loading dose IV over 30 minutes, followed by a 20 mg per day continuous infusion for up to 4 days.[33] If the sodium correction is inadequate, the infusion dose can be increased to 40 mg per day.[33] Conivaptan is a nonselective vasopressin receptor antagonist, which means that it blocks V_1 receptors in the vasculature and V_2 receptors in the kidney. The patient must be observed carefully to avoid hypotension (caused by V_1 receptor blockade). Hypovolemia is a contraindication. Tolvaptan (Samsca) is an oral medication in the same class. This mediation should be initiated in the hospital, where serum sodium levels can be monitored to avoid a too-rapid rise in serum sodium following aquadiuresis.

Nursing Management

Nursing management of the patient with SIADH incorporates a variety of nursing diagnoses (Box 24-17). Nursing management is directed toward restriction of fluids, surveillance for complications, and provision of patient education.

Restriction of Fluids

Thorough, astute nursing assessments are required for care of the patient with SIADH while an attempt is made to correct the fluid and sodium imbalance; the systemic effects of hyponatremia occur rapidly and can be lethal. Fluids are restricted to between 800 and 1200 mL per day.[35] Accurate measurement of I&O is required. Frequent assessment of the patient's hydration status is accomplished with serial measurements of urine output, serum sodium levels, and serum osmolality. Frequent mouth care (moistening of the buccal membrane) may give comfort during the period of fluid restriction. The patient is weighed daily to gauge fluid retention or loss. Weight gain signifies continual fluid retention, whereas weight loss indicates loss of body fluid.

BOX 24-18 PATIENT EDUCATION PRIORITIES: SYNDROME OF INAPPROPRIATE SECRETION OF ANTIDIURETIC HORMONE

Acute Phase

- Explain reasons for admission to the critical care unit.
- Explain reasons for neurologic changes.

Predischarge

- Assess knowledge level.
- Causes of inappropriate secretion of antidiuretic hormone (SIADH)
- Disease process of SIADH
- Measuring intake and output
- Measuring urine specific gravity
- Signs and symptoms to report to health care professional

Patient Education

Rapidly occurring changes in the patient's neurologic status may worry visiting family members. Sensitivity to the family's unspoken fears can be shown by words that express empathy and by providing time for the patient and family to ask questions and express their concerns. The nurse may discuss the course of SIADH, its effect on water balance, and the reasons for fluid restrictions (Box 24-18).

Collaborative Management

At this time, there are no published guidelines that discuss acute collaborative care management of the patient with SIADH. This is a complex condition, and effective clinical management requires the skills of many health care professionals working as a team, with goals that are clearly communicated to all team members.

CASE STUDY Patient with an Endocrine Disorder

Brief Patient History

Ms. S is a 72-year-old woman with a history of hypertension treated with an angiotensin-converting enzyme (ACE) inhibitor and thiazide diuretics. She has a past 100-pack/year history of tobacco abuse but quit 2 years ago. Ms. S lives independently in a senior apartment. She was brought to the hospital by friends because of a fall. Ms. S states that she has a severe headache but cannot recall whether she hit her head during the fall. She is also having difficulty recalling recent events.

Clinical Assessment

Ms. S is admitted to the critical care unit from the emergency department because of nonspecific ECG changes suggestive of inferior wall ischemia and electrolyte abnormalities. She is awake; alert; oriented to person, time, place; and unable to recall the events leading to her hospitalization. She states that her headache is severe and feels like someone is hitting her head with a hammer. Her skin is warm and dry. Ms. S's gait is visibly unsteady.

Diagnostic Procedures

Ms. S's vital signs include the following: blood pressure of 180/92 mm Hg, heart rate of 100 beats/min (sinus rhythm), respiratory rate of 24 breaths/min, and temperature of 98.8° F.

Ms. S reports that her headache is a 10 on the Baker-Wong faces scale. Laboratory findings include the following: sodium

CASE STUDY **Patient with an Endocrine Disorder—cont'd**

level of 116 mmol/L, potassium level of 3.3 mmol/L, chloride level of 88 mmol/L, carbon dioxide level of 22 mEq/L, magnesium level of 1.8 mg/dL, urinary sodium level of 30 mmol/L, and urine osmolality value of 118 mOsm/L. The test result for troponin I on admission was negative. ECG testing shows a normal sinus rhythm, T-wave inversion in leads II, III, and AVF, and a change from prior ECG findings, suggestive of inferior wall ischemia. Chest radiography identified a mass in the right upper lobe that strongly suggested a neoplasm.

Medical Diagnosis

Ms. S is diagnosed with syndrome of inappropriate diuretic hormone (SIADH).

Questions

1. What major outcomes do you expect to achieve for this patient?
2. What problems or risks must be managed to achieve these outcomes?
3. What interventions must be initiated to monitor, prevent, manage, or eliminate the problems and risks identified?
4. What interventions should be initiated to promote optimal functioning, safety, and well-being of the patient?
5. What possible learning needs do you anticipate for this patient?
6. What cultural and age-related factors may have a bearing on the patient's plan of care?

REFERENCES

1. Dellinger RP, et al: Surviving Sepsis Campaign: international guidelines for management of severe sepsis and septic shock: 2012, *Crit Care Med* 41(2):580, 2013.
2. Moghissi ES, et al: American Association of Clinical Endocrinologists and American Diabetes Association consensus statement on inpatient glycemic control, *Diabetes Care* 32(6):1119, 2009.
3. Dünser MW, Hasibeder WR: Sympathetic overstimulation during critical illness: adverse effects of adrenergic stress, *J Intensive Care Med* 24(5):293, 2009.
4. Moraes RB, et al: Comparison of low and high dose cosyntropin stimulation tests in the diagnosis of adrenal insufficiency in septic shock patients, *Horm Metab Res* 44(4):296, 2012.
5. Marik PE, et al: Recommendations for the diagnosis and management of corticosteroid insufficiency in critically ill adult patients: consensus statements from an international task force by the American College of Critical Care Medicine, *Crit Care Med* 36(6):1937, 2008.
6. Fahy BG, et al: Glucose control in the intensive care unit, *Crit Care Med* 37(5):1769, 2009.
7. Van den Berghe G, et al: Intensive insulin therapy in critically ill patients, *N Engl J Med* 345(19):1359, 2001.
8. Van den Berghe G, et al: Intensive insulin therapy in the medical ICU, *N Engl J Med* 354(5):449, 2006.
9. Finfer S, et al: Intensive versus conventional glucose control in critically ill patients, *N Engl J Med* 360(13):1283, 2009.
10. Jacobi J, et al: Guidelines for the use of an insulin infusion for the management of hyperglycemia in critically ill patients, *Crit Care Med* 40(12):3251, 2012.
11. McDonnell ME, Umpierrez GE: Insulin therapy for the management of hyperglycemia in hospitalized patients, *Endocrinol Metab Clin North Am* 41(1):175, 2012.
12. Dombrowski NC, Karounos DG: Pathophysiology and management strategies for hyperglycemia for patients with acute illness during and following a hospital stay, *Metabolism* 62(3):326, 2013.
13. Rodbard HW, et al: American Association of Clinical Endocrinologists medical guidelines for clinical practice for the management of diabetes mellitus, *Endocr Pract* 13 (Suppl 1):1, 2007.
14. McCall AL: Insulin therapy and hypoglycemia, *Endocrinol Metab Clin North Am* 241(1):57, 2012.
15. Evert AB, et al: Nutrition Therapy Recommendations for the management of adults with diabetes, *Diabetes Care* 37 (Suppl 1):S120, 2014.
16. American Diabetes Association: Standards of medical care in diabetes–2014, *Diabetes Care* 37(Suppl 1):S14, 2014.
17. American Diabetes Association: Diagnosis and classification of diabetes mellitus, *Diabetes Care* 37 (Suppl 1):S81, 2014.
18. Nathan DM, et al: Medical management of hyperglycemia in type 2 diabetes: a consensus algorithm for the initiation and adjustment of therapy: a consensus statement of the American Diabetes Association and the European Association for the Study of Diabetes, *Diabetes Care* 32(1):193, 2009.
19. Inzucchi SE, et al: Management of hyperglycemia in type 2 diabetes: a patient-centered approach: position statement of the American Diabetes Association (ADA) and the European Association for the Study of Diabetes (EASD), *Diabetes Care* 35(6):1364, 2012.
20. Qaseem A, et al: Oral pharmacologic treatment of type 2 diabetes mellitus: a clinical practice guideline from the American College of Physicians, *Ann Intern Med* 156(3):218, 2012.
21. Nathan DM, et al: Management of hyperglycemia in type 2 diabetes: a consensus algorithm for the initiation and adjustment of therapy: update regarding thiazolidinediones: a consensus statement from the American Diabetes Association and the European Association for the Study of Diabetes, *Diabetes Care* 31(1):173, 2008.
22. Derosa G, Maffioli P: Efficacy and safety profile evaluation of acarbose alone and in association with other antidiabetic drugs: a systematic review, *Clin Ther* 34(6):1221, 2012.
23. Phillips LK, Prins JB: Update on incretin hormones, *Ann N Y Acad Sci* 1243:E55, 2011.
24. Kitabchi AE, et al: Hyperglycemic crises in adult patients with diabetes, *Diabetes Care* 32(7):1335, 2009.
25. Nyenwe EA, Kitabchi AE: Evidence-based management of hyperglycemic emergencies in diabetes mellitus, *Diabetes Res Clin Pract* 94(3):340, 2011.
26. Newton CA, Raskin P: Diabetic ketoacidosis in type 1 and type 2 diabetes mellitus: clinical and biochemical differences, *Arch Intern Med* 164(17):1925, 2004.

27. Hannon MJ, et al: Pituitary dysfunction following traumatic brain injury or subarachnoid haemorrhage, *Best Pract Res Clin Endocrinol Metab* 25(5):783, 2011.
28. Schreckinger M, et al: Diabetes insipidus following resection of pituitary tumors, *Clin Neurol Neurosurg* 115(2):121, 2013.
29. Fenske W, Allolio B: Current state and future perspectives in the diagnosis of diabetes insipidus: a clinical review, *J Clin Endocrinol Metab* 97(10):3426, 2012.
30. Loh JA, Verbalis JG: Disorders of water and salt metabolism associated with pituitary disease, *Endocrinol Metab Clin North Am* 37(1):213, 2008.
31. Devin JK: Hypopituitarism and central diabetes insipidus: perioperative diagnosis and management, *Neurosurg Clin N Am* 23(4):679, 2012.
32. Esposito P, et al: The syndrome of inappropriate antidiuresis: pathophysiology, clinical management and new therapeutic options, *Nephron Clin Pract* 119(1):c62, 2011.
33. Verbalis JG, et al: Hyponatremia treatment guidelines 2007: expert panel recommendations, *Am J Med* 120(11 Suppl 1):S1, 2007.
34. Gilbar PJ, et al: Syndrome of inappropriate antidiuretic hormone secretion induced by a single dose of oral cyclophosphamide, *Ann Pharmacother* 46(9):e23, 2012.
35. Crawford A, Harris H: SIADH: fluid out of balance, *Nursing* 42(9):50, 2012.

CHAPTER 25

Trauma

Mary E. Lough

Be sure to check out the bonus material, including review questions, on the Evolve website at http://evolve.elsevier.com/Urden/priorities/.

Trauma is the leading cause of death for all age groups younger than 44 years. Injury costs the United States hundreds of billions of dollars annually. It is one of the most pressing health issues in the United States today, but continues to go largely unrecognized.

Injury as a result of trauma is no longer considered to be an accident. The term *motor vehicle accident* (MVA) has been replaced with *motor vehicle crash* (MVC), and the term *accident* has been replaced with *unintentional injury.* Unintentional injury is no accident. Accident traditionally has implied an act of God or an unpredictable event. Domestic violence and alcohol-related issues are priority prevention areas with which health care providers must be actively involved.

Intimate partner violence (IPV) constitutes a major public health issue in the United States. IPV is the leading cause of injury to women; in the United States it is estimated that 4.8 million women and 2.9 million men every year are raped or physically assaulted.[1] Up to one-third of injuries from IPV result in medical attention being sought, and 21% of those who present with acute injuries require emergency surgery.[2]

The Joint Commission has a standard of practice that all patients must be screened for IPV as part of the health history. Studies have shown that screening for IPV in health care settings is effective in identifying women who are victims and that patients are not offended when asked about current or past IPV. Key interventions for the victim of IPV are listed in Box 25-1.

In 2010, 10,228 people were killed in alcohol-impaired driving crashes, which account for 31% of the total motor vehicle traffic fatalities in the United States.[3] Each year, alcohol-related crashes in the United States cost about $51 billion.[3] Alcohol screening and intervention are routine components of trauma care. The Alcohol Use Disorders Identification Test (AUDIT) (Table 25-1) is a screening questionnaire that can be used to identify frequency of alcoholic drinking and problem drinking.[4]

Over the past few decades, major advances have been made in the management of patients with traumatic injuries in the prehospital, emergency department, and critical care settings. Patients with complex, multisystem trauma are admitted to critical care units, and these patients require complex nursing care. This chapter reviews nursing management of patients with traumatic injuries in the critical care setting.

MECHANISMS OF INJURY

Trauma occurs when an external force of energy impacts the body and causes structural or physiologic alterations, or *injuries.* External forces can be radiation, electrical, thermal, chemical, or mechanical forms of energy. This chapter focuses on trauma from mechanical energy. Mechanical energy can produce blunt or penetrating traumatic injuries. Understanding the mechanism of injury helps health care providers anticipate and predict potential internal injuries.

Blunt Trauma

Blunt trauma is seen most often with MVCs, contact sports, blunt force injuries (e.g., trauma caused by a baseball bat), or falls. Injuries occur because of the forces sustained during a rapid change in velocity (deceleration). To estimate the amount of force sustained in an MVC, multiply the person's weight by the miles per hour (speed) the vehicle was traveling. A 130-pound woman in a vehicle traveling at 60 miles per hour that hits a brick wall, for example, would sustain 7800 pounds of force within milliseconds. As the body stops suddenly, tissues and organs continue to move forward. This sudden change in velocity causes injuries that result in lacerations or crush injuries of internal body structures.

Penetrating Trauma

Penetrating injuries occur with stabbings, firearms, or impalement—injuries that penetrate the skin and result in damage to internal structures. Damage is created along the path of penetration. Penetrating injuries can be misleading inasmuch as the condition of the outside of the wound does not determine the extent of internal injury. Bullets can create internal cavities 5 to 30 times larger than the diameter of the bullet.[5]

BOX 25-1 Interventions with Victims of Intimate Partner Violence

Provide Validation
- Listen non-judgmentally
- "I am concerned for your safety (and the safety of your children)."
- "You are not alone and help is available."
- "You don't deserve the abuse and it is not your fault."
- "Stopping the abuse is the responsibility of your partner not you."

Provide Information
- "Domestic violence is common and happens in all kinds of relationships."
- "Violence tends to continue and often becomes more frequent and severe."
- "Abuse can impact your health in many ways."
- "You are not to blame, but exposure to violence in the home can emotionally and physically hurt your children or other dependent loved ones."

Respond to Safety Issues
- Offer a brochure about safety planning and explain contents to the patient.

From *Futures without Violence* (formerly The Family Violence Prevention Fund). National consensus guidelines on identifying and responding to domestic violence victimization in healthcare settings. http://www.futureswithoutviolence.org/userfiles/file/Consensus.pdf Accessed August 17, 2014.

Several factors determine the extent of damage sustained as a result of penetrating trauma. Different weapons cause different types of injuries. The severity of a gunshot wound depends on the type of gun, type of ammunition used, and the distance and angle from which the gun was fired. Pellets from a shotgun blast expand on impact and cause multiple injuries to internal structures. Handgun bullets usually damage what is directly in the bullet's path. Inside the body, the bullet can ricochet off bone and create further damage along its pathway. With penetrating stab wounds, factors that determine the extent of injury include the type and length of object used and the angle of insertion.

PHASES OF TRAUMA CARE

Care of trauma victims during wartime enhanced principles of triage and rapid transport of the injured to medical facilities. The military experience has demonstrated that decreasing the time from injury to definitive care can save more lives. It also has enhanced incentives and models for improvements in civilian trauma care, such as emergency medical service (EMS) systems and trauma care centers. The goal with critically injured patients is to minimize the time from initial insult to definitive care and to optimize prehospital care so that the patient arrives at the hospital alive. Care of the seriously injured trauma patient is a continuum that includes six phases: prehospital resuscitation, hospital resuscitation, definitive care and operative phase, critical care, intermediate care, and rehabilitation.

TABLE 25-1 Audit Alcohol Screening Questionnaire

QUESTION	SCORE*
How often do you have a drink containing alcohol?	Never Monthly or less 2-4 times per month 2-3 times per week 4 or more times per week
How many standard drinks containing alcohol do you have on a typical day when drinking?	1 or 2 3 or 4 5 or 6 7 to 9 10 or more
How often do you have six or more drinks on one occasion?	
During the past year, how often have you found that you were not able to stop drinking once you had started?	Never
During the past year, how often have you failed to do what was normally expected of you because of drinking?	Less than monthly Monthly
During the past year, how often have you needed a drink in the morning to get yourself going after a heavy drinking session?	Weekly Daily or almost daily
During the past year, how often have you had a feeling of guilt or remorse after drinking?	
During the past year, have you been unable to remember what happened the night before because you had been drinking?	
Have you or someone else been injured as a result of your drinking?	No
Has a relative or friend, doctor or other health worker been concerned about your drinking or suggested you cut down?	Yes, but not in the past year Yes, during the past year

*Scores for each question range from 0 to 4, with the first response for each question (never) scoring 0, the second (less than monthly) scoring 1, the third (monthly) scoring 2, the fourth (weekly) scoring 3, and the fifth response (daily or almost daily) scoring 4. For the last two questions, which only have three responses, the scoring is 0, 2, and 4. A score of 8 or more is associated with harmful or hazardous drinking, and a score of 13 or more by women or 15 or more by men is likely to indicate alcohol dependence.
AUDIT, Alcohol Use Disorders Identification Test.

Prehospital Resuscitation

The golden hour of trauma care is a 60-minute time frame that incorporates activation of the EMS system, stabilization in the prehospital setting, transportation to a medical facility, rapid resuscitation on arrival in the emergency department, and provision of definitive care. The goal of prehospital care is immediate stabilization and transportation. This is achieved through airway maintenance, control of external bleeding and shock, immobilization of the patient, and immediate transport (ground or air) to the closest appropriate medical facility.[5] Prehospital personnel should communicate information needed for triage at the hospital. Advanced planning for the injured patient is essential.

Emergency Department Resuscitation

The American College of Surgeons developed guidelines named *Advanced Trauma Life Support* (ATLS) for rapid assessment, resuscitation, and definitive care for trauma patients in the emergency department.[5] The Emergency Nurses Association (ENA) have similar guidelines which are taught in the Trauma Nursing Core Course (TNCC).[6] These guidelines delineate a systematic approach to care of the trauma patient: rapid primary survey, resuscitation of vital functions, more detailed secondary survey, and initiation of definitive care. This process constitutes the ABCDEs of trauma care and assists in identifying injuries.[5,6]

Primary Survey

On arrival of the trauma patient in the emergency department, the primary survey is initiated.[5,6] During this assessment, life-threatening injuries are discovered and treated. The five steps in the trauma primary survey are performed in ABCDE sequence (Table 25-2):

A Airway and Alertness with cervical spine protection
B Breathing and ventilation
C Circulation with hemorrhage control
D Disability: neurologic status, use the the Glasgow Coma Scale
E Exposure and environmental control

Resuscitation Phase

After the primary survey, the resuscitation phase begins. Hypovolemic shock is the most common type of shock that occurs in trauma patients.[5] Hemorrhage must be identified and treated rapidly. Two large-bore (14- to 16-gauge) peripheral intravenous catheters, an intraosseous catheter, may be inserted.[5,6] Central venous catheters are not normally inserted at this stage because of patient acuity and time constraints. During the initiation of intravenous lines, blood samples are drawn (Box 25-2).

Resuscitation is aimed at ensuring adequate perfusion of tissues with oxygen, using volume (blood or crystalloid) to support cellular function. Resuscitation end point parameters must be viewed across the continuum of resuscitation from shock. During resuscitation from traumatic hemorrhagic shock, normalization of vital signs such as blood pressure, heart rate, and urine output are important but are not the only monitoring tools used. Trending of base deficit and serum lactate are essential to determine adequacy of cellular oxygenation during trauma resuscitation.[7] Normalization of base deficit and serum lactate, in conjunction with normalized vital signs, are used as resuscitation end-point targets.[7] The fluid resuscitation strategy begins in the field and continues through the emergency department, operating rooms, and critical care units.

Massive transfusion protocols. Given the emphasis on use of blood products over crystalloids and correction of traumatic coagulopathy, many trauma centers have developed massive transfusion protocols for the 1% to 3% of all trauma patients who require massive transfusion in traumatic shock.[8] Having a defined protocol serves as a system-based strategy to facilitate early, timely release of blood products in what can often be a chaotic situation. The institution-specific massive transfusion protocol outlines the ratio of packed red blood cells, fresh frozen plasma, platelets, and cryoprecipitate to be administered.[8]

BOX 25-2 Blood Samples to Obtain with Intravenous Placement

- Complete blood cell (CBC) count.
- Electrolyte profile (Na^+, K^+, Cl^-, CO_2, glucose, blood urea nitrogen [BUN], creatinine [Cr])
- Coagulation parameters: prothrombin time (PT); partial thromboplastin time (PTT)
- Type and screen (ABO compatibility)
- Amylase
- Toxicology screens
- Liver function studies
- Pregnancy test (for females of childbearing age)
- Lactate

Secondary Survey

The secondary survey begins when the primary survey is completed, resuscitation is well- established, and vital signs are normalizing. During the secondary survey, a head-to-toe approach is used to examine each body region thoroughly. The secondary survey is also categorized alphabetically; this helps with consistency and ensures a systematic process to identify any evolving injuries[6]:

F Full set of vital signs and facilitate family presence
G Get resuscitation adjuncts (listed under L, M, N, O, P below)
  L Laboratory studies, including blood type and cross-match
  M Monitor (apply ECG leads) for continuous rate and rhythm assessment
  N Naso- or oro-gastric tube consideration
  O Oxygenation and ventilation assessment
  P Pain (assessment and pharmacologic and non-pharmacologic interventions)
H History (defer until after "L" while resuscitation interventions are ongoing)

The history (**H** in the secondary survey) is an important aspect of the secondary survey. Often, head injury, shock, or the use of drugs or alcohol may preclude a good history, so the history must be pieced together from other sources. The prehospital providers (paramedics, emergency medical technicians) usually can provide most of the vital information pertaining to the *unintentional injury.* Specific information that must be elicited pertaining to the mechanism of injury is summarized in Box 25-3. This information can help predict

TABLE 25-2 Primary Survey of the Trauma Patient

SURVEY COMPONENT	NURSING ASSESSMENT, CARE
Airway	Immobilize cervical spine. Look: • Is there obvious airway trauma, tachypnea, accessory muscle use, tracheal shift? Listen: • Stridor, hyperresonance, dullness to percussion? Feel: • For air exchange over the mouth; insert finger sweep to clear foreign bodies. Secure airway: • Oropharyngeal • Nasopharyngeal • Endotracheal tube • Cricothyrotomy
Alertness	Use the mnemonic: AVPU A Alert and responsive V Responds to verbal stimulation P Responds only to painful stimulation U Unresponsive
Breathing	Assess for: • Spontaneous breathing • Respiratory rate, depth, symmetry • Chest wall integrity For absent breathing: • Intubate, mechanical ventilation If breathing but ineffective: • Assess life-threatening conditions (e.g., tension pneumothorax, flail chest). • Administer supplemental oxygen. • Initiate pulse oximetry.
Circulation	Assess pulse quality and rate. Use ECG monitoring. If no pulse: • Initiate ACLS. If pulse but ineffective: • Assess and treat life-threatening conditions (uncontrolled bleeding, shock). Initiate two large-bore IVs or central catheter; obtain serum samples for laboratory tests. Provide fluid replacement. **Control of Hemorrhage is Essential and Paramount**
Disability	Determine Glasgow Coma Scale score. Assess pupil size and reactivity.
Exposure and environmental control	Remove all clothing to inspect all body regions. Prevent hypothermia.

ACLS, Advanced cardiac life support; *ECG*, electrocardiogram; *IV*, intravenous line.

internal injuries and facilitate rapid intervention. The patient's pertinent past history can be assessed by use of the mnemonic AMPLE:

*A*llergies,
*M*edications currently used,
*P*ast medical illnesses/pregnancy,
*L*ast meal, and
*E*vents/environment related to the injury.

During the secondary survey the nurse ensures the completion of special procedures, such as an ECG, radiographic studies (chest, cervical spine, thorax, and pelvis), and ultrasonography. Throughout this survey the nurse continuously monitors the patient's vital signs and response to medical therapies. Emotional support to the patient and family is also imperative.

Definitive Care and Operative Phase

After the secondary survey has been completed, specific injuries usually have been diagnosed. Definitive care related to specific injuries is described throughout this chapter. Trauma is sometimes referred to as a "surgical disease" because the nature and extent of injuries usually requires operative management. After surgery, depending on the patient's status, transfer to the critical care unit may be indicated.

Critical Care Phase

Critically ill trauma patients are admitted into the critical care unit as direct transfers from the emergency department or operating room. Information the nurse must obtain from the emergency department or operating room nurse, or both, is summarized using the **SBAR** method: **S**ituation, **B**ackground,

BOX 25-3 History of Mechanism of Injury

Penetrating Trauma
- Weapon used (handgun, shotgun, rifle, knife)
- Caliber of weapon
- Number of shots fired
- Gender of assailant
- Position of victim and assailant when injury occurred

Blunt Trauma
- Height of fall
- Motor vehicle crash extrication time
- Ejection
- Steering wheel deformation
- Location in automobile (passenger, driver, front seat, back seat)
- Restraint status (lap belt, shoulder harness, or combination; unrestrained)
- Speed of automobiles, direction of impact
- Occupants (number and morbidity status)

Assessment, and Recommendations (Box 25-4). This information must be obtained before the patient's admission to the critical care unit to ensure availability of needed personnel, equipment, and supplies. This information also helps the nurse to assess the impact of trauma resuscitation on the patient's presentation and course. Table 25-3 summarizes the prehospital, emergency department, and operating room resuscitative measures that can affect the trauma patient's care.

After the patient's arrival in the critical care unit, the nurse uses the primary and secondary surveys and resuscitative measures in accordance with ATLS/TNCC guidelines to assess the trauma patient's status. Priority nursing care during the critical care phase includes ongoing physical assessments and monitoring the patient's response to medical therapies. The nurse constantly is aware that the third peak of the trimodal distribution of trauma deaths occurs in the critical care setting as a result of complications, including acute respiratory distress syndrome (ARDS), sepsis, prolonged shock states, and MODS. Ongoing nursing assessments are imperative for early detection and treatment of complications.

One of the most important nursing roles is assessment of the balance between oxygen delivery and oxygen demand. Oxygen delivery must be optimized to prevent further system damage. The trauma patient is at high risk for impaired oxygenation as a result of a variety of factors (Table 25-4). Risk factors must be promptly identified and treated to prevent life-threatening sequelae. Prevention and treatment of hypoxemia depend on accurate assessment of the adequacy of pulmonary gas exchange, oxygen delivery, and oxygen consumption.

SPECIFIC TRAUMA INJURIES

Traumatic Brain Injuries

In 2010 more than 2.5 million traumatic brain injuries (TBIs) occurred annually either as an isolated injury or in combination with other injuries.[9]

BOX 25-4 Nursing Report from a Referring Area Using the SBAR Method

S: Situation	Age Gender Mechanism of injury/injuries sustained Admission diagnosis/chief complaint; any loss of consciousness and its duration with current Glasgow Coma Scale score Diagnostic tests and procedures completed Diagnostic test results and laboratory results Medications administered (opiates, sedatives) Current issues, including derangements in any physical assessments requiring acute interventions
B: Background	Significant medical and surgical history Home medications
A: Assessments	Current assessment findings, including vital signs, level of consciousness, established airway, and mechanical ventilation settings Family members present and their assessment of coping and current knowledge of nature and extent of injuries and treatment plan
R: Recommendations	Description of the plan, including fluid volume and blood products

Mechanism of Injury

TBIs occur when mechanical forces are transmitted to brain tissue. Mechanisms of injury include penetrating or blunt trauma to the head. The leading causes of TBI include falls, MVCs, being struck by or against objects, and assaults. Penetrating trauma can result from the penetration of a foreign object such as a bullet, which causes direct damage to cerebral tissue. Blunt trauma can be the result of deceleration, acceleration, or rotational forces. *Deceleration injury* causes the brain to crash against the skull after it has hit a hard surface such as the dashboard of a car. *Acceleration injury* occurs when the brain has been forcefully hit, such as with a baseball bat. In many instances, TBIs can be caused by acceleration and deceleration. Acceleration injuries occur when the skull is hit by a force that causes the brain to move forward toward the point of impact. Then as the brain reverses direction, the brain hits the other side of the skull, and deceleration injuries occur. This is described as a coup–contrecoup injury (Figure 25-1).

Pathophysiology

Review of the pathophysiology of a TBI can be divided into two categories: primary injury and secondary injury. The critical care nurse must understand this pathophysiology because goals of care focus on reducing morbidity and mortality from primary and secondary injuries.

Primary injury. The primary injury occurs at the moment of impact as a result of mechanical forces to the head. The extent of and recovery from injury are related to whether the primary injury was localized to an area or whether it was diffuse (widespread) throughout the brain. Primary injuries may include direct damage to the parenchyma or as injury to the vessels that causes hemorrhage, compressing nearby structures. Examples of primary injuries include contusion, laceration, shearing injuries, and hemorrhage. The primary injury may be mild, with little or no neurologic damage, or severe, with major tissue damage. Immediately

TABLE 25-3 Trauma Resuscitation Impact on Critical Care Management

ASPECT OF INJURY OR RESUSCITATION	IMPACT ON CRITICAL CARE MANAGEMENT
Prolonged extrication time	Gives an indication of length of time patient may have been hypotensive and/or hypothermic before medical care
Period of respiratory or cardiac arrest	Effects of loss of perfusion to brain (anoxic injury), kidneys, and other vital organs
Time on backboard	Potentiates risk of sacral or occipital breakdown
Number of units of blood; whether any were not fully cross-matched; packed cells versus whole blood used	Potentiates risk of ARDS, MODS

ARDS, Acute respiratory distress syndrome; *MODS*, multiple organ dysfunction syndrome.

TABLE 25-4 Factors Predisposing the Trauma Patient to Impaired Oxygenation

FACTOR	IMPAIRMENT
Impaired ventilation	Injury to airway structures, loss of central nervous system regulation of breathing, impaired level of consciousness
Impaired pulmonary gas diffusion	Pneumothorax, hemothorax, aspiration of gastric contents
	Shifts to the left of the oxyhemoglobin dissociation curve (can result from infusion of large volumes of banked blood, hypocarbia or alkalosis, or hypothermia)
Decreased oxygen supply	Reduced hemoglobin (from hemorrhage)
	Reduced cardiac output (cardiovascular injury, decreased preload)
Increased oxygen supply	Increased metabolic demands (associated with the stress response to injury)

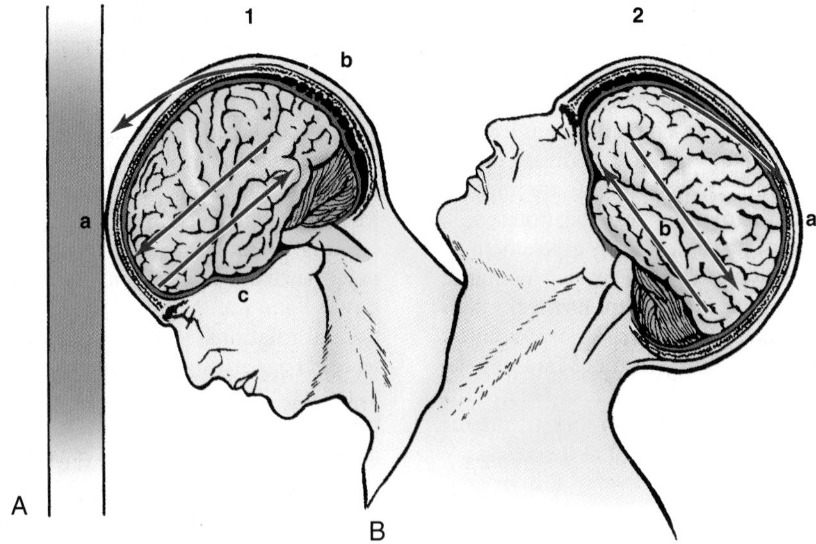

FIG 25-1 **Coup and Contrecoup Head Injury After Blunt Trauma.** *A*, Coup injury: impact against object, showing the site of impact and direct trauma to brain *(a)*, shearing of subdural veins *(b)*, and trauma to the base of the brain *(c)*. *B*, Contrecoup injury: impact within skull, showing the site of impact from brain hitting opposite side of skull *(a)* and shearing forces throughout brain *(b)*. These injuries occur in one continuous motion; the head strikes the wall (coup) and then rebounds (contrecoup).

after the injury, a cascade of neural and vascular processes is activated.

Secondary injury. Secondary injury is the biochemical and cellular response to the initial trauma that can exacerbate the primary injury and cause loss of brain tissue not originally damaged. Secondary injury can be caused by ischemia, hypercapnia, hypotension, cerebral edema, sustained hypertension, calcium toxicity, or metabolic derangements. Hypoxia or hypotension, the best known culprits for secondary injury, typically are the result of extracranial trauma.[10] A self-perpetuating cycle develops that may cause the expansion of a relatively focal primary injury as a result of uncontrolled refractory secondary injury.[10]

Tissue ischemia. Tissue ischemia occurs in areas of poor cerebral perfusion as a result of hypotension or hypoxia. The cells in ischemic areas become edematous. Extreme vasodilation of the cerebral vasculature occurs in an attempt to supply oxygen to the cerebral tissue. This increase in blood volume increases intracranial volume and raises intracranial pressure (ICP).

Hypotension. Even a single episode of hypotension (systolic BP below 90 mm Hg) is associated with a worsened neurologic outcome, because hypotension results in inadequate perfusion to brain tissue. Hypotension typically is not caused by brain injury unless terminal brain stem failure of the medulla oblongata occurs. If a trauma patient is unconscious and hypotensive, a detailed assessment of the chest, abdomen, and pelvis is performed to rule out internal injuries.

Hypercapnia. Hypercapnia is a powerful vasodilator of cerebral vessels. Most often caused by hypoventilation in an unconscious patient, hypercapnia results in cerebral vasodilation, increased cerebral blood volume, and raised ICP.

Brain edema. Cerebral edema occurs as a result of the changes in the cellular environment caused by contusion, loss of autoregulation, and increased permeability of the blood–brain barrier. Cerebral edema can be focal, as it localizes around the area of contusion, or diffuse, as a result of hypotension or hypoxia. The extent of cerebral edema can be minimized by optimiziing other factors that may potentiate secondary injury, including oxygenation, ventilation, and perfusion.

Initial hypertension in the patient with severe TBI is common. As a result of the loss of autoregulation, increased blood pressure results in increased intracranial blood volume and elevates ICP. Every effort must be made to control hypertension to prevent the secondary injury caused by increased ICP (see "Intracranial Pressure Monitoring" in Chapter 17 and "Intracranial Hypertension" in Chapter 18). The effects of increased ICP are varied. As pressure increases inside the closed skull vault, cerebral perfusion decreases, which further compromises the brain. The combined effects of increasing pressure and decreasing perfusion precipitate a downward spiral of events.

Classification of Brain Injuries

Injuries of the brain are described by the functional changes or losses that occur. Some of the major functional abnormalities seen in head injury are described here.

Skull fracture. Skull fractures are common, but they do not by themselves cause neurologic deficits. Skull fractures can be classified as open (dura is torn) or closed (dura is not torn), or they can be classified as those of the vault or those of the base. Common vault fractures occur in the parietal and temporal regions. Basilar skull fractures usually are not visible on conventional skull films, and a computed tomography (CT) scan is required. Assessment findings may include cerebrospinal fluid (CSF) loss—described as rhinorrhea (from nose) or otorrhea (from ear), Battle sign (ecchymosis overlying the mastoid process behind the ear), "raccoon eyes" (subconjunctival and periorbital ecchymosis), or palsy of the seventh cranial nerve.

The significance of a skull fracture is that it identifies the patient with a higher probability of having or developing an intracranial hematoma. Open skull fractures require surgical intervention to remove bony fragments and to close the dura. The major complications of basilar skull fractures are cranial nerve injury and leakage of CSF. The leakage of CSF may result in a fistula, which increases the possibility of bacterial contamination and resultant meningitis. Because fistula formation may be delayed, patients with a basilar skull fracture are admitted to the hospital for observation and possible surgical intervention.

Concussion. A concussion is a brain injury accompanied by a brief loss of neurologic function, especially loss of consciousness. When loss of consciousness occurs, it may last for seconds to an hour. The neurologic dysfunctions include confusion, disorientation, and sometimes a period of antegrade or retrograde amnesia. Other clinical manifestations that occur after concussion are headache, dizziness, nausea, irritability, inability to concentrate, impaired memory, and fatigue. The diagnosis of concussion is based on the loss of consciousness inasmuch as the brain remains structurally intact despite functional impairment. There is increased awareness of long-term risk of concussion and of the need to protect the brain following a concussion during sports activities.[11]

Contusion. Contusion, or "bruising" of the brain, usually is related to acceleration–deceleration injuries, which result in hemorrhage into the superficial parenchyma. Frontal or temporal lobe contusions are most common and can be seen in a coup–contrecoup mechanism of injury (Figure 25-1). Coup injury affects the cerebral tissue directly under the point of impact. Contrecoup injury occurs in a line directly opposite the point of impact.

The clinical manifestations of contusion are related to the location of the contusion, the degree of contusion, and the presence of associated lesions. Contusions can be small, in which localized areas of dysfunction result in a focal neurologic deficit. Larger contusions can evolve over 2 to 3 days after injury as a result of edema and further hemorrhaging. A large contusion can produce a mass effect that can cause a significant increase in ICP. Contusions (parenchymal injury) are almost always associated with subdural hematoma (SDH).[5]

Contusions of the tips of the temporal lobe are a common occurrence and are of particular concern. Because the inner aspects of the temporal lobe surround the opening in the tentorium where the midbrain enters the cerebrum, edema in this area can cause rapid deterioration in level of consciousness and can lead to herniation. Because of the location, this deterioration can occur with little or no warning at a deceptively low ICP.

Diagnosis of brain contusion is made by CT scan. If the CT indicates contusion, especially in the temporal area, the nurse must pay specific attention to neurologic assessments and look for subtle changes in pupillary signs or vital signs, in spite of a stable ICP.

Management of cerebral contusions may consist of medical or surgical therapies. Because a contusion can progress over 3 to 5 days after injury, secondary injury may occur. If contusions are small, focal, or multiple, they are treated medically with serial neurologic assessments and possibly with ICP monitoring. Larger contusions that produce considerable mass effect require surgical intervention to prevent the increased edema and elevations in ICP as the contusion matures. Outcome of cerebral contusion varies, depending on the location and the size of the contused area.

Cerebral hematomas. Extravasation of blood creates a space-occupying lesion within the cranial vault that can lead to increased ICP. Three types of hematomas are discussed here (Figure 25-2). The first two, epidural and SDH, are extraparenchymal (outside of brain tissue) and produce injury by pressure effect and displacement of intracranial contents. The third type, intracerebral hematoma, directly damages neural tissue and can produce further injury as a result of pressure and displacement of intracranial contents.

Epidural hematoma. Epidural hematoma (EDH) is a collection of blood between the inner skull and the outermost layer of the dura (Figure 25-2A). EDHs are most often associated with patients with skull fractures and middle meningeal artery lacerations.[5] A blow to the head that causes a linear skull fracture on the lateral surface of the head may tear the middle meningeal artery. As the artery bleeds, it pulls the dura away from the skull, creating a pouch that expands into the intracranial space.

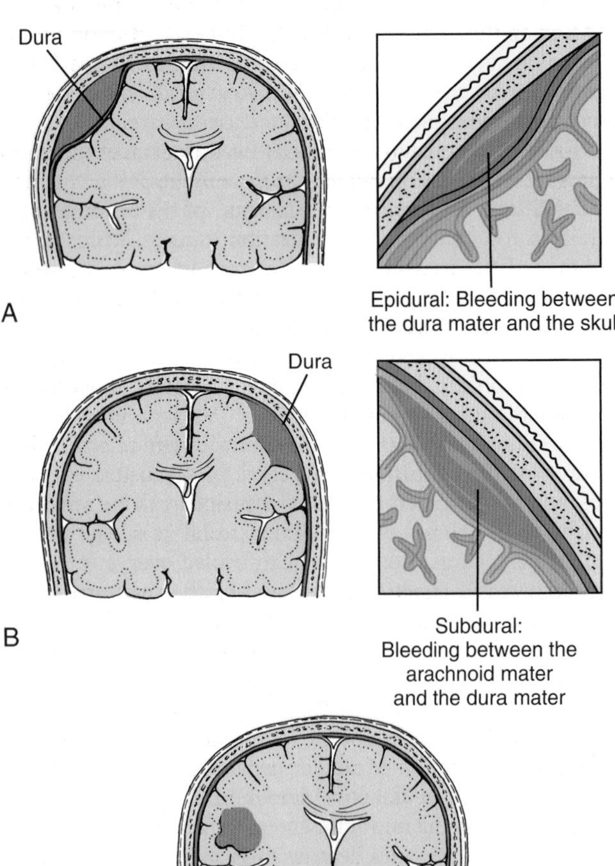

FIG 25-2 Types of Hematomas. *A*, Epidural hematoma. *B*, Subdural hematoma. *C*, Intracerebral hematoma.

The incidence of EDH is relatively low. EDH can occur as a result of low-impact injuries (e.g., falls) or high-impact injuries (e.g., MVCs). EDH occurs from trauma to the skull and meninges, rather than from the acceleration–deceleration forces seen in other types of head trauma.

The classic clinical manifestations of EDH with concussion, include brief loss of consciousness followed by a period of lucidity. Rapid deterioration in the level of consciousness should be anticipated because arterial bleeding into the epidural space can occur quickly. A dilated and fixed pupil on the same side as the impact area is a hallmark of EDH. The patient may complain of a severe, localized headache and may be sleepy. Diagnosis of EDH is based on clinical symptoms and evidence of a collection of epidural blood identified on the CT scan. Treatment of EDH requires surgical intervention to remove the blood and to cauterize the bleeding vessels.

Sub-arachnoid hemorrhage. Traumatic sub-arachnoid hemorrhage can occur after blunt head trauma. Significant amounts of blood may be released into the sub-arachnoid space, between the arachnoid and pia membranes. The blood will circulate with the cerebral spinal fluid (CSF) and causes significant irritation to the cerebral arteries. This results in cerebral vasospasm causing the brain tissue to become ischemic.

Subdural hematoma. Subdural hematoma (SDH), which is the accumulation of blood between the dura and underlying arachnoid membrane, most often is related to a rupture in the bridging veins between the cerebral cortex and the dura (Figure 25-2B). Acceleration–deceleration and rotational forces are the major causes of SDH, which often is associated with cerebral contusions and intracerebral hemorrhage. SDH is common, representing about 30% of severe head injuries. The three types of SDH—acute, subacute, and chronic—are based on the timeframe from injury to clinical symptoms.

Acute subdural hematoma. Acute SDHs are hematomas that occur after a severe blow to the head. The clinical presentation of acute SDH is determined by the severity of injury to the underlying brain at the time of impact and the rate of blood accumulation in the subdural space. In other situations, the patient has a lucid period before deterioration. Careful observation for deterioration of the level of consciousness or lateralizing signs, such as inequality of pupils or motor movements, is essential. Rapid surgical intervention, including *craniectomy* (where bone is removed to accommodate brain swelling following a TBI), *craniotomy* (bone removed only during surgery) or burr hole evacuation, and aggressive medical management can reduce mortality.

Subacute subdural hematoma. Subacute SDHs are hematomas that develop symptomatically 2 days to 2 weeks after trauma. In subacute SDHs, the expansion of the hematoma occurs at a rate slower than that in acute SDH, and it takes longer for symptoms to become obvious. Clinical deterioration of the patient with a subacute SDH usually is slower than with an acute SDH, but treatment by surgical intervention, when appropriate, is the same.

Chronic subdural hematoma. Chronic SDH is diagnosed when symptoms appear days or months after injury. Most

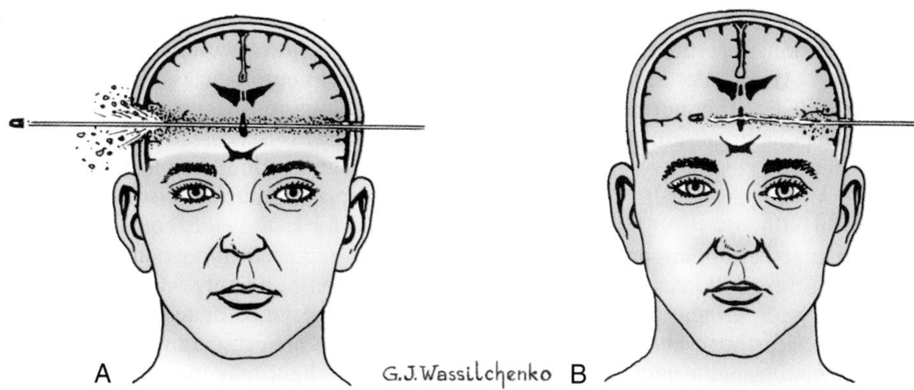

FIG 25-3 **Bullet Wounds of the Head.** A bullet wound or other penetrating missile wounds cause an open (compound) skull fracture and damage to brain tissue. Shock wave effects are transmitted throughout the brain. *A*, Perforating injury. *B*, Penetrating injury.

patients with chronic SDH usually are in late middle age or older adults. Individuals at risk for chronic SDH include those with coordination or balance disturbances and those receiving anticoagulation therapy. Clinical manifestations of chronic SDH are insidious. The patient may report a variety of symptoms such as lethargy, absent-mindedness, headache, vomiting, stiff neck, and photophobia and may show signs of transient ischemic attack, seizures, pupillary changes, or hemiparesis. Because a history of trauma often is not significant enough to be recalled, chronic SDH seldom is seen as an initial diagnosis. CT evaluation can confirm the diagnosis of chronic SDH.

If surgical intervention is required, evacuation of the chronic SDH may occur by craniotomy, burr holes, or catheter drainage. Evacuation by burr hole involves drilling a hole in the skull over the site of the chronic SDH and draining the fluid. Drains or catheters are left in place for at least 24 hours to facilitate total drainage. Outcome after chronic SDH evacuation varies. Return of neurologic status often depends on the degree of neurologic dysfunction before removal. Because this condition is most common in the older or debilitated patient, recovery is a slow process. Recurrence of chronic SDH is not infrequent.

Intracerebral hematoma. Intracerebral hematoma (ICH) results when bleeding occurs within cerebral tissue. Traumatic causes of ICH include depressed skull fractures, penetrating injuries (bullet, knife), or sudden acceleration–deceleration motion. The ICH can act as a rapidly expanding lesion; however, late ICH into the necrotic center of a contused area also is possible (Figure 25-2C). Sudden clinical deterioration of a patient 6 to 10 days after trauma may be the result of ICH.

Medical management of ICH may include surgical or nonsurgical management. It is thought that hemorrhages that do not cause a significant rise in ICP should be treated without surgery. Over time, the hemorrhage may be reabsorbed. If significant problems with elevated ICP occur as a result of the ICH producing a mass effect, surgical removal is necessary. The outcome of a patient with an ICH depends greatly on the location of the hemorrhage. Size, mass effect, and displacement of other intracranial structures also affect the outcome.

Missile injuries. Missile injuries are caused by objects that penetrate the skull and produce a significant focal damage but little acceleration–deceleration or rotational injury. The injury may be depressed, penetrating, or perforating (Figure 25-3). Depressed injuries are caused by fractures of the skull, with penetration of bone into cerebral tissue. Penetrating injury is described as a missile that enters the cranial cavity but does not exit. A low-velocity penetrating injury (knife) may involve only focal damage and no loss of consciousness. A high-velocity missile (bullet) can produce shock waves that are transmitted throughout the brain in addition to the injury caused by the bullet. Perforating injuries are missile injuries that enter and then exit the brain. Perforating injuries have much less ricochet effect but are still responsible for significant injury.

Risk of infection and cerebral abscess is a concern in cases of missile injuries. If fragments of the missile are embedded within the brain, careful consideration of the location and risk of increasing neurologic deficit is weighed against the risk of abscess or infection. The outcome after missile injury is based on the degree of penetration, the location of the injury, and the velocity of the missile.

Diffuse axonal injury. Diffuse axonal injury (DAI) is a term used to describe prolonged posttraumatic coma that is not caused by a mass lesion, although DAI with mass lesions has been reported. DAI covers a wide range of brain dysfunction typically caused by acceleration–deceleration and rotational forces. DAI occurs as a result of damage to the axons or disruption of axonal transmission of the neural impulses.

The pathophysiology of DAI is related to the stretching and tearing of axons as a result of movement of the brain inside the cranium at the time of impact. The stretching and tearing of axons result in microscopic lesions throughout the brain, but especially deep within cerebral tissue and the base of the cerebrum. Disruption of axonal transmission of impulses results in loss of consciousness. Unless surrounding tissue areas are significantly injured, causing small hemorrhages, DAI may not be visible on CT or magnetic resonance imaging (MRI). DAI can be classified as one of three grades based on the extent of lesions: mild, moderate, or severe. The patient with mild DAI may be in a coma for 24 hours and may exhibit periods of decorticate and decerebrate posturing. Patients with moderate DAI may be in a coma for longer than 24 hours and exhibit periods of decorticate and decerebrate posturing. Severe DAI usually manifests as a prolonged, deep coma with periods of hypertension, hyperthermia, and excessive sweating. Treatment of DAI includes support of vital functions and maintenance of ICP within normal limits. The outcome after severe DAI is poor because of the extensive dysfunction of cerebral pathways.

Neurologic Assessment of Traumatic Brain Injury

The neurologic assessment is the most important tool for evaluating the patient with a severe TBI because it can indicate the severity of injury, provide prognostic information, and dictate the speed with which further evaluation and treatment must proceed. The cornerstone of the neurologic assessment is the Glasgow Coma Scale (GCS) as described in chapter 17 (Table 17-1). The GCS is not a complete neurologic examination. Pupils and motor strength assessment must be incorporated into the early and ongoing assessments. After injuries are specifically identified, a more thorough, focused neurologic assessment, such as examination of the cranial nerves, is warranted. To assist with the initial assessment, TBIs are divided into three descriptive categories—mild, moderate, or severe—on the basis of the patient's GCS score and duration of the unconscious state.

Degree of injury

Mild brain injury. Mild TBI is described as a GCS score of 13 to 15, with a loss of consciousness that lasts up to 15 minutes. Patients with mild injury often are seen in the emergency department and discharged home with a family member who is instructed to evaluate the patient routinely and to bring the patient back to the hospital if any further neurologic symptoms appear.

Moderate brain injury. Moderate TBI is described as a GCS score of 9 to 12, with a loss of consciousness for up to 6 hours. Patients with this type of TBI usually are hospitalized. They are at high risk for deterioration from increasing cerebral edema and ICP, and serial clinical assessments are important. Hemodynamic and ICP monitoring and ventilatory support may not be required for these patients unless other systemic injuries make them necessary. A CT scan usually is obtained on admission. Repeat CT scans are indicated if the patient's neurologic status deteriorates.

Severe brain injury. Patients with a GCS score of 8 or less after resuscitation or those who deteriorate to that level within 48 hours of admission have a severe TBI. Patients with severe TBI often receive ventilatory support along with ICP and hemodynamic monitoring. A CT scan is performed to rule out any mass lesions that can be surgically ameliorated. Patients are placed in a critical care setting for continual assessment, monitoring, and management.

Nursing Assessment of the Patient with Traumatic Brain Injury

As in all traumatic injuries, evaluation of the airway, breathing, and circulation (ABCs) is the first step in the assessment of the patient with TBI in the critical care unit. Patients with moderate primary injury may deteriorate as a result of diffuse swelling or bleeding. A patient with severe TBI who is breathing spontaneously may require prophylactic endotracheal or nasotracheal intubation with mechanical ventilatory support to reduce the risk of hypoxia and hypercapnia. After stabilization of the ABCs is assured, a neurologic assessment is performed.

Level of consciousness, motor movements, pupillary response, respiratory function, and vital signs are all part of a complete neurologic assessment of the patient with a TBI. Level of consciousness can be elicited to assess wakefulness. Consciousness is assessed by obtaining the patient's response to verbal and painful stimuli. Determination of orientation to person, place, and time assesses mental alertness. Pupils are assessed for size, shape, equality, and reactivity. Asymmetry must be reported immediately. Pupils are also assessed for constriction to a light source (parasympathetic innervation) or dilation (sympathetic innervation). Because parasympathetic fibers are present in the brainstem, pupils that are slow to react to light may indicate a brainstem injury. A "blown" pupil can be caused by compression of the third cranial nerve as a result of transtentorial herniation. Bilateral fixed pupils can indicate midbrain involvement (see "Pupillary Function" in Chapter 17).

Neurologic assessments are ongoing throughout the patient's critical care stay as part of the initial shift assessment and as part of ongoing assessments to detect subtle deterioration. Serial assessments include monitoring hemodynamic status and ICP. The use of muscle relaxants and sedation for ICP control may mask neurologic signs in the patient with a severe head injury. In these situations, observations for changes in pupils and vital signs become extremely important. Newer shorter-acting sedatives with a very short half-life, such as propofol, can be turned off, and within minutes, a neurologic examination can be performed.

Diagnostic Procedures

The cornerstone of initial diagnostic procedures for evaluation of TBI is the CT scan. CT is a rapid, noninvasive procedure that can provide invaluable information about the presence of mass lesions and cerebral edema. Serial CT scans may be used over a period of several days to assess areas of contusion and ischemia and to detect delayed hematomas. A nurse must always remain with a TBI patient during a CT scan to provide continued observation and monitoring and during transport to and from the scanner. Transporting the patient, moving the patient from the bed to the CT table, and positioning the head flat during the CT scan are all stressful events and can cause severe increases in ICP. Continuous monitoring of ICP enables rapid intervention during these particularly vulnerable times.

Medical Management

Surgical management. If a lesion identified on CT is causing a shift of intracranial contents or increasing ICP, surgical intervention is necessary. A craniotomy is performed to remove the EDH, SDH, or large ICH. Patients may also undergo a *decompressive craniectomy* specifically for elevated ICP. This procedure involves removal of the overlying area of skull to allow the underlying brain tissue to expand and swell. This surgical strategy has demonstrated some benefits but remains controversial.[12]

Nonsurgical management. Most of the management of TBI occurs in the critical care unit. Nonsurgical management includes management of ICP, maintenance of adequate cerebral perfusion pressure (CPP) and oxygenation, and treatment of any complications (e.g., pneumonia, infection). The decision of when to initiate ICP monitoring is critical. ICP monitoring may be required for patients with a GCS score

BOX 25-5 NURSING DIAGNOSES PRIORITIES: TRAUMATIC BRAIN INJURY

- Ineffective Breathing Pattern related to neuromuscular impairment, p. 598
- Risk for Aspiration: impaired laryngeal sensation or reflex; impaired pharyngeal peristalsis or tongue function; impaired laryngeal closure or elevation; increased gastric volume; decreased lower esophageal sphincter pressure, p. 602
- Impaired Gas Exchange related to ventilation–perfusion mismatching, p. 594
- Imbalanced Nutrition: Less Than Body Requirements related to lack of exogenous nutrients and increased metabolic demand, p. 593
- Powerlessness related to lack of control over current situation, p. 600
- Decreased Intracranial Adaptive Capacity related to failure of normal compensatory mechanisms, p. 582
- Risk for Ineffective Cerebral Tissue Perfusion, p. 604

less than 8 and abnormal findings on a head CT scan.[13] Brain tissue oxygen monitoring may also be used.

Nursing Management

Nursing priorities in management of traumatic brain injury focus on 1) ongoing assessments of vital signs and hemodynamics, 2) reducing increased intracranial pressure and maintaining adequate cerebral perfusion pressure

Nursing diagnoses priorities for the patient with TBI are listed in Box 25-5.

Ongoing nursing assessments are the cornerstone of care of the patient with a TBI. These assessments are the primary mechanism for determining secondary brain injury from cerebral edema and increased ICP. If secondary injury is to be prevented, the nurse must respond immediately to hypotensive events and, in collaboration with physicians, maximize CPP through reduction of ICP and restoration of an adequate mean arterial pressure.[13]

All aspects of care, including hemodynamic management, pulmonary care, maintenance of body temperature, fluid volume management and control of the environment, can impact outcome after TBI.[13]

Arterial blood pressure should be monitored because hypotension in a patient with TBI is uncommon and may indicate additional injuries. Hypotension will reduce blood flow to the brain. CPP should be maintained at a minimum of 60 mm Hg.[13] In the absence of cerebral ischemia, aggressive attempts to keep CPP above 70 mm Hg with intravenous fluids and vasopressors should be avoided secondary to the risk of ARDS.[13]

Capnography (monitoring of exhaled carbon dioxide levels) is suggested to prevent inadvertent hypocapnia or hypercapnia.[13] Aggressive pulmonary care must be instituted. However, endotracheal suctioning can elevate ICP. Techniques to counter elevation in ICP with suctioning are outlined in Box 25-6. Cerebral oxygen consumption is increased during periods of increased body temperature, and therefore euthermia (36° to 37° C) may be achieved with early workup and intervention for infection, use of antipyretics, and cooling measures such as evaporative cooling.

BOX 25-6 Recommendations for Suctioning Patients with Traumatic Brain Injury

- Pass the suction catheter for no longer than 10 seconds.
- Limit the number of suction catheter passes, preferably to no more than two passes per suctioning episode.
- Hyperoxygenate the patient before and after each passage of the suction catheter (e.g., deliver 4 ventilator breaths at 135% of the patient's tidal volume on 100% FiO_2, at a rate of 4 breaths in 20 seconds).
- Minimize airway stimulation (e.g., stabilize endotracheal tube, avoid passing the suction catheter all the way to the carina).

From McQuillan KA, Thurman P. Traumatic brain injuries. In: McQuillan K, et al, eds. *Trauma: from Resuscitation Through Rehabilitation*. St. Louis: Elsevier; 2009.

A tremendous catecholamine surge after TBI has been associated potentially preventable mortality.[14] The use of beta-blockers to suppress this catecholamine surge in patients with TBI has been shown to decrease inhospital mortality.[14]

Multisensory Stimulation Program

In the early postinjury phase, the patient's environment must be controlled. Stimuli that produce pain, agitation, or discomfort can increase ICP. Analgesics and sedatives should be administered, and patients should be given rest periods. After ICP stabilization, stimulation programs for patients in a coma may be employed. These programs provide stimulation to the tactile, kinesthetic, olfactory, gustatory, auditory, and visual senses. Several methods have been used to stimulate coma patients with various degrees of intensity:

- Intense Multisensory Stimulation Program: stimulatory cycles lasting approximately 15 to 20 minutes, repeated every hour for 12 to 14 hours per day, 6 days per week
- Formalized Not-Intensive Stimulation Program: cycles of stimulation of 10 to 60 minutes twice daily
- Sensory Regulation Program: single brief sessions of stimulation in a quiet environment completely free of noise

Whatever program is used, a stimulation schedule should be established, and accurate documentation of the stimulus and response is essential. Coma stimulation programs should be individualized and family members encouraged to participate.

Spinal Cord Injuries

Approximately 12,000 new spinal cord injuries (SCIs) occur annually. As the population has aged since the 1970s, the median age at injury has increased from 28 to the current median age of 42 years.[15] The diagnosis of SCI begins with a detailed history of events surrounding the incident, precise evaluation of sensory and motor function, and radiographic studies of the spine.

Mechanism of Injury

The type of primary injury sustained depends on the mechanism of injury. The greatest cause of SCI is MVCs (36.5%), followed by falls (28.5%), violence (14.3%), other or unknown causes (9.2%), and sports (11.4%).[15]

Hyperflexion. Hyperflexion injury is most often seen in the cervical area, especially at the level of C5 to C6, because this is the most mobile portion of the cervical spine. This type of injury most often is caused by sudden deceleration motion, as in head-on collisions. Injury occurs from compression of the cord as a result of fracture fragments or dislocation of the vertebral bodies. Instability of the spinal column occurs because of the rupture or tearing of the posterior muscles and ligaments.

Hyperextension. Hyperextension injuries involve backward and downward motion of the head. With this injury, often seen in rear-end collisions or MVCs, the spinal cord is stretched and distorted. Neurologic deficits associated with this injury are often caused by contusion and ischemia of the cord without significant bony involvement. A mild form of hyperextension is the whiplash injury.

Rotation. Rotation injuries often occur in conjunction with a flexion or extension injury. Severe rotation of the neck or body results in tearing of the posterior ligaments and displacement (rotation) of the spinal column.

Axial loading. Axial loading, or vertical compression, injuries occur from vertical force along the spinal cord. This most commonly is seen in a fall from a height in which the person lands on the feet or buttocks. Compression injuries cause burst fractures of the vertebral body that often send bony fragments into the spinal canal or directly into the spinal cord (Figure 25-4).

Penetrating injuries. Penetrating injury to the spinal cord can be caused by a bullet, knife, or any other object that penetrates the cord. These types of injury cause permanent damage by anatomically transecting the spinal cord.

Pathophysiology

SCIs are the result of a mechanical force that disrupts neurologic tissue or its vascular supply, or both. Much like the pathophysiology of TBI, the injury process includes primary and secondary injury mechanisms. Primary injury is the neurologic damage that occurs at the moment of impact. Secondary injury refers to the complex biochemical processes affecting cellular function. Secondary injury can occur within minutes of injury and can last for days to weeks.

Several events after SCI lead to spinal cord ischemia and loss of neurologic function. A cascade of events is initiated that includes systemic and local vascular changes, electrolyte and biochemical changes, neurotransmitter accumulation, and local edema (Box 25-7). Collectively, these pathophysiologic events result in worsening of the injury, potentially extending the level of functional deficit and worsening long-term outcome. Knowledge of the pathophysiology of secondary processes has led to the development of new medications, which target the cellular changes contributing to injury. Despite ongoing research efforts at repairing the primary injury, minimizing damage by reducing secondary injury has shown the most promise.

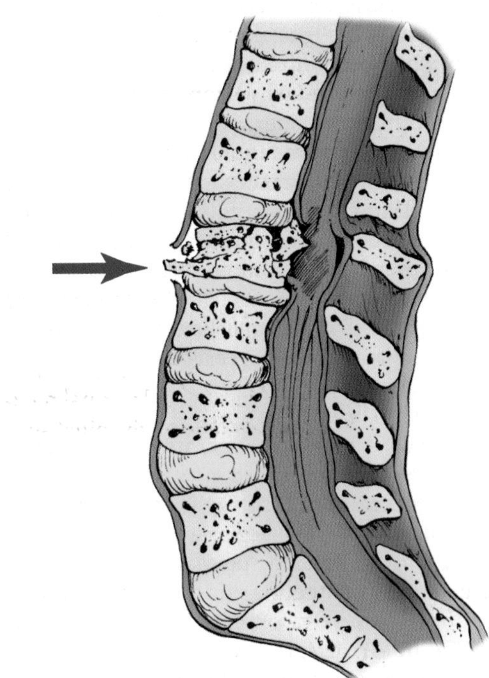

FIG 25-4 Spinal Cord Compression Burst Fracture. Compression injuries cause burst fractures of the vertebral body that often send bony fragments into the spinal canal or directly into the spinal cord. Include hyperflexion, hyperextension, rotation, axial loading (vertical compression), and missile or penetrating injuries.

Functional Injury of the Spinal Cord

Functional injury of the spinal cord refers to the degree of disruption of normal spinal cord function. This depends on what specific sensory and motor structures are damaged. SCIs are classified as complete or incomplete. The most frequent categories at hospital discharge are incomplete tetraplegia (40%) and incomplete paraplegia (18%),[15] followed by complete paraplegia (18%) and complete tetraplegia (11%).[15] SCI cannot be classified until spinal shock has resolved.

Complete injury. Complete SCI is a complete dissection of the spinal cord that results in a total loss of sensory and motor function below the level of injury.

Tetraplegia. With tetraplegia, the injury occurs from the C1 to T1 level. Residual muscle function depends on the specific cervical segments involved. The potential functional status resulting from different neurologic levels of injury is described in Table 25-5.

Paraplegia. With paraplegia, the injury occurs in the thoracolumbar region (T2 to L1). Patients with injuries in this area may have full use of the arms and may need a wheelchair, although some may have limited ability to ambulate short distances with crutches and orthoses (custom external support devices). Thoracic L1 and L2 injuries produce paraplegia with variable innervation to intercostal and abdominal muscles.

Incomplete injury. Incomplete SCI results in a mixed loss of voluntary motor activity and sensation below the level of the lesion. Incomplete SCI exists if any function remains below the level of injury. Incomplete injuries can result in a variety of syndromes, which are classified according to the degree of motor and sensory loss below the level of injury.

Brown-séquard syndrome. The Brown-Séquard syndrome is associated with damage to only one side of the cord. This produces loss of voluntary motor movement on the same side as the injury, with loss of pain, temperature, and sensation on the opposite side. Functionally, the side of the body with the best motor control has little or no sensation, whereas the side of the body with sensation has little or no motor control.

Central cord syndrome. Central cord syndrome is associated with cervical hyperextension–hyperflexion injury and hematoma formation in the center of the cervical cord. This

BOX 25-7 Primary and Secondary Mechanisms of Acute Spinal Cord Injury

Primary Injury Mechanisms
- Acute compression
- Impact
- Missile
- Distraction
- Laceration
- Shear

Secondary Injury Mechanisms
- Systemic effects
- Heart rate: brief increase, then prolonged bradycardia
- Blood pressure: brief hypertension, then prolonged hypotension
- Decreased
- Peripheral resistance
- Decreased cardiac output
- Increased catecholamines, then decreased
- Hypoxia
- Hyperthermia
- Injudicious movement of the unstable spine leading to worsening compression
- Local vascular changes
- Loss of autoregulation
- Systemic hypotension (neurogenic shock)
- Hemorrhage (especially gray matter)
- Loss of microcirculation
- Reduction in blood flow
- Vasospasm
- Thrombosis
- Electrolyte changes
- Increased intracellular calcium
- Increased intracellular sodium
- Increased sodium permeability
- Increased intracellular potassium

Biochemical Changes
- Neurotransmitter accumulation
- Catecholamines (e.g., norepinephrine, dopamine)
- Excitotoxic amino acids (e.g., glutamate)
- Arachidonic acid release
- Free radical production
- Eicosanoid production
- Prostaglandins
- Lipid peroxidation
- Endogenous opioids
- Cytokines
- Edema
- Loss of energy metabolism
- Decreased adenosine triphosphate production
- Apoptosis

Adapted from Sekhon LHS, Fehlings MG. Epidemiology, demographics, and pathophysiology of acute spinal cord injury. *Spine*. 2001: 26(24S):S2.

TABLE 25-5 Quadriplegia Functional Status

NEUROLOGIC LEVEL (VERTEBRAE) OF COMPLETE INJURY	FUNCTIONAL ABILITY
C1-C4	Requires electric wheelchair with breath, head, or shoulder controls
C5	Needs electric wheelchair with hand control and/or manual wheelchair with rim projections; may require adaptive devices to assist with ADLs
C6	Independent in manual wheelchair on level surface; may need hand controls; adaptive devices may be needed for ADLs
C7	Requires manual wheelchair on most surfaces
C8-T1	May need adaptive devices

ADLs, Activities of daily living.

injury produces a motor and sensory deficit more pronounced in the upper extremities than in the lower extremities. Various degrees of bowel and bladder dysfunction may be present.

Anterior cord syndrome. The anterior cord syndrome is associated with injury to the anterior gray horn cells (motor), the spinothalamic tracts (pain), anterior spinothalamic tract (light touch), and the corticospinal tracts (temperature). The result is a loss of motor function and loss of the sensations of pain and temperature below the level of injury. However, below the level of injury, position sense and sensations of pressure and vibrations remain intact. Anterior cord syndrome is commonly caused by flexion injuries or acute herniation of an intervertebral disk.

Posterior cord syndrome. Posterior cord syndrome is associated with cervical hyperextension injury with damage to the posterior column. This results in the loss of position sense, pressure, and vibration below the level of injury. Motor function and sensation of pain and temperature remain intact. These patients may not be able to ambulate because the loss of position sense impairs spontaneous movement.

Spinal shock. Spinal shock is a condition that can occur shortly after traumatic injury to the spinal cord. Spinal shock is the complete loss of all muscle tone and normal reflex activity below the level of injury.[5] Patients with spinal shock may appear completely flaccid, without neurological function below the area of the injury, although all of the area may not necessarily be destroyed.

Neurogenic shock. Neurogenic shock results from injury to the descending sympathetic pathways in the spinal cord. This results from loss of vasomotor tone and sympathetic innervation to the heart. A relative hypovolemia and hypovolemic shock ensues, causing hypotension and decreased systemic vascular resistance. Patients with SCI at T6 or above may have profound neurogenic shock as a result of interruption of the sympathetic nervous system and loss of vasoconstrictor response below the level of the injury. Blood vessels cannot constrict, and the heart rate is slow, which results in hypotension, venous pooling, and decreased cardiac output.

Cellular oxygenation is threatened as cardiac output declines because of a decrease in stroke volume (hypovolemia) and heart rate (bradycardia). The duration of this shock state can persist for up to 1 month after injury. Blood pressure support may be required with the use of sympathomimetic medications. Because hypotension is a problem, the nurse must be cautious when adjusting backrest position or when repositioning a patient in bed because orthostatic blood pressure changes can occur (see "Neurogenic Shock" in Chapter 26).

Autonomic dysreflexia. Autonomic dysreflexia is a life-threatening complication that may occur with SCI. This condition is caused by a massive sympathetic response to a noxious stimuli (e.g., full bladder, line insertions, fecal impaction) that results in bradycardia, hypertension, facial flushing, and headache. Immediate intervention is needed to prevent cerebral hemorrhage, seizures, and acute pulmonary edema. Treatment is aimed at alleviating the noxious stimuli. A clinical algorithm for treatment of autonomic dysreflexia is provided in Box 25-8. If symptoms persist, antihypertensive agents can be administered to reduce blood pressure. Prevention of autonomic dysreflexia is imperative and can be accomplished through the use of a rehabilitative bowel and bladder program.

Assessment in Spinal Cord Injury

On admission to the critical care unit, attention to the ABCs is imperative in the patient with known or suspected SCI. Stabilization of the spinal cord is mandatory to prevent further injury, and spinal precautions are maintained until the spine is cleared of injury. Stabilization may include the use of bedrest with log-rolling maneuvers and a hard cervical collar until definitive stabilization is achieved. After the ABCs have been evaluated and interventions for life-threatening complications have been initiated, a full physical assessment is made to determine the extent of injury.

Airway. Assessment of ABCs is essential to ensure optimal oxygenation and perfusion to all vital organs, including the spinal cord. Complete cardiovascular and respiratory assessments are essential to the patient's survival and prognosis. The primary assessment begins with an evaluation of airway clearance. In an unresponsive person, an oral airway is inserted while the patient's neck is maintained in a neutral position. The patient must undergo intubation before severe hypoxia can occur, which could further damage the spinal cord.

Breathing. Assessment of breathing patterns and gas exchange is made after an airway has been secured. The level of injury dictates the degree of altered breathing patterns and gas exchange (Table 25-6). Because complete injuries above the C3 level result in paralysis of the diaphragm, patients with these injuries require ventilatory assistance.

Circulation. Assessment of cardiac output and tissue perfusion is imperative to detect life-threatening injuries and promote recovery of injured spinal cord tissue. The patient with SCI is at high risk for developing alterations in cardiac output and tissue perfusion because the cardiovascular system is subjected to a variety of serious and potential physiologic alterations, including dysrhythmias, cardiac arrest, orthostatic hypotension, emboli, and thrombophlebitis.

The patient with SCI is assessed for adequate tissue perfusion by means of invasive and noninvasive hemodynamic monitoring techniques. Cardiac monitoring is required to detect bradycardia and other dysrhythmias that occur in response to reflex vagus activity mediated by the dominant parasympathetic nervous system, as well as changes in ECG rhythm as a result of hypothermia or hypoxia.

Neurologic assessment for spinal cord injury. The initial neurologic assessment may not be an accurate indication of eventual motor and sensory loss. It focuses on the rapid and accurate identification of present, absent, or impaired functioning of the motor, sensory, and reflex systems that

BOX 25-8 Autonomic Dysreflexia

- If patient is supine, immediately sit the patient up.
- Begin frequent vital sign monitoring and perform every 5 minutes.
- Survey for instigating causes; begin with urinary system.
- Loosen clothing, constrictive devices.
- If indwelling catheter is not placed, catheterize the patient.
  - Lidocaine jelly may be instilled 5 minutes before catheter insertion.
- If indwelling catheter is present, do the following:
  - Check system for kinks and obstructions to flow.
  - Irrigate the bladder with small sterile amount of fluid, utilizing strict aseptic technique.
  - If not draining, remove the catheter and replace.
- If systolic blood pressure is greater than 150 mm Hg, consider rapid-onset, short-duration antihypertensive agent.
- If acute symptoms persist, suspect fecal impaction:
  - Instill lidocaine jelly into rectum; wait at least 5 minutes.
  - Perform digital examination to check for presence of stool; if present, gently remove. If signs of autonomic dysreflexia persist, stop examination; instill additional lidocaine jelly and wait 20 minutes to reexamine.
  - If no stool is found and the abdomen is distended, consider administration of laxative.

TABLE 25-6 Effects of Spinal Cord Injury on Ventilatory Functions

NEUROLOGIC LEVEL (VERTEBRAE) OF COMPLETE INJURY	RESPIRATORY FUNCTION	COMMENT
C1-C2	Paralysis of diaphragm	Ventilator-dependent
C3-C5	Various degrees of diaphragm paralysis	Some diaphragm control; may need ventilatory support; weaning depends on preinjury pulmonary status.
C6-T11	Various degrees of impaired intercostal muscles and abdominal muscles	Compromised respiratory function; reduced inspiratory ability; paradoxical breathing patterns; ineffective cough, sneeze

coordinate and regulate vital functions. A detailed motor and sensory examination includes the assessment of all 32 spinal nerves for evidence of dysfunction. Carefully mapped pathways for the sensory portion of the spinal nerves, called dermatomes, can assist in localizing the functional sensory level of injury. Muscle strength may be graded on a 6-point scale (Table 25-7). Initial assessment must be performed correctly and findings documented in detail so that subsequent serial assessments can rapidly identify deterioration. The American Spinal Injury Association (ASIA) has developed a form that outlines the required assessments for initial and ongoing classification of SCIs (Figure 25-5). Ongoing spinal cord assessments must be documented during the critical care phase.

Diagnostic procedures. Diagnostic radiographic evaluations can identify the severity of damage to the spinal cord. Initial evaluation includes anteroposterior and lateral views for all areas of the spinal cord. CT scan of all seven cervical vertebrae and the top of T1 must be obtained to rule out cervicothoracic junction injury. Flexion and extension views can identify subtle ligament injuries. CT, tomography, myelography, and MRI also may be used.

TABLE 25-7 Muscle Strength Scale

5. Active movement against maximal resistance
4. Active movement through range of motion against resistance
3. Active movement through range of motion against gravity
2. Active movement through range of motion with gravity eliminated
1. Visible or palpable muscle contraction
0. No contraction; total paralysis

Screening for spinal cord injury. Screening of the spinal cord for injury becomes an integral part of the assessment for all trauma patients. The degree of trauma, alteration in mentation, intoxication, and distracting injuries dictate the type and extent of examination required to clear the cervical spine. The Eastern Association of Surgeons in Trauma (EAST) has published guidelines for the clearance of the cervical spine (Table 25-8).[16] In these guidelines CT scan has replaced plain radiography as the principal modality for cervical spine assessment following trauma.[16] On admission, the spine is palpated for obvious deformity, and the patient is assessed for the subjective response of pain to palpation.[16] If the patient has distracting injuries, such as rib fractures, is intoxicated, or has received analgesics, examination of the spinal cord may be deferred.[16] MRI may be warranted to diagnose SCI definitively when the patient's hemodynamic condition is stabilized.[16]

Medical Management

After assessment and diagnosis of the SCI, medical management begins. The primary treatment goal is to preserve remaining neurologic function with pharmacologic, surgical, and nonsurgical interventions.

Pharmacologic management. Previously methylprednisolone was administered in the first 8 hours after SCI,[17] However, per current guidelines, this medication is no longer recommended.[18]

Surgical management. Surgical intervention provides spinal column stability in the presence of an unstable injury. Unstable injuries include disrupted ligaments and tendons and a vertebral column that cannot maintain normal alignment. Identification and immobilization of unstable injuries are particularly important for the patient with incomplete neurologic deficit. Without adequate stabilization, movement and dislocation of the vertebral column may cause a complete

TABLE 25-8 East Guidelines for Cervical Spine Clearance

TRAUMA PATIENT POPULATION	RECOMMENDATION
Trauma patients that are awake, alert, not intoxicated, neurologically normal, no complaints of neck pain or tenderness with full range of motion of the cervical spine	Neck is palpated in all directions for tenderness or pain. If physical examination is negative for pain or tenderness, CT imaging of the cervical spine is not required, and the cervical collar may be removed.
All other trauma patients with suspected cervical injury must be radiologically evaluated. This includes patients with neck pain or tenderness, whether alert or with altered mental status/neurological deficit, or distracting injury.	Axial CT from occiput to T1 with sagittal and coronal reconstructions If CT is positive for injury, continue cervical collar, obtain spine consultation, and obtain MRI. In the neurologically intact awake patient with neck pain, if the CT is negative (no injury seen), MRI is negative, and adequate flexion/extension films are negative, discontinue cervical collar.
Trauma patients that are obtunded with gross motor function of extremities	Axial CT from occiput to T1 with sagittal and coronal reconstructions If the CT is negative (no injury seen), the risk/benefit of an additional MRI must be determined in each hospital. Options are A. Continue cervical collar until a clinical exam can be performed. B. Remove the cervical collar on the basis of negative CT alone. C. Obtain MRI. If MRI is negative, collar can be safely removed. Flexion/extension radiography should not be performed.

CT, Computed tomography; *EAST*, Eastern Association of Surgeons in Trauma; *MRI*, magnetic resonance imaging.
From Como, et al. Practice management guidelines for identification of cervical spine injuries following trauma: update from the Eastern Association for the Surgery of Trauma Practice Management Guidelines Committee. *J Trauma.* 2009: 67(3):651.

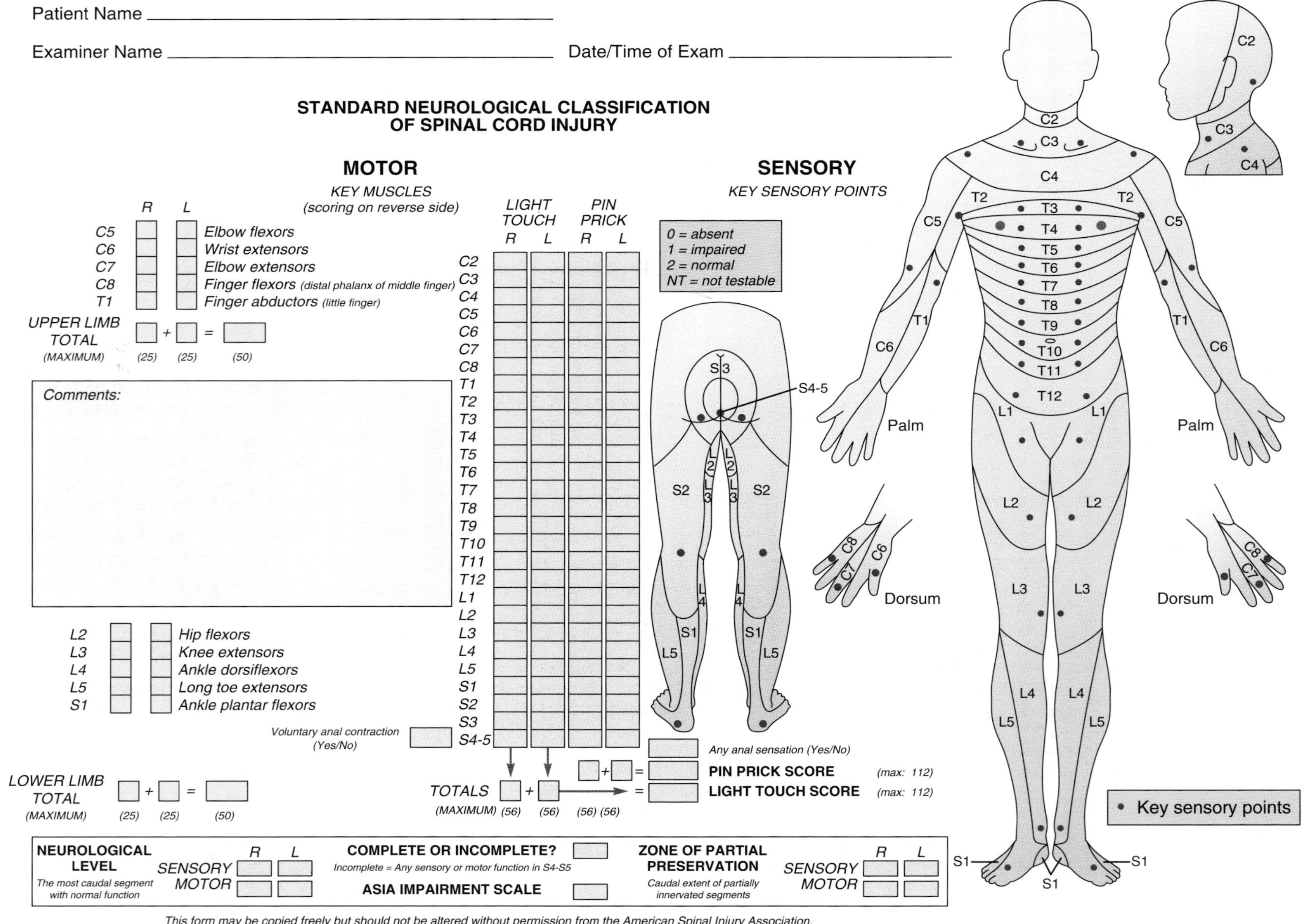

Patient Name ____________________

Examiner Name ____________________ Date/Time of Exam ____________________

STANDARD NEUROLOGICAL CLASSIFICATION OF SPINAL CORD INJURY

MOTOR

KEY MUSCLES (scoring on reverse side)

	R	L	
C5			Elbow flexors
C6			Wrist extensors
C7			Elbow extensors
C8			Finger flexors (distal phalanx of middle finger)
T1			Finger abductors (little finger)

UPPER LIMB TOTAL (MAXIMUM) ☐ + ☐ = ☐ (25) (25) (50)

Comments:

	R	L	
L2			Hip flexors
L3			Knee extensors
L4			Ankle dorsiflexors
L5			Long toe extensors
S1			Ankle plantar flexors

Voluntary anal contraction (Yes/No) ☐

LOWER LIMB TOTAL (MAXIMUM) ☐ + ☐ = ☐ (25) (25) (50)

SENSORY

KEY SENSORY POINTS

	LIGHT TOUCH R	LIGHT TOUCH L	PIN PRICK R	PIN PRICK L
C2				
C3				
C4				
C5				
C6				
C7				
C8				
T1				
T2				
T3				
T4				
T5				
T6				
T7				
T8				
T9				
T10				
T11				
T12				
L1				
L2				
L3				
L4				
L5				
S1				
S2				
S3				
S4-5				

TOTALS (MAXIMUM) ☐ + ☐ (56) (56) (56) (56)

0 = absent
1 = impaired
2 = normal
NT = not testable

Any anal sensation (Yes/No) ☐

PIN PRICK SCORE (max: 112)

LIGHT TOUCH SCORE (max: 112)

NEUROLOGICAL LEVEL The most caudal segment with normal function — SENSORY R ☐ L ☐; MOTOR R ☐ L ☐

COMPLETE OR INCOMPLETE? ☐ Incomplete = Any sensory or motor function in S4-S5

ASIA IMPAIRMENT SCALE ☐

ZONE OF PARTIAL PRESERVATION Caudal extent of partially innervated segments — SENSORY R ☐ L ☐; MOTOR R ☐ L ☐

This form may be copied freely but should not be altered without permission from the American Spinal Injury Association.

FIG 25-5 American Spinal Injury Association (ASIA) Classification of Spinal Cord Injuries.

MUSCLE GRADING

0 total paralysis

1 palpable or visible contraction

2 active movement, full range of motion, gravity eliminated

3 active movement, full range of motion, against gravity

4 active movement, full range of motion, against gravity and provides some resistance

5 active movement, full range of motion, against gravity and provides normal resistance

5* muscle able to exert, in examiner's judgment, sufficient resistance to be considered normal if identifiable inhibiting factors were not present

NT not testable. Patient unable to reliably exert effort or muscle unavailable for testing due to factors such as immobilization, pain on effort, or contracture.

ASIA IMPAIRMENT SCALE

☐ **A = Complete**: No motor or sensory function is preserved in the sacral segments S4-S5.

☐ **B = Incomplete:** Sensory but not motor function is preserved below the neurological level and includes the sacral segments S4-S5.

☐ **C = Incomplete:** Motor function is preserved below the neurological level, and more than half of key muscles below the neurological level have a muscle grade less than 3.

☐ **D = Incomplete:** Motor function is preserved below the neurological level, and at least half of key muscles below the neurological level have a muscle grade of 3 or more.

☐ **E = Normal:** Motor and sensory function are normal.

CLINICAL SYNDROMES (OPTIONAL)

☐ Central Cord
☐ Brown-Séquard
☐ Anterior Cord
☐ Conus Medullaris
☐ Cauda Equina

STEPS IN CLASSIFICATION

The following order is recommended in determining the classification of individuals with SCI.

1. Determine sensory levels for right and left sides.
2. Determine motor levels for right and left sides.
   Note: in regions where there is no myotome to test, the motor level is presumed to be the same as the sensory level.
3. Determine the single neurological level.
   This is the lowest segment where motor and sensory function is normal on both sides, and is the most cephalad of the sensory and motor levels determined in steps 1 and 2.
4. Determine whether the injury is Complete or Incomplete (sacral sparing).
   If voluntary anal contraction = **No** *AND all S4-5 sensory scores =* **0** *AND any anal sensation =* **No**, *then injury is COMPLETE. Otherwise injury is incomplete.*
5. Determine ASIA Impairment Scale (AIS) Grade:

Is injury Complete? If **YES**, AIS=A Record ZPP
(For ZPP, record lowest dermatome or myotome on each side with some [non-zero score] preservation.)

NO ↓

Is injury motor incomplete? If **NO**, AIS=B
(Yes=voluntary anal contraction OR motor function more than three levels below the motor level on a given side.)

YES ↓

Are at least half of the key muscles below the (single) neurological level graded 3 or better?

NO ↓ AIS=C

YES ↓ AIS=D

If sensation and motor function is normal in all segments, AIS=E.
Note: AIS E is used in follow up testing when an individual with a documented SCI has recovered normal function. If at initial testing no deficits are found, the individual is neurologically intact; the ASIA Impairment Scale does not apply.

FIG 25-5, cont'd

neurologic deficit. A variety of surgical procedures may be performed to achieve decompression and stabilization. The question of when surgery should be performed remains controversial.

Nonsurgical management. If the injury to the spinal cord is stable, nonsurgical management is the treatment of choice. Nonsurgical management for cervical and thoracolumbar injuries is discussed in the following sections.

Cervical injury. Management of cervical injuries involves the immobilization of the fracture site and realignment of any dislocation. This is accomplished through skeletal traction that involves the use of two-point tongs, which are inserted into the skull through shallow burr holes and are connected to traction weights. Several types of cervical tongs are used. Gardner-Wells and Crutchfield tongs are the most common. These tongs can be applied at the bedside with the use of a local anesthetic.

After the procedure, the patient can be immobilized on a kinetic therapy bed or a regular bed. The kinetic therapy bed is the most popular method used for cervical immobilization because it maintains spinal column alignment while providing constant turning motion to reduce pulmonary and skin breakdown. Use of cervical skeletal traction on a regular bed makes it difficult to provide adequate care to the pulmonary system and skin because of the extensive degree of immobility.

After the spinal column has been adequately realigned by means of skeletal traction, a halo traction brace often is applied. The halo vest consists of a metal ring secured to the skull with two occipital and two temporal screws. Steel bars anchor the screws to the vest to provide cervical immobilization (Figure 25-6). The halo traction brace immobilizes the cervical spine, which allows the patient to ambulate and participate in self-care.

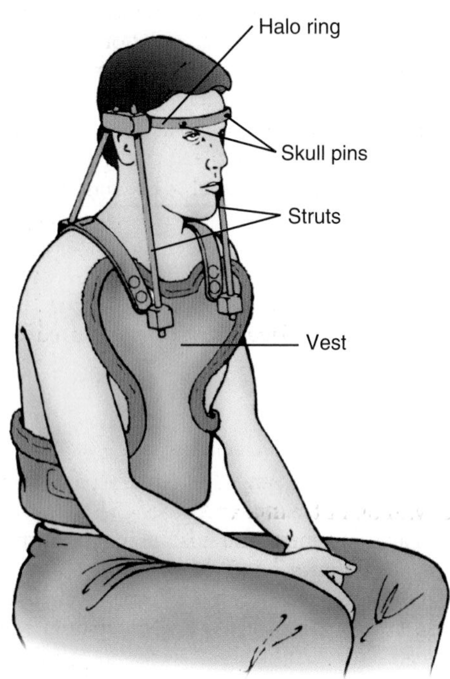

FIG 25-6 Halo Vest. The halo traction brace immobilizes the cervical spine, which allows the patient to ambulate and participate in self-care.

Thoracolumbar injury. Nonsurgical management of the patient with a thoracolumbar injury also involves immobilization. Skeletal traction may be used in high thoracic injury. For the most part, misalignment of the spinal canal does not occur in stable injuries of the thoracolumbar spine. Immobilization to allow fractures to heal is accomplished by bedrest (with the bed flat) and the use of a plastic or fiberglass jacket, a body cast, or a brace.

Nursing Management

Nursing priorities for the patient with SCI are aimed at 1) preventing secondary damage to the spinal cord, 2) managing cardiovascular and pulmonary complications, and 3) coaching the patient to overcome the psychosocial challenges associated with severe neurological deficit.

Nursing diagnoses priorities for the patient with SCI are summarized in Box 25-9. The goal during the critical care phase is to prevent life-threatening complications while maximizing the function of all organ systems. Nursing interventions are aimed at preventing secondary damage to the spinal cord and managing the complications of the neurologic deficit. Because almost all body systems are affected by SCI, nursing management must include interventions that optimize nutrition, elimination, skin integrity, and mobility. Patients with SCIs have complex psychosocial needs that require a great deal of emotional support from the critical care nurse.

Thoracic Injuries

Thoracic injuries involve trauma to the chest wall, lungs, heart, great vessels, and esophagus. Thoracic trauma most commonly is the result of a violent crime or an MVC.

Mechanism of Injury

Blunt thoracic trauma. Blunt trauma to the chest is often caused by an MVC or fall. Thoracic injuries account for 25% of trauma deaths.[19] The underlying mechanism of injury tends to be a combination of acceleration–deceleration injury and direct transfer mechanics, as in a crush injury. Various mechanisms of blunt trauma are associated with specific injury patterns. After head-on collisions, drivers have a higher

BOX 25-9 NURSING DIAGNOSES PRIORITIES: SPINAL CORD INJURY

- Decreased Cardiac Output related to sympathetic blockade, p. 581
- Autonomic Dysreflexia related to excessive autonomic response to noxious stimuli, p. 577
- Impaired Gas Exchange related to alveolar hypoventilation, p. 593
- Ineffective Breathing Pattern related to decreased lung expansion, p. 598
- Ineffective Breathing Pattern related to musculoskeletal fatigue or neuromuscular impairment, p. 598
- Disturbed Body Image related to actual change in body structure, function, or appearance, p. 586
- Ineffective Coping related to situational crisis and personal vulnerability, p. 599

frequency of injury than do backseat passengers because the driver comes in contact with the steering wheel assembly. Severe thoracic injuries often are seen in patients who are unrestrained. Falls from greater than 20 feet are typically associated with thoracic injury.

Penetrating thoracic injuries. The penetrating object involved determines the damage sustained from penetrating thoracic trauma. Low-velocity weapons (e.g., .22-caliber gun, knife) usually damage only what is in the weapon's direct path. Of particular concern, however, are stab wounds that involve the anterior chest wall between the midclavicular lines, the angle of Louis, and the epigastric region because of the proximity of the heart and great vessels.

Thoracic Traumatic Injuries

Chest wall injuries

Rib fractures. Fractures of the ribs can be serious, even life-threatening, particularly when there are three or more rib fractures, there is the presence of preexisting disease (especially cardiopulmonary disease), or the patient is 65 years old or older.[20] Fractures of the first and second ribs are associated with intrathoracic vascular injuries (e.g., brachial plexus, great vessels), and because they are protected by the scapula, clavicle, humerus, and muscles, they signify a very high degree of force applied to the thorax. Fractures to the lower ribs (7th to 12th) may be associated with abdominal injuries, such as spleen and liver injuries. Fractures to the middle ribs may be associated with lung injury, including pulmonary contusion and pneumothorax. Lack of bone calcification in pediatric trauma patients means the chest wall is more compliant, and rib fractures need not have occurred for a tremendous amount of force to have been absorbed by the underlying organs.

The pain associated with rib fractures can be aggravated by respiratory excursion. The patient often splints, takes shallow breaths, and refuses to cough, which can result in atelectasis and pneumonia. Localized pain that increases with respiration or that is elicited by rib compression may indicate rib fractures. Definitive diagnosis can be made with a chest radiograph. Interventions include aggressive pulmonary physiotherapy and pain control to improve chest expansion efforts and gas exchange. Pain management interventions must be tailored to the patient's response to therapy. The primary goal of pain management in patients with rib fractures is prevention of pulmonary complications and patient comfort. Nonsteroidal antiinflammatory drugs (NSAIDs), intercostal nerve blocks, thoracic epidural analgesia, and opiates may be considered to assist with pain control.[19] Epidural analgesia can help increase the functional residual capacity, dynamic lung compliance, and vital capacity; decrease the airway resistance, and increase PaO_2.[19] External splints are not recommended because they further limit chest wall expansion and may add to atelectasis.[19] The patient's preexisting pulmonary status and age may dictate the course of recovery.[19] Patients should also have incentive spirometry values monitored, as a reduction in volume could indicate increasing pain.[20]

Flail chest. Flail chest, which is caused by blunt trauma, disrupts the continuity of chest wall structures. Typically, a flail segment occurs when two or more ribs are fractured in two or more places and are no longer attached to the thoracic cage, producing a free-floating segment of the chest wall. A flail chest is a clinical diagnosis in which the flail segment (or floating segment) moves paradoxically compared to the rest of the chest wall (Figure 25-7).[19] During inspiration, the intact portion of the chest wall expands, while the injured part is sucked in. During expiration, the chest wall moves in, and the flail segment moves out. Although the flail segment increases the work of breathing, the main cause of hypoxemia is the underlying pulmonary contusion.[21] The physiologic effects of the impaired chest wall motion of a flail chest include decreased tidal volume and vital capacity and impaired cough, which lead to hypoventilation and atelectasis.

Inspection of the chest reveals paradoxical movement. Palpation of the chest may indicate crepitus and tenderness near fractured ribs. A chest radiograph that reveals multiple rib fractures and evidence of hypoxia demonstrated by ABG values aids in the diagnosis. Interventions focus on ensuring adequate oxygenation, judicious administration of fluids, and analgesia to improve ventilation.[19] Intubation and mechanical ventilation may be required to prevent further hypoxia.

Ruptured diaphragm. Diagnosis of a diaphragmatic rupture is often missed in trauma patients because of the subtle and nonspecific symptoms this injury produces. The mechanism of injury appears to be a rapid rise in intraabdominal pressure as a result of compression force applied to the lower part of the chest or upper region of the abdomen. This injury can occur when a person is thrown forward over the edge of the steering wheel in a high-speed MVC involving deceleration forces. The diaphragm, which offers little resistance to the force, can rupture or tear. Abdominal viscera then can gradually enter the thoracic cavity, moving from the positive pressure of the abdomen to the negative pressure in the thorax. Diaphragmatic rupture can be a life-threatening event. Massive herniation of abdominal contents into the thoracic cavity can compress the lungs and mediastinum, which hampers venous return and leads to decreased cardiac output. Herniated bowel can become strangulated and perforate.

Diaphragmatic herniation may produce significant compromise and changes in respiratory effort. Auscultation of bowel sounds in the chest or unilateral breath sounds may indicate a ruptured diaphragm. The patient may complain of shoulder pain, shortness of breath, or abdominal tenderness. Thoracoscopy may be helpful in evaluating the diaphragm in indeterminate cases, and CT analysis is helpful in the evaluation of diaphragmatic injuries. A chest radiograph may reveal the tip of a nasogastric tube above the diaphragm, a unilaterally elevated hemidiaphragm, a hollow or solid mass above the diaphragm, and a shift of the mediastinum away from the affected side. Treatment of a ruptured diaphragm includes its immediate repair.

Lung Injuries

Pulmonary contusion. A pulmonary contusion is fundamentally a bruise of the lung. Pulmonary contusion often is associated with blunt trauma and other chest injuries, such as rib fractures and flail chest, and it is the most common potentially lethal chest injury.[19] Pulmonary contusions can occur unilaterally or bilaterally. A contusion manifests initially as a hemorrhage, followed by alveolar and interstitial edema. The edema can remain rather localized in the contused area or can spread to other lung areas. Inflammation affects alveolar-capillary units. As more units are affected by inflammation, further pathophysiologic events can occur, including decreased compliance, increased pulmonary vascular resistance, and

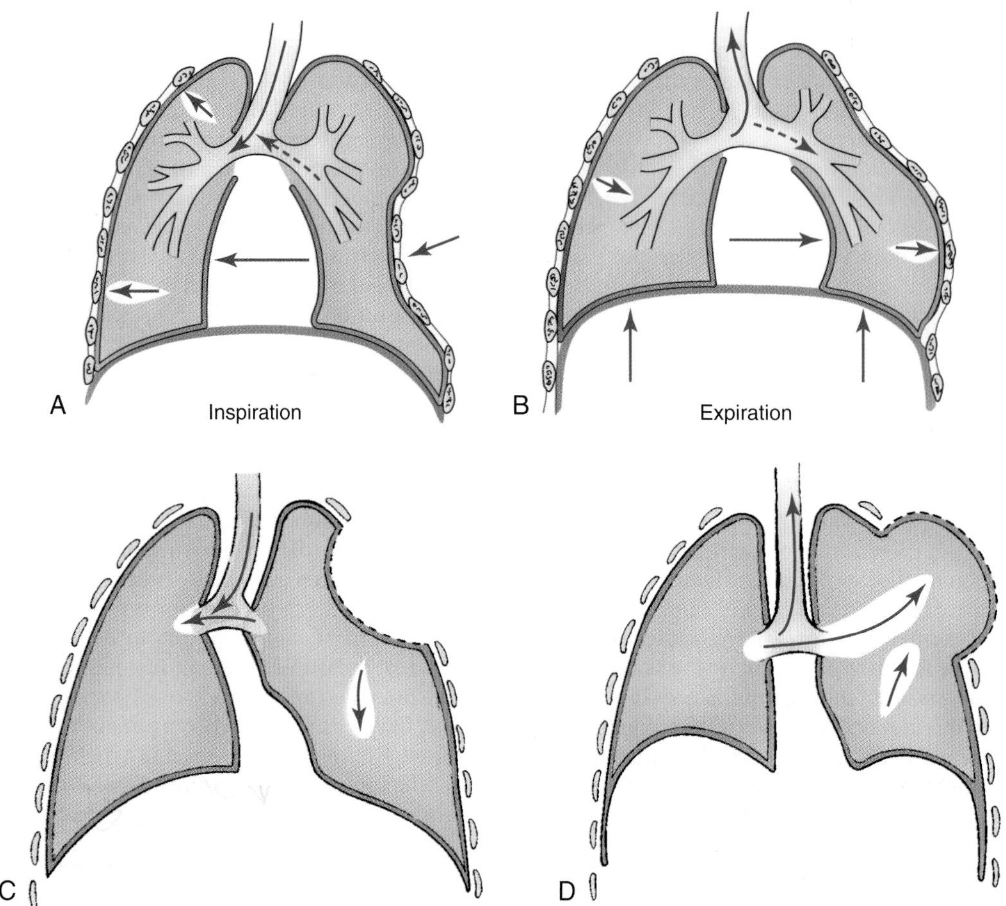

FIG 25-7 Flail Chest. *A*, Normal inspiration. *B*, Normal expiration. *C*, The area of lung underlying the unstable chest wall sucks in on inspiration. *D*, The same area balloons out on expiration. Notice the movement of mediastinum toward opposite lung on inspiration.

decreased pulmonary blood flow. These processes result in a ventilation–perfusion imbalance that results in progressive hypoxemia and poor ventilation over a 24- to 48-hour period.

Clinical manifestations of pulmonary contusion may take up to 24 to 48 hours to develop. Inspections of the chest wall may reveal ecchymosis at the site of impact. Moist crackles may be auscultated in the contused lung. The patient may have a cough and blood-tinged sputum. Abnormal lung function can manifest as systemic arterial hypoxemia. The diagnosis is made primarily by radiography studies consistent with pulmonary infiltrate corresponding to the area of external chest impact that manifests within 12 to 24 hours of injury. Pulmonary contusions tend to worsen over a 24- to 48-hour period and then slowly resolve unless complications occur (e.g., infection, ARDS).

Aggressive respiratory care is the cornerstone for care of nonintubated patients with pulmonary contusion. Interventions include ambulation, deep-breathing exercises, turning, and incentive spirometry. Chest physiotherapy is not tolerated if there are coexisting rib fractures. Aggressive removal of airway secretions is important to avoid infection and to improve ventilation. Patients with unilateral contusions are placed with the injured side up and uninjured side down ("down with the good lung"). This positioning maximizes the match between pulmonary ventilation and perfusion. Patients with severe contusions may continue to show decompensation despite aggressive nursing management. Respiratory acidosis, increases in peak airway and plateau pressures, and increased work of breathing may require endotracheal intubation and mechanical ventilation with *positive end-expiratory pressure* (PEEP). Adequate pain control is accomplished with administration of NSAIDs, opiates, intercostal nerve blocks, or thoracic epidural analgesia.[19]

Complications resulting from pulmonary contusions include pneumonia, ARDS, lung abscesses, emphysema, and pulmonary embolism. Factors that contribute to increased mortality rates include shock, coexisting head injury, flail chest, falls from heights greater than 20 feet, advanced age, and preexisting disease (e.g., coronary artery disease, chronic obstructive pulmonary disease).

Tension pneumothorax. A tension pneumothorax usually is caused by an injury that perforates the chest wall or pleural space. Air flows into the pleural space with inspiration and becomes trapped. As pressure in the pleural space increases, the lung on the injured side collapses and causes the mediastinum to shift to the opposite side (Figure 25-8). As pressure continues to build, the shift exerts pressure on the heart and thoracic aorta, which results in decreased venous return and decreased cardiac output. Tissue perfusion with oxygenated

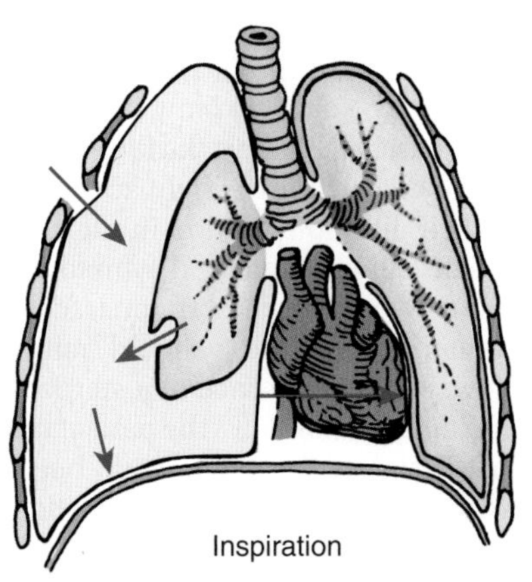

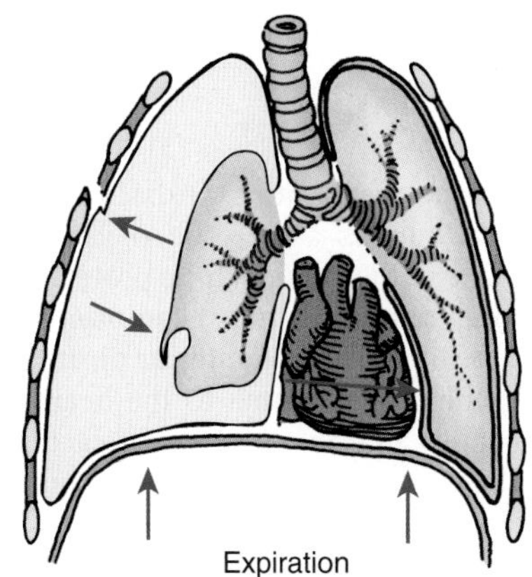

FIG 25-8 A tension pneumothorax usually is caused by an injury that perforates the chest wall or pleural space. Air flows into the pleural space with inspiration and becomes trapped. As pressure in the pleural space increases, the lung on the injured side collapses and causes the mediastinum to shift to the opposite side. (From Marx J, et al. *Rosen's Emergency Medicine: Concepts and Clinical Practice*. 8th ed. St. Louis: Mosby; 2013.)

blood is further hampered because the collapsed lung cannot participate in gas exchange.

Clinical manifestations of a tension pneumothorax include dyspnea, tachycardia, hypotension, and sudden chest pain extending to the shoulders. Tracheal deviation can be observed as the trachea shifts away from the injured side. On the injured side, breath sounds may be decreased or absent. Percussion of the chest reveals a hyperresonant sound over the affected side. Diagnosis of tension pneumothorax is made by clinical assessment.

In a hemodynamically unstable patient with a tension pneumothorax, there is no time for a chest radiograph because this potentially lethal condition must be treated immediately.[5] A large-bore (14-gauge) needle or chest tube is inserted into the affected lung. This procedure allows immediate release of air from the pleural space. A hissing sound is heard as the tension pneumothorax is converted to a simple pneumothorax.

Open pneumothorax. An open pneumothorax ("sucking chest wound") usually is caused by penetrating trauma. Open communication between the atmosphere and intrathoracic pressure results in immediate lung deflation. Air moves in and out of the hole in the chest, producing a sucking sound heard on inspiration. An open pneumothorax produces the same symptoms as a tension pneumothorax. Subcutaneous emphysema may be palpated around the wound.

Initial management of an open pneumothorax is accomplished by promptly closing the wound at end expiration with a sterile occlusive dressing (plastic wrap or petroleum gauze) large enough to overlap the wound's edges.[5] This dressing should be taped securely on three sides to create a "flutter valve" effect.[5] As the patient breathes in, the dressing gets sucked in to occlude the wound and prevent air from entering. A chest tube is placed as soon as possible. Surgical intervention may be required to close the wound.

Hemothorax. Blunt or penetrating thoracic trauma can cause bleeding into the pleural space, resulting in a hemothorax (Figure 25-9). A massive hemothorax results from the accumulation of more than 1500 mL of blood in the chest cavity.[5,22] The source of bleeding may be the intercostal or internal mammary arteries, lungs, heart, or great vessels.

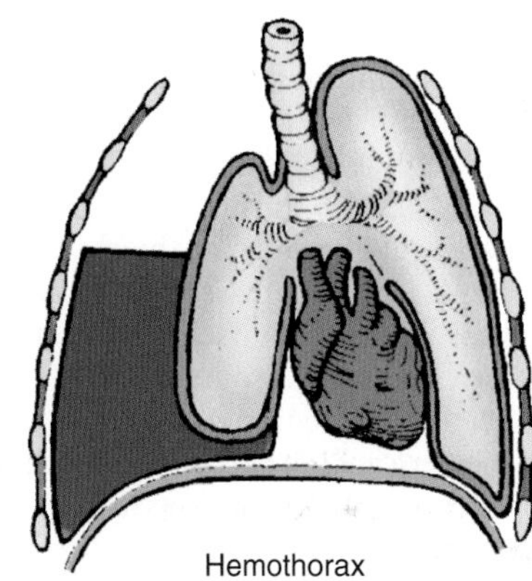

FIG 25-9 Blunt or Penetrating Thoracic Trauma Can Cause Bleeding into the Pleural Space to Form a Hemothorax.

Lacerations to the lung parenchyma are low-pressure bleeds and typically stop bleeding spontaneously.[22] Arterial bleeding from major pulmonary vessels usually requires immediate surgical intervention. In either case, increasing intrapleural pressure results in a decrease in vital capacity. Increasing vascular blood loss into the pleural space causes decreased venous return and decreased cardiac output.

Assessment findings for patients with a hemothorax include hypovolemic shock. Breath sounds may be diminished or absent over the affected lung. With hemothorax, the neck veins are collapsed, and the trachea is at midline. Massive hemothorax can be diagnosed on the basis of clinical manifestations of hypotension associated with the absence of breath sounds or dullness to percussion on one side of the chest.[5,22]

This life-threatening condition must be treated immediately. Resuscitation with intravenous fluids is initiated to treat the hypovolemic shock. A chest tube is placed on the affected side to allow drainage of blood. An autotransfusion device can be attached to the chest tube collection chamber. Thoracotomy may be necessary for patients who require persistent blood transfusions or who have significant bleeding (200 mL/hr for 2 to 4 hours or more than 1500 mL on initial tube insertion) or when there are injuries to major cardiovascular structures.[22]

Heart and Vascular Injuries

Penetrating cardiac injuries. Penetrating cardiac trauma can occur from mechanical injuries as a result of bullets, knives, or impalements. The chest wall offers little protection to the heart from penetrating trauma. The most common site of injury is the right ventricle because of its anterior position. The mortality rate from penetrating trauma to the heart is high. The prehospital mortality rate for penetrating cardiac injuries is very high, and most deaths occur within minutes after injury as a result of exsanguination or tamponade.

Cardiac tamponade. Cardiac tamponade is the progressive accumulation of blood in the pericardial sac (Figure 25-10). With cardiac tamponade, progressive accumulation of 120 to 150 mL of blood increases the intracardiac pressure and compresses the atria and ventricles. An increase in intracardiac pressure leads to decreased venous return and decreased filling pressure, which leads to decreased cardiac output, myocardial hypoxia, heart failure, and cardiogenic shock.

Classic assessment findings associated with cardiac tamponade are called *Beck's triad*—presence of elevated central venous pressure with neck vein distention, muffled heart sounds, and hypotension. Pulsus paradoxus may occur. Pulseless electrical activity (PEA) in the absence of hypovolemia and tension pneumothorax suggests cardiac tamponade.[5] Bedside ultrasonography is useful in penetrating cardiac injury to identify a hemopericardium.[23]

Immediate treatment is required to remove the accumulation of fluid in the pericardial sac. Pericardiocentesis involves aspiration of fluid from the pericardium by use of a large-bore needle. The inherent risk in this procedure is potential laceration of the coronary artery. Other approaches include surgical procedures such as thoracotomy or median sternotomy. The goal of these procedures is to locate and control the source of bleeding.

Blunt cardiac injury. The most common causes of blunt cardiac trauma include high-speed MVCs, direct blows to the chest, and falls. Because of its mobility and its location between the sternum and thoracic vertebrae, the heart is susceptible to blunt traumatic injury. Sudden acceleration (as from contact with a steering wheel) can cause the heart to be thrown against the sternum (Figure 25-11). Sudden deceleration can cause the heart to be thrown against the thoracic vertebrae by a direct blow to the chest, such as blows caused by a baseball, animal kick, or fall. The most often injured chambers include the right atrium and right ventricle because of their anterior position in the chest.[24]

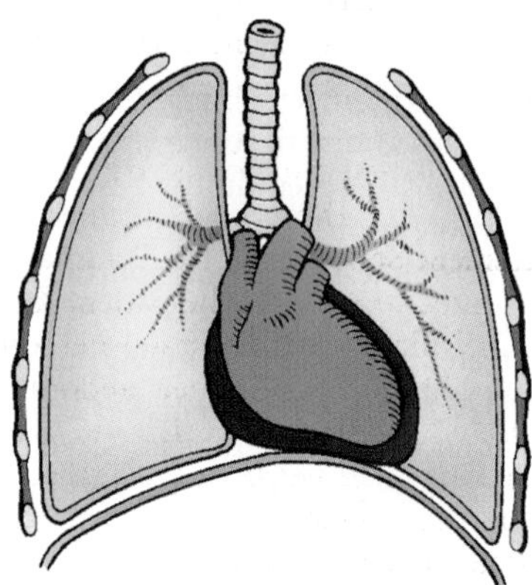

FIG 25-10 Cardiac Tamponade is the Progressive Accumulation of Blood in the Pericardial Sac.

Few clinical signs and symptoms are specific for BCI. Evidence of external chest trauma, such as steering wheel imprint or sternal fractures, should raise the suspicion for BCI. However, the presence of a sternal fracture does not predict the incidence of BCI. The patient may complain of chest pain that is similar to angina pain, but it is not typically relieved with nitroglycerin.[24] The chest pain is usually caused by associated injuries. The EAST guidelines for screening of BCI are listed in Box 25-10.[25] The ECG may reveal dysrhythmias, ST changes, heart block, or unexplained sinus tachycardia.

Medical management is aimed at preventing and treating complications. This approach may include administration of antidysrhythmic medications, treatment of heart failure, or insertion of a temporary pacemaker to control conduction abnormalities. Assessment of fluid and electrolyte balance is imperative to ensure adequate cardiac output and myocardial conduction.

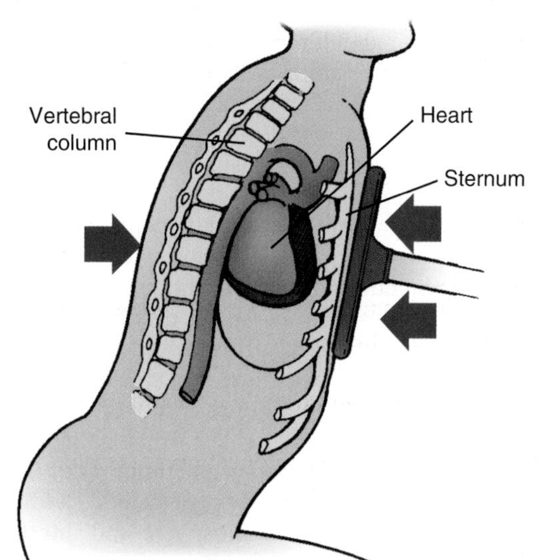

FIG 25-11 Blunt Cardiac Trauma. Sudden acceleration (as from contact with the steering wheel) can cause the heart to be thrown against the sternum.

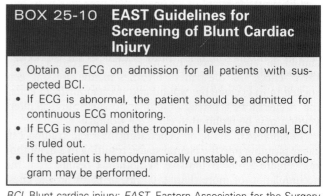

BOX 25-10 EAST Guidelines for Screening of Blunt Cardiac Injury

- Obtain an ECG on admission for all patients with suspected BCI.
- If ECG is abnormal, the patient should be admitted for continuous ECG monitoring.
- If ECG is normal and the troponin I levels are normal, BCI is ruled out.
- If the patient is hemodynamically unstable, an echocardiogram may be performed.

BCI, Blunt cardiac injury; *EAST*, Eastern Association for the Surgery of Trauma; *ECG*, electrocardiogram.

Aortic injury. Blunt aortic injury (BAI) is one of the most lethal blunt thoracic injuries. While BAI occurs in less than 1% of MVCs, it represents 16% of the deaths.[26] Sudden deceleration from speeds of 20 mph are most commonly associated with aortic injury.[26] Injuries associated with aortic injury include a first or second rib fracture, high sternal fracture, left clavicular fracture at the level of the sternal margin, and massive hemothorax. Blunt aortic injury should be suspected in all victims of trauma with a rapid deceleration or acceleration mechanism of injury.

The thoracic aorta is relatively mobile and tears at fixed anatomic points within the thorax. Sites of aortic disruption (in order of frequency) include the aortic isthmus, just distal to the subclavian artery (where the vessel is fixed to the chest by the ligamentum arteriosum); at the ascending aorta (where the aorta leaves the pericardial sac); at the descending aorta (where the aorta enters the diaphragm), and avulsion of the innominate artery from the aortic arch.[27]

The nurse assesses blood pressure in both arms because a tear in the aortic arch may create a pressure gradient resulting in blood pressure changes between upper extremities. If aortic disruption is suspected, blood pressure is also compared between upper and lower extremities. Baroreceptors are stimulated, resulting in upper extremity hypertension with relative lower extremity hypotension. Additional clinical assessment findings include a pulse deficit at any site, unexplained hypotension, sternal pain, precordial systolic murmur, hoarseness, dyspnea, and lower extremity sensory deficits.

Abdominal Injuries

Abdominal injuries often are associated with multisystem trauma. Abdominal injuries are the third leading cause of traumatic death. Injuries to the abdomen are the result of blunt or penetrating trauma. Two major life-threatening conditions that occur after abdominal trauma are hemorrhage and hollow viscus perforation with associated peritonitis. Death occurring after 48 hours following injury is the result of sepsis and its complications. The critical care nurse must pay particular attention to complication prevention strategies throughout the trauma cycle.

Mechanism of Injury

Blunt trauma to the abdomen. Blunt abdominal injuries are common. They result most often from MVCs, falls, and assaults. In MVCs, abdominal injury is more likely to occur when a vehicle is struck from the side. In the passenger position of the front seat, liver injury is likely when the point of impact is on the same side as the passenger. A driver is likely to sustain injury to the spleen when the impact is on the driver's side. Pedestrians hit by motor vehicles are at risk for serious abdominal injuries. Blunt trauma to the thorax can produce injuries to the liver, spleen, and diaphragm. Deceleration and direct forces can produce retroperitoneal hematomas. Blunt abdominal injuries often are hidden, requiring careful assessment and reassessment. Unrecognized abdominal trauma is a common cause of preventable death, and blunt abdominal injury deaths are more likely to be fatal than are penetrating abdominal injuries.

Penetrating trauma in the abdomen. Penetrating abdominal trauma is often caused by knives or bullets. The danger of penetrating abdominal trauma is that the outside appearance of the wound does not reflect the extent of internal injury. Commonly injured organs from knife wounds are the colon, liver, spleen, and diaphragm. Gunshot wounds to the abdomen usually are more serious than are stab wounds. A bullet destroys tissue along its path. Inside the abdomen, a bullet can travel in erratic paths and ricochet off bone. Death from penetrating injuries depends on the injury to major vascular structures and resultant intraabdominal hemorrhage.

Assessment of the Injured Abdomen

The initial assessment of the trauma patient, whether in the emergency department or the critical care unit, follows the primary and secondary survey techniques as outlined by ATLS and TNCC guidelines.[5,6] The initial physical assessment may be unreliable given the confounding influences of alcohol, illicit drugs, analgesics, and an altered level of consciousness.

Physical assessment. The location of entry and exit sites associated with penetrating trauma are assessed and documented. Inspection of the patient's abdomen may reveal purplish discoloration of the flanks or umbilicus (Cullen sign), which indicates blood in the abdominal wall. Ecchymosis in the flank area (Grey Turner sign) may indicate retroperitoneal bleeding or a pancreatic injury. A hematoma in the flank area suggests kidney injury. A distended abdomen may indicate the accumulation of blood, fluid, or gas resulting from a perforated organ or ruptured blood vessel. Auscultation of the abdomen may reveal friction rubs over the liver or spleen and may indicate rupture. The abdomen is assessed for rebound tenderness and rigidity. These assessment findings indicate peritoneal inflammation. Referred pain to the left shoulder (Kehr sign) may indicate a ruptured spleen or irritation of the diaphragm from bile or other material in the peritoneum. Subcutaneous emphysema palpated on the abdomen suggests free air as a result of a ruptured bowel.

Diagnostic procedures. Insertion of a nasogastric tube and urinary catheter serves as a useful diagnostic and therapeutic aid. A nasogastric tube can decompress the stomach, and the contents can be checked for blood. Urine obtained from the urinary catheter can also be tested for the presence of blood.

Serial laboratory test results may be nonspecific for the patient with abdominal trauma. Because of hemoconcentration, hemoglobin and hematocrit results may not reflect actual values. Serial values are more valuable in diagnosing abdominal injuries.

Because of the unreliability of physical examination alone in the patient suspected of having abdominal trauma, diagnostic testing may occur simultaneously during the primary and secondary surveys. Noninvasive tests include bedside ultrasound, CT, and chest and abdominal radiographs.

Bedside ultrasound. The bedside ultrasound, called the Focused Assessment Sonography for Trauma (FAST examination) is performed to evaluate the patient for the presence of intraabdominal blood, free fluid and hemoperitoneum.[28] Typically, the right and left upper abdominal quadrant areas are examined, the pericardial sac and the pelvis (Figure 25-12). An initial negative FAST result may be followed by serial ultrasound examinations, abdominal CT. Hemodynamically unstable patients with a positive FAST, specifically free fluid noted in the abdomen, generally undergo emergency surgery to achieve hemostasis.

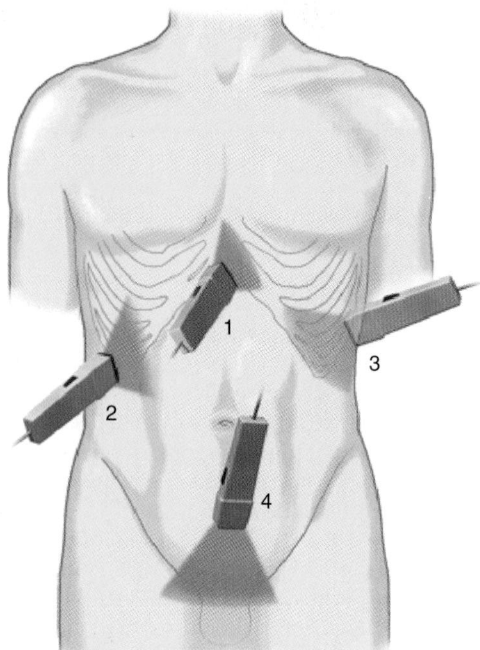

FIG 25-12 **The Focused Assessment Sonography for Trauma (FAST) Quadrants are Examined for the Presence of Free Fluid.** (From Moore FA, Moore EE. Initial management of life-threatening trauma. In: Ashley SW, editorial chair. *ACS Surgery: Principles and Practice.* Hamilton, Ontario, Canada: Decker Publishing; 2012.)

BOX 25-11 Damage Control Sequence

Initial Operation
- Control contamination.
- Control hemorrhage.
- Intraabdominal packing
- Temporary closure

Critical Care Unit Resuscitation
- Correct coagulopathy.
- Rewarming
- Maximize hemodynamics.
- Ventilatory support
- Injury identification

Planned Reoperation
- Pack removal
- Definitive repair

Abdominal CT scanning is the mainstay of diagnostic evaluation in the hemodynamically stable trauma patient.[28] Abdominal CT provides information about specific organ injury, pelvic injury, and retroperitoneal hemorrhage.

Combined Abdominal Organ Injuries

Patients with multiple visceral injuries may require surgical intervention that uses somewhat nontraditional techniques such as "damage control" surgery. The three phases of this treatment strategy are the 1) initial operation (damage control laparotomy), 2) critical care unit resuscitation, and 3) definitive reoperation also known as Staged Abdominal Reconstruction or STAR (Box 25-11).[29] The duration of the initial operation is kept to a minimum. The decision to abbreviate the initial operation is made early during surgery. Damage control laparotomy may be considered if some clinical parameters are met: acidosis (pH less than 7.2), hypothermia (temperature less than 35° C), and clinical coagulopathy and/or if the patient is receiving a massive transfusion.[28] Hypothermia induced by an open visceral cavity in conjunction with massive blood transfusion can lead to coagulopathy and continued bleeding, which results in shock and metabolic acidosis. The triad of hypothermia, coagulopathy, and acidosis creates a self-propagating cycle that can eventually lead to an irreversible physiologic insult. The initial operation must be completed quickly to terminate this self-propagating cycle. Reconstruction and formal closure of the wound may not be completed before the patient is transferred to the critical care unit.

TABLE 25-9 Interventions for Rewarming the Trauma Patient

INTERVENTION	EXTERNAL REWARMING PROCEDURES	INTERNAL REWARMING PROCEDURES
Passive	Maintain a warm room temperature.	Administer warmed, humidified oxygen.
	Remove all wet clothing and linen.	Administer warmed intravenous fluids.
	Cover the patient with blankets.	
	Avoid bathing patient until normothermia achieved.	
Active	Use radiant heat lamps, heating blankets or pads, and hot water bottles.	Perform gastrointestinal irrigation with warmed solutions.
		Perform extracorporeal rewarming for profound hypothermia.
		Use esophageal rewarming tubes.

Adapted from Flarity K. Environmental emergencies. In: Kunz Howard P, Steinmann R, eds. *Sheehy's Emergency Nursing: Principles and Practice.* 6th ed. St. Louis: Mosby; 2010.

The goal of the critical care phase of this strategy is to continue aggressive resuscitation and correct hypothermia, coagulopathy, and acidosis. Rewarming techniques, described in Table 25-9, are used to correct hypothermia. Coagulation factors and platelets may be administered to correct coagulopathies.

Abdominal compartment syndrome. The patient is assessed for additional complications, including ongoing hemorrhage, intraabdominal hypertension (IAH), and abdominal compartment syndrome. Abdominal compartment syndrome is defined as end-organ dysfunction caused by intraabdominal hypertension.[29] The increased pressure can be caused by bleeding, ileus, edema, or a noncompliant abdominal wall. Increased abdominal cavity pressure can impinge on diaphragmatic excursion and can affect ventilation. Clinical manifestations of abdominal compartment syndrome include decreased cardiac output, increased pulmonary vascular resistance, increased peak pulmonary pressures, decreased urine output, and hypoxia.[29] Intraabdominal pressure can be measured through a urinary catheter after the injection of 25 mL of sterile saline.[29] Intraabdominal hypertension (IAH) is defined as an intraabdominal pressure greater than or equal to 12 mm Hg (normal 5 to 7 mm Hg).[30] IAH may be graded: grade I (12 to 15 mm Hg), grade II (16 to 20 mm Hg), grade III (21 to 25 mm Hg), and grade IV (greater than 25 mm Hg).[30] The abdominal perfusion pressure may be calculated (MAP—IAP), with a normal value being greater than 60 mm Hg.

Surgical decompression of the abdomen may be required for abdominal pressures greater than 20 to 25 mm Hg that are associated with signs of organ dysfunction, such as decompensating heart, lung, and kidney status.[30] After surgical decompression is completed and the pressure relieved, the patient may receive a temporary abdominal closure ("open abdomen"), wherein the skin and abdominal fascia are left open. This involves temporarily closing the abdomen with a sterile perforated plastic sheet, clips, vacuum-assisted techniques, and many other options. In some cases closed suction drains are brought out through a sterile plastic drape over the entire wound. The wound is closed permanently in the days, weeks, and months following the surgery or it is allowed to heal by secondary intention and eventual skin grafting.

Specific Organ Injuries

Physical assessment findings and CT scans aid in making a diagnosis of specific abdominal organ injury. The medical and nursing management vary according to specific organ injuries. Liver, spleen, and bowel injuries, which are seen more commonly, are discussed here.

Liver injuries. The liver is the primary organ injured in penetrating trauma and the second most often injured organ in blunt trauma. Abdominal CT is considered to be the most reliable diagnostic tool to identify and assess the severity of the injury to the liver. The severity of liver injuries is graded to provide a mechanism for determining the amount of trauma sustained by that organ, the care needed, and the possible outcomes (Table 25-10). Nonoperative management is considered the standard of care for hemodynamically stable patients with liver injury.[31]

TABLE 25-10 Liver Injury Scale

	GRADE*	INJURY DESCRIPTION
I	Hematoma	Subcapsular, <10% surface area
	Laceration	Capsular tear, <1 cm parenchymal depth
II	Hematoma	Subcapsular, 10%-50% surface area; intraparenchymal <10 cm in diameter
	Laceration	Capsular tear, 1-3 cm parenchymal depth, <10 cm long
III	Hematoma	Subcapsular, >50% surface area or expanding; ruptured subcapsular or parenchymal hematoma; intraparenchymal hematoma >10 cm or expanding
	Laceration	>3 cm parenchymal depth
IV	Laceration	Parenchymal disruption involving 25%-75% of hepatic lobe or 1-3 Couinaud's segments within a single lobe
V	Laceration	Parenchymal disruption involving >75% of hepatic lobe or >3 Couinaud's segments within a single lobe
	Vascular	Juxtahepatic venous injuries (retrohepatic vena cava, central major hepatic veins)
VI	Vascular	Hepatic avulsion

*Advance one grade for multiple injuries up to grade II.
Modified from Trunkey DD. Hepatic trauma: contemporary management. *Surg Clin North Am.* 2004: 84:437.

Hemodynamically unstable patients with liver trauma or who have peritonitis require surgical intervention.[31] Hemodynamic instability can result from hemorrhage and hypovolemic shock, leading to fluid volume deficit, decreased cardiac output, and decreased tissue perfusion. A massive transfusion protocol may be implemented to restore blood volume and correct coagulopathies. A crucial nursing responsibility is to monitor the patient's response to medical therapies. Continued hemodynamic instability (e.g., hypotension, decreased cardiac output) despite aggressive medical intervention may indicate continued hemorrhage, in which case an exploratory laparotomy may be required to determine and correct the source of bleeding. The patient's postoperative course may be complicated by coagulopathy, acidosis, and hypothermia. Jaundice may occur as a sign of liver dysfunction, but it may also be caused by reabsorption of hematomas or breakdown of transfused red blood cells.

Spleen injuries. The spleen is the organ most commonly injured by blunt abdominal trauma and is second to the liver as a source of life-threatening hemorrhage. Spleen injuries, like liver injuries, are graded for the purpose of determining the amount of trauma sustained, the care needed, and the possible outcomes (Table 25-11). Hemodynamically stable patients may be monitored in the critical care unit by means of serial hematocrit values and vital signs.

Patients who exhibit hemodynamic instability require operative intervention with urgent laparotomy.[31] Patients who have had a splenectomy are at risk for the development of overwhelming postsplenectomy sepsis with streptococcal pneumonia. These patients require the polyvalent pneumococcal vaccine (Pneumovax) to help promote immunity against most pneumococcal bacteria. Patients with isolated spleen injuries that require surgical intervention rarely are admitted to the critical care unit. Complications after splenic trauma include wound infection, sepsis, subdiaphragmatic abscess, and fistulas of the colon, pancreas, and stomach.

Hollow viscus injuries. The term hollow viscus refers to the hollow organs in the abdomen, such as the stomach, small intestine, and large intestine. Hollow viscus injury (HVI) can result from blunt or penetrating trauma. The diagnosis of HVI is challenging, as injuries may not show up on CT or ultrasound. A delay in the time to diagnosis contributes to

TABLE 25-11 **Spleen Injury Scale**

GRADE*		INJURY DESCRIPTION
I	Hematoma	Subcapsular, <10% surface area
	Laceration	Capsular tear, <1 cm, parenchymal depth
II	Hematoma	Subcapsular, 10%-50% surface area; intraparenchymal <5 cm in diameter
	Laceration	Capsular tear: 1-3 cm parenchymal depth, which does not involve a trabecular vessel
III	Hematoma	Subcapsular, >50% surface area or expanding; ruptured subcapsular or parenchymal hematoma; intraparenchymal hematoma >5 cm or expanding
IV	Laceration	>3 cm parenchymal depth or involving trabecular vessels
	Laceration	Laceration involving segmental or hilar vessels producing major devascularization (>25% of spleen)
V	Laceration	Completely shattered spleen
	Vascular	Hilar vascular injury that devascularizes spleen

*Advance one grade for multiple injuries up to grade II.

complications. One study demonstrated that serial measurements of the white blood cell (WBC) count can help determine the presence or absence of HVI.[32] Regardless of the mechanism of injury, intestinal contents (e.g., bile, stool, enzymes, bacteria) can leak into the peritoneum and cause peritonitis. Surgical resection and repair is almost always required. The patient's postoperative course is dictated by the amount of spillage of intestinal contents. The patient is observed for signs of sepsis and for abscess or fistula formation.

Genitourinary Injuries

Trauma to the genitourinary tract seldom occurs as an isolated injury. A genitourinary injury must be suspected in any patient with penetrating trauma to the torso; pelvic fracture; blunt trauma to the lower chest or flank; contusions, hematoma, tenderness over the flank, lower abdomen, or perineum; genital swelling or discoloration; blood at the urethral meatus; hematuria after urinary drainage catheter placement; or difficulty with micturition.

Mechanism of Injury

Genitourinary injuries, like all other traumatic injuries, can result from blunt or penetrating trauma. In one study, approximately 5% of patients with pelvic fractures had concomitant genitourinary injury, with men experiencing genitourinary trauma more frequently than women.[33]

Assessment

Evaluation of genitourinary trauma begins after the primary survey has been conducted and immediate life-threatening conditions have been effectively managed. The conscious patient may complain of flank pain or colic pain. Rebound tenderness can be elicited if intraperitoneal extravasation of urine has occurred. Inspection may reveal blood at the urethral meatus. Bluish discoloration of the flanks may indicate retroperitoneal bleeding, whereas perineal discoloration may indicate a pelvic fracture and possible bladder or urethral injury. Hematuria is the most common assessment finding with genitourinary trauma; however, the absence of gross or microscopic hematuria does not exclude a urinary tract injury.

Specific Genitourinary Injuries

Kidney trauma. The kidney is most often injured by blunt trauma, resulting in contusions or lacerations without urinary extravasation. Injury to the kidneys may be reflected by flank ecchymosis and fracture of inferior ribs or spinous processes. Gross or microscopic hematuria may be present; however, the extent of kidney damage is often incongruous with the degree of hematuria. Gross hematuria can exist with minor injuries and usually clears within a few hours. CT is the most accurate modality available for diagnosing kidney injury because it can assess the extent of parenchymal laceration, urine extravasation, surrounding hemorrhage, and the presence of vascular injury.

Contusions and minor lacerations can usually be treated with observation. The success of nonoperative management may be enhanced by using angiographic embolization. Nonoperative treatment of patients with major lacerations and vascular injuries may be achieved in those who are hemodynamically stable. Operative interventions may be performed in patients with kidney injuries with a devascularized segment of the kidney. Postoperative and postinjury complications can include infection, hemorrhage, infarction, extravasation, calcification, acute kidney injury, and hypertension.

Bladder trauma. A large percentage of bladder injuries result from pelvic fractures.[33] Physical findings may include lower abdominal bruising, distention, pain and urinary retention. Bladder injuries are classified as contusions, extraperitoneal ruptures, intraperitoneal ruptures, or combined injuries. The type of injury depends on the location and strength of the blunt force and volume of urine in the bladder at the time of injury. Extraperitoneal rupture of the bladder may be managed conservatively with catheterization and antibiotics for 7 to 10 days. Unresolved extravasation may require surgical intervention.

Nursing Management

Nursing priorities for the patient with genitourinary trauma include **1) assessment for hemorrhage, 2) maintenance of fluid and electrolyte balance, and 3) maintaining patency of drains and tubes.**

After the patient is admitted to the critical care unit, the nurse makes an assessment according to the ATLS guidelines. After the patient's condition has stabilized, nursing management of postoperative kidney trauma is similar to that for genitourinary surgery. The primary nursing interventions include assessment for hemorrhage, maintenance of fluid and electrolyte balance, and maintenance of patency of drains and tubes. Measurement of urinary output includes drainage from the urinary catheter and rarely nephrostomy or suprapubic tubes. Drainage from these areas is recorded separately.

Urine output is measured frequently until bloody drainage and clots have cleared. Gentle irrigation of drainage tubes may be required to clear clots and maintain the patency of the tubes.

COMPLICATIONS OF TRAUMA

Hypermetabolism

Nutritional support is an essential component in the care of critically ill trauma patients. Within 24 to 48 hours after traumatic injury, a predictable hypermetabolic response occurs. The metabolic response to injury mobilizes amino acids and accelerates protein synthesis to support wound healing and the immunologic response to invading organisms. Stress hypermetabolism occurs after any major injury and is characterized by increases in metabolic rate and oxygen consumption. Energy requirements accelerate to promote immune function and tissue repair. The goal of early aggressive nutrition is to maintain host defenses by supporting this hypermetabolism and to preserve lean body mass.

Most nutrition experts advocate beginning enteral nutrition as early as possible. Current guidelines recommend enteral feedings be initiated within 72 hours for patients with blunt and penetrating abdominal injuries and those with severe head injuries.[34] Enteral feeding sites can include the gastric route or any site beyond the pylorus of the stomach, including the duodenum and jejunum. Prompt feeding tube placement by the critical care nurse must be a priority, unless contraindicated. Diminished or absent bowel sounds do not mean the small bowel is not working. Small bowel function and the ability to absorb nutrients remain intact, despite the presence of gastroparesis and absent bowel sounds. Because access to the stomach can be obtained more quickly and easily than the duodenum, early provision of nutrition is possible.[34] Patients at risk for pulmonary aspiration due to gastric retention or gastroesophageal reflux should receive enteral feedings into the jejunum.[34]

Infection

Infection remains a major source of mortality and morbidity in critical care units. The trauma patient is at risk for infection because of contaminated wounds, invasive therapeutic and diagnostic catheters, intubation and mechanical ventilation, host susceptibility, and the critical care environment. Nursing management must include interventions to decrease and eliminate the trauma patient's risk of infection. The patient with multiple trauma is at risk for infection because of host susceptibility (including preexisting medical conditions) and the adverse effect of trauma on the immune system.

Wound contamination poses an infection risk for the trauma patient, especially with injuries resulting from deep or penetrating trauma. Exogenous bacteria (from the external environment) can enter through open wounds. Exogenous bacteria can be introduced by dirt, grass, and debris inoculated into the wound at the time of injury or be introduced by personnel during wound care. Endogenous bacteria (from the internal environment) can be released as a result of gastrointestinal or genitourinary perforation, which spills bacteria into the internal environment.

Meticulous wound care is essential. The goals of wound care include minimizing infection risks, removing dead and devitalized tissue, allowing for wound drainage, and promoting wound epithelialization and contraction. Wound healing also is accomplished through interventions that promote tissue perfusion of well-oxygenated blood and that ensure adequate nutritional support for wound healing.

Standard interventions for the prevention of ventilator-associated pneumonia, catheter-associated urinary tract infections, and central–line-associated bloodstream infection apply to the trauma patient. Proper hand hygiene, invasive catheter care, prompt removal of unnecessary tubes and lines, patient positioning, and medical asepsis or sterile technique for all invasive procedures are paramount to optimal patient outcome.

Severe Sepsis and Septic Shock

The patient with multiple injuries is at risk for overwhelming infections, sepsis and septic shock. The source of sepsis in the trauma patient can be invasive therapeutic and diagnostic catheters or wound contamination with exogenous or endogenous bacteria. The source of the sepsis must be promptly evaluated. Gram stain and cultures of blood, urine, sputum, invasive catheters, and wounds are obtained (see Chapter 26).

Pulmonary Complications

Respiratory Failure

Posttraumatic respiratory failure is often due to the development of ARDS.[35] ARDS can be caused by direct injury to the lungs or indirect injury (see "Acute Respiratory Distress Syndrome" in Chapter 15). Primary direct injuries in the trauma patient can include aspiration, inhalation, and pulmonary contusion. The indirect injuries include sepsis, massive transfusion, fat emboli, and missed injury. ARDS in the trauma patient can develop 24 to 72 hours after initial injury. The patient receiving multiple blood products, particularly fresh-frozen plasma, must also be monitored for *transfusion-related acute lung injury* (TRALI). Signs of TRALI are similar to those of ARDS, although there is a temporal relationship between the new onset of respiratory distress and the transfusion of blood products.[36]

Fat Embolism Syndrome

Fat embolism syndrome can occur as a complication of orthopedic trauma. The clinical onset of fat embolism syndrome ranges from 12 to 72 hours after injury.[37] Fat embolism syndrome appears to develop as a result of fat droplets that leak from fractured bone and embolize to the lungs. The droplets are broken down into free fatty acids that are toxic to the pulmonary microvascular membranes. Pulmonary fat emboli alter pulmonary hemodynamics and pulmonary vascular permeability. The lung becomes highly edematous and hemorrhagic. The clinical presentation is almost indistinguishable from that of ARDS. Early stabilization of unstable extremity fractures may limit the seeding of fat droplets into the pulmonary system.[37]

Pain

Pain may come from many sources, including surgery, procedures, and trauma. Trauma may contribute to cellular death and inflammation that leads to pain. Relief of pain is a major component in the care of trauma patients.

An issue that often complicates pain management is the high incidence of substance abuse among patients who sustain traumatic injury. Trauma patients, regardless of

BOX 25-12 Etiologic Factors in Post-Traumatic Acute Kidney Injury

- Preexisting disease
  - Hypertension
  - Heart failure
  - Diabetes
  - Chronic kidney disease
  - Chronic liver disease
- Prolonged shock states
- Profound acidosis
- SIRS or reperfusion injury
- Abdominal compartment syndrome
- Muscle ischemia; myoglobinuria
- Microemboli
- Nephrotoxic medications
- Radiocontrast dye

SIRS, Systemic inflammatory response syndrome.

substance use history, require multimodal acute pain management (see Chapter 8).

Kidney Complications

Acute Kidney Injury Post-Trauma

Assessment and ongoing monitoring of kidney function is critical to the survival of the trauma patient. The cause of posttraumatic acute kidney injury is complex and may involve a variety of factors, as listed in Box 25-12.

Prevention of kidney failure is the best treatment, and it begins with ensuring adequate volume to provide adequate renal artery perfusion. Serial assessments of blood urea nitrogen (BUN) and creatinine levels commonly are used to evaluate kidney function. Progressive kidney failure requires prompt diagnosis and treatment (see "Acute Kidney Injury" in Chapter 20).

Rhabdomyolysis and Myoglobinuria

Patients with a crush injury are susceptible to the development of rhabdomyolysis, with subsequent secondary kidney failure. Crush injuries can compromise blood flow. Loss of arterial blood flow, particularly to the extremities, results in the loss of oxygen transport to distal tissues and ischemia. This initiates a cascade of events that leads to the necrosis of skeletal muscle cells. As cells die, intracellular contents—particularly potassium and myoglobin—are released. Myoglobin, a muscular pigment, is a large molecule that gets lodged in the glomerulus, resulting in presence of myoglobinuria. Circulating myoglobin can lead to the development of kidney failure by three mechanisms: decreased renal perfusion, cast formation with tubular obstruction, and direct toxic effects of myoglobin in the kidney tubules.[38]

Dark tea-colored urine suggests myoglobinuria. Testing for myoglobin in the urine can be done but may take several days, depending on laboratory resources available for this test. The most rapid screening test is a serum creatine kinase level. Urine output and serial creatine kinase levels should be monitored.

Rhabdomyolysis should be suspected in all patients who experience crush injuries in which blood flow to the muscle is interrupted for a prolonged amount of time. Prevention of kidney dysfunction is paramount through the administration of IV fluids.[38] If rhabdomyolysis is diagnosed, treatment is aimed at prevention of subsequent kidney failure. Aggressive administration of intravenous fluids increases renal blood flow and decreases the concentration of nephrotoxic pigments.[38] Alkalinization of the urine and administration of diuretics have been studied, but their roles in the prevention or management of rhabdomyolysis are not firmly established.[38] Nursing management is directed toward achievement of fluid and electrolyte balance. The patient should be assessed for hypernatremia, hyperosmolarity, acute kidney injury, and volume status.

Vascular Complications

Compartment Syndrome

Compartment syndrome is a condition in which increased pressure within a limited space compromises circulation, resulting in ischemia and necrosis of tissues within that space. Among those at high risk for the development of compartment syndrome are patients with lower extremity trauma, including fractures, penetrating trauma, vascular ruptures, massive tissue injuries, or venous obstruction. Clinical manifestations of compartment syndrome include obvious swelling and tightness of an extremity, paresis, and pain of the affected extremity. Diminished pulses and decreased capillary refill do not reliably identify compartment syndrome because they may be intact until after irreversible changes have occurred. Elevated intracompartmental pressures confirm the diagnosis. The treatment can consist of simple interventions, such as removing an occlusive dressing, to more complex interventions, including a fasciotomy.

Venous Thromboembolism

Despite improvements in the care of the trauma patient, venous thromboembolism (VTE), which includes both DVT and pulmonary emboli, remains an important cause of morbidity and mortality in the multiply injured trauma patient. Major trauma patients are at very high risk for VTE.[39] The factors that form the basis of VTE pathophysiology are blood stasis, injury to the intimal surface of the vessel, and hypercoagulopathy. Trauma patients are at risk for VTE because of endothelial injury, coagulopathy, and immobility.

Trauma patients are at the greatest risk for developing thromboembolism early in their hospitalization. Prevention is key. Routine thromboprophylaxis for the high-risk trauma patient includes use of low–molecular-weight heparin starting as soon as it is considered safe to do so and use of a mechanical method of prophylaxis, such as sequential compression devices.[39] For patients in whom the lower leg is inaccessible, foot pumps may act as an effective alternative to lower the rate of VTE.

Missed Injury

Nursing assessment of the multiply injured patient in the critical care unit may reveal missed diseases or missed injuries. Missed injuries have a reported incidence of 1.3% to 39% and are a cause of morbidity and mortality.[38] Missed disorders may include preexisting undiagnosed medical illnesses such as endocrine disorders (diabetes, hypothyroidism), myocardial infarction, hypertension, decreased respiratory reserve, undiagnosed kidney failure, or malnutrition. Patients who have head injuries with a GCS of 8 or less and greater injury

BOX 25-13 Factors Contributing to Missed Injuries

Hemodynamic Instability
- Shock states in the emergency department
- Aggressive resuscitation
- Emergent surgery taking precedence over thorough secondary surveys

Alterations in Consciousness
- Presence of drugs or alcohol intoxication confuses physical assessments and masks physical findings.
- Disoriented patients are challenging to assess.
- Agitation makes diagnostic testing challenging.
- Patients with altered consciousness cannot provide a history of the injury.

severity scores are more likely to have missed injuries or delayed diagnoses.[40]

Occasionally, injuries may not be diagnosed in the precritical care phases. Missed injuries are commonly discovered in the first 24 to 48 hours of the hospital stay during the routine assessments of the trauma tertiary survey. Injuries are missed for a variety of reasons as summarized in Box 25-13. In the critical care unit, a missed injury may be suspected if the patient fails to show appropriate response to medical or surgical intervention. Change in the character of drainage from wounds or catheters may represent biliary or duodenal injuries. Hypotension and a falling hematocrit level despite aggressive fluid administration may indicate an expanding hematoma. As the patient begins to mobilize, small bone fractures and sprains may manifest. The critical care nurse must be alert to the possibility of a missed injury, especially when the patient does not appear to be responding appropriately to interventions. The physician must be notified immediately because potential complications of infection and hemorrhage may be life-threatening. Nurses play a key role in identifying missed injuries, particularly when patients regain consciousness and begin to increase their activity.

Multiple Organ Dysfunction Syndrome

MODS is a clinical syndrome of progressive dysfunction of organ systems. Trauma patients are at high risk for systemic inflammatory response syndrome (SIRS) and MODS. Organ dysfunction can be the result of primary MODS, which is caused by direct traumatic injury, as may occur with acute lung dysfunction because of pulmonary contusion. Organ dysfunction that occurs later in the trauma patient's critical care course, secondary MODS, results from uncontrolled systemic inflammation with resultant organ dysfunction. Trauma patients may experience primary and secondary MODS. Treatment is aimed at controlling or eliminating the source of inflammation, maintenance of oxygen delivery and consumption, and nutritional and metabolic support for individual organs (see Chapter 26).

MEETING THE NEEDS OF FAMILY MEMBERS AND SIGNIFICANT OTHERS

The impact of traumatic injury can be devastating for patients and for family members and significant others. They are faced with a crisis situation for which they have had little time to prepare. Trauma can precipitate a crisis within the family. Families may exhibit physical and sociocultural reactions and a combination of emotional reactions, including anger, fear, powerlessness, confusion, and mistrust. Recovery from traumatic injury can be long and frustrating for families. There may be many peaks and valleys of good days and bad days. During this time, the family may exhaust its social and financial support systems. Nurses should recognize this and facilitate supportive relationships for families.

A trend has evolved to move away from a paternalistic model of care to one that incorporates the family into all aspects of care, including resuscitation. Family members wish to remain close to their loved ones during these times, and there has been demonstrated benefit to the patient and the family in this model of care delivery.[41] One study demonstrated that family members present during trauma resuscitation suffered no ill psychologic effects and scored equivalent to those family members who were not present on anxiety, satisfaction, and well-being measures.[41] Regardless of the specific system of care delivery, the nurse ensures the family is supported during all aspects of care.

A valuable intervention is to bring families of trauma patients together in support groups. Trauma family support groups can offer sharing of experiences, expression of emotions, mutual support, sharing of coping strategies, and education about hospital and community services.

TRAUMA IN THE OLDER PATIENT

Trauma affects people of all ages. Older patients are predisposed to traumatic injuries because of the inevitable consequences of aging. The ability to react to or avoid environmental hazards is impaired because of age-related deterioration of the senses and changes in motor strength, postural stability, balance, and coordination (see Chapter 7).

Older persons experience most of the falls that result in injuries, and these falls are likely to occur from level surfaces or steps.[42] Factors that predispose older persons to falls are summarized in Box 25-14. Because many of the falls may be caused by an underlying medical condition (e.g., syncope, myocardial infarction, dysrhythmias), management of the older patient who has fallen must include an evaluation of events and conditions immediately preceding the fall.

The exposure of older adults to MVC trauma is a consequence of the increasing growth of the older population and the growing number of older drivers and occupants of motor vehicles. Factors that predispose older adults to MVCs are summarized in Box 25-15. Many deaths of older individuals occur in crosswalks. Physiologic deterioration of cerebral and motor skills and alterations in visual and auditory acuity cause older pedestrians to walk directly into the path of oncoming vehicles.

Trauma in older adults can be associated with higher mortality rates, even when the injuries are less severe. Older adults have a higher complication rate and a higher mortality rate, starting at age 65 years, because of preexisting medical conditions, decreased physiologic reserves, and decreased ability to compensate for severe injury.[43] Older patients who do survive traumatic injury are often faced with changes in their preinjury functional status. Relatively minor trauma can be the event that changes the lifestyle of an older person from

BOX 25-14 Risk Factors for Falls in Older Adults

Acute Illness
- Cerebrovascular accidents
- Dysrhythmias
- Syncope
- Diabetes

Cognitive Impairment
- Dementia

Neuromuscular Disorders
- Arthritis
- Lower extremity weakness
- Unstable gait

Medications
- Antidepressants
- Benzodiazepines
- Diuretics
- Phenothiazines

BOX 25-15 Factors that Predispose Older Adults to Motor Vehicle Crashes

- Alterations in visual and auditory acuity
- Deterioration in strength and slower reaction times
- Diminution of cerebral skills
- Diminution of motor skills
- Exacerbation of acute or chronic medical conditions
- Medications that may interfere with safe driving

one of relative independence to one that requires prolonged rehabilitation or skilled nursing care. Discharge planning early in the patient's hospitalization is necessary.

The concept of *limited physiologic reserve* in the older trauma patient highlights the key difference between the younger trauma patient with normal physiologic reserve and the older patient with underlying physiologic derangements. Age-related changes that occur in virtually every organ system may not produce evidence of organ dysfunction in the resting state. However, the ability of organs to augment function in response to traumatic stress may be greatly compromised. Fluid resuscitation is an integral part of trauma resuscitation. Patients on chronic diuretic therapy may require more volume and potassium supplementation as a result of chronic volume and potassium depletion. The assessment and management of hypovolemic shock is more complex in the older trauma patient. Many older adults are taking beta-blocker medications, thereby limiting an increase in heart rate in response to blood loss; this obscures one of the earliest signs of hypovolemia—tachycardia.[5] Loss of physiologic reserve and the presence of preexisting medical conditions are likely to produce further conflicting hemodynamic data. The older patient's lack of physiologic reserve makes it imperative that early nutritional support is initiated.

CASE STUDY Patient with Trauma

Brief Patient History
Mr. G is a 21-year-old man. He was traveling in the back of a pickup truck that collided with another vehicle. He was ejected onto the side of the road and now is not awake and is barely breathing. He was intubated by emergency services, placed in a collar, and immobilized.

Clinical Assessment
Mr. G is admitted to the emergency department with minimal signs of external injury except for some small abrasions to the side of his face.

Diagnostic Procedures
Admission CT scan shows a large subdural hematoma.

Radiography confirms appropriate placement of the endotracheal tube.

Baseline vital signs are blood pressure (BP) 110/60, heart rate (HR) 108 (sinus tachycardia), respiratory rate (RR) 30, temperature (T) 98.3°F, O_2 saturation 88%, Glasgow Coma Scale 7.

Medical Diagnosis
Mr. G is diagnosed with subdural hematoma secondary to trauma.

Questions
1. What major outcomes do you expect to achieve for this patient?
2. What problems or risks must be managed to achieve these outcomes?
3. What interventions must be initiated to monitor, prevent, manage, or eliminate the problems and risks identified above?
4. What interventions should be initiated to promote optimal functioning, safety, and well-being of the patient?
5. What possible learning needs would you anticipate for this patient?
6. What cultural and age-related factors might have a bearing on the patient's plan of care?

Many older adults take daily anticoagulants and/or antiplatelet medications to prevent thrombotic or embolic complications from preexisting medical conditions. Traumatic injury in conjunction with a prolonged International Normalized Ratio (INR) greatly increases the risk of major hemorrhage. It is essential that systemic anticoagulation be corrected as soon as possible after admission, and when head injury is suspected, a CT of the head is urgently obtained.[43]

Trauma protocols are well-established for the management of young patients after injury. Clinicians increasingly are recognizing that these protocols must be individualized for the older trauma patient. The best outcomes for this patient population have been achieved through early, appropriate, aggressive trauma care, with admission to a trauma center with resources and protocols to provide excellent care to injured adults regardless of age.[43] Clinical practice guidelines that discuss trauma diagnostic tests and procedures can be obtained on the websites of the major professional organizations that are listed in the Internet Resources Box 25-16.

BOX 25-16 TRAUMA INTERNET RESOURCES

American College of Surgeons (ACS): https://www.facs.org/
ACS—Advanced Trauma Life Support (ATLS): https://www.facs.org/quality-programs/trauma/atls
Emergency Nurses Association (ENA): www.ena.org
ENA—Trauma Nurse Core Course (TNCC): http://www.ena.org/education/ENPC-TNCC/tncc/Pages/aboutcourse.aspx
Eastern Association for the Surgery of Trauma (EAST): https://www.east.org/resources/treatment-guidelines

REFERENCES

1. Centers for Disease Control and Prevention: Preventing violence against women: program activities guide. http://www.cdc.gov/violenceprevention/pdf/IPV-SV_Program_Activities_Guide-a.pdf. Accessed August 17, 2014.
2. Wu V, Huff H, Bhandari M: Pattern of physical injury associated with intimate partner violence in women presenting to the emergency department: A systematic review and meta-analysis, *Trauma Violence Abuse* 11(2):71, 2010.
3. Centers for Disease Control and Prevention: Impaired Driving: Get the Facts. http://www.cdc.gov/motorvehiclesafety/impaired_driving/impaired-drv_factsheet.html. Accessed August 17, 2014.
4. Neumann T, et al: Does the alcohol use disorders identification test–consumption identify the same patient population as the full 10-item Alcohol Use Disorders Identification Test? *J Subst Abuse Treat* 43:80, 2012.
5. American College of Surgeons: *Advanced Trauma Life Support*, ed 9, Chicago, IL, 2012, American College of Surgeons.
6. Emergency Nurses Association: *Trauma Nursing Core Course Provider Manual*, ed 7, Des Plaines, IL, 2014, Emergency Nurses Association.
7. Hodgman EI, et al: Base deficit as a marker of survival after traumatic injury: consistent across changing patient populations and resuscitation paradigms, *J Trauma* 72(4):844, 2012.
8. Elmer J, Wilcox SR, Raja AS: Massive transfusion in traumatic shock, *J Emerg Med* 44(4):829, 2013.
9. Centers for Disease Control and Prevention: National Center on Injury Prevention and Control. Traumatic brain injury. http://www.cdc.gov/ncipc/tbi/TBI.htm. Accessed August 17, 2014.
10. Spiotta AM, et al: Brain tissue oxygen–directed management and outcome in patients with severe traumatic brain injury, *J Neurosurg* 113:571, 2010.
11. Giza CC, et al: Summary of evidence-based guideline update: evaluation and management of concussion in sports: report of the Guideline Development Subcommittee of the American Academy of Neurology, *Neurology* 80(24):2250, 2013.
12. Cooper JD, et al: Decompressive craniectomy in diffuse traumatic brain injury, *N Engl J Med* 364:1493, 2010.
13. Brain Trauma Foundation: Guidelines for the management of severe traumatic brain injury, *J Neurotrauma* 24(Suppl 1):1, 2007.
14. Alali AS, et al: Beta blockers for acute traumatic brain injury: a systematic review and meta-analysis, *Neurocrit Care* 20(3):514, 2014.
15. National Spinal Cord Injury Statistical Center: Spinal cord injury facts and figures at a glance, 2013. https://www.nscisc.uab.edu/PublicDocuments/fact_figures_docs/Facts%202013.pdf. Accessed August 17, 2014.
16. Como JJ, et al: Practice management guidelines for identification of cervical spine injuries following trauma: update from the Eastern Association for the Surgery of Trauma practice management guidelines committee, *J Trauma* 67:651, 2009.
17. Bracken MB: Steroids for acute spinal cord injury, *Cochrane Database Syst Rev* (18):CD001046, 1, 2012.
18. Walters BC, et al: Guidelines for the management of acute cervical spine and spinal cord injuries: 2013 update, *Neurosurgery* 60(Suppl 1):82, 2013.
19. Kiraly L, Schreiber M: Management of the crushed chest, *Crit Care Med* 38(9):S469, 2010.
20. Battle CE, Hutchings H, Evans PA: Risk factors that predict mortality in patients with blunt chest wall trauma: a systematic review and meta-analysis, *Injury* 43:8, 2012.
21. Simon B, et al: Management of pulmonary contusion and flail chest: an Eastern Association for the Surgery of Trauma practice management guideline, *J Trauma Acute Care Surg* 73(5, Suppl 4):S351, 2012.
22. Mowery NT, et al: Practice management guidelines for management of hemothorax and occult pneumothorax, *J Trauma* 70(2):510, 2011.
23. Press GM, Miller S: Utility of the cardiac component of FAST in blunt trauma, *J Emerg Med* 44(1):9, 2013.
24. Bock JS, Benitez M: Blunt cardiac injury, *Cardiol Clin* 30:545, 2012.
25. Clancy K, et al: Screening for blunt cardiac injury: An Eastern Association for the Surgery of Trauma practice management guideline, *J Trauma Acute Care Surg* 73(5 Suppl 4):S301, 2012.
26. Neschis DG, Scalea TM, Flinn WR, Griffith BP: Blunt aortic injury, *N Engl J Med* 359:1708, 2008.
27. Kwolek CJ, Blazick E: Current Management of traumatic thoracic aortic injury, *Semin Vasc Surg* 23:215, 2011.
28. Moore CL, Copel JA: Point-of-care ultrasonography, *N Engl J Med* 364(8):749, 2011.
29. De Waele JJ, De Laet I, Kirkpatrick AW, Hoste E: Intra-abdominal hypertension and abdominal compartment syndrome, *Am J Kidney Dis* 57(1):159, 2010.
30. Stassen NA, et al: Nonoperative management of blunt hepatic injury: an Eastern Association for the Surgery of Trauma practice management guideline, *J Trauma Acute Care Surg* 73(5 Suppl 4):S288, 2012.
31. Stassen NA, et al: Selective nonoperative management of blunt splenic injury: an Eastern Association for the Surgery of Trauma practice management guideline, *J Trauma Acute Care Surg* 73(5, Suppl 4):S294, 2012.
32. Schnüriger B, et al: Serial white blood cell counts in trauma: Do they predict a hollow viscus injury? *J Trauma* 69:302, 2010.
33. Bjurlin MA, Fantus RJ, Mellett MM, Goble SM: Genitourinary injuries in pelvic fracture morbidity and mortality using the National Trauma Data Bank, *J Trauma* 67:1033, 2010.

34. Jacobs DG, et al: Practice management guidelines for nutritional support of the trauma patient, *J Trauma* 57(3):660, 2004.
35. Chirag SV, et al: The impact of development of acute lung injury on hospital mortality in critically ill trauma patients, *Crit Care Med* 36:2309, 2008.
36. Alexander V, et al: Risk factors and outcome of transfusion-related acute lung injury in the critically ill: a nested case-control study, *Crit Care Med* 38(3):771, 2010.
37. Sara S, et al: Fat emboli syndrome in a nondisplaced tibia fracture, *J Orthop Trauma* 25(2):e27, 2011.
38. Bosch X, Poch E, Grau JM: Rhabdomyolysis and acute kidney injury, *N Engl J Med* 361:62, 2009.
39. Muntz JE, Michota FA: Prevention and management of venous thromboembolism in the surgical patient: options by surgery type and individual patient risk factors, *Am J Surg* 199:S11, 2010.
40. Pfeifer R, Pape HC: Missed injuries in trauma patients: a literature review, *Patient Saf Surg* 2:20, 2011.
41. Pasquale MA, et al: Family presence during trauma resuscitation: ready for primetime? *J Trauma* 69(5):1092, 2010.
42. Konstantinos S, et al: Ground level falls are associated with significant mortality in elderly patients, *J Trauma* 69(4):821, 2010.
43. Calland JF, et al: Evaluation and management of geriatric trauma: an Eastern Association for the Surgery of Trauma practice management guideline, *J Trauma Acute Care Surg* 73(5, Suppl 4):S345, 2012.

CHAPTER 26

Shock, Sepsis, and Multiple Organ Dysfunction Syndrome

Beverly Carlson

Be sure to check out the bonus material, including review questions, on the Evolve website at http://evolve.elsevier.com/Urden/priorities/.

SHOCK SYNDROME

Description and Etiology

Shock is a complex pathophysiologic process that often results in MODS and death. All types of shock involve ineffective tissue perfusion and acute circulatory failure. The shock syndrome is a pathway involving a variety of pathologic processes that may be categorized as four stages: initial, compensatory, progressive, and refractory. Progression through each stage varies with the patient's prior condition, duration of initiating event, response to therapy, and correction of underlying cause (Figure 26-1).

Shock can be classified as hypovolemic, cardiogenic, or distributive, depending on the pathophysiologic cause and hemodynamic profile. Hypovolemic shock results from a loss of circulating or intravascular volume. Cardiogenic shock results from the impaired ability of the heart to pump. Distributive shock results from maldistribution of circulating blood volume and can be further classified as septic, anaphylactic, or neurogenic. Septic shock is the result of microorganisms entering the body. Anaphylactic shock is the result of a severe antibody–antigen reaction. Neurogenic shock is the result of the loss of sympathetic tone.

Pathophysiology

During the initial stage, cardiac output (CO) is decreased, and tissue perfusion is threatened. Almost immediately, the compensatory stage begins as the body's homeostatic mechanisms attempt to maintain CO, blood pressure, and tissue perfusion. The compensatory mechanisms are mediated by the sympathetic nervous system (SNS) and consist of neural, hormonal, and chemical responses. The neural response includes an increase in heart rate and contractility, arterial and venous vasoconstriction, and shunting of blood to the vital organs. Hormonal compensation includes activation of the renin response and stimulation of the anterior pituitary and adrenal medulla. Activation of the renin response results in the production of angiotensin II, which causes vasoconstriction and the release of aldosterone and antidiuretic hormone (ADH), leading to sodium and water retention. Stimulation of the anterior pituitary results in the secretion of adrenocorticotropic hormone (ACTH), which stimulates the adrenal cortex to produce glucocorticoids, causing a rise in blood glucose levels. Stimulation of the adrenal medulla causes the release of epinephrine and norepinephrine, which further enhance the compensatory mechanisms.

During the progressive stage, the compensatory mechanisms begin failing to meet tissue metabolic needs, and the shock cycle is perpetuated. As tissue perfusion becomes ineffective, the cells switch from aerobic to anaerobic metabolism to produce energy. Anaerobic metabolism produces small amounts of energy but large amounts of lactic acid, producing lactic acidemia. Vasodilation and increased vascular permeability from endothelial and epithelial hypoxia and inflammatory mediators results in intravascular hypovolemia, tissue edema, and further decline in tissue perfusion.[1,2,3] A systemic release of inflammatory mediators in response to tissue hypoxia, especially in gut tissue, produces microcirculatory impairment and derangement of cellular metabolism, facilitating progression of the shock cycle.[1-4] The patient is experiencing systemic inflammatory response syndrome (SIRS), and irreversible damage begins to occur. Some cells die as a result of apoptosis, an injury-activated, preprogrammed cellular suicide. Others die as the sodium–potassium pump in the cell membrane fails, causing the cell and its organelles to swell. Cellular energy production comes to a complete halt as the mitochondria swell and rupture. At this point, the problem becomes one of oxygen use instead of oxygen delivery. Even if the cell were to receive more oxygen, it would be unable to use it because of damage to the mitochondria. The cell's digestive organelles swell and leak destructive enzymes into the cell, accelerating cell death.[4]

Every system in the body is affected by this process (Box 26-1). Cardiac dysfunction develops as a result of the release of myocardial depressant cytokines.[1-3] Ventricular failure eventually occurs, further perpetuating the entire process. Central nervous system (CNS) dysfunction develops as a result of cerebral hypoperfusion, leading to failure of the SNS, cardiac and respiratory depression, and thermoregulatory failure. Endothelial injury from hypoxia and inflammatory cytokines and impaired blood flow result in microvascular thrombosis. Hematologic dysfunction occurs as a result of consumption of clotting factors, release of inflammatory cytokines, and dilutional thrombocytopenia. Disseminated intravascular coagulation (DIC) eventually may develop. Pulmonary dysfunction occurs as a result of increased pulmonary capillary membrane permeability, pulmonary microemboli, and pulmonary vasoconstriction. Ventilatory failure and acute respiratory distress syndrome (ARDS) develop.

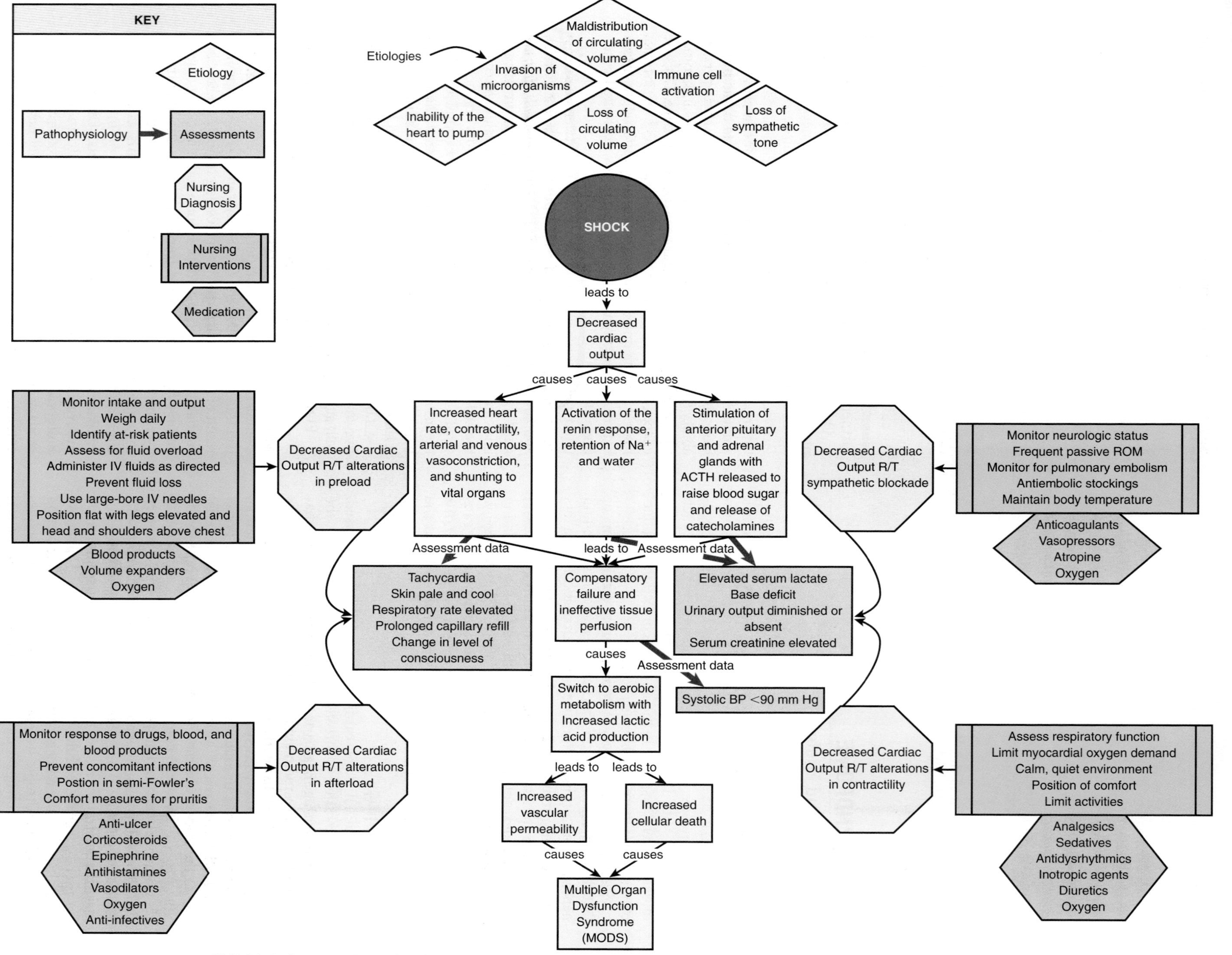

FIG 26-1 Concept Map for Shock. (Concept map illustration created by: Elaine Bishop Kennedy, EdD, RN.)

BOX 26-1 Consequences of Shock

Cardiovascular
- Ventricular failure
- Microvascular thrombosis

Neurologic
- Sympathetic nervous system dysfunction
- Cardiac and respiratory depression
- Thermoregulatory failure
- Coma

Pulmonary
- Acute lung failure (ALF)
- Acute respiratory distress syndrome (ARDS)

Renal
- Acute kidney injury (AKI)

Hematologic
- Disseminated intravascular coagulation (DIC)

Gastrointestinal
- Gastrointestinal tract failure
- Liver failure
- Pancreatic failure

Renal dysfunction develops as a result of renal vasoconstriction and renal hypoperfusion, leading to acute kidney injury (AKI). Gastrointestinal dysfunction occurs as a result of splanchnic vasoconstriction and hypoperfusion and leads to failure of the gut organs. Disruption of the intestinal epithelium releases gram-negative bacteria into the system, which further perpetuates the entire shock syndrome.[5]

During the refractory stage, shock becomes unresponsive to therapy and is considered irreversible. As the individual organ systems die, MODS—defined as failure of two or more body systems—occurs. Death is the final outcome. Regardless of the etiologic factors, death occurs from ineffective tissue perfusion because of the failure of the circulation to meet the oxygen needs of the cell.[4]

Assessment and Diagnosis

The patient with a mean arterial blood pressure (MAP) less than 60 mm Hg or with evidence of global tissue hypoperfusion is considered to be in a shock state.[1,3] Because shock is a dynamic physiologic phenomenon, hypotension may occur late in the process or may normalize even when tissue perfusion is still inadequate.[6-9] Clinical manifestations vary according to the underlying cause of shock, the stage of the shock, and the patient's response to shock.

Compensatory mechanisms may produce normal hemodynamic values even when tissue perfusion is compromised.[3,5,8,10-11] Global indicators of systemic perfusion and oxygenation include serum lactate, arterial base deficit, serum bicarbonate, and central or mixed venous oxygen saturation levels. Inadequate cellular oxygenation with anaerobic metabolism and increased metabolic lactate production increase the serum lactate level.[8,12] The level and duration of this hyperlactatemia are predictive of morbidity and mortality,[7,10-12] and management guided by lactate levels has been effective in improving outcomes.[13-14] The base deficit derived from arterial blood gas (ABG) values also reflects global tissue acidosis and is useful to assess the severity of shock.[6,9-11] Studies have demonstrated serum bicarbonate to be an equivalent alternative to arterial base deficit in predicting mortality in surgical and trauma patients.[15-16] The use of mixed venous oxygen saturation (SvO_2) measured by means of a pulmonary artery catheter or central venous oxygen saturation ($ScvO_2$) measured with a central venous catheter allows assessment of the balance of oxygen delivery and oxygen consumption and the ratio of oxygen extraction.[3,17-19] After years of recommended use to guide the care of patients with severe sepsis, this measure of global oxygen balance is being evaluated for use in other critically ill populations.[17-21] Noninvasive indicators of regional tissue perfusion or oxygenation, such as sublingual capnometry and subcutaneous or skeletal muscle tissue oxygen saturation (StO_2) measured with near-infrared spectroscopy, are also being evaluated.[3,8,19] The sections on different types of shock discuss clinical assessment and diagnosis of the patient in shock.

Medical Management

The major focus of the treatment of shock is the improvement and preservation of tissue perfusion. Adequate tissue perfusion depends on an adequate supply of oxygen being transported to the tissues and the cell's ability to use it. Oxygen transport is influenced by pulmonary gas exchange, CO, and hemoglobin level. Oxygen use is influenced by the internal metabolic environment and mitochondrial function. Management of the patient in shock focuses on supporting oxygen delivery.[1,3]

Adequate pulmonary gas exchange is critical to oxygen transport. Establishing and maintaining an adequate airway are the first steps in ensuring adequate oxygenation. After the airway is patent, emphasis is placed on improving ventilation and oxygenation. Therapies include administration of supplemental oxygen and mechanical ventilatory support.

An adequate CO and hemoglobin level are crucial to oxygen transport. CO depends on heart rate, preload, afterload, and contractility. A variety of fluids and medications are used to manipulate these parameters. The types of fluids used include crystalloids and colloids. The categories of medications used include vasoconstrictors, vasodilators, positive inotropes, and antidysrhythmics.

Fluid administration is indicated for decreased preload related to intravascular volume depletion, and it can be accomplished by use of a crystalloid or colloid solution, or both. Crystalloids are balanced electrolyte solutions that may be hypotonic, isotonic, or hypertonic. Examples of crystalloid solutions used in shock situations are normal saline and lactated Ringer solution. Colloids are protein- or starch-containing solutions. Examples of colloid solutions are blood and blood components, such as albumin, and pharmaceutical plasma expanders, such as hetastarch, dextran, and mannitol.

The quantity and choice of fluid is a subject of debate and depends on the situation.[3,22-27] Excessive volume expansion, more than what increases preload and stroke volume (SV), worsens organ function and may produce coagulopathy, cytokine activation, and abdominal compartment syndrome.[3,24] Methods to measure preload responsiveness include respiratory or positional variation in pulse pressure, systolic pressure, and SV and are more accurate than central venous pressure (CVP).[3] Fluid resuscitation with normal saline or with albumin produces similar outcomes regardless of baseline serum albumin level.[26,28] Crystalloid solutions are inexpensive and effective. Advantages of colloids include faster restoration of intravascular volume and use of smaller amounts. Colloids are believed to stay in the intravascular space, unlike crystalloids, which readily leak into the extravascular space. Disadvantages include expense, allergic reactions, and difficulties in typing and cross-matching blood. Colloids also can leak out of damaged capillaries and cause a variety of additional problems, particularly in the lungs. Hypertonic or hyperoncotic fluids offer no additional benefit over isotonic crystalloids and are not recommended.[3,22,27,29-30]

Blood should be considered to augment oxygen transport if the patient's hemoglobin level is critically low, although what threshold value should be used is still undetermined.[3,5,31] Transfusion of stored red blood cells does not substantially increase oxygen consumption and has been associated with immunosuppression, infection, impairment of microcirculatory flow, increased pulmonary vascular resistance, coagulopathy, and increased mortality. Restrictive transfusion practice has demonstrated lower mortality.[3,5,17,31-32] Transfusion-related acute lung injury (TRALI) resulting from immune and nonimmune neutrophil activation has become the leading cause of transfusion-related death and may occur with transfusion of any plasma-containing blood or blood product.[32-35]

Vasoconstrictor agents are used to increase afterload by increasing the systemic vascular resistance (SVR) and improving the patient's blood pressure level. Vasodilator agents are used to decrease preload or afterload, or both, by decreasing venous return and SVR. Positive inotropic agents are used to increase contractility. Antidysrhythmic agents are used to influence heart rate. Box 26-2 provides examples of each of these agents.

Sodium bicarbonate is not recommended in the treatment of shock-related lactic acidosis.[17,36-37] No overall benefit has been found, and the risks associated with its use are significant. They include shifting of the oxyhemoglobin dissociation curve to the left, rebound increase in lactic acid production, development of hyperosmolar state, fluid overload resulting from excessive sodium, and rapid cellular electrolyte shifts.[36-37]

The critically ill patient should be started on enteral nutritional support therapy within 24 to 48 hours.[38] The type of nutritional supplementation initiated varies according to the cause of shock, and it should be tailored to the individual patient's needs, as indicated by the underlying condition, laboratory data, and treatment. When enteral feeding is contraindicated, parenteral nutrition should be considered, though a delay of 7 days is recommended for better outcomes.[38-41] Supplementation of enteral feeding with parenteral nutrition to increase caloric intake is a subject of debate but has not been shown to improve patient outcomes.[38,41-42] A delay of 1 week is recommended before consideration of this strategy.[38]

Glucose control to a target level of 140 to 180 mg/dL is recommended for all critically ill patients.[43-44] Benefits of glucose control in the critically ill include lower incidences of infection, renal failure, sepsis, and death.[43-46]

BOX 26-2 Agents Used in the Treatment of Shock

Vasoconstrictors
- Epinephrine (Adrenalin)
- Norepinephrine (Levophed)
- Alpha-range dopamine (Intropin)
- Phenylephrine (Neo-Synephrine)
- Vasopressin (Pitressin)

Vasodilators
- Nitroprusside (Nipride, Nitropress)
- Nitroglycerin (Nitrol, Tridil)
- Hydralazine (Apresoline)
- Labetalol (Normodyne, Trandate)

Inotropes
- Beta-range dopamine (Intropin)
- Dobutamine (Dobutrex)
- Epinephrine (Adrenalin)
- Norepinephrine (Levophed)
- Milrinone (Primacor)

Antidysrhythmics
- Amiodarone (Cordarone)
- Adenosine (Adenocard)
- Procainamide (Pronestyl)
- Labetalol (Normodyne, Trandate)
- Verapamil (Calan, Isoptin)
- Esmolol (Brevibloc)
- Diltiazem (Cardizem)
- Lidocaine (Xylocaine)

Nursing Management

The nursing management of a patient in shock is a complex and challenging responsibility. It requires an in-depth understanding of the pathophysiology of the disease and the anticipated effects of each intervention, as well as a solid understanding of the nursing process. Later sections discuss specific interventions for the patient in shock.

The psychosocial needs of the patient and family dealing with shock are extremely important. These needs are based on situational, familial, and patient-centered variables. **Nursing priorities in managing the psychosocial stress of critical illness include 1) providing information on patient status, 2) explaining procedures and routines, 3) supporting the family, 4) encouraging the expression of feelings, 5) facilitating problem solving and shared decision making, 6) individualizing visitation schedules, 7) involving the family in the patient's care, and 8) establishing contacts with necessary resources.** The consensus of all relevant professional organizations is that patients and families should be given the option of family presence during invasive procedures and resuscitation.[47-50] Collaborative management of the patient with shock is outlined in Box 26-3.

HYPOVOLEMIC SHOCK

Description and Etiology

Hypovolemic shock occurs from inadequate fluid volume in the intravascular space. The lack of adequate circulating

BOX 26-3 Collaborative Management

Shock

- Support oxygen transport.
  - Establish a patent airway.
  - Initiate mechanical ventilation.
  - Administer oxygen.
  - Administer fluids (crystalloids, colloids, blood and other blood products).
  - Administer vasoactive medications.
  - Administer positive inotropic medications.
  - Ensure sufficient hemoglobin and hematocrit.
- Support oxygen use.
  - Identify and correct cause of lactic acidosis.
  - Ensure adequate organ and extremity perfusion.
  - Initiate nutritional support therapy.
- Identify underlying cause of shock and treat accordingly.
- Provide comfort and emotional support.
- Institute evidence-based practice protocols to prevent complications.
- Assess response to therapy.
- Prevent and maintain surveillance for complications.

volume leads to decreased tissue perfusion and initiation of the general shock response. Hypovolemic shock is the most commonly occurring form of shock (Figure 26-2). Hypovolemic shock can result from absolute or relative hypovolemia. Absolute hypovolemia occurs when there is a loss of fluid from the intravascular space. This can result from an external loss of fluid from the body or from internal shifting of fluid from the intravascular space to the extravascular space. Fluid shifts can result from a loss of intravascular integrity, increased capillary membrane permeability, or decreased colloidal osmotic pressure. Relative hypovolemia occurs when vasodilation produces an increase in vascular capacitance relative to circulating volume (Box 26-4).

Pathophysiology

Hypovolemia results in a loss of circulating fluid volume. A decrease in circulating volume leads to a decrease in venous return, which results in a decrease in end-diastolic volume or preload. Preload is a major determinant of stroke volume (SV) and CO. A decrease in preload results in a decrease in SV and CO. The decrease in CO leads to inadequate cellular oxygen supply and ineffective tissue perfusion.

Assessment and Diagnosis

The clinical manifestations of hypovolemic shock depend on the severity of fluid loss and the patient's ability to compensate for it. Clinical classes developed by the American College of Surgeons to describe the levels of severity of hypovolemic shock in the trauma setting have been widely accepted, but a recent test of the validity of these classes suggests that modifications are necessary.[51] A simpler approach of classifying hypovolemic shock as mild, moderate, or severe is also commonly used. Class I, or mild shock, indicates a fluid volume loss up to 15% or an actual volume loss up to 750 mL. Compensatory mechanisms maintain CO, and the patient appears free of symptoms other than possibly slight anxiety.[1,5,51]

Class II hypovolemia occurs with a fluid volume loss of 15% to 30% or an actual volume loss of 750 to 1500 mL. As volume loss worsens, the patient moves from mild to moderate hypovolemic shock. Falling CO activates more intense compensatory responses. Anxiety increases.[1] The heart rate may increase to more than 100 beats/minute in response to increased SNS stimulation unless blocked by preexisting beta-blocker therapy. The pulse pressure narrows as the diastolic blood pressure increases because of vasoconstriction. Postural hypotension develops.[1] The respiratory rate increases as blood loss worsens, and ABG specimens drawn during this phase may reveal respiratory alkalosis, as evidenced by a low partial pressure of carbon dioxide ($PaCO_2$). Urine output starts to decline to 20 to 30 mL/hour as renal perfusion decreases. The urine sodium level decreases, whereas urinary osmolality and specific gravity increase as the kidneys start to conserve sodium and water. The patient's skin becomes pale and cool with delayed capillary refill because of peripheral vasoconstriction. Jugular veins appear flat as a result of decreased venous return.[1,5]

Hypovolemic shock that is class III occurs with a fluid volume loss of 30% to 40% or an actual volume loss of 1500 to 2000 mL. This level of severity may produce the progressive stage of shock as compensatory mechanisms become overwhelmed and ineffective tissue perfusion develops. Blood pressure decreases, but often after tissue hypoperfusion is already significant.[6,9] The heart rate may increase to more than 120 beats/minute, and dysrhythmias may develop as myocardial ischemia ensues. During this phase serum lactate levels increase, and ABG values reveal metabolic acidosis evidenced by a low bicarbonate (HCO_3^-) and elevated base deficit. Decreased renal perfusion results in the development of oliguria. Blood urea nitrogen (BUN) and serum creatinine levels start to rise as the kidneys begin to fail. The patient's skin becomes ashen, cold, and clammy, with marked delayed capillary refill. The patient may appear confused as cerebral perfusion decreases.[1,5,51]

Class IV hypovolemic shock is severe shock and usually refractory in nature. It occurs with a fluid volume loss of greater than 40% or an actual volume loss of more than 2000 mL. As the compensatory mechanisms of the body become insufficient, tachycardia and hemodynamic instability worsen, and hypotension ensues. Severe lactic acidosis is present. Peripheral pulses and capillary refill become absent because of marked peripheral vasoconstriction. The skin may appear cyanotic, mottled, and extremely diaphoretic. Organ failure occurs. Urine output ceases. The patient may be confused and agitated, eventually becoming unresponsive. Various clinical manifestations associated with failure of the different body systems will develop.[1,5]

Assessment of the hemodynamic parameters of a patient in hypovolemic shock varies by stage but commonly reveals a decreased CO and cardiac index (CI). Loss of circulating volume leads to a decrease in venous return to the heart, which results in a decrease in the preload of the right and left ventricles. This is evidenced by a decline in the CVP or right atrial pressure (RAP) and pulmonary artery occlusion pressure (PAOP). Vasoconstriction of the arterial system results in an increase in the afterload of the heart, as evidenced by an increase in the SVR. This vasoconstriction may produce inaccurate systolic and diastolic blood pressure values when measured by arterial catheter or noninvasive oscillometry. MAP is more accurate in this low-flow state.[18]

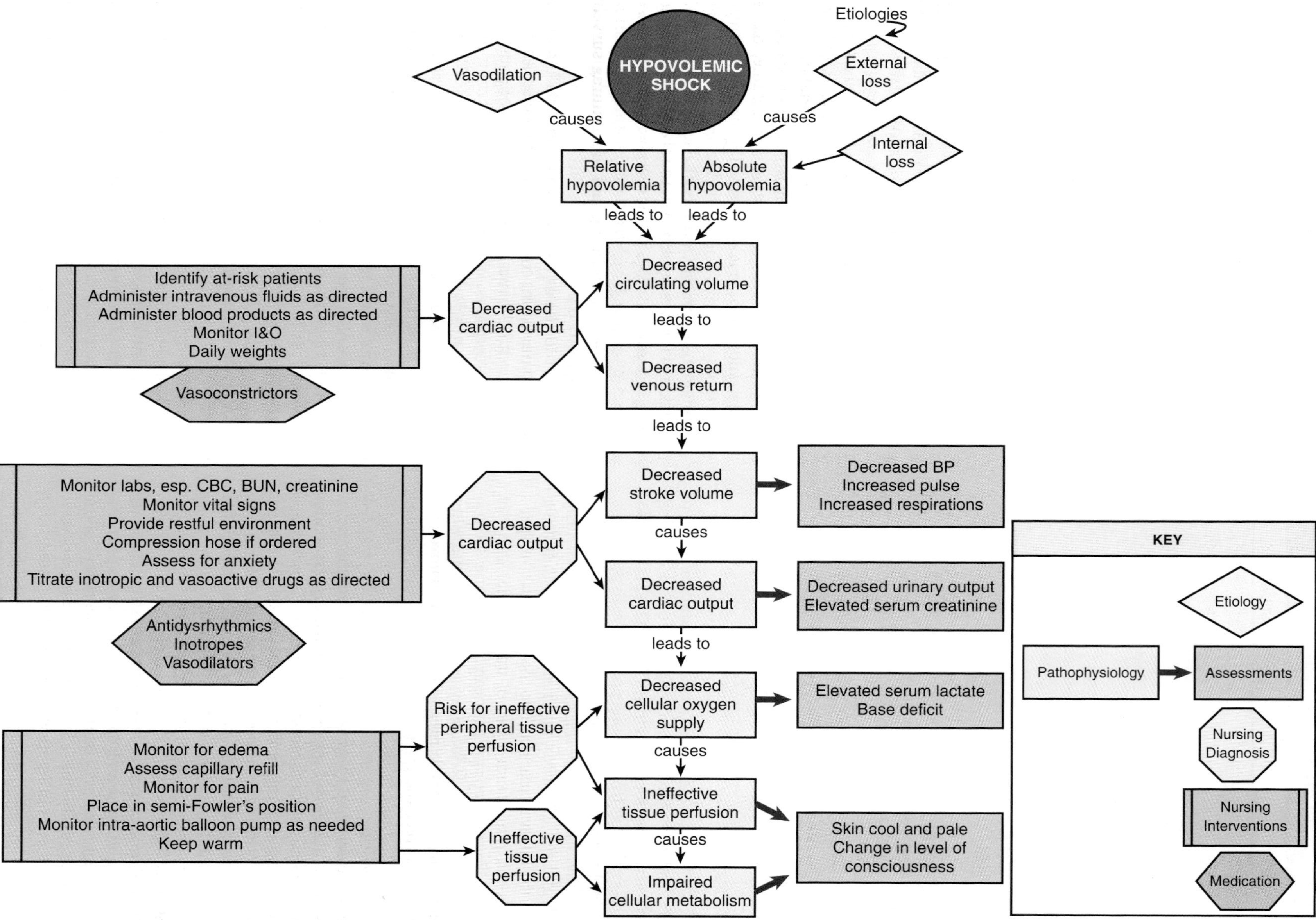

FIG 26-2 Concept Map for Hypovolemic Shock. (Concept map illustration created by Elaine Bishop Kennedy, EdD, RN.)

BOX 26-4 Etiologic Factors in Hypovolemic Shock

Absolute Factors
- Loss of whole blood
  - Trauma or surgery
  - Gastrointestinal bleeding
- Loss of plasma
  - Thermal injuries
  - Large lesions
- Loss of other body fluids
  - Severe vomiting or diarrhea
  - Massive diuresis
  - Loss of intravascular integrity
  - Ruptured spleen
  - Long bone or pelvic fractures
  - Hemorrhagic pancreatitis
  - Hemothorax or hemoperitoneum
  - Arterial dissection or rupture

Relative Factors
- Vasodilation
  - SIRS/sepsis
  - Anaphylaxis
  - Loss of sympathetic stimulation
- Increased capillary membrane permeability
  - SIRS/sepsis
  - Anaphylaxis
  - Thermal injuries
- Decreased colloidal osmotic pressure
  - Severe sodium depletion
  - Hypopituitarism
  - Cirrhosis
  - Intestinal obstruction

Medical Management

The major goals of therapy for the patient in hypovolemic shock are to correct the cause of the hypovolemia, restore tissue perfusion, and prevent complications. This approach includes identifying and stopping the source of fluid loss and administering fluid to replace circulating volume. Fluid administration can be accomplished with use of a crystalloid solution, a colloid solution, blood products, or a combination of fluids. The type of solution used depends on the type of fluid lost, the degree of hypovolemia, the severity of hypoperfusion, and the cause of hypovolemia.

Aggressive fluid resuscitation in trauma and surgical patients is the subject of great debate. The benefit of limited or hypotensive (systolic blood pressure 60 to 80 mm Hg or MAP 40 to 60 mm Hg) volume resuscitation in patients with uncontrolled hemorrhage is postulated to lessen bleeding and improve survival[22,52-54] and has been demonstrated in the preliminary results of a randomized controlled trial.[53] The type and amount of solutions used for fluid resuscitation and the rate of administration influence immune function, inflammatory mediator release, coagulation, and the incidence of cardiac, pulmonary, renal, and gastrointestinal complications.[3,22,24-25,27] Consensus on the optimal resuscitative strategy for hypovolemic shock is lacking and is likely situation-specific.[18,22,24,52,54]

BOX 26-5 NURSING DIAGNOSIS PRIORITIES

Hypovolemic Shock

- Deficient Fluid Volume related to active blood loss, p. 584
- Deficient Fluid Volume related to interstitial fluid shift, p. 583
- Decreased Cardiac Output related to alterations in preload, p. 579
- Anxiety related to threat to biologic, psychologic, and/or social integrity, p. 576

Nursing Management

Prevention of hypovolemic shock is one of the primary responsibilities of the nurse in the critical care area. Preventive measures include the identification of patients at risk and frequent assessment of the patient's fluid balance. Accurate monitoring of intake and output and daily weights are essential components of preventive nursing care. Early identification and treatment result in decreased mortality.

Management of the patient in hypovolemic shock requires continuous evaluation of intravascular volume, tissue perfusion, and response to therapy. The patient in hypovolemic shock may have any number of nursing diagnoses, depending on the progression of the process (Box 26-5). **Nursing priorities are directed toward 1) minimizing fluid loss, 2) administering volume replacement, 3) assessing response to therapy, 4) providing comfort and emotional support, and 5) preventing and maintaining surveillance for complications.**

Measures to minimize fluid loss include limiting blood sampling, observing lines for accidental disconnection, and applying direct pressure to bleeding sites. Measures to facilitate the administration of volume replacement include insertion of large-bore peripheral intravenous catheters, rapid administration of prescribed fluids, and positioning the patient with the legs elevated, trunk flat, and head and shoulders above the chest. Monitoring the patient for clinical manifestations of fluid overload or complications related to fluid and blood product administration is essential for preventing further problems. It is also essential to monitor the patient for SIRS, which may occur for up to several days after resuscitation.[55]

CARDIOGENIC SHOCK

Description and Etiology

Cardiogenic shock is the result of failure of the heart to pump blood forward effectively. It can occur with dysfunction of the right or the left ventricle, or both. The lack of adequate pumping function leads to decreased tissue perfusion and circulatory failure (Figure 26-3). It occurs in approximately 5% to 8% of the patients with an ST-segment myocardial infarction (MI), and it is the leading cause of death of patients hospitalized with MI.[56-58] The mortality rate for cardiogenic shock has decreased with the advent of early revascularization therapy and is currently about 47% to 65%.[56-60]

Cardiogenic shock can result from problems affecting the muscular function or the mechanical function of the heart or

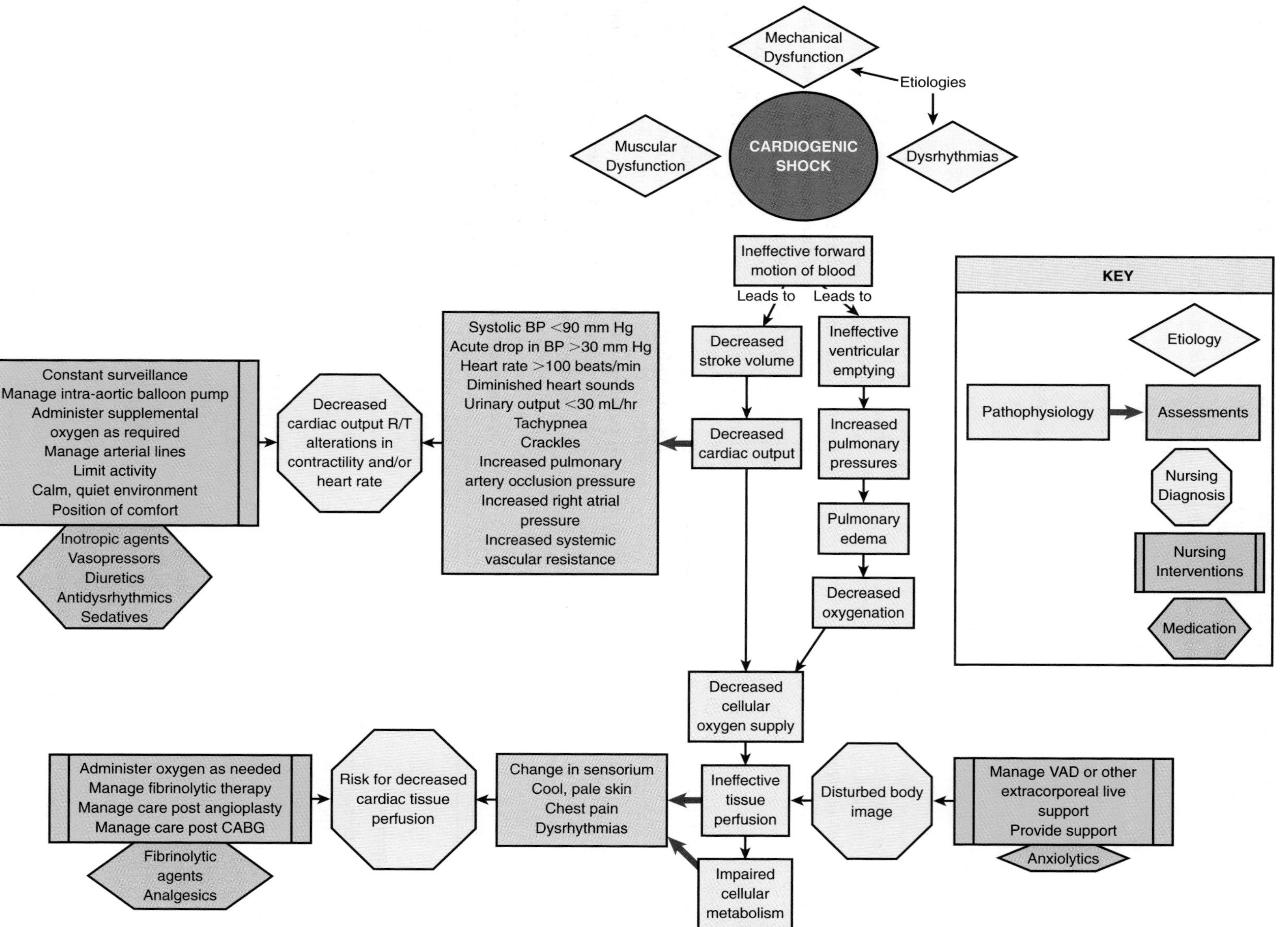

FIG 26-3 **Concept Map for Cardiogenic Shock.** (Concept map illustration created by Elaine Bishop Kennedy, EdD, RN.)

the cardiac rhythm.[57-59,61] The most common cause is acute MI resulting in the loss of 40% or more of the functional myocardium. It can occur with ST-elevation or non–ST-elevation MI.[57-59] The damage to the myocardium may occur after one massive MI (usually of the anterior wall), or it may be cumulative as a result of several smaller MIs or a small MI in a patient with preexisting ventricular dysfunction.[56-57] Cardiomyopathy may cause cardiogenic shock as left ventricular function becomes unable to maintain adequate CO. Examples of problems affecting the mechanical function of the heart to fill and eject adequately include severe valvular disease; acute papillary muscle, chordal, or septal rupture; cardiac tamponade, and massive pulmonary embolus (Box 26-6).[57-59,61]

Pathophysiology

Cardiogenic shock results from the impaired ability of the ventricle to pump blood forward, which leads to a decrease in SV and an increase in the blood left in the ventricle at the end of systole. The decrease in SV results in a decrease in CO, which leads to decreased cellular oxygen supply and ineffective tissue perfusion. Typically, myocardial performance spirals downward as compensatory vasoconstriction increases myocardial afterload and low blood pressure worsens myocardial ischemia. As left ventricular contractility declines and ventricular compliance decreases, an increase in end-systolic volume results in blood backing up into the pulmonary system and the subsequent development of pulmonary edema. Pulmonary edema causes impaired gas exchange and decreased oxygenation of the arterial blood, which further impair tissue perfusion. In a substantial number of patients, the pathophysiology may follow a different course due to activation of inflammatory cytokines. A SIRS response results with systemic vasodilation and, possibly, normalization of the CO.[57-58,62] Whether this process contributes to the genesis or the outcome of cardiogenic shock is uncertain, but it is thought to be activated by acute MI and to facilitate development of sepsis.[57,62] Death due to cardiogenic shock results from cardiopulmonary collapse or multiple organ failure.[59]

BOX 26-6 Etiologic Factors in Cardiogenic Shock

Muscular

- Ischemic injury
  - Acute myocardial infarction
  - Cardiopulmonary arrest
- Acute decompensated heart failure
- Cardiomyopathy
- Acute myocarditis
- Myocardial contusion
- Prolonged cardiopulmonary bypass
- Septic shock
- Hemorrhagic shock
- Medications (beta-adrenergic blockers, calcium-channel antagonists, cytotoxic agents)

Mechanical

- Valvular dysfunction
- Papillary muscle dysfunction or rupture
- Septal wall rupture
- Free wall rupture
- Ventricular aneurysm
- Obstructive hypertrophic cardiomyopathy
- Intracardiac tumor
- Pulmonary embolus
- Atrial thrombus
- Cardiac tamponade
- Massive pulmonary embolus
- Constrictive pericarditis

Rhythmic

- Bradydysrhythmias
- Tachydysrhythmias

Assessment and Diagnosis

A variety of clinical manifestations occur in the patient in cardiogenic shock, depending on etiologic factors, the patient's underlying medical status, and the severity of the shock state. Some clinical manifestations are caused by failure of the heart as a pump, whereas many are related to the overall shock response (Box 26-7).

Initially, clinical manifestations reflect the decline in CO. These signs and symptoms include systolic blood pressure less than 90 mm Hg or an acute drop in systolic or mean blood pressure of 30 mm Hg or more; decreased sensorium; cool, pale, moist skin; and urine output of less than 30 mL/hour.[57,59,63] The patient also may complain of chest pain. Tachycardia develops to compensate for the decrease in CO. A weak, thready pulse develops, and diminished S_1 and S_2 heart sounds may occur as a result of the decreased contractility. The respiratory rate increases to improve oxygenation. ABG values at this point indicate respiratory alkalosis, as evidenced by a decrease in $PaCO_2$. Urinalysis findings demonstrate a decrease in urine sodium level and an increase in urine osmolality and specific gravity as the kidneys start to conserve sodium and water. Serum B-type natriuretic peptide (BNP) levels will likely be elevated.

As the left ventricle fails, auscultation of the lungs may disclose crackles and rhonchi, indicating the development of

BOX 26-7 Clinical Manifestations of Cardiogenic Shock

- Systolic blood pressure <90 mm Hg
- Acute drop in blood pressure >30 mm Hg
- Heart rate >100 beats/min
- Weak, thready pulse
- Diminished heart sounds
- Change in sensorium
- Cool, pale, moist skin
- Urine output <30 mL/hr
- Chest pain
- Dysrhythmias
- Tachypnea
- Crackles
- Decreased cardiac output
- Cardiac index <2.2 L/min/m^2
- Increased pulmonary artery occlusion pressure
- Increased right atrial pressure
- Variable systemic vascular resistance

pulmonary edema. Hypoxemia occurs, as evidenced by a fall in PaO_2 and SaO_2 as measured by ABG values. Heart sounds may reveal an S_3 and S_4. Jugular venous distention is evident with right-sided failure. The patient also may experience dysrhythmias in response to tissue hypoxia, the underlying problem, and drug therapy.[58-59]

Assessment of the hemodynamic parameters of a patient in cardiogenic shock reveals a decreased CO with a CI less than 2.2 L/min/m^2 in the presence of an elevated PAOP of more than 15 mm Hg.[57,59,63] A proportional pulse pressure (systolic BP/pulse pressure) less than 25% is indicative of left ventricular failure and a CI less than 2.2 and may be useful when direct measurement of CI is unavailable.[64] Increased filling pressures are necessary to rule out hypovolemia as the cause of circulatory failure. The increase in PAOP reflects an increase in the left ventricular end-diastolic pressure (LVEDP) and left ventricular end-diastolic volume (LVEDV) resulting from decreased SV. With right ventricular failure, the RAP also increases. Compensatory vasoconstriction typically results in an increase in the afterload of the heart, as evidenced by an increase in the SVR, unless SIRS produces vasodilation and a normal or decreased SVR. Echocardiography confirms the diagnosis of cardiogenic shock, provides noninvasive estimates of PAOP and ejection fraction, and often clarifies etiologic factors.[57-59]

As compensatory mechanisms fail and ineffective tissue perfusion develops, other clinical manifestations appear. Myocardial ischemia progresses, as evidenced by continued increases in heart rate, dysrhythmias, and chest pain. Pulmonary function deteriorates, which leads to respiratory distress. ABG values during this phase reveal respiratory and metabolic acidosis and hypoxemia, as indicated by a high $PaCO_2$, low HCO_3^-, and low PaO_2, respectively. Renal failure occurs, as exhibited by the development of anuria and increases in BUN and serum creatinine levels. Cerebral hypoperfusion manifests as a decreasing level of consciousness.

Medical Management

Treatment of the patient in cardiogenic shock requires an aggressive approach. The major goals of therapy are to treat the underlying cause, enhance the effectiveness of the pump, and improve tissue perfusion. This approach includes identifying and treating the etiologic factors of heart failure and administering pharmacologic agents or using mechanical devices to enhance CO. Inotropic agents are used to increase contractility and maintain adequate blood pressure and tissue perfusion. A vasopressor may be necessary to maintain blood pressure when hypotension is severe.[57-59] As both of these therapies increase myocardial oxygen demand, the lowest possible doses should be used.[57,59] Diuretics may be used for preload reduction. After blood pressure has been stabilized, vasodilating agents are used for preload and afterload reduction. Antidysrhythmic agents should be used to suppress or control dysrhythmias that can affect CO. Intubation and mechanical ventilation are usually necessary to support oxygenation.

Intraaortic balloon pump (IABP) support should be instituted quickly if drug therapy does not immediately reverse the shock state.[57-58] The IABP is a temporary mechanical device used to decrease myocardial workload by improving myocardial supply and decreasing myocardial demand. It achieves this goal by improving coronary artery perfusion and reducing left ventricular afterload. Chapter 16 provides more information about IAPB therapy.

As soon as the cause of pump failure has been identified, measures should be taken to correct the problem, if possible. In the setting of acute MI, early and complete revascularization by percutaneous coronary intervention or coronary artery bypass surgery provides significant survival benefit.[57-60] Fibrinolytic agents may be used in select patients. Procedural or surgical intervention may be necessary to remedy mechanical etiology. When conventional therapies fail, a ventricular assist device (VAD) or extracorporeal life support with a membrane oxygenator (ECMO) may be used to support the patient in acute cardiogenic shock.[57-59] These mechanical circulatory assist devices provide an external means to sustain effective organ perfusion, allowing time for the patient's ventricle to heal or for cardiac transplantation to take place.

Nursing Management

Prevention of cardiogenic shock is one of the primary responsibilities of the nurse in the critical care area. Preventive measures include the identification of patients at risk, facilitation of early reperfusion therapy for acute MI, and frequent assessment and management of the patient's cardiopulmonary status.

The patient in cardiogenic shock may have any number of nursing diagnoses, depending on the progression of the process (Box 26-8). **Nursing priorities are directed toward 1) limiting myocardial oxygen demand, 2) enhancing myocardial oxygen supply, 3) maintaining adequate tissue perfusion, 4) providing comfort and emotional support, and 5) preventing and maintaining surveillance for complications.** Measures to limit myocardial oxygen demand include administering analgesics, sedatives, and agents to control afterload and dysrhythmias, positioning the patient for comfort, limiting activities, providing a calm and quiet environment and offering support to reduce anxiety, and teaching the patient about the condition. Measures to enhance myocardial oxygen supply include administering supplemental oxygen, monitoring the patient's respiratory status, administering prescribed medications, and managing device therapy.

Effective nursing management of cardiogenic shock requires precise monitoring and management of heart rate, preload, afterload, and contractility. This is accomplished through accurate measurement of hemodynamic variables and controlled administration of fluids and inotropic and

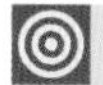

BOX 26-8 NURSING DIAGNOSIS PRIORITIES

Cardiogenic Shock

- Ineffective Cardiopulmonary Tissue Perfusion related to acute myocardial ischemia, p. 581
- Decreased Cardiac Output related to alterations in contractility, p. 580
- Decreased Cardiac Output related to alterations in heart rate, p. 581
- Disturbed Body Image related to functional dependence on life-sustaining technology, p. 587
- Compromised Family Coping related to a critically ill family member, p. 578

vasoactive agents. Close assessment and management of respiratory function is also essential to maintain adequate oxygenation. Dysrhythmias are common and require immediate recognition and treatment.

Patients who require mechanical device (IABP, LVAD, or ECMO) therapy need to be observed frequently for complications. Complications of cardiac mechanical-assist devices may include infection, bleeding, thrombocytopenia, hemolysis, embolus, stroke, device malfunction, circulatory compromise of a cannulated extremity, SIRS, and sepsis.[63]

ANAPHYLACTIC SHOCK

Description and Etiology

Anaphylactic shock, a type of distributive shock, is the result of an immediate hypersensitivity reaction. It is a life-threatening event that requires prompt intervention. The severe and systemic response leads to decreased tissue perfusion and initiation of the general shock response (Figure 26-4). Anaphylaxis is a serious allergic reaction caused by an immunologic antibody–antigen response or nonimmunologic activation of mast cells and basophils.[65-69] A number of triggers have been identified that, when introduced by injection or ingestion or through the skin or respiratory tract, can cause a reaction. This list includes foods, food additives, diagnostic agents, biologic agents, environmental agents, medications, and venoms (Box 26-9).[67-69] Anaphylaxis can also be triggered by physical factors and can even be idiopathic in nature with no known trigger.[67-68] In the hospital environment, latex was once an extremely problematic antigen for patients and health care providers, but efforts to limit and prevent exposure have been highly successful.[68]

Pathophysiology

Both immunologic and nonimmunologic activation of the mast cells and basophils result in the release of biochemical mediators. These mediators include histamine, tryptase, chymase, carboxypeptidase A3, platelet-activating factor (PAF), heparin, leukotrienes, prostaglandins, and cytokines such as IL-6, IL-33, and TNF-alpha, among others.[68-69] The activation of the biochemical mediators causes vasodilation, increased capillary permeability, laryngeal edema, bronchoconstriction, excessive mucus secretion, coronary vasoconstriction, inflammation, cutaneous reactions, and constriction of the smooth muscle in the intestinal wall, bladder, and uterus. Coronary vasoconstriction causes severe myocardial depression. Cutaneous reactions cause stimulation of nerve endings, followed by itching and pain.[68]

Peripheral vasodilation results in relative hypovolemia and decreased venous return. Increased capillary membrane permeability results in the loss of intravascular volume into the interstitial space, as much as 35% within 10 minutes, worsening the hypovolemic state.[67] Decreased venous return results in decreased end-diastolic volume and SV. The decline in SV leads to decreased CO and ineffective tissue perfusion. Death may result from airway obstruction or cardiovascular collapse, or both.[65-66,68,70]

Assessment and Diagnosis

Anaphylactic shock is a severe systemic reaction that can affect multiple organ systems. A variety of clinical manifestations occur in the patient in anaphylactic shock, depending on the extent of multisystem involvement. The symptoms usually start to appear within minutes of exposure to the antigen, but they may not occur for hours (Box 26-10).[65-66,68] Symptoms may also reappear after a 1- to 72-hour window of resolution in what is termed a biphasic *reaction*.[68,71-72] These late-phase reactions may be similar to the initial anaphylactic response, milder, or more severe.[72] In *protracted anaphylaxis*, symptoms may last up to 32 hours.[67]

The cutaneous effects may appear first and include pruritus, generalized erythema, urticaria, and angioedema. Commonly seen on the face and in the oral cavity and lower pharynx, angioedema develops as a result of fluid leaking into the interstitial space. The patient may appear restless, uneasy, apprehensive, and anxious and may complain of being warm. Respiratory effects include the development of laryngeal edema, bronchoconstriction, and mucous plugs. Clinical manifestations of laryngeal edema include inspiratory stridor, hoarseness, a sensation of fullness or a lump in the throat, and dysphagia. Bronchoconstriction causes dyspnea, wheezing, and chest tightness.[68,70] Gastrointestinal and genitourinary manifestations, which may develop as a result of smooth muscle contraction, include vomiting, diarrhea, cramping, and abdominal pain.

Hypotension and reflex tachycardia may develop quickly. This occurs in response to massive vasodilation and rapid loss of circulating volume. Jugular veins appear flat as right ventricular end-diastolic volume is decreased. The eventual outcome is circulatory failure and ineffective tissue perfusion.[68,70] The patient's level of consciousness may deteriorate to unresponsiveness.

Assessment of the hemodynamic parameters of a patient in anaphylactic shock reveals a decreased CO and CI. Venous vasodilation and massive volume loss lead to a decrease in preload, which results in a decline in the RAP and PAOP. Vasodilation of the arterial system results in a decrease in the afterload of the heart, as evidenced by a decrease in the SVR. Box 26-11 outlines the clinical criteria for diagnosing anaphylaxis.

Medical Management

Treatment of anaphylactic shock requires an immediate and direct approach to prevent death. The goals of therapy are to remove the offending antigen, reverse the effects of the biochemical mediators, and promote adequate tissue perfusion. When the hypersensitivity reaction occurs as a result of administration of medications, dye, blood, or blood products, the infusion should be immediately discontinued. Often, it is not possible to remove the antigen because it is unknown or has already entered the patient's system.

Reversal of the effects of the biochemical mediators involves the preservation and support of the patient's airway, ventilation, and circulation. This is accomplished through oxygen therapy, intubation, mechanical ventilation, and administration of medications and fluids.

Epinephrine is the first-line treatment of choice for anaphylaxis and should be administered when initial signs and symptoms occur.[65,67] It promotes bronchodilation, vasoconstriction, and increased myocardial contractility and inhibits further release of biochemical mediators. In mild cases of anaphylaxis, 0.2 to 0.5 mg (0.3 to 0.5 mL) of a 1 : 1000 dilution of epinephrine is administered by intramuscular injection into the anterolateral thigh and repeated every 5 to 15 minutes

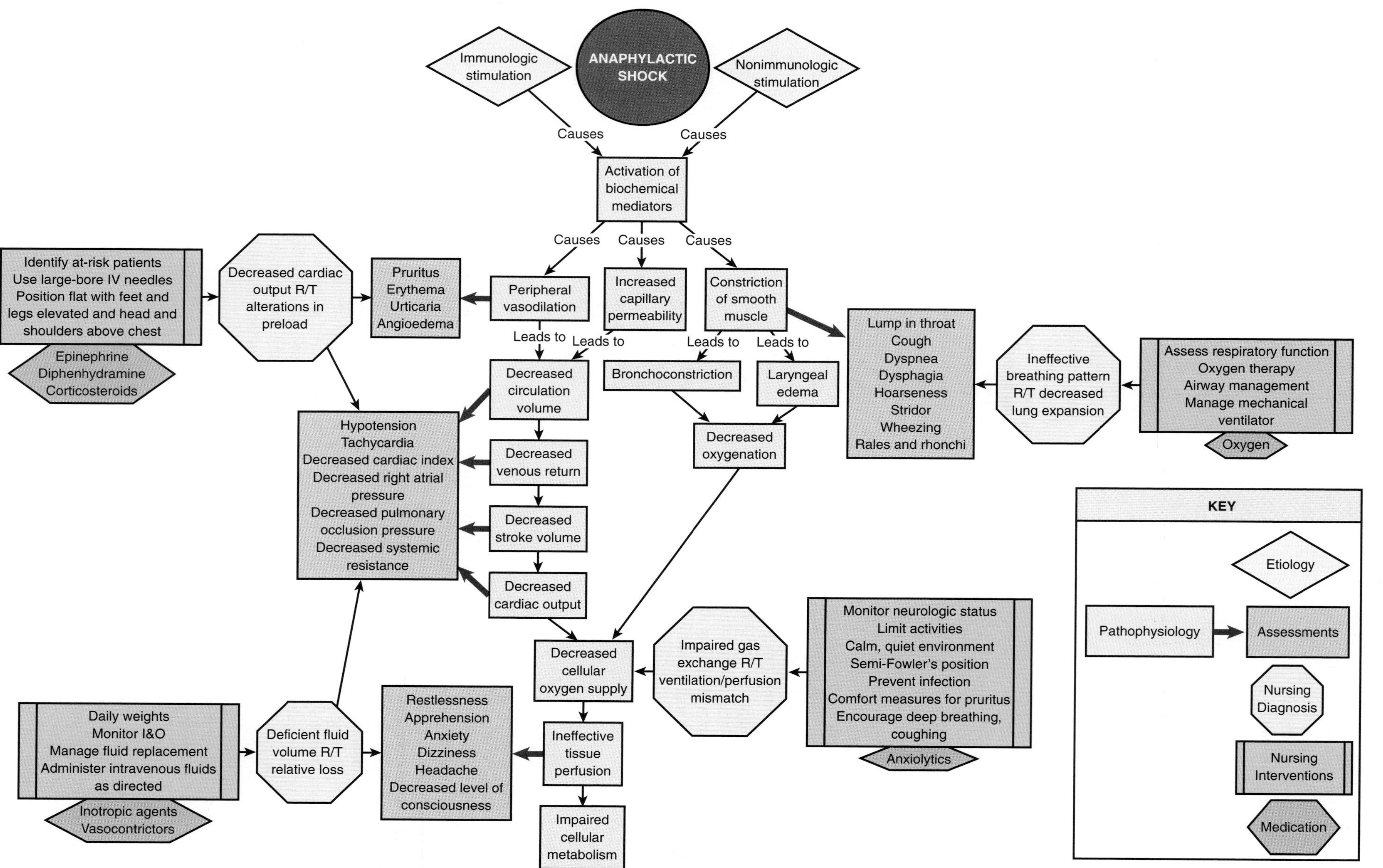

FIG 26-4 Concept Map for Anaphylactic Shock. (Concept map illustration created by Elaine Bishop Kennedy, EdD, RN.)

BOX 26-9 Etiologic Factors in Anaphylactic Shock

Foods
- Eggs and milk
- Fish and shellfish
- Nuts and seeds
- Legumes and cereals
- Soy
- Wheat
- Strawberries
- Avocados
- Any

Food Additives
- Food coloring
- Preservatives

Diagnostic Agents
- Radiocontrast media
- Dehydrocholic acid (Decholin)
- Iopanoic acid (Telepaque)

Biologic Agents
- Blood and blood components
- Insulin and other hormones
- Gammaglobulin
- Seminal fluid
- Vaccines and antitoxins

Environmental Agents
- Pollens, molds, and spores
- Sunlight
- Cold or heat
- Animal dander
- Latex

Drugs
- Antibiotics
- Aspirin
- Nonsteroidal antiinflammatory drugs
- Opioids
- Dextran
- Vitamins
- Muscle relaxants
- Neuromuscular blocking agents
- Barbiturates
- Nonbarbiturate hypnotics
- Protamine
- Infliximab (Remicade)
- Ethanol
- Other

Venoms
- Bees, hornets, yellow jackets, and wasps
- Snakes, jellyfish
- Deer flies
- Fire ants

Physical
- Exercise

BOX 26-10 Clinical Manifestations of Anaphylactic Shock

Cardiovascular
- Hypotension
- Tachycardia
- Bradycardia
- Chest pain

Respiratory
- Lump in throat
- Cough
- Dyspnea
- Dysphagia
- Hoarseness
- Stridor
- Wheezing
- Rhinitis
- Chest tightness

Cutaneous
- Pruritus
- Erythema
- Urticaria
- Angioedema
- Sense of warmth

Neurologic
- Restlessness
- Uneasiness
- Apprehension
- Anxiety
- Dizziness
- Headache
- Sense of impending doom
- Confusion
- Syncope or near syncope

Gastrointestinal
- Nausea
- Vomiting
- Diarrhea
- Cramping abdominal pain

Genitourinary
- Incontinence

Hemodynamic Parameters
- Decreased cardiac output (CO)
- Decreased cardiac index (CI)
- Decreased right atrial pressure (RAP)
- Decreased pulmonary occlusion pressure (PAOP)
- Decreased systemic vascular resistance (SVR)

BOX 26-11 Clinical Criteria for Diagnosing Anaphylaxis

Anaphylaxis is highly likely when one of the following three criteria is fulfilled:

1. Acute onset of an illness (minutes to several hours) with involvement of the skin or mucosal tissue, or both (e.g., generalized hives; pruritus or flushing; swollen lips, tongue, and uvula) *and at least one of the following:*
   a. Respiratory compromise (e.g., dyspnea, wheeze [bronchospasm], stridor, reduced peak expiratory flow, hypoxemia)
   b. Reduced blood pressure or associated symptoms of end-organ dysfunction (e.g., hypotonia [collapse], syncope, incontinence)
2. Two or more of the following that occur rapidly after exposure *to a likely allergen for that patient* (minutes to several hours):
   a. Involvement of the skin-mucosal tissue (e.g., generalized hives; pruritus or flushing; swollen lips, tongue, and uvula)
   b. Respiratory compromise (e.g., dyspnea, wheeze [bronchospasm], stridor, reduced peak expiratory flow, hypoxemia)
   c. Reduced blood pressure or associated symptoms of end-organ dysfunction (e.g., hypotonia [collapse], syncope, incontinence)
   d. Persistent gastrointestinal symptoms (e.g., crampy abdominal pain, vomiting)
3. Reduced blood pressure after exposure *to known allergen for that patient* (minutes to several hours):
   a. Infants and children: low systolic blood pressure (age-specific) or greater than 30% decrease in systolic blood pressure*
   b. Adults: systolic blood pressure of less than 90 mm Hg or greater than 30% decrease for the person's baseline

From Sampson HA, et al. Second symposium on the definition and management of anaphylaxis: summary report—second National Institute of Allergy and Infectious Disease/Food Allergy and Anaphylaxis Network symposium. *J Allergy Clin Immunol.* 2006; 117:391.

*Low systolic blood pressure is defined as less than 70 mm Hg for children 1 month to 1 year old, less than (70 mm Hg + [2 × age]) for children 1 to 10 years old, and less than 90 mm Hg for children 11 to 17 years old.

until anaphylaxis is resolved.[65-68,70-71] Subcutaneous injection is no longer recommended.[71] For anaphylactic shock with hypotension, epinephrine is administered intravenously. The intravenous dose is 0.05 to 0.1 mg (1 mL) of a 1 : 10,000 dilution administered over 5 minutes.[70] If hypotension persists, a continuous infusion of epinephrine is recommended, administered at 1 to 4 mcg/min with titration up to 15 mcg/min as needed.[67,70] Patients receiving beta-blockers may have a limited response to epinephrine. Intravenous glucagon administered as a 20 to 30 mcg/kg bolus over 5 minutes followed by continuous infusion at 5 to 15 mcg/minute is recommended to treat bronchospasm and hypotension in these patients.[66-67,71]

Rapid volume replacement with crystalloid or colloid solutions is also used for patients with hypotension.[66-67,71] Up to 1 L in 5 to 10 minutes is suggested if needed to restore perfusion.[68] Vasopressors may be necessary to reverse the vasodilation and increase blood pressure.[65-66,68,71]

Several medications are used as second-line adjunctive therapy. Inhaled beta-adrenergic agents are used to treat bronchospasm unresponsive to epinephrine.[67-68,70] Diphenhydramine (Benadryl) given 1 to 2 mg/kg (25 to 50 mg) by a slow intravenous is used to block histamine response.[65,67,71] Ranitidine, given in conjunction with diphenhydramine at a dose of 1mL/kg intravenously over 10 to 15 minutes, has been found helpful.[65,67] Corticosteroids are not effective in the immediate treatment of acute anaphylaxis[67,73] but may be given with the goal of preventing a prolonged or delayed reaction.[66,70-71]

BOX 26-12 NURSING DIAGNOSIS PRIORITIES

Anaphylactic Shock

- Deficient Fluid Volume related to relative loss, p. 584
- Decreased Cardiac Output related to alterations in preload, p. 579
- Ineffective Breathing Pattern related to decreased lung expansion, p. 598
- Impaired Gas Exchange related to ventilation/perfusion mismatching or intrapulmonary shunting, p. 594
- Ineffective Coping related to situational crisis and personal vulnerability, p. 599

Nursing Management

Prevention of anaphylactic shock is one of the primary responsibilities of the nurse in the critical care area. Preventive measures include the identification of patients at risk and cautious assessment of the patient's response to the administration of medications, blood, and blood products. A complete and accurate history of the patient's allergies is an essential component of preventive nursing care. In addition to a list of the allergies, a detailed description of the type of response for each one should be obtained.

The patient in anaphylactic shock may have any number of nursing diagnoses, depending on the progression of the process (Box 26-12). **Nursing priorities are directed toward 1) administering epinephrine, 2) facilitating ventilation, 3) administering volume replacement, 4) providing comfort and emotional support, 5) maintaining surveillance for recurrent reactions, and 6) preventing and maintaining surveillance for complications.**

Measures to facilitate ventilation include positioning the patient to assist with breathing and instructing the patient to breathe slowly and deeply. Airway protection through prompt administration of prescribed medications is essential. Measures to facilitate the administration of volume replacement include inserting large-bore peripheral intravenous catheters, rapidly administering prescribed fluids, and positioning the patient in a supine position with the legs elevated. Measures to promote comfort include administering medications to relieve itching and applying warm soaks to skin. Observing the patient for clinical manifestations of a delayed or recurrent reaction is critical. Patient education about how to avoid the precipitating allergen is essential for preventing future episodes of anaphylaxis. Education about how to recognize and respond to a future episode including self-administration of epinephrine is essential to prevent a future life-threatening event.

NEUROGENIC SHOCK

Description and Etiology

Neurogenic shock, another type of distributive shock, is the result of the loss or suppression of sympathetic tone. The lack of sympathetic tone leads to decreased tissue perfusion and initiation of the general shock response (Figure 26-5). Neurogenic shock is the most uncommon form of shock. Neurogenic shock can be caused by anything that disrupts the SNS. The problem can occur as the result of interrupted impulse transmission or blockage of sympathetic outflow from the vasomotor center in the brain.[74-75] The most common cause is spinal cord injury (SCI). Neurogenic shock may mistakenly be referred to as *spinal shock*. The latter condition refers to loss of neurologic activity below the level of SCI, but it does not necessarily involve ineffective tissue perfusion.[74-76]

Pathophysiology

Loss of sympathetic tone results in massive peripheral vasodilation, inhibition of the baroreceptor response, and impaired thermoregulation. Arterial vasodilation leads to a decrease in SVR and a fall in blood pressure. Venous vasodilation leads to relative hypovolemia and pooling of blood in the venous circuit. The decreased venous return results in a decrease in end-diastolic volume or preload, causing a decrease in SV and CO. The fall in blood pressure and CO leads to inadequate or ineffective tissue perfusion. Loss of sympathetic tone and inhibition of the baroreceptor response result in bradycardia.[74-75,77-78] The slow heart rate worsens CO, which further compromises tissue perfusion. Impaired thermoregulation occurs because of loss of vasomotor tone in the cutaneous blood vessels that dilate and constrict to maintain body temperature. The patient becomes poikilothermic, or dependent on the environment for temperature regulation.

Assessment and Diagnosis

The patient in neurogenic shock characteristically presents with hypotension, bradycardia, and warm, dry skin.[74-75,78-79] The decreased blood pressure results from massive peripheral vasodilation. The decreased heart rate is caused by inhibition of the baroreceptor response and unopposed parasympathetic control of the heart.[74-75,78] Consensus on the specific blood pressure and heart rate thresholds for the diagnosis of neurogenic shock has not been established.[74-75] Hypothermia develops from uncontrolled peripheral heat loss. The warm, dry skin occurs as a consequence of pooling of blood in the extremities and loss of vasomotor control in surface vessels of the skin that control heat loss.

Assessment of the hemodynamic parameters of a patient in neurogenic shock reveals a decreased CO and CI. Venous vasodilation leads to a decrease in preload, which results in a decline in the RAP and PAOP. Vasodilation of the arterial system causes a decrease in the afterload of the heart, as evidenced by a decrease in the SVR.[75,78]

Medical Management

Treatment of neurogenic shock requires a careful approach. The goals of therapy are to treat or remove the cause, prevent cardiovascular instability, and promote optimal tissue perfusion. Cardiovascular instability can result from hypovolemia, bradycardia, and hypothermia. Specific treatments are aimed at preventing or correcting these problems as they occur.

Hypovolemia is treated with careful fluid resuscitation. The minimal amount of fluid is administered to ensure adequate tissue perfusion. Volume replacement is initiated for systolic blood pressure lower than 90 mm Hg or evidence of inadequate tissue perfusion. Base deficit or lactate levels are recommended to guide fluid resuscitation in patients with SCI.[77] The patient is carefully observed for evidence of fluid overload. Vasopressors are used as necessary to maintain blood pressure and organ perfusion.[74,76-79] Higher than typical MAPs are commonly needed for patients with acute SCI to prevent cord ischemia, but optimal pressures have not been determined.[74,77] Bradycardia associated with neurogenic shock rarely requires specific treatment, but atropine, intravenous infusion of a beta-adrenergic agent, or electrical pacing can be used when necessary.[78,80] Hypothermia is treated with warming measures and environmental temperature regulation.

Nursing Management

Prevention of neurogenic shock is one of the primary responsibilities of the nurse in the critical care area. This includes the identification of patients at risk and constant assessment of the neurologic status. Vigilant immobilization of spinal cord injuries and slight elevation of the head of the patient's bed after spinal anesthesia are essential components of preventive nursing care. Early identification allows for early treatment and decreased mortality.

The patient in neurogenic shock may have any number of nursing diagnoses, depending on the progression of the process (Box 26-13). **Nursing priorities are directed toward 1) treating hypovolemia and maintaining tissue perfusion, 2) maintaining normothermia, 3) monitoring for and treating dysrhythmias, 4) providing comfort and emotional support, and 5) preventing and maintaining surveillance for complications.**

Venous pooling in the lower extremities promotes the formation of deep vein thrombosis (DVT), which can result in a pulmonary embolism. All patients at risk for DVT should be started on prophylaxis therapy. DVT-prophylactic measures include monitoring of passive range-of-motion exercises, application of sequential pneumatic stockings, and administration of prescribed anticoagulation therapy.

SEVERE SEPSIS AND SEPTIC SHOCK

Description and Etiology

Sepsis occurs when microorganisms invade the body and initiate a systemic inflammatory response. This host response often results in perfusion abnormalities with organ dysfunction (severe sepsis) and eventually hypotension (septic shock). The primary mechanism of this type of shock is the maldistribution of blood flow to the tissues (Figure 26-6).[4] Severe sepsis is estimated to result in more than 700,000 hospitalizations annually in the United States, with an estimated hospital mortality rate of 23% to 50%.[81-84] It is the leading cause of inhospital death, and the eleventh leading cause of all deaths in the United States.[82,85]

Specific terms are used to describe the continuum of conditions that the patient with an infection may experience. In 1991 at the American College of Chest Physicians/Society of Critical Care Medicine (ACCP/SCCM) Consensus

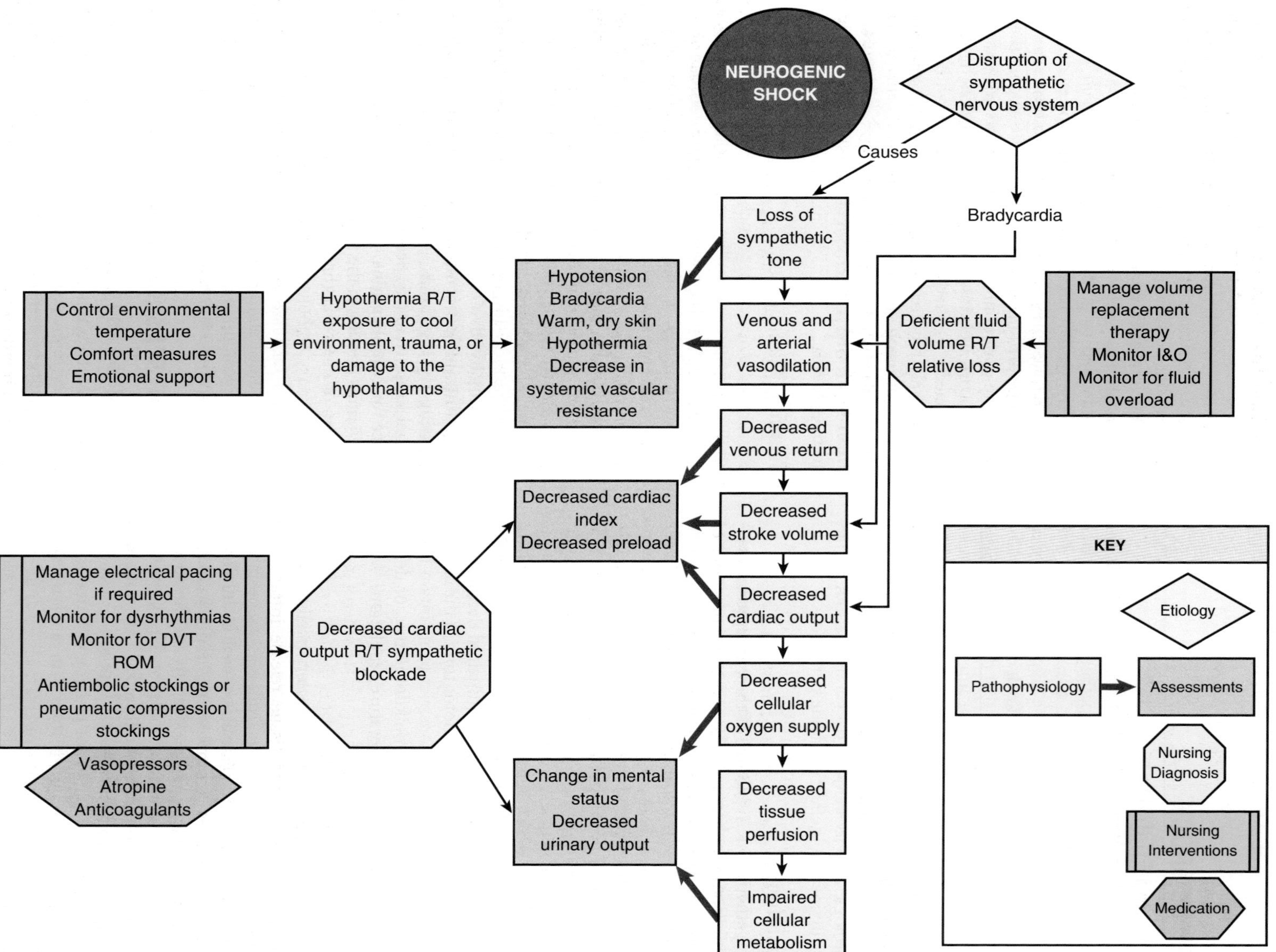

FIG 26-5 Concept Map for Neurogenic Shock. (Concept map illustration created by Elaine Bishop Kennedy, EdD, RN.)

 BOX 26-13 **NURSING DIAGNOSIS PRIORITIES**

Neurogenic Shock

- Deficient Fluid Volume related to relative loss, p. 584
- Decreased Cardiac Output related to sympathetic blockade, p. 581
- Hypothermia related to exposure to cold environment, trauma, or damage to the hypothalamus, p. 592
- Anxiety related to threat to biologic, psychologic, or social integrity, p. 576

Conference, definitions were developed to describe and differentiate these conditions (Box 26-14).[86] These definitions were clarified, reinforced, and updated in subsequent conferences in 2001, 2004, 2008, and 2012.[17,87-88] This discussion focuses on severe sepsis and septic shock.

Sepsis is caused by a wide variety of microorganisms, including gram-negative and gram-positive aerobes, anaerobes, fungi, and viruses. The source of these microorganisms varies. The respiratory system is the most common site of infection producing severe sepsis and septic shock, followed by the genitourinary and gastrointestinal systems.[82,83] Gram-positive bacteria are the predominant cause of sepsis.[83,89] Sepsis and septic shock are associated with a wide variety of intrinsic and extrinsic precipitating factors (Box 26-15). All of these factors interfere directly or indirectly with the body's anatomic and physiologic defense mechanisms. Several of the intrinsic factors are not modifiable or are very difficult to control. Several of the extrinsic factors may be required for diagnosis and management. All critically ill patients are therefore at risk for septic shock.

Pathophysiology

The syndrome encompassing severe sepsis and septic shock is a complex systemic response that is initiated when a microorganism enters the body and stimulates the inflammatory/immune system. In a host-pathogen interaction, both the invading organism and injured tissue release intracellular proteins activating neutrophils, monocytes, lymphocytes, macrophages, mast cells, and platelets as well as numerous plasma enzyme cascades (complement, kinin/kallikrein, coagulation, and fibrinolytic factors). When this reaction is localized, infection is contained and eradicated. But when the magnitude of the infectious insult is great or the patient is physiologically unable to generate an effective host response, containment fails.[90] The result is a systemic release of the pathogen, activated cells, and mediators, including cytokines, which initiate a chain of complex interactions leading to an uncontrolled SIRS.[90-94]

With systemic activation, a variety of physiologic and pathophysiologic events occur that affect clotting, the distribution of blood flow to the tissues and organs, capillary membrane permeability, and the metabolic state of the body. Subsequently, a systemic imbalance between cellular oxygen supply and demand develops that results in cellular hypoxia, damage, hibernation, and death.[5,91,93-94]

Hallmarks of severe sepsis are endothelial damage and coagulation dysfunction.[91-92,95-96] Tissue factor (TF) is released from endothelial cells and monocytes in response to stimulation by inflammatory cytokines.[91,95-97] Release of TF initiates the coagulation cascade, producing widespread microvascular thrombosis and further stimulation of the systemic inflammatory pathways.[91-92,95-97] Diffuse endothelial damage impairs endogenous anticlotting mechanisms.[91-92,95,97] Mediator-induced suppression of fibrinolysis slows clot breakdown. The result is DIC with eventual consumption of coagulation factors, bleeding, and hemorrhage.[92,96-97]

Significant alterations in cardiovascular hemodynamics are caused by the activation of inflammatory cytokines and endothelial damage.[90-92] Massive peripheral vasodilation results in the development of relative hypovolemia. Increased capillary permeability produces a loss of intravascular volume to the interstitium, which accentuates the reduction in preload and CO. These changes, coupled with the microvascular thrombosis, produce maldistribution of circulating blood volume, decreased tissue perfusion, and inadequate oxygen delivery to the cells. Microcirculatory shunting is a key feature of this distributive shock.[91,98] Impaired ventricular contractility results from cytokine activity.[5,91-92,96]

Activation of the central nervous and endocrine systems also occurs as part of the response to invading microorganisms. This activation leads to stimulation of the SNS and the release of ACTH. These events trigger the release of epinephrine, norepinephrine, glucocorticoids, aldosterone, glucagon, renin, and growth hormone, resulting in the development of a hypermetabolic state and contributing to vasoconstriction of the renal, pulmonary, and splanchnic beds. Selective vasoconstriction in the splanchnic bed may contribute to hypoperfusion of the gastrointestinal mucosal barrier, an area particularly vulnerable to the effects of inflammatory cytokines.[92,99] The resulting gut injury propagates the inflammatory response.[2,99]

Several metabolic alterations occur as a result of CNS, endocrine system, and cytokine activation. The hypermetabolic state increases energy expenditure and oxygen demand, and it contributes to cellular hypoxia. Lactic acid is produced as a result of increased metabolic lactate production and hypoxic anaerobic metabolism. Glucocorticoids, ACTH, epinephrine, glucagon, and growth hormone are all catabolic hormones that are released as part of this response. In conjunction with the inflammatory cytokines, these hormones stimulate catabolism of protein stores in the visceral organs and skeletal muscles to fuel glucose production in the liver, hyperglycemia, and insulin resistance.[94,100] The cytokines also stimulate the use of fats for energy production (lipolysis).[94,100-101]

Metabolic derangements in severe sepsis and septic shock include an inability of the cells to use oxygen even if blood flow is adequate. Mitochondrial dysfunction is thought to be the underlying mechanism.[91,94,101-102] This bioenergetic failure plays an important role in the development of tissue ischemia and multiple organ dysfunction.[91,94,101-102] These complex and interrelated pathophysiologic changes produce a pathologic imbalance between cellular oxygen demand and cellular oxygen supply and consumption.

The exaggerated systemic inflammatory response associated with severe sepsis and septic shock results in cell death via both ischemic necrosis and, to a large degree, apoptosis. Apoptosis is a programmed cell death or cellular suicide mediated by caspase-3, a cysteine protease, and affecting endothelial, gastrointestinal epithelial, and immune cells in

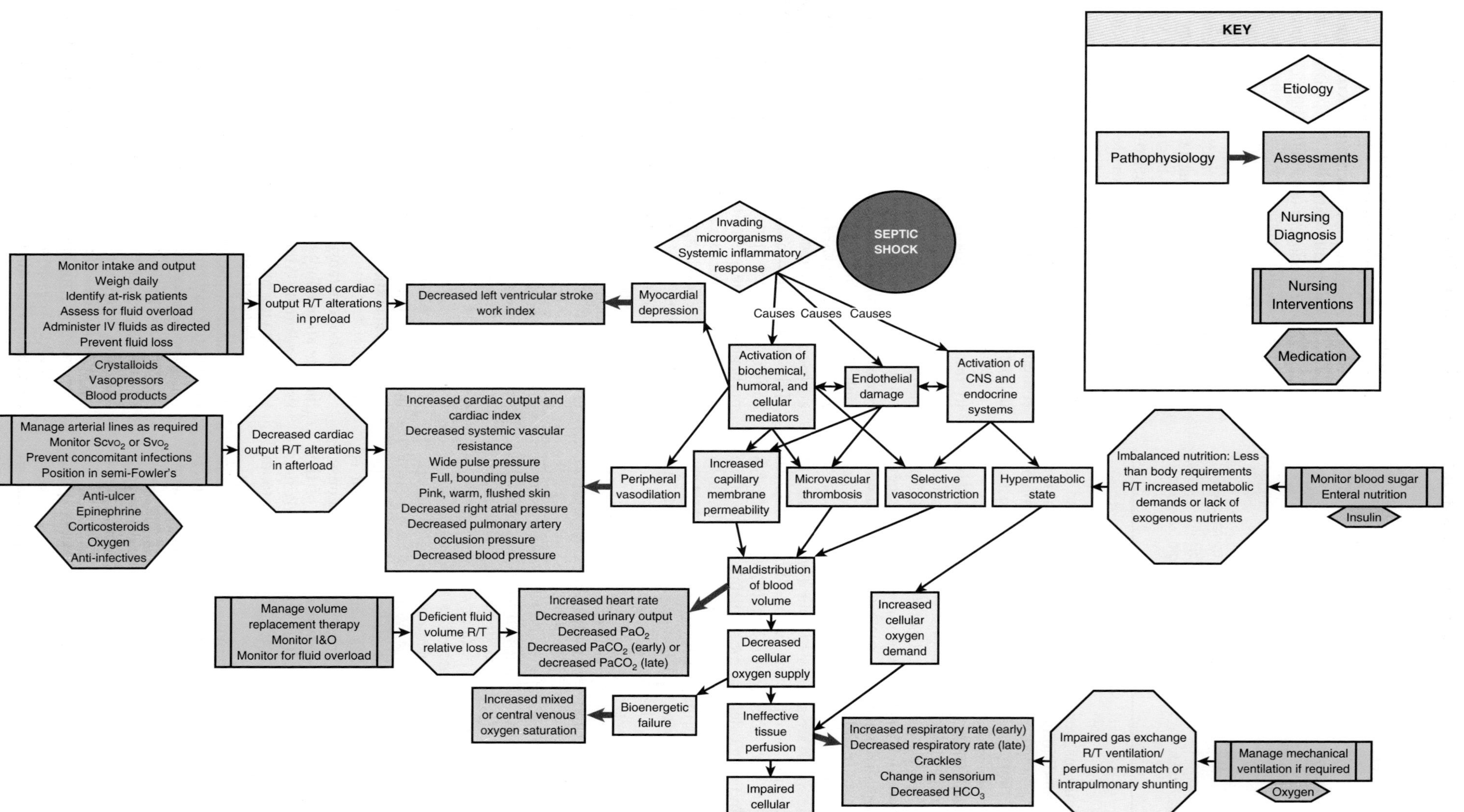

FIG 26-6 **Concept Map for Septic Shock.** (Concept map illustration created by Elaine Bishop Kennedy, EdD, RN.)

BOX 26-14 Definitions for Sepsis and Organ Failure

- *Infection:* Microbial phenomenon characterized by an inflammatory response to the presence of microorganisms or the invasion of normally sterile host tissue by those organisms.
- *Bacteremia:* Presence of viable bacteria in the blood.
- *Systemic inflammatory response syndrome (SIRS):* Systemic inflammatory response to a variety of severe clinical insults, manifested by two or more of the following conditions: 1) temperature >38° C or <36° C; 2) heart rate >90 beats/min; 3) respiratory rate >20 breaths/min or $PaCO_2$ <32 mm Hg; and 4) white blood cell count >12,000/mm^3, <4000/mm^3, or >10% immature (band) forms.
- *Sepsis:* Presence (probable or document) of infection together with systemic manifestations of infection.
- *Severe sepsis:* Sepsis plus sepsis-induced organ dysfunction or tissue hypoperfusion.
- *Sepsis-induced tissue hypoperfusion:* Infection-induced hypotension, elevated lactate, or oliguria.
- *Septic shock:* Sepsis-induced hypotension persisting despite adequate fluid resuscitation.
- *Sepsis-induced hypotension:* A systolic blood pressure <90 mm Hg or mean arterial pressure (MAP) <70 mm Hg, or a SBP decrease of >40 mm Hg or less than 2 standard deviations below normal for age in the absence of other causes for hypotension.
- *Multiple organ dysfunction syndrome (MODS):* Altered organ function in an acutely ill patient such that homeostasis cannot be maintained without intervention.

Adapted from Dellinger RP, Levy MM, Rhodes A, et al. Surviving Sepsis Campaign: international guidelines for management of severe sepsis and septic shock: 2012. *Crit Care Med.* 2013:41(2):585 and American College of Chest Physicians/Society of Critical Care Medicine Consensus Conference. Definitions for sepsis and organ failure and guidelines for the use of innovative therapies in sepsis. *Crit Care Med.* 1992; 20:864.

BOX 26-15 Precipitating Factors Associated with Septic Shock

Intrinsic Factors
- Extreme of age
- Coexisting diseases
  - Malignancies
  - Burns
  - Acquired immunodeficiency syndrome (AIDS)
  - Diabetes
  - Substance abuse
  - Dysfunction of one or more of the major body systems
- Malnutrition

Extrinsic Factors
- Invasive devices
- Medication therapy
- Fluid therapy
- Surgical and traumatic wounds
- Surgical and invasive diagnostic procedures
- Immunosuppressive therapy

particular.[91-92,94,96] Apoptosis of immune cells results in immunosuppression and secondary infection as well as release of immune cell toxins. Both ischemic necrosis and apoptosis stimulate further inflammation, propagating an ongoing cycle of infection, tissue injury, and SIRS.[90,96] If unabated, this situation ultimately results in MODS and death.

Assessment and Diagnosis

Effective treatment of severe sepsis and septic shock depends on timely recognition. The diagnosis of severe sepsis is based on the identification of three conditions: known or suspected infection, systemic manifestations of and evidence of sepsis-induced tissue hypoperfusion. or organ dysfunction. Clinical indications of systemic inflammatory response and sepsis were included in the original ACCP/SCCM consensus definitions and are listed in Box 26-14. The second consensus conference expanded this list to facilitate prompt clinical recognition (Box 26-16).[88]

Signs of individual organ dysfunction are discussed later in the chapter. The two most common organs to demonstrate dysfunction in severe sepsis are the cardiovascular system and the lungs. The patient with persistent hypotension requiring vasopressor therapy despite adequate volume resuscitation is demonstrating cardiovascular dysfunction. Pulmonary dysfunction is manifested by a PaO_2/FIO_2 (fraction of oxygen in inspired air) ratio of less than 300, indicating ARDS.[17,103] Signs indicating septic shock are hypotension despite adequate fluid resuscitation and the presence of perfusion abnormalities such as lactic acidosis, oliguria, or acute change in mentation.

The patient in severe sepsis or septic shock may present with a variety of clinical manifestations that may change dynamically as the condition progresses (Box 26-17). During the initial stage, massive vasodilation occurs in the venous and arterial beds. Dilation of the venous system leads to a decrease in venous return to the heart, which results in a decrease in the preload of the right and left ventricles. This is evidenced by a decline in the RAP and PAOP. Dilation of the arterial system results in a decrease in the afterload of the heart, as evidenced by a decrease in the SVR. The patient's skin becomes pink, warm, and flushed as a result of the massive vasodilation. Myocardial contractility is decreased, as evidenced by a decline in the left ventricular stroke work index (LVSWI) and ejection fraction.

The heart rate rises in response to increased SNS, metabolic, and adrenal gland stimulation. If circulating volume and preload are adequate, this results in a normal-to-high CO and CI despite impaired contractility. The pulse pressure widens as the diastolic blood pressure decreases because of the vasodilation, and the systolic blood pressure increases because of the elevated CO. A full, bounding pulse develops. The net result of these changes is a relatively normal blood pressure in severe sepsis. However, as the reduction in preload and afterload becomes overwhelming and contractility fails, hypotension ensues, resulting in septic shock.

In the lungs, ventilation/perfusion mismatching develops as a result of pulmonary vasoconstriction and the formation of pulmonary microemboli. Hypoxemia occurs, and the respiratory rate increases to compensate for the lack of oxygen. Crackles develop as increased pulmonary capillary membrane permeability leads to pulmonary edema.[103]

The level of consciousness starts to change as a result of decreased cerebral perfusion, immune mediator activation,

BOX 26-16 Diagnostic Criteria for Sepsis

General Variables
- Fever (>38.3° C)
- Hypothermia (core temperature < 36° C)
- Heart rate > 90/min^{-1} or more than two SD above the normal value for age
- Tachypnea
- Altered mental status
- Significant edema or positive fluid balance (>20 mL/kg over 24 hr)
- Hyperglycemia (plasma glucose > 140 mg/dL or 7.7 mmol/L) in the absence of diabetes

Inflammatory Variables
- Leukocytosis (WBC count > 12,000 μL^{-1})
- Leukopenia (WBC count < 4000 μL^{-1})
- Normal WBC count with greater than 10% immature forms
- Plasma C-reactive protein more than two SD above the normal value
- Plasma procalcitonin more than two SD above the normal value

Hemodynamic Variables
- Arterial hypotension (SBP < 90 mm Hg, MAP < 70 mm Hg, or an SBP decrease >40 mm Hg in adults or less than two SD below normal for age)

Organ Dysfunction Variables
- Arterial hypoxemia (PaO_2/FiO_2 < 300)
- Acute oliguria (urine output < 0.5 mL/kg/hr for at least 2 hrs despite adequate fluid resuscitation)
- Creatinine increase > 0.5 mg/dL or 44.2 μmol/L
- Coagulation abnormalities (INR > 1.5 or aPTT > 60 s)
- Ileus (absent bowel sounds)
- Thrombocytopenia (platelet count < 100,000 μL^{-1})
- Hyperbilirubinemia (plasma total bilirubin > 4 mg/dL or 70 μmol/L)

Tissue Perfusion Variables
- Hyperlactatemia (>1 mmol/L)
- Decreased capillary refill or mottling

WBC, White blood cell; *SBP*, systolic blood pressure; *MAP*, mean arterial pressure; *INR*, international normalized ratio; *aPTT*, activated partial thromboplastin time.

Adapted from Adapted from Levy MM, et al.: 2001 SCCM/ESICM/ACCP/ATS/SIS International Sepsis Definitions Conference. Crit Care Med. 2003; 31:1250.

Modified from Dellinger RP, et al. Surviving Sepsis Campaign: international guidelines for management of severe sepsis and septic shock: 2012. *Crit Care Med.* 2013:41(2):585.

hyperthermia, and lactic acidosis. This septic encephalopathy is demonstrated by acute onset of impaired cognitive functioning, or delirium, which may fluctuate during its course.[104] The patient may appear disoriented, confused, combative, or lethargic.

ABG values initially reveal hypocarbia, hypoxemia, and metabolic acidosis. This is demonstrated by a low PaO_2, low $PaCO_2$, and low HCO_3^- level, respectively. The respiratory alkalosis is caused by the patient's increased respiratory rate.

BOX 26-17 Clinical Manifestations of Septic Shock

- Increased heart rate
- Decreased blood pressure
- Wide pulse pressure
- Full, bounding pulse
- Pink, warm, flushed skin
- Increased respiratory rate (early) or decreased respiratory rate (late)
- Crackles
- Change in sensorium
- Decreased urine output
- Increased temperature
- Increased cardiac output and cardiac index
- Decreased systemic vascular resistance
- Decreased right atrial pressure
- Decreased pulmonary artery occlusion pressure
- Decreased left ventricular stroke work index
- Decreased PaO_2
- Decreased $PaCO_2$ (early) or increased $PaCO_2$ (late)
- Decreased HCO_3^-
- Increased SvO_2 or $ScvO_2$

$PaCO_2$, Partial pressure of carbon dioxide; *PaO_2*, partial pressure of oxygen; *$ScvO_2$*, central venous oxygen saturation; *SvO_2*, mixed venous oxygen saturation.

As pathologic pulmonary changes progress and the patient becomes fatigued, the effectiveness of respirations decreases and the $PaCO_2$ increases, resulting in respiratory acidosis. The metabolic acidosis is the result of a lack of oxygen to the cells and the development of lactic acidemia. Serum lactate levels increase above 2 mmol/L because of anaerobic metabolism. The mixed venous oxygen saturation (SvO_2) may increase because of microcirculatory shunting or decrease because of inadequate oxygen delivery.[91,98] The white blood cell (WBC) count is elevated as part of the immune response to the invading microorganisms. The WBC differential count reveals an increase in immature neutrophils (shift to the left). This occurs because the body has to mobilize increasing numbers of WBCs to fight the infection. An elevated procalcitonin level is a valuable biomarker of significant bacterial infection, and procalcitonin levels have been used in clinical trials to guide antibiotic therapy with positive outcomes.[91,105] Serum glucose levels increase as part of the hypermetabolic response and the development of insulin resistance. The patient's temperature is elevated in response to pyrogens released from the invading microorganisms, immune mediator activation, and increased metabolic activity. Urine output declines because of decreased perfusion of the kidneys. As impaired tissue perfusion develops, a variety of other clinical manifestations appear that indicate the development of MODS.

Medical Management

Treatment of the patient in severe sepsis or septic shock requires a multifaceted approach. The goals of treatment are to reverse the pathophysiologic responses, control the infection, and promote metabolic support. This approach includes supporting the cardiovascular system and enhancing tissue perfusion, identifying and treating the infection, limiting the

BOX 26-18 Surviving Sepsis Campaign Bundles

To be Completed within 3 Hours:

1. Measure serum lactate.
2. Obtain blood cultures prior to administration of antibiotics.
3. Administer broad-spectrum antibiotics.
4. Administer 30 mL/kg crystalloid for hypotension or lactate ≥ 4 mmol/L.

To be Completed within 6 Hours:

5. Apply vasopressors (for hypotension that does not respond to initial fluid resuscitation) to maintain a mean arterial pressure (MAP) ≥65 mm hg.
6. In the event of persistent arterial hypotension despite volume resuscitation (septic shock) or initial lactate ≥4 mmol/L (36 mg/dl):
   - Measure adequate central venous (CVP).*
   - Measure central venous oxygen saturation ($ScvO_2$).
7. Remeasure lactate if initial lactate was elevated.

*Targets for quantitative resuscitation included in the guidelines are CVP of ≥ 8 mm Hg, $ScvO_2$ of ≥ 70%, and normalization of lactate.

From Dellinger RP, et al.: Surviving sepsis campaign: international guidelines for management of severe sepsis and septic shock: 2012. Crit Care Med 2013; 41:580-637.

systemic inflammatory response, restoring metabolic balance, and initiating nutritional therapy. Dysfunction of the individual organ systems must be prevented. Early treatment reduces mortality.[17,106-107] Guidelines for the management of severe sepsis and septic shock have been developed and updated under the auspices of the Surviving Sepsis Campaign (SSC), an international effort of more than 11 organizations to improve patient outcomes.[17,87] From these guidelines, a group ("bundle") of selected interventions was identified as having the most impact on patient outcomes. There is a 3-hour bundle and a 6-hour bundle (Box 26-18). More information regarding these interventions is available at the SSC website (http://www.survivingsepsis.org).

The patient in severe sepsis or septic shock requires immediate resuscitation of the hypoperfused state. Specific interventions are aimed at increasing cellular oxygen supply and decreasing cellular oxygen demand. These treatments include administration of fluids, vasopressors, and positive inotropic agents. Early goal-directed therapy during the first 6 hours of resuscitation improves survival[84,106] and is recommended as a protocalized quantitative resuscitation in the SSC guidelines.[17] This therapy includes aggressive fluid resuscitation to augment intravascular volume and increase preload until a CVP of 8 to 12 mm Hg (12 to 15 mm Hg in mechanically ventilated patients) is achieved. Crystalloids are the initial fluid of choice.[17] A fluid challenge for hypovolemia should be initiated with at least 30 mL per kilogram of crystalloids. Albumin may be added when substantial amounts of crystalloids are required. The guidelines recommend against use of hydroxethyl starches. Vasopressors should be administered as necessary to maintain a MAP of 65 mm Hg. These agents reverse the massive peripheral vasodilation and increase SVR. Norepinephrine is recommended as the first-choice agent, as recent evidence strongly indicates superiority of norepinephrine in lowering mortality rates and a higher risk of dysrhythmias when dopamine is used.[108-109] Epinephrine is recommended in addition or as an alternative agent if response to norepinephrine is poor.[17] Dopamine is an alternative only in highly selected patients defined as those with low risk for tachyarrhythmias and absolute or relative bradycardia.[17] Phenylephine is not recommended except in very specific circumstances.[17] Arterial line placement is recommended for any patient requiring vasopressor therapy. Intermittent or continuous monitoring of central venous or mixed venous oxygen saturation ($ScvO_2$ or SvO_2) allows evaluation of the effectiveness of oxygen delivery. If the $ScvO_2$ is less than 70% or the SvO_2 is less than 65% after the CVP goal is achieved, administration of packed red cells to achieve a hematocrit of at least 30% or inotropic stimulation with dobutamine (administered to a maximum of 20 mcg/kg/minute) to counteract myocardial depression and maintain adequate CO are recommended options to obtain this goal.[17,106] The dobutamine infusion should be reduced or discontinued if a tachycardia greater than 120 beats/minute develops.[106]

Intubation and mechanical ventilatory support are usually required to optimize oxygenation and ventilation for the patient in severe sepsis or septic shock. Ventilation with lower than traditional tidal volumes (6 versus 12 mL/kg) in patients with ARDS decreases mortality.[110] SSC guidelines recommend the goals of 6 mL/kg of predicted body weight and plateau pressures no more than 30 cm H_2O for patients with severe sepsis or septic shock with ARDS.[17] Increased $PaCO_2$ may result from this therapy and is acceptable if tolerated as evidenced by hemodynamic stability. Ventilator settings should include positive end-expiratory pressure (PEEP) and be adjusted to provide the patient with a PaO_2 greater than 70 mm Hg. Patients receiving mechanical ventilation should be maintained in a semirecumbent position with the head of the bed raised to 30 to 45 degrees to decrease the incidence of ventilator-associated pneumonia.[17] Prone positioning is suggested for use in the septic patient with ARDS with a paO_2/FiO_2 ratio of 100 mm Hg or less.[17] Sedation protocols using intermittent bolus or continuous infusion using a standardized sedation scale and specific goals are recommended for all patients requiring mechanical ventilation. Daily interruption of sedative infusions to allow wakefulness and reevaluation of sedation needs reduces duration of mechanical ventilation and is recommended.[17] Neuromuscular blocking agents should be avoided, if possible, to prevent prolonged blockade after discontinuation except for a short course of 48 hours or less for patients with ARDS and a PaO_2/FiO_2 ratio of less than 150 mm Hg.[17]

A key measure in the treatment of septic shock is finding and eradicating the cause of the infection. At least two blood cultures plus urine, sputum, and wound cultures should be obtained to find the location of the infection before antibiotic therapy is initiated unless doing so would delay antimicrobial initiation by more than 45 minutes.[17] Antibiotic therapy should be started within 1 hour of recognition of severe sepsis without delay for cultures.[17] Each hour of delay is associated with a substantial drop in the survival rate.[107] If the microorganism is unknown, anti-infective therapy with one or more agents known to be effective against likely pathogens should be initiated, with daily reassessment of the regimen. Low procalcitonin levels are recommended to identify patients to be considered for discontinuation of empiric antiobiotics.[17] Combination therapy is recommended for known or suspected *Pseudomonas* or Acinetobacter infection and for neutropenic patients but should be limited to less than 3 to 5 days.[17] Intervention for a specific source of infection should be undertaken within 12 hours of presentation.[17] Surgical intervention to débride infected or necrotic tissue or to drain abscesses may be necessary to facilitate removal of the septic source.[17] Intravascular devices that may be the source of the infection should be removed after establishment of alternative vascular access.

Only one medication has been brought to market specifically for the treatment of severe sepsis and septic shock, recombinant human activated protein C (rhAPC), marketed as drotrecogin alfa [activated] under the trade name Xigris. This medication was recommended only for patients at high risk for death.[17] However, a Cochrane review found that none of the results of subsequent randomized clinical trials supported the beneficial findings in mortality demonstrated in the original trials used for drug approval both in the United States and Europe.[111] Following failure to show a survival benefit in a major clinical trial launched to reassess the medication, Xigris was voluntarily withdrawn from the market by the manufacturer in October 2011.[112-113] Studies of numerous other medications thought to block or alter the effects of immune mediators have failed to demonstrate effectiveness or have been associated with unacceptable adverse effects.[90,96]

Low-dose intravenous corticosteroids reduce mortality in a select group of catecholamine-dependent septic shock patients.[114-115] Therefore, intravenous hydrocortisone as a continuous infusion of 200 mg per day is recommended *only* for the patient in septic shock who remains hypotensive despite adequate fluid resuscitation and vasopressor therapy.[17,116] Steroid therapy should be weaned when vasopressors are no longer required.

Continuous infusion of intravenous insulin is recommended by SSC guidelines when blood glucose level exceeds 180 mg/dL with a goal blood glucose level equal to or less than 180 mg/dL.[17,117] Glucose levels should be monitored every 1 to 2 hours until stable and then every 4 hours. Low glucose levels measured by capillary testing may be inaccurate in this population.[17] Platelets should be administered when counts are $<10,000/mm^3$ or when counts are <20,000 if a significant risk of bleeding is present. Red blood cell transfusions are recommended when the hemoglobin level is less than 7.0 g/dL to obtain a target value of 7 to 9 g/dL.[17] Stress ulcer prophylaxis using H_2-receptor antagonists or proton pump inhibitors and DVT prophylaxis are recommended for all patients with severe sepsis or septic shock. The SCCM guidelines recommend against the use of intravenous immunoglobulins or selenium and sodium bicarbonate for lactic acidemia if the pH is equal to or greater than 7.15.[17] Low-dose dopamine infusion for renal protection is not beneficial and should not be used.[17] Setting goals of care with the patient and family, including use of palliative care principles when appropriate, are recommended within 72 hours of ICU admission.[17]

The initiation of nutritional therapy is critical in the management of the patient in severe sepsis or septic shock, and enteral feeding is recommended within 48 hours of diagnosis.[17] The goal is to improve the patient's overall nutritional status, enhance immune function, and promote wound healing. A daily caloric intake of 20 to 30 kcal/kg of usual body weight is recommended for critically ill patients, but low-dose feeding, up to 500 calories per day, is recommended for patients in severe sepsis or septic shock in the first week.[17] When compared to enteral nutrition, parenteral nutrition or a combination of both methods has been associated with higher mortality in patients with severe sepsis or septic shock and is not recommended during the first 7 days after diagnosis.[118]

Sufficient protein needs to be provided because of the metabolic derangements that develop in the hypermetabolic state. A range of 1.2 to 2.0 g/kg actual body weight per day is recommended for patients with a body mass index (BMI) less than 30, with progressively larger amounts for those with higher BMI.[38] Specific nutritional therapies to reduce the inflammatory and hypermetabolic responses associated with sepsis, such as antioxidant supplementation and feeding with long-chain n-3 polyunsaturated fatty acids, are the source of much debate and evaluation.[100,119] Glutamine is considered by some to be an essential amino acid in critically ill patients and has the most empirical support,[91,119] but others may actually worsen outcomes. Current SSC recommendations stress not using any immune-modulating supplementation in patients with severe sepsis.[17,38]

Nursing Management

Nursing recommendations to complement the SSC guidelines have recently been published and focus on infection prevention and transmission, early recognition and treatment of severe sepsis and septic shock and its progression, and supportive nursing care.[120] Prevention of severe sepsis and septic shock is one of the primary responsibilities of the nurse in the critical care area. These measures include the identification of patients at risk and reduction of their risk factors, including exposure to invading microorganisms. Hand washing, aseptic technique, and an understanding of evidence-based practice to reduce nosocomial infection in critically ill patients are essential components of preventive nursing care. Early identification allows for early treatment and decreases mortality. Figure 26-7 is a simple screening tool for identifying patients with severe sepsis. Subsequent continual observation to detect subtle changes that indicate the progression of the septic process is vitally important, as is evidence-based practice to prevent further infection. Immunosuppression is common as sepsis progresses,[96] and recent research has found that a resurgence in opportunistic infection in patients with severe sepsis and septic shock occurs in the later stages, more than 2 weeks after initial diagnosis and treatment.[121] Evidence-based practice to prevent complications of critical illness and prolonged bed rest are essential to prevent further compromise and negative short- and long-term outcomes. Ongoing mortality and impaired quality-of-life persist in the months and years after hospital discharge for survivors of sepsis.[122]

The patient in septic shock may have any number of nursing diagnoses, depending on the progression of the process (Box 26-19). **Nursing priorities are directed toward 1) early identification of sepsis syndrome, 2) administering prescribed fluids, medications, and nutrition, 3) providing comfort and emotional support, and 4) preventing and maintaining surveillance for complications.** Evidence-based guidelines for the management of the patient with severe sepsis or septic shock are listed in Box 26-20.

Evaluation for Severe Sepsis Screening Tool

Instructions: Use this optional tool to screen patients for severe sepsis in the emergency department, on the wards, or in the ICU.

1. Is the patient's history suggestive of a new infection?

❑ Pneumonia, empyema
❑ Urinary tract infection
❑ Acute abdominal infection
❑ Meningitis
❑ Skin/soft tissue infection
❑ Bone/joint infection
❑ Wound infection
❑ Bloodstream catheter infection
❑ Endocarditis
❑ Implantable device infection
❑ Other ____________

___ **Yes** ___ **No**

2. Are any two of the following signs & symptoms of infection both present and new to the patient? Note: laboratory values may have been obtained for inpatients but may not be available for outpatients.

❑ Hyperthermia > 38.3° C (101.0° F)
❑ Hypothermia < 36° C (96.8° F)
❑ Tachycardia > 90 bpm
❑ Tachypnea > 20 bpm
❑ Acutely altered mental status
❑ Leukocytosis (WBC count >12,000 mcg-1)
❑ Leukopenia (WBC count < 4000 mcg-1)
❑ Hyperglycemia (plasma glucose >120 mg/dL) in the absence of diabetes

___ **Yes** ___ **No**

If the answer is yes to both either question 1 and 2, *suspicion of infection* is present:

✓ Obtain: **lactic acid, blood cultures,** CBC with differential, basic chemistry labs, bilirubin.
✓ At the physician's discretion obtain: UA, chest x-ray, amylase, lipase, ABG, CRP, CT scan.

3. Are any of the following organ dysfunction criteria present at a site remote from the site of the infection that are not considered to be chronic conditions? Note: the remote site stipulation is waived in the case of bilateral pulmonary infiltrates.

❑ SBP < 90 mm Hg or MAP < 65 mm Hg
❑ SBP decrease > 40 mm Hg from baseline
❑ Bilateral pulmonary infiltrates with a new (or increased) oxygen requirement to maintain SpO_2 > 90%
❑ Bilateral pulmonary infiltrates with PaO_2/FiO_2 ratio < 300
❑ Creatinine > 2.0 mg/dL (176.8 mmol/L) or Urine Output < 0.5 mL/kg/hour for > 2 hours
❑ Bilirubin > 2 mg/dL (34.2 mmol/L)
❑ Platelet count < 100,000
❑ Coagulopathy (INR > 1.5 or aPTT > 60 secs)
❑ Lactate > 2 mmol/L (18.0 mg/dL)

___ **Yes** ___ **No**

If *suspicion of infection* is present AND *organ dysfunction* is present, the patient meets the criteria for SEVERE SEPSIS and should be entered into the severe sepsis protocol.

Date: ___/___/___ (circle: dd/mm/yy or mm/dd/yy) Time: ___:___ (24 hr. clock)

Version 7.12.2005 © 2005 Surviving Sepsis Campaign and the Institute for Healthcare Improvement

FIG 26-7 Evaluation for Severe Sepsis Screening Tool. (Redrawn from the Institute for Healthcare Improvement, Cambridge, MA. Copyright 2005 Surviving Sepsis Campaign and the Institute for Healthcare Improvement.)

MULTIPLE ORGAN DYSFUNCTION SYNDROME

Description and Etiology

MODS results from progressive physiologic failure of two or more separate organ systems in an acutely ill patient such that homeostasis cannot be maintained without intervention.[86] MODS is the major cause of death in patients cared for in critical care units. Mortality is closely linked to the number of organ systems involved. Dysfunction or failure of two or more organ systems is associated with an estimated mortality rate of 54%, which rises to 100% when five organ systems fail.[123] MODS survivors may develop generalized polyneuropathy and a chronic form of pulmonary disease from ARDS, complicating recovery. These patients often require prolonged, expensive rehabilitation.[124]

BOX 26-19 NURSING DIAGNOSIS PRIORITIES

Septic Shock

- Deficient Fluid Volume related to relative loss, p. 584
- Decreased Cardiac Output related to alterations in preload, p. 579
- Decreased Cardiac Output related to alterations in contractility, p. 580
- Impaired Gas Exchange related to ventilation/perfusion mismatching or intrapulmonary shunting, p. 594
- Imbalanced Nutrition: Less Than Body Requirements related to increased metabolic demands or lack of exogenous nutrients, p. 593
- Anxiety related to threat to biologic, psychologic, or social integrity, p. 576

Trauma patients are particularly vulnerable to developing MODS because they often experience ischemia-reperfusion events resulting from hemorrhage, blunt trauma, or SNS-induced vasoconstriction.[125] Other high-risk patients include those who have experienced infection, a shock episode, various ischemia-reperfusion events, acute pancreatitis, sepsis, burns, aspiration, multiple blood transfusions, or surgical complications.[86] Patients age 65 years or older are at increased risk because of their decreased organ reserve and comorbidities.[126]

Organ dysfunction may be the direct consequence of an initial insult (Primary MODS) or can manifest latently and involve organs not directly affected in the initial insult (Secondary MODS). Patients can experience both Primary and Secondary MODS (Figure 26-8).

Primary MODS results from a well-defined insult in which organ dysfunction occurs early and is directly attributed to the insult itself. Direct insults initially cause localized

BOX 26-20 EVIDENCE-BASED PRACTICE (QSEN)

Severe Sepsis and Septic Shock Management Guidelines

A. **Initial Resuscitation**
1. Protocolized, quantitative resuscitation of patients with sepsis-induced tissue hypoperfusion. Goals during first 6 hrs of resuscitation:
   a) Central venous pressure 8-12 mm Hg
   b) Mean arterial pressure (MAP) ≥ 65 mm Hg
   c) Urine output ≥ 0.5 mL/kg/hr
   d) Central venous (superior vena cava) or mixed venous oxygen saturation 70% or 65%, respectively (grade 1C).
2. In patients with elevated lactate levels, targeting resuscitation to normalize lactate (grade 2C).

B. **Screening for Sepsis and Performance Improvement**
1. Routine screening of potentially infected seriously ill patients for severe sepsis to allow earlier implementation of therapy (grade 1C).
2. Hospital–based performance improvement efforts in severe sepsis (UG).

C. **Diagnosis**
1. Cultures before antimicrobial therapy if delay is <45 min in the start of antimicrobial(s) (grade 1C). ≥2 sets of blood cultures (aerobic and anaerobic) with at least 1 drawn percutaneously and 1 drawn through each vascular access device, unless the device was inserted <48 hrs (grade 1C).
2. 1,3 beta-D-glucan assay (grade 2B), mannan and anti-mannan antibody assays (2C), if available and invasive candidiasis is in differential diagnosis.
3. Imaging studies to confirm a potential source of infection (UG).

D. **Antimicrobial Therapy**
1. Goal: IV antimicrobials within first hour of septic shock (grade 1B) and severe sepsis without septic shock (grade 1C).

2a. Initial empiric antiinfective therapy of drug(s) active against all likely pathogens and that penetrate inadequately into sepsis source tissues (grade 1B).

2b. Antimicrobial regimen reassessed daily for potential deescalation (grade 1B).

3. Low procalcitonin levels or similar biomarkers assist clinicians in discontinuation of therapy in patients who initially appeared septic, but have no subsequent evidence of infection (grade 2C).

4a. Combination therapy for neutropenic patients with severe sepsis (grade 2B) and for patients with difficult-to-treat, multi-drug-resistant bacterial pathogens (grade 2B). For patients with severe infections associated with respiratory failure and septic shock, combination therapy with an extended spectrum beta-lactam and either an aminoglycoside or a fluoroquinolone (for *P. aeruginosa* bacteremia) (grade 2B). A combination of beta-lactam and macrolide for patients with septic shock from bacteremic *Streptococcus pneumoniae* infections (grade 2B).

4b. Combination therapy should not be administered for >3-5 days. Deescalation to most appropriate single therapy should be performed as soon as the susceptibility profile is known (grade 2B).

5. Duration of therapy typically 7-10 days; longer courses may be appropriate in patients who have a slow clinical response, undrainable foci of infection, bacteremia with *S. aureus,* and some fungal and viral infections or immunologic deficiencies (grade 2C).
6. Antiviral therapy initiated as early as possible in patients with severe sepsis or septic shock of viral origin (grade 2C).
7. Antimicrobial agents should not be used in patients with severe inflammatory states determined to be of noninfectious cause (UG).

E. **Source Control**
1. Specific anatomical diagnosis and emergent source control should be diagnosed or excluded as rapidly as possible; source control intervention should be undertaken <12 hr after diagnosis, if feasible (grade 1C).
2. When source is potentially infected peripancreatic necrosis, definitive intervention is best delayed until after adequate demarcation of viable tissues (grade 2B).

BOX 26-20 **EVIDENCE-BASED PRACTICE—cont'd**

Severe Sepsis and Septic Shock Management Guidelines

3. For source control in severely septic patients, effective interventions associated with the least physiologic insult should be used (UG).
4. If IV access devices are possible sources, they should be removed promptly after other vascular access has been established (UG).

F. **Infection Prevention**

1a. Selective oral and digestive decontamination should be considered to reduce the incidence of ventilator-associated pneumonia; this can be instituted in settings where it is effective (grade 2B).

1b. Oral chlorhexidine gluconate should be used to reduce risk of ventilator-associated pneumonia in ICU patients with severe sepsis (grade 2B).

G. **Fluid Therapy of Severe Sepsis**

1. Crystalloids initially in resuscitation of severe sepsis and septic shock (grade 1B).
2. Against hydroxyethyl starches for resuscitation of severe sepsis and septic shock (grade 1B).
3. Albumin in resuscitation of severe sepsis and septic shock when patients require substantial crystalloids (grade 2C).
4. Initial fluid challenge (to a minimum of 30 mL/kg of crystalloids) in patients with sepsis-induced tissue hypoperfusion with suspicion of hypovolemia. More rapid administration and greater amounts may be needed in some (grade 1C).
5. Fluid challenge technique may be applied wherein fluid administration is continued if there is hemodynamic improvement based on dynamic or static variables (UG).

H. **Vasopressors**

1. Vasopressor therapy initially to target mean arterial pressure (MAP) of 65 mm Hg (grade 1C).
2. Norepinephrine (NE) as first choice vasopressor (grade 1B).
3. Epinephrine (added to and potentially substituted for norepinephrine) when additional agent is needed to maintain adequate BP (grade 2B).
4. Vasopressin 0.03 units/minute can be added to NE to raise MAP or decrease NE dosage (UG).
5. Low-dose vasopressin not recommended as the single initial vasopressor for treatment of sepsis-induced hypotension. Vasopressin doses >0.03-0.04 units/minute should be reserved for salvage therapy (UG).
6. Dopamine as an alternative to norepinephrine only in highly selected patients (grade 2C).
7. Phenylephrine not recommended in the treatment of septic shock except where a) norepinephrine is associated with serious arrhythmias, b) cardiac output is high and BP persistently low, or c) as salvage therapy when combined inotrope/vasopressor drugs and low-dose vasopressin have failed to achieve MAP target (grade 1C).
8. Low-dose dopamine should not be used for renal protection (grade 1A).
9. All patients requiring vasopressors have an arterial catheter placed as soon as practical (UG).

I. **Inotropic Therapy**

1. A trial of dobutamine infusion up to 20 mcg/kg/min be administered or added to vasopressor (if in use) in the presence of a) myocardial dysfunction or b) ongoing signs of hypoperfusion, despite adequate intravascular volume and adequate MAP (grade 1C).
2. Not using a strategy to increase cardiac index to predetermined supranormal levels (grade 1B).

J. **Corticosteroids**

1. Do not use IV hydrocortisone to treat adults if adequate fluid resuscitation and vasopressor therapy are able to restore hemodynamic stability. Otherwise, IV hydrocortisone alone at a dose of 200 mg per day (grade 2C) is suggested.
2. Do not use ACTH stimulation test to identify adults who should receive hydrocortisone (grade 2B).
3. If used, hydrocortisone tapered when vasopressors no longer required (grade 2D).
4. Do not use corticosteroids for treatment of sepsis without shock (grade 1D).
5. When hydrocortisone is given, use continuous flow (grade 2D).

K. **Blood Product Administration**

1. Once tissue hypoperfusion has resolved (in absence of extenuating circumstances), red blood cell transfusion is recommended only when Hgb decreases to <7.0 g/dL to target an Hgb concentration of 7.0-9.0 g/dL in adults (grade 1B).
2. Do not use erythropoietin to treat anemia associated with severe sepsis (grade 1B).
3. Do not use fresh frozen plasma to correct laboratory clotting abnormalities in the absence of bleeding or planned invasive procedures (grade 2D).
4. Do not use antithrombin for treatment of severe sepsis and septic shock (grade 1B).
5. In patients with severe sepsis, administer platelets prophylactically when <10,000/mm^3 (10 × 10^9/L) in absence of apparent bleeding. Prophylactic platelet transfusion suggested when <20,000/mm^3 (20 × 10^9/L) if patient has significant risk of bleeding. Higher platelet counts (≥50,000/mm^3 [50 × 10^9/L]) advised for active bleeding, surgery, or invasive procedures (grade 2D).

L. **Immunoglobulins**

1. Do not use IV immunoglobulins in adults with severe sepsis or septic shock (grade 2B).

M. **Selenium**

1. Do not use IV selenium for treatment of severe sepsis (grade 2C).

N. **Mechanical Ventilation of Sepsis-Induced Acute Respiratory Distress Syndrome (ARDS)**

1. Target tidal volume of 6 mL/kg predicted body weight in patients with sepsis-induced ARDS (grade 1A vs. 12 mL/kg).
2. Measure plateau pressures in patients with ARDS. Initial upper limit goal in a passively inflated lung is ≤30 cm H_2O (grade 1B).
3. Apply positive end-expiratory pressure (PEEP) to avoid alveolar collapse at end expiration (grade 1B).

Continued

BOX 26-20 **EVIDENCE-BASED PRACTICE—cont'd**

Severe Sepsis and Septic Shock Management Guidelines

4. Use strategies based on higher levels of PEEP for patients with sepsis-induced moderate or severe ARDS (grade 2C).
5. Use recruitment maneuvers in sepsis patients with severe refractory hypoxemia (grade 2C).
6. Use prone positioning in sepsis-induced ARDS patients with a PaO_2/FiO_2 ratio ≤100 mm Hg (grade 2B).
7. Maintain mechanically ventilated sepsis patients with head of bed elevated 30-45° to limit aspiration risk and prevent development of ventilator-associated pneumonia (grade 1B).
8. Use noninvasive mask ventilation (NIV) in that minority of sepsis-induced ARDS patients in whom the benefits of NIV have been carefully considered (grade 2B).
9. Put a weaning protocol in place. Mechanically ventilated patients with severe sepsis should undergo spontaneous breathing trials regularly to evaluate ability to discontinue mechanical ventilation when they a) are arousable, b) are hemodynamically stable (without vasopressor agents), c) have no new potentially serious conditions, d) have low ventilator and end-expiratory pressure requirements, and e) have low FiO_2 requirements that can be met with a face mask or nasal cannula. If spontaneous breathing trial is successful, consider extubation (grade 1A).
10. Do not routinely use pulmonary artery catheter for patients with sepsis-induced ARDS (grade 1A).
11. Use a conservative fluid strategy for patients with established sepsis-induced ARDS who do not have evidence of tissue hypoperfusion (grade 1C).
12. In the absence of specific indications, do not use beta 2-agonists for treatment of sepsis-induced ARDS (grade 1B).

O. **Sedation, Analgesia, and Neuromuscular Blockade in Sepsis**

1. Continuous or intermittent sedation should be minimized in mechanically ventilated sepsis patients, targeting specific titration endpoints (grade 1B).
2. Avoid neuromuscular blocking agents (NMBAs) if possible in septic patients *without ARDS* due to risk of prolonged neuromuscular blockade following discontinuation. If NMBAs must be maintained, use either intermittent bolus as required or continuous infusion with train-of-four monitoring (grade 1C).
3. Use a short course of NMBA ≤48 hours for patients *with* early sepsis-induced ARDS and $PaO_2/FiO_2 < 150$ mm Hg (grade 2C).

P. **Glucose Control**

1. A protocolized approach to management in ICU patients with severe sepsis commencing insulin dosing when 2 consecutive blood glucose levels are >180 mg/dL. Approach should target an upper blood glucose ≤180 mg/dL (grade 1A).
2. Blood glucose values should be monitored every 1-2 hrs until glucose values and insulin infusion rates stabilize, then every 4 hr, thereafter (grade 1C).
3. Glucose levels obtained with point-of-care testing of capillary blood should be interpreted with caution (UG).

Q. **Renal Replacement Therapy**

1. Continuous renal replacement therapies and intermittent hemodialysis are equivalent in severe sepsis and acute renal failure (grade 2B).
2. Use continuous therapies to facilitate management of fluid balance in hemodynamically unstable septic patients (grade 2D).

R. **Bicarbonate Therapy**

1. Do not use sodium bicarbonate therapy for improving hemodynamics or reducing vasopressor requirements in patients with hypoperfusion-induced lactic acidemia with pH ≥7.15 (grade 2B).

S. **Deep Vein Thrombosis Prophylaxis**

1. Patients with severe sepsis should receive daily pharmacoprophylaxis against venous thromboembolism (grade 1B). Accomplish with daily subcutaneous low–molecular-weight heparin (LMWH) (grade 1B vs. twice daily UFH, grade 2C vs. three times daily UFH). If creatinine clearance <30 mL/min, use dalteparin (grade 1A) or another form of LMWH that has a low degree of renal metabolism (grade 2C) or UFH (grade 1A).
2. Treat patients with severe sepsis with combination of pharmacologic therapy and intermittent pneumatic compression devices if possible (grade 2C).
3. Do not use pharmacoprophylaxis in septic patients who have a contraindication for heparin use (grade 1B). Use mechanical prophylactic treatment (grade 2C), unless contraindicated. When risk decreases, start pharmacoprophylaxis (grade 2C).

T. **Stress Ulcer Prophylaxis**

1. Give stress ulcer prophylaxis using H2 blocker or proton pump inhibitor to patients with severe sepsis/septic shock who have bleeding risk factors (grade 1B).
2. If used, proton pump inhibitors preferred over H2RA (grade 2D)
3. Patients without risk factors do not receive prophylaxis (grade 2B).

U. **Nutrition**

1. Administer oral or enteral feedings rather than either complete fasting or provision of only IV glucose within the first 48 hours after diagnosis of severe sepsis/septic shock (grade 2C).
2. Avoid mandatory full caloric feeding in first week. Suggest low-dose feeding, advancing only as tolerated (grade 2B).
3. Use IV glucose and enteral nutrition rather than total parenteral nutrition alone or parenteral nutrition in conjunction with enteral feeding in the first 7 days after diagnosis of severe sepsis/septic shock (grade 2B).
4. Use nutrition with no specific immunomodulating supplementation in patients with severe sepsis (grade 2C).

V. **Setting Goals of Care**

1. Discuss goals and prognosis with patients and families (grade 1B).
2. Incorporate goals into treatment and end-of-life care planning (grade 1B).
3. Address goals as early as feasible, but no later than within 72 hours of ICU admission (grade 2C).

UG, Ungraded.

Data from Dellinger RP, Levy MM, Rhodes A, et al. Surviving Sepsis Campaign: international guidelines for management of severe sepsis and septic shock: 2012. *Crit Care Med.* 2013: 41(2):580.

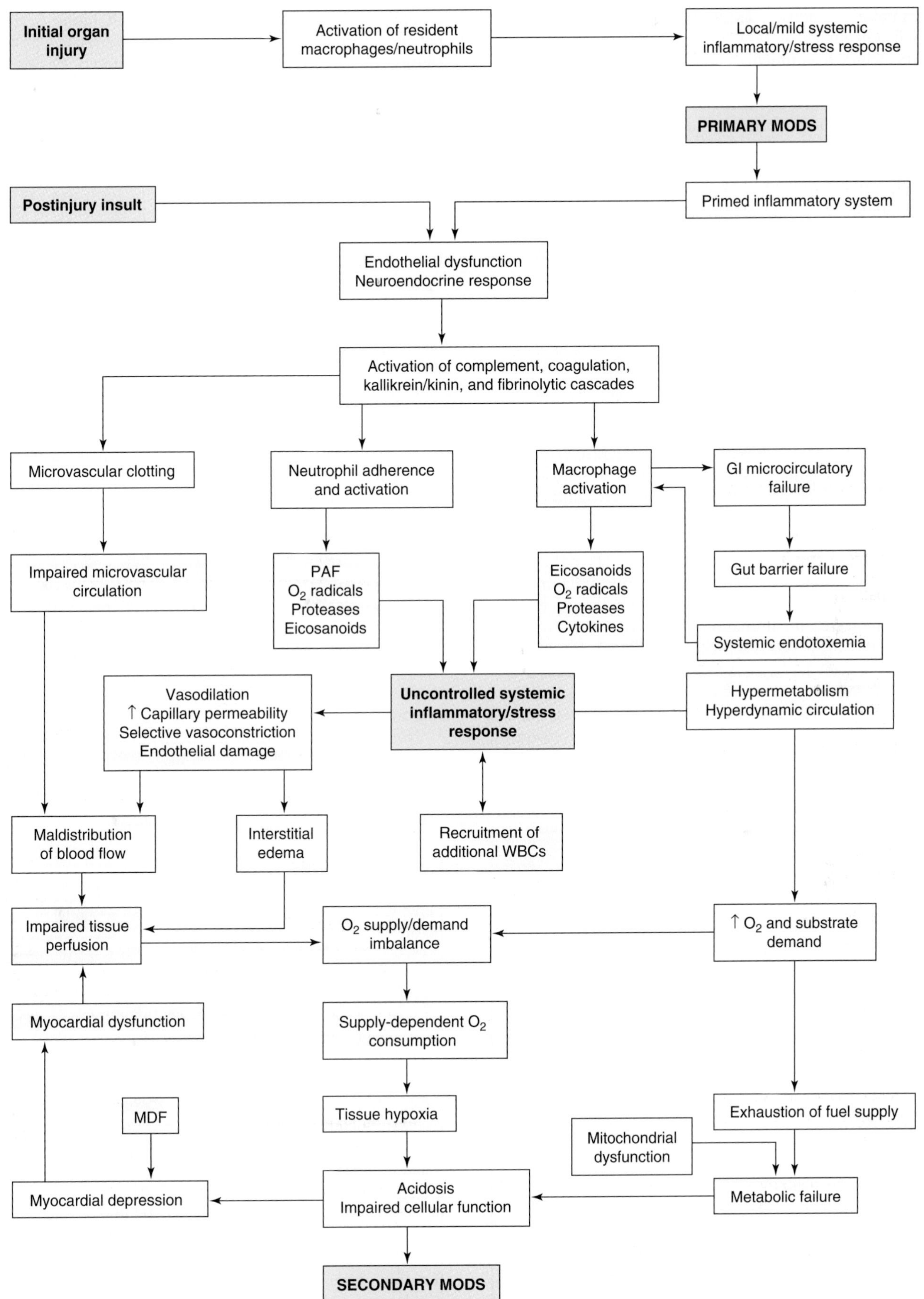

FIG 26-8 Pathogenesis of Multiple Organ Dysfunction Syndrome. *GI,* Gastrointestinal; *MDF,* myocardial depressant factor; *MODS,* multiple organ dysfunction syndrome; *PAF,* platelet activating factor; *WBCs,* white blood cells. (From McCance KL, Huether SE, eds. *Pathophysiology: The Biological Basis for Disease in Adults and Children.* 7th ed. St. Louis: Elsevier; 2014.)

inflammatory responses. Primary MODS accounts for only a small percentage of MODS cases. Examples of Primary MODS include the immediate consequences of posttraumatic pulmonary failure, thermal injuries, AKI, or invasive infections.[86] These cellular or microcirculatory insults may lead to a loss of critical organ function induced by failure of delivery of oxygen and substrates, coupled with the inability to remove end-products of metabolism. The inflammatory response in Primary MODS has a less apparent presentation and may resolve without long-term implications. However, Primary MODS may "prime" physiologic systems for a more sustained exaggerated inflammatory response that leads to Secondary MODS.

Secondary MODS is a consequence of widespread sustained systemic inflammation that results in dysfunction of organs not involved in the initial insult. Secondary MODS develops latently after an initial insult.[86] The early impairment of organs normally involved in immunoregulatory function, such as the liver and the GI tract, intensifies the host response to the insult.[127] The initial insult may prime the inflammatory system in such a way that even a mild second insult (hit) may perpetuate a sustained hyperinflammatory response. This "two-hit hypothesis" has been increasingly recognized as an important contributor to morbidity and mortality in patients with Secondary MODS.[128]

SIRS and sepsis are common initiating events in the development of Secondary MODS. The systemic inflammatory response is an intense host response characterized by sustained generalized inflammation in organs remote from the initial insult. SIRS is widespread inflammation or clinical responses to inflammation that occur in patients suffering a variety of insults. Clinical conditions and manifestations associated with SIRS are listed in Box 26-21. These insults produce similar or identical systemic inflammatory responses, even in the absence of infection. The diagnostic criteria for SIRS have been previously addressed (Figure 26-7). Manifestations of SIRS must represent an acute alteration from the patient's normal baseline and must not be related to other causes (e.g., neutropenia from chemotherapy). Organ dysfunction, such as ARDS, AKI, and MODS, is a complication of SIRS.[86,123] In epidemiologic studies, SIRS was found to occur in one-third of all hospitalized patients, in 50% to 93% of all patients in critical care units, and in about 80% of all patients in surgical critical care units.[129-130]

When SIRS is a result of infection, the term *sepsis* is used. SIRS, sepsis, severe sepsis, and septic shock represent a hierarchical continuum of the inflammatory response to infection.[17] Infection and shock are the most common precipitating factors; however, any disease that induces a major inflammatory response can initiate the events that lead to MODS.

When inflammation is not contained locally, consequences occur systemically that lead to organ dysfunction, including intense, uncontrolled activation of inflammatory cells, direct damage of vascular endothelium, disruption of immune cell function, persistent hypermetabolism, and maldistribution of circulatory volume to organ systems. Inflammation becomes a systemic, self-perpetuating process that is inadequately controlled and results in organ dysfunction.[123]

During hypermetabolism, changes occur in cellular anabolic and catabolic function, resulting in autocatabolism. Autocatabolism manifests as a severe decrease in lean body mass, severe weight loss, anergy, and increased CO and VO_2 resulting from profound alterations in carbohydrate, protein, and fat metabolism.[123] Concurrently, GI, hepatic, and immunologic dysfunction may occur, which intensifies systemic inflammation.[131] Clinical consequences may affect gut function, wound healing, muscles wasting, host response, respiratory function, and continued promotion of the hypermetabolic response.

Not all patients develop MODS from SIRS. The development of MODS appears to be associated with failure to control the source of inflammation or infection, persistent hypoperfusion, flow-dependent oxygen consumption (VO_2), or the continued presence of necrotic tissue.[125]

BOX 26-21 Clinical Conditions and Manifestations Associated with SIRS

Clinical Conditions

- Infection
- Infection of vascular structures (heart and lungs)
- Pancreatitis
- Tissue ischemia or hypoxia
- Multiple trauma with massive tissue injury
- Hemorrhagic shock
- Immune-mediated organ injury
- Exogenous administration of tumor necrosis factor or other cytokines
- Aspiration of gastric contents
- Massive transfusion
- Host defense abnormalities

Clinical Manifestations

- Temperature >38° C or <36° C
- Heart rate >90 beats/min
- Respiratory rate >20 breaths/min or $PaCO_2$ <32 mm Hg
- WBC >12,000 cells/mm^3 or <4000 cells/mm^3 or >10% immature (band) forms

WBC, White blood cell count.

Pathophysiology

Secondary MODS results from altered regulation of the patient's acute immune and inflammatory responses. Dysregulation, or failure to control the host inflammatory response, leads to the excessive production of inflammatory cells and biochemical mediators that cause widespread damage to vascular endothelium and organ damage.[123,132] The critically ill patient's compromised immune state also fosters an environment conducive to organ failure.

The definitive clinical course of Secondary MODS has not been completely identified. Organ dysfunction may occur in a sequential or progressive pattern. Organ dysfunction may begin in the lungs, the most commonly affected major organ, and progress to the liver, gut, and kidneys. Cardiac and bone marrow dysfunction may follow. Neurologic and autonomic system impairment may occur and propagate the progression of organ failure and is associated with illness severity and mortality.[133] Organs may fail simultaneously; for example, kidney dysfunction may occur concurrently with hepatic dysfunction. After the initial insult and resuscitation, patients develop persistent hypermetabolism, a metabolic consequence of sustained systemic inflammation and physiologic stress, followed closely by pulmonary dysfunction, manifested as ARDS.

BOX 26-22 Inflammatory Mediators

Inflammatory Cells
- Neutrophils
- Macrophages or monocytes
- Mast lymphocytes
- Endothelial

Biochemical Mediators
- Reactive oxygen species
  - Superoxide radical
  - Hydroxyl radical
  - Hydrogen peroxide
- Tumor necrosis factor
- Interleukins
- Platelet activating factor
- Arachidonic acid metabolites
  - Prostaglandins
  - Leukotrienes
  - Thromboxanes
- Proteases

Plasma Protein Systems
- Complement
- Kinin
- Coagulation

Certain cellular and biochemical activity evoke the inflammatory and immune responses implicated in SIRS and MODS. The mediators associated with SIRS and MODS can be classified as inflammatory cells, biochemical mediators, or plasma protein systems (Box 26-22). Activation of one mediator often leads to activation of another. The biologic activity of inflammatory cells, biochemical mediators, and plasma protein systems and how they work in concert to cause SIRS and MODS have not been totally determined.

Assessment and Diagnosis

Secondary MODS is a systemic disease with organ-specific manifestations. Organ dysfunction is influenced by numerous factors, including organ host defense function, response time to the injury, metabolic requirements, organ vasculature response to vasoactive medications, organ sensitivity to damage, and physiologic reserve. The responses of the gastrointestinal, hepatobiliary, cardiovascular, pulmonary, renal, and hematologic systems are discussed in the following paragraphs. Clinical manifestations of organ dysfunction are outlined in Box 26-23.

Gastrointestinal Dysfunction

The gastrointestinal tract plays an important role in MODS. Gastrointestinal organs normally have immunoregulatory functions, and the gastrointestinal tract contains about 70% to 80% of the immunologic tissue of the entire body. A normally functioning gastrointestinal tract prevents bacteria from entering the systemic circulation.[123] Normal gut flora and gut environment are altered in patients with severe SIRS. Healthy probiotics (e.g., *Bifidobacterium, Lacto bacillus)* are decreased in a SIRS state, and pathogenic organisms (e.g., *Staphylococcus, Pseudomonas)* proliferate.[131]

With microcirculatory failure to the gastrointestinal tract, the gut's barrier function may be lost, which leads to bacterial translocation, sustained inflammation, endogenous endotoxemia, and MODS.[123,132] Hypoperfusion and shocklike states damage the normal gastrointestinal mucosa barrier by decreasing mesenteric blood flow, leading to hypoperfusion of the villi, mucosal edema, ischemic necrosis, sloughing of the mucosa, and malabsorption. The gastrointestinal tract is extremely vulnerable to oxygen metabolite-induced reperfusion injury. Endothelial injury and gastrointestinal lesions occur in response to mediator-induced tissue damage. Ischemic events and the absence of feedings can disrupt the normal metabolism of the gastric or intestinal lumen and the normal protective function of the gut barrier.[119,127]

The translocation of gastrointestinal bacteria through a "leaky gut" into the systemic circulation initiates and perpetuates an inflammatory focus in the critically ill patient.[127] The gastrointestinal tract harbors organisms that present an inflammatory focus when carried from the gut via the intestinal lymphatics. After hemorrhagic shock, trauma, or a major burn injury, gut-released proinflammatory and tissue-injurious factors may lead to acute lung injury, bone marrow failure, myocardial dysfunction, neutrophil activation, RBC injury, and endothelial cell activation and injury. These factors, released from the gut and carried in the mesenteric lymphatics, are capable of causing a septic state and Secondary MODS. In summary, the "gut-lymph hypothesis" proposes that gut ischemia-reperfusion injury leads to loss of a gut-protective barrier, bacterial translocation, and a gut inflammatory response. Gut-derived inflammatory factors are carried in the mesenteric lymph leading to a septic state and distant organ failure and MODS.[2]

Lastly, the oropharynx of the critically ill patient also becomes colonized with potentially pathogenic organisms from the gastrointestinal tract. Pulmonary aspiration of colonized secretions presents an inflammatory focus that can contribute to concomitant pulmonary dysfunction.[134]

Hepatobiliary Dysfunction

The liver plays a vital role in host homeostasis related to the acute inflammatory response. The liver responds to sustained inflammation by selectively altering carbohydrate, fat, and protein metabolism. Consequently, hepatic dysfunction threatens the patient's survival. The liver normally controls the inflammatory response by several mechanisms. Kupffer cells, which are hepatic macrophages, detoxify substances that may normally induce systemic inflammation and vasoactive substances that cause hemodynamic instability. Failure to detoxify gram-negative bacteria causes endotoxemia, perpetuates SIRS, and may lead to MODS. The liver also produces proteins and antiproteases to control the inflammatory response; however, hepatic dysfunction limits this response.

Common causes of liver failure in critically ill patients are infection-related cholestasis and hepatocellular injury in response to toxins and to toxins themselves. In infection-related cholestasis, bacterial toxins and released cytokines affect the uptake and excretion of bilirubin leading to jaundice. In hepatocellular injury, endotoxins and bacteria are phagocytized by Kupffer cells that release hepatotoxic substances that cause cellular damage. Hepatic dysfunction may also occur with organ hypoperfusion, hemolysis, and with hepatotoxic medications. Measurements of liver enzymes, bilirubin, ammonia, and liver-produced proteins should be carefully monitored.[135]

BOX 26-23 Clinical Manifestations of Organ Dysfunction

Gastrointestinal
- Abdominal distention and ascites
- Intolerance to enteral feedings
- Paralytic ileus
- Upper or lower gastrointestinal bleeding
- Diarrhea
- Ischemic colitis
- Mucosal ulceration
- Decreased bowel sounds
- Bacterial overgrowth in stool

Liver
- Jaundice
- Hepatomegaly
- Increased serum bilirubin (hyperbilirubinemia)
- Increased liver enzymes
- Increased serum ammonia
- Decreased serum albumin
- Decreased serum transferrin

Gallbladder
- Right upper quadrant tenderness or pain
- Abdominal distention
- Unexplained fever
- Decreased bowel sounds

Metabolic and Nutritional
- Decreased lean body mass
- Muscle wasting
- Severe weight loss
- Negative nitrogen balance
- Hyperglycemia
- Hypertriglyceridemia
- Increased serum lactate
- Decreased serum albumin, serum transferrin, prealbumin
- Decreased retinol-binding protein

Immune
- Infection
- Decreased lymphocyte count
- Anergy

Pulmonary
- Tachypnea
- Acute adult respiratory distress pattern of respiratory failure (dyspnea, patchy infiltrates, refractory hypoxemia, respiratory acidosis, abnormal O_2 indexes)
- Pulmonary hypertension

Kidney
- Decreased glomerular filtration rate/creatinine clearance
- Increased serum creatinine, blood urea nitrogen levels
- Oliguria, anuria, or polyuria consistent with prerenal azotemia or acute kidney injury
- Urinary indexes consistent with prerenal azotemia or acute kidney injury
- Electrolyte imbalance

Cardiovascular

Hyperdynamic
- Decreased pulmonary capillary occlusion pressure
- Decreased systemic vascular resistance
- Decreased right atrial pressure
- Decreased left ventricular stroke work index
- Increased oxygen consumption
- Increased cardiac output, cardiac index, heart rate

Hypodynamic
- Increased systemic vascular resistance
- Increased right atrial pressure
- Increased left ventricular stroke work index
- Decreased oxygen delivery and consumption
- Decreased cardiac output and cardiac index

Central Nervous System
- Lethargy
- Altered level of consciousness
- Fever
- Hepatic encephalopathy

Coagulation or Hematologic
- Thrombocytopenia
- Disseminated intravascular coagulation

The liver and gallbladder are extremely vulnerable to ischemic injury from organ hypoperfusion. Ischemic hepatitis occurs after a prolonged period of physiologic shock and is associated with centrilobular hepatocellular necrosis. The degree of hepatic damage is related directly to the severity and duration of the shock episode. Anoxic and reperfusion injuries damage hepatocytes and the vascular endothelium. Patients at high risk for ischemic hepatitis after a hypotensive event include those with a history of heart failure or cardiac dysrhythmias. Clinical manifestations of hepatic insufficiency are evident 1 to 2 days after the insult. Jaundice and transient elevations in serum transaminase and bilirubin levels occur. Hyperbilirubinemia results from hepatocyte anoxic injury and an increased production of bilirubin from hemoglobin catabolism. Ischemic hepatitis may resolve spontaneously or progress to acute liver failure. Although ischemic hepatitis is not a life-threatening complication, it can contribute to morbidity and mortality as a component of MODS. Acute liver failure is discussed further in Chapter 22.

Acalculous cholecystitis manifests 3 to 4 weeks after an insult. Its pathogenesis is unclear, but it may be related to ischemic reperfusion injury, PEEP greater than 5 cm H_2O, volume depletion, total parenteral nutrition (TPN), opioids, and cystic duct obstruction as a result of hyperviscous bile.[136] Visceral hypotension and vasoactive medication use may decrease perfusion of the gallbladder mucosa contributing to ischemia. Bacterial invasion may stimulate activation of factor XII and initiate the coagulation pathway.[136] Clinical manifestations of acalculous cholecystitis may mimic acute cholecystitis with gallstones. However, patients may demonstrate vague symptoms, including right upper quadrant pain and tenderness. Critical to the detection of acalculous cholecystitis is the recognition of abdominal distention, unexplained fever, loss of bowel sounds, and a sudden deterioration in the patient's condition. About 50% of patients with acalculous cholecystitis have gallbladder gangrene, and 10% have gallbladder perforation, requiring a cholecystectomy.[136]

Pulmonary Dysfunction

The lungs are frequent and early target organs for mediator-induced injury and are usually the first organs affected in the progression of SIRS to MODS.[137] ARDS is the pulmonary manifestation of MODS. Patients who develop MODS usually have pulmonary symptoms; however, not all patients with ARDS develop Secondary MODS. ARDS patients who develop SIRS or sepsis concurrently with acute respiratory failure are at the greatest risk for MODS.[138]

ARDS associated with MODS usually occurs 24 to 72 hours after the initial insult. Patients initially exhibit a low-grade fever, tachycardia, dyspnea, and mental confusion. As dyspnea progresses, hypoxemia, and the work of breathing increase, intubation and mechanical ventilation are required. ARDS results in refractory hypoxemia caused by intrapulmonary shunting, decreased pulmonary compliance, and altered airway mechanics; there usually is radiographic evidence of noncardiogenic pulmonary edema.[139]

Mediators associated with ARDS include inflammatory cells, such as polymorphonuclear cells, macrophages, monocytes, endothelial cells, and mast cells, and biochemical mediators, such as AA metabolites, toxic oxygen metabolites, proteases, TNF, platelet activating factor (PAF), and interleukins. Intense mediator activity damages the pulmonary vascular endothelium and the alveolar epithelium, resulting in surfactant deficiency, mild pulmonary hypertension, and increased pulmonary capillary permeability leading to increased lung water (noncardiogenic pulmonary edema).[103,139] ARDS is discussed further in Chapter 15.

Kidney Dysfunction

Acute kidney injury (AKI) is a common manifestation of MODS. The kidney is highly vulnerable to hypoperfusion and reperfusion injury. Consequently, kidney ischemic-reperfusion injury may be a major cause of kidney dysfunction in MODS. Mechanisms of cellular death may differ in septic versus non–septic-induced AKI. Acute tubular apoptosis may occur in septic AKI, while nonseptic AKI may be associated with necrosis.[140]

The patient with AKI may demonstrate oliguria or anuria resulting from decreased renal perfusion and relative hypovolemia. Early oliguria is likely caused by decreases in renal perfusion related to shocklike states; late oliguria is typically a sign of evolving kidney injury and ischemia. Renal function may become refractory to diuretics, fluid challenges, and vasoactive medications. Prerenal oliguria may progress to AKI, necessitating continuous renal replacement therapies. The frequent use of nephrotoxic medications also intensifies the risk of AKI.

Early recognition of AKI is imperative. However, the lack of early and reliable biomarkers for AKI leads to a delay in initiating treatment. The instability of kidney function in the critically ill patient decreases the validity of measures that are based on creatinine assessment. An elevated serum creatinine level is usually a late sign, but it is typically accepted as the index for renal dysfunction. However, serum creatinine concentrations can vary for reasons other than renal function in organ failure patients and are rarely at a steady state.[140] It may be preferable to use either 8-, 12-, or 24-hr urinary creatinine clearance values to estimate GFR in critically ill patients especially when determining medication dosages.[135] Additional signs of kidney impairment may include decreased erythropoietin-induced anemia, vitamin D malabsorption, and altered fluid and electrolyte balance. AKI is discussed further in Chapter 20.

Cardiovascular Dysfunction

The initial cardiovascular response in SIRS or sepsis is myocardial depression, decreased RAP and SVR, and increased venous capacitance, CO, and heart rate. Despite an increased CO, myocardial depression occurs and is accompanied by decreased SVR, increased heart rate, and ventricular dilation. These compensatory mechanisms help maintain CO during the early phase of SIRS or sepsis. An inability to increase CO in response to a low SVR may indicate myocardial failure or inadequate fluid resuscitation, and it is associated with increased mortality. VO_2 may be twice that of normal and may be flow-dependent.[141]

As MODS progresses, heart failure develops. Cardiac dysfunction is characterized by ventricular dilation, decreased diastolic compliance, and decreased systolic contractile function. Cardiovascular function becomes vasopressor-dependent. Heart failure may be caused by immune mediators, TNF-alpha, acidosis, or myocardial depressant factor, a substance secreted by the pancreas. Myocardial depression is exacerbated by myocardial hypoperfusion from a low CO state and persistent lactic acidosis. Cardiogenic shock and biventricular failure occur and lead to death.[141] Heart failure is discussed further in Chapter 12, and more information on cardiogenic shock can be found earlier in this chapter.

Hemotologic Dysfunction

The most common manifestations of hematologic dysfunction in sepsis or MODS are thrombocytopenia, coagulation abnormalities, and anemia.[142] The most severe is coagulation system dysfunction manifesting as DIC. DIC is a complex, consumptive coagulopathy that occurs in patients with a variety of disorders, including sepsis, tissue injury, and shock; it is overstimulation of the normal coagulation process. DIC results simultaneously in microvascular clotting and hemorrhage in organ systems, leading to thrombosis and fibrinolysis in life-threatening proportions. Clotting factor derangement leads to further inflammation and further thrombosis. Microvascular damage leads to further organ injury. Cell injury and damage to the endothelium activate the intrinsic or extrinsic coagulation pathways.[97,143] Low platelet counts and elevated D-dimer concentrations and fibrinogen degradation products are clinical indicators of DIC. DIC is discussed further in Chapter 27.

Medical Management

The patient with MODS requires multidisciplinary collaboration in clinical management, including fluid resuscitation and hemodynamic support (when appropriate), prevention and treatment of infection, maintenance of tissue oxygenation, nutritional and metabolic support, comfort and emotional support, and support for individual organ function. The use of investigational therapies may be part of the patient's clinical management.

Identification and Treatment of Infection

Identification and treatment of the underlying source of inflammation or infection are important ways to reduce mortality. Medical and surgical intervention to remove sources of infection or contamination may limit the inflammatory response and improve chances of recovery. Surgical procedures such as early fracture stabilization, removal of infected organs or tissue, and burn excision are helpful. Appropriate antibiotics are needed if the cause cannot be removed by surgical débridement or incision and draining.[137]

Antibiotic management in septic patients with MODS remains a challenge.[135] Ulldemolins and colleagues have provided antibiotic dosing recommendation for critically ill patients with MODS. They purport that tissue hypoperfusion during the early phases of sepsis/septic shock may lead to decreased antibiotic tissue concentrations. Therefore, "higher-than-standard" front-loading doses of *hydrophilic* antibiotics may be considered in the initial course of treatment because their volume of distribution will be significantly increased with tissue hypoperfusion. Hydrophilic antibiotics include beta-lactams, aminoglycosides, and glycopeptides. Hydrophilic antibiotics are cleared mostly by glomerular filtration and tubular secretion. Therefore, patients with renal dysfunction will require maintenance dose reductions or extended dosing intervals to prevent nephrotoxicity due to decreased drug elimination.[135]

Commonly administered *lipophilic* antibiotics include fluoroquinolones, lincosamides, and nitroimidazoles. As these antibiotics are cleared by the liver, kidney, or by both organs, attention to renal and hepatic function for initial and maintenance dosing is needed. In addition, total body weight, especially with obese patients, should be considered with front-loading administration of fluoroquinolones and lincosamides. Macrolides are *lipophilic* antibiotics and allow normal initial and maintenance dosing.

Underdosing of antibiotics may occur with tissue hypoperfusion and with decreased protein binding of highly bound antibiotics in patients with hepatic dysfunction. Overdosing may occur in patients with renal dysfunction due to decreased elimination of *hydrophilic* antibiotics and in hepatic dysfunction due to decreased metabolism of *lipophilic* antibiotics.

Other timely interventions, such as prevention of skin ulceration and early nutritional support, may improve outcomes. Regardless of the identification of potential risk factors, clinical markers, bacterial contaminants, and investigative approaches for detection and prevention, treatment remains largely supportive, and little improvement in the mortality rate has been appreciated.[90]

Maintenance of Tissue Oxygenation

Normally under steady state conditions, VO_2 is relatively constant and independent of oxygen delivery (DO_2) unless delivery becomes severely impaired. The relationship is called *supply-independent oxygen consumption.* Consequently, a percentage of oxygen is not used (physiologic reserve). Patients with SIRS/MODS often develop supply-dependent oxygen consumption in which VO_2 becomes dependent on DO_2, rather than demand, at a normal or high DO_2. When VO_2 does not equal demand, a tissue oxygen debt develops, subjecting organs to failure.[137]

Hypoperfusion and resultant organ hypoxemia often occur in patients at high risk for MODS, subjecting essential organs to failure. Effective fluid resuscitation and early recognition of flow-dependent VO_2 are essential, and patients at risk for MODS require hemodynamic monitoring, frequent measurements or surrogate measurements of DO_2 and VO_2, and serum lactate levels to guide therapy. Serum lactate levels provide information regarding the severity of impaired perfusion and the presence of lactic acidosis and differ significantly in MODS survivors and nonsurvivors. Failure to maintain adequate oxygenation to vital organs results in organ dysfunction. Despite adequate DO_2, VO_2 may not meet the needs of the body during MODS.

Patients with ARDS, MODS, or SIRS frequently manifest supply-dependent oxygen consumption and are unable to use oxygen appropriately despite normal delivery.[137] Interventions that decrease oxygen demand and increase oxygen delivery are essential. Sedation, mechanical ventilation, rest, and temperature and pain control may be able to decrease oxygen demand.[133] Oxygen delivery may be increased by maintaining normal hematocrit and PaO_2 levels, using PEEP, increasing preload or myocardial contractility to enhance CO, or reducing afterload to increase CO. Various methods of kinetic or prone therapies are available and may enhance alveolar recruitment, improve oxygenation delivery, and decrease other potential complications.

Nutritional and Metabolic Support

Hypermetabolism in SIRS or MODS results in profound weight loss, cachexia, and loss of organ function. The goal of nutritional support is the preservation of organ structure and function. Although nutritional support may not definitely alter the course of organ dysfunction, it prevents generalized nutritional deficiencies and preserves gut integrity. Enteral nutrition may exert a physiologic effect that down-regulates the systemic immune response and reduces oxidative stress.[144] The enteral route is preferable to parenteral support.[38] Enteral feedings are given distal to the pylorus to reduce the risk of pulmonary aspiration. Enteral feedings may limit bacterial translocation. In addition to early nutritional support, the pharmacologic properties of enteral feeding formulas may limit SIRS for selected critical care populations. Supplementation of enteral feedings with glutamine may be beneficial.[91,119,138] However, the optimum formulation of nutritional support and the use of immune-modulating supplements to improve outcomes in patients with or at risk for MODS continues to be the subject of much debate and study.[38,91,119] Nutritional support is discussed further in Chapter 8.

Nursing Management

Preventive measures include a multitude of assessment strategies to detect early organ manifestations of this syndrome. Patients who continue to experience sites of inflammation, septic foci, and inadequate tissue perfusion may be at higher risk. Hand hygiene, aseptic technique, and an understanding of how microorganisms can invade the body are essential components of preventive nursing care.

Nursing management of the patient with MODS incorporates a variety of nursing diagnoses (Box 26-24). **Nursing priorities are directed toward 1) preventing development of infection, 2) facilitating oxygen delivery and limiting tissue oxygen demand, 3) facilitating nutritional support, 4) providing comfort and emotional support, and 5) preventing and maintaining surveillance for complications.**

 BOX 26-24 **NURSING DIAGNOSIS PRIORITIES**

Multiple Organ Dysfunction Syndrome

- Decreased Cardiac Output related to alterations in preload, p. 579
- Decreased Cardiac Output related to alterations in afterload, p. 580
- Decreased Cardiac Output related to alterations in contractility, p. 580
- Impaired Gas Exchange related to ventilation/perfusion mismatching or intrapulmonary shunting, p. 594
- Imbalanced Nutrition: Less Than Body Requirements related to increased metabolic demands or lack of exogenous nutrients, p. 593
- Compromised Family Coping related to a critically ill family member, p. 578

Patients are assessed closely for inflammation and infection. Subtle expressions of infection warrant investigation. Nursing measures include strict adherence to standards of practice to prevent infection. Practices related to infection control with invasive hemodynamic monitoring, urinary catheters, endotracheal tubes, intracranial pressure monitoring devices, TPN, and wound care must be stringent to prevent further infection. Prevention of a concomitant ventilator-associated pneumonia or aspiration pneumonia is a priority.[17,145]

Measures to limit tissue oxygen consumption include administering analgesics and sedatives, positioning the patient for comfort, limiting activities, offering support to reduce anxiety, providing a calm and quiet environment, and educating the patient and family about the condition. Measures to enhance tissue oxygen supply include administering supplemental oxygen, monitoring the patient's respiratory status, and administering prescribed fluids and medications. Collaborative management of the patient with MODS is outlined in Box 26-25. See Box 26-26 for Internet Resources.

BOX 26-25 **Collaborative Management**

Multiple Organ Dysfunction Syndrome

- Support oxygen transport:
  - Establish a patent airway.
  - Initiate mechanical ventilation.
  - Administer oxygen.
  - Administer fluids (crystalloids, colloids, blood, and other blood products).
  - Administer vasoactive medications.
  - Administer positive inotropic medications.
  - Administer antidysrhythmic medications.
  - Ensure sufficient hemoglobin and hematocrit.
- Support oxygen use:
  - Identify and correct cause of lactic acidosis.
  - Ensure adequate organ and extremity perfusion.
- Decrease oxygen demand:
  - Administer sedation or paralytics.
  - Administer antipyretics and external cooling measures.
  - Administer pain medications.
- Identify the underlying cause of inflammation and treat accordingly:
  - Remove infected organs or tissue.
  - Administer antibiotics.
- Initiate nutritional support.
- Treat individual organ dysfunction:
  - Gastrointestinal
  - Hepatobiliary
  - Pulmonary
  - Renal
  - Cardiovascular
  - Coagulation system
- Prevent and maintain surveillance for complications, particularly infection.
- Provide comfort and emotional support.

BOX 26-26 **INTERNET RESOURCES**

- American Association of Critical-Care Nurses: http://www.aacn.org/
- Society of Critical Care Medicine: http://www.sccm.org/
- the heart.org: http://www.theheart.org/
- Trauma.org: http://www.trauma.org/
- The Food Allergy & Anaphylaxis Network: http://www.foodallergy.org/
- Anaphylaxis Campaign: http://www.anaphylaxis.org.uk/
- Neurogenic Shock Resource Blog: http://www.neurogenicshock.net/
- Surviving Sepsis Campaign: http://www.survivingsepsis.org
- Advances in Sepsis: http://www.advancesinsepsis.com/
- European Society of Intensive Care Medicine: http://www.esicm.org/
- International Sepsis Forum: http://sepsisforum.org/
- Survive Sepsis: http://www.survivesepsis.org/
- Sepsis Know From Day 1: http://www.sepsisknowfromday1.com
- American College of Physicians: http://www.acponline.org/
- American College of Surgeons: http://www.facs.org/
- American Medical Association: http://www.ama-assn.org/
- National Digestive Diseases Information Clearinghouse: http://digestive.niddk.nih.gov/
- National Institutes for Health: http://www.nih.gov/
- PubMed Health: http://www.ncbi.nlm.nih.gov/pubmedhealth/
- American Society for Parenteral and Enteral Nutrition: http://www.nutritioncare.org/

CASE STUDY Patient with Systemic Inflammatory Response Syndrome

Brief Patient History

Mr. Z is a 38-year-old Hispanic construction worker who sustained a liver laceration after falling from a roof. He required an exploratory laparotomy for splenectomy and repair of the liver laceration 4 days earlier. His medical history reveals no chronic health problems, although he smokes 20 packs of cigarettes per year.

Clinical Assessment

Mr. Z is admitted to the medical intensive care unit from the telemetry unit with acute respiratory insufficiency and hypotension. He is using his accessory muscles to breathe. He is speaking Spanish. Mr. Z's abdomen is distended, and there are no bowel sounds. Small amounts of dark green drainage are visible in the nasogastric tube. There is no sign of redness or drainage around his surgical wound.

Diagnostic Procedures

Vital signs were as follows: blood pressure of 78/55 mm Hg, heart rate of 142 beats/min (sinus tachycardia), respiratory rate of 35 breaths/min, temperature of 103.1° F, and urine output of 20 mL over the past 8 hours. ABG values on a 100% nonrebreather mask were as follows: pH of 7.22, PaO_2 of 54 mm Hg, $PaCO_2$ of 69 mm Hg, HCO_3^- level of 18 mEq/L, and O_2 saturation of 88%. The chest radiograph revealed infiltrates in the right lower lobe. Laboratory data revealed a hemoglobin level of 9.8 g/dL, hematocrit of 25%, and WBC count of 18,000/mm^3.

Medical Diagnosis

Mr. Z is diagnosed with severe sepsis.

Questions

1. What major outcomes do you expect to achieve for this patient?
2. What problems or risks must be managed to achieve these outcomes?
3. What interventions must be initiated to monitor, prevent, manage, or eliminate the problems and risks identified?
4. What interventions should be initiated to promote optimal functioning, safety, and well-being of the patient?
5. What possible learning needs do you anticipate for this patient?
6. What cultural and age-related factors may have a bearing on the patient's plan of care?

REFERENCES

1. Rivers EP: Approach to the patient with shock. In Goldman L, Schafer AI, editors: *Goldman's cecil medicine*, ed 24, Philadelphia, 2012, Elsevier.
2. Deitch EA, et al: Role of the gut in the development of injury and shock induced SIRS and MODS: the gut-lymph hypothesis, a review, *Front Biosci* 11:520, 2006.
3. Pieracci FM, et al: Current concepts in resuscitation, *J Intensive Care Med* 27:79, 2012.
4. Wilmot LA: Shock: early recognition and management, *J Emerg Nurs* 36:134, 2010.
5. Hameed SM, et al: Oxygen delivery, *Crit Care Med* 31(Suppl 12):S658, 2003.
6. Parks JK, et al: Systemic hypotension is a late marker of shock after trauma: a validation study of Advanced Trauma Life Support principles in a large national sample, *Am J Surg* 192:727, 2006.
7. Barbee RW, et al: Assessing shock resuscitation strategies by oxygen debt repayment, *Shock* 33:113, 2010.
8. Holley A, et al: Review article: part two: goal-directed resuscitation—which goals? Perfusion targets, *Emerg Med Australas* 24:127, 2012.
9. Martin JT, et al: Normal vital signs belie occult hypoperfusion in geriatric trauma patients, *Am Surg* 76:65, 2010.
10. Neville AL, et al: Mortality risk stratification in elderly trauma patients based on initial arterial lactate and base deficit levels, *Am Surg* 77:1337, 2011.
11. Vandromme MJ, et al: Lactate is a better predictor than systolic blood pressure for determining blood requirement and mortality: could prehospital measures improve trauma triage? *J Am Coll Surg* 210:861, 2010.
12. Jansen TC, et al: Blood lactate monitoring in critically ill patients: a systematic health technology assessment, *Crit Care Med* 37:2827, 2009.
13. Jansen TC, et al: Early lactate-guided therapy in intensive care unit patients: A multicenter, open-label, randomized controlled trial, *Am J Respir Crit Care Med* 182:752, 2010.
14. Jones AE, et al: Lactate clearance vs central venous oxygen saturation as goals of early sepsis therapy: a randomized clinical trial, *JAMA* 303:739, 2010.
15. FitzSullivan E, et al: Serum bicarbonate may replace the arterial base deficit in the trauma intensive care unit, *Am J Surg* 190:961, 2005.
16. Surbatovic M, et al: Predictive value of serum bicarbonate, arteral base deficit/excess and SAPS III score in critically ill patients, *Gen Physiol Biophys* 28(Spec No):271, 2009.
17. Dellinger RP, et al: Surviving Sepsis Campaign: international guidelines for management of severe sepsis and septic shock: 2012, *Crit Care Med* 41:580, 2013.
18. Holley A, et al: Review article: part one: goal-directed resuscitation—which goals? Haemodynamic targets, *Emerg Med Australas* 24:14, 2012.
19. Nebout S, Pirracchio R: Should we monitor $ScVO_2$ in critically ill patients, *Cardiol Res Pract* 2012:370697, 2012.
20. Collaborative Study Group on Perioperative ScVO2 Monitoring: Multicentre study on peri- and postoperative central venous oxygen saturation in high-risk surgical patients, *Crit Care* 10:R158, 2006.
21. Vallet B, et al: Physiologic transfusion triggers, *Best Pract Res Clin Anaesthesiol* 21:173, 2007.
22. Alam HB: Advances in resuscitation strategies, *Int J Surg* 9:5, 2011.
23. Bunn F, Trivedi D: Colloid solutions for fluid resuscitation, *Cochrane Database Syst Rev* (6):CD001319, 2012.
24. Cotton BA, et al: The cellular, metabolic, and systemic consequences of aggressive fluid resuscitation strategies, *Shock* 26:115, 2006.
25. Niemi TT, et al: Colloid solutions: a clinical update, *J Anesth* 24:913, 2010.
26. Perel P, Roberts I: Colloids versus crystalloids for fluid resuscitation in critically ill patients, *Cochrane Database Syst Rev* (3):CD000567, 2011.

27. Reinhart K, et al: Consensus statement of the ESICM task force on colloid volume therapy in critically ill patients, *Intensive Care Med* 38:368, 2012.
28. SAFE Study Investigators: Effect of baseline serum albumin concentration on outcome of resuscitation with albumin or saline in patients in intensive care units: analysis of data from the saline versus albumin fluid evaluation (SAFE) study, *BMJ* 333:1044, 2006.
29. Bulger EM, et al: Out-of-hospital hypertonic resuscitation after traumatic hypovolemic shock, *Ann Surg* 253:431, 2011.
30. Patanwala AE, et al: Use of hypertonic saline injection in trauma, *Am J Health Syst Pharm* 67:1920, 2010.
31. Carson JL, et al: Transfusion thresholds and other strategies for guiding allogenic red blood cell transfusion, *Cochrane Database Syst Rev* (4):CD002042, 2012.
32. Vlaar AP, Juffermans NP: Transfusion-related acute lung injury: a clinical review, *Lancet* 382:984, 2013.
33. Federico A: Transfusion-related acute lung injury, *J Perianesth Nurs* 24:35, 2009.
34. Kopko PM: Transfusion-related acute lung injury, *J Infus Nurs* 33:32, 2010.
35. Murad MH, et al: The effect of plasma transfusion on morbidity and mortality: a systematic review and meta-analysis, *Transfusion* 50:1370, 2010.
36. Boyd JH, Walley KR: Is there a role for sodium bicarbonate in treating lactic acidosis from shock? *Curr Opin Crit Care* 14:379, 2008.
37. Rachoin JS, et al: Treatment of lactic acidosis: appropriate confusion, *J Hosp Med* 5:E1, 2010.
38. Martindale RG, et al: Guidelines for the provision and assessment of nutrition support therapy in the adult critically ill patient: Society of Critical Care Medicine and American Society for Parenteral and Enteral Nutrition: executive summary, *Crit Care Med* 37:1757, 2009.
39. Cahill NE, et al: When early enteral feeding is not possible in critically ill patients: results of a multicenter observational study, *J Parenter Enteral Nutr* 35:160, 2011.
40. Casaer MP, et al: Early versus late parenteral nutrition in critically ill adults, *N Engl J Med* 365:506, 2011.
41. Wenerman J: Combined enteral and parenteral nutrition, *Curr Opin Clin Nutr Metab Care* 15:161, 2012.
42. Kutsogiannis J, et al: Early use of supplemental parenteral nutrition in critically ill patients: results of an international multicenter observational study, *Crit Care Med* 39:2691, 2011.
43. American Diabetes Association: Standards of medical care in diabetes—2012, *Diabetes Care* 35(Suppl 1):S11. 2012.
44. Moghissi ES, et al: American Association of clinical endocrinologists and American diabetes association consensus statement on inpatient glycemic control, *Endocr Pract* 15:1, 2009.
45. Schetz M, et al: Tight blood glucose control is renoprotective in critically ill patients, *J Am Soc Nephrol* 19:571, 2008.
46. Wiener RS, et al: Benefits and risks of tight glucose control in critically ill adults: a meta-analysis, *JAMA* 300:933, 2008.
47. American Association of Critical-Care Nurses: Family presence during resuscitation and invasive procedures. http://www.aacn.org/WD/Practice/Docs/PracticeAlerts/Family%20Presence%2004-2010%20final.pdf. Accessed May 10, 2014.
48. Davidson JE, et al: Clinical practice guidelines for support of the family in the patient-centered intensive care unit: American College of Critical Care Medicine Task force 2004-2005, *Crit Care Med* 35:605, 2007.
49. Egging D, et al: Emergency nursing resource: family presence during invasive procedures and resuscitation in the emergency department, *J Emerg Nurs* 37:469, 2011.
50. Morrison LJ, et al: Part 3: Ethics: 2010 American Heart Association Guidelines for Cardiopulmonary Resuscitation and Emergency Cardiovascular Care, *Circulation* 122(18 Suppl 3):S665, 2010.
51. Guly HR, et al: Vital signs and estimated blood loss in patients with major trauma: Testing the validity of the ATLS classification of hypovolaemic shock, *Resuscitation* 82:556, 2011.
52. Kwan I, et al: Timing and volume of fluid administration for patients with bleeding, *Cochrane Database Syst Rev* (1):CD002245, 2009.
53. Morrison CA, et al: Hypotensive resuscitation strategy reduces transfusion requirements and severe postoperative coagulopathy in trauma patients with hemorrhagic shock: preliminary results of a randomized controlled trial, *J Trauma* 70:652, 2011.
54. Roppolo LP, et al: Intravenous fluid resuscitation for the trauma patient, *Curr Opin Crit Care* 16:283, 2010.
55. Szopinski J, et al: Microcirculatory responses to hypovolemic shock, *J Trauma* 71:1779, 2011.
56. Goldberg RJ, et al: Thirty-year trends (1975 to 2005) in the magnitude of, management of, and hospital death rates associated with cardiogenic shock in patients with acute myocardial infarction, *Circulation* 119:1211, 2009.
57. Reynolds HR, Hochman JS: Cardiogenic shock: current concepts and improving outcomes, *Circulation* 117:686, 2008.
58. Topalian S, et al: Cardiogenic shock, *Crit Care Med* 36(Suppl 1):S66, 2008.
59. Buerke M, et al: Pathophysiology, diagnosis, and treatment of infarction-related cardiogenic shock, *Herz* 36:73, 2011.
60. Hussain F, et al: The ability to achieve complete revascularization is associated with improved in-hospital survival in cardiogenic shock due to myocardial infarction: Manitoba cardiogenic SHOCK Registry investigators, *Catheter Cardiovasc Interv* 78:540, 2011.
61. Chatterjee K, et al: Analytic reviews: cardiogenic shock with preserved systolic function: a reminder, *J Intensive Care Med* 23:355, 2008.
62. Shpektor A: Cardiogenic shock: the role of inflammation, *Acute Card Care* 12:115, 2010.
63. Brown JL, et al: Short-term mechanical management of cardiogenic shock, *Curr Treat Options Cardiovasc Med* 13:343, 2011.
64. Stevenson LW, Perloff JK: The limited reliability of physical signs for estimating hemodynamics in chronic heart failure, *JAMA* 261:884, 1989.
65. Kemp SF, et al: Epinephrine: the drug of choice for anaphylaxis. A statement of the World Allergy Organization, *Allergy* 63:1061, 2008.
66. Kim H, Fischer D: Anaphylaxis, *Allergy Asthma Clin Immunol* 7(Suppl 1):S6, 2011.
67. Lieberman P, et al: The diagnosis and management of anaphylaxis practice parameter: 2010 update, *J Allergy Clin Immunol* 126:477, 2010.
68. Simons FE: Anaphylaxis, *J Allergy Clin Immunol* 125(2 Suppl 2):S161, 2010.

69. Simons FE: Anaphylaxis: recent advances in assessment and treatment, *J Allergy Clin Immunol* 124:625, 2009.
70. American Heart Association: 2010 American Heart Association Guidelines for cardiopulmonary resuscitation and emergency cardiovascular care. Part 12.2: Cardiac arrest associated with anaphylaxis, *Circulation* 122(Suppl 3):S832, 2010.
71. Sampson HA, et al: Second symposium on the definition and management of anaphylaxis: summary report—second National Institute of Allergy and Infectious Disease/Food Allergy and Anaphylaxis Network symposium, *J Allergy Clin Immunol* 117:391, 2006.
72. Tole JW, Lieberman P: Biphasic anaphylaxis: review of incidence, clinical predictors, and observation recommendations, *Immunol Allergy Clin North Am.* 27:309, 2007.
73. Choo KJL, et al: Glucocorticoids for the treatment of anaphylaxis, *Cochrane Database Syst Rev* (4):CD007596, 2012.
74. Furlan JC, Fehlings MG: Cardiovascular complications after acute spinal cord injury: pathophysiology, diagnosis, and management, *Neurosurg Focus* 25:1, 2008.
75. Guly HR, et al: The incidence of neurogenic shock in patients with isolated spinal cord injury in the emergency department, *Resuscitation* 76:57, 2008.
76. Krassioukov A, Claydon VE: The clinical problems in cardiovascular control following spinal cord injury: an overview, *Prog Brain Res* 152:223, 2006.
77. Consortium for Spinal Cord Medicine: Early acute management in adults with spinal cord injury: a clinical practice guideline for health-care professionals. http://www.pva.org/site/apps/ka/ec/product.asp?c=ajIRK9NJLcJ2E&b=6423003&en=8hIFLROvG7LOL1PyF6JLKYMJJlIQIXPAJfKRL8OQJvG&ProductID=895972. Accessed May 10, 2014.
78. Popa C, et al: Vascular dysfunctions following spinal cord injury, *J Med Life* 3:275, 2010.
79. Young WF: Shock. In Stone CK, Humphries RL, editors: *Current diagnosis & treatment: emergency medicine*, ed 6, New York, 2008, McGraw-Hill.
80. American Heart Association: 2010 American Heart Association Guidelines for cardiopulmonary resuscitation and emergency cardiovascular care. Part 8: Adult advanced cardiovascular resuscitation and emergency cardiovascular care, *Circulation* 122:S729, 2010.
81. Beale R, et al: Promoting global research excellence in severe sepsis (PROGRESS): lessons from an international sepsis registry, *Infection* 37:222, 2009.
82. Lagu T, et al: Hospitalizations, costs, and outcomes of severe sepsis in the United States 2003 to 2007, *Crit Care Med* 40:754, 2012.
83. Mann EA, et al: Comparison of mortality associated with sepsis in the burn, trauma, and general intensive care unit patient: a systematic review of the literature, *Shock* 37:4, 2012.
84. Sivayoham N, et al: Outcomes from implementing early goal-directed therapy for severe sepsis and septic shock: a 4-year observational cohort study, *Eur J Emerg Med* 19:235, 2012.
85. Hoyert DL, Xu J: *Deaths: preliminary data for 2011*, National Vital Statistics Reports; vol 61, no 6, Hyattsville, MD, 2012, National Center for Health Statistics. http://www.cdc.gov/nchs/data/nvsr/nvsr61/nvsr61_06.pdf. Accessed May 10, 2014.
86. American College of Chest Physicians/Society of Critical Care Medicine Consensus Conference: Definitions for sepsis and organ failure and guidelines for the use of innovative therapies in sepsis, *Crit Care Med* 20:864, 1992.
87. Dellinger RP, et al: Surviving Sepsis Campaign guidelines for management of severe sepsis and septic shock, *Crit Care Med* 32:858, 2004.
88. Levy MM, et al: 2001 SCCM/ESICM/ACCP/ATS/SIS International Sepsis Definitions Conference, *Crit Care Med* 31:1250, 2003.
89. Seymour CW, et al: Marital status and the epidemiology and outcomes of sepsis, *Chest* 137:1289, 2010.
90. Fry DE: Sepsis, systemic inflammatory response, and multiple organ dysfunction: the mystery continues, *Am Surg* 78:1, 2012.
91. Cinel I, Dellinger RP: Advances in pathogenesis and management of sepsis, *Curr Opin Infect Dis* 20:345, 2007.
92. Nduka OO, Parrillo JE: The pathophysiology of septic shock, *Crit Care Nurs Clin North Am* 23:41, 2011.
93. Rivers EP, et al: The influence of early hemodynamic optimization on biomarker patterns of severe sepsis and septic shock, *Crit Care Med* 35:2016, 2007.
94. Singer M: Mitochondrial function in sepsis: acute phase versus multiple organ failure, *Crit Care Med* 35(Suppl 9):S441, 2007.
95. Levi M, et al: Systemic versus localized coagulation activation contributing to organ failure in critically ill patients, *Semin Immunopathol* 34:167, 2012.
96. Stearns-Kurosawa DJ, et al: The pathogenesis of sepsis, *Annu Rev Pathol* 6:19, 2011.
97. Semeraro N, et al: Sepsis, thrombosis and organ dysfunction, *Thromb Res* 129:290, 2012.
98. Trzeciak S, et al: Early microcirculatory perfusion derangements in patients with severe sepsis and septic shock: relationship to hemodynamics, oxygen transport, and survival, *Ann Emerg Med* 49:88, 2007.
99. Vollmar B, Menger MD: Intestinal ischemia/reperfusion: microcirculatory pathology and functional consequences, *Langenbecks Arch Surg* 396:13, 2011.
100. Tappy L, Chiolero R: Substrate utilization in sepsis and multiple organ failure, *Crit Care Med* 35(Suppl 9):S531, 2007.
101. Baumgart K, et al: Pathophysiology of tissue acidosis in septic shock: blocked microcirculation or impaired cellular respiration? *Crit Care Med* 36:640, 2008.
102. Garrabou G, et al: The effects of sepsis on mitochondria, *J Infect Dis* 205:392, 2012.
103. Perl M, et al: Pathogenesis of indirect (secondary) acute lung injury, *Expert Rev Respir Med* 5:115, 2011.
104. Jacob A, et al: Septic encephalopathy: inflammation in man and mouse, *Neurochem Int* 58:472, 2011.
105. Jensen JU, et al: Procalcitonin-guided interventions against infections to increase early appropriate antibiotics and improve survival in the intensive care unit: a randomized trial, *Crit Care Med* 39:2048, 2011.
106. Rivers E, et al: Early goal-directed therapy in the treatment of severe sepsis and septic shock, *N Engl J Med* 345:1368, 2001.
107. Kumar A, et al: Duration of hypotension before initiation of effective antimicrobial therapy is the critical determinant of survival in human septic shock, *Crit Care Med* 34:1589, 2006.

108. De Backer D, et al: Dopapmine versus norepinephrine in the treatment of septic shock: a meta-analysis, *Crit Care Med* 40:725, 2012.
109. Vasu TS, et al: Norepinephrine or dopamine for septic shock: a systematic review of randomized clinical trials, *J Intensive Care Med* 27:172, 2012.
110. The Acute Respiratory Distress System Network: Ventilation with lower tidal volumes as compared with traditional tidal volumes for acute lung injury and the acute respiratory distress syndrome, *N Engl J Med* 342:1301, 2000.
111. Marti-Carvajal AJ, et al: Human recombinant activated protein C for severe sepsis, *Cochrane Database Syst Rev* (3):CD004388, 2012.
112. Mullard A: Drug withdrawal sends critical care specialists back to basics, *Lancet* 378:1769, 2011.
113. FDA. FDA Drug Safety Communication: Voluntary market withdrawal of Xigis [drotrecogin alfa (activated)] due to failure to show a survival benefit. http://www.fda.gov/Drugs/DrugSafety/ucm277114.htm. Accessed May 10, 2014.
114. Annane D, et al: Effect of treatment with low doses of hydrocortisone and fludrocortisone on mortality in patients with septic shock, *JAMA* 288:862, 2002.
115. Annane D, et al: Corticosteroids for treating severe sepsis and septic shock, *Cochrane Database Syst Rev* (12):CD002243, 2010.
116. Sprung CL, et al: Steroid therapy of septic shock, *Crit Care Nurs Clin North Am* 23:171, 2011.
117. Finfer S: Clinical controversies in the management of critically ill patients with severe sepsis: resuscitation fluids and glucose control, *Virulence* 5:200, 2014.
118. Elke G, et al: Current practice in nutritional support and its association with mortality in septic patients—results from a national, prospective, multicenter study, *Crit Care Med* 36:1762, 2008.
119. Beale RJ, et al: Early enteral supplementation with key pharmaconutrients improves Sequential Organ Failure Assessment score in critically ill patients with sepsis: outcome of a randomized, controlled, double-blind trial, *Crit Care Med* 36:131, 2008.
120. Aitken LM, et al: Nursing considerations to complement the surviving sepsis campaign guidelines, *Crit Care Med* 39:1800, 2011.
121. Otto GP, et al: The late phase of sepsis is characterized by an increased microbiological burden and death rate, *Crit Care* 15:R183, 2011.
122. Winters BD, et al: Long-term mortality and quality of life in sepsis: a systematic review, *Crit Care Med* 38:1276, 2010.
123. Martin LL, et al: Shock, multiple organ dysfunction syndrome, and burns in adults. In McCance KL, et al, editors: *Pathophysiology: the biologic basis for disease in adults and children*, ed 7, St Louis, 2014, Elsevier.
124. Fan E: Critical illness neuromyopathy and the role of physical therapy and rehabilitation in critically ill patients, *Respir Care* 57:933, 2012.
125. Cohn SM, et al: Tissue oxygen saturation predicts the development of organ dysfunction during traumatic shock resuscitation, *J Trauma* 62:44, 2007.
126. Epstein CD, et al: Oxygen transport and organ dysfunction in the older trauma patient, *Heart Lung* 31:315, 2002.
127. Clark JA, Coopersmith CM: Intestinal crosstalk: a new paradigm for understanding the gut as the "motor" of critical illness, *Shock* 28:384, 2007.
128. Tschoeke SK, et al: The early second hit in trauma management augments the proinflammatory immune response to multiple injuries, *J Trauma* 62:1396, 2007.
129. Dulhunty JM, et al: Does severe non-infectious SIRS differ from severe sepsis? Results from a multi-centre Australian and New Zealand intensive care unit study, *Intensive Care Med* 34:1654, 2008.
130. Sankoff J, et al: Validation of the Mortality in Emergency Department Sepsis (MEDS) score in patients with the systemic inflammatory response syndrome (SIRS), *Crit Care Med* 36:421, 2008.
131. Shimizu K, et al: Altered gut flora and environment in patients with severe SIRS, *J Trauma* 60:126, 2006.
132. Rote NS, et al: Innate immunity: inflammation. In McCance K, et al, editors: *Pathophysiology: the biologic basis for disease in adults and children*, ed 7, St. Louis, 2014, Elsevier.
133. Schmidt H, et al: The alteration of autonomic function in multiple organ dysfunction syndrome, *Crit Care Clin* 24:149, 2008.
134. Marshall JC, et al: The gastrointestinal tract. The "undrained abscess" of multiple organ failure, *Ann Surg* 218:111, 1993.
135. Ulldemolins M, et al: Antibiotic dosing in multiple organ dysfunction syndrome, *Chest* 139:1210, 2011.
136. Barie PS, Eachempati SR: Acute acalculous cholecystitis, *Gastroenterol Clin North Am* 39:343, 2010.
137. Krau SD: Making sense of multiple organ dysfunction syndrome, *Crit Care Nurs Clin North Am* 19:87, 2007.
138. Vincent JL, Zambon M: Why do patients who have acute lung injury/acute respiratory distress syndrome die from multiple organ dysfunction syndrome? Implications for management, *Clin Chest Med* 27:725, 2006.
139. Crouser ED, et al: Acute lung injury, pulmonary edema, and multiple system organ failure. In Wilkins RL, et al, editors: *Egan's fundamentals of respiratory care*, ed 10, St. Louis, 2013, Elsevier.
140. Honore PM, et al: Septic AKI in ICU patients, diagnosis, pathophysiology, and treatment type, dosing, and timing: a comprehensive review of recent and future developments, *Ann Intensive Care* 1:32, 2011.
141. Zanotti-Cavazzoni SL, Hollenberg SM: Cardiac dysfunction in severe sepsis and septic shock, *Curr Opin Crit Care* 15:392, 2009.
142. Dhainaut JF, et al: Dynamic evolution of coagulopathy in the first day of severe sepsis: relationship with mortality and organ failure, *Crit Care Med* 33:341, 2005.
143. Gando S: Microvascular thrombosis and multiple organ dysfunction syndrome, *Crit Care Med* 38(Suppl 2):S35, 2010.
144. McClave SA, Heyland DK: The physiologic response and associated clinical benefits from provision of early enteral nutrition, *Nutr Clin Pract* 24:305, 2009.
145. Hillier B, et al: Preventing ventilator-associated pneumonia through oral care, production selection, and application methdo, *AACN Adv Crit Care* 24:38, 2013.

Hematologic Disorders and Oncologic Emergencies

Mary Russell, Carol A. Suarez

Ⓔ Be sure to check out the bonus material, including review questions, on the Evolve website at http://evolve.elsevier.com/Urden/priorities/.

DISSEMINATED INTRAVASCULAR COAGULATION

Description and Etiology

Disseminated intravascular coagulation (DIC) is a syndrome that arises as a complication of other serious or life-threatening conditions. Although DIC is not seen often, it can seriously hamper diagnostic and treatment efforts for the critically ill patient. An understanding of the etiologic and pathophysiologic mechanisms of DIC can assist in anticipating the syndrome's occurrence, recognizing the signs and symptoms, and prompting intervention. Also known as consumptive *coagulopathy*, DIC is characterized by bleeding and thrombosis, both of which result from depletion of clotting factors, platelets, and RBCs. If not treated quickly, DIC will progress to multiple organ failure and death.[1]

Many clinical events can prompt the development of DIC in the critically ill patient, but the exact underlying trigger may not be identifiable (Box 27-1). There are, however, some commonly known conditions associated with the development of DIC.

Sepsis, particularly that caused by gram-negative organisms, can be identified as the culprit in as many as 20% of cases, making it the most common cause of DIC. In this instance, endotoxins serve as a trigger for activation of tissue factor and the extrinsic coagulation pathway. Metabolic acidosis and hypoperfusion associated with shock syndromes can result in increased formation of free radicals and damage to tissues. Tissue factor is activated, resulting in DIC. Massive trauma or burns are frequently associated with DIC. Direct tissue damage activates the extrinsic coagulation pathway, and damage to endothelial surfaces activates the intrinsic pathway.[2] Obstetric emergencies, such as abruptio placenta, retained placenta, or incomplete abortion, are also associated with the development of DIC. Tissue factor is concentrated in the placenta, and damage or disruption of this structure can activate coagulation pathways, resulting in coagulopathy.[2]

Pathophysiology

Regardless of the cause, the common thread in the development of DIC is damage to the endothelium that results in activation of the coagulation mechanism (Figure 27-1).[3] The extrinsic coagulation pathway plays a major role in the development of DIC. Direct damage to the endothelium results in the release of tissue factor and activation of this pathway. The secondary surge of thrombin formation as a result of activation of the intrinsic coagulation pathway leads to the massive disruption of the delicate balance that is hemostasis. Excessive thrombin formation results in rapid consumption of coagulation factors and depletion of regulatory substances—protein C, protein S, and antithrombin.[4] With no checks and balances, thrombi continue to form along damaged epithelial walls, resulting in occlusion of the vessels. As occlusion reaches a critical level, tissue ischemia ensues, leading to further tissue damage and perpetuating the process. Eventually, end-organ function is affected by the ischemia, and failure is evident.[3]

In response to the formation of clots, the fibrinolytic system is activated. As plasmin breaks down the fibrin clots, fibrin split products are released, and they act as anticoagulants.[2] Coupled with depletion of circulating clotting factors, activation of fibrinolysis results in excessive bleeding. The end result is shock and further tissue ischemia that aggravate end-organ dysfunction and failure. Death is imminent if this destructive cycle is not interrupted.[5]

Assessment and Diagnosis

Favorable outcomes for patients with DIC depend on accurate and timely diagnosis of the condition. Realization of the role underlying pathology plays, recognition of clinical manifestations, and assessment of appropriate laboratory values are key steps in this process.

Clinical Manifestations

Clinical manifestations are related to the two primary pathophysiologic mechanisms of DIC: the formation of thrombi and bleeding. Thrombi in peripheral capillaries can lead to cyanosis, particularly in the fingers, toes, ears, and nose. In severe, untreated cases, this peripheral ischemia may progress to gangrene.[1,2] As the condition progresses, ischemia worsens, and end organs are affected. The result of this more central ischemia can be respiratory insufficiency and failure, acute kidney injury, bowel infarction, and ischemic stroke. The tissue damage that results perpetuates the anomalies of DIC.[2]

As coagulation factors are depleted, bleeding from intravenous and other puncture sites is observed. Ecchymosis may result from even routine interventions such as the use of a manual blood pressure cuff, bathing, or turning.[1,2] Bloody drainage may also occur from surgical sites, drains, and

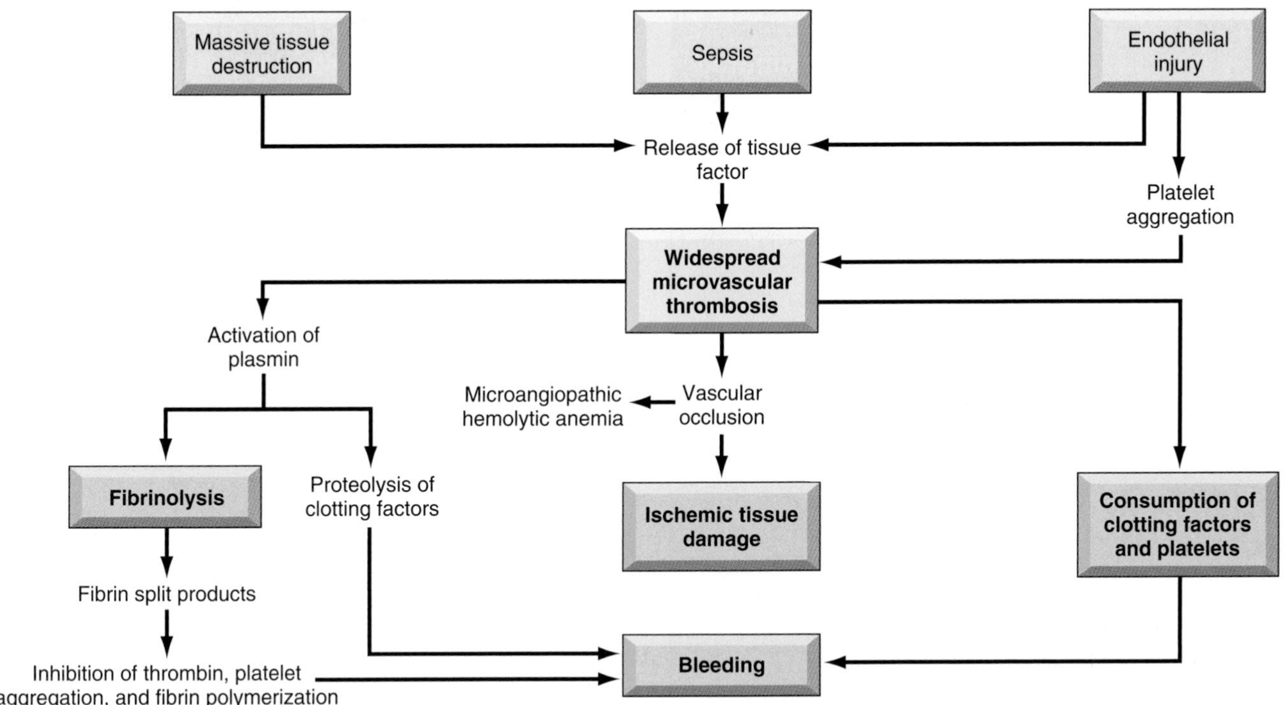

FIG 27-1 Pathophysiology of Disseminated Intravascular Coagulation. (From Kumar V, et al. Red blood cell and bleeding disorders. In: Kumar V, et al, eds. Robbins and Cotran Pathologic Basis of Disease. 8th ed. Philadelphia: Saunders; 2010.)

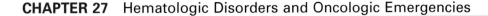

BOX 27-1 Causes of Disseminated Intravascular Coagulation

Obstetric Complications
- Abruptio placenta
- Placenta previa
- Retained dead fetus
- Septic abortion
- Amniotic fluid embolism
- Toxemia of pregnancy

Infections
- Gram-negative sepsis
- Gram-positive sepsis
- Meningococcemia
- Rocky Mountain spotted fever
- Histoplasmosis
- Aspergillosis
- Malaria

Neoplasms
- Carcinomas of pancreas, prostate, lung, and stomach
- Acute promyelocytic leukemia
- Tumor lysis syndrome
- Chemotherapy

Massive Tissue Injury
- Traumatic
- Crush injuries
- Burns
- Extensive surgery
- Heat stroke
- Acute transplant rejection

Miscellaneous
- Acute intravascular hemolysis
- Snakebite
- Giant hemangioma
- Shock
- Heat stroke
- Vasculitis
- Aortic aneurysm
- Liver disease
- Cardiac arrest

Modified from Cotran RS, et al. *Robbins Pathologic Basis of Disease*. 6th ed. Philadelphia: Saunders; 1999.

urinary catheters. With progression of DIC, the patient is at risk for severe gastrointestinal or subarachnoid hemorrhage.[1,2] Table 27-1 lists many of the common signs and symptoms of DIC.

Laboratory Findings

Laboratory tests used to diagnose DIC essentially assess the four basic characteristics of this syndrome: 1) increased coagulant activity, 2) increased fibrinolytic activity, 3) impaired regulatory function, and 4) end-organ failure.[2]

Continuous activation of the coagulation pathways results in consumption of coagulation factors. Because of this, the prothrombin time (PT), the activated partial thromboplastin time (aPTT), and the international normalized ratio (INR) values are elevated. Although the platelet count may fall within normal ranges, serial examination reveals a declining

TABLE 27-1 Common Signs and Symptoms of Disseminated Intravascular Coagulation

SYSTEM	SIGNS RELATED TO HEMORRHAGE	SIGNS RELATED TO THROMBI
Integumentary	Bleeding from gums, venipunctures, and old surgical sites; epistaxis; ecchymosis	Peripheral cyanosis, gangrene
Cardiopulmonary	Hemoptysis	Dysrhythmias, chest pain, acute myocardial infarction, pulmonary embolus, respiratory failure
Renal	Hematuria	Oliguria, acute kidney injury, renal failure
Gastrointestinal	Abdominal distention, hemorrhage	Diarrhea, constipation, bowel infarct
Neurologic	Subarachnoid hemorrhage	Altered level of consciousness, ischemic stroke

trend in values. An unexpected drop of at least 50% in the platelet count, particularly in the presence of known contributing factors and associated signs and symptoms, strongly indicates DIC.[3] Fibrinogen levels drop as more and more clots are formed. Thrombus formation in small vessels narrow the vessel lumen, forcing RBCs to squeeze through. The resulting damage and fragmentation of these cells can be seen on microscopic examination of blood samples. Damaged, fragmented RBCs are called *schistocytes.*[1,2]

In response to the excess clotting activity, the fibrinolytic process accelerates, and levels of byproducts increase. This is reflected in markedly elevated levels of fibrin degradation products. Another key laboratory test used to evaluate the degree of clot dissolution—and therefore the severity of the coagulopathy—is the D-dimer level.[1] D-dimers exclusively indicate clot degradation because, unlike fibrin degradation products, which also result from the breakdown of free circulating fibrin, D-dimers result only from dissolution of clots.[2] With progression of the coagulopathy, normal regulatory mechanisms are disrupted, as reflected in decreasing levels of inhibitory factors such as protein C, factor V, and antithrombin III.[1,2,6]

Unchecked DIC resulting in occlusion of vessels and tissue ischemia leads to end-organ dysfunction. Respiratory failure, indicated by abnormal arterial blood gas (ABG) levels; liver failure, indicated by increasing liver enzymes, and renal impairment, indicated by rising blood urea nitrogen (BUN) and creatinine levels, are common findings in advanced DIC.[6]

TABLE 27-2 Key Laboratory Studies in Disseminated Intravascular Coagulation

TEST	VALUE
Prothrombin time (PT)	>12.5 sec
Platelets	<50,000/mm^3 or at least 50% drop from baseline
Activated partial thromboplastin time (aPTT)	>40 sec
D-dimer	>250 ng/mL
Fibrin degradation products (FDP)	>40 mg/mL
Fibrinogen	<100 mg/dL

No single laboratory study can confirm the diagnosis of DIC, but several key results are strong indicators of the condition (Table 27-2). The International Society of Thrombosis and Hemostasis emphasizes early detection of DIC through observation of abnormal trends in laboratory values.[4]

Medical Management

Without question, the primary intervention in DIC is prevention. Being aware of the conditions that commonly contribute to the development of DIC and treating them vigorously and without delay provide the best defense against this devastating condition.[1-3,6] After DIC is identified, maintaining organ perfusion and slowing consumption of coagulation factors are paramount to achieving a favorable outcome.[1,2]

Multiple organ dysfunction syndrome (MODS) frequently results from DIC and exacerbates the underlying pathology.[5] It is essential to prevent end-organ ischemia and damage by supporting blood pressure and circulating volume. Administration of intravenous fluids and inotropic agents and, if overt hemorrhaging is evident, infusion of packed RBCs are appropriate interventions to replace blood volume and essential, oxygen-carrying RBCs.

In the presence of severe platelet depletion (less than 50,000/mm^3) and severe hemorrhage, platelet transfusions are often indicated.[1,4] However, caution must be used when administering platelets because antiplatelet antibodies may be formed. These antibodies may become activated during future platelet transfusions and elicit DIC.[7]

Replacement of clotting factors in the patient with DIC is thought by some authorities to perpetuate the coagulopathy; however, there is little scientific evidence to support this theory.[3] Fibrinogen levels less than 100 mg/dL indicate the appropriateness of administering cryoprecipitate. A prolonged PT indicates the need for fresh-frozen plasma.[1,2,4]

Slowing consumption of coagulation factors by inhibiting the processes involved in clot formation is another strategy used in treating DIC. The use of heparin, particularly low-molecular-weight heparin (LMWH), to prevent formation of future clots is controversial.[1] It is contraindicated in patients with DIC associated with recent surgery or with gastrointestinal or central nervous system (CNS) bleeding. However, heparin has been beneficial in obstetric emergencies such as retained placenta or incomplete abortion, severe arterial occlusions, or MODS caused by microemboli.[3,6] Inhibitors such as aminocaproic acid may be used in conjunction with heparin.[1,2]

The use of recombinant activated protein C is gaining popularity in treating DIC, especially in the setting of severe sepsis. Activated protein C acts as an anticoagulant and works to restore normal inhibition of coagulation pathways. However, it has been associated with an increased incidence of intracerebral bleeding and must be used with caution in patients with severely decreased platelets.[2,4]

Thrombin production in DIC surpasses that of antithrombins and other regulatory factors that would normally be present to inactivate thrombin and its subsequent actions. The use of antithrombin III has recently been approved in the United States. Ongoing research is yielding mixed results in the treatment of DIC.[4] One interesting area of research is the use of protease inhibitors. Protease molecules normally inhibit the conversion of fibrinogen to fibrin in the coagulation mechanism, but in DIC, this inhibitory mechanism is impaired. The introduction of protease inhibitors by intravenous infusion may be advantageous in arresting DIC.[2]

Nursing Management

Nursing management of the patient with DIC incorporates a variety of nursing diagnoses (Box 27-2). Assessment and monitoring are the primary weapons in the critical care nurse's arsenal against DIC. Knowing the diseases and conditions that are most often associated with DIC and understanding the pathophysiologic mechanisms involved enable the critical care nurse to anticipate its development and intervene quickly. **Nursing priorities are directed toward 1) supporting the patient's vital functions, 2) initiating bleeding precautions, 3) providing comfort and emotional support, and 4) maintaining surveillance for complications.**

Supporting Patient's Vital Functions

Frequent assessments should include parameters for neurologic status, renal function, cardiopulmonary function, and skin integrity that indicate impaired tissue or organ perfusion. Particular parameters to include are mental status, BUN and creatine levels, urine output, vital signs, hemodynamic values, cardiac rhythm, arterial blood gas and pulse oximetry values, skin breakdown, ecchymoses, or hematomas.[1]

The critical care nurse must recognize and support the patient's vital physiologic functions. Administration of intravenous fluids, blood products, and inotropic agents to provide adequate hemodynamic support and tissue oxygenation is essential in preventing or combating end-organ damage. Close monitoring of vital signs, hemodynamic parameters, intake and output, and appropriate laboratory values assists the critical care nurse in administering and titrating appropriate agents.[2]

Initiating Bleeding Precautions

Awareness of the patient's bleeding potential necessitates adjustments to normal nursing interventions. The nurse avoids unnecessary venipunctures that may result in bleeding, bruising, or hematomas by drawing blood from and administering medications through existing arterial or venous lines. The use of manual or automatic blood pressure cuffs is avoided whenever possible. If tracheal or oral suctioning is necessary, the use of low-level suction is recommended.[6] Meticulous skin care is advised, keeping the skin moist and using specialty mattresses and beds as appropriate to prevent breakdown. Gentle care should be used when bathing or turning the patient to prevent bruising or hematoma formation.

Providing Comfort and Emotional Support

The development of DIC in the already critically ill patient can be stressful for the patient and his or her significant others. It is imperative to provide psychosocial support throughout this crisis. Calm reassurance and uncomplicated explanations of the care the patient is receiving can help to allay much of the anxiety experienced. The critical care nurse must answer all questions and provide information in terms best understood by all parties. The use of an interpreter when English is not the primary language can enhance understanding and help avoid misconceptions. Providing spiritual support as requested may also be of assistance. Collaborative management of the patient with DIC is outlined in Box 27-3.

BOX 27-2 NURSING DIAGNOSIS PRIORITIES

Disseminated Intravascular Coagulation

- Deficient Fluid Volume related to active blood loss, p. 584
- Decreased Cardiac Output related to alterations in preload, p. 579
- Risk for Infection, p. 607
- Anxiety related to threat to biologic, psychologic, or social integrity, p. 576
- Compromised Family Coping related to a critically ill family member, p. 578

HEPARIN-INDUCED THROMBOCYTOPENIA

Description and Etiology

Another form of thrombocytopenia seen in critical care patients is heparin-induced thrombocytopenia (HIT). There are two distinct types of HIT. The most common form is non–immune-mediated HIT, formally known as type 1 HIT.[8] Seen in up to 30% of patients receiving heparin therapy, this nonautoimmune condition manifests within a few days of initiation of therapy. Platelet depletion is moderate, counts are usually less than 100,000/mm^3, and the condition is transient, often resolving spontaneously. Discontinuation of heparin is not required. The second form is type 2 HIT, or immune-mediated HIT,[8] which is less commonly encountered but has more severe consequences.[9-11] This discussion is limited to immune-mediated HIT.

Immune-mediated HIT is a response to the administration of heparin therapy. It has been observed in 0.5% to 5% of patients treated with unfractionated heparin and has occurred after exposure to LMWH, although to a lesser degree.[8] The disorder is characterized by severe thrombocytopenia during heparin therapy. Diagnostically, it is identified by a platelet count less than 50,000/mm^3 or at least a 50% decrease from the baseline platelet count from the initiation of therapy. Onset usually occurs 5 to 14 days from the first

BOX 27-3 COLLABORATIVE MANAGEMENT

Disseminated Intravascular Coagulation

- Identify and eliminate the underlying cause.
- Provide hemodynamic support to prevent end-organ ischemia.
  - Intravenous fluids
  - Positive inotropic agents
- Administer blood and blood components.
  - Fresh-frozen plasma
  - Platelets
  - Cryoprecipitate
  - Antithrombin III
- Administer medications.
  - Heparin
  - Aminocaproic acid
  - Protein C
  - Antithrombin III
- Initiate bleeding precautions.
- Maintain surveillance for complications.
  - Hypovolemic shock
  - Peripheral ischemia
  - Central ischemia
  - Multiple organ dysfunction syndrome (MODS)
- Provide comfort and emotional support.

exposure to heparin, but the onset can occur within hours of a reexposure to heparin.[9-12] Depending on the source of the disorder, reported mortality rates are as high as 30%.[8]

Pathophysiology

The thrombocytopenia that occurs with immune-mediated HIT is related to the formation of heparin-antibody complexes. These complexes release a substance known as platelet factor 4 (PF4). PF4 attracts heparin molecules, forming immunogenic complexes that adhere to platelet and endothelial surfaces (Figure 27-2). Activation of platelets stimulates the release of thrombin and the subsequent formation of platelet clumps.[9]

Patients with immune-mediated HIT are at greater risk for thrombosis than bleeding. Vessel occlusion can result in the need for limb amputation, stroke, acute myocardial infarction, and even death.[9-12] The resultant formation of fibrin-platelet-rich thrombi is the primary characteristic of HIT that distinguishes it from other forms of thrombocytopenia and gives rise to its more descriptive name: white clot syndrome.[10]

Assessment and Diagnosis

HIT can be associated with severe consequences. Rapid recognition of risk factors and subsequent development of signs and symptoms is essential in treating this condition.

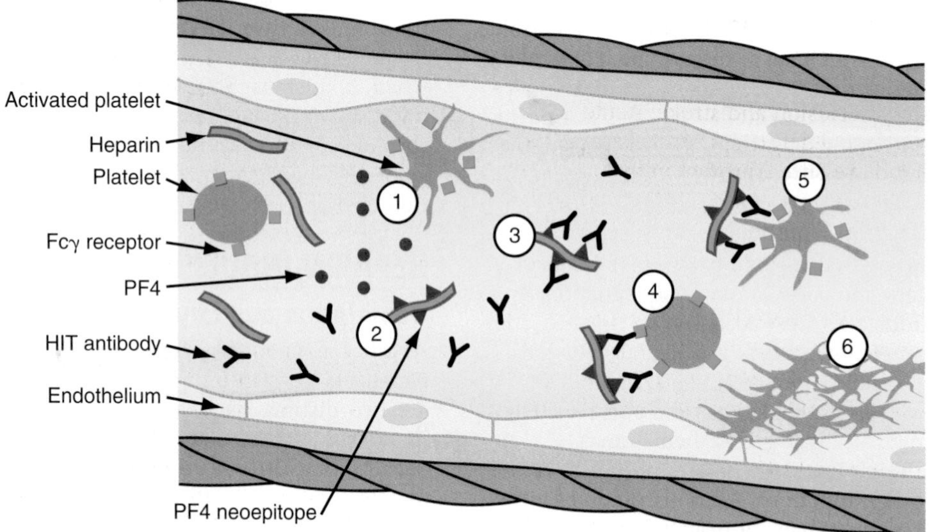

FIG 27-2 Pathogenesis of Heparin-Induced Thrombocytopenia (HIT). *(1)* Activated platelets release procoagulant proteins from α-granules, including platelet factor 4 (PF4). Administered heparin binds PF4 *(2)*, which undergoes a conformation change and expresses a new antigen (neoepitope). Individuals with HIT produce an immunoglobulin G (IgG) antibody that specifically reacts *(3)* with multiple identical neoepitopes on the heparin-PF4 complex. The reaction forms heparin-PF4-IgG immune complexes. Platelets express FcγRIIa receptors (Fcγ receptor) that react *(4)* with the Fc portion of IgG in immune complexes. Cross-linking of Fc receptors *(5)* results in FcγRIIa-dependent platelet activation. The activated platelets mediate a series of events that lead to further activation of the coagulation cascade, resulting in thrombin generation. Further release of PF4 from newly activated platelets leads to a cycle of continuing platelet activation and *(6)* formation of a primary clot. The reaction can be enhanced by the release of platelet-derived microparticles that are rich in surface phosphatidylserine and increase activation of coagulation and by the binding of heparin-PF4 complexes and HIT-IgG to the vascular endothelium (not shown). (From McCance KL et al, eds. Pathophysiology: The Biologic Basis for Disease in Adults and Children. 7th ed. St. Louis: Elsevier; 2014.)

TABLE 27-3 Heparin-Induced Thrombocytopenia: Signs, Symptoms, and Laboratory Data

SYSTEM OR STUDY	SIGNS AND SYMPTOMS
Cardiac	Chest pain, diaphoresis, pallor, alterations in blood pressure, dysrhythmias
Vascular	Arterial: pain, pallor, pulselessness, paresthesia, paralysis
	Venous: pain, tenderness, unilateral leg swelling, warmth, erythema, a palpable cord, pain on passive dorsiflexion of the foot, and spontaneous maintenance of the relaxed foot in abnormal plantar flexion (Homans sign)
Pulmonary	Dyspnea, pleuritic pain, rales, chest pain, chest wall tenderness, back pain, shoulder pain, upper abdominal pain, syncope, hemoptysis, shortness of breath, wheezing
Renal	Thirst, decreased urine output, dizziness, orthostatic hypotension
Gastrointestinal	Abdominal pain, vomiting, bloody diarrhea, abnormal bowel sounds
Neurologic	Confusion, headache, impaired speech patterns, hemiparesis or hemiplegia, vision disturbances, dysarthria, aphasia, ataxia, vertigo, nystagmus, sudden decrease in consciousness
Laboratory	Platelets <50,000/mm^3 or sudden drop of 30%-50% from baseline; positive results for HIPA, SRA, ELISA

ELISA, Enzyme-linked immunosorbent assay; *HIPA*, heparin-induced platelet aggregation; *SRA*, serotonin release assay.

Clinical Manifestations

Common signs and symptoms are listed in Table 27-3. The clinical manifestations of HIT are related to the formation of thrombi and subsequent vessel occlusion.[8] Most thrombotic events are venous, although both venous and arterial thrombosis can occur. Thrombotic events typically include deep vein thrombosis, pulmonary embolism, limb ischemia thrombosis, thrombotic stroke, and myocardial infarction.[8,12] The presence of blanching and the loss of peripheral pulses, sensation, or motor function in a limb indicate peripheral vascular thrombi. Neurologic signs and symptoms such as confusion, headache, and impaired speech can signal the onset of cerebral artery occlusion and stroke. Acute myocardial infarction may be heralded by dyspnea, chest pain, pallor, and alterations in blood pressure. Thrombi in the pulmonary vasculature may be evidenced by pleuritic pain, rales, and dyspnea.[9,10]

Laboratory Findings

The key indicator for identifying HIT is the platelet count. General consensus in the literature considers a platelet count of less than 100,000/mm^3 or a sudden drop of 50% from the patient's baseline after initiation of heparin therapy strongly to indicate HIT.[10-12]

Two types of assays have become available to assist in confirming the diagnosis of HIT: activation assays, based on platelet aggregation or the release of granular contents such as serotonin, and assays that identify the HIT antigen. Activation assays are highly sensitive in detecting the presence of HIT. The most common assay used is heparin-induced platelet aggregation (HIPA). Serotonin-release assay (SRA) is used by a few institutions. The enzyme-linked immunosorbent assay (ELISA) identifies the presence of the HIT antigen.[10]

Medical Management

Early identification is critical to managing the effects of immune-mediated HIT. Current guidelines suggest that for high-risk patients platelet count monitoring be performed every 2 or 3 days from day 4 to day 14.[13] When a decrease in the platelet count is detected, heparin therapy should be discontinued immediately, and the patient should be tested for the presence of heparin antibodies.[9,11-13] If the original

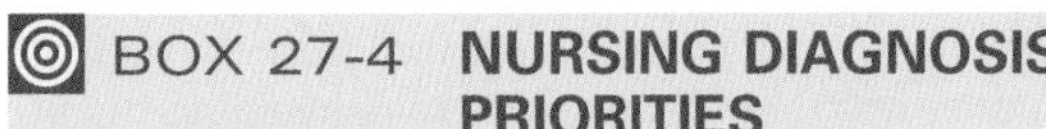

BOX 27-4 NURSING DIAGNOSIS PRIORITIES

Heparin-Induced Thrombocytopenia

- Risk for Decreased Cardiac Tissue Perfusion, p. 603
- Risk for Ineffective Peripheral Tissue Perfusion, p. 605
- Risk for Ineffective Renal Tissue Perfusion, p. 606
- Risk for Ineffective Gastrointestinal Tissue Perfusion, p. 605
- Risk for Ineffective Cerebral Tissue Perfusion, p. 604
- Powerlessness related to lack of control over the current situation or disease progression, p. 600
- Deficient Knowledge related to lack of previous exposure to information, p. 585 (see Box 27-5, Patient Education for Heparin-Induced Thrombocytopenia)

indication for heparin still exists or new thrombosis occurs, an alternative form of anticoagulation is usually necessary.[13]

Direct Thrombin Inhibitors

Direct thrombin inhibitors (DTIs) are being used with increasing frequency to treat HIT. DTIs bind directly to the thrombin molecule, thereby inhibiting its action.[12] Currently, the only medication approved for use in the United States is argatroban. Warfarin, although commonly used to treat deep vein thrombosis, is not indicated as a sole agent in treating HIT because of its prolonged onset of action. Studies have shown that the use of warfarin without concomitant use of DTIs can significantly increase the incidence of thrombosis in patients with HIT.[8,10-12]

Nursing Management

Nursing management of the patient with HIT incorporates a variety of nursing diagnoses (Box 27-4). **Nursing priorities are directed toward 1) decreasing the incidence of heparin exposure, 2) maintaining surveillance for complications, 3) providing comfort and emotional support, and 4) initiating patient education.** The critical care nurse plays a pivotal role in prevention and detection of HIT. Initial assessment is crucial to identifying those patients at risk for HIT. Ascertaining a medical history that includes previous heparin therapy, deep vein thrombosis, or cardiovascular surgery that

BOX 27-5 PATIENT EDUCATION PRIORITIES

Heparin-Induced Thrombocytopenia

- Pathophysiology of disease
- Purpose of heparin
- Measures to avoid future exposure to heparin
- Identify different types of heparin (unfractionated and low–molecular-weight forms).
- Encourage purchase of medical alert bracelet or similar type of warning device.
- Tell any new health care provider about the heparin allergy and previous reaction.

included the use of cardiopulmonary bypass can alert the nurse to potential problems.

Decreasing the Incidence of Heparin Exposure

Ensuring that all heparin has been removed from the patient's hemodynamic pressure monitoring system, avoiding the use of heparin-coated catheters, and discontinuing heparin flushes to maintain the patency of other intravenous lines are essential elements of nursing management.

Maintaining Surveillance for Complications

Patients with HIT remain at high risk for thrombotic complications for several days or weeks after cessation of heparin. Vigilant monitoring, early recognition of signs and symptoms, deep vein thrombosis prevention strategies, and prompt notification of the physician are key roles of the critical care nurse.

Educating the Patient and Family

Prevention of subsequent episodes in patients sensitized to heparin incudes education of the patient and family (Box 27-5). Education should include measures to avoid future exposure to heparin. The use of medical alert bracelets and listing heparin allergies in the medical record are necessary to avoid this serious complication in the future. Collaborative management of the patient with HIT is outlined in Box 27-6.

BOX 27-6 COLLABORATIVE MANAGEMENT

Heparin-Induced Thrombocytopenia

- Stop all heparin exposure.
  - Unfractionated and low–molecular-weight heparin by any route
  - Heparin flushes
  - Heparin-coated vascular access devices
- Begin therapy with an alternative anticoagulant.
  - Argatroban
- Maintain surveillance for complications.
  - Deep vein thrombosis
  - Pulmonary emboli
  - Acute limb ischemia
  - Ischemic stroke
  - Acute myocardial infarction
- Administer antifibrinolytic therapy (as indicated) if thrombosis occurs.
- Prepare patient for surgical embolectomy (as indicated) if thrombosis occurs.
- Provide comfort and emotional support.

SICKLE CELL ANEMIA

Description and Etiology

Sickle cell anemia (SCA) is a disease passed down through families in which RBCs form an abnormal sickle or crescent shape. RBCs carry oxygen to the body and are normally shaped like a disk.[3] The sickle-shaped cells have a shortened life span, are unable to carry adequate oxygen to tissues, and due to their shape become trapped in the vasculature, and can cause severe pain, increased risk of infection, and life-threatening complications.[14]

SCA is an autosomal recessive genetic disorder. An individual with normal hemoglobin has two copies of hemoglobin A (Hb A) gene. An individual with SCA has two copies of hemoglobin S (Hb S) gene. Individuals who have one gene for Hb S and one gene for Hb A are known as "carriers" of the sickle cell trait (Hb AS). When two "carriers" have a child, there is a 25% chance that they will have a child with SCA (Hb SS), a 50% chance of having a child with sickle cell trait (Hb AS), and a 25% chance of having a child with entirely normal hemoglobin (Hb AA).[15,16]

This genetic trait is primarily found in people of West African descent. The disease has also been linked to persons of sole European or Middle Eastern ancestry; however, this is extremely rare. The disease is not prevalent in persons of Asian or Pacific Islander descent.[15] SCA is usually diagnosed during the first few years of life due to manifestation of initial symptoms. Prenatal screening is now available for at-risk couples.[16] This consists of DNA analysis from fetal cells. This should be offered as part of their prenatal counseling. There are more than 40 states that undergo universal neonatal screening for hemoglobinopathies.[16]

Pathophysiology

Sickle cell disease (SCD) is a chronic inflammatory condition characterized by hemolysis and vasoocclusion. The cause of SCA is a mutation in the genetic sequence in the beta chain gene of the hemoglobin. This results in a sequence of the replacement of valine with glutamic acid at the N-terminal amino acid position 6 of the protein chain.[15,16] This substitution leads to the production of hemoglobin S.

Normal RBCs contain hemoglobin that are flexible, biconcave disks. When deoxygenated, RBCs containing predominantly Hb S distort into a crescent or sickle shape. In this form, the hemoglobin becomes rigid and friable, causing vasoocclusion in the small vessels of the circulatory system. This tends to happen during times of physiologic stress, such as physical overexertion, muscle tissue ischemia, dehydration, infection, or extreme temperatures.[16] Even though these conditions have a tendency to exacerbate the condition, the majority of the sickling events have no identifying cause.[15]

The RBCs become lodged in the vasculature and the microcirculation causing stasis and obstruction of blood flow and damage to the surrounding organs, tissue ischemia, infarction, and if not corrected eventually, necrosis (Figure 27-3).[16] In addition, hemolysis of the RBCs occurs, resulting in anemia.

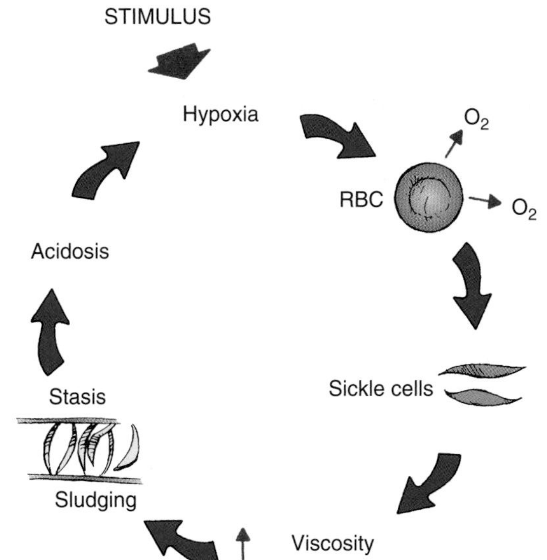

FIG 27-3 Cycle Causing Vasoocclusive Episodes in Sickle Cell Anemia. (From Hockenberry M, Coody D, eds. Pediatric Oncology and Hematology: Perspectives on Care. St. Louis: Mosby; 1986.)

Assessment and Diagnosis

SCA can be associated with severe consequences. Rapid recognition of signs and symptoms is essential in treating this condition.

Clinical Manifestations

There are a variety of clinical manifestations associated with SCA (Figure 27-4). The patient may present with a low-grade fever, bone or joint pain, pinpoint pupils, inability to follow commands, photophobia, tachycardia, tachypnea, decreased respiratory excursion, hepatomegaly, nonpalpable spleen, and pretibial ulcers.[17]

Laboratory Studies

Initial laboratory studies include a complete blood count (CBC), a peripheral blood smear, and a quantitative hemoglobin electrophoresis. Sickle cells constitute 5% to 10% of the blood smear. The elevated reticulocyte count (greater than 10%) is characteristically accompanied by the presence of Howell-Jolly bodies. Howell-Jolly bodies are small remnants of nuclear material from hemolyzed erythrocytes reflective of hyposplenia or autoinfarction and target cells (an erythrocyte with a deeply stained core surrounded by a lighter-stained margin; it resembles a target with a bull's eye).[16] Typically an elevated WBC count occurs during and following a crisis. Other tests might include an indirect bilirubin level, which will be elevated following hemolysis. The haptoglobin level will be low or absent because it cannot be replaced quickly enough after severe hemolysis. Haptoglobin, a glycoprotein, exists to bind free hemoglobin that is released from hemolyzed erythrocytes.[16]

Medical Management

SCA is not a curable disease; however, there are treatment options available for management of symptoms and complications. Bone marrow transplant offers a cure in a limited number of cases.[14] Medical interventions are aimed at preventing infections, managing pain, transfusing RBCs, and administering hydroxyurea. Patients with chronic disease are more effectively managed through a multidisciplinary approach.[14] It is also important to look at other issues that may exacerbate the patient disease process such as diet, inadequate housing, lack of education, poor access to services, and poor lifestyle choices.

Prevent Infection

Both children and adults with SCA are more prone to infection and have a more difficult time fighting off infection.[17] This can result in damage to the spleen from constant sickling of the RBCs. Damage to the spleen can prevent the destruction of bacteria in the blood. Prophylactic administration of oral antibiotics starting at 2 months old can decrease the chances of a pneumococcal infection and early death. Proper vaccinations against pneumococcal infections, meningitis, hepatitis, and influenza are important to prevent future infections.[17]

Pain Management

Pain associated with SCA can be acute or chronic in nature. The most common type of pain associated with SCA is vasoocclusive pain. It is commonly treated with an antiinflammatory and opioid or nonopioid analgesics.[17,18] The pain associated with SCA can vary enormously; therefore, a number of different approaches may be required. The medication of choice should be influenced by the patient's history of analgesia use. Some patients may have extremely intricate medication regimes.[17] Paracetamol and nonsteroidal antiinflammatory drugs (NSAIDs) are used for mild to moderate pain relief. If this is not effective, oral or parenteral opiates may be an alternative.[17,18]

For those who wish to try the nonpharmacologic route, there are other approaches such as psychological support, massage, acupuncture, and transcutaneous electrical nerve stimulation. Distraction can be another valuable tool to use. The use of television, video games, repeating inspirational phrases and mental calculations can also be a form of distraction. Studies suggested that cognitive behavioral therapy can help teach patients coping strategies for acute and chronic pain.[17]

Transfusion Therapy

RBC transfusion therapy in SCD is an important life-saving treatment option but should be done with careful consideration. Transfusion therapy is primarily used for treatment of patients who are experiencing complications due to SCD or as an emergency measure.[18] Transfusion therapy should be used with extreme caution due to risks such as iron overload, exposure to hepatitis, HIV and other infectious agents, alloimmunization, induction of hyperviscosity, and limitations on resources. The indication for having a blood transfusion are recurrent painful vasoocclusive crises with long hospital admissions, acute chest syndrome, stroke, priapism, and leg ulcers. Blood transfusions can also be performed before major operations, such as hip replacement because of avascular necrosis of the hip bone.[17]

Administration of Hydroxyurea

Hydroxyurea is an oral agent that is a safe and effective treatment for children and adults that suffer from SCA. It works by increasing the level of fetal hemoglobin in the RBCs,

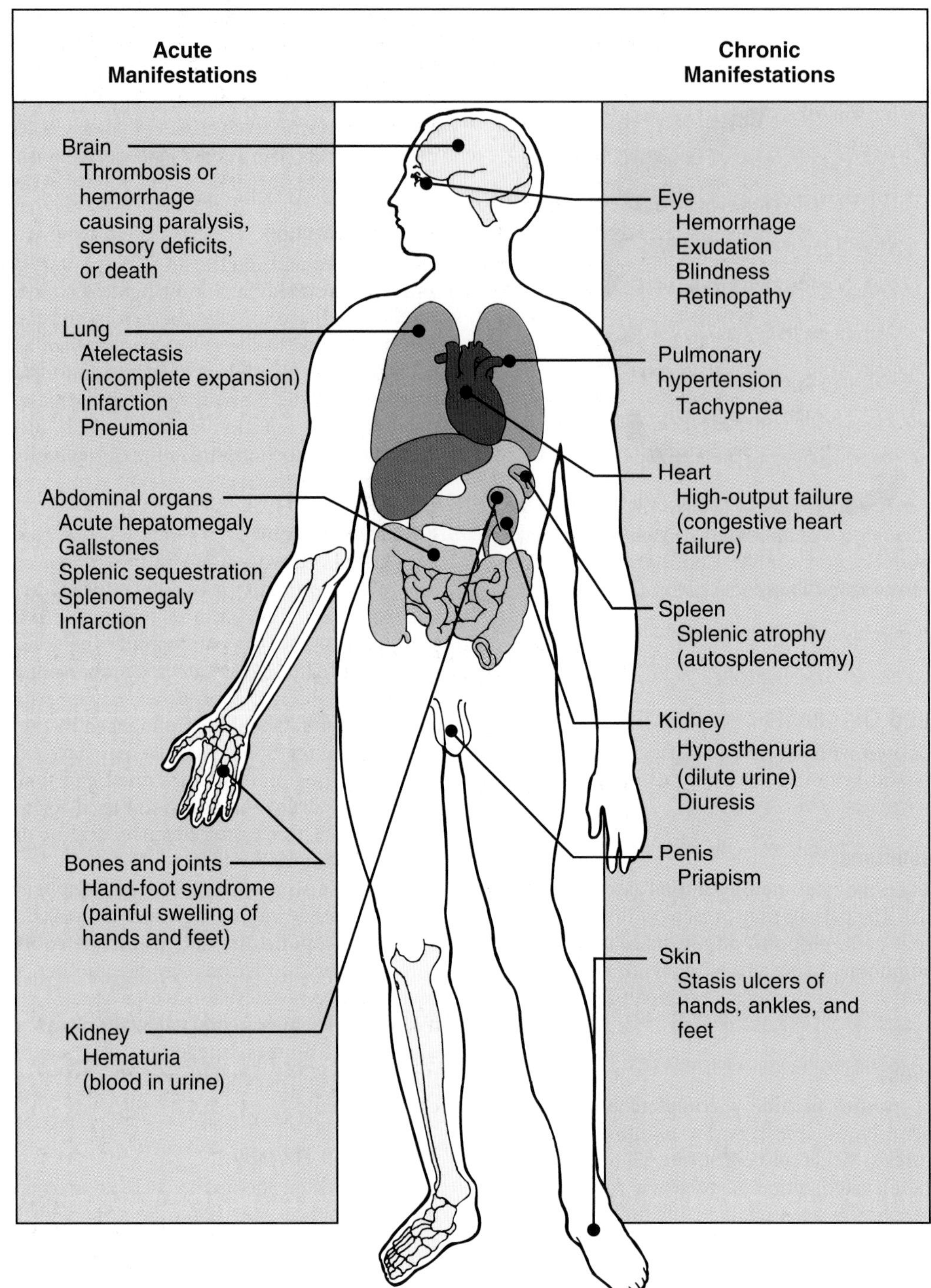

FIG 27-4 Clinical Manifestations of Sickle Cell Disease. (From McCance KL et al, eds. Pathophysiology: The Biologic Basis for Disease in Adults and Children. 7th ed. St. Louis: Elsevier; 2014.)

thereby reducing the concentration of sickle hemoglobin and sickling itself.[17] The patient is usually started at a dose of 15 mg/kg PO once a day. The dose is increased by 5 mg/kg every 12 weeks until 35 mg/kg is reached, providing the patient's blood count remains within an acceptable range. Research shows patients receiving hydroxyurea had lower episodes of pain and acute chest syndrome and also had a decreased need for blood transfusion and hospitalizations compared to those that received no treatment. Research states that hydroxyurea can be used as an alternative to regular blood transfusions.[18]

Nursing Management

Nursing management of the patient with SCA incorporates a variety of nursing diagnoses (Box 27-7). **Nursing priorities are directed toward 1) supporting the patient's vital functions, 2) providing comfort and emotional support, 3) maintaining surveillance for complications, and 4) educating the patient and family.**

Supporting Patient's Vital Functions

Frequent assessments should include parameters for neurologic status, renal function, cardiopulmonary function, and

BOX 27-7 NURSING DIAGNOSIS PRIORITIES

Sickle Cell Anemia

- Acute Pain related to transmission and perception of cutaneous, visceral, muscular, or ischemic impulses, p. 574
- Risk for Ineffective Peripheral Tissue Perfusion, p. 605
- Risk for Ineffective Renal Tissue Perfusion, p. 606
- Risk for Ineffective Gastrointestinal Tissue Perfusion, p. 605
- Risk for Ineffective Cerebral Tissue Perfusion, p. 604
- Powerlessness related to lack of control over the current situation or disease progression, p. 600
- Deficient Knowledge related to lack of previous exposure to information, p. 585 (see Box 27-8, Patient Education for Sickle Cell Anemia)

skin integrity that indicate impaired tissue or organ perfusion. Particular parameters to include are mental status, BUN and creatine levels, urine output, vital signs, hemodynamic values, cardiac rhythm, arterial blood gas and pulse oximetry values, skin breakdown, ecchymosis, or hematomas.[18]

The critical care nurse must recognize and support the patient's vital physiologic functions. Administration of intravenous fluids, blood products, and inotropic agents to provide adequate hemodynamic support and tissue oxygenation is essential in preventing or combating end-organ damage. Close monitoring of vital signs, hemodynamic parameters, intake and output, and appropriate laboratory values assists the critical care nurse in administering and titrating appropriate agents.[18]

Maintaining Surveillance for Complications

The critical care nurse needs to be vigilant for signs of life-threatening complications such as septicemia, acute myocardial infarction, priapism, ischemic stroke, and shock.[14] If there are any significant concerns, these must be reported immediately. Other issues that may arise are dehydration, hypoxia, infection, skin and tissue viability, and decreased hemoglobin levels.

Educating the Patient and Family

Even though there is no cure for SCA, the focus of care is prevention. Early in the patient's hospital stay, the patient and family should be taught about SCA, its etiologies, and treatment options available (Box 27-8). Patient and family education focuses on measures to help prevent painful reoccurring episodes. If the patient smokes, he or she should be encouraged to stop smoking and be referred to a smoking cessation program. In addition, the importance of continuous medical follow-up should be stressed. While research continues to try to find a cure, nurses must continue to be sensitive to the effects of the disease on the patient and the family as well as the need to be culturally sensitive.[20] Collaborative management of the patient with SCA is outlined in Box 27-9.

TUMOR LYSIS SYNDROME

Description and Etiology

Tumor lysis syndrome (TLS) refers to a variety of metabolic disturbances that may be seen with the treatment of cancer.

BOX 27-8 PATIENT EDUCATION PRIORITIES

Sickle Cell Anemia

- Pathophysiology of disease
- Precipitating factor modification
- Importance of taking medications
- Maintenance of adequate hydration (especially during febrile periods and hot weather)
- Use of pharmacologic and nonpharmacologic methods of pain management
- Avoidance of situations that can precipitate condition such as extreme cold
- Smoking cessation and avoidance of secondhand smoke
- Get plenty of rest and relaxation and avoid exhaustive exercise.
- Genetic screening
- Encourage purchase of medical alert bracelet or similar type of warning device.

BOX 27-9 COLLABORATIVE MANAGEMENT

Sickle Cell Anemia

- Prevent infection.
  - Prophylactic antibiotics
  - Vaccinations
- Manage pain.
  - Pharmacologic management
  - Nonpharmacologic management
- Administration of blood
- Administration of hydroxyurea
- Maintain surveillance for complications.
  - Septicemia
  - Acute kidney injury
  - Acute myocardial infarction
  - Acute limb ischemia
  - Ischemic stroke
  - Anemia
- Provide comfort and emotional support.

A potentially lethal complication of various forms of cancer treatment, TLS occurs when large numbers of neoplastic cells are rapidly killed, resulting in the release of large amounts of potassium, phosphate, and uric acid into the systemic circulation. It is most commonly seen in patients with lymphoma, leukemia, or multiple metastatic conditions.[19]

Although most often associated with the use of chemotherapeutic medications, biologic agents, and irradiation used in the treatment of malignant disorders, TLS can in rare instances occur spontaneously. The development of TLS has been linked to other pathophysiologic conditions such as elevated WBC counts, large tumors, multiple organ involvement by malignancy, and renal insufficiency.[19]

Pathophysiology

The primary mechanism involved in the development of TLS is the destruction of massive numbers of malignant cells by chemotherapy or radiation therapy (Figure 27-5). Massive

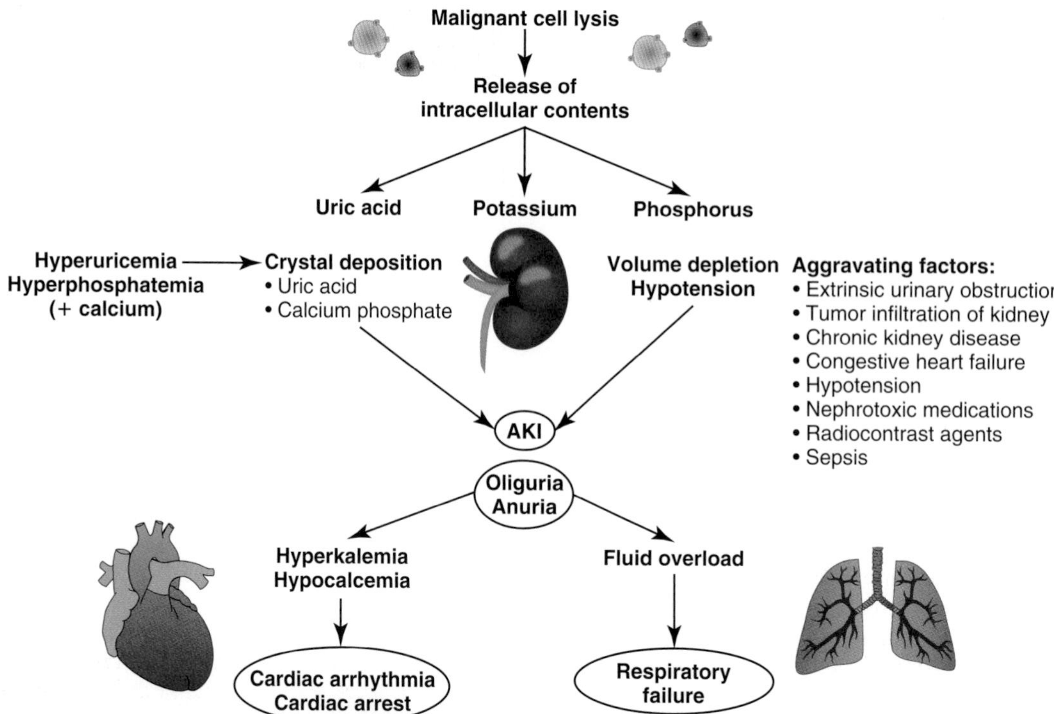

FIG 27-5 Metabolic Abnormalities in Tumor Lysis Syndrome and Clinical Consequences. *AKI*, Acute kidney injury. (From Abu-Alfa AK, Younes A. Tumor lysis syndrome and acute kidney injury: evaluation, prevention and management. Am J Kidney Dis. 2010;55[5 suppl 3]:S1.)

TABLE 27-4 Electrolyte Abnormalities Encountered in Tumor Lysis Syndrome and Their Clinical Consequences

ELECTROLYTE	PATHOPHYSIOLOGY	CLINICAL CONSEQUENCE	TREATMENT OPTIONS
Potassium	Rapid expulsion of intracellular K^+ into the circulation due to cell lysis	Adverse skeletal and cardiac manifestations (e.g., ventricular dysrhythmias, weakness, paresthesias)	Insulin/glucose, sodium bicarbonate, inhaled beta-agonist, K^+-binding resins, dialysis, calcium gluconate
Phosphate	Release of intracellular PO_4^- due to cell lysis		
May be compounded by renal dysfunction	Muscle cramps, tetany, dysrhythmias, seizures	Dialysis, phosphate binders	
Calcium	Precipitation of the calcium phosphate complex because of the rapid increase in the phosphorous concentration	Muscle cramps, tetany, dysrhythmias, seizures, renal failure (acute nephrocalcinosis)	Calcium gluconate (Treatment should be reserved for those with neuromuscular irritability.)
Uric acid	Cell lysis leads to increased levels of purine nucleic acids into the circulation that are metabolized to uric acid.	Renal failure (uric acid nephropathy)	Hydration, dialysis, xanthine oxidase inhibitors, alkalization of urine, urate oxidase

From Davidson MB, et al. Pathophysiology, clinical consequences, and treatment of tumor lysis syndrome. *Am J Med.* 2004; 116:546.

destruction of cells releases large amounts of potassium, phosphorus, and nucleic acids, leading to severe metabolic disturbances such as hyperuricemia, hyperkalemia, hyperphosphatemia, and hypocalcemia (Table 27-4). Vomiting, diarrhea, and other insensible fluid losses from fever or tachypnea also contribute to these electrolyte disturbances.[19] Death of patients with TLS is most often caused by complications of renal failure or cardiac arrest.[19-21]

Hyperuricemia

Hyperuricemia occurs 48 to 72 hours after the initiation of anticancer therapy.[19] Tumor cells undergo rapid growth and development, and large amounts of nucleic acids are present within them. When therapy is initiated, tumor cell destruction releases nucleic acids, which are metabolized into uric acid. Metabolic acidosis ensues, resulting in crystallization of the uric acid in the distal tubules of the kidney and leading to obstruction of urine flow. Glomerular filtration rates drop as the kidneys are unable to clear the increasing amounts of uric acid. Consequently, acute kidney injury eventually occurs.[22] Acute kidney injury is discussed further in Chapter 20.

Hyperuricemia associated with TLS can be potentiated by several other factors, including elevated uric acid levels before the initiation of therapy. Other causes of increased uric acid production are elevated WBC counts, destruction of WBCs, and enlargement of the lymph nodes, spleen, or liver.[19]

Hyperkalemia

Hyperkalemia occurs within 6 to 72 hours after the initiation of chemotherapy. This is the most deleterious of all the manifestations of TLS.[19] In addition to the release of nucleic acids, tumor cell destruction also results in the release of potassium. Renal insufficiency related to hyperuricemia prevents adequate excretion of potassium, and levels rise. The resultant hyperkalemia may have a profound effect on intracellular and extracellular fluid levels.[23] Left untreated, hyperkalemia can have devastating consequences, including cardiac arrest and death.[19]

Hyperphosphatemia and Hypocalcemia

Hyperphosphatemia and hypocalcemia occur 24 to 48 hours after the initiation of therapy.[19] Phosphorus levels also rise as a consequence of tumor cell destruction. Calcium ions then bind with the excess phosphorus, creating calcium phosphate salts and bringing about hypocalcemia. These salts precipitate in the kidney tubules, worsening renal insufficiency. Hypocalcemia causes tetany and cardiac dysrhythmias, which can result in cardiac arrest and death.[22,23]

Assessment and Diagnosis

Detection and recognition of TLS is accomplished through assessment of clinical manifestations, evaluation of laboratory findings, and other diagnostic tests. Table 27-5 summarizes common findings in TLS.[19,21]

Clinical Manifestations

Clinical manifestations are related to the metabolic disturbances associated with TLS.[21] The patient's history reveals an unexplained weight gain after initiation of chemotherapy or radiation therapy. The weight gain is associated with fluid retention due to electrolyte disturbances. Other early signs heralding the onset of TLS include diarrhea, lethargy, muscle cramps, nausea, vomiting, paresthesias, and weakness.[20]

Physical examination reveals positive Chvostek and Trousseau signs related to hypocalcemia. Hyperactive deep tendon reflexes indicate hyperkalemia and hypocalcemia.[21] Potassium and calcium disturbances result in changes that can be seen on the electrocardiogram (ECG), such as peaked or inverted T waves, altered QT intervals, widened QRS complexes, and dysrhythmias.[19]

Laboratory Findings

Laboratory findings demonstrate electrolyte disturbances such as elevated potassium and phosphorus levels and a decreased calcium level. Uric acid levels are increased. Elevated levels of BUN and creatinine and a decreased creatinine clearance also indicate TLS. Metabolic acidosis is confirmed by the presence of decreased pH, bicarbonate levels, and partial pressure of carbon dioxide ($PaCO_2$) on arterial blood gas measurements.[20]

TABLE 27-5 Common Findings in Tumor Lysis Syndrome

DIAGNOSTIC PARAMETER	FINDINGS
Clinical	Weight gain, edema, diarrhea, lethargy, muscle cramps, nausea and vomiting, paresthesia, weakness, oliguria, uremia, seizures
Laboratory	↑ Potassium, phosphorus, uric acid, BUN, Cr ↓ Calcium, creatinine clearance, pH, bicarbonate, $PaCO_2$
Diagnostic	Positive Chvostek and Trousseau signs, hyperactive deep tendon reflexes, dysrhythmias, ECG changes

BUN, Blood urea nitrogen; *Cr*, creatinine; *ECG*, electrocardiogram; *$PaCO_2$*, partial pressure of carbon dioxide; ↑ increased; ↓ decreased.

Medical Management

Medical interventions are aimed at maintaining adequate hydration, treating metabolic imbalances, and preventing life-threatening complications (Table 27-4).[20,23]

Adequate Hydration

Administration of intravenous fluids may be necessary early in the course of treatment if inadequate hydration exists. The administration of isotonic saline (0.9% normal saline) reduces serum concentrations of uric acid, phosphate, and potassium.[21] The use of nonthiazide diuretics to maintain adequate urine output may be required. If renal failure occurs, hemodialysis should be considered.[21]

Metabolic Imbalances

Electrolytes and arterial blood gases are closely monitored. Dietary restrictions of potassium and phosphorus may be necessary. The goals in treating hyperuricemia are to inhibit uric acid formation and to increase renal clearance.[23] This can be accomplished through the administration of sodium bicarbonate to increase the pH of the urine to above 7.0, which increases the solubility of uric acid, preventing subsequent crystallization. Allopurinol administration can also inhibit uric acid formation.[21]

Life-Threatening Complications

If potassium levels rise dangerously, Kayexalate (sodium polystyrene sulfonate) may be given orally, or if the patient is unable to tolerate oral medications due to nausea and vomiting, rectal instillation may be used. If the patient is oliguric, glucose and insulin infusions may be given to facilitate lowering the potassium levels. A 10% solution of calcium gluconate may be administered to stabilize cardiac tissue membranes to prevent life-threatening dysrhythmias.[24] Phosphorus-binding antacids can be used for treating hyperphosphatemia. Stool softeners may be necessary to treat the constipation often associated with the administration of these antacids. Calcium gluconate may be required to replace calcium, but it should be used judiciously.[19]

Nursing Management

Nursing management of the patient with TLS incorporates a variety of nursing diagnoses (Box 27-10). **Nursing priorities are directed toward 1) monitoring fluid and electrolytes, 2) providing comfort and emotional support, 3) maintaining surveillance for complications, and 4) initiating patient education.**

Monitoring Fluid and Electrolytes

Assessment and continued monitoring of the patient is an important role of the critical care nurse when caring for the patient with TLS. Recognizing critical laboratory changes or development of symptoms and notifying the physician in a timely manner are essential. Insertion of a urinary catheter and maintenance of the intravenous line site are necessary to ensure adequate intake and output. Vital signs should be monitored frequently, and weight should be monitored daily.

Maintaining Surveillance for Complications

Nursing interventions are aimed at preventing complications. Seizure precautions should be instituted, especially if calcium levels are disrupted. Insertion of a nasogastric tube is appropriate if nausea or vomiting occurs. Dietary adjustments are necessary, such as potassium and phosphorus restrictions in the presence of elevated serum levels and providing additional fiber to combat the constipation associated with the administration of antacids.[24]

Educating the Patient and Family

Education of the patient and family is a primary role of the critical care nurse. All treatments and interventions should be explained before carrying them out, and questions should be answered at a level understandable to the patient and family. Before discharge, potential risk factors and identification of early signs and symptoms should be reviewed. Collaborative management of the patient with TLS is outlined in Box 27-11.

BOX 27-10 NURSING DIAGNOSES

Tumor Lysis Syndrome

- Excess Fluid Volume related to renal dysfunction, p. 590
- Decreased Cardiac Output related to alterations in contractility, p. 580
- Anxiety related to threat to biologic, psychologic, and/or social integrity, p. 576
- Ineffective Coping related to a situational crisis and personal vulnerability, p. 599

BOX 27-11 COLLABORATIVE MANAGEMENT

Tumor Lysis Syndrome

- Facilitate adequate renal function.
  - Volume hydration with 0.9% normal saline
  - Nonthiazide diuretics
- Treat hyperkalemia.
  - Kayexalate
  - Glucose and insulin
- Treat hyperuricemia.
  - Sodium bicarbonate
  - Allopurinol
- Treat hyperphosphatemia.
  - Dietary restrictions
  - Phosphorus-binding antacids
- Treat hypocalcemia.
  - Calcium gluconate
- Maintain surveillance for complications.
  - Acute kidney injury
  - Cardiac dysrhythmias
- Provide comfort and emotional support.

CASE STUDY Patient with Hematologic Disorders and Oncologic Emergencies

Brief Patient History

Mr. L is an otherwise healthy, 23-year-old African American man who presents with a week-long history of diarrhea, nausea, and vomiting after attending a barbecue last weekend.

Clinical Assessment

Mr. L is admitted to the critical care unit from the emergency department with hypotension, fever, and leukocytosis.

Diagnostic Procedures

His vital signs are as follows: blood pressure of 65/42 mm Hg, heart rate of 145 beats/min (sinus tachycardia), respiratory rate of 35 breaths/min, and temperature of 102.4°F. His white blood cell count is 25,000/mm^3 with 15% bands, lactate level is 7 mmol/L, prothrombin time is 25 seconds, and platelet count is 22,000/mm^3. Blood cultures reveal gram-negative bacilli.

Medical Diagnosis

Mr. L is diagnosed with severe sepsis and disseminated intravascular coagulation.

Questions

1. What major outcomes do you expect to achieve for this patient?
2. What problems or risks must be managed to achieve these outcomes?
3. What interventions must be initiated to monitor, prevent, manage, or eliminate the problems and risks identified?
4. What interventions should be initiated to promote optimal functioning, safety, and well-being of the patient?
5. What possible learning needs do you anticipate for this patient?
6. What cultural and age-related factors may have a bearing on the patient's plan of care?

REFERENCES

1. Kitchens CS: Thrombocytopenia and thrombosis in disseminated intravascular coagulation (DIC), *Hematology Am Soc Hematol Educ Program* 2009:240, 2009.
2. Levi M, van der Poll T: Disseminated intravascular coagulation: a review for the internist, *Intern Emerg Med* 8:23, 2013.
3. Rote NS, McCance KL: Structure and function of the hematologic system. In McCance KL, et al, editors: *Pathophysiology: the biologic basis for disease in adults and children*, ed 7, St. Louis, 2014, Mosby.
4. Castoldi E, Hackeng TM: Regulation of coagulation by protein S, *Curr Opin Hematol* 15:529, 2008.
5. Gando S: Microvascular thrombosis and multiple organ dysfunction, *Crit Care Med* 38(Suppl 2):S35, 2010.
6. Blaisdell FW: Causes, prevention, and treatment of intravascular coagulation and disseminated intravascular coagulation, *J Trauma Acute Care Surg* 72:1719, 2012.
7. Furie B, Furie BC: Mechanisms of thrombus formation, *N Engl J Med* 359:938, 2008.
8. Shantsila E, et al: Heparin-induced thrombocytopenia. A contemporary clinical approach to diagnosis and management, *Chest* 135:1651, 2009.
9. Marques MB: Thrombotic thrombocytopenic purpura and heparin-induced thrombocytopenia: two unique causes of life-threatening thrombocytopenia, *Clin Lab Med* 29:321, 2009.
10. Warkentin TE: Heparin-induced thrombocytopenia, *Hematol Oncol Clin North Am* 21:589, 2007.
11. Selleng K, et al: Heparin-induced thrombocytopenia in intensive care patients, *Crit Care Med* 35:1165, 2007.
12. Donavan JL, et al: An overview of heparin-induced thrombocytopenia, *J Pharm Pract* 23:226, 2010.
13. Linkins LA, et al: Treatment and prevention of heparin-induced thrombocytopenia: Antithrombotic Therapy and Prevention of Thrombosis, 9th ed.: American College of Chest Physicians Evidence-Based Clinical Practice Guidelines, *Chest* 141(2 Suppl):e495S, 2012.
14. De D: Acute nursing care and management of patients with sickle cell, *Br J Nurs* 17:818, 2012.
15. Pack-Mabien A, Haynes J Jr: A primary care provider's guide to preventive and acute care management of adults and children with sickle cell disease, *J Am Acad Nurse Pract* 21:250, 2009.
16. Porter B, et al: Hematologic and immune problems. In Dunphy L, et al, editors: *Primary care: the art and science of advanced practice nursing*, ed 3, Philadelphia, 2011, FA Davis.
17. Addis G: Sickle cell disease, part 1: Understanding the condition, *Br J Nurs* 5:231, 2010.
18. Brown M: Managing the acutely ill adult with sickle cell disease, *Br J Nurs* 21:90, 2012.
19. Robison J: Metabolic emergencies: tumor lysis syndrome. In Newton S, et al, editors: *Oncology nursing advisor: a comprehensive guide to clinical practice*, St. Louis, 2009, Mosby.
20. Tosi P, et al: Consensus conferences on the management of tumor lysis syndrome, *Haemtologica* 93:1877, 2008.
21. Behl D, et al: Oncologic emergencies, *Crit Care Clin* 26:181, 2010.
22. Shelton BK: Tumor lysis syndrome. In Chernecky CC, Murphy-Ende K, editors: *Acute care oncology*, ed 2, St. Louis, 2009, Mosby.
23. Abu-Alfa AK, Younes A: Tumor lysis syndrome and acute kidney injury: evaluation, prevention and management, *Am J Kidney Dis* 55(5 Suppl 3):S1, 2010.
24. Myers JS: Complications of cancer and cancer treatment. In Langhorne ME, et al, editors: *Oncology nursing*, ed 5, St. Louis, 2007, Mosby.

A APPENDIX

Nursing Management Plans of Care

ACTIVITY INTOLERANCE

Definition: Insufficient physiologic or psychologic energy to endure or complete required or desired daily activities.

Activity Intolerance Related to Cardiopulmonary Dysfunction

Defining Characteristics

- Chest pain with activity
- Electrocardiographic changes with activity
- Heart rate is >15 beats/min above baseline with activity for patients on beta-blockers or calcium channel blockers.
- Heart rate remains elevated above baseline 5 minutes after activity.
- Breathlessness with activity
- SpO_2 <92% with activity
- Postural hypotension when moving from supine to upright position
- Patient reports fatigue with activity.

Outcome Criteria

- Heart rate is <20 beats/min above baseline with activity and is <10 beats/min above baseline with activity for patients on beta-blockers or calcium channel blockers.
- Heart rate returns to baseline 5 minutes after activity.
- Chest pain with activity is absent.
- Patient reports tolerance to activity.

Nursing Interventions and Rationale

1. Encourage active or passive range-of-motion exercises while the patient is in bed ***to keep joints flexible and muscles stretched.***
2. Teach patient to refrain from holding breath while performing exercises and ***to avoid the Valsalva maneuver.***
3. Encourage performance of muscle-toning exercises at least three times daily, ***because a toned muscle uses less oxygen when performing work than an untoned muscle.***
4. Progress ambulation ***to increase tolerance to activity.***
5. Teach patient to take pulse ***to determine activity tolerance:*** Take pulse for a full minute before exercise and then for 10 seconds and multiply by 6 at exercise peak.
6. Consult with physician regarding the administration of fluids to ensure that the patient is hydrated to 24-hour fluid requirements per body surface area (BSA) ***to increase preload and thereby increase stroke volume and cardiac output.***

Activity Intolerance Related to Prolonged Immobility or Deconditioning

Defining Characteristics

- Decrease in systolic blood pressure is >20 mm Hg.
- Increase in heart rate is >20 beats/min with postural change.
- Syncope with postural change
- Patient reports lightheadedness with postural change.

Outcome Criteria

- Decrease in systolic blood pressure is <10 mm Hg.
- Increase in heart rate is <10 beats/min with postural change.
- Syncope or lightheadedness is absent with postural change.
- Absence of hypoxemia
- Patient reports tolerance to activity.

Nursing Interventions and Rationale

1. Collaborate with physician regarding patient's activity level and the need for physical therapy ***to ensure patient's safety.***
2. Collaborate with physical therapist to develop progressive activity plan for patient ***to return to prior level of function.***

For Patient on Bed Rest

1. Instruct the patient how to perform straight-leg raises, dorsiflexion or plantar flexion, and quadriceps-setting and gluteal-setting exercises ***to increase muscular and vascular tone.***
2. Reposition patient incrementally ***to avoid syncope:***
   a. Head of bed to 45 degrees and hold until symptom free
   b. Head of bed to 90 degrees and hold until symptom free
   c. Dangle until symptom free
   d. Stand until symptom free and ambulate

For Patient on Ventilator

1. Collaborate with physician, respiratory care practitioner, and physical therapist regarding patient's eligibility for early progressive mobility ***to ensure patient is ready and able to participate***.
2. Initiate early progressive mobility program when patient is ready ***to limit the effects of prolonged immobility.***
   a. Elevation of the head of the bed
   b. Turn patient every 2 hours.

ACTIVITY INTOLERANCE—cont'd

c. Perform passive range of motion at least 3 times/day.
d. Progress patient to active range of motion when ready.
e. Place bed in chair position to position patient in upright/leg-down position.
f. Initiate bed mobility activities such as sitting on the edge of the bed (dangling).
g. Initiate transfer training.
h. Implement pre-gait activities such as standing at the side of the bed and marching in place.
i. Progress patient to ambulation.

3. Monitor patient's response to activity and discontinue activity if patient shows signs of intolerance ***to ensure patient safety:***
   a. Hypoxemia
   b. Hypotension
   c. Dysrhythmias or electrocardiographic changes

ACUTE CONFUSION

Definition: Abrupt onset of reversible disturbances of consciousness, attention, cognition, and perception that develop over a short period of time.

Acute Confusion Related to Sensory Overload, Sensory Deprivation, and Sleep Pattern Disturbance

Defining Characteristics

Early Symptoms

- Sudden onset of global cognitive function impairment (hours to days)
- Restlessness, agitation, and combative behavior
- Drowsiness (can lead to loss of consciousness)
- Slurring of speech, inappropriate statements or "word salad," mumbling, or inappropriate gestures
- Short attention span (needs questions repeated); inability to learn new material
- Disordered sleep/wake cycle
- Disorientation to person, time, place, and situation
- Difficulty in separating dreams from reality (may experience bizarre dreams or nightmares)
- Anger at staff for continued questions about his or her orientation

Later Symptoms

- Symptoms that tend to fluctuate throughout the day and night
- Continuations of early symptoms, which may be more frequent or of longer duration
- Illusions
- Hallucinations
- Extreme agitation (e.g., attempts to climb out of bed, pull out catheters, rip off dressings)
- Calling out in loud voice, swearing, or attempting to bite or hit people who approach patient

Nursing Interventions and Rationale

1. Determine and document the patient's dominant spoken language, his or her literacy, and the languages in which he or she is literate. ***Sometimes, people are not literate in their spoken language, or, less commonly, they are literate only in their second language.***
2. Determine and document patient's premorbid degree of orientation, cognitive capabilities, and any sensory/perceptual deficits.

For Sensory Overload

1. Initiate each nurse/patient encounter by calling the patient by name and identifying yourself by name. ***This fosters reality orientation and assists the patient in filtering irrelevant or impersonal conversation.***
2. Assess the patient's immediate physical environment from his or her viewpoint and explain equipment, its sounds, and its therapeutic purpose. Demonstrate audible and visual alarms and explain possible alarm conditions. ***This decreases alienation of the patient from the technologic environment and reduces the inherent sense of fear and urgency accompanying alarm conditions.***
3. Provide preparatory sensory information by explaining procedures in relation to the sensations the patient will experience, including duration of sensations. ***Preparatory sensory information enhances learning and lessens anticipatory anxiety.***
4. Limit noise levels. ***Audible alarms cannot and must not be silenced, and many critical but noisy activities must take place in the critical care area. It has been shown, however, that noise levels produced by clinical personnel exceed those levels designated as acceptable and are often greater than those generated by technologic devices.***
   a. Keep staff conversations soft enough that they are inaudible to the patient whenever possible.
   b. Assume that everything said at or around a patient's bedside is intended for that patient's awareness and that it will be interpreted as pertaining to him or her. ***As in the discussion that follows, conversations about the patient but not to him or her foster depersonalization and delusions of reference.***
   c. Enforce nighttime noise limits.
5. Readjust alarm limits on physiologic monitoring devices as the patient's condition changes (improves or deteriorates) ***to lessen unnecessary alarm states.***
6. Consider use of headphones and digital music player with patient's favorite and/or subliminal or classical music. ***This can effectively filter out assaultive noise of the critical care environment and supplant it with familiar, soothing sounds and rhythms.***
7. Modify lighting. ***Day and night cycles need to be simulated with environmental lighting.***
   a. Never turn on overhead fluorescent lights abruptly without warning the patient, assisting him or her out of

Continued

ACUTE CONFUSION—cont'd

the supine position, and/or shielding his or her eyes with gauze or a face cloth. ***Continuous bright lighting sustains anxiety and promotes circadian rhythm desynchronization.***

8. Shield patients from viewing urgent and emergent events in the critical care unit. ***Resuscitation efforts, albeit difficult to conceal, engender fear in the patient and a sense of instability and vulnerability (e.g., "I'm next").***
   a. When such an event occurs, elicit the patient's cognitive and emotional reaction; ***thoughts, impressions, and feelings need to be shared and misconceptions clarified.***
9. Ensure patients' privacy, modesty, and dignity. ***Physical exposure and nudity, although they seemingly pale in importance compared with priorities such as physiologic assessment and stabilization, are primal indignities for all individuals.***
   a. Keep the patient minimally exposed. When it becomes necessary to expose the patient, verbally apologize for this necessity. ***To be naked is to feel vulnerable; to be vulnerable is to feel fearful.***

For Sensory Deprivation

1. Provide reality orientation in four spheres (personal, place, time, and situation) at more frequent intervals than when testing.
   a. Convey this information in the context of routine conversation. *Sample statements*: "Mr. Clark, this is Tuesday morning, and you're in University Hospital. Your heart surgery was yesterday morning, and you're doing well. My name is Joe, and I'm your nurse today." ***The patient is made to feel patronized by repetitions, such as "Do you know where you are?" Given the effects of general anesthesia, opioid analgesics, sedatives, and sleep, it is expected that some degree of disorientation will exist normally.***
2. Ensure the patient's visual access to a calendar.
3. Apprise the patient of daily news events and the weather.
4. Touch patients for the express purpose of communicating caring. Hold their hands, stroke their brows, and rub the skin on an aspect of the arms. ***Touch is the universal language of caring. In the setting of critical care, in which there is considerable physical body manipulation, it is useful and important to contrast assaultive touch with comforting touch. Touch can be used as a technique for distraction from painful stimuli when used in conjunction with uncomfortable procedures.*** *(NOTE: See later discussion of the use of touch in management of the patient experiencing hallucinations.)*
5. Foster liberal visitation by family and significant others. Encourage significant others to touch the patient as consistent with their individual comfort level and cultural norms.
6. Structure and identify opportunities for the patient to exercise decision-making skills, however small. ***Although not so designated, patients with sensory alterations also experience a type of cognitive deprivation.***
7. Assist patients to find meaning in their experiences. ***Patients need to find meaning and to identify their roles in the experience of critical illness and critical care.***
   a. Explain the therapeutic purpose of all they are asked to do for themselves and all that is done with them and for them.
   b. Avoid statements such as "Will you turn to that side for me?" or "I need you to swallow this medication." ***These statements implicitly convey that the maneuver has some value for the nurses instead of the patients.***
   c. Similarly, use "thank you" judiciously. ***This simple salutation, when used indiscriminately, suggests something was done to benefit the nurses, not the patients.***

For Hallucinations

1. Approach the patient with a calm, matter-of-fact demeanor. ***The goal of this interaction is for the nurse to demonstrate external control. This helps decrease the anxiety and fear that generally accompany hallucinations and allows the patient to feel safe. Anxiety is transferable.***
2. Address the patient by name. ***This is a useful presentation of reality because self-identity is the last sphere of orientation to vanish.***
3. In responding to the patient's description of the hallucination, do not deny, argue, or attempt to disprove the existence of the perceived event. Statements such as "There are no voices coming from that air vent" or "Look, I'm brushing my hand across the wall, and there are no bugs" confuse the patient further, ***because the hallucination, although frightening, is his or her perceived reality.***
4. Express to the patient that your experiences are dissimilar and acknowledge how frightening his or hers must be. *Sample statements*: "I don't hear (see, etc.) what you do, but I know how frightening such an experience must be to you. I'm Joe, your nurse, and I'm going to stay with you until the voices (visions, etc.) go away." ***Validating the patient's feelings demonstrates acceptance and sensitivity to the experience and promotes trust.***
5. Remain with any patient who is experiencing a hallucination. ***Feelings of fear and anxiety often accelerate when a patient is left alone. He or she needs someone to represent a nonthreatening reality.***
6. Do not explore the content of the hallucination with the patient by asking about its nature or character. ***The nurse is the patient's link with reality. Pursuit of a detailed description of a hallucination may signify to the patient that the nurse accepts his or her sensory distortion as factual. This may further confuse the patient and distance him or her more from reality.***
   a. Ascertain that the voices are not telling the patient to harm himself or herself, by asking simply and concretely, "What are the voices saying?" ***The nurse can help bridge the gap between the patient's misperception and reality by addressing the feelings (e.g., fear, anxiety) and/or meanings (e.g., danger, death) engendered by the hallucination.***
   b. Determine how the misperception affects the patient emotionally, acknowledge those feelings, and use a calm, controlled, matter-of-fact approach to provide the trust and comfort the patient needs to tolerate this

ACUTE CONFUSION—cont'd

frightening experience. ***In other words, the nurse should deal with the intent more than the content of the hallucination. The resultant decrease in anxiety will enable the patient to focus more accurately on his or her immediate environment.***

7. Talk concretely with the patient about things that are really happening. *Sample statements*: "How does your chest incision feel this afternoon, Mr. Clark?" "Your sister Kate was here to see you, but you were sleeping. She went down to the cafeteria and will be back." "Your secretions are a little easier for you to cough up today." ***Interpretation of reality-based stimuli by the nurse encourages the patient to focus on actual circumstances and discourages a preoccupation with sensory misperceptions.***
8. Distract the patient by changing the topic. ***This tactic is useful in situations of escalating anxiety and confusion or when all else fails. Topics need to consist of basic themes that are universally understood and culturally congruent, such as music, food, or weather or topics of special interest to the patient, such as hobbies, crafts, or sports.***
   a. Avoid topics that evoke strong emotions, such as politics, religion, or sexuality. ***This is especially true of the patient with reality distortions; sometimes, hallucinations and delusions are expressions of repressed conflicts associated with religious, sexual, or aggressive issues. Pursuit of such subjects could increase confusion and anxiety.***
9. Avoid the use of touch as an intervention strategy for any patient who demonstrates escalating anxiety or paranoid, suspicious, or mistrustful thoughts. ***While touch can be useful in the management of patients with sensory alterations, for patients experiencing hallucinations (as well as delusions and illusions), touch can be readily misinterpreted as aggression or pain, and it can actually provide the basis for a tactile illusion.***
10. For auditory hallucinations:
    a. *Patient behaviors*: Head cocked as if listening to an unseen presence; lips moving.
    b. *Therapeutic nurse responses*: "Mr. Clark, you appear to be listening to something." If the patient acknowledges voices: "I don't hear any voices, but I know this is troubling you. The voices will go away. Nothing is going to harm you. I'm Joe, your nurse, and I'll be here with you."
    c. *Nontherapeutic nurse responses*: "Tell me about your conversations with these voices." "To whom do these voices belong—anyone you know?"
11. For visual hallucinations:
    a. *Patient behaviors*: Staring into space as if focused on an unseen object; startled movements and anxious facial expression.
    b. *Therapeutic nurse responses*: "Mr. Clark, something seems to be troubling you. Tell me what it is." If patient states he visualizes people, images, or the devil in his environment and implies a sense of danger, respond, "There are only nurses and doctors here, Mr. Clark. I know this must be upsetting, but these images will go away. We're here with you in the hospital. Nothing will happen to you."
    c. *Nontherapeutic nurse responses*: "Describe the people you see. What are they wearing?" "What does the devil mean in your life? What about God?"

For Delusions

1. Explain all unseen noises, voices, and activity simply and clearly. ***They readily feed a delusional system.*** *Sample statements*: "That is Dr. Smith. He's come to see you and other patients here in the hospital." "The voices and activity you hear are from the bedside of the patient behind this curtain. He's being helped by one of the nurses."
2. Avoid the "negative challenge" of the patient's delusions (e.g., "Nobody here stole your belongings" or "Doctors and nurses do not harm people"). Similarly, avoid defending the referents of the patient's belief: "Nurses are good" and "Doctors mean well." ***A delusion is a belief, albeit false, that cannot be changed with logic. To attempt this change is to challenge the patient's belief system and thereby escalate his or her anxiety, further blurring the boundaries between reality and the patient's internally based "logic."***
3. For the patient with persecutory delusions who refuses food, fluids, or medications because of a belief that he or she has been poisoned or the medications are tainted, permit the refusal unless it is a life-threatening event. Try again in 20 minutes; allow the patient to choose an alternative selection of food or to read the label on the unit's medication. ***Coercion, show of force, or engagement in complicated, logical justifications will only heighten the patient's suspiciousness and possibly reinforce the delusional belief. When the patient feels more in control, he or she need not rely on the "paradoxical" quality of the delusion to equip him or her with a false sense of power. His or her power instead is derived from making reality-based decisions.***
4. Staff members should be particularly careful not to engage in unnecessary laughter or whispering within view of the delusional patient. ***The delusional patient is hypervigilant, scanning the environment for evidence to corroborate or confirm his or her belief that staff members are colluding against him or her; laughter and whispers easily suggest this belief, this delusion of reference. This rationale also pertains to the patient experiencing hallucinations and/or illusions.***
5. Observe the principles detailed in the third intervention in the *For Hallucinations* section.

For Illusions

1. Interpret a reality-based stimulus for the patient in a calm, matter-of-fact manner. ***Seen and unseen noises, voices, activity, and people can provide the stimulus for a sensory misinterpretation, an illusion.***
2. Minimize stimulation in the patient's immediate environment. *Nursing interventions detailed previously under "Sensory Overload" are especially relevant here.*

Continued

ACUTE CONFUSION—cont'd

3. Address the feeling and meaning associated with the experience, not the content of the sensory misinterpretation.
   a. *Patient behaviors*: Eyes darting, startled movements, frightened facial expression. "I know who you are. You're the devil come to take me to hell."
   b. *Therapeutic nurse responses*: "I'm Joe, your nurse. I know this experience is troubling for you. You're in the hospital, and no one here will harm you."
   c. Nontherapeutic nurse responses: "There are no such things as devils and angels." "Do you think the devil would be dressed in white?" ***The first nontherapeutic nurse response carries a parental tone (i.e., "You know better than that"), infantilizing the patient and adding to his or her feelings of powerlessness over the environment. The second nontherapeutic response reflects obvious logic, which is not in the patient's sensory domain; it cannot be processed and only adds to his or her confused state.***
4. Observe the principles detailed in the fifth intervention of the *For Hallucinations* section.

ACUTE PAIN

Definition: Unpleasant sensory and emotional experience arising from actual or potential tissue damage or described in terms of such damage (International Association for the Study of Pain); sudden or slow onset of any intensity from mild to severe with an anticipated or predictable end and a duration of less than 6 months.

Acute Pain Related to Transmission and Perception of Cutaneous, Visceral, Muscular, or Ischemic Impulses

Defining Characteristics

Subjective
- Patient verbalizes presence of pain.
- Patient rates pain on a scale of 1 to 10 using a visual analog scale.

Objective
- Increase in blood pressure, heart rate, and respiratory rate
- Pupillary dilation
- Diaphoresis, pallor
- Skeletal muscle reactions (e.g., grimacing, clenching fists, writhing, pacing, guarding or splinting of affected part)
- Apprehension, fearful appearance
- May not exhibit any physiologic change

Outcome Criteria
- Patient verbalizes that pain is reduced to a tolerable level or is totally relieved.
- Patient's pain rating is lower on a scale of 1 to 10.
- Blood pressure, heart rate, and respiratory rate return to baseline 5 minutes after administration of an intravenous opioid analgesic or 20 minutes after administration of intramuscular opioid analgesic.

Nursing Interventions and Rationale
1. Modify variables that heighten the patient's experience of pain.
   a. Explain to the patient that frequent, detailed, and seemingly repetitive assessments will be conducted to allow the nurse better to understand the patient's pain experience, not because the existence of pain is in question.
   b. Explain the factors responsible for pain production in the individual. Estimate the expected duration of the pain, if possible.
   c. Explain diagnostic and therapeutic procedures to the patient in relation to sensations the patient should expect to feel.
   d. Reduce the patient's fear of addiction by explaining the difference between drug tolerance and drug dependence. ***Drug tolerance is a physiologic phenomenon in which a medication begins to lose effectiveness after repeated doses; drug dependence is a psychologic phenomenon in which opioids are used regularly for emotional, not medical, reasons.***
   e. Instruct the patient to ask for pain medication when pain is beginning and not to wait until it is intolerable.
   f. Explain that the physician will be consulted if pain relief is inadequate with the present medication.
   g. Instruct the patient in the importance of adequate rest, especially when it reduces pain ***to maintain strength and coping abilities and to reduce stress.***
2. Collaborate with the physician regarding pharmacologic interventions.
   - **For postoperative or posttraumatic cutaneous, muscular, or visceral pain,** perform the following:
     a. Medicate with an opioid analgesic to break the pain cycles as long as level of consciousness and vital signs are stable.
     b. Check patient's previous response to similar dosage and opioids.
     c. Establish optimal analgesic dose that brings optimal pain relief.
     d. Offer pain medication at prescribed regular intervals rather than making patient ask for it ***to maintain more steady blood levels.***
     e. Consider waking patient to avoid loss of opiate blood levels during sleep.
     f. If administering medication on as-necessary (PRN) basis, give it when the patient's pain is just beginning rather than at its peak.
        (1) Advise the patient to intercept pain, not endure it, or several hours and higher doses of opioid analgesics may be necessary to relieve pain, leading to a cycle of undermedication and pain alternating with overmedication and drug toxicity.

ACUTE PAIN—cont'd

g. Perform rehabilitation exercises (turn, deep breathe, leg exercises, ambulate) shortly before peak of drug effect ***because this will be the optimal time for the patient to increase activity with the least risk of increasing pain.***
h. When making the transition from one drug to another or from intravenous to oral medication, use an equianalgesic chart. ***Equianalgesic means approximately the same pain relief. The patient's response should be closely monitored to determine if the right analgesic choice was made.***
i. To assess effectiveness of pain medication, do the following:
   (1) Reevaluate pain 15 to 30 minutes after intravenous and 30 to 60 minutes after oral medication administration, observe the patient's behavior, and ask the patient to rate pain on a scale of 1 to 10.
   (2) Collaborate with the physician to add or delete other medications that potentiate the action of analgesics, such as antiemetics, hypnotics, sedatives, or muscle relaxants.
   (3) Observe for indicators of undertreatment: report of pain not relieved; observed restlessness, sleeplessness, irritability, and anorexia; decreased activity level.
j. Evaluate the patient's level of sedation and respiratory rate at regular intervals ***to avoid oversedation***.
   (1) Respirations should be counted for a full minute and qualified according to rhythm and depth of chest excursion.
   (2) Consider the use of capnography (end-tidal CO_2 monitoring) ***as an early indicator of hypoventilation and oversedation.***
k. If patient-controlled analgesia (PCA) is used, perform the following:
   (1) Instruct the patient on what the drug is, the dose, and how often it can be self-administered by pushing the button to activate the PCA machine. For example, "When you have pain, instead of asking the nurse to bring medication, push the button that activates the machine, and a small dose of the pain medicine will be injected into your IV line. You can keep your pain under control by administering additional medicine as soon as your pain begins to return or increases. Push the button before undertaking a painful activity, such as ambulation. Try to balance your pain relief against sleepiness and don't activate the machine if you start to feel sleepy. If your pain medicine seems to stop working despite pushing the button several times, call the nurse to check your IV. If you are not receiving adequate pain relief, the nurse will call your doctor."
   (2) Monitor vital signs, especially blood pressure and respiratory rate, every hour for the first 4 hours and assess postural heart rate and blood pressure before initial ambulation.
   (3) Monitor respiratory rate every 2 hours while patient is on patient-controlled analgesia.
   (4) If patient's respiratory rate decreases to <10/min or if patient is overly sedated, anticipate administration of naloxone.
l. If epidural opioid analgesia is used, do the following:
   (1) Keep patient's head elevated 30 to 45 degrees after injection ***to prevent respiratory depressant effects.***
   (2) Observe closely for respiratory depression up to 24 hours after injection. Monitor respiratory rate every 15 minutes for 1 hour, every 30 minutes for 7 hours, and every hour for the remaining 16 hours.
   (3) Assess for adequate cough reflex.
   (4) Avoid use of other central nervous system depressants, such as sedatives.
   (5) Observe for reports of pruritus, nausea, and vomiting.
   (6) Anticipate administration of naloxone for respiratory depression (and smaller doses of naloxone for pruritus).
   (7) Assess for and treat urinary retention.
   (8) Assess epidural catheter site for local infection. Keep the catheter taped securely ***to prevent catheter migration.***

- For peripheral vascular ischemic pain (hypothetic vascular occlusion of leg), do the following:
   a. Correctly identify and differentiate ischemic pain from other types of pain. ***(NOTE: Ischemic pain is usually a burning, aching pain made worse by exercise and lessened or relieved by rest. Eventually, the pain occurs at rest. Coldness and pallor of extremity may be noted, especially if the limb is elevated above the heart level. Rubor and mottling of the skin may be evident from prolonged tissue anoxia and inability of damaged vessels to constrict. Eventually, cyanosis and gangrenous tissue will be evident. Chronic ischemia leads to visible changes in the limb, such as flaking skin, brittle nails and hair, leg ulcers, and cellulitis.)***
   b. Administer pain medications and evaluate their effectiveness as previously described. ***Remember that the pain of ischemia is chronic and continuous and can make the patient irritable and depressed.***
   c. Treat the cause of the ischemic pain and institute measures ***to increase circulation to the affected part.***

3. Initiate nonpharmacologic interventions.
   a. Treat contributing factors; b. Apply comfort measures.
      (1) Use relaxation techniques, such as back rubs, massage, warm baths, music, and aromatherapy.
         (a) Use blankets and pillows to support the painful part and reduce muscle tension.
         (b) Encourage slow, rhythmic breathing.
      (2) Encourage progressive muscle relaxation techniques.
         (a) Instruct patient to inhale and tense (tighten) specific muscle groups and then relax the muscles as exhalation occurs.

Continued

ACUTE PAIN—cont'd

(b) Suggest an order for performing the tension and relaxation cycle (e.g., start with facial muscles and move down body, ending with toes).

(3) Encourage guided imagery.

(a) Ask patient to recall an experienced image that is very pleasurable and relaxing and involves at least two senses.

(b) Have patient begin with rhythmic breathing and progressive relaxation and then travel mentally to the scene.

(c) Have patient slowly experience the scene (e.g., how it looks, sounds, smells, feels).

(d) Ask patient to practice this imagery in private.

(e) Instruct patient to end the imagery by counting to three and saying, "Now I'm relaxed." If the person does not end the imagery and falls asleep, the purpose of the technique is defeated.

ANXIETY

Definition: Vague uneasy feeling of discomfort or dread accompanied by an autonomic response (the source often nonspecific or unknown to the individual); a feeling of apprehension caused by anticipation of danger. It is an alerting signal that warns of impending danger and enables the individual to take measures to deal with threat.

Anxiety Related to Threat to Biologic, Psychologic, or Social Integrity

Defining Characteristics

Subjective

- Verbalizes increased muscle tension
- Expresses frequent sensation of tingling in hands and feet
- Relates continuous feeling of apprehension
- Expresses preoccupation with a sense of impending doom
- Reports difficulty falling asleep
- Repeatedly expresses concerns about changes in health status and outcome of illness

Objective

- Psychomotor agitation (fidgeting, jitteriness, restlessness)
- Tightened, wrinkled brow
- Strained (worried) facial expression
- Hypervigilance (scans environment)
- Startles easily
- Distractibility
- Sweaty palms
- Fragmented sleep patterns
- Tachycardia
- Tachypnea

Outcome Criteria

- Patient effectively uses learned relaxation strategies.
- Patient demonstrates significant decrease in psychomotor agitation.
- Patient verbalizes reduction in tingling sensations in hands and feet.
- Patient is able to focus on the tasks at hand.
- Patient expresses positive, future-based plans to family and staff.
- Patient's heart rate and rhythm remain within limits commensurate with physiologic status.

Nursing Interventions and Rationale

1. Instruct the patient in the following simple, effective relaxation strategies:
   a. If not contraindicated for cardiovascular reasons, tense and relax all muscles progressively from toes to head. ***Progressive toe-to-head relaxation releases the muscular tension that may be a stress-related effect resulting from the threat or change in the patient's health status and outcome of illness.***
   b. Perform slow deep-breathing exercises. ***Deep-breathing exercises provide slow, rhythmic, controlled breathing patterns that relax the patient and distract him or her from the effects of his or her illness and hospitalization.***
   c. Focus on a single object or person in the environment. ***Focusing on a single object or person helps the patient dismiss myriad disorienting stimuli from his or her visual-perceptual field, which can have a dizzying, distorted effect. A clear sensorium allows him or her to feel more in control of his or her environment.***
   d. Listen to soothing music or relaxation tapes with eyes closed. ***Music or words expressed in soft, low tones tend to produce soothing, relaxing effects that counteract or inhibit escalating anxiety and provide respites from the patient's situational crisis. Closed eyes eliminate distracting visual stimuli and promote a more restful environment.***
2. Actively listen to and accept the patient's concerns regarding the threats from his or her illness, outcome, and hospitalization. ***Active listening and unconditional acceptance validate the patient as a worthwhile individual and assure him or her that his or her concerns, no matter how great, will be addressed. Knowledge that he or she has an avenue for ventilation will assuage anxiety.***
3. Help the patient distinguish between realistic concerns and exaggerated fears through clear, simple explanations. *Sample statements*: "Your lab results show that you're doing okay right now." "The shortness of breath you're experiencing is not unusual." "The pain you described is expected, and this medication will relieve it." ***A patient who is informed about his or her progress and is reassured about expected symptoms and management***

ANXIETY—cont'd

of care will be better equipped to maintain a more realistic perspective of his or her illness and its outcome. Anxiety emanating from imagined or exaggerated fears will likely be assuaged or averted.

4. Provide simple clarification of environmental events and stimuli that are not related to the patient's illness and care. *Sample statements*: "That loud noise is coming from a machine that is helping another patient." "The visitor behind the curtain is crying because she's had an upsetting day." "That gurney is here to take another patient to x-ray." ***Clarification of events and stimuli that are unrelated to the patient helps to disengage him or her from the extant anxiety-provoking situations surrounding him or her, avoiding further anxiety and apprehension.***
5. Assist the patient in focusing on building on prior coping strategies to deal with the effects of his or her illness and care. *Sample statements*: "What methods have helped you get through difficult times in the past?" "How can we help you use those methods now?" (See the nursing management plan for Ineffective Coping for interventions that assist patients to use coping strategies effectively.) ***Use of previously successful coping strategies in conjunction with newly learned techniques arms the patient with an arsenal of weapons against anxiety, providing him or her with greater control over the situational crisis and decreased feelings of doom and despair.***
6. Give the patient permission to deny or suppress the effects of his or her illness and hospitalization with which he or she cannot cope or control. *Sample statements*: "It's perfectly okay to ignore things you can't handle right now." "How can we help ease your mind during this time?" "What are some things or tasks that may help distract you?" ***Adaptive denial can be helpful in reducing feelings of anxiety in patients with life-threatening illness.***

AUTONOMIC DYSREFLEXIA

Definition: Life-threatening, uninhibited sympathetic response of the nervous system to a noxious stimulus after a spinal cord injury at T7 or above.

Autonomic Dysreflexia Related to Excessive Autonomic Response to Noxious Stimuli

Defining Characteristics

- Paroxysmal hypertension (sudden increase in both systolic and diastolic blood pressure >20 mm Hg above patient's normal blood pressure); for many spinal cord injury patients, a normal blood pressure may be only 90/60 mm Hg.
- Pounding headache
- Bradycardia (may be a relative slowing so the heart rate may still appear within the normal range)
- Profuse sweating (above the level of the injury) especially in the face, neck, and shoulders
- Pilomotor erection (goose bumps) above the level of the injury
- Cardiac dysrhythmias (atrial fibrillation, premature ventricular contractions, and atrioventricular conduction abnormalities)
- Flushing of the skin (above the level of the injury) especially in the face, neck, and shoulders
- Blurred vision
- Appearance of spots in the visual fields
- Nasal congestion
- Feelings of apprehension or anxiety

Outcome Criteria

- Blood pressure returns to patient's baseline level.
- Heart rate and rhythm return to patient's baseline level.
- Absence of headache
- Absence of sweating, flushing, and piloerection above level of injury
- Absence of visual disturbances and nasal congestion
- Absence of feelings of apprehension or anxiety

Nursing Interventions and Rationale

1. Place the patient on cardiac monitor and assess for bradycardia or other dysrhythmias. ***Disturbances of cardiac rate and rhythm can occur because of autonomic dysfunction associated with dysreflexia.***
2. Check the patient's blood pressure every 3 to 5 minutes ***as blood pressure may fluctuate very quickly.***
3. Sit the patient upright and lower the legs if possible ***to decrease venous return and blood pressure.***
4. Loosen any clothing or constrictive devices ***to decrease venous return and blood pressure.***
5. Investigate for and remove instigating cause of dysreflexia:
   a. Bladder
      (1) If indwelling catheter not in place, catheterize patient immediately.
         (a) Prior to inserting the catheter, instill 2% lidocaine jelly into the urethra and wait 2 minutes, if possible.
         (b) Drain 500 mL of urine and recheck BP.
         (c) If BP is still elevated, drain another 500 mL of urine.
         (d) If BP declines after the bladder is empty, serial BP must be monitored closely because the bladder can go into severe contractions causing hypertension to recur.
      (2) If indwelling catheter is in place, check the catheter and tubing for kinks, folds, constrictions, or obstructions and for correct placement. If problem is found, correct it immediately.
      (3) If catheter is plugged, irrigate it gently with no more than 10-15 mL of sterile normal saline solution at body temperature.
      (4) If unable to irrigate catheter, remove it and prepare to reinsert a new catheter: proceed with its lubrication, drainage, and observation as outlined above.

Continued

AUTONOMIC DYSREFLEXIA—cont'd

(5) Avoid manually compressing or tapping on the bladder.

b. Bowel: if systolic blood pressure is >150 mm Hg, proceed to no. 6 prior to checking for a fecal impaction.
   (1) With a gloved hand, instill a topical anesthetic agent (2% lidocaine jelly), generously into the rectum ***to decrease flow of impulses from bowel.***
   (2) Wait 2 minutes if possible ***for sensation in area to decrease.***
   (3) With a gloved hand, insert a lubricated finger into the rectum and check for the presence of stool.
   (4) If stool is felt, gently remove, if possible.

c. Skin
   (1) Loosen clothing or bed linens as indicated.
   (2) Inspect skin for pimples, boils, pressure ulcers, and ingrown toenails and treat as indicated.

6. If symptoms of dysreflexia do not subside, collaborate with physician regarding the administration of antihypertensive medications (e.g., nifedipine [immediate-release form], nitrates [sodium nitroprusside, isosorbide dinitrate, or nitroglycerin ointment], hydralazine, mecamylamine, diazoxide, phenoxybenzamine, captopril, prazosin).
   a. Administer medications and monitor their effectiveness.
   b. Assess blood pressure and heart rate.
7. Instruct patient about causes, symptoms, treatment, and prevention of dysreflexia.
8. Encourage patient to carry medical bracelet or informational card to present to medical personnel in the event dysreflexia may be developing.

COMPROMISED FAMILY COPING

Definition: Usually, supportive primary person (family member or close friend) provides insufficient, ineffective, or compromised support, comfort, assistance, or encouragement that may be needed by the patient to manage or master adaptive tasks related to his or her health challenge.

Compromised Family Coping Related to Critically Ill Family Member

Defining Characteristics

- Disruption of usual family functions and roles
- Inability to accept or deal with crisis situation; use of defense mechanisms (e.g., denial, anger); unrealistic expectations of patient's outcome and care provided; judgmental toward health care providers
- Nonrecognition that family is in state of crisis
- Inappropriate emotional outbursts; arguments among family and with others; inability to respond to each other's feelings or support each other
- Misinterpretation of information; short attention span with repeated questions about information already provided; members not sharing information with each other
- Inability to make decisions regarding changes in family structure or about course of care for ill member; noncooperation among family members
- Expressions of grief, hopelessness, powerlessness, and isolation; do not seek or respond to support services
- Hesitancy to spend time with ill person in the critical care unit or inappropriate behavior when visiting (may upset patient)
- Neglect of own personal health; fatigue, apathy; refusal of offers for respite time

Outcome Criteria

- The family will express an understanding of course/prognosis of illness, therapies, and alternative measures.
- The family will diminish or resolve conflicts and cooperate in decision making.
- The family will develop trust and mutual support for each member and form a cohesive unit.
- The family will support ill person in making decisions (if capable) or respect prior wishes regarding provision of health care.
- Family efforts will be directed toward a purpose and readjust to changes in life patterns and role function. Members will accept responsibility for changes.
- The family will identify and use effective coping strategies.
- The family will identify and use available resources as needed to facilitate resolution of the crisis.
- The family will have a sense of control and confidence in meeting personal and collective needs.

Nursing Interventions and Rationale

1. Identify family's perception of the crisis situation. ***All initial nursing interventions should be directed toward resolving the crisis situation. Understanding and using family theory principles will facilitate this process and individualize care.***
   a. Determine family structure, roles' developmental phase, and ethnic, cultural, and belief factors that may affect communication with family and the plan of care.
   b. Identify strengths of the family.
2. Provide honest and accurate information in language persons can understand. Give updated information as appropriate. Listen! ***This facilitates open communication among family and health care providers, projects a caring attitude and concern for them and patient, and assists family in making decisions and being involved with the plan and goals of care.***
3. Encourage liberal visitation with patient.
   a. Before the visit, prepare family members for what they will observe in a technical environment. ***This prevents a strong emotional reaction to an unfamiliar and frightening situation.***
      (1) Inform them about patient's appearance, behaviors (etc.) that may be distressing to them.

COMPROMISED FAMILY COPING—cont'd

(2) Explain the etiology of patient responses to stimuli (e.g., pain, trauma, surgery, medication) and explain that these behaviors are being monitored and are usually temporary.

b. Encourage them to touch the patient and let the patient know of their presence.

4. Identify and support effective coping behaviors. ***This aids in the family's sense of control and resolution of helplessness/powerlessness.***
5. Observe for signs of fatigue and the need for emotional/spiritual support and respite from hospital waiting routine. ***This provides support and comfort, facilitates hope, resolves sense of isolation, gives sense of security, and diminishes guilt feeling for attending to personal needs.***
   a. Encourage family to verbalize feelings.
   b. Provide information on available resources.
   c. Alert interdisciplinary team members (social, psychologic, spiritual) to family needs.
   d. Provide pager device (if available) or obtain phone numbers when family leaves the hospital premises.
6. Instruct family in simple caregiving techniques and encourage participation in patient's care. ***This facilitates giving a sense of normalcy to the experience, self-confidence, and assurance that good care is being provided.***
7. Serve as advocate for patient and family. Teach family how to negotiate with the health care delivery system and include them in health care team conferences when appropriate. ***This facilitates informed decision making, promotes control and satisfaction, and permits mutual goal-setting.***
8. Consider nonbiologic or nonlegal family relationships. Encourage contact with patient and participation in care. ***This facilitates holistic care and support of emotional ties and demonstrates respect for the family unit and relationships.***
9. Provide emotional support and compassion when patient's condition worsens or deteriorates. ***The use of touch and expression of concern for the patient and family convey comfort and trust in the health care provider and respect and assurance that the family's loved one will receive appropriate care and attention.***

DECREASED CARDIAC OUTPUT

Definition: Inadequate blood pumped by the heart to meet the metabolic demands of the body.

Decreased Cardiac Output Related to Alterations in Preload

Defining Characteristics

- Cardiac output is <4.0 L/min.
- Cardiac index is <2.5 L/min/m^2.
- Heart rate is >100 beats/min.
- Urine output is <30 mL/hr or 0.5 mL/kg/hr.
- Decreased mentation, restlessness, agitation, confusion
- Diminished peripheral pulses
- Blue, gray, or dark purple tint to tongue and sublingual area
- Systolic blood pressure is <90 mm Hg.
- Subjective complaints of fatigue

Reduced Preload

- Right atrial pressure is <2 mm Hg.
- Pulmonary artery occlusion pressure is <6 mm Hg.

Excessive Preload

- Right atrial pressure is >8 mm Hg.
- Pulmonary artery occlusion pressure is >12 mm Hg.

Outcome Criteria

- Cardiac output is 4-8 L/min.
- Cardiac index is 2.5-4 L/min/m^2.
- Right atrial pressure is 2-8 mm Hg.
- Pulmonary artery occlusion pressure is 6-12 mg Hg.

Nursing Interventions and Rationale

1. Collaborate with physician regarding the administration of oxygen to maintain an SpO_2 >92% ***to prevent tissue hypoxia.***
2. Maintain surveillance for signs of decreased tissue perfusion and acidosis ***to facilitate the early identification and treatment of complications.***
3. Monitor fluid balance and daily weights to facilitate regulation of the patient's fluid balance.

For Reduced Preload Resulting from Volume Loss

1. Collaborate with physician regarding the administration of crystalloids, colloids, blood, and blood products ***to increase circulating volume.***
2. Limit blood sampling, observe intravenous lines for accidental disconnection, apply direct pressure to bleeding sites, and maintain normal body temperature ***to minimize fluid loss.***
3. Position patient with legs elevated, trunk flat, and head and shoulders above the chest ***to enhance venous return.***
4. Encourage oral fluids (as appropriate), administer free water with tube feedings, and replace fluids that are lost through wound or tube drainage ***to promote adequate fluid intake.***
5. Maintain surveillance for signs of fluid volume excess and adverse effects of blood and blood product administration ***to facilitate the early identification and treatment of complications.***

For Reduced Preload Resulting from Venous Dilation

1. Collaborate with physician regarding the administration of vasoconstrictors ***to increase venous return.***

Continued

DECREASED CARDIAC OUTPUT—cont'd

2. Maintain surveillance for adverse effects of vasoconstrictor therapy ***to facilitate the early identification and treatment of complications.***
3. If patient is hyperthermic, administer tepid bath, hypothermia blanket, and/or ice bags to axilla and groin ***to decrease temperature and promote vasoconstriction.***

For Excessive Preload Resulting from Volume Overload

1. Collaborate with physician regarding the administration of the following:
   a. Diuretics to remove excessive fluid
   b. Vasodilators to decrease venous return
   c. Inotropes to increase myocardial contractility
2. Restrict fluid intake and double concentrate intravenous drips ***to minimize fluid intake.***
3. Position patient in semi-Fowler's or high-Fowler's position ***to reduce venous return.***
4. Maintain surveillance for signs of fluid volume deficit and adverse effects of diuretic, vasodilator, and inotropic therapies ***to facilitate the early identification and treatment of complications.***

For Excessive Preload Resulting from Venous Constriction

1. Collaborate with physician regarding the administration of vasodilators ***to promote venous dilation.***
2. Maintain surveillance for adverse effects of vasodilator therapy ***to facilitate the early identification and treatment of complications.***
3. If patient is hypothermic, wrap him or her in warm blankets or administer hyperthermia blanket ***to increase temperature and promote vasodilation.***

Decreased Cardiac Output Related to Alterations in Afterload

Defining Characteristics

- Cardiac output is <4 L/min.
- Cardiac index is <2.5 L/min/m^2.
- Heart rate is >100 beats/min.
- Urine output is <30 mL/hr.
- Decreased mentation, restlessness, agitation, confusion
- Diminished peripheral pulses
- Blue, gray, or dark purple tint to tongue and sublingual area
- Systolic blood pressure is <90 mm Hg.
- Subjective complaints of fatigue

Reduced Afterload

- Pulmonary vascular resistance is <100 dyn·sec·cm^{-5}.
- Systemic vascular resistance is <800 dyn·sec·cm^{-5}.

Excessive Afterload

- Pulmonary vascular resistance is >250 dyn·sec·cm^{-5}.
- Systemic vascular resistance is >1200 dyn·sec·cm^{-5}.

Outcome Criteria

- Cardiac output is 4-8 L/min.
- Cardiac index is 2.5-4 L/min/m^2.
- Pulmonary vascular resistance is 80-250 dyn·sec·cm^{-5}.
- Systemic vascular resistance is 800-1200 dyn·sec·cm^{-5}.

Nursing Interventions and Rationale

1. Collaborate with physician regarding the administration of oxygen to maintain an SpO_2 >92% ***to prevent tissue hypoxia.***
2. Maintain surveillance for signs of decreased tissue perfusion and acidosis ***to facilitate the early identification and treatment of complications.***

For Reduced Afterload

1. Collaborate with physician regarding the administration of vasoconstrictors ***to promote arterial vasoconstriction and prevent relative hypovolemia.*** If decreased preload is present, implement nursing management plan for Decreased Cardiac Output Related to Alterations in Preload.
2. Maintain surveillance for adverse effects of vasoconstrictor therapy ***to facilitate the early identification and treatment of complications.***
3. If patient is hyperthermic, administer tepid bath, hypothermia blanket, and/or ice bags to axilla and groin ***to decrease temperature and promote vasoconstriction.***

For Excessive Afterload

1. Collaborate with physician regarding the administration of vasodilators ***to promote arterial vasodilation.***
2. Collaborate with physician regarding initiation of intraaortic balloon pump ***to facilitate afterload reduction.***
3. Promote rest and relaxation and decrease environmental stimulation ***to minimize sympathetic stimulation.***
4. Maintain surveillance for adverse effects of vasodilator therapy ***to facilitate the early identification and treatment of complications.***
5. If patient is hypothermic, wrap patient in warm blankets or administer hyperthermia blanket ***to increase temperature and promote vasodilation.***
6. If patient is in pain, treat pain ***to reduce sympathetic stimulation.*** Implement nursing management plan for Acute Pain Related to Transmission and Perception of Cutaneous, Visceral, Muscular, or Ischemic Impulses.

Decreased Cardiac Output Related to Alterations in Contractility

Defining Characteristics

- Cardiac output is <4 L/min.
- Cardiac index is <2.5 L/min/m^2.
- Heart rate is >100 beats/min.
- Urine output is <30 mL/hr.
- Decreased mentation, restlessness, agitation, confusion
- Diminished peripheral pulses
- Blue, gray, or dark purple tint to tongue and sublingual area
- Systolic blood pressure is <90 mm Hg.
- Subjective complaints of fatigue
- Right ventricular stroke work index is <7 g/m^2/beat.
- Left ventricular stroke work index is <35 g/m^2/beat.

DECREASED CARDIAC OUTPUT—cont'd

Outcome Criteria
- Cardiac output is 4-8 L/min.
- Cardiac index is 2.5-4 L/min/m^2.
- Right ventricular stroke work index is 7-12 g/m^2/beat.
- Left ventricular stroke work index is 35-85 g/m^2/beat.

Nursing Interventions and Rationale
1. Collaborate with physician regarding the administration of oxygen to maintain an SpO_2 >92% ***to prevent tissue hypoxia.***
2. Maintain surveillance for signs of decreased tissue perfusion and acidosis ***to facilitate the early identification and treatment of complications.***
3. Ensure preload is optimized. If preload is reduced or excessive, implement nursing management plan for Decreased Cardiac Output Related to Alterations in Preload.
4. Ensure afterload is optimized. If afterload is reduced or excessive, implement nursing management plan for Decreased Cardiac Output Related to Alterations in Afterload.
5. Ensure electrolytes are optimized. Collaborate with physician regarding the administration of electrolyte replacement therapy ***to enhance cellular ionic environment.***
6. Collaborate with physician regarding the administration of inotropes ***to enhance myocardial contractility.***
7. Monitor ST segment continuously ***to determine changes in myocardial tissue perfusion.*** If myocardial ischemia is present, implement nursing management plan for Ineffective Cardiopulmonary Tissue Perfusion.

Decreased Cardiac Output Related to Alterations in Heart Rate or Rhythm

Defining Characteristics
- Cardiac output is <4 L/min.
- Cardiac index is <2.5 L/min/m^2.
- Heart rate is >100 beats/min or <60 beats/min.
- Urine output is <30 mL/hr or 0.5 mL/kg/hr.
- Decreased mentation, restlessness, agitation, confusion
- Diminished peripheral pulses
- Blue, gray, or dark purple tint to tongue and sublingual area
- Systolic blood pressure is <90 mm Hg.
- Subjective complaints of fatigue
- Dysrhythmias

Outcome Criteria
- Cardiac output is 4-8 L/min.
- Cardiac index is 2.5-4 L/min/m^2.
- Absence of dysrhythmias or return to baseline
- Heart rate is >60 beats/min or <100 beats/min.

Nursing Interventions and Rationale
1. Collaborate with physician regarding the administration of oxygen to maintain an SpO_2 >92% ***to prevent tissue hypoxia.***
2. Ensure electrolytes are optimized. Collaborate with physician regarding the administration of electrolyte therapy ***to enhance cellular ionic environment and avoid precipitation of dysrhythmias.***
3. Collaborate with physician and pharmacist regarding patient's current medications and their effect on heart rate and rhythm ***to identify any prodysrhythmic or bradycardic side effects.***
4. Maintain surveillance for signs of decreased tissue perfusion and acidosis ***to facilitate the early identification and treatment of complications.***
5. Monitor ST segment continuously ***to determine changes in myocardial tissue perfusion.*** If myocardial ischemia is present, implement nursing management plan for Altered Cardiopulmonary Tissue Perfusion.

For Lethal Dysrhythmias or Asystole
1. Initiate Advanced Cardiac Life Support interventions and notify physician immediately.

For Nonlethal Dysrhythmias
1. Collaborate with physician regarding administration of antidysrhythmic therapy, synchronized cardioversion, and/or overdrive pacing ***to control dysrhythmias.***
2. Maintain surveillance for adverse effects of antidysrhythmic therapy ***to facilitate the early identification and treatment of complications.***

For Heart Rate <60 Beats/Min
1. Collaborate with physician regarding the initiation of temporary pacing ***to increase heart rate.***

Decreased Cardiac Output Related to Sympathetic Blockade

Defining Characteristics
- Decreased cardiac output and cardiac index
- Systolic blood pressure is <90 mm Hg or below patient's baseline.
- Decreased right atrial pressure and pulmonary artery occlusion pressure
- Decreased systemic vascular resistance
- Bradycardia
- Cardiac dysrhythmias
- Postural hypotension

Outcome Criteria
- Cardiac output and cardiac index are within normal limits.
- Systolic blood pressure is >90 mm Hg or returns to baseline.
- Right atrial pressure and pulmonary artery occlusion pressure are within normal limits.
- Systemic vascular resistance is within normal limits.
- Sinus rhythm is present.
- Dysrhythmias are absent.
- Fainting or dizziness with position change is absent.

Continued

DECREASED CARDIAC OUTPUT—cont'd

Nursing Interventions and Rationale

1. Implement measures to prevent episodes of postural hypertension:
   a. Change patient's position slowly ***to allow the cardiovascular system time to compensate.***
   b. Apply pneumatic compression stockings ***to promote venous return.***
   c. Perform range-of-motion exercises every 2 hours ***to prevent venous pooling.***
   d. Collaborate with the physician and physical therapist regarding the use of a tilt table ***to progress the patient from supine to upright position.***
2. Collaborate with the physician regarding the administration of the following:
   a. Crystalloids and/or colloids to increase the patient's circulating volume, ***which increases stroke volume and subsequently cardiac output***
   b. Vasopressors if fluids are ineffective to constrict the patient's vascular system, ***which increases resistance and subsequently blood pressure***
3. Monitor cardiac rhythm for bradycardia and/or dysrhythmias, ***which can further decrease cardiac output.***
4. Avoid any activity that can stimulate the vagal response ***because bradycardia can result.***
5. Treat symptomatic bradycardia and symptomatic dysrhythmias according to unit's emergency protocol or advanced cardiac life support (ACLS) guidelines.

DECREASED INTRACRANIAL ADAPTIVE CAPACITY

Definition: Intracranial fluid dynamic mechanisms that normally compensate for increases in intracranial volumes are compromised, resulting in repeated disproportionate increases in intracranial pressure (ICP) in response to a variety of noxious and non-noxious stimuli.

Decreased Intracranial Adaptive Capacity Related to Failure of Normal Intracranial Compensatory Mechanisms

Defining Characteristics

- Intracranial pressure is >15 mm Hg, sustained for 15-30 minutes.
- Headache
- Vomiting, with or without nausea
- Seizures
- Decrease in Glasgow Coma Scale score of 2 or more points from baseline
- Alteration in level of consciousness, ranging from restlessness to coma
- Change in orientation: disoriented to time and/or place and/or person
- Difficulty or inability to follow simple commands
- Increasing systolic blood pressure of more than 20 mm Hg with widening pulse pressure
- Bradycardia
- Irregular respiratory pattern (e.g., Cheyne-Stokes, central neurogenic hyperventilation, ataxic, apneustic)
- Change in response to painful stimuli (e.g., purposeful to inappropriate or absent response)
- Signs of impending brain herniation:
  - Hemiparesis or hemiplegia
  - Hemisensory changes
  - Unequal pupil size (1 mm or more difference)
  - Failure of pupil to react to light
  - Disconjugate gaze and inability to move one eye beyond midline if third, fourth, or sixth cranial nerves involved
  - Loss of oculocephalic or oculovestibular reflexes
  - Possible decorticate or decerebrate posturing

Outcome Criteria

- Intracranial pressure is <15 mm Hg.
- Cerebral perfusion pressure is >60 mm Hg.
- Clinical signs of increased intracranial pressure are absent.

Nursing Interventions and Rationale

1. Maintain adequate cerebral perfusion pressure.
   a. Collaborate with physician regarding the administration of volume expanders, vasopressors, or antihypertensives ***to maintain the patient's blood pressure within normal range.***
   b. Implement measures to reduce intracranial pressure.
      (1) Elevate head of bed 30-45 degrees ***to facilitate venous return.***
      (2) Maintain head and neck in neutral plane (avoid flexion, extension, or lateral rotation) ***to enhance venous drainage from the head.***
      (3) Avoid extreme hip flexion.
      (4) Collaborate with the physician regarding the administration of steroids, osmotic agents, and diuretics and need for drainage of cerebrospinal fluid if a ventriculostomy is in place.
      (5) Assist patient to turn and move self in bed (instruct patient to exhale while turning or pushing up in bed) ***to avoid isometric contractions and Valsalva maneuver.***
2. Maintain patent airway and adequate ventilation and supply oxygen ***to prevent hypoxemia and hypercarbia.***
3. Monitor arterial blood gas values and maintain PaO_2 >80 mm Hg, $PaCO_2$ >35 mm Hg, and pH at 7.35-7.45 ***to prevent cerebral vasodilation.***
4. Avoid suctioning beyond 10 seconds at a time; hyperoxygenate and hyperventilate before and after suctioning ***to avoid hypoxemia.***
5. Plan patient care activities and nursing interventions around patient's intracranial pressure response. Avoid unnecessary additional disturbances and allow patient up to 1 hour of rest between activities as frequently as

DECREASED INTRACRANIAL ADAPTIVE CAPACITY—cont'd

possible. ***Studies have shown the direct correlation between nursing care activities and increases in intracranial pressure.***

6. Maintain normothermia with external cooling or heating measures as necessary. Wrap hands, feet, and male genitalia in soft towels before cooling measures ***to prevent shivering and frostbite.***
7. With physician's collaboration, control seizures with prophylactic and PRN anticonvulsants. ***Seizures can greatly increase the cerebral metabolic rate.***
8. Collaborate with the physician regarding the administration of sedatives, barbiturates, or paralyzing agents ***to reduce cerebral metabolic rate.***
9. Counsel family members to maintain calm atmosphere and avoid disturbing topics of conversation (e.g., patient condition, pain, prognosis, family crisis, financial difficulties).
10. If signs of impending brain herniation are present, implement the following:
    a. Notify the physician at once.
    b. Ensure that head of bed is elevated 45 degrees and that patient's head is in neutral plane.
    c. Administer mainline intravenous infusion slowly to keep-open rate.
    d. Drain cerebrospinal fluid as ordered if a ventriculostomy is in place.
    e. Prepare to administer osmotic agents and/or diuretics.
    f. Prepare patient for emergency computed tomography head scan and/or emergency surgery.

DEFICIENT FLUID VOLUME

Definition: Decreased intravascular, interstitial, and/or intracellular fluid. This refers to dehydration, water loss alone without a change in sodium concentration.

Deficient Fluid Volume Related to Absolute Loss

Defining Characteristics

- Cardiac output is <4 L/min.
- Cardiac index is <2.2 L/min.
- Pulmonary artery occlusion pressure is <6 mm Hg.
- Right atrial pressure is <2 mm Hg.
- Tachycardia
- Narrowed pulse pressure
- Systolic blood pressure is <100 mm Hg.
- Urinary output is <30 mL/hr.
- Pale, cool, moist skin
- Apprehensiveness

Outcome Criteria

- Cardiac output is >4 L/min, and cardiac index is >2.2 L/min.
- Pulmonary artery occlusion pressure is >6 mm Hg or returns to baseline level.
- Right atrial pressure is >2 mm Hg or returns to baseline level.
- Heart rate is normal or returns to baseline level.
- Systolic blood pressure is >90 mm Hg.
- Urinary output is >30 mL/hr.

Nursing Interventions and Rationale

1. Secure airway and administer oxygen to maintain SpO_2 >92%.
2. Place patient in supine position with legs elevated ***to increase preload.*** For patient with head injury, consider using low-Fowler's position with legs elevated.
3. For fluid repletion, use the 3:1 rule, replacing three parts of fluid for every unit of blood lost.
4. Administer crystalloid solutions using the fluid challenge technique: infuse precise boluses of fluid (usually 5-20 mL/min) over 10-minute periods; monitor hemodynamic pressures serially ***to determine successful challenging.*** If the pulmonary artery occlusion pressure elevates more than 7 mm Hg above beginning level, the infusion should be stopped. If the pulmonary artery occlusion pressure rises only to 3 mm Hg above baseline or falls, another fluid challenge should be administered.
5. Replete fluids first before considering use of vasopressors ***because vasopressors increase myocardial oxygen consumption out of proportion to the reestablishment of coronary perfusion in the early phases of treatment.***
6. When blood replacement is indicated, replace it with fresh packed red cells and fresh frozen plasma ***to keep clotting factors intact.***
7. Move or reposition patient minimally to decrease or limit tissue oxygen demands.
8. Evaluate patient's anxiety level and intervene through patient education or sedation ***to decrease tissue oxygen demands.***
9. Maintain surveillance for signs and symptoms of fluid overload.

Deficient Fluid Volume Related to Decreased Secretion of Antidiuretic Hormone (ADH)

Defining Characteristics

- Confusion and lethargy
- Decreased skin turgor
- Thirst
- Weight loss over short period
- Decreased pulmonary artery occlusion pressure
- Decreased right atrial pressure
- Urinary output is >6 L/day.
- Serum sodium is >148 mEq/L.
- Serum osmolality is >295 mOsm/kg.
- Urine osmolality is <100 mOsm/kg.
- Urine specific gravity is <1.005.

Continued

DEFICIENT FLUID VOLUME—cont'd

Outcome Criteria

- Weight returns to baseline.
- Urinary output is >30 mL/hr and <200 mL/hr.
- Serum osmolality is 280-295 mOsm/kg.
- Urine specific gravity is 1.010-1.030.

Nursing Interventions and Rationale

1. Record intake and output every hour, noting color and clarity of urine ***because color and clarity are an indication of urine concentration.***
2. Monitor cardiac rhythm continuously for dysrhythmias ***caused by electrolyte imbalance.***
3. Collaborate with physician regarding administration of vasopressin or desmopressin ***to replace ADH.***
   a. Monitor patient for adverse effects of medications (e.g., headache, chest pain, abdominal pain) ***caused by vasoconstriction.***
   b. Report adverse effects to physician immediately.
4. Collaborate with physician regarding intravenous fluid and electrolyte replacement therapy ***to restore fluid balance, correct dehydration, and maintain electrolyte balance.***
   a. Administer hypotonic saline ***to replace free water deficit.***
5. Provide oral fluids low in sodium, such as water, coffee, tea, or orange juice, ***to decrease sodium intake.***
6. Weigh patient daily at same time, in same amount of clothing, and preferably with same scale ***to ensure accuracy of readings.***
7. Reposition patient every 2 hours to prevent skin integrity issues caused by dehydration.
8. Provide mouth care every 4 hours to prevent breakdown of oral mucous membranes.
9. Collaborate with physician regarding administration of medications to prevent constipation ***caused by dehydration.***
10. Maintain surveillance for symptoms of hypernatremia (muscle twitching, irritability, seizures), hypovolemic shock (hypotension, tachycardia, decreased CVP and PAOP), and deep vein thrombosis (calf pain, tenderness, swelling).

Deficient Fluid Volume Related to Relative Loss

Defining Characteristics

- Pulmonary artery occlusion pressure is <6 mm Hg.
- Right atrial pressure is <2 mm Hg.
- Tachycardia
- Narrowed pulse pressure
- Systolic blood pressure is <100 mm Hg.
- Urinary output is <30 mL/hr.
- Increased hematocrit level

Outcome Criteria

- Pulmonary artery occlusion pressure is >6 mm Hg or returns to baseline level.
- Right atrial pressure is >2 mm Hg or returns to baseline level.
- Systolic blood pressure is >90 mm Hg.
- Urinary output is >30 mL/hr.
- Hematocrit level is normal.

Nursing Interventions and Rationale

1. Collaborate with the physician regarding the administration of intravenous fluid replacements (usually normal saline solution or lactated Ringer solution) at a rate sufficient to maintain urinary output >30 mL/hr. Colloid solutions are avoided in the initial phases (but can be used later) because of the possibility of increased edema formation ***as a result of the increased capillary permeability.***

DEFICIENT KNOWLEDGE

Definition: Absence or deficiency of cognitive information related to a specific topic.

Deficient Knowledge Related to Cognitive or Perceptual Learning Limitations

Defining Characteristics

- Verbalized statement of inadequate knowledge of skills
- Verbalization of inadequate recall of information
- Verbalization of inadequate understanding of information
- Evidence of inaccurate follow-through of instructions
- Inadequate demonstration of a skill
- Lack of compliance with prescribed behavior

Outcome Criteria

- Patient participates actively in necessary and prescribed health behaviors.
- Patient verbalizes adequate knowledge or demonstrates adequate skills.

Nursing Interventions and Rationale

1. Determine specific cause of patient's cognitive or perceptual limitation.
2. Provide uninterrupted rest period before teaching session to decrease fatigue and encourage optimal state for learning and retention.
3. Manipulate environment as much as possible to provide quiet and uninterrupted learning sessions.
   a. Ensure that lights are bright enough to see teaching aids but not too bright.
   b. Schedule care and medications to allow uninterrupted teaching periods.

DEFICIENT KNOWLEDGE—cont'd

   c. Move patient to quiet, private room for teaching, if possible.
4. Adapt teaching sessions and materials to patient's and family's levels of education and ability to understand.
   a. Provide printed material appropriate to reading level.
   b. Use terminology understood by the patient.
   c. Provide printed materials in patient's primary language, if possible.
   d. Use interpreters during teaching sessions *when necessary*.
5. Teach only present-tense focus during periods of sensory overload.
6. Determine potential effects of medications on ability to retain or recall information. Avoid teaching critical content while patient is taking sedatives, analgesics, or other medications that affect memory.
7. Reinforce new skills and information in several teaching sessions. Use several senses when possible in teaching session (e.g., see a film, hear a discussion, read printed information, demonstrate skills related to self-injection of insulin).
8. Reduce patient's anxiety.
   a. Listen attentively and encourage verbalization of feelings.
   b. Answer questions as they arise in a clear and succinct manner.
   c. Elicit patient's concerns and address those issues first.
   d. Give only correct and relevant information.
   e. Continually assess response to teaching session and discontinue if anxiety increases or physical condition becomes unstable.
   f. Provide nonthreatening information before more anxiety-producing information is presented.
   g. Plan for several teaching sessions so information can be divided into small, manageable packages.

Deficient Knowledge Related to Lack of Previous Exposure to Information

Defining Characteristics
- Verbalized statement of inadequate knowledge or skills
- New diagnosis or health problem requiring self-management or care
- Lack of prior formal or informal education about the specific health problem
- Demonstration of inappropriate behaviors related to management of health problem

Outcome Criteria
- Patient verbalizes adequate knowledge about or performs skills related to disease process, its causes, factors related to onset of symptoms, and self-management of disease or health problem.
- Patient actively participates in health behaviors required for performance of a procedure or in those behaviors enhancing recovery from illness and preventing recurrence or complications.

Nursing Interventions and Rationale
1. Determine existing level of knowledge or skill.
2. Assess factors that affect the knowledge deficit:
   a. Learning needs, including patient's priorities and the necessary knowledge and skills for safety
   b. Learning ability of patient, including language skills, level of education, ability to read, preferred learning style
   c. Physical ability to perform prescribed skills or procedures; consider effect of limitations imposed by treatment such as bed rest, restriction of movement by intravenous or other equipment, or effect of sedatives or analgesics.
   d. Psychologic effect of stage of adaptation to disease
   e. Activity tolerance and ability to concentrate
   f. Motivation to learn new skills or gain new knowledge
3. Reduce or limit barriers to learning:
   a. Provide consistent nurse–patient contact to encourage development of trusting and therapeutic relationship.
   b. Structure environment to enhance learning and control unnecessary noise or interruptions.
   c. Individualize teaching plan to fit patient's current physical and psychologic status.
   d. Delay teaching until patient is ready to learn.
   e. Conduct teaching sessions during period of day when patient is most alert and receptive.
   f. Meet patient's immediate learning needs as they arise (e.g., give brief explanation of procedures when they are performed).
4. Promote active participation in the teaching plan by the patient and family:
   a. Solicit input during development of plan.
   b. Develop mutually acceptable goals and outcomes.
   c. Solicit expression of feelings and emotions related to new responsibilities.
   d. Encourage questions.
5. Conduct teaching sessions, using the most appropriate teaching methods.
6. Use the "teach-back" method ***to confirm that you have explained to the patient what they need to know in a manner that the patient understands.***
   a. Use simple lay language; explain the concept or demonstrate the process to the patient/caregiver.
      (1) Avoid technical terms to avoid misunderstandings.
      (2) If the patient/caregiver has limited English proficiency, use a professional translator to reduce miscommunication.
   b. Ask the patient/caregiver to repeat in his or her own words how he or she understands the concept explained. If a process was demonstrated to the patient, ask the patient/caregiver to demonstrate it independent of assistance.
   c. Identify and correct misunderstandings of or incorrect procedures by the patient/caregiver.
   d. Ask the patient/caregiver to demonstrate his or her understanding or procedural ability again ***to ensure the above-noted misunderstandings are now corrected.***
   e. Repeat steps until convinced the patient/caregiver comprehends the concept or possesses the ability to perform the procedure accurately and safely.

Continued

DEFICIENT KNOWLEDGE—cont'd

7. Provide written materials that enhance health literacy:
   a. Limit content to one or two key objectives. Don't provide too much information or try to cover everything at once.
   b. Limit content to what patients really need to know. Avoid information overload.
   c. Use only words that are well known to individuals without medical training.
   d. Make certain content is appropriate for age and culture of the target audience.
   e. Write at or below the 6th-grade level.
   f. Use one- or two-syllable words.
   g. Use short paragraphs.
   h. Use active voice.
   i. Avoid all but the most simple tables and graphs. Clear explanations (legends) should be placed adjacent to the table or graph and also in the text.
   j. Use large font (minimum 12 point) with serifs. (Serif text has the little horizontal lines that you see at the bottoms of letters like f, x, n, and others.)
   k. Don't use more than two or three font styles on a page. ***Consistency in appearance is important.***
   l. Use upper- and lower-case text. ALL UPPER-CASE TEXT IS HARD TO READ.
   m. Ensure a good amount of empty space on the page. Don't clutter the page with text or pictures.
   n. Use headings and subheadings to separate blocks of text.
   o. Bulleted lists are preferable to blocks of text in paragraphs.
   p. Illustrations are useful if they depict common, easy-to-recognize objects. Images of people, places, and things should be age-appropriate and culturally appropriate to the target audience. Avoid complex anatomical diagrams.
8. Initiate referrals for follow-up if necessary:
   a. Health educators
   b. Home health care
   c. Rehabilitation programs
   d. Social services
9. Evaluate effectiveness of teaching plan, based on patient's ability to meet preset goals and objectives ***to determine need for further teaching.***

DISTURBED BODY IMAGE

Definition: Confusion in mental picture of one's physical self.

Disturbed Body Image Related to Actual Change in Body Structure, Function, or Appearance

Defining Characteristics
- Actual change in appearance, structure, or function
- Avoidance of looking at body part
- Avoidance of touching body part
- Hiding or overexposing body part (intentional or unintentional)
- Trauma to nonfunctioning part
- Change in ability to estimate spatial relationship of body to environment
- Verbalization of the following:
  - Fear of rejection or reaction by others
  - Negative feeling about body
  - Preoccupation with change or loss
  - Refusal to participate in or to accept responsibility for self-care of altered body part
- Personalization of part or loss with a name
- Depersonalization of part or loss by use of impersonal pronouns
- Refusal to verify actual change

Outcome Criteria
- Patient verbalizes the specific meaning of the change to him or her.
- Patient requests appropriate information about self-care.
- Patient completes personal hygiene and grooming daily with or without help.
- Patient interacts freely with family or other visitors.
- Patient participates in the discussions and conferences related to planning his or her medical and nursing management in the critical care unit and transfer from the unit.
- Patient talks with trained visitors (support-group representatives) at least twice about his or her loss.

Nursing Interventions and Rationale
1. Evaluate patient's mental, physical, and emotional state; recognize assets, strengths, response to illness, coping mechanisms, past experience with stress, and support system.
2. Appraise the response of family and significant others. ***Body image is derived from the "reflected appraisals" of family and significant others.***
3. Determine the patient's goals and readiness for learning.
4. Provide the necessary information to help the patient and family adapt to the change. Clarify misconceptions about future limitations.
5. Permit and encourage the patient to express the significance of the loss or change; note nonverbal behavior responses.
6. Allow and encourage the patient's expression of anxiety. ***Anxiety is the most predominant emotional response to a body image disturbance.***
7. Recognize and accept the use of denial as an adaptive defense mechanism when used early and temporarily.
8. Recognize maladaptive denial as that which interferes with the patient's progress and/or alienates support systems. Use confrontation.

DISTURBED BODY IMAGE—cont'd

9. Provide an opportunity for the patient to discuss sexual concerns.
10. Touch the affected body part ***to provide the patient with sensory information about altered body structure and/or function.***
11. Encourage and provide movement of altered body part ***to establish kinesthetic feedback. This enables the person to know his or her body as it now exists.***
12. Prepare the patient to look at the body part. Call the body part by its anatomic name (e.g., stump, stoma, limb) as opposed to "it" or "she." ***The use of impersonal pronouns increases a sense of fantasy and depersonalization of the body part.***
13. Allow the patient to experience excellence in some aspect of physical functioning—walking, turning, deep breathing, healing, self-care—and point out progress and accomplishment. ***This helps to balance the patient's sense of dysfunction with function.***
14. Avoid false reassurance. Acknowledge the difficulty of incorporating the altered body part or function into one's body image. ***This evidences the nurse's sensitivity and promotes trust.***
15. Talk with the patient about his or her life, generativity, and accomplishments. ***Patients with disturbances in body image frequently see themselves in a distortedly "narrow" sense. Encouraging a wider focus of themselves and their life reduces this distortion.***
16. Help the patient explore realistic alternatives.
17. Recognize that incorporating a body change into one's body image takes time. Avoid setting unrealistic expectations and ***thereby inadvertently reinforcing a low self-esteem.***
18. Suggest the use of additional resources such as trained visitors who have mastered situations similar to those of the patient.
    a. Refer the patient to a psychiatric nurse, psychologist, or psychiatrist if needed.

Disturbed Body Image Related to Functional Dependence on Life-Sustaining Technology

Defining Characteristics
- Actual change in function requiring permanent or temporary replacement
- Refusal to verify actual loss
- Verbalization of the following: feelings of helplessness, hopelessness, powerlessness, fear of failure to wean from technology

Outcome Criteria
- Patient verifies actual change in function.
- Patient does not refuse or fight technologic intervention.
- Patient verbalizes acceptance of expected change in lifestyle.

Nursing Interventions and Rationale
1. Evaluate patient's response to the technologic intervention.
2. Assess responses of family and significant others. ***Body image is derived from the "reflected appraisals" of family and significant others.***
3. Provide information needed by patient and family.
4. Promote trust, security, comfort, and privacy.
5. Recognize anxiety. Allow and encourage its expression. ***Anxiety is the most predominant emotion accompanying body image alterations.*** Implement nursing management plan for Anxiety Related to Threat to Biologic, Psychologic, or Social Integrity.
6. Assist patient to recognize his or her own functioning and performance in the face of technology. For example, assist patient to distinguish spontaneous breaths from mechanically delivered breaths. ***The activity will assist in weaning patient from the ventilator when feasible. To establish realistic, accurate body boundaries, a patient needs help to separate himself or herself from the technology that is supporting his or her functioning. Any participation or function on the part of the patient during periods of dependency is helpful in preventing and/or resolving an alteration in body image.***
7. Plan for discontinuation of the treatment (e.g., weaning from ventilator). Explain procedure that will be followed and be present during its initiation.
8. Plan for transfer from the critical care environment.
9. Document care, ensuring an up-to-date management plan is available to all involved caregivers.

DISTURBED SLEEP PATTERN

Definition: Time-limited disruption of sleep amount and quality due to external factors.

Disturbed Sleep Pattern Related to Fragmented Sleep

Defining Characteristics
- Decreased sleep during one block of sleep time
- Daytime sleepiness
- Decreased sleep
    - Less than one-half of normal total sleep time
    - Decreased slow-wave or rapid-eye-movement (REM) sleep
- Anxiety
- Fatigue
- Restlessness
- Disorientation and hallucinations
- Combativeness
- Frequent awakenings

Outcome Criteria
- Patient's total sleep time approximates patient's normal.
- Patient can complete sleep cycles of 90 minutes without interruption.

Continued

DISTURBED SLEEP PATTERN—cont'd

- Patient has no delusions or hallucinations.
- Patient has reality-based thought content.

Nursing Interventions and Rationale

1. Assess normal sleep pattern on admission and any history of sleep disturbance or chronic illness that may affect sleep or sedative/hypnotic use.
   a. Promote normal sleep activity while patient is in critical care unit.
   b. Assess sleep effectiveness by asking patient how his or her sleep in the hospital compares with sleep at home.
2. Promote comfort, relaxation, and a sense of well-being.
   a. Treat pain; change, smooth, or refresh bed linens at bedtime, and provide oral hygiene.
   b. Eliminate stressful situations before bedtime.
   c. Use relaxation techniques, imagery, music, massage, or warm blankets.
   d. Have a close family member sit beside the bed and provide the patient with his or her own garments or coverings.
   e. Provide quiet or background noise of the television or music (patient preference) ***to best promote sleep.***
   f. Provide a comfortable room temperature.
3. Minimize noise, particularly that of the staff and noisy equipment.
   a. Reduce the level of environmental stimuli.
   b. Dim the lights at night.
4. Foods containing tryptophan (e.g., milk, turkey) may be appropriate ***because these promote sleep.***
5. Plan nap times to assist in approximating the patient's normal 24-hour sleep time.
6. Minimize awakenings ***to allow for at least 90-minute sleep cycles.***
   a. Continually assess the need to awaken the patient, particularly at night. Distinguish between essential and nonessential nursing tasks.
   b. Organize nursing management to allow for maximal amount of uninterrupted sleep while ensuring close monitoring of the patient's condition. Whenever possible, monitor physiologic parameters without waking the patient.
   c. Coordinate awakenings with other departments, such as laboratory and radiography, ***to minimize sleep interruptions.***
7. Be aware of the effects of commonly used medications on sleep. ***Many sedative and hypnotic medications decrease REM sleep.***
   a. Use sedative and analgesic medications that minimally disrupt sleep to complement comfort measures, with dosages reduced gradually as the medication is no longer necessary.
   b. Do not abruptly withdraw REM-suppressing medications ***because this can result in REM rebound.***
8. Document amount of uninterrupted sleep per shift, especially sleep episodes lasting longer than 2 hours. ***Sleep pattern disturbance is diagnosed, treated, and resolved more efficiently when formally documented in this manner.***

DYSFUNCTIONAL VENTILATORY WEANING RESPONSE

Definition: Inability to adjust to lowered levels of mechanical ventilator support that interrupts and prolongs the weaning process.

Dysfunctional Ventilatory Weaning Response (DVWR) Related to Physical, Psychosocial, or Situational Factors

Defining Characteristics

Mild DVWR

- Responds to lowered levels of mechanical ventilator support with:
  - Restlessness
  - Slightly increased respiratory rate from baseline
  - Expressed feelings of increased need for oxygen, breathing discomfort, fatigue, warmth
  - Queries about possible machine malfunction
  - Increased concentration on breathing

Moderate DVWR

- Responds to lowered levels of mechanical ventilator support with:
  - Slight baseline increase in blood pressure is <20 mm Hg.
  - Slight baseline increase in heart rate is <20 beats/min.
  - Baseline increase in respiratory rate is <5 breaths/min.
  - Hypervigilance to activities
  - Inability to respond to coaching
  - Inability to cooperate
  - Apprehension
  - Diaphoresis
  - Eye widening ("wide-eyed look")
  - Decreased air entry on auscultation
  - Color changes: pale, slight cyanosis
  - Slight respiratory accessory muscle use

Severe DVWR

- Responds to lowered levels of mechanical ventilator support with:
  - Agitation
  - Deterioration in arterial blood gases from current baseline
  - Baseline increase in blood pressure is >20 mm Hg.
  - Baseline increase in heart rate is >20 beats/min.
  - Respiratory rate increases significantly from baseline.
  - Profuse diaphoresis
  - Full respiratory accessory muscle use
  - Shallow, gasping breaths
  - Paradoxic abdominal breathing
  - Discoordinated breathing with the ventilator
  - Decreased level of consciousness

DYSFUNCTIONAL VENTILATORY WEANING RESPONSE—cont'd

- Adventitious breath sounds, audible airway secretions
- Cyanosis

Outcome Criteria

- Airway is clear.
- Underlying disorder is resolving.
- Patient is rested, and pain is controlled.
- Nutritional status is adequate.
- Patient has feelings of perceived control, situational security, and trust in the nurses.
- Patient is able to adapt to selected levels of ventilator support without undue fatigue.

Nursing Interventions and Rationale

1. Communicate interest and concern for the patient's well-being and demonstrate confidence in ability to manage weaning process ***to instill trust in the patient.***
2. Use normalizing strategies (e.g., grooming, dressing, mobilizing, social conversation) ***to reinforce the patient's self-esteem and feeling of identity.***
3. Identify parameters of the patient's usual functioning before the weaning process begins ***to facilitate early identification of problems.***
4. Identify the patient's strengths and resources that can be mobilized ***to enhance the patient's coping and maximize weaning effort.***
5. Note concerns that adversely affect the patient's comfort and confidence and manage them discreetly ***to facilitate the patient's ease.***
6. Praise successful activities, encourage a positive outlook, and review the patient's positive progress ***to increase the patient's perceived self-efficacy.***
7. Inform the patient of his or her situation and weaning progress ***to permit the patient as much control as possible.***
8. Teach the patient about the weaning process and how he or she can participate in the process.
9. Negotiate daily weaning goals with the patient ***to gain cooperation.***
10. Position the patient with the head of the bed elevated ***to optimize respiratory efforts.***
11. Coach the patient in breath control by regular demonstrations of slow, deep, rhythmic patterns of breathing ***to assist with dyspnea.***
12. Remain visible in the room and reassure the patient that help is immediately available if needed ***to reduce the patient's anxiety and fearfulness.***
13. Encourage the patient to view weaning trials as a form of training, regardless of whether the weaning goal is achieved, ***to avoid discouragement.***
14. Encourage the patient to maintain emotional calmness by reassuring, being present, comforting, talking down if emotionally aroused, and reinforcing the idea that he or she can and will succeed.
15. Monitor the patient's status frequently ***to avoid undue fatigue and anxiety.***
16. Provide regular periods of rest by reducing activities, maintaining or increasing ventilator support, and providing oxygen as needed before fatigue advances.
17. Provide distraction (e.g., visitors, radio, television, conversation) when the patient's concentration starts to create tension and increases anxiety.
18. Ensure adequate nutritional support, sufficient rest and sleep time, and sedation or pain control ***to promote the patient's optimal physical and emotional comfort.***
19. Start weaning early in the day ***when the patient is most rested.***
20. Restrict unnecessary activities and visitors who do not cooperate with weaning strategies ***to minimize energy demands on the patient during the weaning process.***
21. Coordinate necessary activities to promote adequate time for rest and relaxation. Implement the nursing management plan for Activity Intolerance Related to Prolonged Immobility or Deconditioning.
22. Monitor the patient's underlying disease process ***to ensure it is stabilized and under control.***
23. Advocate for additional resources (e.g., sedation, analgesia, rest) needed by the patient ***to maximize comfort status.***
24. Develop and adhere to an individualized plan of care ***to promote the patient's feelings of control.***

EXCESS FLUID VOLUME

Definition: Increased isotonic fluid retention.

Excess Fluid Volume Related to Increased Secretion of Antidiuretic Hormone (ADH)

Defining Characteristics

- Headache
- Decreased sensorium
- Weight gain over short period
- Intake greater than output
- Increased pulmonary artery occlusion pressure
- Increased right atrial pressure
- Urine output is <30 mL/hr.
- Serum sodium is <120 mEq/L.
- Serum osmolality is <275 mOsm/kg.
- Urine osmolality greater than serum osmolality
- Urine sodium is >200 mEq/L.
- Urine specific gravity is >1.03.

Outcome Criteria

- Weight returns to baseline.
- Urine output is >30 mL/hr.
- Serum sodium is 135-145 mEq/L.
- Urine specific gravity is 1.005-1030.

Continued

EXCESS FLUID VOLUME—cont'd

Nursing Interventions and Rationale

1. Monitor cardiac rhythm continuously for dysrhythmias ***caused by electrolyte imbalance.***
2. Restrict patient's fluids to 500 mL less than output per day ***to decrease fluid retention.***
3. Provide patient chilled beverages high in sodium content such as tomato juice or broth ***to increase sodium intake.***
4. Collaborate with physician regarding administration of demeclocycline, lithium, and/or opioid agonists ***to inhibit renal response to ADH.***
5. Collaborate with physician regarding administration of hypertonic saline and furosemide ***for rapid correction of severe sodium deficit and diuresis of free water.***
   a. Administer hypertonic saline at a rate of 1-2 mL/kg/hr until the patient's serum sodium is increased no greater than 1-2 mEq/L/hr.
6. Weigh patient daily at same time, in same amount of clothing, and preferably with same scale ***to ensure accuracy of readings.***
7. Provide frequent mouth care to prevent breakdown of oral mucous membranes.
8. Initiate seizure precautions because patient is at high risk as a result of hyponatremia.
   a. Pad side rails of bed to protect patient from injury.
   b. Remove any objects from immediate environment that could injure patient in the event of a seizure.
   c. Keep appropriate-size oral airway at bedside to assist with airway management after the seizure.
9. Collaborate with physician regarding administration of medications to prevent constipation ***caused by decreased fluid intake and immobility.***
10. Maintain surveillance for symptoms of hyponatremia (e.g., headache, abdominal cramps, weakness) and congestive heart failure (e.g., dyspnea, rales, increased central venous pressure, and pulmonary artery occlusion pressure).

Excess Fluid Volume Related to Renal Dysfunction

Defining Characteristics

- Weight gain that occurs during a 24- to 48-hour period
- Dependent pitting edema
- Ascites in severe cases
- Fluid crackles on lung auscultation
- Exertional dyspnea
- Oliguria or anuria
- Hypertension
- Engorged neck veins
- Decrease in urinary osmolality as renal failure progresses
- Right atrial pressure is >8 mm Hg.
- Pulmonary artery occlusion pressure is >12 mm Hg.

Outcome Criteria

- Weight returns to baseline.
- Edema or ascites is absent or reduced to baseline.
- Lungs are clear to auscultation.
- Exertional dyspnea is absent.
- Blood pressure returns to baseline.
- Heart rate returns to baseline.
- Neck veins are flat.
- Mucous membranes are moist.

Nursing Interventions and Rationale

1. Promote skin integrity of edematous areas by frequent repositioning and elevation of areas where possible. Avoid massaging pressure points or reddened areas of skin ***because this results in further tissue trauma.***
2. Plan patient care to provide rest periods ***so as not to heighten exertional dyspnea.***
3. Weigh patient daily at same time, in same amount of clothing, and preferably with same scale.
4. Instruct the patient about the correlation between fluid intake and weight gain, using commonly understood fluid measurements; for example, ingesting 4 cups (1000 mL) of fluid results in an approximate 2-pound weight gain in the anuric patient.

HYPERTHERMIA

Definition: Body temperature elevated above normal range.

Hyperthermia Related to Increased Metabolic Rate

Defining Characteristics

- Increased body temperature above normal range
- Seizures
- Flushed skin
- Increased respiratory rate
- Tachycardia
- Skin warm to touch
- Diaphoresis

Outcome Criteria

- Temperature is within normal range.
- Respiratory rate and heart rate are within patient's baseline range.
- Skin is warm and dry.

HYPERTHERMIA—cont'd

Nursing Interventions and Rationale

1. Monitor temperature every 15 minutes to 1 hour until within normal range and stable, then every 4 hours ***to maintain close surveillance for temperature fluctuations and evaluate effectiveness of interventions.***
   a. Use temperature taken from pulmonary artery catheter or bladder catheter if available ***because these methods closely reflect core body temperature.***
   b. Use tympanic membrane temperature if core body temperature devices are unavailable.
   c. Use rectal temperature if none of the methods listed above are available.
2. Collaborate with physician regarding administration of antithyroid medications ***to block the synthesis and release of thyroid hormone.***
3. Collaborate with physician regarding the use of cooling blanket ***to facilitate heat loss by conduction.***
   a. Wrap hands, feet, and genitalia to protect them from maceration during cooling and to decrease chance of shivering.
   b. Avoid rapidly cooling the patient and overcooling the patient because this initiates the heat-conserving response (i.e., shivering).
4. Place ice packs in patient's groin and axilla ***to facilitate heat loss by conduction.***
5. Maintain patient on bedrest ***to decrease the effects of activity on the patient's metabolic rate.***
6. Provide tepid sponge baths ***to facilitate heat loss by evaporation.***
7. Decrease the patient's room temperature ***to facilitate radiant heat loss.***
8. Place fan near patient to circulate cool air ***to facilitate heat loss by convection.***
9. Provide patient with nonrestrictive gown and lightweight bed coverings ***to allow heat to escape from the patient's trunk.***
10. Collaborate with physician and respiratory care practitioner on the administration of oxygen to maintain SpO_2 >90% ***because patient has increased oxygen consumption resulting from an increased metabolic rate.***
11. Collaborate with physician regarding use of antipyretic medications ***to facilitate patient comfort.***
12. Collaborate with physician regarding use of intravenous and oral fluids ***to maintain adequate hydration of the patient.***

HYPOTHERMIA

Definition: Body temperature below normal range.

Hypothermia Related to Decreased Metabolic Rate

Defining Characteristics

- Reduction in body temperature below normal range
- Shivering
- Pallor
- Piloerection
- Hypertension
- Skin cool to touch
- Tachycardia
- Decreased capillary refill

Outcome Criteria

- Temperature is within normal range.
- Heart rate is within patient's baseline range.
- Skin is warm and dry.
- Capillary refill is normal.

Nursing Interventions and Rationale

1. Monitor temperature every 15 minutes to 1 hour until within normal range and stable, then every 4 hours ***to maintain close surveillance for temperature fluctuations and evaluate effectiveness of interventions.***
   a. Use temperature taken from pulmonary artery catheter or bladder catheter if available ***because these methods closely reflect core body temperature.***
   b. Use tympanic membrane temperature ***if core body temperature devices are unavailable.***
   c. Use rectal temperature if none of the methods listed above are available.
2. Collaborate with physician regarding administration of thyroid medications ***to replace lacking thyroid hormone.***
3. Collaborate with physician regarding the use of fluid-filled heating blanket ***to facilitate rewarming by conduction.***
4. Initiate forced air-warming therapy ***to facilitate convective heat gain.***
5. Provide patient with warm blankets ***to facilitate heat transfer to the patient.***
6. Increase the patient's room temperature ***to decrease radiant heat loss.***
7. Replace wet patient gown and bed linen promptly ***to decrease evaporative heat loss.***
8. Warm intravenous fluids and blood products ***to facilitate rewarming by conduction.***

Continued

HYPOTHERMIA—cont'd

Hypothermia Related to Exposure to Cold Environment, Trauma, or Damage to the Hypothalamus

Defining Characteristics

- Core body temperature below 35° C (95° F)
- Skin cold to touch
- Slurred speech, incoordination
- At temperature below 33° C (91.4° F):
  - Cardiac dysrhythmias (atrial fibrillation, bradycardia)
  - Cyanosis
  - Respiratory alkalosis
- At temperatures below 32° C (89.6° F):
  - Shivering replaced by muscle rigidity
  - Hypotension
  - Dilated pupils
- At temperatures below 28° to 29° C (82.4° to 84.2° F):
  - Absent deep tendon reflexes
  - 3-4 breaths/min to apnea
  - Ventricular fibrillation possible
- At temperatures below 26° to 27° C (78.8° to 80.6° F):
  - Coma
  - Flaccid muscles
  - Fixed, dilated pupils
  - Ventricular fibrillation to cardiac standstill
  - Apnea

Outcome Criteria

- Core body temperature is greater than 35° C (95° F).
- Patient is alert and oriented.
- Cardiac dysrhythmias are absent.
- Acid–base balance is normal.
- Pupils are normoreactive.

Nursing Interventions and Rationale

1. Monitor core body temperature continuously.
2. Collaborate with the physician regarding the need for intubation and mechanical ventilation.
   a. Heated air or oxygen can be added ***to help rewarm the body core.***
   b. Do not hyperventilate the hypothermic patient ***because carbon dioxide production is low and this action may induce severe alkalosis and precipitate ventricular fibrillation.***
3. Maintain cardiopulmonary resuscitation and advanced cardiac life support (ACLS) until core body temperature is up to at least 29.5° C (85.1° F) before determining that patients cannot be resuscitated. ***Electrical defibrillation is usually successful in terminating ventricular fibrillation if the temperature is greater than 28° C (82.4° F).***
4. Administer cardiac resuscitation drugs sparingly ***because as the body warms, peripheral vasodilation occurs. Drugs that remain in the periphery are suddenly released, leading to a bolus effect that may cause fatal dysrhythmias.***
5. Monitor arterial blood gas values ***to direct further therapy and ensure that the pH, PaO_2, and $PaCO_2$ are corrected for temperature.***
6. Rewarm patient rapidly ***because the pathophysiologic changes associated with chronic hypothermia have not had time to evolve.***
   a. Institute rapid, active rewarming by immersion in warm water (38° to 43° C) (100.4° to 109.4° F).
   b. Apply thermal blanket at 36.6° to 37.7° C (97.9° to 99.9° F). Some researchers suggest rewarming only the torso or trunk first, leaving the extremities exposed to room temperature. ***This is done to prevent early peripheral vasodilation with abrupt redistribution of intravascular volume. This also prevents colder blood trapped in the extremities from returning to the body core before the heart is rewarmed.***
   c. Perform rapid core rewarming with heated (37° to 43° C; 98.6° to 109.4° F) intravenous infusion, hemodialysis, peritoneal dialysis, and colonic or gastric irrigation fluids.
7. Monitor peripheral circulation ***because gangrene of the fingers and toes is a common complication of accidental hypothermia.***

IMBALANCED NUTRITION: LESS THAN BODY REQUIREMENTS

Definition: Intake of nutrients insufficient to meet metabolic needs.

Imbalanced Nutrition: Less Than Body Requirements Related to Lack of Exogenous Nutrients and Increased Metabolic Demand

Defining Characteristics

- Unplanned weight loss of 20% of body weight within the past 6 months
- Serum albumin is <3.5 g/dL.
- Total lymphocytes are <1500/mm^3.
- Anergy
- Negative nitrogen balance
- Fatigue; lack of energy and endurance
- Nonhealing wounds
- Daily caloric intake less than estimated nutritional requirements
- Presence of factors known to increase nutritional requirements (e.g., sepsis, trauma, multiple organ dysfunction syndrome)
- Maintenance of nothing by mouth (NPO) status for >7-10 days
- Long-term use of 5% dextrose intravenously
- Documentation of suboptimal calorie counts
- Drug or nutrient interaction that might decrease oral intake (e.g., chronic use of bronchodilators, laxatives, anticonvulsives, diuretics, antacids, opioids)
- Physical problems with chewing, swallowing, choking, and salivation and presence of altered taste, anorexia, nausea, vomiting, diarrhea, or constipation

Outcome Criteria

- Patient exhibits stabilization of weight loss or weight gain of one-half pound daily.
- Serum albumin is >3.5 g/dL.
- Total lymphocytes are <1500/mm^3.
- Patient has positive response to cutaneous skin antigen testing.
- Patient is in positive nitrogen balance.
- Wound healing is evident.
- Daily caloric intake equals estimated nutritional requirements.
- Increased ambulation and endurance are evident.

Nursing Interventions and Rationale

1. Inquire if patient has any food allergies and food preferences ***to ensure the food provided to the patient is not contraindicated.***
2. Monitor patient's caloric intake and weight daily ***to ensure adequacy of nutritional interventions.***
3. Collaborate with dietitian regarding patient's nutritional and caloric needs ***to determine the appropriateness of the patient's diet to meet those needs.***
4. Monitor patient for signs of nutritional deficiencies ***to facilitate evaluation of extent of nutritional deficient.***
5. Provide patient with oral care before eating ***to ensure optimal consumption of diet.***
6. Assist patient to eat as appropriate ***to ensure optimal consumption of diet.***
7. Collaborate with physician and dietitian regarding the administration of parenteral and enteral nutrition as needed.

IMPAIRED GAS EXCHANGE

Definition: Excess or deficit in oxygenation and/or carbon dioxide elimination at the alveolar–capillary membrane.

Impaired Gas Exchange Related to Alveolar Hypoventilation

Defining Characteristics

- Abnormal arterial blood gas values (decreased PaO_2, increased $PaCO_2$, decreased pH, decreased SaO_2)
- Somnolence
- Neurobehavioral changes (e.g., restlessness, irritability, confusion)
- Tachycardia or dysrhythmias
- Central cyanosis

Outcome Criteria

- Arterial blood gas values are within patient's baseline.
- Central cyanosis is absent.

Nursing Interventions and Rationale

1. Initiate continuous pulse oximetry or monitor SpO_2 every hour.
2. Collaborate with physician and respiratory care practitioner on the administration of oxygen to maintain an SpO_2 >90%.
    a. Administer supplemental oxygen by an appropriate oxygen-delivery device ***to increase driving pressure of oxygen in the alveoli.***
    b. If supplemental oxygen alone is not effective, administer high-flow oxygen via high-flow nasal cannula, BiPAP via noninvasive ventilation (NIV), or positive end-expiratory pressure (PEEP) via invasive mechanical ventilation ***to open collapsed alveoli and increase the surface area for gas exchange.***
3. Prevent hypoventilation.
    a. Position patient in high-Fowler's position or semi-Fowler's position ***to promote diaphragmatic descent and maximal inhalation.***

Continued

IMPAIRED GAS EXCHANGE—cont'd

b. Assist with deep-breathing exercises and/or incentive spirometry with sustained maximal inspiration 5-10 times/hr ***to help reinflate collapsed portions of the lung.*** See the nursing management plan for Ineffective Breathing Pattern Related to Decreased Lung Expansion for further instructions.

c. Treat pain, if present, ***to prevent hypoventilation and atelectasis.*** Implement the nursing management plan for Acute Pain Related to Transmission and Perception of Cutaneous, Visceral, Muscular, or Ischemic Impulses.

4. Assist physician with intubation and initiation of mechanical ventilation as indicated.

Impaired Gas Exchange Related to Ventilation/Perfusion Mismatching or Intrapulmonary Shunting

Defining Characteristics

- Abnormal arterial blood gas values (decreased PaO_2, decreased SaO_2)
- Somnolence
- Neurobehavioral changes (restlessness, irritability, confusion)
- Central cyanosis

Outcome Criteria

- ABG values are within patient's baseline.
- Central cyanosis is absent.

Nursing Interventions and Rationale

1. Initiate continuous pulse oximetry or monitor SpO_2 every hour.
2. Collaborate with physician and respiratory care practitioner on the administration of oxygen to maintain an SpO_2 >90%.
   a. Administer supplemental oxygen by an appropriate oxygen-delivery device ***to increase driving pressure of oxygen in the alveoli.***
   b. If supplemental oxygen alone is not effective, administer high-flow oxygen via high-flow nasal cannula, BiPAP via noninvasive ventilation (NIV), or positive end-expiratory pressure (PEEP) via invasive mechanical ventilation ***to open collapsed alveoli and increase the surface area for gas exchange.***
3. Position patient to optimize ventilation/perfusion matching.
   a. For patient with unilateral lung disease, position with the good lung down ***because gravity will improve perfusion to this area, and this will best match ventilation with perfusion.***
   b. For patient with bilateral lung disease, position with the right lung down ***because this lung is larger than the left and affords a greater area for ventilation and perfusion*** or change position every 2 hours, favoring positions that improve oxygenation.
   c. For patient with diffuse bilateral disease, collaborate with the physician regarding the use of prone positioning ***to encourage perfusion to the anterior region of the lungs, which are usually less damaged than the posterior region.***
   d. Avoid any position that seriously compromises oxygenation status.
4. Perform procedures only as needed and provide adequate rest and recovery time in between ***to prevent desaturation.***
5. Collaborate with the physician regarding the administration of the following:
   a. Sedatives ***to decrease ventilator asynchrony and facilitate patient's sense of control***
   b. Neuromuscular blocking agents ***to prevent ventilator asynchrony and decrease oxygen demand***
   c. Analgesics ***to treat pain if present.*** Implement the nursing management plan for Acute Pain Related to Transmission and Perception of Cutaneous, Visceral, Muscular, or Ischemic Impulses.
6. Evaluate patient for the presence of secretions. If present, implement the nursing management plan for Ineffective Airway Clearance Related to Excessive Secretions or Abnormal Viscosity of Mucus.

IMPAIRED SPONTANEOUS VENTILATION

Definition: Decreased energy reserves result in an individual's inability to maintain breathing adequate to support life.

Impaired Spontaneous Ventilation Related to Respiratory Muscle Fatigue or Metabolic Factors

Defining Characteristics

- Dyspnea and apprehension
- Increased metabolic rate
- Increased restlessness
- Increased use of accessory muscles
- Decreased tidal volume
- Increased heart rate
- Abnormal arterial blood gas values (decreased PaO_2, increased $PaCO_2$, decreased pH, decreased SaO_2)
- Decreased cooperation

Outcome Criteria

- Metabolic rate and heart rate are within patient's baseline.
- Patient experiences eupnea.
- ABG values are within patient's baseline.

Nursing Interventions and Rationale

1. Collaborate with the physician regarding the application of pressure support to the ventilator ***to assist patient in overcoming the work of breathing imposed by the ventilator and endotracheal tube.***

IMPAIRED SPONTANEOUS VENTILATION—cont'd

2. Carefully snip excess length from the proximal end of the endotracheal ***tube to decrease dead space and thereby decrease the work of breathing.***
3. Collaborate with the physician and dietitian to ensure that at least 50% of the diet's nonprotein caloric source is in the form of fat rather than carbohydrates ***to prevent excess carbon dioxide production.***
4. Collaborate with the physician and respiratory care practitioner regarding the best method of weaning for individual patients ***because each situation is different and a variety of weaning options are available.***
    a. Consider initiating daily spontaneous awakening trial ("sedation vacation") and spontaneous breathing trial.
    b. Monitor patient for signs of weaning intolerance.
5. Collaborate with the physician and physical therapist regarding a progressive ambulation and conditioning plan ***to promote overall muscle conditioning and respiratory muscle functioning.*** Implement the nursing management plan for Activity Intolerance Related to Prolonged Immobility or Deconditioning.
6. Determine the most effective means of communication for the patient ***to promote independence and reduce anxiety.***
7. Develop a daily schedule and post it in patient's room ***to coordinate care and facilitate patient's involvement in the plan.***
8. Treat pain, if present, ***to prevent respiratory splinting and hypoventilation.*** Implement the nursing management plan for Acute Pain Related to Transmission and Perception of Cutaneous, Visceral, Muscular, or Ischemic Impulses.
9. Ensure that patient receives at least 2- to 4-hr intervals of uninterrupted sleep in a quiet, dark room. Collaborate with the physician and respiratory care practitioner regarding the use of full ventilatory support at night ***to provide respiratory muscle rest.***
10. Place patient in semi-Fowler's position or in a chair at the bedside ***for best use of ventilatory muscles and to facilitate diaphragmatic descent.***
11. Explain the weaning procedure to the patient before the trial ***so that patient will understand what to expect and how to participate.***
12. Monitor patient during the weaning trial for evidence of respiratory muscle fatigue ***to avoid overtiring the patient.***
13. Collaborate with physician and occupational therapist to provide diversional activities during the weaning trial ***to reduce the patient's anxiety.***
14. Collaborate with physician and respiratory care practitioner regarding the removal of the ventilator and artificial airway ***when patient has been successfully weaned.***

IMPAIRED SWALLOWING

Definition: Abnormal functioning of the swallowing mechanism associated with deficits in oral, pharyngeal, or esophageal structure or function.

Impaired Swallowing Related to Neuromuscular Impairment, Fatigue, and Limited Awareness

Defining Characteristics

- Evidence of difficulty swallowing:
    - Drooling
    - Difficulty handling oral secretions
    - Absence of gag, cough, and/or swallow reflex
    - Moist, wet, gurgling voice quality
    - Decreased tongue and mouth movements
    - Presence of dysarthria
- Difficulty handling solid foods:
    - Uncoordinated chewing or swallowing
    - Stasis of food in the oral cavity
    - Wet-sounding voice or change in voice quality
    - Sneezing, coughing, or choking with eating
    - Delay in swallowing of more than 5 seconds
    - Change in respiratory patterns
- Difficulty handling liquids:
    - Momentary loss of voice or change in voice quality
    - Nasal regurgitation of liquids
    - Coughing with drinking
- Evidence of aspiration:
    - Hypoxemia
    - Productive cough
    - Frothy sputum
    - Wheezing, crackles, or rhonchi
    - Temperature elevation

Outcome Criteria

- Evidence of swallowing difficulties is absent.
- Evidence of aspiration is absent.

Nursing Interventions and Rationale

1. Collaborate with physician and speech therapist regarding swallowing evaluation and rehabilitation program ***to decrease the incidence of aspiration.***
2. Collaborate with physician and dietitian regarding a nutritional assessment and nutritional plan ***to ensure that the patient is receiving enough nutrition.***
3. Place the patient in an upright position with the head midline and the chin slightly down ***to keep food in the anterior portion of the mouth and to prevent it from falling over the base of the tongue into the open airway.***
4. Provide patient with single-textured soft foods (e.g., cream cereals) that maintain their shape ***because these foods require minimal oral manipulation.***
5. Avoid particulate foods (e.g., hamburger) and foods containing more than one texture (e.g., stew) ***because these foods require more chewing and oral manipulation.***

Continued

IMPAIRED SWALLOWING—cont'd

6. Avoid dry foods (e.g., popcorn, rice, crackers) and sticky foods (e.g., peanut butter, bananas) ***because these foods are difficult to manipulate orally.***
7. Provide patient with thick liquids (e.g., fruit nectar, yogurt) ***because thick liquids are more easily controlled in the mouth.***
8. Thicken thin liquids (e.g., water, juice) with a thickening preparation or avoid them ***because thin liquids are easily aspirated.***
9. Place foods in the uninvolved side of the mouth ***because oral sensitivity and function are greatest in this area.***
10. Avoid the use of straws ***because they can deposit the liquid too far back in the mouth for the patient to handle.***
11. Serve foods and liquids at room temperature ***because the patient may be overly sensitive to heat or cold.***
12. Offer solids and liquids at different times ***to avoid swallowing solids before being properly chewed.***
13. Provide oral hygiene after meals ***to clear food particles from the mouth that could be aspirated.***
14. Collaborate with physician and pharmacist regarding oral medication administration ***to adjust medication regimen to prevent aspiration and choking and to ensure all prescribed medications are swallowed.***
15. Crush tablets (if appropriate) and mix with food that is easily formed into a bolus, use thickened liquid medications (if available), and/or embed small capsules into food ***to facilitate oral medication administration.***
16. Inspect mouth for residue after all medication administration ***to ensure medication has been swallowed.***
17. Educate patient and family on the swallowing problem, rehabilitation program, and emergency measures for choking.

IMPAIRED VERBAL COMMUNICATION

Definition: Decreased, delayed, or absent ability to receive, process, transmit, and use a system of symbols.

Impaired Verbal Communication Related to Cerebral Speech Center Injury

Defining Characteristics

- Inappropriate or absent speech or responses to questions
- Inability to speak spontaneously
- Inability to understand spoken words
- Inability to follow commands appropriately through gestures
- Difficulty or inability to understand written language
- Difficulty or inability to express ideas in writing
- Difficulty or inability to name objects

Outcome Criterion

- Patient is able to make basic needs known.

Nursing Interventions and Rationale

1. Consult with physician and speech pathologist ***to determine the extent of the patient's communication deficit (e.g., whether fluent, nonfluent, or global aphasia is involved).***
2. Have the speech therapist post a list of appropriate ways to communicate with the patient in the patient's room ***so that all nursing personnel can be consistent in their efforts.***
3. Assess the patient's ability to comprehend, speak, read, and write.
   a. Ask questions that can be answered with "yes" or "no." If a patient answers "yes" to a question, ask the opposite (e.g., "Are you hot?" "Yes." "Are you cold?" "Yes."). ***This may help determine whether the patient understands what is being said.***
   b. Ask simple, short questions and use gestures, pantomime, and facial expressions to give the patient additional clues.
   c. Stand in the patient's line of vision, giving a good view of your face and hands.
   d. Have the patient try to write with a pad and pencil. Offer pictures and alphabet letters at which to point.
   e. Make flash cards with pictures or words depicting frequently used phrases (e.g., glass of water, bedpan).
4. Maintain an uncluttered environment and decrease external distractions ***to enhance communication.***
5. Maintain a relaxed and calm manner and explain all diagnostic, therapeutic, and comfort measures before initiating them.
6. Do not shout or speak in a loud voice. ***Hearing loss is not a factor in aphasia, and shouting will not help.***
7. Have only one person talk at a time. ***It is more difficult for the patient to follow a multisided conversation.***
8. Use direct eye contact and speak directly to the patient in unhurried, short phrases.
9. Give one-step commands and directions and provide cues through pictures and gestures.
10. Try to ask questions that can be answered with a "yes" or a "no" and avoid topics that are controversial, emotional, abstract, or lengthy.
11. Listen to the patient in an unhurried manner and wait for his or her attempt to communicate.
    a. Expect a time lag from when you ask the patient something until the patient responds.
    b. Accept the patient's statement of essential words without expecting complete sentences.
    c. Avoid finishing the sentence for the patient if possible.
    d. Wait approximately 30 seconds before providing the word the patient may be attempting to find (except when the patient is very frustrated and needs something quickly, such as a bedpan).
    e. Rephrase the patient's message aloud ***to validate it.***
    f. Do not pretend to understand the patient's message if you do not.

IMPAIRED VERBAL COMMUNICATION—cont'd

12. Encourage the patient to speak slowly in short phrases and to say each word clearly.
13. Ask the patient to write the message, if able, or draw pictures if only verbal communication is affected.
14. Observe the patient's nonverbal clues for validation (e.g., answers "yes" but shakes head "no").
15. When handing an object to the patient, state what it is ***because hearing language spoken is necessary to stimulate language development.***
16. Explain what has happened to the patient and offer reassurance about the plan of care.
17. Verbally address the problem of frustration over the inability to communicate and explain that both the nurse and the patient need patience.
18. Maintain a calm, positive manner and offer reassurance (e.g., "I know this is very hard for you, but it will get better if we work on it together").
19. Talk to the patient as an adult. Be respectful and avoid talking down to the patient.
20. Do not discuss the patient's condition or hold conversations in the patient's presence without including him or her in the discussion. ***This may be the reason some aphasic patients develop paranoid thoughts.***
21. Do not exhibit disapproval of emotional utterances or spontaneous use of profanity; instead, offer calm, quiet reassurance.
22. If the patient makes an error in speech, do not reprimand or scold but try to compliment the patient by saying, "That was a good try."
23. Delay conversation if the patient is tired. ***The symptoms of aphasia worsen if the patient is fatigued, anxious, or upset.***
24. Be prepared for emotional outbursts and tears from patients who have more difficulty in expressing themselves than with understanding. ***The patient may become depressed, refuse treatment and food, ignore relatives, and push objects away.*** Comfort the patient with statements such as "I know it's frustrating and you feel sad, but you are not alone. Other people who have had strokes have felt the way you do. We will be here to help you get through this."

INEFFECTIVE AIRWAY CLEARANCE

Definition: Inability to clear secretions or obstructions from the respiratory tract to maintain a clear airway.

Ineffective Airway Clearance Related to Excessive Secretions or Abnormal Viscosity of Mucus

Defining Characteristics

- Abnormal breath sounds (displaced normal sounds, adventitious sounds, diminished or absent sounds)
- Ineffective cough with or without sputum
- Tachypnea, dyspnea
- Verbal reports of inability to clear airway

Outcome Criteria

- Cough produces thin mucus.
- Lungs are clear to auscultation.
- Respiratory rate, depth, and rhythm return to baseline.

Nursing Interventions and Rationale

1. Assess sputum for color, consistency, and amount.
2. Assess for clinical manifestations of pneumonia.
3. Provide for maximal thoracic expansion by repositioning, deep breathing, splinting, and pain management ***to avoid hypoventilation and atelectasis.*** If hypoventilation is present, implement the nursing management plan for Ineffective Breathing Pattern Related to Decreased Lung Expansion.
4. Maintain adequate hydration by administering oral and intravenous fluids (as ordered) ***to thin secretions and facilitate airway clearance.***
5. Provide humidification to airways by an oxygen-delivery device or artificial airway ***to thin secretions and facilitate airway clearance.***
6. Administer bland aerosol every 4 hours ***to facilitate expectoration of sputum.***
7. Collaborate with the physician regarding the administration of the following:
   a. Bronchodilators ***to treat or prevent bronchospasms and facilitate expectoration of mucus***
   b. Mucolytics and expectorants ***to enhance mobilization and removal of secretions***
   c. Antibiotics ***to treat infection***
8. Assist with directed coughing exercises ***to facilitate expectoration of secretions.*** If patient is unable to perform cascade cough, consider using huff cough (patients with hyperactive airways), end-expiratory cough (patient with secretions in distal airway), or augmented cough (patient with weakened abdominal muscle).
   a. Cascade cough—instruct patient to do the following:
      (1) Take a deep breath and hold it for 1-3 seconds.
      (2) Cough out forcefully several times until all air is exhaled.
      (3) Inhale slowly through the nose.
      (4) Repeat once.
      (5) Rest and then repeat as necessary.
   b. Huff cough—instruct patient to do the following:
      (1) Take a deep breath and hold it for 1-3 seconds.
      (2) Say the word "huff" while coughing out several times until air is exhaled.
      (3) Inhale slowly through the nose.
      (4) Repeat as necessary.
   c. End-expiratory cough—instruct patient to do the following:
      (1) Take a deep breath and hold it for 1-3 seconds.
      (2) Exhale slowly.

Continued

INEFFECTIVE AIRWAY CLEARANCE—cont'd

(3) At the end of exhalation, cough once.
(4) Inhale slowly through the nose.
(5) Repeat as necessary or follow with cascade cough.

d. Augmented cough—instruct patient to do the following:
(1) Take a deep breath and hold it for 1-3 seconds.
(2) Perform one or more of the following maneuvers to increase intraabdominal pressure:
(a) Tighten knees and buttocks.
(b) Bend forward at the waist.
(c) Place a hand flat on the upper abdomen just under the xiphoid process and press in and up abruptly during coughing.
(d) Keep hands on the chest wall and press inward with each cough.
(3) Inhale slowly through the nose.
(4) Rest and repeat as necessary.

9. Suction nasotracheally or endotracheally as necessary ***to assist with secretion removal.***
10. Reposition patient at least every 2 hours or use kinetic therapy ***to mobilize and prevent stasis of secretions.***
11. Allow rest periods between coughing sessions, suctioning, or any other demanding activities ***to promote energy conservation.***

INEFFECTIVE BREATHING PATTERN

Definition: Inspiration and/or expiration that does not provide adequate ventilation.

Ineffective Breathing Pattern Related to Decreased Lung Expansion

Defining Characteristics

- Abnormal respiratory patterns (hypoventilation, hyperventilation, tachypnea, bradypnea, obstructive breathing)
- Abnormal arterial blood gas values (increased $PaCO_2$, decreased pH)
- Unequal chest movement
- Shortness of breath, dyspnea

Outcome Criteria

- Respiratory rate, rhythm, and depth return to baseline.
- Minimal or absent use of accessory muscles
- Chest expands symmetrically.
- Arterial blood gas values return to baseline.

Nursing Interventions and Rationale

1. Treat pain, if present, ***to prevent hypoventilation and atelectasis.*** Implement the nursing management plan for Acute Pain Related to Transmission and Perception of Cutaneous, Visceral, Muscular, or Ischemic Impulses.
2. Position patient in high-Fowler's or semi-Fowler's position ***to promote diaphragmatic descent and maximal inhalation.***
3. Assist with deep-breathing exercises and incentive spirometry with sustained maximal inspiration 5-10 times/hr ***to help reinflate collapsed portions of the lung.***
a. Deep breathing—instruct patient to do the following:
(1) Sit up straight or lean forward slightly while sitting on edge of bed or chair (if possible).
(2) Take in a slow, deep breath.
(3) Pause slightly or hold breath for at least 3 seconds.
(4) Exhale slowly.
(5) Rest and repeat.
b. Incentive spirometry—instruct patient to do the following:
(1) Exhale normally.
(2) Place lips around the mouthpiece and close mouth tightly around it.
(3) Inhale slowly and as deeply as possible, noting the maximal volume of air inspired.
(4) Hold maximal inhalation for 3 seconds.
(5) Take the mouthpiece out of mouth and slowly exhale.
(6) Rest and repeat.
4. Assist physician with intubation and initiation of mechanical ventilation as indicated.

Ineffective Breathing Pattern Related to Musculoskeletal Fatigue or Neuromuscular Impairment

Defining Characteristics

- Unequal chest movement
- Shortness of breath, dyspnea
- Use of accessory muscles
- Tachypnea
- Thoracoabdominal asynchrony
- Abnormal arterial blood gas values (increased $PaCO_2$, decreased pH)
- Nasal flaring
- Assumption of 3-point position

Outcome Criteria

- Respiratory rate, rhythm, and depth return to baseline.
- Use of accessory muscles is minimal or absent.
- Chest expands symmetrically.
- Arterial blood gas values return to baseline.

Nursing Interventions and Rationale

1. Prevent unnecessary exertion ***to limit drain on patient's ventilatory reserve.***

INEFFECTIVE BREATHING PATTERN—cont'd

2. Instruct patient in energy-saving techniques ***to conserve patient's ventilatory reserve.***
3. Assist with pursed-lip and diaphragmatic breathing techniques ***to facilitate diaphragmatic descent and improved ventilation.***
   a. Diaphragmatic breathing—instruct the patient to do the following:
      (1) Sit in the upright position.
      (2) Place one hand on the abdomen just above the waist and the other on the upper chest.
      (3) Breathe in through the nose and feel the lower hand push out; the upper hand should not move.
      (4) Breathe out through pursed lips and feel the lower hand move in.
4. Position patient in high-Fowler's or semi-Fowler's position ***to promote diaphragmatic descent and maximal inhalation.***
5. Assist physician with intubation and initiation of mechanical ventilation as indicated.

INEFFECTIVE COPING

Definition: Inability to form a valid appraisal of the stressors, inadequate choices of practiced responses, and/or inability to use available resources.

Ineffective Coping Related to Situational Crisis and Personal Vulnerability

Defining Characteristics

- Verbalization of inability to cope. *Sample statements*: "I can't take this anymore." "I don't know how to deal with this."
- Ineffective problem solving (problem lumping). *Sample statements*: "I have to eliminate salt from my diet. They tell me I can no longer mow the lawn. This hospitalization is costing a mint. What about my kids' future? Who's going to change the oil in the car? This is an incredible amount of time away from work."
- Ineffective use of coping mechanisms
  - Projection: blames others for illness or pain
  - Displacement: directs anger and/or aggression toward family
    - *Sample statements*: "Get out of here. Leave me alone."
    - Cursing, shouting, or demanding attention; striking out or throwing objects
  - Denial of severity of illness and need for treatment
- Noncompliance. *Examples*: activity restriction; refusal to allow treatment or to take medications
- Suicidal thoughts (verbalizes desire to end life)
- Self-directed aggression. *Examples*: disconnects or attempts to disconnect life-sustaining equipment; deliberately tries to harm self
- Failure to progress from dependent to more independent state (refusal or resistance to care for self)

Outcome Criteria

- Patient verbalizes beginning ability to cope with illness, pain, and hospitalization. *Sample statements*: "I'm trying to do the best I can." "I want to help myself get better."
- Patient demonstrates effective problem solving (lists and prioritizes problems from most to least urgent).
- Patient uses effective behavioral strategies to manage the stress of illness and care.
- Patient demonstrates interest or involvement in illness or environment. *Examples*: patient does the following:
  - Requests medications when anticipating pain
  - Questions course of treatment, progress, and prognosis
  - Asks for clarification of environmental stimuli and events
  - Seeks out supportive individuals in his or her environment
  - Uses coping mechanisms and strategies more effectively to manage situational crisis
  - Demonstrates significant reduction in impulsive, angry, or aggressive outbursts (projection, shouting, cursing) directed toward family
  - Verbalizes future-based plans, with cessation of self-directed aggressive acts and suicidal thoughts
  - Willingly complies with treatment regimen
  - Begins to participate in self-care

Nursing Interventions and Rationale

1. Actively listen and respond to patient's verbal and behavioral expressions. ***Active listening signifies unconditional respect and acceptance for the patient as a worthwhile individual. It builds trust and rapport, guides the nurse toward problem areas, encourages the patient to express concerns, and promotes compliance.***
2. Offer effective coping strategies to help the patient better tolerate the stressors related to his or her illness and care. Give permission to vent feelings in a safe setting. *Sample statements:* "I don't blame you for feeling angry or frustrated." "Others who are ill like you have expressed similar feelings." "I will listen to anything you want to share with me." "We don't have to talk; I'd like to sit here with you." "It's perfectly okay to cry." ***Individuals who are provided with opportunities to express their feelings will be better able to release pent-up emotions and derive a greater sense of relief and comfort. They are less likely to resort to overly impulsive, aggressive acts, which may harm self or others.***
3. Inform the family of the patient's need to displace anger occasionally but that you will be working with the patient to help him or her release his or her feelings in a more constructive, effective way. ***Family members who are well informed are better equipped to cope with their loved one's emotional anguish and outbursts. They are less likely to waste energy on feelings of guilt, fear,***

Continued

INEFFECTIVE COPING—cont'd

anger, or despair and can use their strength to help the patient in more constructive ways. The knowledge that their loved one is being cared for emotionally as well as physically provides family members with a greater sense of comfort and understanding. They will feel nurtured and respected by the nurse's attempt to include them in the process.

4. With the patient, list and number problems from the most to least urgent. Assist him or her in finding immediate solutions for most urgent problems, postpone those that can wait, delegate some to family members, and help him or her to acknowledge problems that are beyond his or her control. ***Listing and numbering problems in an organized fashion helps to break them down into more manageable "pieces" so that the patient is better able to identify solutions for those that are solvable and to suppress those that are less relevant or not amenable to interventions.***
5. Identify individuals in the patient's environment who best help him or her to cope and identify those who do not. Validate your observations with the patient. *Sample statements:* "I notice you seemed more relaxed during your daughter's visit." "After the clergy left, you were able to sleep a bit longer than usual; would you like to see him more often?" "Your grandson was a bit upset today; I'll be glad to talk to him if you like." ***Supportive persons can invoke a calming effect on the patient's physiologic and psychologic states. Conversely, well-meaning but nonsupportive individuals can have a deleterious effect on the patient's ability to cope and must be carefully screened and counseled by the nurse.***
6. Teach the patient effective cognitive strategies to help him or her better manage the stress of critical illness and care. Help him or her construct pleasant thoughts, situations, or images that can simultaneously inhibit unpleasant realities. Examples: a day at the beach, a walk in the park, drinking a glass of wine, or being with a loved one. ***Pleasant thoughts and images constructed during critical illness and care tend to inhibit or reduce the intensity of the unpleasant, stressful effects of the experience.***
7. Assist the patient in using coping mechanisms more effectively so he or she can better manage his or her situational crisis.
   a. Suppression of problems beyond his or her control
   b. Compensation for illness and its effects; focusing on his or her strengths, interests, family, and spiritual beliefs
   c. Adaptive displacement of anger, fear, or frustration through healthy, verbal expressions to staff. ***Effective use of coping mechanisms helps to assuage the patient's painful feelings in a safe setting. The patient is strengthened and need not resort to the use of more ineffective defenses to eliminate anxiety.***
8. Initiate a suicidal assessment if the patient verbalizes the desire to die, states that life is not worth living, or exhibits self-directed aggression. *Sample statement*: "We know that this is a bad time for you. You're saying repeatedly that you want to die. Are you planning to harm yourself?" If the response is "yes," remain with the patient, alert staff members, and provide for psychiatric consultation as soon as possible. Continue to express concern to the patient and protect him or her from harm. ***Suicidal thoughts as a result of ineffective coping or exhaustion of coping devices are not an uncommon occurrence in critically ill patients. If the mood state is distressing enough, a patient may seek relief by attempting a self-destructive act. Although the patient may not imminently have the energy to succeed in his or her attempt, voicing a specific plan signifies a depressed mood state and depletion of coping strategies. Immediate intervention is needed, because the attempt may be successful when the patient's energy is restored.***
9. Encourage the patient to participate in self-care activities and treatment regimen in accordance with his or her level of progress. Offer praise for his or her efforts toward self-care. ***Patients who take an active role in their own treatment and progress are less apt to feel like helpless or powerless victims. This greater sense of control over their illness and environment will guide them more swiftly toward becoming as independent as possible.***

POWERLESSNESS

Definition: Perception that one's own action cannot significantly affect an outcome; a perceived lack of control over a current situation or immediate happening.

Powerlessness Related to Lack of Control over Current Situation or Disease Progression

Defining Characteristics

Severe

- Verbal expressions of having no control or influence over situation
- Verbal expressions of having no control or influence over outcome
- Verbal expressions of having no control over self-care
- Depression over physical deterioration that occurs despite patient's compliance with regimens
- Apathy

Moderate

- Nonparticipation in care or decision making when opportunities are provided
- Expressions of dissatisfaction and frustration about inability to perform previous tasks and/or activities
- Lack of progress monitoring
- Expressions of doubt about role performance
- Reluctance to express true feelings, fearing alienation from caregivers
- Passivity

POWERLESSNESS—cont'd

- Inability to seek information about care
- Dependence on others that may result in irritability, resentment, anger, and guilt
- No defense of self-care practices when challenged

Low
- Passivity

Outcome Criteria
- Patient verbalizes increased control over situation by wanting to do things his or her way.
- Patient actively participates in planning care.
- Patient requests needed information.
- Patient chooses to participate in self-care activities.
- Patient monitors progress.

Nursing Interventions and Rationale
1. Evaluate the patient's feelings and perception of the reasons for lack of power and sense of helplessness.
2. Determine as far as possible the patient's usual response to limited control situations. Determine through ongoing assessment the patient's usual locus of control (i.e., believes that influence over his or her life is exerted by luck, fate, powerful persons [external locus of control] or that influence is exerted through personal choices, self-effort, self-determination [internal locus of control]).
3. Support patient's physical control of the environment by involving him or her in care activities; knock before entering room, if appropriate; ask permission before moving personal belongings. Inform the patient that, although an activity may not be to his or her liking, it is necessary. ***This gives the patient permission to express dissatisfaction with the environment and the regimen.***
4. Personalize the patient's care using his or her preferred name. ***This supports the patient's psychologic control.***
5. Provide therapeutic rationale for all the patient is asked to do for himself or herself and for all that is being done for and with him or her. Reinforce the physician's explanations; clarify misconceptions about the illness situation and treatment plans. ***This supports the patient's cognitive control.***
6. Include the patient in care planning by encouraging participation and allowing choices wherever possible (e.g., timing of personal care activities; deciding when pain medicines are needed). Point out situations in which no choices exist.
7. Provide opportunities for the patient to exert influence over himself or herself and his or her body, thereby affecting an outcome. For example, share with the patient the nurse's assessment of his or her breath sounds and explain that they can be improved by self-initiated deep-breathing exercises. ***Feedback that the patient has been successful in helping clear his or her lungs reinforces the influence he or she does retain.***
8. Encourage family to permit patient to do as much independently as possible ***to foster perception of personal power.***
9. Assist the patient to establish realistic short-term and long-term goals. ***Setting unrealistic or unattainable goals inadvertently reinforces the patient's perception of powerlessness.***
10. Document care to provide for continuity ***so that the patient can maintain appropriate control over the environment.***
11. Assist the patient to regain strength and activity tolerance as appropriate, ***increasing a sense of control and self-reliance.***
12. Increase the sensitivity of the health team members and significant others to the patient's sense of powerlessness. Use power over the patient carefully. Use the words *must, should,* and *have to* with caution ***because they communicate coercive powers and imply that the objects of "musts" and "shoulds" are of benefit to the nurse instead of the patient.***
13. Plan with the patient for transfer from the critical care unit to the intermediate unit and eventually to home.

RELOCATION STRESS SYNDROME

Definition: Physiologic and/or psychologic disturbances after transfer from one environment to another.

Relocation Stress Syndrome Related to Transfer Out of the Critical Care Unit

Defining Characteristics
- Alienation
- Aloneness
- Anger
- Anxiety
- Concern over relocation
- Dependency
- Depression
- Fear of an unknown environment
- Frustration
- Increased illness
- Increased physical symptoms
- Increased verbalization of needs
- Insecurity
- Loneliness
- Loss of identify
- Loss of self-esteem
- Loss of self-worth
- Move from critical care unit to another environment
- Pessimism
- Sleep disturbance
- Unwillingness to move
- Withdrawal
- Worry

Continued

RELOCATION STRESS SYNDROME—cont'd

Outcome Criteria
- Patient will express willingness to move to new environment.
- Absence of anxiety

Nursing Interventions and Rationale
1. Initiate pretransfer teaching as soon as appropriate during the patient's stay in the critical care unit ***to ease the transition from critical care to the next environment.*** Teaching should focus on the differences in the environment and the care they would receive.
2. Provide the patient and family written information regarding the transfer (if available) ***to enhance effectiveness of teaching.***
3. Help the patient see that progress is being made ***in preparation for transfer.*** Each time a tube is removed or a treatment frequency is decreased, reinforce with the patient and family that the patient is progressing.
4. Remove monitoring and supportive equipment from the patient's room when no longer needed ***to allow the patient to experience the loss of technology while still in the critical care unit.***
5. Encourage patient and family to discuss concerns regarding relocation.
6. Assist patient and family members to develop and maintain a positive perception of the transfer.
7. Arrange for the patient's family to have a tour of the new unit ***as a means of familiarizing them with the unit before the patient's transfer.***

RISK FOR ASPIRATION

Definition: At risk for entry of gastrointestinal secretions, oropharyngeal secretions, solids, or fluids into tracheobronchial passages.

Risk Factors

- Impaired laryngeal sensation or reflex
  - Reduced level of consciousness
  - Extubation
- Impaired pharyngeal peristalsis or tongue function
  - Neuromuscular dysfunction
  - Central nervous system dysfunction
  - Head or neck injury
- Impaired laryngeal closure or elevation
  - Laryngeal nerve dysfunction
  - Artificial airways
  - Gastrointestinal tubes
- Increased gastric volume
  - Delayed gastric emptying
  - Enteral feedings
  - Medication administration
- Increased intragastric pressure
- Upper abdominal surgery
  - Obesity
  - Pregnancy
  - Ascites
- Decreased lower esophageal sphincter pressure
  - Increased gastric acidity
  - Gastrointestinal tubes
- Decreased antegrade esophageal propulsion
  - Trendelenburg or supine position
  - Esophageal dysmotility
  - Esophageal structural defects or lesions

Outcome Criteria

- Breath sounds are normal, or there is no change in patient's baseline breath sounds.
- Arterial blood gas values remain within patient's baseline.
- There is no evidence of gastric contents in lung secretions.

Nursing Interventions and Rationale

1. Assess gastrointestinal function ***to rule out hypoactive peristalsis and abdominal distention.***
2. Position patient with head of bed elevated 30 degrees ***to prevent gastric reflux through gravity.*** If head elevation is contraindicated, position patient in right lateral decubitus position ***to facilitate passage of gastric contents across the pylorus.***
3. Maintain patency and functioning of nasogastric suction apparatus ***to prevent accumulation of gastric contents.***
4. Provide frequent and scrupulous mouth care ***to prevent colonization of the oropharynx with bacteria and inoculation of the lower airways.***
5. Ensure that the endotracheal or tracheostomy cuff is properly inflated ***to limit aspiration of oropharyngeal secretions.***
6. Treat nausea promptly; collaborate with physician on an order for antiemetic ***to prevent vomiting and resultant aspiration.***

Additional Interventions for Patient Receiving Continuous or Intermittent Enteral Tube Feedings

7. Position patient with head of bed elevated 45 degrees ***to prevent gastric reflux.*** If a head-down position becomes necessary at any time, interrupt the feeding 30 minutes before the position change.
8. Check placement of feeding tube by auscultation or radiographically at regular intervals (e.g., before administering intermittent feedings and after position changes, suctioning, coughing episodes, or vomiting) ***to ensure proper placement of the tube.***

RISK FOR ASPIRATION—cont'd

9. Monitor patient for signs of delayed gastric emptying ***to decrease potential for vomiting and aspiration.***
   a. For large-bore tubes, check residuals of tube feedings before intermittent feedings and every 4 hours during continuous feedings. Consider withholding feedings for residuals greater than 150% of the hourly rate (continuous feeding) or greater than 50% of the previous feeding (intermittent feeding).
   b. For small-bore tubes, observe abdomen for distention, palpate abdomen for hardness or tautness, and auscultate abdomen for bowel sounds.

RISK FOR DECREASED CARDIAC TISSUE PERFUSION

Definition: At risk for a decrease in cardiac (coronary) circulation that may compromise health.

Risk Factors

- Hypovolemia
- Hypoxemia
- Hypertension
- Hypotension
- Vasoconstriction
- Vasodilation
- Embolism
- Stenosis
- Coronary artery disease
- Trauma
- Cardiac tamponade

Outcome Criteria

- Systolic blood pressure is >90 mm Hg.
- Mean arterial pressure is >60 mm Hg.
- Heart rate is <100 beats/min.
- Pulmonary artery pressures are within normal limits or back to baseline.
- Cardiac index is >2.2 L/min/m^2.
- Urine output is >0.5 mL/kg/hr or >30 mL/hr.
- 12-lead ECG is normalized without new Q waves.
- Chest pain is absent.
- CK-MB enzymes, troponin I, and myoglobin levels are within normal range.

Nursing Interventions and Rationale

1. Collaborate with the physician regarding the administration of fibrinolytic therapy or the preparation of the patient for percutaneous coronary intervention (PCI) ***to restore myocardial blood flow.***
2. Collaborate with physician regarding the administration of oxygen at 2 L/min to achieve SpO_2 >90% ***to maximize myocardial oxygen supply.***
3. Collaborate with physician regarding the administration of sublingual nitroglycerin and/or intravenous nitroglycerine infusion ***to augment coronary blood flow and reduce cardiac work by decreasing preload and afterload.***
   a. Do not administer nitrates to patients who have taken phosphodiesterase inhibitors for erectile dysfunction within the last 24 to 48 hours (depending on the medication) ***as severe hypotension may occur.***
4. Collaborate with physician regarding the administration of morphine ***to control pain.***
5. Collaborate with the physician regarding the administration of aspirin, antiplatelet therapy, and heparin ***to prevent recurrent thrombosis and inhibit platelet function.***
6. Collaborate with the physician regarding the administration of beta-blockers ***to decrease myocardial oxygen demand and prevent recurrent ischemia.***
7. Collaborate with the physician regarding the administration of angiotensin-converting enzyme (ACE) inhibitors ***to block the conversion of angiotensin I to angiotensin II, a potent vasoconstrictor.***
8. Maintain the patient on bed rest with bedside commode privileges ***to minimize myocardial oxygen demand.***
9. Monitor patient's hemodynamic and cardiac rhythm status:
   a. Select cardiac monitoring leads based on infarct location and rhythm to obtain the best rhythm for monitoring.
   b. Evaluate cardiac rhythm for presence of dysrhythmias, which are common complications of myocardial ischemia.
   c. Collaborate with physician regarding the administration of antidysrhythmic medications.
   d. Assess serum electrolytes (potassium and magnesium) and arterial blood gases.
   e. Collaborate with physician regarding the administration of electrolytes to correct any imbalances.
   f. Monitor ST segment continuously to determine changes in myocardial tissue perfusion.
   g. Monitor patient's blood pressure at least every hour as many conditions (e.g., drugs, dysrhythmias, myocardial ischemia) may cause hypotension (systolic blood pressure <90 mm Hg).
   h. Treat symptomatic dysrhythmias according to unit's emergency protocol or advanced cardiac life support (ACLS) guidelines.
10. Instruct patient to avoid the Valsalva maneuver as forced expiration against a closed glottis causes sudden and intense changes in systolic blood pressure and heart rate.

RISK FOR INEFFECTIVE CEREBRAL TISSUE PERFUSION

Definition: At risk for a decrease in cerebral tissue circulation that may compromise health.

Risk Factors

- Hypovolemia
- Hypoxemia
- Hypertension
- Hypotension
- Vasoconstriction
- Vasodilation
- Embolism
- Stenosis
- Hemorrhage
- Vascular disease
- Trauma

Outcome Criteria

- Patient is oriented to time, place, person, and situation.
- Pupils are equal and normoreactive.
- Blood pressure is within baseline or ordered parameters.
- Motor function is bilaterally equal.
- Headache, nausea, and vomiting are absent.
- Patient verbalizes importance of and displays compliance with reduced activity.
- Absence of neurologic deficits.

Nursing Interventions and Rationale

For Ischemia

1. Collaborate with physician regarding the administration of fibrinolytic therapy ***to facilitate lysis of the clot and restoration of blood flow to affected area.***
2. Monitor the patient for alterations in blood pressure, oxygenation, temperature, rhythm, and glucose levels.
3. Collaborate with physician regarding the administration of vasodilators for hypertension ***to maintain the patient's blood pressure within desired range.*** Use caution in lowering blood pressure ***as hypotension decreases cerebral blood flow.***
   a. Patients receiving fibrinolytic therapy—keep systolic blood pressure <185 mm Hg and diastolic blood pressure <110 mm Hg.
   b. Patients not receiving fibrinolytic therapy—keep systolic blood pressure <220 mm Hg and diastolic blood pressure <120 mm Hg.
4. Collaborate with physician regarding the administration of intravenous fluids and vasoconstrictors for hypotension ***as hypotension decreases cerebral blood flow.***
5. Collaborate with physician regarding the administration of oxygen to maintain SpO_2 >95% ***to prevent hypoxemia and potential worsening of the neurologic injury.***
6. Collaborate with physician regarding administration of acetaminophen for elevated temperature ***because hyperthermia is associated with increased morbidity in the stroke patient.***
7. Collaborate with the physician regarding the treatment of dysrhythmias ***due to increased sympathetic nervous system stimulation.***
8. Collaborate with the physician regarding the administration of insulin for hyperglycemia ***as elevated blood glucose has been linked to an increase in the area of infarct.***
9. Collaborate with the speech therapist regarding the patient's ability to swallow before initiating oral feedings ***to ensure patient is not at risk for aspirating.***
10. Collaborate with the physical therapist to assess the patient's ability to ambulate safely ***to ensure the patient is not at risk for falling*** and ability to perform activities of daily living ***to facilitate discharge home.***
11. Maintain surveillance for complications such as increased intracranial pressure, seizures, and acute lung failure.
12. Collaborate with the physician and rehabilitation specialist regarding the patient's need for rehabilitation ***to maximize the patient's independence.***

For Hemorrhage

1. Assess for indicators of increased intracranial pressure and brain herniation (see the nursing management plan for Decreased Intracranial Adaptive Capacity Related to Failure of Normal Intracranial Compensatory Mechanism).
2. Collaborate with the physician regarding the administration of anticonvulsant medications ***to prevent the onset of seizures or to control seizures.***
3. Collaborate with physician regarding the administration of vasodilators for hypertension ***to avoid further bleeding.*** Use caution in lowering blood pressure ***as hypotension decreases cerebral blood flow.***
   a. If systolic blood pressure is >200 mm Hg or mean arterial pressure is >150 mm Hg, aggressive reduction in blood pressure is indicated.
   b. If systolic blood pressure is >180 mm Hg or mean arterial pressure is >130 mm Hg in the presence of increased intracranial pressure, cautious reduction in pressure is indicated maintaining cerebral perfusion pressure >60-80 mm Hg.
   c. If systolic blood pressure is >180 mm Hg or mean arterial pressure is >130 mm Hg in the absence of elevated intracranial pressure, reduction in blood pressure is indicated with a target of 160/90 mm Hg.
4. Collaborate with the physician regarding the administration of insulin for hyperglycemia ***as elevated blood glucose has been linked to an increase in the area of infarct.***
5. Collaborate with physician regarding administration of acetaminophen for elevated temperature ***because hyperthermia is associated with increased morbidity in the stroke patient.***
6. Initiate precautions ***to prevent rebleeding.***
   a. Ensure bed rest in a quiet environment ***to lessen external stimuli.***

RISK FOR INEFFECTIVE CEREBRAL TISSUE PERFUSION—cont'd

b. Maintain a darkened room to lessen symptoms of photophobia.
c. Restrict visitors and instruct them to keep conversation as nonstressful as possible.
d. Administer sedatives as prescribed ***to reduce anxiety to promote rest.***
e. Administer analgesics as prescribed ***to relieve or lessen headache.***
f. Provide a soft, high-fiber diet and stool softeners to prevent constipation, which can lead to straining and increased risk of rebleeding.
g. Assist with activities of daily living (feeding, bathing, dressing, toileting).
h. Avoid any activity that could lead to increased intracranial pressure; ensure that patient does not flex hips beyond 90 degrees and avoids neck hyperflexion, hyperextension, or lateral hyperrotation ***that could impede jugular venous return.***

7. Collaborate with the physical therapist to assess the patient's ability to ambulate safely ***to ensure the patient is not at risk for falling*** and ability to perform activities of daily living ***to facilitate discharge home.***
8. Collaborate with the physician and rehabilitation specialist regarding the patient's need for rehabilitation ***to maximize the patient's independence.***

RISK FOR INEFFECTIVE GASTROINTESTINAL PERFUSION

Definition: At risk for decrease in gastrointestinal circulation that may compromise health.

Risk Factors

- Hypovolemia
- Hypoxemia
- Hypertension
- Hypotension
- Vasoconstriction
- Vasodilation
- Embolism
- Stenosis
- Vascular disease
- Trauma

Outcome Criteria

- Normal bowel sounds
- Absence of abdominal pain, distention, and guarding
- Vital signs at baseline

Nursing Interventions and Rationales

1. Collaborate with physician regarding the administration of crystalloids, colloids, blood, and blood products ***to maintain adequate circulating volume.*** Implement the nursing management plan for Deficit Fluid Volume Related to Absolute Loss.
2. Collaborate with physician regarding pain management. Implement the nursing management plan for Acute Pain Related to Transmission and Perception of Cutaneous, Visceral, Muscular, or Ischemic Impulses.
3. Collaborate with physician regarding the administration of oxygen to maintain SpO_2 >92% ***to prevent hypoxemia and potential worsening of the gastrointestinal injury.***
4. Collaborate with physician regarding the administration of electrolyte replacement therapy ***to maintain adequate electrolyte balance.***
5. Collaborate with dietitian regarding administration of nutrition ***because patient will be unable to eat.*** Implement the nursing management plan for Imbalanced Nutrition: Less Than Body Requirements.
6. Maintain surveillance for complications such as gastrointestinal hemorrhage, hypovolemic shock, and septic shock.
7. Collaborate with physician regarding preparation for surgery ***to remove infarcted bowel.***

RISK FOR INEFFECTIVE PERIPHERAL TISSUE PERFUSION

Definition: At risk for a decrease in blood circulation to the periphery that may compromise health.

Ineffective Peripheral Tissue Perfusion

Risk Factors

- Hypovolemia
- Hypoxemia
- Hypertension
- Hypotension
- Vasoconstriction
- Vasodilation
- Embolism
- Stenosis
- Iatrogenic (arterial catheters, intraaortic balloon pump catheters)
- Vascular disease
- Trauma

Continued

RISK FOR INEFFECTIVE PERIPHERAL TISSUE PERFUSION—cont'd

Outcome Criteria

- Peripheral pulses are full and equal bilaterally.
- Capillary refill is equal bilaterally.
- Ischemic pain is absent.
- Skin temperature is equal in both extremities.
- Skin is pink and warm in both extremities.
- Paresthesias are absent.

Nursing Interventions and Rationale

1. Collaborate with physician regarding the administration of antiplatelet, anticoagulant, and/or fibrinolytic therapy.
2. Collaborate with physician regarding pain management. Implement the nursing management plan for Acute Pain Related to Transmission and Perception of Cutaneous, Visceral, Muscular, or Ischemic Impulses.
3. Ensure patient is adequately hydrated ***to decrease blood viscosity.***
4. Maintain affected extremity in dependent position if possible ***to enhance blood flow.***
5. Keep affected extremity warm and protect it from injury. ***Do not apply heat directly to the affected extremity because this can result in injury.***
6. Maintain surveillance for pain, pallor, pulselessness, paresthesia, paralysis, and poikilothermia ***as indicators of abrupt change in blood flow.***
7. Maintain surveillance for tissue breakdown and arterial ulcers ***as indicators of injury.***
8. Prepare patient for possible surgery or interventional procedure to restore blood flow.

RISK FOR INEFFECTIVE RENAL PERFUSION

Definition: At risk for a decrease in blood circulation to the kidney that may compromise health.

Risk Factors

- Hypovolemia
- Hypoxemia
- Hypertension
- Hypotension
- Vasoconstriction
- Vasodilation
- Embolism
- Stenosis
- Nephrotoxic medications
- Vascular disease
- Trauma

Outcome Criteria

- Electrolytes are within normal range.
- Serum creatinine and BUN are within normal range.
- Normal acid–base balance
- Urinary output is within normal limits, or patient is stable on dialysis.
- Hemoglobin and hematocrit values are stable.

Nursing Interventions and Rationale

1. Monitor intake and output, urine output, and patient weight.
2. Collaborate with physician regarding the administration of crystalloids, colloids, blood, and blood products ***to increase circulating volume and maintain mean arterial pressure >70 mm Hg.***
3. Collaborate with physician regarding the administration of inotropes ***to enhance myocardial contractility and increase cardiac index to >2.5 L/min.***
4. Collaborate with physician regarding the administration of diuretics to the oliguric patient ***to flush out cellular debris and increase urine output.***
5. Minimize the patient's exposure to nephrotoxic medications ***to decrease damage to kidneys.***
6. Monitor blood levels of drugs cleared by kidneys ***to avoid accumulation.***
7. Monitor patient for signs of electrolyte imbalance ***due to impaired electrolyte regulation.***
8. Maintain surveillance for signs and symptoms of fluid overload.
9. Monitor patient's clinical status and response to dialysis therapy ***to ensure the patient is receiving safe and effective dialytic therapy.***

RISK FOR INFECTION

Definition: At increased risk for being invaded by pathogenic organisms.

Risk Factors

- Inadequate primary defenses (e.g., broken skin, traumatized tissue, decreased ciliary action, stasis of body fluids, change in pH secretions, altered peristalsis)
- Inadequate secondary defenses (e.g., decreased hemoglobin, leukopenia, suppressed inflammatory or immune response)
- Immunocompromise
- Inadequate acquired immunity
- Tissue destruction and increased environmental exposure
- Chronic disease
- Invasive procedures
- Malnutrition
- Pharmacologic agents (e.g., antibiotics, steroids)

Outcome Criteria

- Total lymphocyte count is >1000/mm^3.
- White blood cell count is within normal limits.
- Temperature is within normal limits.
- Blood, urine, wound, and sputum culture results are negative.

Nursing Interventions and Rationale

1. Perform proper hand hygiene before and after patient care ***to reduce the transmission of microorganisms.***
2. Use appropriate personal protective equipment in accordance with CDC guidelines.
   a. Ensure physician uses maximum barrier precautions when inserting lines.
      (1) Ensure sterile gloves, gown, and mask are worn.
      (2) Drape patient completely with a sterile sheet.
3. Use aseptic technique for insertion and manipulation of invasive monitoring devices, intravenous (IV) lines, and urinary drainage catheters ***to maintain sterility of environment.***
   a. Ensure physician uses maximum barrier precautions when inserting lines.
      (1) Ensure sterile gloves, gown, and mask are worn.
      (2) Drape patient completely with a sterile sheet.
4. Stabilize all invasive lines and catheters ***to avoid unintentional manipulation and contamination.***
5. Use aseptic technique for dressing changes ***to prevent contamination of wounds or insertion sites.***
6. Change any line placed under emergent conditions within 24 hours ***because aseptic technique is usually breached during an emergency.***
7. Collaborate with the physician to change any dressing that is saturated with blood or drainage ***because these are mediums for microorganism growth.***
8. Minimize use of stopcocks and maintain caps on all stopcock ports ***to reduce the ports of entry for microorganisms.***
9. Avoid the use of nasogastric tubes, nasotracheal tubes, and nasopharyngeal suctioning in the patient with a suspected cerebrospinal fluid leak ***to decrease the incidence of central nervous system infection.***
10. Change ventilator circuits with humidifiers when visibly soiled or mechanically malfunctioning ***to avoid introducing microorganisms into the system.*** Do not change routinely.
11. Provide the patient with a clean manual resuscitation bag ***to avoid cross-contamination between patients.***
12. Provide oral care to patient with artificial airway or unresponsive patient every 2-4 hours and PRN ***to decrease the incidence of hospital-acquired pulmonary infections.***
    a. Swab mouth and moisten lips every 4 hours.
    b. Brush teeth with in-line suction toothbrush every 12 hours. Rinse or swab patient's mouth with chlorhexidine after brushing.
    c. Suction subglottic secretions (secretions pooling above the cuff of the endotracheal [ET] or tracheostomy tube) every 12 hours and before repositioning the tube or deflation of the cuff.
    d. Provide lip balm to keep patient's lips moistened PRN.
    e. Provide mouth moisturizer to keep patient's mouth moistened PRN.
13. Cleanse in-line suction catheters with sterile saline according to the manufacturer's instructions ***to avoid accumulation of secretions within the catheter.***
14. Maintain the head of the bed elevated at 30 to 45 degrees in patients with an artificial airway ***to decrease the incidence of aspiration.***
15. Use disposable sterile scissors, forceps, and hemostats ***to reduce the transmission of microorganisms.***
16. Maintain a closed urinary drainage system ***to decrease incidence of urinary infections.***
17. Keep the urinary drainage tubing and bag below the level of the patient's bladder ***to prevent the backflow of urine.***
18. Assess the urinary drainage tubing for kinks ***to prevent stasis of urine.***
19. Protect all access device sites from potential sources of contamination (nasogastric reflux, draining wounds, ostomies, sputum).
20. Refrigerate parenteral nutrition solutions and opened enteral nutrition formulas ***to inhibit bacterial growth.***
21. Maintain daily surveillance of invasive devices for signs and symptoms of infection.
22. Notify physician of elevated temperature or if any signs or symptoms of infection are present.

Additional Interventions for Patient Receiving Immunosuppressive Drugs

23. Obtain blood, urine, and sputum cultures for temperature elevations >38° C (100.4° F) ***inasmuch as elevation likely***

Continued

RISK FOR INFECTION—cont'd

is caused by bacteremia or bladder or pulmonary infection.

24. Auscultate breath sounds at least every 6 hours. ***Pulmonary infection is the most common type of infection, and changes in breath sounds might be an early indication.***
25. Inspect wounds at least every 8 hours for redness, swelling, and/or drainage, ***which may indicate infection.***
26. Inspect overall skin integrity and oral mucosa for signs of breakdown, ***which place the patient at risk for infection.***
27. Notify physician of new-onset cough. ***Even a nonproductive cough may indicate pulmonary infection.***
28. Monitor white blood cell count daily and report leukocytosis or sudden development of leukopenia, ***which may indicate an infectious process.***
29. Protect patient from exposure to any staff or family member with contagious lesion (e.g., herpes simplex) or respiratory infections.
30. Collaborate with dietitian regarding the patient's nutritional status and need for augmentation of nutritional intake as necessary ***to prevent debilitation and increased susceptibility to infection.***
31. Collaborate with physician to remove invasive lines and catheters as soon as possible ***to decrease potential portals of entry.***
32. Teach patient the clinical manifestations of infection. ***A knowledgeable patient will seek medical attention promptly, which will result in earlier treatment and a decreased risk that infection will become life-threatening.***

SITUATIONAL LOW SELF-ESTEEM

Definition: Development of a negative perception of self-worth in response to a current situation.

Situational Low Self-Esteem Related to Feelings of Guilt about Physical Deterioration

Defining Characteristics
- Inability to accept positive reinforcement
- Lack of follow-through
- Nonparticipation in therapy
- Not taking responsibility for self-care (i.e., self-neglect)
- Self-destructive behavior
- Lack of eye contact

Outcome Criteria
- Patient verbalizes feelings of self-worth.
- Patient maintains positive relationships with significant others.
- Patient manifests active interest in appearance by completing personal grooming daily.

Nursing Interventions and Rationale
1. Evaluate the meaning of health-related situation. How does the patient feel about himself or herself, the diagnosis, and the treatment? How does the present fit into the larger context of his or her life?
2. Assess the patient's emotional level, interpersonal relationships, and feeling about himself or herself. Recognize the patient's uniqueness (e.g., how the hair is worn, preference for name used).
3. Help the patient discover and verbalize feelings and understand the crisis by listening and providing information.
4. Assist the patient to identify strengths and positive qualities that increase the sense of self-worth. Focus on past experiences of accomplishment and competency. Help the patient with positive self-reinforcement. Reinforce the obvious love and affection of family and significant others.
5. Assess coping techniques that have been helpful in the past. Help the patient decide how to handle negative or incongruent feedback about the situation.
6. Encourage visits from family and significant others. Facilitate interactions and ensure privacy. Help family members entering the critical care unit by explaining what they will see. Increase visitors' comfort with equipment; offer chairs and other courtesies.
7. Encourage the patient to pursue interest in individual or social activities, even though difficult in the critical care unit.
8. Reflect caring, concern, empathy, respect, and unconditional acceptance in nurse–patient relationships.
9. Remember that for the patient the nurse is a significant other who provides important appraisals of the patient and who can facilitate the change process.
10. Help the family support the patient's self-esteem.
11. Provide for continuity of nurse assignment to ensure consistent contacts that can ***facilitate support of the patient's self-esteem.***

PLAN UNILATERAL NEGLECT

Definition: Impairment in sensory and motor response, mental representation and spatial attention of the body, and the corresponding environment characterized by inattention to one side and over-attention to the opposite side. Left-side neglect is more severe and persistent than right-side neglect.

Unilateral Neglect Related to Perceptual Disruption

Defining Characteristics
- Neglect of involved body parts and/or extrapersonal space
- Denial of existence of the affected limb or side of body
- Denial of hemiplegia or other motor and sensory deficits
- Left homonymous hemianopia
- Difficulty with spatial–perceptual tasks
- Left hemiplegia

Outcome Criteria
- Patient is safe and free from injury.
- Patient is able to identify safety hazards in the environment.
- Patient recognizes disability and describes physical deficits present (e.g., paralysis, weakness, numbness).
- Patient demonstrates ability to scan the visual field to compensate for loss of function or sensation in affected limbs.

Nursing Interventions and Rationale
1. Adapt environment to patient's deficits ***to maintain patient safety.***
   a. Position the patient's bed with the unaffected side facing the door.
   b. Approach and speak to the patient from the unaffected side. If the patient must be approached from the affected side, announce your presence as soon as entering the room ***to avoid startling the patient.***
   c. Position the call light, bedside stand, and personal items on the patient's unaffected side.
   d. If the patient will be assisted out of bed, simplify the environment ***to eliminate hazards*** by removing unnecessary furniture and equipment.
   e. Provide frequent reorientation of the patient to the environment.

Continued

PLAN UNILATERAL NEGLECT—cont'd

f. Observe the patient closely and anticipate his or her needs. ***In spite of repeated explanation, the patient may have difficulty retaining information about the deficits.***
g. When patient is in bed, elevate his or her affected arm on a pillow ***to prevent dependent edema and support the hand in a position of function.***

2. Assist the patient to recognize the perceptual defect.
   a. Encourage the patient to wear any prescriptive corrective glasses or hearing aids ***to facilitate communication.***
   b. Instruct the patient to turn the head past midline ***to view the environment on the affected side.***
   c. Encourage patient to look at the affected side and to stroke the limbs with the unaffected hand. Encourage handling of the affected limbs ***to reinforce awareness of the affected side.***
   d. Instruct the patient to look for the affected extremity when performing simple tasks ***to know where it is at all times.***
   e. After pointing to them, have the patient name the affected parts.
   f. Encourage the patient to use self-exercises (e.g., lifting the affected arm with the unaffected hand).
   g. If the patient is unable to discriminate between the concepts of *right* and *left,* use descriptive adjectives such as "the weak arm," "the affected leg," or "the good arm" to refer to the body. Use gestures, not just words, to indicate right and left.
3. Collaborate with the patient, physician, and rehabilitation team ***to design and implement a beginning rehabilitation program for use during the critical care unit stay.***
   a. Use adaptive equipment (braces, splints, slings) as appropriate.
   b. Teach the patient the individual components of any activity separately, then proceed to integrate the component parts into a completed activity.
   c. Instruct the patient to attend to the affected side, if able, and to assist with the bath or other tasks.
   d. Use tactile stimulation to reintroduce the arm or leg to the patient. Rub the affected parts with different textured materials to stimulate sensations (e.g., warm, cold, rough, soft).
   e. Encourage activities that require the patient to turn the head toward the affected side and retrain the patient to scan the affected side and environment visually.
   f. If the patient is allowed out of bed, cue him or her with reminders to scan visually when ambulating. Assist and remain in constant attendance ***because the patient may have difficulty maintaining correct posture, balance, and locomotion.*** There may be vertical–horizontal perceptual problems, with the patient leaning to the affected side to align with the perceived vertical. Provide sitting, standing, and balancing exercises before getting the patient out of bed.
4. Assist patient with oral feedings.
   a. Avoid giving patient any very hot food items that could cause injury.
   b. Place the patient in an upright sitting position, if possible.
   c. Encourage the patient to feed himself or herself; if necessary, guide the patient's hand to the mouth.
   d. If the patient is able to feed himself or herself, place one dish at a time in front of the patient. When the patient is finished with the first, add another dish. Tell the patient what he or she is eating.
   e. Initially, place food in patient's visual field, then gradually move the food out of the field of vision and teach the patient to scan the entire visual field.
   f. When the patient has learned visually to scan the environment, offer a tray of food with various dishes.
   g. Instruct the patient to take small bites of food and to place the food in the unaffected side of the mouth.
   h. Teach the patient to sweep out pockets of food with the tongue after every bite ***to eliminate retained food in the affected side of the mouth.***
   i. After meals or oral medications, check the patient's oral cavity for pockets of retained material.
5. Initiate patient and family health teaching.
   a. Assess to ensure that the patient and the family understand the nature of the neurologic deficits and the purpose of the rehabilitation plan.
   b. Teach the proper application and use of any adaptive equipment.
   c. Teach the importance of maintaining a safe environment and point out potential environmental hazards.
   d. Instruct family members how to facilitate relearning techniques (e.g., cueing, scanning visual fields).

Physiologic Formulas for Critical Care

HEMODYNAMIC FORMULAS

Mean (Systemic) Arterial Pressure (MAP)

$$MAP = \frac{(Diastolic \times 2) + (Systolic \times 1)}{3}$$

Systemic Vascular Resistance (SVR)

$$\frac{MAP - RAP}{CO} = SVR \text{ in units}$$

Normal range is 10-18 units.

$$\frac{MAP - RAP}{CO} \times 80 = SVR \text{ in dyn} \cdot \text{sec} \cdot \text{cm}^{-5}$$

Normal range is 800-1400 dyn·sec·cm^{-5}.

Systemic Vascular Resistance Index (SVRI)

$$\frac{MAP - RAP}{CO} \times 80 = SVR \text{ in dyn} \cdot \text{sec} \cdot \text{cm}^{-5}/\text{m}^2$$

Normal range is 2000-2400 dyn·sec·cm^{-5}/m^2.

Pulmonary Vascular Resistance (PVR)

$$\frac{PAP \text{ mean} - RAP}{CO} = PVR \text{ in units}$$

Normal range is 1.2-3 units.

$$\frac{PAP \text{ mean} - RAP}{CO} \times 80 = PVR \text{ in dyn} \cdot \text{sec} \cdot \text{cm}^{-5}$$

Normal range is 100-250 dyn·sec·cm^{-5}.

Pulmonary Vascular Resistance Index (PVRI)

$$\frac{PAP \text{ mean} - PAOP}{CI} \times 80 = PVR \text{ in dyn} \cdot \text{sec} \cdot \text{cm}^{-5}/\text{m}^2$$

Normal range is 225-315 dyn·sec·cm^{-5}/m^2.

CI, Cardiac index; *CO*, cardiac output; *PAOP*, pulmonary arterial occlusion pressure (wedge pressure); *PAP*, pulmonary arterial pressure; *RAP*, right atrial pressure.

Left Cardiac Work Index (LCWI)

Step 1. MAP × CO × 0.0136 = LCW

Step 2. $\frac{LCW}{BSA} = LCWI$

Normal range is 3.4-4.2 kg-m/m^2.

Left Ventricular Stroke Work Index (LVSWI)

Step 1. MAP × SV × 0.0136 = LVSW

Step 2. $\frac{LVSW}{BSA} = LVSWI$

Normal range is 50-62 g-m/m^2.

Right Cardiac Work Index (RCWI)

Step 1. PAP mean × CO × 0.0136 = RCW

Step 2. $\frac{RCW}{BSA} = RCWI$

Normal range is 0.54-0.66 kg-m/m^2.

Right Ventricular Stroke Work Index (RVSWI)

Step 1. PAP mean × SV × 0.0136 = RVSW

Step 2. $\frac{RVSW}{BSA} = RVSWI$

Normal range is 7.9-9.7 g-m/m^2.

Corrected QT Interval (QTc)

$$\frac{QT}{\sqrt{(RR \text{ interval})}} = QTc$$

Body Surface Area (BSA)

Many hemodynamic formulas can be indexed or adjusted to body size by use of a BSA nomogram (Fig. B-1). To calculate BSA:

1. Obtain height and weight.
2. Mark height on the left scale and weight on the right scale.
3. Draw a straight line between the two points marked on the nomogram.

The number where the line crosses the middle scale is the BSA value.

PULMONARY FORMULAS

Shunt Equation (Qs/Qt)

CcO_2 = Pulmonary capillary oxygen content (calculated value)
CaO_2 = Arterial oxygen content (calculated value)
CvO_2 = Venous oxygen content (calculated value)
Normal range is less than 5%.

Pulmonary Capillary Oxygen Content (CcO_2)

Hgb = hemoglobin (measured via laboratory sample or arterial blood gas)
ScO_2 = Pulmonary capillary oxygen saturation
PcO_2 = Partial pressure of oxygen in capillary blood
Normal range is greater than 19 mL/dL.

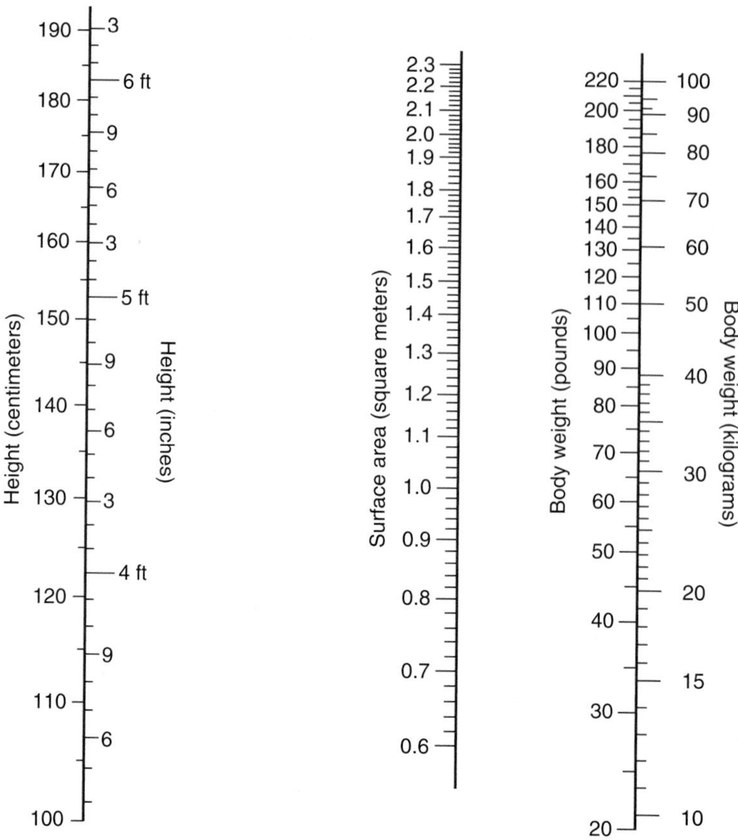

FIG B-1 Body surface area (BSA) nomogram.

Arterial Oxygen Content (CO_2)

Hgb = Hemoglobin (measured via laboratory sample or arterial blood gas)
SaO_2 = Arterial oxygen saturation (measured via arterial blood gas)
PaO_2 = Partial pressure of oxygen in arterial blood (measured via arterial blood gas)
Normal range is 17 to 20 mL/dL.

Venous Oxygen Content (CvO_2)

Hgb = Hemoglobin (measured via laboratory sample or arterial blood gas)
SvO_2 = Mixed venous oxygen saturation (measured via mixed venous blood gas)
PvO_2 = Partial pressure of oxygen in mixed venous blood (measured via mixed venous blood gas)
Normal range is 12 to 15 mL/dL.

Alveolar Pressure of Oxygen (P_AO_2)

F_IO_2 = Fraction of inspired oxygen (obtained from oxygen settings)
Pb = Barometric pressure (assumed to be 760 mm Hg at sea level)
pH_2O = Water pressure in the lungs (assumed to be 47 mm Hg)
$PaCO_2$ = Partial pressure of carbon dioxide in arterial blood (measured via arterial blood gas)
RQ = Respiratory quotient (assumed to be 0.8)
Normal range is 60 to 100 mm Hg.

Arterial/Inspired Oxygen Ratio

PaO_2 = Partial pressure of oxygen in arterial blood (measured via arterial blood gas)
F_IO_2 = Fraction of inspired oxygen (obtained from oxygen settings)
Normal range is greater than 300.

Arterial/Alveolar Oxygen Ratio

PaO_2 = Partial pressure of oxygen in arterial blood (measured via arterial blood gas)
P_AO_2 = Partial pressure of oxygen in alveoli (calculated value)
Normal range is greater than 0.75 (75%).

Alveolar-Arterial Gradient

P_AO_2 = Partial pressure of oxygen in alveoli (calculated value)
PaO_2 = Partial pressure of oxygen in arterial blood (measured via arterial blood gas)
Normal range is 25 to 65 mm Hg.

Dead Space Equation (Vd/Vt)

$PaCO_2$ = Partial pressure of carbon dioxide in arterial blood (measured via arterial blood gas)
$P_{ET}CO_2$ = Partial pressure of carbon dioxide in exhaled gas (measured via end-tidal CO_2 monitor)
Normal range is 0.2 to 0.4 (20% to 40%).

Static Compliance (C_{ST})

This value is calculated for mechanically ventilated patients.

$$C_{ST} = \frac{V_T}{PP} - PEEP$$

V_T = Tidal volume (obtained from ventilator)
PP = Plateau pressure (measured via ventilator)
PEEP = Positive end-expiratory pressure (obtained from ventilator)
Normal value is 60 to 100 mL/cm H_2O.

Dynamic Compliance (C_{DY})

Also called *characteristic,* this value is calculated for mechanically ventilated patients.

$$C_{DY} = \frac{V_T}{PIP} - PEEP$$

V_T = Tidal volume (obtained from ventilator)
PIP = Peak inspiratory pressure (obtained from ventilator)
PEEP = Positive end-expiratory pressure (obtained from ventilator)
Normal value is 40 to 80 mL/cm H_2O.

NEUROLOGIC FORMULAS

Cerebral Perfusion Pressure (CPP)

$$CCP = MAP - ICP$$

MAP = Mean arterial pressure (measured via arterial line or blood pressure cuff)
ICP = Intracranial pressure (measured via ICP monitoring device)
Normal range is 60 to 150 mm Hg.

Arteriojugular Oxygen Difference ($AjDO_2$)

SaO_2 = Arterial oxygen saturation (measured via arterial blood gas)
$SjvO_2$ = Jugular venous oxygen saturation (measured via jugular blood gas or jugular venous catheter)
Hgb = Hemoglobin (measured via laboratory sample or arterial blood gas)
Normal range is 5 to 7.5 mL/dL.

ENDOCRINE FORMULAS

Serum Osmolality

$$\text{Serum osmolality} = 2(Na^+ + K^+) + \frac{\text{Glucose}}{18} + \frac{\text{BUN}}{2.8}$$

Na^+ = Sodium
K^+ = Potassium
BUN = Blood urea nitrogen
Normal range is 275 to 295 mOsm/kg of water.

Fluid Volume Deficit in Liters

$$\text{Fluid volume deficit} = \frac{0.6(\text{kg/weight}) \times (Na^+ - 140)}{140}$$

Na^+ = Sodium

KIDNEY FORMULAS

Anion Gap

$$[Na^+] - ([Cl^-] + [HCO_3^-])$$

Normal range is 8 to 16 mEq.

Clearance

$$\text{Clearance} = U \times \frac{(V)}{(P)}$$

U = Concentration of substance in urine
V = Time
P = Concentration of substance in plasma
Normal range depends on substance measured.

NUTRITIONAL FORMULAS

Resting Metabolic Rate (RMR)

PSU 2003b (Penn State Equation)

When indirect calorimetry is not available, the Penn State Equation is the best equation to use to estimate resting metabolic rate (RMR) in critically ill patients of any age with BMI below 30 or critically ill patients who are younger than 60 years old with BMI over 30. This equation was validated in 2009 by the Academy of Nutrition and Dietetics Evidence Analysis Library.[1]

$$RMR = \text{Mifflin RMR}(0.96) + V_E(31) + T_{max}(167) - 6212 \; *$$

PSU 2010 (Modified Penn State Equation)

For a subset of obese critically ill patients aged 60 years and older, a modified Penn State Equation (PSU 2010) is recommended to estimate RMR. Validated in 2010 by the Academy of Nutrition and Dietetics Evidence Analysis Library.[2]

$$RMR = \text{Mifflin RMR}(0.71) + V_E(64) + T_{max}(85) - 3085 \; *$$

Mifflin-St. Jeor Equation

In non-critically ill populations, the Mifflin-St. Jeor equation performed the best when predicting RMR in non-obese and obese populations, 20 to 82 years of age.[3]

Men: Mifflin RMR

$$= (9.99 \times \text{weight}) + (6.25 \times \text{height}) - (4.92 \times \text{age}) + 5$$

Women: Mifflin RMR

$$= (9.99 \times \text{weight}) + (6.25 \times \text{height}) - (4.92 \times \text{age}) - 161$$

Mifflin-St. Jeor equation uses weight in kg, height in cm, age in years.

Caloric and Protein Needs[4]

Estimating Caloric Needs

Step 1. Calculate resting metabolic rate (RMR) using the appropriate equation from above. This is the energy needed

---

*Where:
Mifflin RMR = Resting metabolic rate as calculated by the MSJ equation
V_E = Minute ventilation in liters per minute (L/min)
T_{max} = Maximum temperature in degrees Celsius

for basic life processes, such as respiratory function and maintenance of body temperature. **Step 2.** Multiply by an appropriate stress factor to meet the needs of the ill or injured patient (see the following table). If the patient has more than one stressor (e.g., burn and pneumonia), use only the stress factor for the highest level of stress.

Type of Stress	Multiply the Value from Step 2 by
Fever	1 + 0.13/1°C above normal (or 0.07/1°F)
Pneumonia	1.2
Major injury	1.3
Severe sepsis, burn of 15%-30% of BSA	1.5
Burn of 31%-49% of BSA content (calculated value)	1.5-2.0
Burn ≥50% of BSA	1.8-2.1

BSA, Body surface area.

Estimating Protein Needs

Protein needs vary with the degree of malnutrition and stress (see the following table).

Condition	Multiply Desirable Body Weight (kg) by
Healthy individual or well-nourished elective surgery patient	0.8-1.0 g protein
Malnourished or catabolic state (e.g., sepsis, major injury)	1.2 to 2+ g protein
Burns	
15%-30% BSA	1.5 g protein
31%-49% BSA	1.5-2.0 g protein
50% or greater BSA	2.0-2.5 g protein

BSA, Body surface area.

Example of a Calculation of Calorie and Protein Needs

A 28-year-old woman has a fracture of the left femur and burns to 40% of her BSA after a motor vehicle crash. Her height is 1.65 m (5 ft 5 in), and her weight is 59.1 kg (130 lb).

Energy needs

1. RMR = (9.99 × 59.1 kg) + (6.25 × 165 cm) − (4.92 × 28 years) − 161 = 1323 calories/day
2. Energy needs for injury = 1323 calories × 1.75 = 2315 calories/day

Protein needs

Protein needs = 59.1 kg × 1.75 g = 103 g/day

REFERENCES

1. *Academy of Nutrition and Dietetics*: Evidence Analysis Library. If indirect calorimetry is unavailable or impractical, what is the best way to estimate resting metabolic rate (RMR) in non-obese adult critically ill patients? http://www.adaevidencelibrary.com. Accessed April 24, 2012.
2. *Academy of Nutrition and Dietetics*: Evidence Analysis Library. If indirect calorimetry is unavailable or impractical, what is the best way to estimate resting metabolic rate (RMR) in obese adult critically ill patients? http://www.adaevidencelibrary.com. Accessed April 24, 2012.
3. *Academy of Nutrition and Dietetics*: Evidence Analysis Library. Estimating RMR with predictive equations: what does the evidence tell us? http://www.adaevidencelibrary.com. Accessed April 24, 2012.
4. Data from Deitch EA: *Crit Care Clin* 11:735, 1995; Owen OE, et al: *Am J Clin Nutr* 4:1, 1986; Owen OE, et al: *Am J Clin Nutr* 46:875, 1987; Garrel DR, Jobin N, de Jonge LH: *Nutr Clin Pract* 11:99, 1996.

A

Page numbers followed by "f" indicate figures, "t" indicate tables, and "b" indicate boxes.

B

C

I

J

K

U

V

W

X

Z

SPECIAL FEATURES

CASE STUDIES

COLLABORATIVE MANAGEMENT

CONCEPT MAPS

DATA COLLECTION

EVIDENCE-BASED PRACTICE

INTERNET RESOURCES